Bailey & Love's
Essential Operations in Hepatobiliary and Pancreatic Surgery

T0303874

Bailey & Love's
Other Titles

Bailey & Love's Essential Operations in Oral & Maxillofacial Surgery (2024)
Peter A. Brennan, Rabindra P. Singh, Kaveh Shakib

Bailey & Love's Short Practice of Surgery, 28th Edition (2023)
Edited by P. Ronan O'Connell, Andrew W. McCaskie, Robert D. Sayers

Bailey & Love's Essential Clinical Anatomy, 2nd Edition (2019)
John Lumley, John Craven, Peter Abrahams, Richard Tunstall

www.baileyandlove.tandf.co.uk

Bailey & Love's
Essential Operations in Hepatobiliary and Pancreatic Surgery

Edited by

Ashley R. Dennison

MBChB, MD, FRCS

Professor of Hepatobiliary and Pancreatic Surgery, University of Leicester
Consultant Hepatobiliary Surgeon, University of Leicester and Leicester General Hospital University
Hospitals of Leicester NHS Trust
Leicester, UK

Guy J. Maddern

PhD, MS, MD, FRACS, FAHMS, FGESA, RP

Jepson Professor of Surgery, Discipline Leader – Surgery
Faculty of Health and Medical Sciences, University of Adelaide
Director of Research, Basil Hetzel Institute for Translational Health Research
The Queen Elizabeth Hospital, Woodville, Australia

Jia Fan

PhD

President of Zhongshan Hospital of Fudan University
Director of Liver Surgery Department, Zhongshan Hospital of Fudan University
Deputy Director of Organ Transplantation Centre of Fudan University
Deputy Director of Oncology Department of Shanghai Medical College of Fudan University
Deputy Director of Shanghai Hepatic Oncology Clinical Centre, Department of Liver Surgery
Zhongshan Hospital of Fudan University, Xuhui District, Shanghai, China

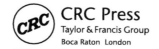

CRC Press
Taylor & Francis Group
Boca Raton London

CRC Press is an imprint of the
Taylor & Francis Group, an **informa** business

First edition published 2025
by CRC Press
2385 NW Executive Center Drive, Suite 320, Boca Raton, FL 33431

and by CRC Press
4 Park Square, Milton Park, Abingdon, Oxon, OX14 4RN

ISBN: 9780367530006 (hbk)
ISBN: 9780367468798 (pbk)
ISBN: 9781003080060 (ebk)
ISBN: 9781032806815 (pbk; restricted territorial availability)

DOI: 10.1201/9781003080060

Typeset in Baskerville MT Pro
by Apex CoVantage, LLC

Contents

Bailey & Love's Essential Operations Bailey & Love's Essential Operatic
Bailey & Love's Essential Operations Bailey & Love's Essential Operatic
Bailey & Love's Essential Operations Bailey & Love's Essential Operatic

Foreword

Surgery continues to become increasingly specialized, and informed, as progress is documented and experience reported from around the world. This new edition in Bailey and Love's Essential Operation Series provides a contemporary overview of the practice of hepatobiliary and pancreatic (HPB) surgery. Treating conditions of the liver and pancreas provide surgical challenges to not only the specialist HPB surgeon but also the more broadly practising abdominal and visceral surgeon. The most apparently straightforward cholecystectomy can become an anatomical nightmare unless careful steps are followed and surgical minefields avoided. New energy devices, instruments and robotic assistance have all helped provide improved outcomes and simplified technical aspects of complex procedures.

The last 30 years has witnessed extraordinary progress in the field of HPB surgery on the back of improved surgical and anaesthetic techniques. The result of which has been improved morbidity and mortality falling to less than 1% for the majority of even the most complex and hazardous procedures. This has been in part built on increased specialization, better anatomical understanding and the remarkable improvements in devices and imaging.

With communication worldwide now so easy to achieve, the need to capture the available international expertise is vital to provide a timely, contemporary view of the stateoftheart in HPB surgery. The Editors have collated an impressive collection of contributions. Not only from established icons of the craft, but also young leaders in this most complex area of surgery. Great surgical outcomes are achieved with meticulous and careful surgical techniques and a reliance on appropriate and sophisticated imaging and biomarkers. This needs to be combined with an understanding of the surgical and non-surgical options available to manage the abnormalities and diseases encountered every day as well as in exceptional situations.

Within its 78 chapters, most challenges encountered by the frequent and occasional HPB surgeon are described. The reader is provided with the essential knowledge required to take on the surgical tasks and understand the steps and backgrounds to best treat the patients presenting to them. The Editors are to be congratulated in marshalling such a diverse and expert collection of authors in this comprehensive handbook that will be of enormous value, particularly to senior trainees and early-stage consultant surgeons.

Perhaps the most important change in recent years in HPB surgery has been the appreciation and acceptance of the move from eminence decisions to evidence-based practice. This extensive text provides details of the practice supported by contemporary evidence.

Bernard Launois MD FACS
Emeritus Professor of Surgery, Hospital Pontchaillou, Université de Rennes, France
Honorary Fellow, American College of Surgeons
Member, Académie Nationale de Médecine, France

Former President
Académie Nationale de Chirurgie, France

ailey & Love's Essential Operations Bailey & Love's Essential Operations
ailey & Love's Essential Operations Bailey & Love's Essential Operations
ailey & Love's Essential Operations Bailey & Love's Essential Operations

Foreword

It is a great pleasure to introduce the first edition of Bailey & Love's (B&L) Essential Operations in Hepatobiliary and Pancreatic Surgery and to congratulate editors Ashley Dennison, Guy Maddern and Jia Fan, their contributing authors and our B&L publishers on this excellent book.

Bailey & Love's Short Practice of Surgery, first published in 1932, has been venerated by generations of medical students and surgeons as a repository of the core knowledge needed for safe surgical practice. However, the editors understand that in the modern era, a parent textbook can only cover knowledge essential for early surgical training and recognise the need for a compendium of texts to take B&L readership to the next level of speciality knowledge. Bailey & Love's Hepatobiliary and Pancreatic Surgery is the first in a planned compendium of operative texts designed to support trainees in higher surgical and sub-specialty training. The current text remains true to the heritage and traditions of the parent textbook. The most up-to-date content in Hepatobiliary and Pancreatic Surgery is presented in a familiar format and style. The text, written by a series of internationally-renowned authors, is clear and concise throughout. Each chapter is richly illustrated with operative photographs and accompanying line diagrams where needed.

I am sure readers will enjoy Bailey & Love's Essential Operations in Hepatobiliary and Pancreatic Surgery and trust that it will be a useful adjunct to their study and clinical practice.

P. Ronan O'Connell
MD FRCSI FRCSGlas (Hon) FRCSEdin (Hon)
RCSEng (Hon) FCSHK (Hon) FRCPSC (Hon)

Editor-in-Chief, *Bailey & Love's Short Practice of Surgery*

Preface

When conceiving this specialist volume of Bailey & Love's Essential Operations we set out to provide an accessible, relevant and authoritative guide on the practice of Hepatobiliary and Pancreatic Surgery (HPB) surgery. The support of over 190 authors provides international perspective on the understanding and solutions currently available to surgeons and their patients.

This is not a book that should be read cover-to-cover, but rather one opened regularly to answer questions of detail, or approach, and provide revision and reassurance for conditions or situations less frequently encountered. We have been keen to ensure it is published and available in surgical tearooms and departmental bookshelves but also in electronic formats, accessible anytime, anywhere, when required.

While it has been aimed at the up-and-coming HPB surgeon, it is also a valuable reference for the experienced surgeon requiring reassurance that their approach and understanding reflects contemporary practice. The need for clear illustrations and clinical images has been a major goal of the book, hoping to save a thousand words with each one selected.

The frustration with any text, such as this one, is that inevitably knowledge progresses even before publication is available. This book aims to lay down the principles and fundamentals of HPB surgery and needs to be supplemented by contemporary advances in molecular biology, chemotherapeutic advances, ablative techniques and interventional refinements. The anatomy and diseases needing surgical care will not change and we are all obliged to be constant students of our specialty, a task that is as exhausting as it is exciting. The views provided from the American, European, Indian, Chinese, Middle Eastern, Asian and Australasian contributors further emphasise how we are all facing the same challenges with varying infrastructure and support. We hope this is a platform that can be built on, over the years, as knowledge increases and ambiguity is replaced with certainty.

Ashley R. Dennison
Guy J. Maddern
Jia Fan

ailey & Love's Essential Operations Bailey & Love's Essential Operations
ailey & Love's Essential Operations Bailey & Love's Essential Operations
ailey & Love's Essential Operations Bailey & Love's Essential Operations

Acknowledgements

Chapter 10, **Energy Devices:** Thanks to Akshay Kanhere, Year 2 Medical Student, University of Adelaide for the contribution of sketches and figures.

Chapter 14, **History of Intraoperative Ultrasound during Open and Laparoscopic Liver Surgery:** We would like to give special thanks to Dr. Akinori Miyata and Prof. Kiyoshi Hasegawa for providing us with images of 3D Vincent and real-time virtual sonography.

Chapter 25, **Pancreas Trauma:** We would like to thank Prof. D. Kruger, Head of the Research Unit Department of Surgery Faculty of Health Sciences, University of the Witwatersrand Johannesburg, for her editing of the chapter and Yanni Massalis for providing some of the photographs used.

Acknowledgement and thanks to Brooke Sivendra for proofreading, problem solving and helping to understand the incomprehensible. We also thank Miranda Bromage and Nora Naughton for helping to bring together the authors from all over the world and gain their valuable contributions.

To Les Blumgart (1931–2022), a pioneer, teacher, mentor, and friend.

Contributors

Jo Etienne Abela
Government of Malta; Mater Dei Hospital
Msida, Malta

Monis Jaleel Ahmed
Mediclinic City Hospital
Dubai, UAE

M. Zeeshan Akhtar
Recanati/Miller Institute for Transplantation
Mount Sinai, NY, USA

Mohamed E. Akoad
Lahey Hospital & Medical Center
Burlington, MA, USA

Wasfi Alrawashdeh
Newcastle University
Newcastle upon Tyne, UK

Donna Marie L. Alvino
Beth Israel Deaconess Medical Center
Harvard Medical School
Boston, MA, USA

Leonidas Apostolidis
National Center for Tumor Diseases (NCT)
Heidelberg University Hospital
Heidelberg, Germany

Prateek Arora
AIG Hospitals,
Hyderabad, India

Ali Arshad
University Hospital Southampton
Southampton, UK

Georgi Atanasov
The University of Adelaide
The Queen Elizabeth Hospital
Adelaide, Australia

Abhirup Banerjee
D. Hinduja Hospital and Medical Research Centre
Mumbai, India

Savio G. Barreto
Flinders University; Flinders Medical Center,
Bedford Park
Adelaide, Australia

Jenifer Barrie
Manchester Royal Infirmary; Sheffield Teaching
Hospitals
Manchester, UK; Sheffield, UK

Claudio Bassi
Verona University Hospital (Borgo Roma)
Verona, Italy

Greg Beilman
University of Minnesota
Minneapolis, MN, USA

Clare Bent
The Royal Bournemouth Hospital
Bournemouth, UK

Zachary Bergman
University of Minnesota
Minneapolis, MN, USA

Marc G. Besselink
Amsterdam UMC
Amsterdam, Netherlands

Debanshu Bhaduri
Sadhu Vaswani Mission's Medical Complex
Maharashtra, India

Neil Bhardwaj
Glenfield Hospital
Leicester, UK

Henri Bismuth
Paul Brousse Hospital
Villejuif, France

Emily Britton
Bristol Royal Infirmary
Bristol, UK

David J. Brough
Royal Brisbane and Women's Hospital
University of Queensland
Queensland, Australia

Marcus W. Büchler
Heidelberg University Hospital
Heidelberg, Germany

Ishtiyaq Bukhari
Peterborough City Hospital
Peterborough, UK

Stefan Burgdorf
Rigshospitalet
Copenhagen, Denmark

Kurt Carabott
Mater Dei Hospital, Malta
Msida, Malta

Noel Cassar
Mater Dei Hospital, Malta
Msida, Malta

Xiao-Ping Chen
Tongji Hospital, Tongji Medical College,
Huazhong
University of Science and Technology
Shanghai, China

John W. Chen
Flinders University; Flinders Medical Center,
Bedford Park
Adelaide, Australia

Daniel Cherqui
Paul Brousse Hospital
Villejuif, France

Christopher Christophi
The University of Melbourne
Melbourne, Australia

Wen-Ning Cong
Shanghai Eastern Hepatobiliary Surgery Hospital
Naval Medical University
People's Republic of China

Kevin C. Conlon
St. Vincent's University Hospital;
University of Dublin
Dublin, Ireland.

Christopher Connelly
Oregon Health & Science University
Portland, OR, USA

Paul M. Cromwell
St. Vincent's University Hospital
Dublin, Ireland

Rebecca Dalli
Mater Dei Hospital
Msida, Malta

Joey de Hondt
Amsterdam UMC; University of Amsterdam
Amsterdam, Netherlands

Ashley R. Dennison
University of Leicester; University Hospitals of
Leicester NHS Trust
Leicester, UK

Rahul Deshpande
Manchester Royal Infirmary
Manchester UK

John W. S. Devar
University of Witwatersrand; Chris Hani
Baragwanath Academic Hospital
Johannesburg, South Africa

Radha Krishna Dhiman
Sanjay Gandhi Post Graduate Institute of Medical
Sciences
Lucknow, India

Tom Diamond
Belfast Health & Social Care Trust
Belfast, N. Ireland

Elijah Dixon
University of Calgary
Alberta, Canada

Jia Fan
Zhongshan Hospital; Fudan University; Shanghai
Hepatic Oncology Clinical Center
Shanghai, China

Michiel F. G. Francken
Amsterdam UMC, University of Amsterdam
Amsterdam, Netherlands

Peter J. Friend
Oxford University Hospitals NHS Foundation Trust
Oxford, UK

Giuseppe Kito Fusai
Royal Free London NHS Foundation Trust;
University College London
London, UK

Jun Gao
Fudan University; Chinese Academy of Medical Sciences
Shanghai, China; Beijing, China

Giuseppe Garcea
University Hospitals of Leicester NHS Trust
Leicester, UK

Mohammad Ghallab
Icahn School of Medicine
Mount Sinai, NY, USA

Philippa Graff-Baker
University Hospitals of Leicester NHS Trust
Leicester, UK

Rachel V. Guest
University of Edinburgh
Edinburgh, UK

Thilo Hackert
Heidelberg University Hospital
Heidelberg, Germany

Fiona Hand
Royal Infirmary of Edinburgh
Edinburgh, UK

Jack A. Helliwell
University of Leeds
Leeds, UK

Jia Hong-Dong
Tsinghua Changgung Hospital
Beijing, China

John Isherwood
University Hospitals of Leicester NHS Trust
Leicester, UK

Eyad Issa
University Hospitals of Leicester NHS Trust
Leicester, UK

Eduard Jonas
University of Cape Town
Cape Town, South Africa

Raja R. Kalayarasan
Jawaharlal Institute of Post-Graduate Medical
Education and Research (JIPMER)
Pondicherry, India

Trisha Kanani
University Hospitals of Leicester
Leicester, UK

Harsh Kanhere
Royal Adelaide Hospital; The Queen Elizabeth
Hospital; University of Adelaide
Adelaide, Australia

Dimitrios Karavias
University Hospital Southampton
Southampton, UK

Vikram Kate
Jawaharlal Institute of Post-Graduate Medical
Education and Research (JIPMER)
Pondicherry, India

Tara S. Kent
Harvard Medical School
Boston, MA, USA

Yazan S. Khaled
University of Leeds
Leeds, UK

Jaekeun Kim
Lahey Hospital & Medical Center
Burlington, MA, USA

David A. Kooby
Emory University
Atlanta, GA, USA

Ahmed Kotb
St James's University Teaching Hospital
Leeds, UK

Jake Krige
Surgical Gastroenterology Unit, Division of General
Surgery, Department of Surgery Groote Schuur
Hospital, Faculty of Health Sciences, University of
Cape Town
Cape Town, South Africa

Li Lian Kuan
The Queen Elizabeth Hospital
Adelaide, Australia

Rohan Kumar
University of Alberta
Alberta, Canada

Pankaj Kundra
Jawaharlal Institute of Postgraduate Medical
Education and Research (JIPMER)
Pondicherry, India

Louise I. T. Lee
University Hospitals of Leicester NHS Trust
Leicester, UK

Major Kenneth Lee
University of Pennsylvania
Philadelphia, PA, USA

Janet W. Y. Li
Oregon Health & Science University
Portland, OR, USA

Leo Lin
Brigham and Women's Hospital
Boston, MA, USA

Hou-Bao Liu
Fudan University
Shanghai, China

Rong Liu
Chinese PLA General Hospital
Beijing, China

Wei-Ren Liu
Fudan University; Chinese Academy of Medical
Sciences
Shanghai, China; Beijing, China

Martin Loos
Heidelberg University Hospital
Heidelberg, Germany

Brendan P. Lovasik
Washington University
St Louis, MO, USA

Thomas MacCabe
Bristol Royal Infirmary
Bristol, UK

Claudia E. Mack
Heidelberg University Hospital
Heidelberg, Germany

Christopher T. J. Madden-McKee
N. Ireland Foundation Training Programme
N. Ireland, UK

Guy J. Maddern
University of Adelaide; Basil Hetzel Institute for
Translational Health Research; University of
Adelaide
Adelaide, Australia

Balaji Mahendran
Newcastle University
Newcastle-upon-Tyne, UK

Masatoshi Makuuchi
Koto Hospital
Tokyo, Japan

Deep Malde
Glenfield Hospital
Leicester, UK

Derek M. Manas
Newcastle University
Newcastle-upon-Tyne, UK

Giovanni Marchegiani
Verona University Hospital (Borgo Roma)
Verona, Italy

John J. McGoran
Western Health and Social Care Trust
Londonderry, N. Ireland, UK

Keno Mentor
Newcastle University
Newcastle upon Tyne, UK

Shreeyash Modak
AIG Hospitals
Hyderabad, India

Samir Mohindra
Post Graduate Institute of Medical Sciences
Lucknow, India

Zaheer Nabi
Asian Institute of Gastroenterology
Hyderabad, India

Raja R. Narayan
Harvard Medical School
Boston, MA, USA

Hossamaldin Nawara
University Hospitals Bristol NHS
Foundation Trust
Bristol, UK

John P. Neoptolemos
Heidelberg University Hospital
Heidelberg, Germany

Alexander Ney
University College London
London, UK

Seok Ling Ong
North West Anglia NHS Foundation Trust
Peterborough, UK

Derek A. O'Reilly
Beijing United Family Hospital (BJU)
Beijing, China

Susan L. Orloff
Oregon Health & Science University
Portland, OR, USA

Nicholas O'Rourke
Royal Brisbane and Women's Hospital;
University of Queensland
Queensland, Australia

Andrew Packham
University Hospitals of Leicester NHS Trust
Leicester, UK

Greg M. Padmore
University of Calgary
Alberta, Canada

Laurent Palazzo
Trocadero Clinic
Paris, France

Maxime Palazzo
European Hospital
Marseille, France

Sanjay Pandanaboyana
Newcastle University
Newcastle-upon-Tyne, UK

Rajesh Panwar
All India Institute of Medical Sciences
New Delhi, India

Rowan W. Parks
University of Edinburgh
Edinburgh, UK

Dave Patel
University Hospitals of Leicester NHS Trust
Leicester, UK

Adam Peckham-Cooper
Leeds Teaching Hospital NHS Trust
Leeds, United Kingdom

Cheng-Hong Peng
Ruijin Hospital; Shaghai Jiao Tong University
Shanghai, China

Stephen P. Pereira
Institute for Liver and Digestive Health, University
College London
London UK

Giampaolo Perri
Verona University Hospital (Borgo Roma)
Verona, Italy

Helen Pham
The University of Sydney
Sydney, Australia

Raaj Praseedom
Cambridge University Hospitals NHS Foundation
Trust
Cambridge, UK

John Primrose
University of Southampton
Southampton, UK

Wei-Feng Qu
Fudan University; Chinese Academy of Medical
Sciences
Shanghai, China; Beijing, China

Arumugam Rajesh
University Hospitals of Leicester NHS Trust
Leicester, UK

G. V. Rao
AIG Hospitals
Hyderabad, India

Dimtri Aristotle Raptis
Royal Free London NHS Foundation Trust
London, UK

Samrat Ray
University of Toronto
Toronto, Canada

D. Nageshwar Reddy
Asian institute of Gastroenterology
Hyderabad, India

Trevor W. Reichman
University of Toronto
Toronto, Canada

Arthur Richardson
The University of Sydney
Sydney, Australia

John Keith Roberts
University Hospitals Birmingham
Birmingham, UK

Francis P. Robertson
Newcastle University
Newcastle upon Tyne, UK

Richard J. Robinson
University Hospitals of Leicester
Leicester, UK

Peush Sahni
All India Institute of Medical Sciences
New Delhi, India

Yoshihiro Sakamoto
Kyorin University Hospital
Tokyo, Japan

Ali Salim
Brigham and Women's Hospital
Boston, MA, USA

Camila Hidalgo Salinas
Royal Free London NHS Foundation Trust
London, UK

Roberto Salvia
Verona University Hospital (Borgo Roma)
Verona, Italy

Ana Sather
University of Minnesota
Minneapolis, MN, USA

Sudeep R. Shah
D. Hinduja Hospital and Medical Research Centre
Mumbai, India

A. M. James Shapiro
University of Alberta
Edmonton, Canada

Ying-Hong Shi
Fudan University
Shanghai, China

Michael Silva
Churchill Hospital
Oxford, UK

Rajneesh Kumar Singh
Sanjay Gandhi Post Graduate Institute of Medical
Sciences
Lucknow, India

Ajith K. Siriwardena
University of Manchester
Manchester, UK

Martin D. Smith
University of Witwatersrand; Chris Hani
Baragwanath Academic Hospital
Johannesburg, South Africa

Steven C. Stain
Tufts University School of Medicine
Burlington, MA, USA

Andrew Strickland
Bristol Royal Infirmary
Bristol, UK

Lulu Tanno
Oxford University Hospitals NHS
Foundation Trust
Oxford, UK

Mark A. Taylor
Mater Hospital
Belfast, N. Ireland

Sarah Thomasset
Royal Infirmary of Edinburgh
Edinburgh, UK

Giles Toogood
Leeds Teaching Hospital NHS Trust
Leeds, United Kingdom

Markus Trochsler
The University of Adelaide, The Queen Elizabeth
Hospital
Adelaide, Australia

Andrew Tsang
North West Anglia NHS Foundation Trust
Peterborough, UK

Richard Tunstall
University of Leeds
Leeds, UK

Shams ul Bari
Sheri-Kashmir Institute of Medical Sciences
Srinagar, India

Hemant Jitendra Vadeyar
Mediclinic City Hospital Dubai, Mohammed
bin Rashid University of Medical and Health
Sciences
Dubai, UAE

Charlotte L. van Veldhuisen
University of Amsterdam
Amsterdam, Netherlands

Stalin Vinayagam
Jawaharlal Institute of Postgraduate Medical
Education and Research (JIPMER)
Pondicherry, India

Brendan C. Visser
Stanford University
Stanford, CA, USA

Charles M. Vollmer Jr
University of Pennsylvania
Philadelphia, PA, USA

Xiao-Ying Wang
Fudan University; Chinese Academy of Medical
Sciences
Shanghai, China; Beijing, China

Steve White
Newcastle University
Newcastle upon Tyne, UK

Colin Wilson
Newcastle University
Newcastle upon Tyne, UK

Rachel Wong
University of Queensland
Queensland, Australia

Xiao-Ling Wu
Fudan University; Chinese Academy of Medical Sciences
Shanghai, China; Beijing, China

Zhen Yang
Shanghai Jiao Tong University
Shanghai, China

Zhai Meng Yao
Beijing United Family Hospital and Clinics
Beijing, China

Muhammad Umar Younis
Mediclinic City Hospital
Dubai, UAE

Jian Zhou
Fudan University; Chinese Academy of
Medical Sciences
Shanghai, China; Beijing, China

Kai Zhu
Fudan University; Chinese Academy of Medical Sciences
Shanghai, China; Beijing, China

Chapter 1

Embryology of the Liver, Pancreas and Biliary System

Richard Tunstall

INTRODUCTION

During the embryonic stage of development and following the folding of the trilaminar embryonic disc (week 4 of gestation), the primitive gut tube extends from the oropharyngeal (buccopharyngeal) membrane to the cloacal membrane and is divided by its three blood supplies into the foregut, midgut and hindgut (*Figure 1.1*). Initially, the gut tube is formed from embryonic endoderm. The endoderm eventually develops into a range of structures including the epithelial linings of the gastrointestinal (GI) canal, biliary system (tree), pancreatic ducts and tracheobronchial tree, hepatocytes and the exocrine and endocrine cells of the pancreas. The connective tissues, vessels and visceral peritoneum associated with the gut tube, liver and pancreas develop from varying parts of the splanchnic mesoderm. Cardiac mesoderm is also essential for inducing liver development.

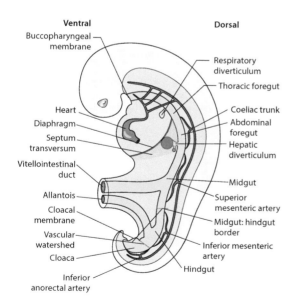

Figure 1.1 Embryo at 4 weeks of gestation (stage 12). The gut tube passes from the buccopharyngeal to the cloacal membrane, and is divided into the foregut, midgut and hindgut by its blood supplies. The early stage of liver development has begun in the region of the septum transversum.

During week 5 of gestation, the entire abdominal part of the gut tube has a dorsal mesentery formed by two thin layers of mesothelium or peritoneum. The dorsal mesentery attaches the gut tube to the posterior wall of the body cavity and conveys the neurovasculature and lymphatics (*Figure 1.2*). The abdominal part of the foregut also has a ventral mesentery derived from septum transversum mesenchyme. Likewise, it consists of two layers of mesothelium or peritoneum that pass from the abdominal part of the oesophagus, lesser curvature of the stomach and first (superior) part of the duodenum to the midline anterior abdominal wall, down to the level of the umbilicus, and to the diaphragm. The ventral mesentery contains the liver, gallbladder, parts of the extrahepatic biliary system, hepatic portal vein, proper hepatic artery and ligamentum teres (umbilical vein *in utero*) and forms the lesser omentum and falciform ligament. In early development, the ventral mesentery also contains the ventral pancreatic bud, and the dorsal mesentery contains the dorsal pancreatic bud, spleen and associated vessels.

LIVER AND BILIARY SYSTEM (TRACT)

The liver starts developing during the middle of week 3 (Carnegie stage 10). The septum transversum, a mass of splanchnic mesenchyme separating the pericardial and peritoneal cavities, together with cardiac mesoderm induce hepatic endodermal proliferation. The hepatic endodermal primordium develops from the endoderm of the ventral region of the distal (duodenal) part of the abdominal foregut. At the end of week 4 (stage 12), proliferation of the hepatic endodermal primordium forms the hepatic diverticulum (*Figure 1.3*). The diverticulum grows ventrally into the mesenchyme of the septum transversum and has caudal and cranial parts. Endodermal cells from the cranial part proliferate rapidly to form interconnected trabeculae of hepatocytes which surround the developing hepatic sinusoids within the septum transversum. These endodermal cells also form the epithelial lining of the intrahepatic biliary system and the left and right hepatic ducts. The extrahepatic biliary system, specifically the gallbladder, cystic duct, common hepatic duct, and bile duct, develops from derived endoderm from the caudal part of the hepatic diverticulum.

Figure labels for Figure 1.1:

Ventral | **Dorsal**

Buccopharyngeal membrane
Respiratory diverticulum
Thoracic foregut
Heart
Coeliac trunk
Diaphragm
Abdominal foregut
Septum transversum
Hepatic diverticulum
Vitellointestinal duct
Midgut
Allantois
Superior mesenteric artery
Cloacal membrane
Midgut: hindgut border
Vascular watershed
Inferior mesenteric artery
Cloaca
Hindgut
Inferior anorectal artery

DOI: 10.1201/9781003080060-1

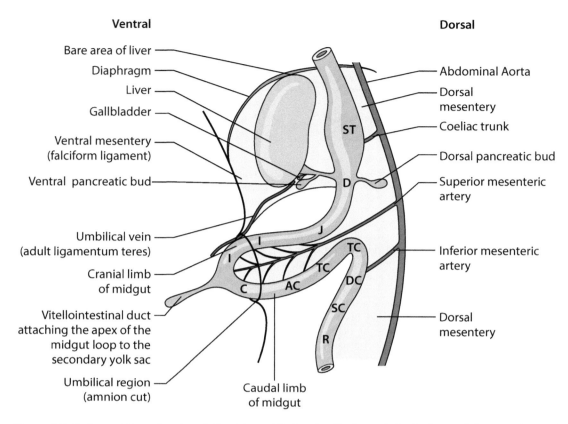

Figure 1.2 Embryo at 5 weeks of gestation (stage 14) showing the intra-abdominal part of the gut tube, and the developing liver, pancreas and gallbladder. The dorsal mesentery is present along the length of the gut tube. The intra-abdominal part of the foregut also has a ventral mesentery derived from the septum transversum. Key: ST: stomach; D: duodenum; J: jejunum; I: ileum; C: caecum; AC: ascending colon; TC: transverse colon; DC: descending colon; SC: sigmoid colon; R: rectum.

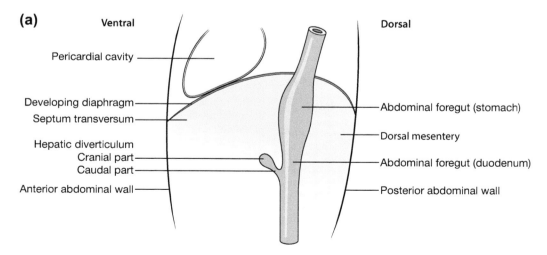

Figure 1.3 Development of the liver from the endoderm of the hepatic diverticulum and the mesenchyme of the septum transversum. All figures show a left lateral view. For simplicity, the concurrent rotation of the gut tube is not shown. (a) Week 4 (stage 12) embryo showing the hepatic diverticulum projecting into the septum transversum. (*Continued*)

(b)

(c)

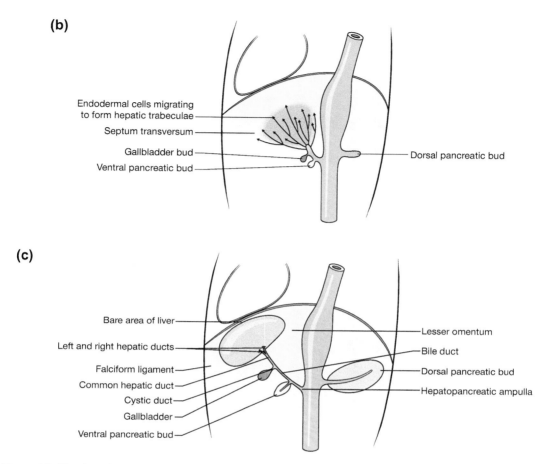

Figure 1.3 *(Continued)* (b) Early week 5 (stage 14) embryo showing migration of endodermal cells from the cranial part of the hepatic diverticulum into the mesenchyme of the septum transversum. The endodermal cells form the interlinked hepatic trabeculae (laminae) around the developing hepatic sinusoids. (c) Late week 5 (stage 15) embryo showing development of the gallbladder, extrahepatic bile ducts, and the ventral and dorsal pancreatic buds within their respective mesenteries.

Mesenchyme derived from the septum transversum forms the connective tissues of the liver, including its thin fibrous capsule (Glisson) and the connective tissues of the intrahepatic vessels (hepatic portal venous system and sinusoids). The mesodermal cells of the liver also give rise two intra-sinusoidal macrophages (Kupffer cells or stellate macrophages) and early haemopoietic cells. *In utero*, red blood cell production occurs in the liver from week 6 of gestation with production later moving to the bone marrow.

Peritoneal formations

The developing liver enlarges quickly and by week 10 of gestation protrudes into the superior (upper) part of the abdominal cavity, within the ventral mesentery. Part of the superior aspect of the developing liver, known as the 'bare area', remains in contact with the part of the septum transversum that forms the central tendon of the diaphragm. The peritoneal reflections around the margins of the bare area, passing from the liver to the diaphragm, form the coronary and triangular hepatic ligaments.

The part of the ventral mesentery passing between the liver and the midline anterior abdominal wall (down to the umbilicus) is known as the falciform ligament, and the parts of the ventral mesentery passing between the liver and stomach (hepatogastric ligament), liver and superior (first) part of the duodenum (hepatoduodenal ligament) and liver and abdominal part of the oesophagus (hepato-oesophageal ligament) are collectively known as the lesser omentum. If present, the hepatocolic and hepatophrenic ligaments also contribute to the lesser omentum. *In utero,* the inferior (lower) free-edge of the falciform ligament contains the (left) umbilical vein as it passes from the umbilicus to porta hepatis. After birth, the umbilical vein fibroses to form the ligamentum teres (round ligament of the liver). Portal hypertension may recanalize the ligamentum teres, resulting in dilated portosystemic anastomoses around the umbilicus, which may be seen as caput medusae. The inferior border of the ventral mesentery passing between the liver and superior part of the duodenum (hepatoduodenal ligament), is commonly termed the free edge (border) of the lesser omentum. It provides a conduit from the retroperitoneal region of the posterior abdominal wall to the porta hepatis, and contains the bile duct, proper hepatic artery and hepatic portal vein.

Vascular system

Due to its central location, inferior to the developing heart, the developing liver is located adjacent to several major embryonic vessels (*Figure 1.4a–e*). The left and right horns of the sinus venosus of the developing heart each receive blood from the left or right (respectively) umbilical, vitelline and common cardinal veins. The vitelline and umbilical veins pass through the region of liver development and parts of these vessels will eventually contribute to the hepatic vascular system. The vitelline veins bring blood from the extraembryonic secondary yolk sac and developing gut tube, the proper hepatic artery brings blood from coeliac trunk, and the left and right umbilical veins bring blood from the placenta. As development progresses, the venous supply to the liver undergoes numerous and significant changes; initially four veins (two umbilical and two vitelline) supply the developing liver, this soon reduces to two veins (umbilical and hepatic portal), and following birth one vein (hepatic portal). The right umbilical vein briefly supplies the developing liver, but soon regresses.

Hepatic sinusoids

Development of the hepatic sinusoids is prompted by the formation of the endodermal hepatic trabeculae (laminae). The hepatocytes forming the hepatic trabeculae eventually surround the hepatic sinusoids. Interaction between the early vitelline veins and the tissue of the septum transversum creates a plexus of hepatic veins. These veins interconnect with endothelium-lined spaces within the mesenchyme of the septum transversum to form the network of hepatic sinusoids. During early development, the hepatic sinusoids receive venous blood from branches of the left and right vitelline (deoxygenated) and the left and right umbilical (oxygenated) veins, collectively known as the venae advehentes. Venous blood leaves the hepatic sinusoidal system via the terminal ends of the left and right umbilical and vitelline veins, known as the venae revehentes or hepatocardiac channels (veins). These drain into the sinus venosus.

(a)

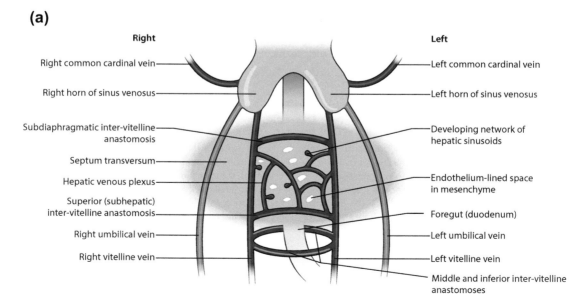

Figure 1.4 Anterior view of the developing liver and associated vasculature, from week 5 of gestation (stage 13) to neonate. (a) Three paired embryonic vessels enter the left and right horns of the sinus venosus (week 5, stage 13). The vitelline veins are forming a venous plexus and hepatic sinusoids within the septum transversum. (*Continued*)

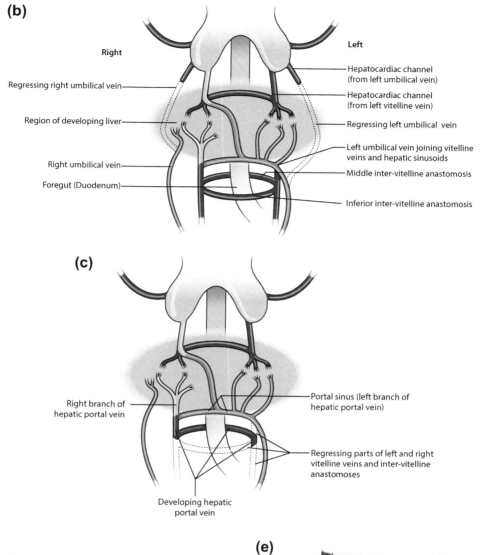

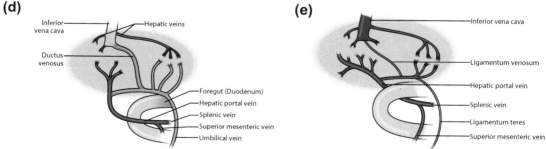

Figure 1.4 (*Continued*) (b) Vascular remodelling and regression continue (week 6, stage 15). The developing hepatic sinusoids receive blood from branches of the vitelline and umbilical veins (venae advehentes) and drain blood to the sinus venosus via four hepatocardiac channels (venae revehentes), two left and two right. (c) The prehepatic inter-vitelline anastomoses are remodelling to form the hepatic portal vein and portal sinus (week 6, stage 16). The subdiaphragmatic inter-vitelline anastomosis is draining blood from the left side of the liver to the right. (d) The hepatic portal vein has formed from parts of the left and right vitelline veins (week 8, stage 20). The umbilical vein mostly bypasses the liver via the ductus venosus. (e) Following birth, the umbilical vein and ductus venosus close, forming the ligamentum teres and ligamentum venosum, respectively. The hepatic portal vein supplies the hepatic sinusoids, and the hepatic veins drain them.

Vitelline veins

The left and right vitelline veins drain the extraembryonic secondary yolk sac of the embryo and the developing gut tube. By week 6 (stage 15), they interconnect via three prehepatic (inferior, middle and superior [subhepatic]) and one subdiaphragmatic inter-vitelline anastomoses. The inferior and middle inter-vitelline anastomoses form a vascular ring around the duodenum. As development progresses, parts of the anastomoses and the vitelline veins regress and remodel. The proximal part of the left vitelline vein (hepatocardiac channel) also regresses and loses its connection with the left horn of the sinus venosus. The proximal part of the right vitelline vein (hepatocardiac channel) eventually forms the hepatocardiac part, or hepatic segment, of the inferior vena cava. The hepatic portal vein is formed by a more distal part of the right vitelline vein, the middle prehepatic inter-vitelline anastomosis (posterior to the duodenum) and a more distal part of the left vitelline vein. The hepatic portal vein connects with the presumptive splenic vein and superior mesenteric vein, and drains the gut tube. The portal sinus, a vascular channel within the liver, is formed by the superior (subhepatic) inter-vitelline anastomosis.

The right and left intrahepatic branches of the hepatic portal vein are derived from a remnant of the right vitelline vein and the portal sinus, respectively. Functional segmentation of the liver is determined by the distribution of the hepatic portal venous system, with each segment supplied by a major branch. Developmental defects of the hepatic portal venous system include; hepatic portal vein hypoplasia, atresia or stenosis; congenital absence of the hepatic portal vein with either partial or full extrahepatic portosystemic shunting; intrahepatic portosystemic shunting; and congenital absence of hepatic portal vein branches, with agenesis of the dependent part of the liver.

Umbilical veins

During early development, the left and right umbilical veins bring oxygenated blood from the placenta to both the liver and sinus venosus of the developing heart. As development progresses parts of the right and left umbilical veins regress. The remaining caudal part of the left umbilical vein enlarges, connects with the subhepatic (superior) inter-vitelline anastomosis and provides the majority blood supply to the hepatic sinusoids (hepatic capillary plexus). At this stage, the left umbilical vein becomes known as the umbilical vein and conveys all oxygenated blood from the placenta to the developing liver. Eventually, the umbilical vein becomes connected to the inferior vena cava via a venous shunt, the ductus venosus, with only smaller connections remaining to the plexus of hepatic sinusoids. The umbilical vein connects with the portal circulation on the right side of the liver via

the subhepatic inter-vitelline anastomosis, which at this stage is termed the portal sinus.

During the early stage of hepatic development (early week 5), blood flow to the right and left lobes (sides) of the liver is relatively equal. However, as cardiac development progresses, the left horn of the sinus venosus decreases in size, with venous blood from the embryo being returned preferentially to the right horn. Consequently, the left lobe of the liver drains blood via vessels in the right lobe. The umbilical vein provides the majority blood supply to the left lobe of the liver, whereas the right lobe receives a mixed (1:1) supply from the umbilical and hepatic portal veins. During development, the left lobe of the liver has a greater blood supply than the right, and the umbilical vein is the greatest contributor to total hepatic blood supply.

Hepatic artery

The common hepatic artery forms during week 8, as a branch of the coeliac trunk. Development of the arterial system of the liver is linked to development of the intrahepatic biliary system (tree). The proper hepatic artery branches sequentially as it passes into and through the liver, following the intrahepatic branches of the hepatic portal venous system. Extensive arterial branching occurs from week 10 to week 15. The hepatic arterial system supplies the periportal and peribiliary capillary plexuses, the hepatic sinusoids and the hepatic (Glisson) capsule. The cystic artery arises from the proper hepatic artery. Variation in the origin and branching pattern of the hepatic artery, proper hepatic artery and cystic artery are common.

Biliary system

As the liver forms, the caudal part of the hepatic diverticulum narrows and remodels to form the extrahepatic biliary system (tract), which includes the gallbladder, cystic duct, common hepatic duct and bile duct. The region of the bile duct system cranial to the connection of the cystic duct becomes the common hepatic duct and is joined by the left and right cystic ducts, which derive from the cranial part of the hepatic diverticulum. The gallbladder and cystic duct develop from an outpouching (budding) of the bile duct that projects into the ventral mesentery. Developmental defects or anomalies related to the formation of the gallbladder include; Phrygian cap (a commonly encountered folding of the gallbladder fundus); duplication; intrahepatic or left-sided location; septation; agenesis (rare); absence of the cystic duct; and outpouching of the infundibular region (Hartmann pouch).

Variants of the bile duct system, such as accessory hepatic ducts, may occur and can be the cause of unintended high location bile duct injury during operative procedures. Accessory hepatic ducts pass from the liver (mostly from the right side) and join the common hepatic duct, cystic duct or bile duct (*Figure 1.5*). Alternatively,

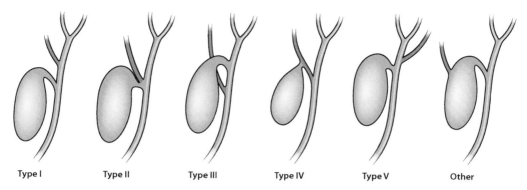

Figure 1.5 Classification of accessory hepatic ducts into Types I–V and Other. Types I–IV arise from the right lobe (side) of the liver, and Type V arises from the left. Type 1 (the most common) joins the common hepatic duct; Type II joins the common hepatic duct in the same location as the cystic duct, via a shared entrance; Type III joins the bile duct; Type 4 joins the cystic duct and their common stem joins the common hepatic duct; and Type 5, joins the common hepatic duct. 'Other' represents a direct connection with the gallbladder. Adapted from Uchiyama et al., 2006 (1).

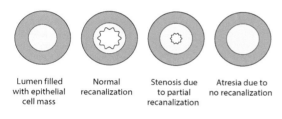

Figure 1.6 The normal process of bile duct occlusion by epithelial cell proliferation, followed by recanalization. Defective recanalization can result in stenosis or atresia.

accessory hepatic ducts pass directly to the gallbladder. Individuals with an accessory hepatic duct may have longer and thinner hepatic ducts. Rarely, accessory bile ducts may be present.

Biliary atresia

As with other regions of the developing gut tube, the endodermal lining of the biliary duct system proliferates rapidly during early development, to occlude the lumen (*Figure 1.6*). Coinciding with bile formation, recanalization of the biliary ducts occurs by week 12. A failure of recanalization can result in stenosis (partial occlusion) or atresia (complete blockage) of the biliary tree, with extrahepatic forms more common than intrahepatic. Biliary atresia is associated with neonatal cholestasis and requires prompt diagnosis and treatment.

PANCREAS

The pancreas develops from two buds (outgrowths) of endoderm that unite during rotation of the developing gut tube (*Figures 1.2, 1.3* and *1.7*). The

dorsal pancreatic bud appears in week 4 (stage 9) and the ventral pancreatic bud in week 5 (stage 12). The ventral pancreatic bud arises from the endoderm of the caudal part of the hepatic diverticulum, caudal to the bud of the developing gallbladder, and grows within the ventral mesentery. Initially the ventral bud consists of two parts, left and right; only the right part develops. The dorsal pancreatic bud arises from the endoderm of the duodenal part of the gut tube, proximal to the hepatic diverticulum, and grows within the dorsal mesentery. Both buds derive splanchnic mesenchyme from the pericardioperitoneal canals. The ventral bud also derives mesenchyme from the septum transversum. The connective tissues of the pancreas, including the interlobular septa and pancreatic capsule (connective tissue covering), develop from the splanchnic mesoderm. Blood vessels within the pancreas develop from angiogenic mesenchyme and are supplied by branches of the nearby coeliac trunk and superior mesenteric artery.

As development continues, the right part of the ventral pancreatic bud and associated bile duct migrate posterior to the duodenal part of the foregut, to assume a position within the dorsal mesentery next to the dorsal pancreatic bud. By week 7 (stage 18) the ventral and dorsal buds are fused. The dorsal pancreatic bud forms a majority of the pancreas, with the ventral pancreatic bud forming posterior parts of the pancreatic head and uncinate process. As development and rotation of the gut tube progresses, the intraperitoneal pancreas is pushed against the posterior abdominal wall and subsequent mesenteric zygosis (*Figure 1.8*) results in most of the pancreas becoming secondarily retroperitoneal.

Congenital defects

Maldevelopment of the pancreatic buds may cause congenital pancreatic hypoplasia or dorsal pancreatic

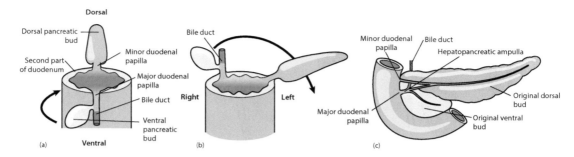

Figure 1.7 Development of the pancreas from the ventral and dorsal pancreatic buds (anterior view). (a) The ventral and dorsal pancreatic buds, and the associated bile duct, begin rotating behind to the duodenum during rightward rotation of the gut tube (week 5, stage 14). (b) The ventral pancreatic bud and bile duct system move behind the duodenum to join the dorsal pancreatic bud in the dorsal mesentery (week 6, stage 16). (c) Fusion of the ventral and dorsal pancreatic buds forms a single pancreas (week 7, stage 18). The main pancreatic duct forms from the duct system of the ventral bud and the distal (dorsal) part of the duct system of the dorsal bud; the accessory pancreatic duct (orange) forms from proximal (ventral) part duct system of the dorsal bud.

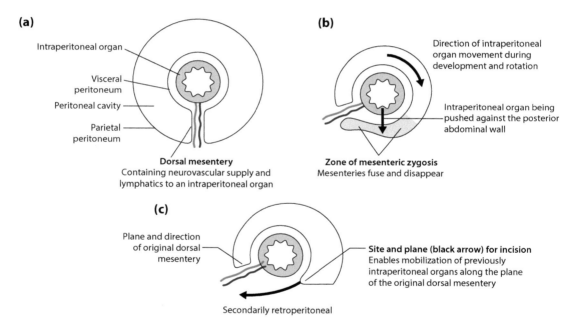

Figure 1.8 Mesenteric zygosis of an intraperitoneal organ. (a) An intraperitoneal organ with its neurovascular supply contained within the dorsal mesentery. (b) An intraperitoneal organ being pushed against the posterior abdominal wall and losing its dorsal mesentery via mesenteric zygosis. (c) A secondarily retroperitoneal organ showing the positioning of its neurovasculature. A knowledge of this process and its direction guides the safe surgical mobilisation of secondarily retroperitoneal organs (black arrow).

(bud) agenesis. A failure of regression of the left part of the ventral pancreatic bud can result in an annular pancreas. In this condition, the left and right parts of the ventral bud pass anterior and posterior, respectively, to the duodenum and surround it (*Figure 1.9*). Annular pancreas can cause duodenal obstruction which may symptomatically mimic duodenal stenosis or atresia.

Circumportal pancreas is a form of annular pancreas, in which pancreatic tissue surrounds the hepatic portal vein, superior mesenteric vein and splenic vein. Ectopic (heterotopic) pancreatic tissue may be found in almost any location within the GI canal, with the commonest being the stomach, duodenum, colon, oesophagus and ileal (Meckel) diverticulum. Less

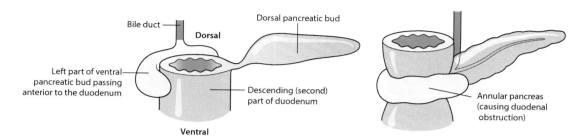

Figure 1.9 Development of an annular pancreas during week 6 (stage 16). (a) A persistent left part of the ventral pancreatic bud abnormally rotates anterior to the duodenum, in addition to the normal rotation of the right part of the ventral pancreatic bud posterior to the duodenum. (b) The left and right parts of the ventral pancreatic bud surround the second part of the duodenum causing either partial or complete obstruction.

common locations include the gallbladder, spleen and mesenteries.

Pancreatic duct system

The main pancreatic ducts remodel such that the distal (or dorsal) section of the main duct system within the dorsal pancreatic bud drains into the duct system within the ventral pancreatic bud. Following its rotation, the duct within the ventral pancreatic bud remains connected to the bile duct, thus forming the hepatopancreatic ampulla (Vater), which opens into the descending (second) part of the duodenum at the major duodenal papilla. An anomalous pancreaticobiliary junction occurs when the main pancreatic duct and bile duct converge within the head of the pancreas, resulting in a single common duct draining into the duodenum. This is associated with an incompetent ampullary sphincter (Oddi) and reflux from the duodenum.

As the pancreas grows, the pancreatic part of the bile duct becomes variably embedded in pancreatic tissue. The remaining proximal (or ventral) part of the main pancreatic duct system within the dorsal pancreatic bud usually persists as a small accessory pancreatic duct, which drains into the duodenum proximal to the hepatopancreatic ampulla via the minor duodenal papilla. In some cases, the pancreatic duct systems may not fuse leaving two separate routes of drainage into the duodenum (pancreas divisum), one for each pancreatic bud. In other cases, the accessory pancreatic duct system may be absent.

The full duct system of the pancreas develops via the sequential branching of endodermal tubules derived from the main pancreatic ducts. This process forms the interlobar, intralobar and intercalated ducts, which are evident from weeks 24–32.

Pancreatic acini and islets

The secretory cells of the pancreas derive from endoderm. The pancreatic acini develop around the ends of the endodermal tubules forming the intercalated ducts. The pancreatic islets (Langerhans) develop during the 3rd month of gestation from pancreatic tubule cells that migrate to sit between the pancreatic acini.

REFERENCE

1. Uchiyama K, Tani M, Kawai M, Ueno T, Hama T, Yamaue H. Preoperative evaluation of the extrahepatic bile duct structure for laparoscopic cholecystectomy. *Surg Endosc* 2006;**20(7)**:1119–23.

Bailey & Love's Essential Operations Bailey & Love's Essential Operatio
Bailey & Love's Essential Operations Bailey & Love's Essential Operatio
Bailey & Love's Essential Operations Bailey & Love's Essential Operatio

SECTION 1 | BASIC PRINCIPLES

Chapter

2

Liver Anatomy and Physiology

Jia Fan and Ashley R. Dennison

INTRODUCTION

The liver is a highly complex organ found only in vertebrates and responsible for over 500 individual functions. It is located in the right upper quadrant, protected by the ribs and weighs on average 1.5 kg (970–1860 g). It is wedge shaped in both coronal and axial planes and divided by the middle hepatic vein into two lobes with the larger right lobe generally representing 60% by volume. The parenchyma is covered by a thin capsule (Glisson's capsule) and visceral peritoneum apart from the posterior surface, known as the 'bare area'. Due to the liver's complexity and lack of anatomical details, performing major surgical procedures required developments in multiple fields (*Table 2.1*).

Pioneering early work by eponymous authors such as Cantlie (1), Langenbuch (2), Healey and Schroy (3) and Couinaud (4) led to the first formal resection in 1952 by Lortat-Jacob and Robert (5). Developments in surgical technique, anaesthesia and intensive care including preoperative and intraoperative imaging, liver transection technology and low central venous pressure (CVP) anaesthesia have facilitated the remarkable further progress in liver surgery to-date. Progress continues with the incorporation of laparoscopic and robotic surgery and training techniques including virtual reality.

ANATOMY OF THE LIVER

Embryology

Liver development begins at 3–4 weeks gestation when a hepatic foregut diverticulum buds into the ventral wall of the primitive midgut. This diverticulum is the anlage for the liver, extrahepatic biliary ducts, gallbladder and ventral pancreas which develop over the next week. The basement membrane surrounding the liver bud is then lost and cords of bipotential hepatoblasts invade the septum transversum and differentiate into hepatocytes and cholangiocytes. For a detailed description of the embryology of the liver (*see* **Chapter 1**).

Ligaments and peritoneal reflections

The liver is covered by visceral peritoneum (serosa), with a layer of connective tissue, the Glisson capsule underneath. At the porta hepatis, the Glisson capsule envelops and travels along the portal tracts (triads)

into the liver, carrying branches of the hepatic artery, portal vein and bile ducts. The liver is fixed in the right upper quadrant by the hepatic veins and ligaments formed from the peritoneal reflections. Dividing the left triangular ligament on the superior surface of the left lobe mobilizes it from the diaphragm exposing the left lateral wall of the IVC. The right triangular ligament similarly fixes the right lobe to the undersurface of the right hemidiaphragm, and division mobilizes the liver sufficiently to allow it to be rotated to the left. Another major supporting structure is the falciform ligament (remnant of the umbilical vein), which runs cephalad from the umbilicus, enters the liver at the interlobar fissure and passes anteriorly on the surface of the liver attaching it to the anterior abdominal wall. Dividing the cephalad leaves of the falciform ligament exposes the suprahepatic IVC within a thin fibrous sheath. The final peritoneal reflection is the lesser omentum between the stomach and the liver which contains the hilar structures in its right free-edge.

The blood supply to the liver

The liver is composed of eight segments (*Figure 2.1*) each supplied by terminal branches of the portal vein (80% of the blood flow) and hepatic artery (20%) and drained by bile ducts and hepatic veins. The shape of the segments varies between individuals, but the configuration remains relatively constant. The arterial blood supply is variable in origin and course but in most individuals is derived from the coeliac trunk which usually divides into left gastric, common hepatic and splenic arteries. After supplying the gastroduodenal artery, the hepatic artery branches at a variable level to produce the right- and left-hepatic arteries; the larger right branch supplying the right lobe. The right lobe may be partly or completely supplied by a right hepatic artery arising directly from the superior mesenteric artery running to the liver on the posterior wall of the bile duct after passing behind the uncinate process and head of the pancreas. Similarly, the left lobe artery may be augmented or replaced by a branch of the left gastric artery running in the lesser omentum from the lesser curve of the stomach.

The porta hepatis is a pronounced transverse fissure on the visceral surface of the liver. It runs between the cephalad end of the fissure for the

DOI: 10.1201/9781003080060-2

Table 2.1 Landmarks in the development of liver surgery

Author and date	Development
Egypt 3000 BCE	Papyri record a number of medical conditions including jaundice
Mesopotamia around 1900 BCE	Priests practiced hepatoscopy and considered the liver to be the 'seed of life'
Greece 400 BCE	Disease recognized as a disorder of healthy tissue not a punishment. The liver was considered central to a wide range of conditions. Galen believed the liver was 'the author of blood and the origin of the veins' and 'a site for repairing the spirit and determining the quality of a man'
Aztecs 1325	The Aztecs believed the liver was the 'repository of the human spirit'
Glisson 1654	Francis Glisson, 1957–1677 Regis Professor of Physic, Cambridge, UK described the capsule of the liver and its blood supply in his book *Anatomia Hepatis* in 1654. Glisson's capsule delineated the lobular structure of the liver
Luis 1886	First recorded formal hepatectomy, fatal haemorrhage after 6 hours
Cantlie 1887	Sir James Cantlie, 1851–1926, a Scottish born physician cofounded the Hong Kong College of Medicine for Chinese (now Hong Kong University School of Medicine). He described Cantlie's line which is the vertical plane that runs from the inferior vena cava (IVC) to the gallbladder fossa and divides the liver into right and left lobes. It is the principal plane used for hepatectomy
Langenbuch 1888	First successful hepatectomy although required further surgery for bleeding
McLane-Tiffany 1890	Tumour resection at Johns Hopkins Hospital
Lucke 1891	Successful removal of malignant tumour
Keen 1899	First formal left lateral segmentectomy
Cattell 1943	Resection of a colorectal metastasis at the Lahey Clinic
Lortat-Jacob and Robert 1952	First formal right hepatectomy in Paris
Quattlebaum 1953	Description of three right hepatectomies; dissection using scalpel handle
Healey and Schroy 1953	John E Healey and Paul C Schroy in 1953 described the anatomy of the biliary ducts within the human liver, defining its lobular structure
Couinaud 1957	Claude Couinaud, 1922–2008, French surgeon and anatomist, described the segmental anatomy of the liver in his seminal book *Le Foie: Études anatomiques et chirurgicales*. He continued to describe new details about liver anatomy until 1991
Lin 1958	Figure fracture technique described
Starzl 1963	First successful liver transplant
Raia July 1989 Broelsch November 1989	First living donor liver transplants: University of Sao Paulo University of Chicago Medical Center

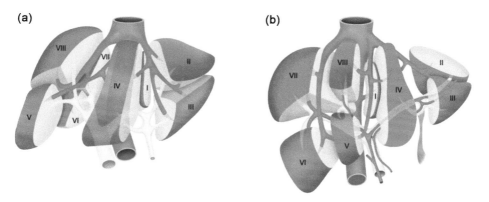

Figure 2.1 The functional division of the liver and of the liver segments according to Couinaud's nomenclature; as seen in the patient (a), in the *ex vivo* position (b).

ligamentum teres and the gall bladder fossa. The neurovascular structures and lymphatics running in the right free-edge of the lesser omentum (the hepatoduodenal ligament) enter at this point and the right- and left-hepatic ducts emerge. There are numerous variations of the hilar structures which are important in the planning and performance of operations on the liver (*Figure 2.2*).

In the most common (traditional) arrangement, the bile duct runs in the free-edge of the hepatoduodenal ligament with the hepatic artery medially and the portal vein posteriorly each dividing into two branches at the hilum. The right- and left-hepatic ducts arise from the hepatic parenchyma and form the common hepatic duct. The cystic duct draining the gallbladder enters the ligament at a variable level joining the common hepatic duct to form the common bile duct (CBD). The right hepatic artery crosses the bile duct anteriorly or posteriorly before giving rise to the cystic artery and multiple branches predominantly from the right hepatic artery supply the bile duct. The portal vein is formed by the confluence of the splenic and superior mesenteric veins behind the neck of the pancreas with the left branch having a longer, approximately 2 cm, extrahepatic course. The portal vein often has two large branches to the right lobe, which are usually outside the liver for a short length, before giving a left-portal vein branch that runs behind the left hepatic duct.

The venous drainage

The IVC occupies a groove on the posterior surface of the liver which drains into it via three large veins immediately below the diaphragm. The suprahepatic IVC immediately traverses the diaphragm to enter the right atrium but below the liver there is a short clear segment above the insertion of the renal veins. A variable number of short inferior hepatic veins pass directly from the liver to the anterior wall of the IVC. The right hepatic vein can be exposed fully outside the liver parenchyma, but the middle and left veins usually terminate in a short common trunk before entering the IVC. The right adrenal gland is adjacent to the retrohepatic IVC and drains into it, usually by a single vein.

Segmental anatomy

The liver is divided into functional right and left units along the line between the gallbladder fossa and the middle hepatic vein (Cantlie's line). Understanding the internal anatomy of the liver, facilitated safe liver surgery and Couinaud, a French anatomist, described the liver as being divided into eight segments (*Figure 2.1a,b*). Each segment can be considered a functional unit supplied by a branch of the hepatic artery, portal vein and bile duct, and drained by a hepatic vein tributary and this concept facilitates anatomical liver resection. Liver segments V–VIII to the right of Cantlie's line

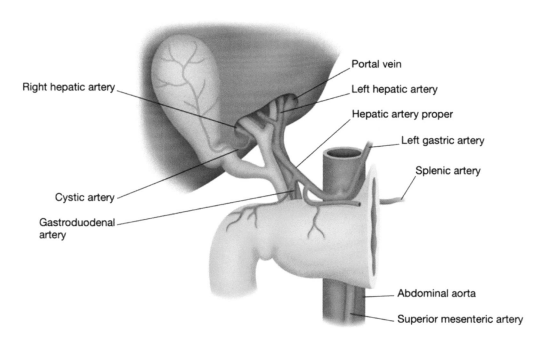

Figure 2.2 Anatomy of the liver hilum. A hilum is a depression or fissure where nerves, vessels or ducts enter a bodily organ.

are supplied by the right hepatic artery and the right branch of the portal vein and biliary drainage is via the right hepatic duct. To the left of Cantlie's line segments, I–IV are supplied by the left hepatic artery and left portal vein and drain via the left hepatic duct. Resections of individual segments, the whole of the left or right hemi-liver, or combinations, are possible.

Microscopic anatomy and structure

The liver comprises ≈100 000 hexagonal functional units known as lobules with a central vein surrounded by six hepatic portal veins and six hepatic arteries. These vessels are connected by capillary-like tubes called sinusoids, which extend to meet the central vein. Lobules are separated by hepatic sinusoids, large-diameter capillaries lined by endothelial cells between rows of plates or cords of hepatocytes. Each sinusoid contains Kupffer cells, a type of macrophage that capture and breaks down effete red blood cells, and hepatocytes which are cuboidal epithelial cells making up the majority of cells in the liver. Karl Wilhelm von Kupffer, 1829–1902, Professor of Anatomy at Kiel (1867), Königsberg (1875) and Munich, Germany (1880), described these 'stellate cells' in 1880 (6).

Hepatocytes perform most liver functions including metabolism, storage, digestion and bile production. Tiny bile canaliculi run parallel to the sinusoids on the contralateral side to the hepatocytes and drain bile in the opposite direction to the blood flow via the bile duct tributaries within portal tracts.

PHYSIOLOGY OF THE LIVER

The physiology of the liver is extremely complex and involves metabolism, excretion and body defense. The liver performs and controls myriad biochemical, metabolic and immunological functions and is the site of a multitude of biochemical reactions essential to the human organism, including synthesis, degradation, interconversion, storage and biotransformation. Anhepatic humans survive for 24–48 hours and it is the only visceral organ in the body that regenerates. The blood supply to the liver is complex due to the dual supply from the hepatic artery and portal vein and liver blood flow is controlled by mechanisms that are independent of extrinsic innervation or vasoactive agents. About three-quarters of the blood flow by volume comes from the portal vein and the rest is from the hepatic artery. The portal vein contains partially deactivated blood from the splanchnic circulation and unlike the volume flow, 50% of the oxygen provided to the liver comes from the portal vein and 50% from the hepatic artery. The hepatic portal system connects the capillaries of the GI tract with the capillaries in the liver. Nutrient-rich blood leaves the GI tract and is first

brought to the liver for processing before being sent to the heart.

Under normal circumstances the total hepatic blood flow ranges between 800 and 1200 mL/min, which is equivalent to approximately 100 mL/min per 100 g liver. Although the liver mass represents only 2.5% of the total body weight, the liver receives almost 25% of the cardiac output.

The portal vein contains no valves and the pressure and resistance are low. The mean pressure ranges from 6–10 mmHg which contrasts sharply with the hepatic artery where the mean pressure is similar to the aorta. Within the liver the sinusoidal pressure is slightly above that of the inferior vena cava at approximately 2–4 mmHg (7).

The functional unit of the liver is the lobule (*Figure 2.3*) which is traditionally hexagonal with a portal triad consisting of a bile duct, hepatic artery and portal vein, situated at each corner. Hepatocytes which account for 60–80% of the liver cell mass comprise the liver parenchyma making up the lobule and are described by their function and blood supply and are described as occupying three distinct zones. Hepatocytes with the best blood supply are located in the periportal region described as zone 1. They are involved in functions which have a high oxygen demand including oxidative metabolism, amino acid turnover, and bile and cholesterol formation. At an intermediate distance from the location of the portal triads is described as zone 2. The function of zone 2 hepatocytes, also called pericentral hepatocytes, is unclear but their position protects them from injury and they are believed to contribute significantly to regeneration following a toxic or ischaemic insult (8).

The perfusion of zone 3 is relatively poor due to its location furthest from a portal triad (although closest to the central vein). Zone 3 hepatocytes are essential for cytochrome p450 drug detoxification, lipogenesis and glycolysis, glutamine formation and glycogen synthesis.

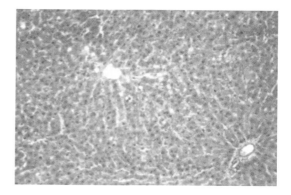

Figure 2.3 Classical appearance of a liver lobule.

A detailed description of all the functions of the liver is beyond the remit of this chapter but the main functions are outlined below:

- Maintaining core body temperature
- pH balance and correction of lactic acidosis
- The liver manages the synthesis of nearly every plasma protein in the body, some examples include albumin, binding globulins, protein C, protein S, and all the clotting factors of the intrinsic and extrinsic pathways besides factor VIII
- Glucose metabolism, glycolysis and gluconeogenesis
- Urea formation from protein catabolism
- Expression of protein coding genes for the production of plasma proteins, liver enzymes proteins involved in synthesis and transporter proteins involved in drug metabolism
- Bilirubin formation from haemoglobin after breakdown of effete red cells in the spleen
- Drug and hormone metabolism and excretion
- The liver plays a role in thyroid hormone function as the site of deiodination of T4 to T3
- Removal of gut endotoxins and foreign antigens
- Vitamin and mineral storage including A, D, E, K and B12
- Immunological function as part of the mononuclear phagocyte system
- Albumin production for the transport of fatty acids, steroids and waste products
- Angiotensin synthesis
- Body temperature through heat production
- Cytochrome p450 detoxifies contaminants and pollutants, insecticides and food additives

Drug metabolism

Hepatic drug metabolism and consequent detoxification is principally through biotransformation which occurs in the smooth endoplasmic reticulum of hepatocytes. The liver converts lipophilic molecules into a hydrophilic form or produces a hydrophilic metabolite.

Drugs can be metabolized by oxidation, reduction, hydrolysis, hydration, conjugation, condensation, or isomerization but whichever process occurs the end result is a molecule that is able to be excreted. All the enzymes involved in metabolism are present throughout the body in most tissues but are significantly more concentrated in the liver. For the majority of drugs, metabolism occurs in 2 phases. Phase 1 reactions involve the formation of a new or modified functional group or cleavage by oxidation, reduction or hydrolysis. Phase 2 reactions are synthetic reactions and drugs are conjugated with an endogenous substance such as glucuronic acid, sulphate or glycine. Due to the metabolic products resulting from phase 2 reactions being more polar they can be excreted in the urine and bile (9).

Bilirubin petabolism

The liver plays a significant role in the breakdown of haem. Haemolysis occurs in the liver, spleen and bone marrow where haem is converted to biliverdin which is then reduced to unconjugated bilirubin and passes albumin bound to the liver. Unconjugated bilirubin is conjugated in the uridine diphosphate glucuronyltransferase (UGT) system and becomes hydrophilic facilitating secretion via bile canaliculi into the bile (10).

Bile production

Bile enables the clearance of metabolites or drugs which can't be excreted by the kidneys and emulsifies ingested fats to facilitate their absorption. Bile is produced by hepatocytes and is principally composed of water, electrolytes, bile salts, bile acids, cholesterol, bile pigment, bilirubin and phospholipids. Bile is secreted from hepatocytes into the bile canaliculi where it travels from smaller calibre ducts to the common hepatic duct, in the opposite direction to the blood flow in the portal vein and hepatic artery, ending up in the duodenum or temporarily in the gallbladder for storage and concentration depending on the contents of the stomach and duodenum and the pressure in the sphincter of Oddi.

Following secretion of bile into the duodenum, it undergoes enterohepatic circulation (EHC) where bile acids and bile components that are secreted by the liver into the GI tract but are not excreted are recycled by absorption in the ileum and returned to the liver via the portal vein. EHC is responsible for the circulation of 20–30 g of bile acids each day and only a very small proportion is lost in the faeces.

Fat-soluble vitamin storage and metabolism

Following absorption from the GI tract, fat-soluble vitamins are transported to the liver as chylomicrons or very low-density lipoproteins (VLDL) where they are metabolized and subsequently stored. Vitamin A is stored in Ito cells which are mesenchymal perisinusoidal fat-storing cells, stellate cells and lipocytes located in the space of Disse (the space between a hepatocyte and a sinusoid). They are the main location for vitamin A storage which appears as characteristic lipid droplets.

Vitamin D3, whether derived from the skin after sun exposure or ingested plant or animal products or therapeutic supplementation, must undergo 25-hydroxylation by cytochrome p450 following which subsequent renal hydroxylation results in the functional form.

Tocopherols are a group of closely related compounds which collectively constitute vitamin E. They are radical scavengers, delivering a hydrogen atom to inactivate free radicals. Vitamin E exists in eight different forms. γ-Tocopherol (γT) is a major form of vitamin E in the diet and the second most abundant vitamin E in the blood and tissues, while α-tocopherol (αT) is the predominant vitamin E in tissues. α-tocopherol is integrated with VLDL or HDL in the liver and secreted back into the circulation. Vitamin K is not stored or metabolized in the liver but it is essential for the gamma-γ-carboxylation of coagulation factors II, VII, IX, X, and proteins C and S (11).

Liver blood tests

The complexity of the liver exposes it to an array of physical, metabolic and infectious insults in addition to problems resulting from systemic and intrinsic disorders. An awareness of currently available liver blood tests and their significance is essential to be able to understand hepatic dysfunction (*Table 2.2*).

Liver dysfunction

Depending on the severity of the liver dysfunction, the aetiology and acute or chronic development, symptoms vary, and combinations occur. The most common include jaundice, drowsiness, abdominal pain/swelling, nausea, tremors, vomiting, malaise, confusion and disorientation, bruising, peripheral oedema and foetor hepaticus (strong musty smell to the breath).

SUMMARY

The liver is located in the right upper quadrant beneath the diaphragm. It is related to the hepatic flexure of the colon, right kidney, duodenum and the stomach. It weighs on average 1.5 kg (970–1860 g) and is wedge shaped in both coronal and axial planes and divided by the middle hepatic vein into two lobes with the larger right lobe generally representing 60% by volume. The liver receives oxygenated blood from the hepatic artery and nutrient rich blood from the portal vein. The liver contains 13% of the systemic blood volume.

There are a vast number and array of functions of the liver involved in the maintenance of homeostasis, the production of proteins, metabolism of drugs and the protection of the body against infection. Hepatic dysfunction results in a wide range of pathologies and illnesses, and unlike the gut or kidney which can be supported or replaced by artificial nutrition or dialysis, without liver transplantation disorders of the liver are often fatal.

Table 2.2 Routinely available blood tests for the assessment of liver function

Test	Normal range	Significance
Bilirubin	5–17 µmol/L [0.3–1.2 mg/dL]	Bilirubin is synthesized in the liver and excreted in bile. Increased levels may be associated with increased haemoglobin breakdown, hepatocellular dysfunction resulting in impaired bilirubin transport and excretion or mechanical biliary obstruction. In patients with known parenchymal liver disease, progressive elevation of bilirubin in the absence of a secondary complication suggests deterioration in liver function
Alkaline phosphatase (ALP)	30–140 IU/L	The serum alkaline phosphatase (ALP) is particularly elevated with cholestatic liver disease or biliary obstruction. It is important to note that routine laboratory analysis of ALP is not isoform specific and so alkaline phosphatase from a skeletal source may also lead to elevation, particularly Paget's disease and prostate cancer
Aspartate transaminase (AST)	5–40 IU/L	Although significant liver injury does occur in the presence of normal liver blood tests, levels of the transaminase (aspartate transaminase (AST), alanine transaminase (ALT) and gamma-glutamyl transpeptidase (GGT)) usually reflect acute hepatocellular damage and GGT is a useful marker of alcohol intake
Alanine transaminase (ALT)	5–40 IU/L	
Gamma-glutamyl transpeptidase (GGT)	10–48 IU/L	
Albumin	35–50 g/L [3.5–5 g/dL]	The synthetic functions of the liver are indicated by the ability to synthesize proteins (albumin level) and clotting factors (prothrombin time) and the standard method of monitoring liver function in patients with chronic liver disease is serial measurement of bilirubin, albumin and prothrombin time
Total protein	60–85 g/L [6–8.5 g/dL]	
Prothrombin time (PT)	12–16 s	

REFERENCES

1. Cantlie J. On a new arrangement of the right and left lobes of the liver. *Proc Anat Soc GT BR Irel* 1897;**32**:4–9.
2. Hardy KJ. Carl Langenbuch and the Lazarus Hospital: Events and circumstances surrounding the first cholecystectomy. *Aust N Z J Surg* 1993;**63(1)**:56–64. doi: 10.1111/j.1445-2197.1993.tb00035.x. PMID: 8466463.
3. Healey JE Jr, Schroy PC. Anatomy of the biliary ducts within the human liver; analysis of the prevailing pattern of branchings and the major variations of the biliary ducts. *AMA Arch Surg* 1953;**66(5)**:599–616. doi: 10.1001/archsurg.1953.01260030616008. PMID: 13039731
4. Couinaud C. Bases anatomique des heatectomies gauche et droite reglees. *J Chir* 1954;**70**:933–66.
5. Lortat-Jacob J-LR. Hepatectomie lobaire droite reglee pour tumeur maligne secondaire. *Arch Mal App Digestif* 1952;**41**:662–7.
6. von Kupffer C. Ueber die sogennanten Sternzellen der S–ugethierleber. *Arch mikr Anat* 1899;**54**:254–88.
7. Eipel C, Abshagen K, Vollmar B. Regulation of hepatic blood flow: The hepatic arterial buffer response revisited. *World J Gastroenterol* 2010;**16**:6046–57.
8. Wei Y, Wang YG, Jia Y, Li L, Yoon J, Zhang S, et al. Liver homeostasis is maintained by midlobular zone 2 hepatocytes. *Science* 2021;**371(6532)**:eabb1625. doi: 10.1126/science.abb1625. PMID: 33632817; PMCID: PMC8496420.
9. Almazroo OA, Miah MK, Venkataramanan R. Drug metabolism in the liver. *Clin Liver Dis* 2017;**21(1)**:1–20. doi: 10.1016/j.cld.2016.08.001 PMID: 27842765.
10. Hansen TWR, Wong RJ, Stevenson DK. Molecular physiology and pathophysiology of bilirubin handling by the blood, liver, intestine, and brain in the newborn. *Physiol Rev* 2020;**100(3)**:1291–346. doi: 10.1152/physrev.00004.2019. PMID: 32401177.
11. Stevens SL. Fat-soluble vitamins. *Nurs Clin North Am* 2021;**56(1)**:33–45. doi: 10.1016/j.cnur.2020.10.003. PMID: 33549284.

Chapter 3

Pancreas Anatomy and Physiology

John Isherwood and Giuseppe Garcea

INTRODUCTION

The pancreas is an important gastrointestinal (GI) organ located in the retroperitoneum between the duodenum and the hilum of the spleen. It is a mixed or heterocrine gland having endocrine and exocrine functions. The endocrine component consists of the islets of Langerhans composed of five different cell types secreting a number of different hormones which are essential for glucose homeostasis and functioning of the GI tract.

PANCREATIC ANATOMY

The word pancreas originates from the Greek '*pan kreas*' meaning 'all flesh'. It is a soft, pale yellow, lobulated racemose gland located in the anterior pararenal space of the retroperitoneum. On average, the pancreas measures between 12–20 cm in length and weighs between 60–125 g (1). To understand the anatomy of the pancreas, it is crucial to understand the embryological development, rotation and fusion of the dorsal and ventral pancreatic buds described in **Chapter 1**. The pancreas is anatomically divided into four parts; the head, neck, body and tail (*Figure 3.1*). Although the divisions are arbitrary, the generally accepted nomenclature is as follows. The pancreatic head is located within the concave curvature of the duodenum and to the right of the superior mesenteric (SMV) and portal veins. The neck is situated ventral to the SMV. The body is situated to the left of the SMV with the tail lying directed towards the splenic hilum. The border between the body and tail can be determined using one-half of the distance between the neck and end of the pancreas (2).

The head of the pancreas is discoid in shape and proceeds inferiorly, continuing medially, as the hook shaped uncinate process. The neck, body and tail are flattened and inversely triangular, being flatter anteriorly. The width and thickness of the pancreas are greatest at the head and narrowest towards the tail. The size of the pancreas varies between patients and assessing abnormalities in the features of the gland (architecture, symmetry, enhancement and duct anatomy) are important for detecting abnormal pathology.

Associated relations and ligaments to the pancreas

The pancreas is a retroperitoneal organ with most of its anterior surface covered by peritoneum which is the posterior wall of the lesser sac. It has a very thin fascial capsule and behind the peritoneum it is covered by connective tissue, blood vessels, lymphatics and nodes. The pancreas is closely related to several important retroperitoneal and peritoneal structures and knowledge of their relationship is important in surgical oncology and during surgical procedures. The pancreas lies in front of the anterior renal fascia and posterior to the peritoneum in the anterior pararenal space. Posterior to the head of the pancreas is the vena cava (at the entry of the left and right renal veins) and aorta. Anteriorly lies the pylorus, the first part of the duodenum and the transverse colon. The uncinate process curves behind the SMV and may end before the SMV, or may continue further, ending between the aorta and superior mesenteric artery (SMA).

Posteriorly, the neck of the pancreas lies on the SMV and portal vein and anteriorly beneath the pylorus. Posterior to the body and tail are the SMA, aorta, splenic vein, inferior mesenteric vein, splenic artery, left adrenal and left kidney. The body of the pancreas lies adjacent to the fourth part of the duodenum and ligament of Trietz and anteriorly the neck and tail are covered by the stomach, gastrocolic ligament and transverse colon.

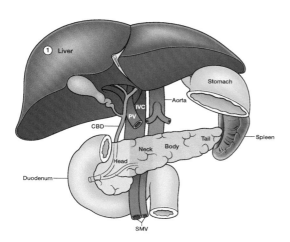

Figure 3.1 Pancreatic anatomy showing the key structural relationships.

DOI: 10.1201/9781003080060-3

Pancreatic ductal system

Aristotle believed the function of the pancreas was to protect the great vessels and four centuries later Galen claimed it to be a cushion for the stomach (3). It was not until the Renaissance that major anatomical descriptions were defined, starting with the pancreatic duct first described by Johann Georg Wirsung on March 2nd 1642, whilst working at San Francesco Hospital. He identified the duct in the pancreas during the dissection of an executed murderer, Zuane Viaro della Badia (4).

The ductal system results from the embryological fusion of the ventral and dorsal pancreatic buds, at approximately 7 weeks (*see* **Chapter 1**). The ventral duct and distal dorsal duct fuse to become the main pancreatic duct (MPD). The proximal part of the dorsal duct may atrophy or persist as an accessory duct of Santorini (5). This fusion can result in a wide variety of ductal anatomical configurations (6) of which there are at least 27 described (7). The failure of the ventral and dorsal buds to fuse results in separate draining fields, called pancreas divisum, and in this case the dorsal and ventral pancreatic tissue may be fused or remain separate. Pancreas divisum occurs in approximately 4–10% of individuals and there are two types described as complete and incomplete (6). In complete divisum, the dorsal duct drains through the minor papilla and the ventral duct drains through major papilla. In incomplete divisum, a small branch of the ventral duct joins the dorsal duct. Pancreas divisum is usually asymptomatic but is seen more frequently in patients with idiopathic pancreatitis and chronic abdominal pain, when compared to the general population (8).

An annular pancreas is an anomaly with a prevalence of 1 in 2000 people (9), where failed rotation of a portion of the ventral pancreas results in a branch of the ventral pancreas passing posteriorly to the descending duodenum, encircling approximately 75% of the bowel. This results in a ring-like narrowing (6) and can lead to gastric outlet obstruction in children and pancreatitis in adults (10,11). Ansa pancreatica is another rare anomalous ductal configuration, where the duct of Santorini forms a sigmoid curve as it courses to the duct of Wirsung. While this does not appear to have any clinical significance, it can make the passage of a wire during endoscopic retrograde cholangiopancreatography (ERCP) particularly challenging.

The main pancreatic duct of Wirsung begins in the tail of the pancreas and ends by emptying into the duodenum through the major papilla. The duct joins the common bile duct (CBD) in the head of the pancreas and forms a common channel at the hepatopancreatic ampulla of Vater. This common channel traverses the sphincter of Oddi, which consists of three separate smooth muscles, separated and distinct from the duodenal smooth muscle adjoining it. The major papilla is normally located at the midpoint of the second part of the duodenum, but variations do exist and it can sometimes be found in the midpoint of the third part of the duodenum. The accessory duct of Santorini drains the anterior and superior portion of the head and terminates in the minor papilla, opening approximately 2 cm superior and anterior to the major papilla (12). The MPD extends the length of the pancreas with a diameter of 3.1–3.5 mm in the head, 2.0–2.5 mm in the body and 0.9–1.5 mm in the tail (13) and deviations from this are a possible indication of pathological change. The MPD has numerous (approximately 20–30) side branches entering the duct at right angles along its length (7). The MPD and CBD unite within the sphincter of Oddi in approximately 80–90% of cases and this common channel can either be short (shaped like a V) or long (shaped like a Y).

An anomalous pancreaticobiliary junction is defined as the fusion of MPD and CBD outside the duodenal wall, forming an unusually long common channel, greater than 15 mm in length (14). It is hypothesized that a high CBD and MPD junction may theoretically allow pancreatic secretions to reflux up the CBD and it is an aetiological hypothesis for the development of some types of choledochal cysts (13). The CBD is completely covered by the pancreatic head in 30% of people, partially covered posteriorly in 51.5% and not covered in 16.5% (15).

Blood supply of the pancreas

The pancreas has a rich and complex blood supply (*Figure 3.2*). The arterial supply is via branches arising from the coeliac and SMA. There are many different arterial anatomical variations and preoperative review of the arterial landscape is essential (16). The arterial supply can be thought of as two separate systems, with

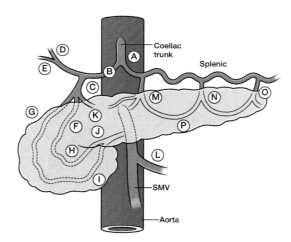

Figure 3.2 Labelled illustration of the arterial blood supply to the pancreas. Diagram arterial guide: A: left gastric; B: common hepatic; C: gastro duodenal; D: left hepatic; E: right hepatic; F: anterior superior pancreatico duodenal; G: posterior superior pancreatico duodenal; H: anterior inferior pancreatico duodenal; I: posterior inferior gastro duodenal; J: inferior pancreatico duodenal; K: right gastro epiploic; L: middle colic; M: dorsal pancreatic; N: pancreatica magna artery; O: caudal pancreatic artery; P: transverse pancreatic artery.

one supplying the head and uncinate process and a further system supplying the body and tail with the neck a potential watershed between these two. The head and neck (and associated duodenum) are supplied by both the coeliac trunk and SMA which are connected by two pancreaticoduodenal arteries that run parallel to the concave curve of the duodenum. These arteries run on the anterior and posterior surface of the pancreas and form an arcade between the superior pancreaticoduodenal artery from the gastroduodenal, and the inferior pancreaticoduodenal artery from the SMA.

The body and tail of the gland are supplied by three dominant arteries, the dorsal pancreatic, pancreatica magna and caudal pancreatic arteries which arise from the splenic artery. The number of these branches is quite variable and there can be up to ten. The dorsal pancreatic artery is the most medial and aberrant and can arise from a number of different vessels including the common hepatic artery. The transverse pancreatic artery runs along the inferior margin of the pancreas and is the left branch of the dorsal pancreatic artery in the majority of cases, and anastomoses with the pancreatica magna and caudal pancreatic arteries.

The venous drainage of the pancreas often runs alongside and in parallel with the arterial supply and drains into the portal system (*Figure 3.3*). The body and tail drain to the splenic vein via multiple short vessels on the posterior aspect of the pancreas (17,18). The drainage of the transverse pancreatic vein is variable and includes the SMV and splenic vein. A double-arched (anterior and posterior) venous arcade similar to the

arterial arcades drains the head and uncinate process. The superior pancreaticoduodenal veins drain into the SMV via the gastrocolic trunk. The inferior pancreaticoduodenal veins drain into the SMV via the first jejunal branch, with numerous tributaries draining between them. The relationship of the pancreas to the SMV, splenic and portal vein is critical during surgical resection. The pancreas can be dissected off the SMV at its neck allowing elevation of the pancreas from the SMV producing a safe tissue plane. Apart from the inferior pancreaticoduodenal veins that enter the SMV at the inferior border of the pancreas it is rare to see veins draining posteriorly from the pancreas to the SMV.

Lymphatic drainage of the pancreas

A network of lymphatic vessels exist within the pancreas with the majority lying in the interlobular septa of connective tissue that divides the pancreas into lobes and lobules (12). The lymph capillaries anastomose to form lymph ducts running along blood vessels, which empty into a ring of regional lymph nodes that intimately surround the pancreas. These subsequently drain into secondary nodes along the coeliac, SMA and aorta (19). A number of classifications are used to define these lymph node stations with the most used being derived from the Japanese Research Society for Gastric Cancer (JRSGC) (20), who divided the upper abdominal regional lymph nodes into 16 stations. The lymphatic drainage of the pancreas is crucial in the surgical workup and resection of the pancreas (21). There has been extensive research into the benefits of an extended lymphadenectomy in pancreatic cancer, with no survival benefit demonstrated over a standard lymphadenectomy, and often with debilitating side effects such as intractable diarrhoea (22–25).

Neuro-anatomy of the pancreas

The pancreas is innervated by both sympathetic and parasympathetic nerves. These nerves interact with hormones to provide a co-ordinated response to stimuli associated with eating and digestion (26). The parasympathetic supply originates from the vagus nerve and, passes through the coeliac plexus distributing itself along the arterial network. Parasympathetic stimulation results in the exocrine secretion of pancreatic digestive secretions. The sympathetic supply arises from the greater and lesser splanchnic nerves to the coeliac plexus and the post-ganglionic nerve fibres pass alongside the parasympathetic nerves to the pancreas. These post-ganglionic nerves innervate blood vessels and islets (12). Importantly, the nerve plexuses serve as a route for perineural extrapancreatic spread of pancreatic ductal adenocarcinoma (27,28).

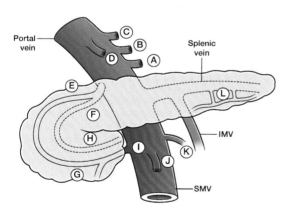

Figure 3.3 Labelled illustration of the venous blood supply. Note that there are numerous venous configurations of Henle's trunk that involve variations of the right gastro-epiploic vein, the superior, right colic vein and the anterior (superior/inferior) pancreaticoduodenal vein. A: coronary vein; B: pyloric vein; C: left gastric; D: right gastric; E: anterior superior pancreatico duodenal; F: posterior superior pancreatico duodenal; G: anterior inferior pancreatico duodenal; H: posterior inferior pancreatico duodenal; I: Henle's trunk (gastrocolic trunk); J: middle colic vein; K: 1st jejunal branch; L: inferior pancreatic vein. SMV – superior mesenteric vein, IMV – inferior mesenteric vein.

PANCREATIC PHYSIOLOGY

The function of the pancreas can be divided into separate exocrine and endocrine roles which are undertaken by structurally distinct but functionally integrated

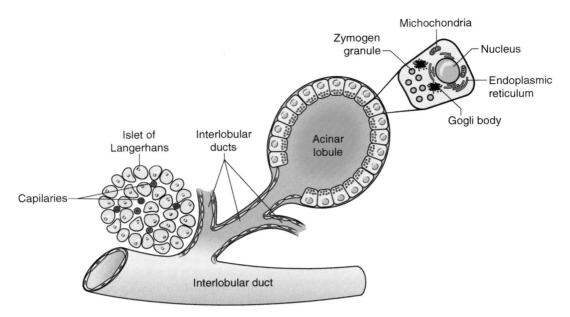

Figure 3.4 Labelled illustration of the acinar cell/ductal system within Islet of Langerhans cell. The exocrine pancreas comprises of approximately 90% of the pancreas and is made up of a ductal tree and pancreatic acini, with each of these acini made up of a cluster of hundreds of acinar cells around a central duct.

anatomy. This is a complex and extensive topic and this chapter will aim to provide a succinct overview of these processes.

Exocrine pancreas

The exocrine pancreas comprises of two structures. A ductal 'tree' and pancreatic acini with each of these acini made up of a cluster of hundreds of acinar cells around a central duct (29). These cells make up approximately 90% of the pancreatic mass (*Figure 3.4*). Acini are further grouped into lobules with a branched network of tubules that converge into interlobular then extralobular ducts and finally the pancreatic duct. The main function of the exocrine pancreas is the production of bicarbonate rich pancreatic secretion and secretory proteins, predominately digestive enzymes (30). The pancreas secretes approximately 1–2.5 L of fluid and 6–20 g of enzyme proteins daily (31).

The alkaline bicarbonate rich fluid from ductal cells neutralizes acidic gastric chyme, protecting the duodenal mucosa and providing an optimal pH for pancreatic enzymes. The concentration of HCO_3^- secretion by the ductal epithelium is astonishingly high at 120–140 mmol/L (32), which is five-fold higher than that in plasma. The secretion of high concentrations of HCO_3^- is under the control of several ion channels, the most notable being the cystic fibrosis transmembrane conductance regulator (CFTR). This is obviously clinically relevant in patients with cystic fibrosis, who have a genetic defect in this anion channel.

The pancreatic acinar cell's main role is to produce, store and secrete three major categories of digestive enzymes, alpha-amylase, protease and lipase, which digest carbohydrates, proteins and lipids, respectively (33). This is evident on histological examination with acinar cells possessing abundant rough endoplasmic reticulum and secretory vesicles containing zymogen granules. These zymogen granules contain numerous enzymes and precursor enzymes including trypsinogen, chymotrypsinogen and procarboxypeptidases. The secretion of precursor enzymes and their activation in the duodenum prevents auto-digestion of the pancreas. The precursor enzyme trypsinogen is activated by the duodenal enzyme enteropeptidase into trypsin, which then is responsible for the activation of other zymogens.

Neuro-hormonal control

Pancreatic exocrine secretions are regulated by various mechanisms and respond to stimuli including food ingestion with the neural hormonal system playing a central role. The response of the exocrine pancreas to a meal involves three phases:

1 The cephalic phase, stimulated by the sight and smell of food
2 The gastric phase triggered by food in the stomach and gastric distention
3 The intestinal phase, initiated by gastric chyme entering the duodenum (31)

The intestinal phase is neuro-hormonally regulated and responsible for pancreatic exocrine secretion. The pancreas is innervated by the central and autonomic nervous system with afferent and efferent signalling with the vagus nerve playing a major role in the regulatory pathway (34,35). A wide variety of neurotransmitters including acetylcholine (ACh), vasoactive intestinal polypeptide (VIP) secretin and cholecystokinin (CCK) regulate the exocrine pancreas through a complex interplay of neurocrine, endocrine and paracrine pathways (33). These neurotransmitters bind to their respective receptors, resulting in the exocytosis of secretory granules through a rise in cytosolic Ca^{2+} (36). Importantly, low or high concentrations of neurotransmitter release will result in varying amounts of calcium release from intracellular stores resulting in specific actions. This reliance on calcium signalling is very finely balanced which is essential to maintain homeostasis. Deviations are potentially hazardous with one example being excessive hyper-stimulation resulting in elevated Ca^{2+} which has the potential to activate the digestive proteases inside the cell through a poorly understood pathway, resulting in acute pancreatitis (37).

Endocrine pancreas

The endocrine pancreas and the islets of Langerhans comprize only approximately 2% of the pancreas, but utilize 20% of the arterial blood entering the gland (34). The main function of islets is to control the body's glucose haemostasis through hormonal control. There are approximately one million islets of Langerhans in the adult human pancreas (38). The islets are located at various points along the pancreatic arterial tree with larger islets being located closer to major arterioles with each islet containing approximately 2000 cells (38). Within these islets there are four types of exocrine cells, alpha (α), beta (β), delta (δ) and pancreatic polypeptide (F or PP) cells which secrete more than 20 hormones (39). Of the four cell types, the β-cells are dominant comprising about 80% of the islet population and are located in the centre of the islets with the α- and δ-cells around the periphery. Blood flow is arranged from the centre to the periphery which ensures a paracrine interaction between cells (33). The β- and δ-cells are distributed throughout the pancreas, while α-cells are located in the superior part of the head, body and tail (dorsal pancreas) and F cells are located in the middle and inferior head of the pancreas (ventral pancreas). Islets of Langerhans are richly innervated by parasympathetic, sympathetic and sensory nerves. Parasympathetic stimulation increases insulin release, sympathetic stimulation inhibits insulin secretion (40).

β-cells and insulin

Insulin is produced and released by β-cells and decreases plasma glucose levels by increasing its uptake into peripheral tissue in addition to supressing hepatic gluconeogenesis. Insulin is assembled in a precursor form as pre-proinsulin in the endoplasmic reticulum

and cleaved to proinsulin. It is subsequently packaged into vesicles in the Golgi body and further develops into mature secretory granules. During granule maturation, proinsulin is cleaved by the prohormone convertase which removes C-peptide resulting in mature insulin. These granules containing mature insulin and C-peptide are released by exocytosis in response to regulated secretion. In insulinomas, insulin is released continuously without the need for external stimuli, often presenting with a classic Whipple triad of episodic hypoglycaemia, central nervous system dysfunction and the reversal of this dysfunction by glucose administration.

Insulin is released from β-cells through a number of pathways including:

1 Neural stimulation including vagal- and β-adrenergic
2 Gut hormones such as glucagon like peptide-1 (GLP-1), gastric inhibitory peptide (GIP), secretin and CCK
3 Plasma levels of glucose, amino acids and fatty acids

Glucose is the most important regulator of insulin release and enters the cell through a glucose transporter called GLUT-2 (*Figure 3.5*). This occurs via a process of phosphorylation, membrane depolarization and calcium influx which results in exocytosis of insulin containing secretory granules (41). Insulin secretion in response to orally administered glucose is 25–50% greater than that after intravenous administration (42,43). This so-called 'incretin effect' is mediated by the gut hormones GLP-1 and GIP demonstrating that the response to eating is the main stimulus to insulin secretion and explains how the treatment of hypoglycaemia is effective with oral glucose.

GLUCAGON AND OTHER ISLET HORMONES

The islets of Langerhans are responsible for secreting a variety of other hormones, including glucagon, somatostatin and pancreatic polypeptide. Alpha cells produce glucagon which functions to regulate hepatic glucose output, accelerating gluconeogenesis and glycogenolysis resulting in increased blood glucose levels. Glucagon secretion is activated by hypoglycaemia but inhibited by hyperglycaemic glucose levels (33). With a total pancreatectomy, patients become profoundly glucagon deficient and prone to hypoglycaemia. Historically this has been associated with brittle diabetes which is characterized by swings in blood glucose levels which can be difficult to control (31). More recent studies have demonstrated that brittle diabetes does not affect all patients undergoing a total pancreatectomy (44).

Somatostatin is produced by the δ-cells and classically acts on the hypothalamic-pituitary axis but exhibits a wide spectrum of secretory and motor

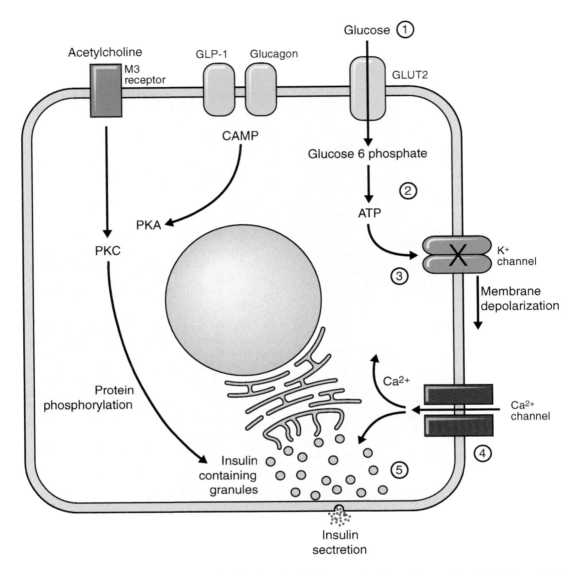

Figure 3.5 Main pathway of insulin secretion from β-cells: **1.** Glucose enters the cell through the GLUT-2 transporter; **2.** Glucose is phosphorylated to glucose-6-phosphate, which is metabolized to convert adenosine diphosphate (ADP) to adenosine triphosphate (ATP); **3.** The increase in ATP to ADP ratio closes the potassium channel resulting in membrane depolarization; **4.** Membrane depolarization results in opening of voltage dependent calcium channels resulting in the increase of intracellular calcium; **5.** The resultant rise in intracellular calcium results in the exocytosis of insulin containing secretory granules. Note the alternative pathways also included explain how the incretins (GIP and GLP-1) and glucagon lead to the rise of cyclic AMP through various pathways result in the activation of protein kinase A (PKA). Acetylcholine released from the vagal afferents, results in the activation of protein kinase C (PKC). PKA and PKC activation leads to protein phosphorylation and the secretion of insulin by exocytosis of insulin granules.

functions which affect the GI system. Somatostatin acts to decrease the assimilation rate of all nutrients from the GI tract and inhibits insulin and glucagon release. Somatostatin analogues are widely used following pancreatic resection, aimed at reducing pancreatic secretions and therefore fistula rates. Although widely used internationally, controversy remains as to the benefit in postoperative fistula rates and the morbidity associated with pancreatic surgery (45–47).

REFERENCES

1. Quinlan RM. Anatomy and embryology of the pancreas. In: Zuidema GD (ed). *Shackelford's Surgery of the Alimentary Tract*, 3rd edn, Volume III. Philadelphia: W B Saunders Co Ltd; 1991, pp. 3–18.
2. Kuroda A. Surgical anatomy of the pancreas. In: Howard J, Idezuki Y, Ihse I, (eds). *Surgical Diseases of the Pancreas*, Baltimore, MD: Williams & Wilkins; 1998, pp. 11–21.

3. Williams JA. The nobel pancreas: A historical perspective. *Gastroenterology* 2013;**144(6)**:1166–9.

4. Garrison F. *Contributions to the History of Medicine.* Philadelphia: Hanfer Publishing Company; 1966.

5. Gavaghan M. The pancreas-hermit of the abdomen. *AORN* 2002;**75(6)**:1109–11.

6. Barkay O, Fogel EL, Watkins JL, Mchenry LEE, Lehman GA, Sherman S. Normal ductal anatomy and variants. *YJCGH* 2009;**7(9)**:931–43.

7. Mortelé KJ, Rocha TC, Streeter JL, Taylor AJ. Multimodality imaging of pancreatic and biliary congenital anomalies. *Radiographics* 2006;**26**:715–31.

8. Cotton PB. Congenital anomaly of pancreas divisum as cause of obstructive pain and pancreatitis. *Gut* 1980; **21(2)**:105–14.

9. Jimenez JC, Emil S, Podnos Y, Nguyen N. Annular pancreas in children: A recent decade's experience. *J Pediatr Surg* 2004;**39(11)**:1654–7.

10. Lehman GA, O'Connor KW. Coexistence of annular pancreas and pancreas divisum–ERCP diagnosis. *Gastrointest Endosc* 1985;**31(1)**:25–8.

11. England RE, Newcomer MK, Leung JWC, Cotton PB. Case report. Annular pancreas divisum – A report of two cases and review of the literature. *Br J Radiol* 1995;**68(807)**:324–8.

12. Pour PM, Konishi Y, Klöppel G, Longnecker DS (eds). Gross anatomy of the Pancreas. In: *Atlas of Exocrine Pancreatic Tumors.* Japan: Springer; 1994, pp. 1–15.

13. Varley PF, Rohrmann CA, Silvis SE, Vennes JA. The normal endoscopic pancreatogram. *Radiology* 1976; **118(2)**:295–300.

14. Sugiyama M, Haradome H, Takahara T, Abe N, Tokuhara M, Masaki T, et al. Case report. Anomalous pancreaticobiliary junction shown on multidetector CT. *Am J Roentgenol* 2003;**180(1)**:173–5.

15. Mortelé KJ, Rocha TC, Streeter JL, Taylor AJ. Multimodality imaging of pancreatic and biliary congenital anomalies. *Radiographics* 2006;**26(3)**:715–31.

16. Murakami G, Hirata K, Takamuro T, Mukaiya M, Hata F, Kitagawa S. Vascular anatomy of the pancreaticoduodenal region: A review. *J Hepatobiliary Pancreat Surg* 1999;**6(1)**:55–68.

17. Mourad N, Zhang J, Rath AM, Chevrel JP. The venous drainage of the pancreas. *Surg Radiol Anat* 1994; **16(1)**:37–45.

18. Ibukuro K. Vascular anatomy of the pancreas and clinical applications. *Int J Gastrointest Cancer* 2001; **30(1)**:87–104.

19. O'Morchoe CCC. Lymphatic system of the pancreas. *Microsc Res Tech* 1997;**37(5–6)**:456–77.

20. Murakami T. The general rules for the gastric cancer study in surgery. *Jpn J Surg* 1973;**3(1)**:61–71.

21. Fink DM, Steele MM, Hollingsworth MA. The lymphatic system and pancreatic cancer. *Cancer Lett* 2016;**381(1)**:217–36.

22. Masui T, Kubota T, Aoki K, Nakanishi Y, Miyamoto T, Nagata J, et al. Long-term survival after resection of pancreatic ductal adenocarcinoma with para-aortic lymph node metastasis: Case report. *World J Surg Oncol* 2013;**11(1)**:195.

23. Pedrazzoli S, DiCarlo V, Dionigi R, Mosca F, Pederzoli P, Pasquali C, et al. Standard versus extended lymphadenectomy associated with pancreatoduodenectomy in the surgical treatment of adenocarcinoma of the head of the pancreas: A multicenter, prospective, randomized study. *Ann Surg* 1998; **228(4)**:508–17.

24. Tol JAMG, Gouma DJ, Bassi C, Dervenis C, Montorsi M, Adham M, et al. Definition of a standard lymphadenectomy in surgery for pancreatic ductal adenocarcinoma: A consensus statement by the International Study Group on Pancreatic Surgery (ISGPS). *Surgery* 2014;**156(3)**:591–600.

25. Farnell MB, Pearson RK, Sarr MG, DiMagno EP, Burgart LJ, Dahl TR, et al. A prospective randomized trial comparing standard pancreatoduodenectomy with pancreatoduodenectomy with extended lymphadenectomy in resectable pancreatic head adenocarcinoma. *Surgery* 2005;**138(4)**:618–30.

26. H Beger, A Warshaw MB, et al (eds). *The Pancreas: An Integrated Textbook of Basic Science, Medicine, and Surgery,* 2nd edn. London: Wiley; 2008.

27. Nagai H, Kuroda A, Morioka Y. Lymphatic and local spread of T1 and T2 pancreatic cancer. A study of autopsy material. *Ann Surg* 1986;**204(1)**:65–71.

28. Liebig C, Ayala G, Wilks JA, Berger DH, Albo D. Perineural invasion in cancer: A review of the literature. *Cancer* 2009;**115(15)**:3379–91.

29. Takahashi H. Scanning electron microscopy of the rat exocrine pancreas. *Arch Histol Jpn* 1984;**47(4)**: 387–404.

30. Heitz PU, Beglinger CGK. Anatomy and Physiology of the Exocrine Pancreas. In: Kloppel G, Heitz PU, (eds). *Pancreatic Pathology.* Edinburgh: Churchill Livingstone; 1984, pp. 3–21.

31. Jarnagin W. *Blumgart's Surgery of the Liver, Biliary Tract, and Pancreas.* Vols. 1–2. London: Elsevier, 2012.

32. Domschke S, Domschke W, Rösch W, Konturek SJ, Sprügel W, Mitznegg P, et al. Inhibition by somatostatin of secretin-stimulated pancreatic secretion in man: A study with pure pancreatic juice. *Scand J Gastroenterol* 1977;**12(1)**:59–63.

33. Leung PS. Physiology of the pancreas. *Adv Exp Med Biol* 2010;**690**:13–27.

34. Pandiri AR. Overview of exocrine pancreatic pathobiology. *Toxicol Pathol* 2014;**42(1)**:207–16.

35. Owyang C, Logsdon CD. New insights into neurohormonal regulation of pancreatic secretion. *Gastroenterology* 2004;**127(3)**:957–69.

36. Petersen OH. Stimulus-secretion coupling: Cytoplasmic calcium signals and the control of ion channels in exocrine acinar cells. *J Physiol* 1992;**448(1)**: 1–51.

37. Petersen OH, Sutton R. Ca2+ signalling and pancreatitis: Effects of alcohol, bile and coffee. *Trends Pharmacol Sci* 2006;**27(2)**:113–20.

38. Moldovan S, Brunicardi FC. Endocrine pancreas: Summary of observations generated by surgical fellows. *World J Surg* 2001;**25(4)**:468–73.

39. Orci L. The microanatomy of the islets of Langerhans. *Metabolism* 1976;**25(11 Suppl 1)**:1303–13.

40. Ahrén B. Autonomic regulation of islet hormone secretion – implications for health and disease. *Diabetologia* 2000;**43(4)**:393–410.

41. Schuit FC, Huypens P, Heimberg H, Pipeleers DG. Glucose sensing in pancreatic beta-cells: A model for the study of other glucose-regulated cells in gut, pancreas, and hypothalamus. *Diabetes* 2001;**50(1)**:1–11.

42. Shapiro ET, Tillil H, Miller MA, Frank BH, Galloway JA, Rubenstein AH, et al. Insulin secretion and clearance. Comparison after oral and intravenous glucose. *Diabetes* 1987;**36(12)**:1365–71.

43. Tillil H, Shapiro ET, Miller MA, Karrison T, Frank BH, Galloway JA, et al. Dose-dependent effects of oral and intravenous glucose on insulin secretion and clearance in normal humans. *Am J Physiol* 1988;**254(3)**:E349–57.

44. Roberts KJ, Blanco G, Webber J, Marudanayagam R, Sutcliffe RP, Muiesan P, et al. How severe is dia-betes after total pancreatectomy? A case-matched analysis. *HPB (Oxford)* 2014;**16(9)**:814–21.

45. Li T, D'Cruz RT, Lim SY, Shelat VG. Somatostatin analogues and the risk of post-operative pancreatic fis-tulas after pancreatic resection – A systematic review & meta-analysis. *Pancreatology* 2020;**20(2)**:158–68.

46. Adiamah A, Arif Z, Berti F, Singh S, Laskar N, Gomez D. The use of prophylactic somatostatin ther-apy following pancreaticoduodenectomy: A meta-analysis of randomised controlled trials. *World J Surg* 2019;**43(7)**:1788–801.

47. Jin K, Zhou H, Zhang J, Wang W, Sun Y, Ruan C, et al. Systematic review and meta-analysis of soma-tostatin analogues in the prevention of postoperative complication after pancreaticoduodenectomy. *Dig Surg* 2015;**32(3)**:196–207.

Chapter

4

Biliary Anatomy

Christopher T. J. Madden-McKee and Tom Diamond

INTRODUCTION

Bile is generated by the hepatocytes and drains via canaliculi within portal triads into an intrahepatic branching ductal system. The extrahepatic biliary tree then takes bile to the gallbladder for storage, before it releases it episodically back into the ductal system. It then drains into the second part of the duodenum via the ampulla of Vater.

INTRAHEPATIC BILIARY ANATOMY

The liver is divided into eight segments each with its own blood supply and biliary drainage (*Figure 4.1*). There are four segments in the right lobe and four in the left. Each lobe is sub-divided into two sectors, each containing two segments. In the right lobe the posterior or lateral sector contains segments VI and VII and the anterior or medial sector contains segments V and VIII. In the left lobe, the medial sector contains segments I and IV. The lateral sector (lateral to the falciform ligament) contains segments II and III. Segment I was traditionally known as the caudate lobe and segment IV as the quadrate lobe

Within the liver, branches of the bile duct, hepatic artery and portal vein (the 'portal trinity') are arranged within Glissonian sheaths with a predictable anatomical course. The normal arrangement is such that the portal vein tends to lie posterior to both the bile duct and the hepatic artery. The bile duct tends to have an elliptical appearance and usually lies superior to the hepatic artery.

The right hepatic ducts unite to form the anterior (medial) sectoral duct and the posterior (lateral) sectoral duct. The anterior sectoral duct has a more vertical course and drains segments V and VIII. The posterior sectoral duct drains segments VI and VII and tends to course more horizontally before curving around the posterior aspect of the anterior sectoral duct and then inserting onto its medial aspect – the so-called 'Hjortsjo's crook' (*Figure 4.2*).

The left hepatic duct drains segments II, III and IV. Segment I usually drains via 2–3 small ducts directly into both the right and left hepatic ducts. In contrast to the right hepatic duct, the left hepatic duct is long and largely extrahepatic, coursing superficially in a groove between segments IV and I. The surgical significance of this is that the left hepatic duct can be exposed relatively easily along its course. It can be utilized for hepaticojejunostomy, if a more distal reconstruction is not possible, for example due to a cholangiocarcinoma or bile duct stricture. Knowledge of the relatively 'vertical' course of the right hepatic duct and the more 'horizontal' course of the left hepatic duct is very helpful in biliary surgery, not only when dissecting these structures but also to aid orientation when visualizing them from within, during choledochoscopy.

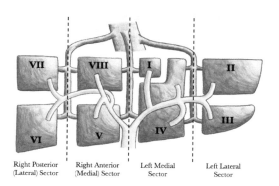

Figure 4.1 The sectoral and segmental anatomy of the liver.

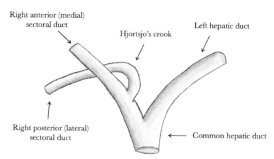

Figure 4.2 Illustration of the right posterior (lateral) sectoral duct curving around the posterior aspect of the right anterior (medial) sectoral duct, demonstrating Hjortso's crook.

DOI: 10.1201/9781003080060-4

EXTRAHEPATIC BILIARY ANATOMY

The right and left hepatic ducts unite to form the common hepatic duct (CHD). The common hepatic duct then unites with the cystic duct, forming the medial and inferior borders of the cystohepatic triangle of Calot, which is bounded superiorly by the inferior surface of the liver and usually contains the right hepatic artery and cystic artery.

Distal to its junction with the cystic duct, the common hepatic duct is known as the common bile duct (CBD). The common hepatic duct and supraduodenal portion of the common bile duct reside in the free-edge of the lesser omentum along with the hepatic artery and the portal vein. The usual anatomical relationship of these structures is for the portal vein to lie posteriorly with the hepatic artery to the left anterior aspect of it and the common bile duct to the right of the artery. These three structures in the free-edge of the lesser omentum are referred to as the hepatic pedicle.

The hepatic pedicle can be occluded (known as the Pringle manoeuvre) to reduce hepatic inflow during liver resection or catastrophic liver haemorrhage. A Pringle manoeuvre is achieved by inserting a finger into the foramen of Winslow, posterior to and around the hepatic pedicle, and then dividing the loose connective tissue of the lesser omentum at the tip of the finger. This then allows application of a non-crushing clamp or compression tape. The supraduodenal artery (branch of gastroduodenal artery) usually crosses anterior to the distal aspect of the common bile duct and may be damaged when performing a choledochotomy or dissecting the lesser omentum.

The distal common bile duct becomes retropancreatic as it passes through a groove or tunnel in the pancreas. It usually runs parallel to the main pancreatic duct for approximately 1–2 cm before joining it and draining into the second part of the duodenum via the ampulla of Vater, with flow controlled by the sphincter of Oddi.

GALLBLADDER

The gallbladder is a pear-shaped biliary storage organ situated on the under-surface of the liver within the cystic or gallbladder fossa between segments IV and V. It has an infundibulum, body and fundus, with the latter usually reaching the free-edge of the liver. A fold or pouch, known as Hartmann's pouch, in the infundibular area is a common site for gallstones to lodge. Variations in gallbladder anatomy are rare but may include diverticulae, septae and duplication. The main blood supply of the gallbladder is via the cystic artery and vein. However, small arteries and veins between the gallbladder and liver bed are often present.

HILAR PLATE

The hilar plate is a term which often confuses surgical trainees. The term 'plate' probably conjures the concept of a flat, covering structure but it is, in fact, more like a single line or reflection of tissue. It is situated where the peritoneum covering the anterior surface of the hepatic pedicle reflects anteriorly to join the liver capsule at the base of segment IV (*see Figure 4.9*). It therefore looks like a white line, reminiscent of the white line between the right colon and abdominal wall, which is divided during a right hemicolectomy. Division of the hilar plate, also commonly referred to as lowering of the hilar plate, exposes the confluence of the right and left hepatic ducts.

CYSTIC PLATE

Unlike the hilar plate, the cystic plate is a flat, covering structure and refers to the fibrous tissue or capsule which is situated between the gallbladder and the liver parenchyma of the gallbladder fossa (*Figure 4.3*). This identifies the ideal plane of dissection between the gallbladder and the cystic plate during cholecystectomy. Dissection which strays deep to the cystic plate, into the liver parenchyma, increases the risk of a bile leak or bleeding.

BLOOD, LYMPHATIC AND NERVE SUPPLY OF THE BILIARY TREE

Arterial

The hilar region of the biliary tree has a rich blood supply from the right and left hepatic arteries. The supraduodenal bile duct is mainly supplied by approximately eight small axial arteries running along its length which are vulnerable to damage and can lead to ischaemia and formation of bile duct strictures. The retropancreatic bile duct has a rich blood supply derived from branches of the posterior pancreaticoduodenal artery.

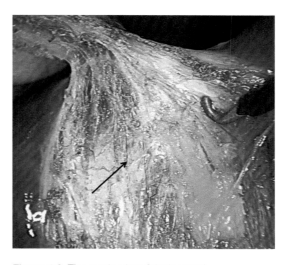

Figure 4.3 The cystic plate (black arrow).

Venous

A venous plexus surrounds the biliary tree and drains into the liver, portal vein and posterior superior pancreaticoduodenal vein. The veins of this plexus may become dilated, known as portal venous collateralization, with increased portal pressure secondary to cirrhosis. This collateralization may be very marked in portal vein thrombosis, known as cavernous transformation.

Lymphatics

Lymph drains from the liver, biliary tree and gallbladder mainly to the coeliac lymph nodes along various branches of the coeliac trunk. Lymph from the distal aspect of the common bile duct and ampulla drains via nodes in the pancreatic head to the mesenteric nodes. The cystic lymph node of Lund usually resides in Calot's triangle and may be closely adherent to the cystic artery or cystic duct. It is often encountered during cholecystectomy.

Nerves

The gallbladder and biliary tree have a rich autonomic nerve supply. The gallbladder and sphincter motility are also controlled by enteric hormones. The parasympathetic supply is via the anterior and posterior vagal trunks. Sympathetic supply arises from the coeliac plexus forming a dense sheath of nerve fibres along the hepatic and gastroduodenal arteries. Parasympathetic stimulation leads to contraction of the gallbladder and ejection of bile into the biliary tree but the cystic duct and bile ducts do not undergo peristalsis themselves.

IMPORTANT ANATOMICAL ANOMALIES AND CONSIDERATIONS FOR CHOLECYSTECTOMY

Sub-vesical ducts

These are small accessory ducts that originate from the right lobe of the liver and pass through the cystic plate to either drain directly into the gallbladder or course along the cystic plate and drain into the extrahepatic biliary system. They are invariably too small to identify during cholecystectomy. Occasionally, a more defined duct can be seen coursing along the cystic plate; this was traditionally referred to as the duct of Lushka. The significance of these small ducts is that they are the second most frequent cause for post-cholecystectomy bile leaks, after cystic duct leaks.

Parallel or long cystic duct

In 75–80% of cases, the cystic duct joins the common hepatic duct approximately 1–2 cm from the confluence of the right and left hepatic ducts. However, in the remaining cases, it may have a longer course passing parallel to the common hepatic duct before merging with it inferiorly or it may pass around the duct posteriorly (*Figure 4.4*). In these anomalous cases, the common bile duct could be damaged if there is excessive dissection to always try to visualize the junction between the cystic duct and common hepatic duct. Occasionally, a long dilated cystic duct, running parallel to the CBD, may be misinterpreted as the CBD during bile duct exploration. In such cases it will be possible to pass a catheter or choledochoscope inferiorly, but not superiorly.

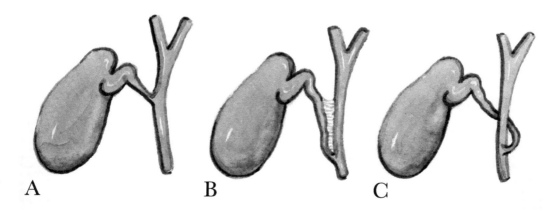

Figure 4.4 Important variations in the anatomy of the cystic duct. **(A)** Normal anatomical relationship of the cystic duct with the common hepatic duct. **(B)** The cystic duct is long and passes parallel to the common hepatic duct for a variable length before merging with it. **(C)** The cystic duct passes around the posterior aspect of the common hepatic duct before merging with it medially.

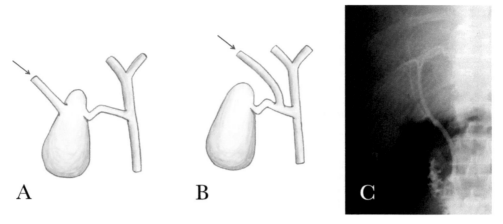

Figure 4.5 Important variations in the anatomy of the posterior sectoral duct, indicated by blue arrows. **(A)** Insertion into the gallbladder. **(B)** Insertion into the cystic duct. **(C)** Intraoperative cholangiogram demonstrating the anomalous posterior sectoral duct inserting into the cystic duct.

Posterior sectoral duct

In 4–8% of cases, the posterior sectoral duct does not unite with the anterior right hepatic duct but instead drains into another part of the biliary tree. It may drain into the gallbladder, the left hepatic duct, the common hepatic duct or into the cystic duct directly (*Figure 4.5*). In the latter scenario, if the anomalous posterior sectoral duct is not recognized at cholecystectomy, division of the cystic duct distal to the insertion of the posterior sectoral duct will result in a bile leak from segments VI and VII and will most likely present in the early post-operative period. Alternatively, clipping of the posterior sectoral duct will lead to elevated obstructive liver enzymes, possible recurrent sepsis in the undrained segments VI and VII and ultimately atrophy of these segments.

Superficial middle hepatic vein

The middle hepatic vein (or a major tributary of it) may be very superficial in 10–15% of cases, running in close relation to the cystic plate in the gallbladder fossa (1–3). It is sometimes referred to in the general surgical literature as a venous sinus. Its relevance in biliary surgery is that opening into it can lead to significant venous haemorrhage when dissecting the gallbladder from the liver bed during cholecystectomy (*Figure 4.6*). To avoid this, the surgeon should keep the dissection plane superficial to the white fibrous tissue of the cystic plate. In cases of very severe cholecystitis, where there is a higher risk of penetrating the cystic plate and entering the liver parenchyma, it may be prudent to perform a sub-total cholecystectomy. In this technique the fundus and body of the gallbladder are removed, leaving the infundibular area but the portion of the gallbladder wall adherent to the cystic plate may

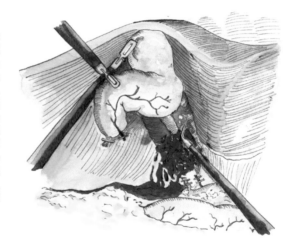

Figure 4.6 Illustration of venous haemorrhage from a superficially located middle hepatic vein, damaged when dissecting the gallbladder from the liver bed during cholecystectomy.

also be left, to reduce the risk of entering the liver parenchyma and the middle hepatic vein.

Anomalies of the right hepatic artery

The right hepatic artery normally arises from the hepatic artery proper, itself arising from the coeliac trunk. It usually passes posterior to the upper bile duct before giving off the cystic artery within Calot's triangle.

In approximately 20% of cases, the right hepatic artery passes anterior to the bile duct. This is more common when the cystic artery arises to the left of the bile

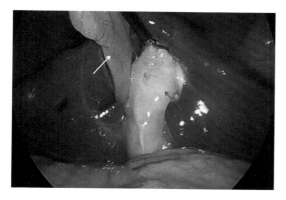

Figure 4.7 Gallbladder to the left (blue arrow) of the falciform ligament (white arrow).

duct, for example from the common hepatic artery. In these cases, the right hepatic artery can appear much more prominent in Calot's triangle and is usually associated with a short cystic duct. This makes it much more susceptible to injury or clipping during dissection of the cystic duct and artery.

In approximately 9% of cases, the right hepatic artery arises from the superior mesenteric artery and runs posterolateral to the bile duct in the free-edge of the hepatic pedicle/lesser omentum. Underlying pathological conditions such as inflammation or tumour may make it difficult to recognize this anomaly intraoperatively, increasing the risk of arterial injury. For example, a large impacted stone in Hartmann's pouch may cause effacement of the hepatic pedicle and may also lead to erosion into the anomalous right hepatic artery and

this can result in significant bleeding during cholecystectomy.

Gallbladder to the left of the falciform ligament

In approximately 0.2–0.3% of the population, the gallbladder is situated to the left of the falciform ligament (*Figure 4.7*). This is more common, but not confined to, individuals with situs inversus. Surgery must proceed with great caution and intraoperative cholangiography may be required to accurately identify the biliary anatomy and unusual variations.

ORIENTATION OF BILIARY ANATOMY DURING SURGERY, PARTICULARLY CHOLECYSTECTOMY

While the anatomical anomalies discussed above are important factors in complications of biliary surgery, such as cholecystectomy, the majority of biliary injuries are due to incorrect orientation and identification of the extrahepatic biliary anatomy. Misinterpretation of the anatomy is a well-recognized phenomenon leading to bile duct injury during cholecystectomy. The most common misinterpretation is to identify the common bile duct as the cystic duct. This results in the common bile duct being dissected and clipped and the dissection proceeding superiorly, so that the common hepatic duct is clipped or divided, with the result that a segment of bile duct is removed in a T-shaped fashion with the gallbladder. This is known as the 'classical bile duct injury' (*Figure 4.8*). This

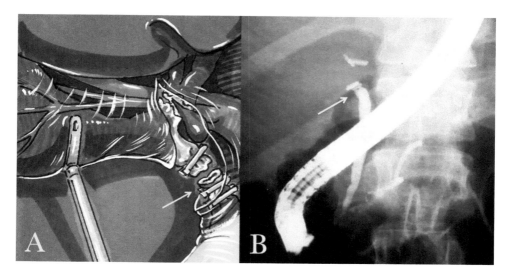

Figure 4.8 Illustration of the 'classical bile duct injury' during cholecystectomy. (A) Shows the erroneous clipping of the common bile duct (yellow arrow) and division of common hepatic duct superiorly. (B) An ERCP image demonstrating clipping of the common bile duct (yellow arrow).

usually occurs when the surgeon commits a perceptual error, is disorientated and commences dissection too far medially and inferiorly so that dissection is on the hepatic pedicle, medial to the CBD, rather than lateral to the hepatic pedicle.

In order to prevent this type of anatomical misinterpretation and subsequent biliary injury many surgeons and centres will have an orientation process which is strictly observed in each case, before dissection commences. We have previously described our anatomical orientation and cross-checking system which involves a wider overall consideration of the segmental liver and biliary anatomy, including the falciform ligament and hepatic pedicle (4). Despite laparoscopic cholecystectomy being one of the most commonly performed procedures, many general surgeons may not be familiar with this anatomy and initially focus too much on the Calot's triangle area.

The orientation commences with identification of the point where the falciform ligament, having passed behind the tissue bridge connecting segments II and IV, inserts into the liver at the medial aspect of the base of segment IV. The hilar plate passes in an arc from this point over to the lateral aspect of the base of segment IV. An imaginary line, known as the line of safety, overlaid between the gallbladder and the lateral edge of segment IV, passing the lateral end of the hilar plate and extending along the lateral edge of the hepatic pedicle divides the operative field into two areas (*Figure 4.9*). Keeping dissection strictly lateral to this line will allow safe dissection of the cystic artery, the cystic duct and the lower third of the gallbladder in order to obtain Strasberg's critical view (5). Dissection that strays medial to this line risks injury to the bile duct or other hepatic pedicle structures.

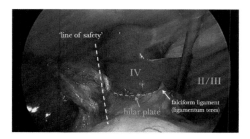

Figure 4.9 Labelled intraoperative demonstration of the line of safety and the hilar plate. During cholecystectomy, the surgeon should keep dissection lateral to the line of safety to avoid inadvertent damage to the bile duct or other hepatic pedicle structures.

REFERENCES

1. Shen BY, Li HW, Chen M, Zheng MH, Zang L, Jiang SM, et al. Color Doppler ultrasonographic assessment of the risk of injury to major branch of the middle hepatic vein during laparoscopic cholecystectomy. *Hepatobiliary Pancreat Dis Int* 2003;**2**:126–30.
2. Ball CG, MacLean AR, Kirkpatrick AW, Bathe OF, Sutherland F, Debru E, et al. Hepatic vein injury during laparoscopic cholecystectomy: The unappreciated proximity of the middle hepatic vein to the gallbladder bed. *J Gastrointest Surg* 2006;**10**:1151–5.
3. Zhang WZ, Shen J, Xie JX, Zhu H. Color Doppler ultrasonographic examination on the relationship between the gallbladder bed and major branch of the middle hepatic vein. *Hepatobiliary Pancreat Dis Int* 2005;**4**:299–301.
4. Diamond T, Mole DJ. Anatomical orientation and cross-checking – the key to safer laparoscopic cholecystectomy. *Br J Surg* 2005;**92**:663–4.
5. Strasberg SM, Hertl M, Soper NJ. An analysis of the problem of biliary injury during laparoscopic cholecystectomy. *J Am Coll Surg* 1995;**180**:101–5.

Chapter
5

Assessment of Pancreatic and Liver Function

Dimitrios Karavias and John Primrose

INTRODUCTION

The pancreas, like the liver, has both endocrine and exocrine functions. In simple terms the endocrine function regulates the homeostasis of glucose and the metabolism of carbohydrates, whereas the exocrine function plays a vital role in digestion by controlling the breakdown of fats, proteins, and sugars.

The liver is the largest internal organ and its function is essential for life. Without any hepatic function, life expectancy is only 1–2 days. The functions of the liver are numerous and beyond the scope of this chapter (*see* **Chapter 2**). In brief it is involved in protein catabolism and urea formation, bilirubin formation, glucose metabolism, pH homeostasis, temperature regulation, formation of clotting factors, metabolism and excretion of hormones and drugs, sequestration of gut-related organisms and antigen removal with presentation to the immune system.

ASSESSMENT OF PANCREATIC FUNCTION

Exocrine pancreatic function

The pancreas secretes around 800 mL of pancreatic juice every day which is a clear, enzyme rich, alkaline fluid. Both the volume and the composition of the pancreatic secretions vary during different phases of digestion and are regulated by several well-orchestrated negative feedback loops. In between meals, during fasting or basal state, the pancreas only secretes a small volume of a protein rich, mildly alkaline fluid with a bicarbonate concentration of around 80 mEq/L. During meals, pancreatic secretions are altered in consistency and increase in volume, both by neuronal pathways and by the effect of two main hormones, secretin and cholecystokinin (CCK). The presence of gastric acid in the duodenum triggers the production of secretin by the S cells of the duodenum and secretin stimulates the secretion of bicarbonate and water from the pancreatic ductal cells, gradually increasing the volume of the pancreatic secretions. As chyme or partly digested food enters the duodenum, CCK is also produced by the enteroendocrine cells of the duodenum and the proximal jejunum. Cholecystokinin stimulates the secretion of pancreatic digestive enzymes and proenzymes from the acinar cells. At this phase, the pancreatic juice is a clear, enzyme rich, watery, and highly alkaline fluid with a bicarbonate concentration of around 120 mEq/L. The high concentration of bicarbonate acts to neutralize the gastric acid in the duodenum, allowing for more effective enzymatic digestion.

A series of digestive enzymes, either in their final activated form or in an inactive state, are present in the pancreatic juice. Enzymes like trypsinogen and chymotrypsinogen, involved in the breakdown of proteins, are secreted in an inactive form to avoid autodigestion of the pancreatic tissue. These proenzymes are activated as they enter the duodenum by enteropeptidase to trypsin and chymotrypsin. Carboxipeptidases A and B, zymogens involved in proteolysis, are also secreted by the acinar cells in an inactive form and are activated by trypsin in the duodenum and small intestine. Similarly, elastase, a serine protease, is secreted as an inactive zymogen by the pancreas and is also activated in the duodenum by trypsin. In contrast, enzymes involved in the digestion of fats and the breakdown of carbohydrates are secreted in their final active state. Amylase (alpha-amylase in humans), produced both by the salivary gland and the pancreas, hydrolyses complex starches to maltose and glucose. Lipase, phospholipase A2 and cholesterol esterase, also produced by the pancreas, are involved in the digestion of fats. This process is aided by bile salts, which emulsify dietary lipids to micelles, exponentially increasing the surface area for these enzymes to work.

The assessment of the pancreatic function requires a good understanding of the normal pancreatic physiology and the exocrine function of the pancreas. Several pancreatic function tests are available nowadays, both invasive and non-invasive. All these tests aim to assess pancreatic function and measure pancreatic secretion, to help discriminate between different causes of malabsorption in clinical practise. Exocrine pancreatic insufficiency is common in diseases like acute and chronic pancreatitis, pancreatic cancer, cystic fibrosis and occurs after pancreatic, gastric, or metabolic surgery. Gradual decline in the exocrine pancreatic function leads to disruption of the normal digestion of proteins, fats and sugars and occurs when over 90% of the pancreatic enzyme secretion is lost (1). Clinically, exocrine pancreatic insufficiency leads to malabsorption presenting with abdominal pain and bloating, weight loss, diarrhoea in the form of steatorrhea and deficiency of the fat-soluble vitamins A, D, E and K (2).

DOI: 10.1201/9781003080060-5

ASSESSMENT OF EXOCRINE PANCREATIC FUNCTION

Pancreatic function can be assessed with imaging studies, endoscopic procedures, and laboratory measurements. The latter involve tests that directly measure pancreatic exocrine function either in the blood or the pancreatic juice itself and indirect tests that assess the effects from the lack of pancreatic enzymes like steatorrhea (*Table 5.1*).

Imaging

Imaging studies provide invaluable information about the pancreatic gland and the pancreatic anatomy. Ease of use and widespread availability has rendered radiologic imaging the principal method of assessing pancreatic function, at least in initial stages. Computed tomography (CT) is very sensitive in detecting chronic pancreatitis especially when gland atrophy has developed or when calcification and/or duct dilatation are present (3), however, when these signs are not present the sensitivity of CT is quite limited. CT scanning can also identify fat replacement, cystic disease, anatomic variations, and other pathologies such as pancreatic cancer. It can also be very helpful in acute pancreatitis and the identification of early complications. Magnetic resonance imaging (MRI) and cholangiopancreatography (MRCP) provide similar diagnostic abilities and sensitivity to CT (4). However, MRCP can better visualize the biliary tree, characterize pancreatic strictures and when combined with secretin improves the visualization of the pancreatic ductal anatomy providing insight into the pancreatic secretion (5). CT and MRI are very helpful as screening tools, but are primarily used to guide further diagnostic planning and investigations.

Endoscopic retrograde cholangiopancreatography (ERCP) is the most sensitive test for assessing the pancreatic ductal anatomy and is generally considered the gold standard in the diagnosis of ductal disease. While it has high sensitivity in diagnosing advanced chronic pancreatitis, its sensitivity in early or mild pancreatitis is significantly lower (6). The invasive nature of the procedure along with the risks involved, including post ERCP pancreatitis, have limited the use of ERCP in the assessment of pancreatic exocrine function. Instead, endoscopic ultrasound (EUS) has gained popularity over the recent years as it offers the ability to identify early changes in the pancreatic parenchyma, well before traditional imaging. EUS can also identify anatomical abnormalities and help with the diagnosis of pancreatic cancer. While operator dependant, the adoption of international guidelines on terminology and diagnostic criteria has improved sensitivity and specificity of EUS diagnosis of chronic pancreatitis (7). Limitations of EUS include widespread availability, interobserver variability and the invasive nature of the procedure.

Indirect pancreatic function tests

Indirect pancreatic function tests are non-invasive tests that measure by-products and metabolites of the pancreatic enzyme activity. They are relatively inexpensive and well tolerated by patients, however they offer lower sensitivity comparing to other tests. Measurement of faecal fat is considered the gold standard for diagnosing malabsorption. The 72-hour faecal fat test is a quantitative test where patients adhere to a high fat diet of 100 g of fat per day followed by a 72-hour collection of stools for a total of 6 days. Measured faecal fat content of greater that 7 g per day is considered abnormal and consistent with steatorrhea (6). While inexpensive, the test is not logistically easy to perform accurately, as it requires the consumption of significant amount of fats and the storage and refrigeration of stools over a period of 3 days. Alternative qualitative tests commonly used in clinical practice are the Sudan stain and the acid steatocrit tests. While these tests are easier to perform, they are not considered as reliable or sensitive (8).

To simplify the process, a series of more practical tests have also been utilized to indirectly assess the pancreatic function. Several breath tests have been explored over the years that indirectly assess the activity of pancreatic lipase (9). In principle, patients consume a ^{13}C- or ^{14}C-labelled triglyceride in the form of butter on toast. The labelled triglycerides are hydrolyzed by pancreatic lipase, metabolized in the liver, and exhaled in the form of labelled CO_2, which can be easily measured with mass spectrometry. The most common labelled substrates used in clinical practice are ^{13}C-mixed triglycerides and ^{14}C-triolein. While promising, these breath tests are not widely available, and their sensitivity and reliability are still under investigation. Historically, two urine tests have also been used to evaluate the pancreatic function. The pancreolauryl test (PLT) evaluates the function of cholesterol esterase and bentiromide tests the function of pancreatic chymotrypsin. In the former, fluorescein dilaurate is administered orally, which is metabolized by cholesterol esterase (10). Fluorescein, a by-product of the enzymatic activity is absorbed by the gut and excreted in urine. In the later, bentiromide (N-benzoyl-L-tyrosyl-p-aminobenzoic acid) is administered orally, which is metabolized by chymotrypsin (11). Para-aminobenzoic acid (PABA) is released, which is metabolized in the liver and also excreted in the urine. Both metabolites can be easily measured in urine, but liver or renal insufficiency can greatly impact the accuracy of results. While serum alternatives were developed, neither test is currently used in clinical practice.

Direct pancreatic function tests

Direct pancreatic function tests measure the levels of pancreatic enzymes in pancreatic fluid, serum, or stools. Tests that measure pancreatic enzyme levels in stools or blood, historically referred to as 'tubeless'

Table 5.1 Summary of pancreatic function tests and their relative advantages and disadvantages

	Advantages	Disadvantages
Radiology		
CT	● Widely available, cost effective ● High specificity for advanced chronic pancreatitis *(i.e. calcification, atrophy, fat replacement)* ● Used for screening *(e.g. cystic disease, pancreatic cancer)*	● Low sensitivity overall
MRI/MRCP	● Widely available, cost effective ● High sensitivity for moderate to severe chronic pancreatitis ● Good visualization of biliary tree ● Ability to characterize pancreatic strictures	● Low sensitivity for mild pancreatitis ● Limited ability to characterize side branch disease
Secretin-enhanced MRI/MRCP	● Improved characterization of pancreatic ductal anatomy ● Non-invasive evaluation of pancreatic exocrine function	● Not widely available ● Lower sensitivity comparing to secretin test
Endoscopy		
ERCP	● 'Gold standard' for assessing ductal disease ● Higher sensitivity for advanced chronic pancreatitis	● Invasive *(i.e. post-ERCP pancreatitis)* ● Low sensitivity for mild pancreatitis ● Operator dependant
EUS	● High sensitivity overall ● Ability to characterize early parenchymal changes	● Low interobserver reliability ● Invasive ● Not widely available
Indirect tests		
Faecal fat assessment		
72-hour faecal fat	● 'Gold standard' for diagnosis of malabsorption	● Complex to perform reliably ● Pancreatic enzyme replacement therapy (PERT) needs to be stopped ● False-positive results with medication like Orlistat
Sudan stain	● Simple to perform ● Inexpensive	● Very low sensitivity for malabsorption ● False-positive results with medication like Orlistat
Acid steatocrit	● Simple to perform ● Inexpensive	● Low sensitivity overall
Urine tests		
Bentiromide test		● Unreliable results in liver or kidney disease
Pancreolauryl test		● Unreliable results in liver or kidney disease. Not available commercially
Direct tests		
Non-invasive 'tubeless'		
Serum amylase	● High sensitivity for acute pancreatitis	● Low specificity overall
Serum lipase	● High sensitivity for acute pancreatitis ● Useful in alcohol-related pancreatitis and late presentation	● Low specificity overall
Serum trypsinogen	● High sensitivity and specificity for pancreatic insufficiency and chronic pancreatitis	

(Continued)

Table 5.1 (*Continued*) Summary of pancreatic function tests and their relative advantages and disadvantages

Non-invasive 'tubeless' (continued)

Faecal chymotrypsin	• High sensitivity for advanced chronic pancreatitis • Can be used to monitor PERT compliance	• Watery diarrhoea and PERT affect results
Faecal elastase 1	• High sensitivity and specificity for pancreatic insufficiency • Correlates well with other tests • Oral PERT doesn't affect results	• Mid-range results can be difficult to interpret • Can't be used to monitor PERT compliance
^{13}C-MTG breath test		• Not widely available • Sensitivity and reliability under investigation
^{14}C-triolein breath test		• Not widely available • Sensitivity and reliability under investigation
Invasive tests		
Lundh test		• Legacy procedure
Secretin test	• High sensitivity for chronic pancreatitis	• Invasive, not well tolerated
CCK test	• High sensitivity for chronic pancreatitis	• Invasive, not well tolerated • Bile secretions impact measurements
Combined secretin-CCK test	• Ability to evaluate acinar and ductal exocrine pancreatic function	• Invasive, not well tolerated • Bile secretions impact measurements

tests, are non-invasive, widely available, and inexpensive. However, their sensitivity can vary significantly in different clinical situations, rendering their clinical interpretation ambiguous. Analysis of the pancreatic juice is the most sensitive and specific method to assess the exocrine pancreatic function. This is achieved by collecting the pancreatic secretions after hormonal stimulation with specialized gastrointestinal (GI) tubes or endoscopic procedures. While directly measuring pancreatic secretions is considered the 'gold standard' assay for evaluating pancreatic function, it involves invasive procedures, is not well tolerated by patients and can be complex to perform.

Serum amylase and lipase measurements are widely available and commonly used in clinical setting, primarily for the diagnosis of acute pancreatitis. Both tests have high sensitivity, with lipase being considered more useful in alcoholic pancreatitis or in late presentation (12). A major disadvantage is the low specificity. Raised levels of amylase and lipase have been reported in several conditions, which limits their use in the investigation of malabsorption. Measuring serum trypsinogen is more helpful in clinical practice. It offers high sensitivity and specificity for diagnosing pancreatic insufficiency and chronic pancreatitis, when levels are <20 mg/mL (13).

Faecal elastase 1 (FE-1) is probably the most commonly used test for the assessment of pancreatic insufficiency, with high sensitivity and specificity (14). Pancreatic elastase doesn't degrade in the GI tract and it can easily be detected in faeces with commercially available enzyme-linked immunosorbent assay (ELISA) kits. Values >200 µg of elastase/gram of stool depicts normal pancreatic exocrine function, and values <100 are indicative of severe pancreatic insufficiency (15). Oral pancreatic enzyme replacement therapy doesn't seem to affect the results, as the preparations don't contain elastase, so the test can't be used to assess response to treatment (15). A major advantage of the FE-1 test is that it correlates well with MRCP and ERCP findings, and other invasive tests like the secretin test (14,16,17). Despite these advantages, false positive results can occur in certain conditions and mid-range results are difficult to interpret.

Measuring faecal chymotrypsin is an alternative test to faecal elastase (18). It is equally available and affordable, but its clinical use is limited due to two major disadvantages. Chymotrypsin degrades as it transits through the GI tract and its levels are affected in the presence of diarrhoea. Furthermore, oral pancreatic enzyme replacement therapy influences the results, so treatment needs to be suspended prior to testing (6).

Invasive, direct pancreatic function tests offer invaluable information for the assessment of pancreatic function. Pancreatic fluid is collected after hormonal stimulation or standardized meals. Historically, several different meal preparations have been proposed, with the Lundh test being the most recognized. As originally proposed, 300 mL of a standardized meal containing a reference non-absorbable, water-soluble substance was administered, the duodenal content was aspirated with a nasojejunal tube and analyzed (19). Presently, pancreatic fluid is collected after hormonal stimulation by secretin, CCK, or a combination of both. The collection was traditionally realized with a Dreiling tube, which is a double-lumen tube placed under fluoroscopy (20). The first tip of the double-lumen tube is positioned at the pylorus, enabling the aspiration of the gastric content. The longer, weighted tip is advanced towards the ligament of Treitz and allows the collection of all duodenal content. Contemporaneously, samples are collected endoscopically.

The secretin stimulation test starts with the administration of a bolus dose of synthetic human secretin intravenously. The test measures bicarbonate levels in duodenal aspirates after four 15-minute collection intervals. Bicarbonate levels <80 mEq/L suggest exocrine pancreatic insufficiency (21). Alternative approaches to using a Dreiling tube involve endoscopic collection under sedation. Researchers previously attempted the collection of pancreatic fluid by directly catheterizing the pancreatic duct during ERCP. While this technique allows for sampling of pure pancreatic juice, it has not proven as effective as traditional collection methods and increases the risk of pancreatitis (22). Instead, pancreatic aspirates are commonly collected using the suction channel of endoscopes. The secretin endoscopic pancreatic function test (ePFT) has proven as effective as traditional methods, and is quicker to perform and better tolerated by patients (23).

CCK tests measure primarily lipase levels in duodenal aspirates over 80 minutes, in four 20-minute collection intervals (24). CCK, or synthetic analogues like ceruletide, are administered as a continuous infusion to stimulate pancreatic secretions (25). A major disadvantage of the test is that CCK increases bile secretions in the duodenum, by stimulating the contraction of the gallbladder, which impacts measurements. Combined secretin-CCK hormonal stimulation offers the ability to evaluate acinar and ductal exocrine pancreatic function simultaneously. Popular in Europe and Japan, it hasn't proved to be more accurate than secretin test alone, while sharing the same limitations as CCK tests (26).

ASSESSMENT OF ENDOCRINE PANCREATIC FUNCTION

Pancreatic islet cells, formerly known as islets of Langerhans, comprise 1–2% of the pancreatic gland and are responsible for the endocrine functions. Four distinct cell types are responsible for the production of glucagon, insulin, somatostatin, and pancreatic polypeptide. Glucagon is produced by α-cells, insulin by β-cells and somatostatin by δ-cells. These hormones are responsible for the homeostasis of glucose, whereas pancreatic polypeptide, produced by the PP (or F) cells, regulates pancreatic secretions. Endocrine functional assessment primarily evaluates the functional capacity of beta cells. Fasting concentrations of insulin,

C-peptide and proinsulin to insulin ratios can easily be measured in plasma and are the first step in assessing endocrine pancreatic function. Oral or intravenous stimulation tests however are more valuable in clinical practice (27). Oral stimulation tests offer a better representation of the normal physiology. Oral glucose tolerance test (OGTT) is considered the 'gold standard' assessment and is widely used. After an overnight fast, 75 g of glucose is administered orally followed by serial blood sampling. Two-hour glucose levels >140 mg/dL indicate impaired tolerance and levels >200 mg/dL confirm the diagnosis of diabetes (28).

ASSESSMENT OF LIVER FUNCTION

The deficiencies of liver function that confront the surgeon are multiple. First, the removal of a large part of the liver compromises its function, and although the liver's capacity to regenerate is exceptional, this takes several weeks. Second, liver function may be disordered by chronic liver disease, in which case the capacity to survive a significant resection is compromised and sometimes resection of any type is impossible. Thirdly, in recent times surgeons have had to operate on patients who have received cytotoxic chemotherapy which is known to induce chemotherapy associated steatohepatitis (CASH). As with chronic liver disease this compromises the liver's capacity to withstand surgery.

Postoperative hepatic failure (PHLF) is the commonest cause of mortality after major hepatectomy. It is therefore unsurprising that assessment of liver function preoperatively has been the subject of numerous studies using a variety of techniques. The fact that so many methodologies are available, each with a large number of advocates, testifies to the fact that there is no 'gold standard' method. All have significant drawbacks.

PHLF is multifactorial, and the factors associated have been described in a systematic review (29). These include patient-related factors (biliary sepsis, diabetes, obesity, frailty), liver-related factors (liver disease including cirrhosis and steatohepatitis and chemotherapy associated liver injury) and surgical factors (large liver resection, inadequate future liver remnant, prolonged operation and blood loss). However, most surgeons who are experienced in major hepatectomy will, from time to time, encounter a patient who suffers from severe PHLF despite apparently having an adequate volume of liver assumed to be of reasonable quality. The need for accurate functional assessment methods is therefore real.

Tests of liver function are useful to a degree in predicting complications and death but will not generally provide a stop/go for resection surgery. This is especially the case in most patients with malignancy as there may be no other worthwhile option. Patients in this setting are often more willing to accept higher levels of mortality than the surgeon.

Table 5.2 Summary of liver function tests and their relative advantages and disadvantages

Functional Test	Advantages	Disadvantages
Routine clinical data including blood tests and elastography and derivations (*Child-Pugh stage and MELD score*)	• Inexpensive as based on clinical data that is universally available • Most useful in patients with chronic liver disease as surgery may be deemed inadvisable	• Not generally useful outside of chronic liver disease • No information of quality or size of any FLR
Metabolic studies (*indocyanine green clearance [ICG] and ^{13}C-methacetin breath test*)	• Useful in assessing global liver function and predicting complications with useful accuracy • ICG clearance is well studied and inexpensive • ^{13}C-methacetin breath test requires more equipment and the advantage over ICG is not proven	• No information on size or function of any FLR
CT-based volumetric studies	• Gives reasonable assessment of volume of the FLR	• May not correspond to the surgical resection • Gives no indication of the function of the remnant
CT/multiparametric MRI-based volumetric and functional analyses	• Combines functional and volumetric analyses	• Very complex analyzes and not widely available • In general benefit unclear
Technetium-99 mebrofenin scintigraphy combined with CT	• Best functional assessment of FLR with good sensitivity and specificity	• Very complex to perform and methodology varies between centres • Not widely available
Hepatic venous pressure gradient	• Gives reliable indication of risk of liver resection possibly with greater sensitivity than ICG clearance • Easily measured postoperatively and predicts liver failure	• Performed preoperatively it is an invasive procedure • Post-resection measurement does not allow mitigation

Assessments of liver function can be grouped into (*see Table 5.2*):

1   Tests based on routine clinical information and elastography
2   Metabolic studies
3   Volumetric, radiological and scintigraphy studies
4   Physiological studies

Tests based on routine clinical information and elastography

Child-Pugh staging and MELD score

There are many systems based on clinical, biochemical and haematological parameters (29). The Child-Pugh staging is the most well-known, but applies only to patients who have chronic liver disease. Based on a 3-point system for each of bilirubin, prothrombin time, albumin and the presence of ascites and hepatic encephalopathy. A total of 5–6 points represent Child-Pugh A, 7–9 B and 10–15 C. The staging was designed to give a prediction of chronic liver disease survival (from 100% at 1 year for A, to 45% for C). In reality, only patients in stage A (or early B) will tolerate major hepatectomy and the volumetric response to portal vein embolization (below) may be informative

in such patients. The MELD (Model for End-Stage Liver Disease) score is less relevant to resectional surgery and more to transplantation, as it is designed to predict mortality in end-stage liver failure. It is based on the international normalized ratio (INR), creatinine, bilirubin and whether, or not, the patient is on renal dialysis.

Elastography

Transient elastography (Fibroscan) is a commonly used, ultrasound-based outpatient assessment of liver stiffness. It is used routinely in most hepatology clinics to screen for and assess liver fibrosis and cirrhosis. It has been assessed in relation to the surgery of HCC and the results strongly correlate with adverse outcomes following surgery (30) and a model has been built on the basis of a multivariate analysis. This incorporates the liver elastography result together with age, albumin and MELD score. This predicts severe complication with reasonable sensitivity and specificity.

Metabolic studies

Indocyanine green clearance (ICG)

This is a simple and easy-to-use method where ICG is taken up by the liver and excreted unchanged in bile.

The plasma disappearance rate, and the retention at 15 minutes, are the most commonly used outputs of the test. In conducting the test ICG is given intravenously (IV) and at a dose of 0.25 mg/kg. Disappearance is measured by pulse spectroscopy. Critical values are variously described in one report with the cut-off being identified as clearance of 19.5% at 1-minute or a 15-minute retention of 5.6% (31). Whilst these cut-offs do identify a higher risk of PHLF by ~2.5-fold, the overlap is considerable and using the result clinically is likely to be problematic in most instances.

Liver maximum capacity (LiMAx) breath test

This breath test uses ^{13}C-methacetin which is metabolized by a liver enzyme CYP1A2 which is not polymorphic and not induced by drugs and other agents. The test employs the measurement of $^{13}CO_2$ in the breath by infrared spectroscopy and the readout is the $^{13}CO_2 : ^{12}CO_2$ ratio (32). Its actual utility in assessing for the likelihood of PHLF appears to be similar to ICG clearance. LiMAx was shown to be higher in patients accepted for hepatectomy compared to those declined (33). In addition, although the preoperative levels were identical between post-hepatectomy survivors and non-survivors, the non-survivors had a much lower-level postoperatively. Unfortunately, this latter observation is of little clinical value.

Volumetry

Assessing the volume of future liver remnant (FLR) after a major hepatectomy is routine, and of particular concern in relation to portal vein embolization and double vein embolization where the FLR was initially considered inadequate. Surgeons involved in these major procedures develop a good subjective sense for the size of the liver but objective measurements are preferred. One clear problem however relates to the definition of FLR by surgeon and radiologist and strict segmental boundaries are fuzzy both surgically and radiologically. Either more liver can be left by the surgeon than may be apparent using strict segmental boundaries or conversely achieving a margin may need a greater resection. All FLR calculation needs to be in the context of the clinical situation and erring on the side of having more remnant is a good strategy. It is also the case that volume is only one component and considering the FLR function is equally important. Some of the methods described below may be of value in this respect.

Various volumetric methods are available from the radiologist drawing round the liver margins manually to various analytical programmes based on the computed tomography (CT) data (34). The software solutions are accurate and in normal circumstances are always used now. For safety, a surgeon will seek a FLR of not much less that 30% depending on the quality of remnant if PHLF is to be avoided.

Volumetry with gadoxetic acid functional MRI

Volumetry will give the volume of the FLR but little information about function. Gadoxetic acid (Primovist®) a calculation of volume and function. In one study (35) the functional FLR (derived combining CT and contrast MRI data) was found to strongly correlate with PHLF (all grades) and the selected cut-off had a sensitivity of 94% and specificity of 76%. It was found to be superior to indocyanine green clearance performed on the same cohort but the analysis unfortunately requires considerable radiological input.

Other MRI-based approaches have been published using multiparametric MRI and proprietary software to assess FLR volume and liver health (36) although these are less studied and validated. It appears to show longer hospital stay and worse postoperative outcomes in patients with adverse scores. The advantage is that the analysis can be done with routine MRI that will be available in most patients having a liver resection as a matter of course.

Technetium-99 mebrofenin scintigraphy

Radionucleotide imaging combined with CT is used routinely in some centres to give information on the functional FLR. Technetium-99 mebrofenin is taken up by the liver to give a measure of function on single-photon emission computed tomography (SPECT) imaging. However, analysis is complex, the methodology is not standardized between centres and a radiation dose is required (37). However, it is reported (38) in one study to have a sensitivity of 92% and specificity of 98% in predicting PHLF.

Measurement of hepatic venous pressure gradient (HVPG)

The HVPG is the pressure difference between the portal vein and the hepatic vein/systemic venous pressure. The normal range is 1–5 mmHg, and 10 mmHg represents significant portal hypertension. Traditionally, this is measured by transjugular delivery of a wedged hepatic venous balloon and the portal pressure indirectly determined following inflation of the balloon. In patients with hepatocellular cancer a pressure difference of greater than 5 mmHg was associated with significantly higher rates of postoperative liver dysfunction, other complications and longer hospital stays (39). Even if useful this technique is not very commonly used, as it is quite invasive. More recently, a technique to assess the HVPG through EUS and direct vein needle puncture (portal and hepatic vein or IVC) has been described which may make allow its more routine use (40).

The measurement of HVPG after liver resection gives a guide to the likelihood of PHLF developing. In one study (41) the critical value was 13.5 mmHg which had a sensitivity of 100% and specificity of 93%, however, as this is following a hepatectomy it's unclear how the result can alter management. It has been suggested that reducing portal pressure by splenectomy or splenic artery ligation (the spleen contributes around 30% of portal flow) may be helpful but this is not widely practiced at present.

SUMMARY

The evaluation of FLR and assessment of the basic clinical and biochemical parameters is used universally. At present, it is difficult to make the case for one of the more complex and expensive means of assessment over the integration of easily measured clinical parameters combined with volumetry, either formally measured or based on clinical experience. What is used often also depends on what is available locally and whether the expertise to interpret the results is available. The best assessed of the complex techniques is probably technetium-99 mebrofenin scintigraphy combined with CT. However, there is potential for single modality methods such as multiparametric MRI but further studies and more data will be needed before they are reliable clinically.

REFERENCES

1. DiMagno EP, Go VL, Summerskill WH. Relations between pancreatic enzyme outputs and malabsorption in severe pancreatic insufficiency. *N Engl J Med* 1973;**288**(**16**):813–15.
2. Levy P, Dominguez-Munoz E, Imrie C, Lohr M, Maisonneuve P. Epidemiology of chronic pancreatitis: Burden of the disease and consequences. *United European Gastroenterol J* 2014;**2**(**5**):345–54.
3. Malfertheiner P, Buchler M, Stanescu A, Ditschuneit H. Exocrine pancreatic function in correlation to ductal and parenchymal morphology in chronic pancreatitis. *Hepatogastroenterology* 1986;**33**(**3**):110–14.
4. Sugiyama M, Haradome H, Atomi Y. Magnetic resonance imaging for diagnosing chronic pancreatitis. *J Gastroenterol* 2007;**42**(**Suppl 17**):108–12.
5. Swensson J, Zaheer A, Conwell D, Sandrasegaran K, Manfredi R, Tirkes T. Secretin-enhanced MRCP: How and why-AJR expert panel narrative review. *AJR Am J Roentgenol* 2021;**216**(**5**):1139–49.
6. Lieb JG 2nd, Draganov PV. Pancreatic function testing: Here to stay for the 21st century. *World J Gastroenterol* 2008;**14**(**20**):3149–58.
7. Kitano M, Gress TM, Garg PK, Itoi T, Irisawa A, Isayama H, et al. International consensus guidelines on interventional endoscopy in chronic pancreatitis. Recommendations from the working group for the international consensus guidelines for chronic pancreatitis in collaboration with the International Association of Pancreatology, the American Pancreatic Association, the Japan Pancreas Society, and European Pancreatic Club. *Pancreatology* 2020;**20**(**6**):1045–55.
8. Simko V. Fecal fat microscopy. Acceptable predictive value in screening for steatorrhea. *Am J Gastroenterol* 1981;**75**(**3**):204–8.
9. Weaver LT, Amarri S, Swart GR. 13C mixed triglyceride breath test. *Gut* 1998;**43**(**Suppl 3**):S13–19.
10. Lankisch PG, Brauneis J, Otto J, Goke B. Pancreolauryl and NBT-PABA tests. Are serum tests more practicable alternatives to urine tests in the diagnosis of exocrine pancreatic insufficiency? *Gastroenterology* 1986;**90**(**2**):350–4.
11. Tanner AR, Fisher D, Ward C, Smith CL. An evaluation of the one-day NBT-PABA/14C-PABA in the assessment of pancreatic exocrine insufficiency. *Digestion* 1984;**29**(**1**):42–6.
12. Yadav D, Agarwal N, Pitchumoni CS. A critical evaluation of laboratory tests in acute pancreatitis. *Am J Gastroenterol* 2002;**97**(**6**):1309–18.
13. Jacobson DG, Curington C, Connery K, Toskes PP. Trypsin-like immunoreactivity as a test for pancreatic insufficiency. *N Engl J Med* 1984;**310**(**20**):1307–9.
14. Loser C, Mollgaard A, Folsch UR. Faecal elastase 1: A novel, highly sensitive, and specific tubeless pancreatic function test. *Gut* 1996;**39**(**4**):580–6.
15. Leeds JS, Oppong K, Sanders DS. The role of fecal elastase-1 in detecting exocrine pancreatic disease. *Nat Rev Gastroenterol Hepatol* 2011;**8**(**7**):405–15.
16. Bilgin M, Bilgin S, Balci NC, Momtahen AJ, Bilgin Y, Klor HU, et al. Magnetic resonance imaging and magnetic resonance cholangiopancreatography findings compared with fecal elastase 1 measurement for the diagnosis of chronic pancreatitis. *Pancreas* 2008;**36**(**1**):e33–9.
17. Hardt PD, Marzeion AM, Schnell-Kretschmer H, Wusten O, Nalop J, Zekorn T, et al. Fecal elastase 1 measurement compared with endoscopic retrograde cholangiopancreatography for the diagnosis of chronic pancreatitis. *Pancreas* 2002;**25**(**1**):e6–9.
18. Durr HK, Otte M, Forell MM, Bode JC. Fecal chymotroypsin: A study on its diagnostic value by comparison with the secretin-cholecystokinin test. *Digestion* 1978;**17**(**5**):404–9.
19. Borgstrom B, Dahlqvist A, Lundh G. On the site of absorption of fat from the human small intestine. *Gut* 1962;**3**:315–17.
20. Dreiling DA, Hollander F. Studies in pancreatic function; preliminary series of clinical studies with the secretin test. *Gastroenterology* 1948;**11**(**5**):714–29.
21. Stevens T, Conwell DL, Zuccaro G Jr, Van Lente F, Purich E, Khandwala F, et al. A randomized crossover study of secretin-stimulated endoscopic and dreiling tube pancreatic function test methods in healthy subjects. *Am J Gastroenterol* 2006;**101**(**2**):351–5.
22. Denyer ME, Cotton PB. Pure pancreatic juice studies in normal subjects and patients with chronic pancreatitis. *Gut* 1979;**20**(**2**):89–97.
23. Stevens T, Parsi MA. Update on endoscopic pancreatic function testing. *World J Gastroenterol* 2011;**17**(**35**):3957–61.
24. Conwell DL, Zuccaro G, Morrow JB, Van Lente F, O'Laughlin C, Vargo JJ, et al. Analysis of duodenal drainage fluid after cholecystokinin (CCK) stimulation in healthy volunteers. *Pancreas* 2002;**25**(**4**):350–4.

25. Gullo L, Costa PL, Fontana G, Labo G. Investigation of exocrine pancreatic function by continuous infusion of caerulein and secretin in normal subjects and in chronic pancreatitis. *Digestion* 1976;**14(2)**:97–107.

26. Del Rosario MA, Fitzgerald JF, Gupta SK, Croffie JM. Direct measurement of pancreatic enzymes after stimulation with secretin versus secretin plus cholecystokinin. *J Pediatr Gastroenterol Nutr* 2000;**31(1)**:28–32.

27. Choi CS, Kim MY, Han K, Lee MS. Assessment of beta-cell function in human patients. *Islets* 2012;**4(2)**:79–83.

28. American Diabetes Association. 2. Classification and diagnosis of diabetes: Standards of medical care in diabetes–2020. *Diabetes Care* 2020;**43(Suppl 1)**:S14-S31.

29. Rahnemai-Azar AA, Cloyd JM, Weber SM, Dillhoff M, Schmidt C, Winslow ER, et al. Update on liver failure following hepatic resection: Strategies for prediction and avoidance of post-operative liver insufficiency. *J Clin Transl Hepatol* 2018;**6(1)**:97–104.

30. Serenari M, Han KH, Ravaioli F, Kim SU, Cucchetti A, Han DH, et al. A nomogram based on liver stiffness predicts postoperative complications in patients with hepatocellular carcinoma. *J Hepatol* 2020;**73(4)**:855–62.

31. Schwarz C, Plass I, Fitschek F, Punzengruber A, Mittlbock M, Kampf S, et al. The value of indocyanine green clearance assessment to predict postoperative liver dysfunction in patients undergoing liver resection. *Sci Rep* 2019;**9(1)**:8421.

32. Stockmann M, Lock JF, Riecke B, Heyne K, Martus P, Fricke M, et al. Prediction of postoperative outcome after hepatectomy with a new bedside test for maximal liver function capacity. *Ann Surg* 2009;**250(1)**:119–25.

33. Stockmann M, Lock JF, Malinowski M, Niehues SM, Seehofer D, Neuhaus P. The LiMAx test: A new liver function test for predicting postoperative outcome in liver surgery. *HPB (Oxford)* 2010;**12(2)**:139–46.

34. Suzuki K, Epstein ML, Kohlbrenner R, Garg S, Hori M, Oto A, et al. Quantitative radiology: Automated CT liver volumetry compared with interactive volumetry and manual volumetry. *AJR Am J Roentgenol* 2011;**197(4)**:W706–12.

35. Asenbaum U, Kaczirek K, Ba-Ssalamah A, Ringl H, Schwarz C, Waneck F, et al. Post-hepatectomy liver failure after major hepatic surgery: Not only size matters. *Eur Radiol* 2018;**28(11)**:4748–56.

36. Mole DJ, Fallowfield JA, Sherif AE, Kendall T, Semple S, Kelly M, et al. Quantitative magnetic resonance imaging predicts individual future liver performance after liver resection for cancer. *PloS one* 2020;**15(12)**:e0238568.

37. Rassam F, Olthof PB, Richardson H, van Gulik TM, Bennink RJ. Practical guidelines for the use of technetium-99m mebrofenin hepatobiliary scintigraphy in the quantitative assessment of liver function. *Nucl Med Commun* 2019;**40(4)**:297–307.

38. Chapelle T, Op De Beeck B, Huyghe I, Francque S, Driessen A, Roeyen G, et al. Future remnant liver function estimated by combining liver volumetry on magnetic resonance imaging with total liver function on (99m)Tc-mebrofenin hepatobiliary scintigraphy: Can this tool predict post-hepatectomy liver failure? *HPB (Oxford)* 2016;**18(6)**:494–503.

39. Stremitzer S, Tamandl D, Kaczirek K, Maresch J, Abbasov B, Payer BA, et al. Value of hepatic venous pressure gradient measurement before liver resection for hepatocellular carcinoma. *Br J Surg* 2011;**98(12)**:1752–8.

40. Huang JY, Samarasena JB, Tsujino T, Lee J, Hu KQ, McLaren CE, et al. EUS-guided portal pressure gradient measurement with a simple novel device: A human pilot study. *Gastrointest Endosc* 2017;**85(5)**:996–1001.

41. Golse N, Joly F, Combari P, Lewin M, Nicolas Q, Audebert C, et al. Predicting the risk of post-hepatectomy portal hypertension using a digital twin: A clinical proof of concept. *J Hepatol* 2021;**74(3)**:661–9.

Chapter

6

Preoperative Assessment

Janet W.Y. Li, Susan L. Orloff and Christopher Connelly

INTRODUCTION

Hepato-pancreatico-biliary (HPB) operations are typically high-risk procedures and can be very morbid, given the risks of significant haemorrhage, vascular and biliary injury. In addition to postoperative complications including infections, biliary and pancreatic leaks, or postoperative liver insufficiency. Mortality for HPB procedures was quite high in the latter-half of the 20th century, but in the current day, mortality is reported to be less than 5%. This trend is certainly multifactorial, with increasingly specialized surgical training programmes, advances in surgical equipment and devices, improvements in patient selection, and more sophisticated and dedicated anaesthesia and care in intensive care units (ICU). Patient selection begins with an understanding of which patients will benefit from surgery, but also includes a better ability to predict which patients will tolerate significant perioperative physiological stress (1). The aim of this chapter is to review the components of a rigorous preoperative assessment to both stratify and mitigate risk in patients undergoing HPB surgery in order to optimize the best outcomes for those patients in need.

HISTORY

Obtaining a thorough history and performing a complete physical examination are the first steps to determine a patient's surgical risk factors. Reported symptomatology, either from history of presenting illness or review of systems, can often raise concerns that may need to be addressed for patient surgical optimization. For example, if the patient has lost significant weight from a liver, biliary or pancreatic malignancy, perioperative nutritional supplementation may be necessary to improve their postoperative recovery. Some presenting symptoms may potentially have multiple aetiologies, such as when a patient reports the worsening, or shortness of breath, and it isn't clear whether the symptoms are due to the mass effect from a large, liver cyst splinting the diaphragm, cardiopulmonary comorbidities or a combination with the HPB pathology having exacerbated an underlying issue.

More recently, geriatric patients are being considered for HPB surgery with increased frequency as the population ages and life expectancy lengthens. Multiple studies have shown that there is no difference in oncologic benefit, based on age (2,3). In the United States, more than half of the cancer diagnoses are in patients who are 70 years or older (4). Estimates predict a 67% increase in cancer incidence in patients older than 65 years compared to an 11% increase in younger patients (5). A patient's chronological and physiological ages can be quite disparate and may impart different clinical significance. Physiological age is related to a patient's comorbidities and functional status, while chronological age can impact liver physiology, and ultimately outcomes after surgery. Liver function decreases over time, as seen by proxy with decreases in serum albumin, liver blood flow, and cytochrome P450 activity (4). Schiergens et al. showed that overall survival for patients who are older than 70 years old, who underwent elective liver resection experienced inferior outcomes than younger patients due to intraoperative estimated blood loss, comorbidities and postoperative complications (6). Reddy et al. in a multi-institution analysis, reported a direct association between an increase in age and an increase in postoperative mortality, independent of their American Society of Anesthesiology (ASA) score (7). Additionally, patients with underlying liver disease and older age, undergo liver regeneration much more slowly and less effectively than younger patients, particularly when the background liver is cirrhotic.

PAST MEDICAL HISTORY

A complete past medical history is another integral part of the preoperative assessment. Careful evaluation of patient comorbidities can determine the optimal treatment strategy and can impact survival during cancer treatment (4). In particular for HPB surgery, cirrhosis, obesity and diabetes can significantly impact postoperative outcomes.

Impaired liver function and cirrhosis, independent of the aetiology of the liver disease, poses a common challenge for patients undergoing liver resection. The inflammatory state and scarring of cirrhosis increase the risk of these patients developing hepatomas requiring surgical intervention discussed in **Chapter 50** (8). However, cirrhotic patients are also less likely to be able to tolerate the physiological stress of a liver resection and have limited potential for liver parenchymal regeneration (8). Also, progression to portal hypertension with elevated portal venous wedge pressures, varices, splenomegaly and thrombocytopenia, significantly increases the risk of postoperative liver decompensation (9). The Child-Turcotte-Pugh (CTP) scoring system was initially

DOI: 10.1201/9781003080060-6

developed to risk stratify patients with portal hypertension who would benefit from a portocaval shunt (10). By using serum laboratory values to approximate liver function, the CTP scoring system categorizes patients into three groups, Child A, B and C (*Table 6.1*). It has been more broadly applied to cirrhotic patients undergoing major abdominal surgery, with mortality rates of 10%, 30% and greater than 70% in Child A, B and C patients, respectively (11). In general, Child A patients can tolerate a major liver resection as long as they have sufficient future liver remnant (FLR) whereas Child B and C generally do not tolerate major resections and are high risk for intraoperative complications, postoperative liver decompensation, liver failure and death (10).

The volume of liver remaining after a resection, known as FLR, is an important aspect of preoperative planning. The FLR is calculated from volume measurements estimated from cross-sectional imaging as a ratio of FLR to total pre-procedure liver volume based on a formula using body surface area (12). The FLR must sustain the patient as the liver organ hypertrophies but the volume required to avoid postoperative hepatic insufficiency differs based on the baseline quality of the liver. The generally accepted sufficient FLR for patients with normal liver function is 20%, for patients who have been treated with preoperative chemotherapy or are obese and have NASH 30%, for patients with underlying liver dysfunction (typically cirrhosis) 40% (13). If the FLR is deemed marginal, there are a number of techniques to augment liver volume such as portal vein embolization, hepatic vein embolization, Yttrium 90 to treat the liver tumour as well as enhance remnant liver regeneration, associating liver partition and portal vein ligation for staged hepatectomy (ALPPS) and hepatic artery embolization.

Analogously, impaired pancreatic function should be assessed preoperatively prior to surgery by taking a thorough history to understand if symptoms of pancreatic insufficiency and/or a diagnosis of diabetes are present. Diabetes mellitus is associated with cardiovascular disease, posing increased perioperative morbidity and mortality. However, pancreatic insufficiency preoperatively can be used to assess the risk of postoperative new-onset diabetes or worsening insulin resistance. In a small study of 27 patients undergoing pancreaticoduodenectomy, preoperative normoglycemia as measured by a normal haemoglobin A1c (HbA1c) resulted in an unlikely development of postoperative diabetes (14). The type of pancreatic resection *per se*, for example pancreaticoduodenectomy or distal pancreatectomy has no significant effect on the risk of developing postoperative diabetes but both are associated with a rate of new-onset diabetes of greater than 35% (15). Exocrine pancreatic insufficiency has been described in 36% of patients after pancreatic resection and can present as late as 14 months following surgery (16). Signs of malabsorption include steatorrhea and malnutrition which resolves with pancreatic enzyme supplementation.

SOCIAL HISTORY

A thorough social history is important to assess for lifestyle and habits that may suggest exposure to substances that may portend the possibility of undiagnosed, well-compensated cirrhosis (heavy alcohol use, intravenous drug use, toxic environmental or occupational exposures). Assessment of the preoperative functional status is another key component of the social history. The two widely-accepted and validated classification schemas of functional status are the Karnofsky Performance Status (KPS) scale and Eastern Cooperative Oncology Group (ECOG) Performance Status Scale (17) (*Table 6.2*). Patients who are functionally fit preoperatively are expected to have decreased postoperative morbidity and mortality. Dolgin et al. demonstrated that liver transplant recipients with moderate and severe disability pre-transplant had worse 1-year mortality rates and graft failure rate compared to recipients with no functional impairment (18). Handgrip strength (HGS) has been proposed as a simple and reproducible way to assess muscle strength, as well as other preoperative parameters of risk, including frailty, level of physical activity, lean body mass with malnutrition, and cardiopulmonary and/or metabolic diseases. Chan et al. sought to use HGS to predict postoperative complications in patients undergoing HPB surgery. Although not predictive of complications, a weaker HGS did predict a more prolonged hospital stay (≥21 days) (19).

Another assessment of social history that has been associated with perioperative outcomes in liver transplantation is the Stanford Integrated Psychosocial Assessment for Transplant (SIPAT). The score

Table 6.1 CTP Classification

	Points		
	1	2	3
Encephalopathy	None	Grade 1-2	Grade 3-4
Ascites	None	Mild-Moderate	Severe
Bilirubin (mg/dL)	<2	2-3	>3
Albumin (g/dL)	>3.5	2.8-3.5	<2.8
INR	<1.7	1.7-2.3	>2.3

Sum the points to determine the CTP class

Child's A: 5–6 points (well-compensated liver disease)

Child's B: 7–9 points (significant functional compromise)

Child's C: 10–15 points (decompensated disease)

Note: The CTP classification is calculated based on the patient's serum laboratories and clinical status. It is useful in understanding their level of liver disfunction and how that may affect their perioperative mortality

Table 6.2 The KPS scale and ECOG performance status scales are useful in quantifying a patient's performance status

ECOG performance status		KPS performance status	
0	Fully active, able to carry on all pre-disease performance without restriction	100	Normal, no complaints; no evidence of disease
		90	Able to carry on normal activity; minor signs or symptoms of disease
1	Restricted in physically strenuous activity but ambulatory and able to carry out work of a light or sedentary nature, e.g. light housework, office work	80	Normal activity with effort, some signs or symptoms of disease
		70	Cares for self but unable to carry on normal activity or to do active work
2	Ambulatory and capable of all self-care but unable to carry out any work activities; up and about more than 50% of waking hours	60	Requires occasional assistance but is able to care for most personal needs
		50	Requires considerable assistance and frequent medical care
3	Capable of only limited self-care; confined to bed or chair more than 50% of waking hours	40	Disabled; requires special care and assistance
		30	Severely disabled; hospitalization is indicated although death not imminent
4	Completely disabled; cannot carry on any self-care; totally confined to bed or chair	20	Very ill; hospitalization and active supportive care necessary
		10	Moribund
5	Dead	0	Dead

culminates a patient's psychosocial risk by assessing four domains. The patient's readiness level, social support system, psychological suitability and psychopathology and lifestyle and effect of substance use (20). The SIPAT score is independently associated with biopsy-proven allograft rejection and immunosuppression nonadherence (21).

NUTRITIONAL ASSESSMENT

Malnutrition or under nutrition is corollary related to a patient's performance status. Reportedly, up to 50% of patients undergoing GI surgery are malnourished (22). Malnutrition increases perioperative morbidity as it is associated with muscle wasting, delayed wound healing and an impaired immune environment (23–25). Although a number of studies have sought to improve outcomes with preoperative nutritional 'prehabilitation', no intervention has shown a clear benefit (26). Also, protein or carbohydrate supplementation in patients with normal nutritional status has shown little to no benefit (27). In a meta-analysis of patients specifically undergoing cancer surgery, prehabilitation decreased the hospital stay but did not improve perioperative morbidity and mortality (26). In the 2022 Enhanced Recovery After Surgery (ERAS®) Society guidelines, preoperative nutritional assessment is a strong recommendation and should be optimized 7–14 days preoperatively in order to improve postoperative outcomes (28). The implementation of ERAS pathways has been shown to decrease length of stay, the risk of postoperative complications and hospital costs (29).

CARDIAC ASSESSMENT

Major adverse cardiac events are a source of significant postoperative mortality and major morbidity (30). Preoperative cardiac risk assessment begins with a history and physical examination to identify any unstable or undiagnosed cardiac conditions. A number of risk calculators are available to determine the risk of major adverse cardiac events (MACE), such as myocardial infarction or death, perioperatively. The most widely used calculators are the Revised Cardiac Risk Index (RCRI), the Gupta Myocardial Infarction and Cardiac Arrest (MICA) calculator or the American College of Surgeons (ACS) National Surgical Quality Improvement Program (NSQIP) surgical risk calculator (30). Patients who are low risk (<1%) do not need further testing before proceeding to surgery. Patients who have intermediate (1–5%) or high (>5%) risk of MACE then proceed to a stepwise approach to preoperative cardiac testing. The urgency of the operation and the surgical risk of the type of surgery are the first considerations. HPB surgery is considered intermediate risk (1–5% risk of MACE) with the exception of liver transplant which is high risk (>5% risk of MACE) (31). All patients undergoing intermediate or high-risk surgeries should proceed to a functional capacity assessment in metabolic equivalents (METs). One MET is defined as the caloric consumption of a person at rest, while 2–4 METs is light walking, housework or equivalent and ten METs is running or climbing (32). Those with a functional capacity of less than four METs should then be considered for additional cardiac stress testing (31). Electrocardiograms (ECGs) are useful in patients with known cardiovascular disease (CVD) to establish a baseline or discover undiagnosed CVD in asymptomatic patients. Echocardiograms and serum brain natriuretic peptide (BNP) are useful in patients with unexplained dyspnoea or a history of heart failure. Angiograms should be performed if vascular compromise is diagnosed during preoperative evaluation. Stress testing, either exercise or chemically-induced, has a limited role in preoperative evaluation. Kaw et al. found that in patients undergoing noncardiac surgery, functional status and RCRI was adequate in predicting the postoperative risk of MACE, with preoperative stress testing only of moderate value (33).

CONSENT

Informed consent is simultaneously an important part of the therapeutic relationship between a physician or surgeon and their patient and is also a legal requirement before performing an invasive procedure or operation. The three key components of informed consent include: 1) The nature of the intervention; 2) The benefits, risks, and likely consequences; and 3) The alternatives and their benefits, risks and consequences. Ensuring patient comprehension of the nature of the treatment is a common problem with informed consent. A patient may enter the discussion with some baseline understanding or expectations, which may or may not be medically accurate. Conversely, a patient may have poor health-literacy requiring more careful consideration during the surgeon's explanation. A number of decision aids have been developed that can help enhance a patient's understanding (34). When a patient's native language is not English, it is imperative to have an appropriate language-specific translator present when explaining the details of the operation as well as when obtaining consent.

When reviewing the risks, benefits and consequences of the treatment, the same attention must be paid to the alternatives. In the treatment of HPB pathologies, the alternative to surgery is often locoregional ablative therapy, palliative chemotherapy, or transition to palliative/hospice care. A discussion of the consequences of each approach to therapy should include the expected median survival and how suggested therapies and support will affect the individual patient's quality of life and longevity (34).

Disclosure of surgeon or hospital experience with a treatment may be ethically desirable but is not legally required. Most patients when making a decision about surgery, consider surgeon experience with highly innovated procedures (35). In addition, patients may wish to know the role of the trainee.

The primary goal of surgical recommendations should be to enhance or maintain patient wellbeing. Patient consent should be voluntary and aligned with their goals and values, as well as those of designated family members. In some cases, where there is no clearly preferred option, the surgeon should help the patient and family deliberate without bias. However, if the patient is clearly acting against their best interest, it is the role of the surgeon to try to explain the rationale for the procedure and attempt to persuade them with involvement of relevant family members as well as those in the advanced directive role (34).

ETHICS

Certain ethical dilemmas are specific to the procedural nature of surgery. Some pertain to the fact that only the surgical team is present during the operation to advocate for the patient. When unexpected intraoperative findings change the operation, the surgeon may consider performing a substantially different procedure than the one discussed during the informed consent. Some surgeons obtain a blanket consent preoperatively allowing for any needed real-time changes to the operation. Others may call the next of kin to discuss the additional procedure in an attempt to ensure the patient's goals and values are preserved. This is distinct from anatomical variation or intraoperative conduct requiring an additional procedure, which should be performed at the discretion of the surgeon and then explained postoperatively.

The role of the trainee is also unique in surgical disclosure. Supervising physicians can guide cognitive-skill development with less risk than technical skills. Trainees performing technical skills may make a mistake before the attending surgeon can intervene. Discussing the supervision of trainees is appreciated by most patients and generally leads to agreement in the involvement of trainees (36). Concurrent surgery, where the attending surgeon is involved in the critical portions of the operation in two different patients, is ethically acceptable and should be differentiated from overlapping surgery.

The invasive nature of surgery and the manual role of the surgeon makes refusal of treatment distinct from that of a physician. A surgeon may refuse to conduct surgery for a number of reasons. The preoperative evaluation may reveal that the patient risk is too high, related to perioperative mortality and morbidity, and the risk outweighs the benefits of surgery. If the patient feels that they are willing to undertake such risks despite the surgeon's caution, referral to a second surgeon may be useful. The surgeon may also deem an operation futile, or not indicated, despite a patient's insistence. Building consensus with the patient, the family, and other support, with a focus on the patient's best interest in mind, should always be the goal.

In other instances, a patient may specify certain (occasionally quite detailed) restrictions during the operation and postoperatively, the most common example being the refusal of blood products. The surgeon may have the legal right to decline to operate and transfer care to another physician if the requests are too restrictive to the successful or safe conduct of the operation. However, most would once again try to approach this circumstance as an opportunity to build consensus. In the example of refusing blood transfusion, a number of measures can be taken to minimize the likelihood of requiring a transfusion including treating anaemia preoperatively, haemodilution, incorporation of synthetic pro-coagulant factors, and utilization of cell saver autotransfusion intraoperatively.

SUMMARY

The preoperative assessment of a candidate for HPB surgery is very important to enable the surgeon or anaesthetist to properly risk-stratify a patient for surgery. This allows for the surgeon and the patient (family) to have a frank conversation about the nature of the surgery, risks, benefits and alternatives, and explore whether undergoing the operation is in line with the patient's goals, values and wishes. A number of risk calculators are available to assess cardiovascular risk for HPB surgery in intermediate- to high-risk surgical candidates. However, to fully evaluate a patient, many patient-specific factors must be taken into account to provide a holistic assessment of risk as well as to provide the best possible outcomes for the patient.

REFERENCES

1. Snowden C, Prentis J. Anesthesia for hepatobiliary surgery. *Anesthesiol Clin* 2015;**33(1)**:125–41.
2. Adam R, Frilling A, Elias D, Laurent C, Ramos E, Capussotti L, et al. Liver resection of colorectal metastases in elderly patients. *Br J Surg* 2010; **97(3)**:366–76.
3. Turrini O, Guiramand J, Moutardier V, Viret F, Bories E, Giovannini M, et al. Major hepatectomy for metastasis of colorectal cancer improves survival in the elderly. *Ann Chir* 2005;**130(9)**:562–5.
4. Pasetto LM, Lise M, Monfardini S. Preoperative assessment of elderly cancer patients. *Crit Rev Oncol Hematol* 2007;**64(1)**:10–18.
5. Smith BD, Smith GL, Hurria A, Hortobagyi GN, Buchholz TA, et al. Future of cancer incidence in the United States: Burdens upon an aging, changing nation. *J Clin Oncol* 2009;**27(17)**:2758–65.
6. Schiergens TS, Stielow C, Schreiber S, Hornuss C, Jauch K-W, Rentsch M, et al. Liver resection in the elderly: Significance of comorbidities and blood loss. *J Gastrointest Surg* 2014;**18(6)**:1161–70.
7. Reddy SK, Barbas AS, Turley RS, Gamblin TC, Geller DA, Marsh JW, et al. Major liver resection in elderly patients: A multi-institutional analysis. *J Am Coll Surg* 2011;**212(5)**:787–95.
8. Schuppan D, Afdhal NH. Liver cirrhosis. *Lancet* 2008;**371(9615)**:838–51.
9. Mizuguchi T, Kawamoto M, Meguro M, Hui TT, Hirata K, et al. Preoperative liver function assessments to estimate the prognosis and safety of liver resections. *Surg Today* 2014;**44(1)**:1–10.
10. Child CG, Turcotte, JG. Surgery and portal hypertension. *Major Probl Clin Surg* 1964;**1**:1–85.
11. Garrison RN, Cryer HM, Howard DA, Polk HC Jr., et al. Clarification of risk factors for abdominal operations in patients with hepatic cirrhosis. *Ann Surg* 1984;**199(6)**:648–55.
12. Vauthey JN, Chaoui A, Do KA, Bilimoria MM, Fenstermacher MJ, Charnsangavej C, et al. Standardized measurement of the future liver remnant prior to extended liver resection: Methodology and clinical associations. *Surgery* 2000;**127(5)**:512–19.
13. Ribero D, Chun YS, Vauthey JN. Standardized liver volumetry for portal vein embolization. *Semin Intervent Radiol* 2008;**25(2)**:104–9.
14. Hamilton L, Jeyarajah DR. Hemoglobin A1c can be helpful in predicting progression to diabetes after Whipple procedure. *HPB (Oxford)* 2007;**9(1)**:26–8.
15. Nguyen A, Demirjian A, Yamamoto M, Hollenbach K, Imagawa DK, et al. Development of postoperative diabetes mellitus in patients undergoing distal pancreatectomy versus Whipple procedure. *Am Surg* 2017;**83(10)**:1050–3.
16. Simon R. Complications after pancreaticoduodenectomy. *Surg Clin North Am* 2021;**101(5)**:865–74.
17. Oken MM, Creech RH, Tormey DC, Horton J, Davis TE, McFadden ET, et al. Toxicity and response criteria of the Eastern Cooperative Oncology Group. *Am J Clin Oncol* 1982;**5(6)**:649–55.
18. Dolgin NH, Movahedi B, Anderson FA, Bruggenwirth IM, Martins PN, Bozorgzadeh A, et al. Impact of recipient functional status on 1-year liver transplant outcomes. *World J Transplant* 2019;**9(7)**:145–57.
19. Chan KS, Chia CLK, Ng FKL, Seow WHJ, Leong DY, Shelat VG. Impaired handgrip strength does not predict postoperative morbidity in major hepatobiliary surgery. *J Surg Res* 2020;**256**:549–56.
20. Maldonado JR, Dubois HC, David EE, Sher Y, Lolak S, Dyal J, et al. The Stanford Integrated Psychosocial Assessment for Transplantation (SIPAT): A new tool for the psychosocial evaluation of pre-transplant candidates. *Psychosomatics* 2012;**53(2)**:123–32.
21. Deutsch-Link S, Weinberg EM, Bittermann T, McDougal M, Dhariwal A, Jones LS, et al. The Stanford Integrated Psychosocial Assessment for Transplant is associated with outcomes before and after liver transplantation. *Liver Transpl* 2021;**27(5)**:652–67.
22. Schwegler I, et al. Nutritional risk is a clinical predictor of postoperative mortality and morbidity in surgery for colorectal cancer. *Br J Surg* 2010; **97(1)**:92–7.
23. Clark MA, Plank LD, Hill GL. Wound healing associated with severe surgical illness. *World J Surg* 2000;**24(6)**:648–54.
24. Vernon DR, Hill GL. The relationship between tissue loss and function: Recent developments. *Curr Opin Clin Nutr Metab Care* 1998;**1(1)**:5–8.
25. Schneider SM, Veyres P, Pivot X, Soummer AM, Jambou P, Filippi J, et al. Malnutrition is an independent factor associated with nosocomial infections. *Br J Nutr* 2004;**92(1)**:105–11.
26. Lambert JE, Hayes LD, Keegan TJ, Subar DA, Gaffney CJ, et al. The impact of prehabilitation

on patient outcomes in hepatobiliary, colorectal, and upper gastrointestinal cancer surgery: A PRISMA-Accordant Meta-analysis. *Ann Surg* 2021; **274(1)**:70–77.

27. MacFie J, Woodcock NP, Palmer MD, Walker A, Townsend S, Mitchell CJ, et al. Oral dietary supplements in pre- and postoperative surgical patients: A prospective and randomized clinical trial. Nutrition 2000;16(9):723–8.

28. Joliat GR, Kobayashi K, Hasegawa K, Thomson J-E, Padbury R, Scott M, et al. Guidelines for perioperative care for liver surgery: Enhanced Recovery After Surgery (ERAS) Society recommendations 2022. *World J Surg* 2023;**47(1)**:11–34.

29. Noba L, Rodgers S, Chandler C, Balfour A, Hariharan D, Yip VS, et al. Enhanced Recovery After Surgery (ERAS) reduces hospital costs and improves clinical outcomes in liver surgery: A systematic review and meta-analysis. *J Gastrointest Surg* 2020;**24(4)**:918–32.

30. Levine GN, Bates ER, Bittl JA, Brindis RG, Fihn SD, Fleisher LA, et al. 2016 ACC/AHA Guideline Focused Update on Duration of Dual Antiplatelet Therapy in Patients With Coronary Artery Disease: A Report of the American College of Cardiology/American Heart Association Task Force on Clinical Practice Guidelines: An Update of the 2011 ACCF/AHA/SCAI Guideline for Percutaneous Coronary Intervention, 2011 ACCF/AHA Guideline for Coronary Artery Bypass Graft Surgery, 2012 ACC/AHA/ACP/AATS/PCNA/SCAI/STS Guideline for the Diagnosis and Management of Patients With Stable Ischemic Heart Disease, 2013 ACCF/AHA Guideline for the Management of ST-Elevation Myocardial Infarction, 2014 AHA/ACC Guideline for the Management of Patients With Non-ST-Elevation Acute Coronary Syndromes, and 2014 ACC/AHA Guideline on Perioperative Cardiovascular Evaluation and Management of Patients Undergoing Noncardiac Surgery. *Circulation* 2016;**134(10)**:e123–55.

31. Raslau D, Bierle DM, Stephenson CR, Mikhail MA, Kebede EB, Mauck KF, et al. Preoperative cardiac risk assessment. *Mayo Clin Proc* 2020;**95(5)**:1064–79.

32. Jette M, Sidney K, Blumchen G. Metabolic equivalents (METs) in exercise testing, exercise prescription, and evaluation of functional capacity. *Clin Cardiol* 1990;**13(8)**:555–65.

33. Kaw R, Nagarajan V, Jaikumar L, Halkar M, Mohananey D, Hernandez AV, et al. Predictive value of stress testing, revised cardiac risk index, and functional status in patients undergoing noncardiac surgery. *J Cardiothorac Vasc Anesth* 2019;**33(4)**:927–32.

34. Lo B. *Resolving Ethical Dilemmas: A Guide for Clinicians*. 6th edn. Philadelphia: Wolters Kluwer; 2019.

35. Lee Char SJ, Hills NK, Lo B, Kirkwood KS, et al. Informed consent for innovative surgery: A survey of patients and surgeons. *Surgery* 2013;**153(4)**:473–80.

36. Arambula A, Bonnet K, Schlundt DG, Langerman A, et al. Patient opinions regarding surgeon presence, trainee participation, and overlappping surgery. *Laryngoscope* 2019;**129(6)**:1337–46.

Bailey & Love's Essential Operations Bailey & Love's Essential Operatic
Bailey & Love's Essential Operations Bailey & Love's Essential Operatic
Bailey & Love's Essential Operations Bailey & Love's Essential Operatic

SECTION 1 | BASIC PRINCIPLES

Chapter 7

Enhanced Recovery after Surgery (ERAS®)

Christopher Christophi

INTRODUCTION

ERAS or 'fast-track surgery' is an evidence-based, multidisciplinary, protocol driven approach to the patient undertaking major surgery. ERAS protocols focus on reducing morbidity, length of hospital stay and costs, compared with conventional treatment, by targeting key therapeutic aspects of the perioperative pathway.

The concept of ERAS protocols was first introduced by Henrik Kehlet in 1997 representing surgeons in northern Europe and focusing on colorectal surgery (1). Since that time and especially over the last 10 years, other surgical specialties, including HPB surgery have adopted the concept of ERAS protocols (2).

ERAS PROTOCOLS AND GENERAL PRINCIPLES IN MAJOR ABDOMINAL SURGERY

The multidisciplinary team includes representatives from Surgery, Anaesthesia and Intensive Care, dieticians, nursing staff and other allied health professionals. The team should meet on a regular basis and conduct regular audits to monitor outcome results.

Clinical goals aim to achieve an expedited and safe recovery by targeting specific aspects of patient care (3). These include reducing the levels of neural and endocrine responses, caused by the stress of surgery, to baseline levels. Other principles include adequate pain relief with non-opioid analgesia, early mobilization, return of early gastrointestinal tract (GIT) function, adequate nutrition, prevention of sepsis and optimization of fluid therapy (4).

PREOPERATIVE PHASE

Education and counselling

The patient needs to be fully counselled and educated in ERAS protocols, especially the role expected of patient participation. This has been shown to increase patient compliance, lower anxiety levels and have a positive impact on postsurgical recovery (5).

Assessment

A comprehensive history and examination should be undertaken with assessment and optimization of any organ dysfunction. The functional status of the patient and risk assessment should be documented using well-validated criteria.

Prehabilitation

For high-risk patients, rehabilitation prior to surgery should be considered for a period of 4–6 weeks. Appropriate exercise intervention improves the functional capacity of the patient resulting in improved outcomes following surgery. Other comorbidities may be corrected. Avoiding smoking or consumption of alcohol (moderate or heavy drinker) for at least 4 weeks prior to surgery will also decrease complications. In addition, issues of nutrition, including sarcopenia, may be addressed during this period.

Nutrition

A detailed nutritional assessment should be undertaken on all preoperative patients. In patients with an adequate nutritional status, there is no significant evidence to support any beneficial effects of pre- or postoperative nutritional supplementation. However, in high-risk patients, nutritional supplementation for 10–14 days prior to surgery have been shown to improve patient outcomes. High-risk patients include those with a history of weight loss of more than 10–15% over the last 6 months, a BMI of less than 18.5 kg/m^2 or a serum albumin less than 30 g/L; they are associated with increased complications following surgery.

Immune nutrition

Giving immune nutrition supplements (arginine, glutamine, nucleotides, omega-3 fatty acids) to the patient during the perioperative period has been suggested. The rationale is to modify the inflammatory processes and the host immune response following surgery and thus improve patient outcomes (especially sepsis and wound healing). Several studies support a positive effect in patients undergoing major surgery. It is difficult to assess these studies however, due to bias, heterogeneity and different regimes of duration and dosage. No authoritative evidence currently supports a significant benefit of immune nutrition in the perioperative phase of major abdominal surgery.

DOI: 10.1201/9781003080060-7

Fasting

The recommended period of fasting prior to surgery has been reduced to 6 hours for semisolids and 2 hours for clear fluids. This maintains gastrointestinal (GI) function, with no increase in pulmonary aspiration rates. Prophylactic use of nasogastric tube (NG) insertion is not recommended.

Thromboembolic prophylaxis

This should commence 2–12 hours preoperatively using appropriate doses of low-molecular weight or unfragmented heparin. This should be complemented by elastic support stockings. The use of mechanical intermittent compression devices should be considered for high-risk patients. Pharmacological prophylaxis should continue until discharge for low-risk patients and up to 1 month post-discharge for high-risk or oncology patients.

Carbohydrate loading

Ingestion of carbohydrate enriched fluids 2–3 hours before surgery has been shown to increase glycogen storage, decrease insulin resistance and minimize protein catabolism. It is safe and leads to improved patient outcomes with decreased recovery times and decreased stress and anxiety levels for the patient. It also promotes early return of GIT function.

Premedication

The use of opiates and long-acting anxiolytic agents should be avoided in the immediate preoperative period. Evidence suggests that these agents are associated with postoperative cognitive dysfunction, decreased mobilization and delayed oral intake.

The future opioid requirements may be reduced by giving a premedication combined dose of a neuromodulator (Gabapentin) and paracetamol. Non-steroidal anti-inflammatory drugs (NSAIDs) or Cox-2 inhibitors may be used in the postoperative period, providing renal function is not impaired.

OPERATIVE PHASE

Analgesia

The main goal is to achieve adequate non-narcotic analgesia using multimodal approaches. Narcotic side effects include nausea and vomiting, drowsiness, respiratory depression, urinary retention and dysmotility of the gut leading to increased postoperative morbidity, a prolonged postoperative recovery period and increased length of stay (LOS). Several of the following strategies discussed have been suggested to minimize opioid requirements, improve patient outcomes and decrease LOS.

Epidural anaesthesia

Thoracic epidural for abdominal operations has long been considered the 'gold standard' of opiate-sparing analgesia. Several studies have confirmed a decreased narcotic use with improvements in patient outcomes. However, a recent multicentre randomized control trial in high-risk patients undergoing major abdominal surgery showed no reduction in adverse morbid outcomes in patients having epidural insertion.

Limiting effects of epidural anaesthesia include the risk of epidural haematoma (especially in coagulopathic patients), prolonged motor blockade affecting mobilization, urinary retention and hypotension. It is also labour intensive and technically demanding to perform.

Locoregional analgesia

Several alternative strategies to epidural anaesthesia should also be considered. These techniques lead to improved pain scores, decreased recovery times and have an opiate-sparing effect. They include regional anaesthesia using field blocks covering the incision and local infiltration or continuous irrigation of the surgical wound using catheters. Infusion of local anaesthetic by preperitoneal approach under ultrasound (US) guidance between internal oblique and transverse abdominis (TAP) leads to decreased pain scores, decreased GI side effects and greater opioid-sparing effects. No comparative data on the efficacy of thoracic epidural, versus the latter techniques in an ERAS® setting, are available.

Intrathecal morphine

A single dose of intrathecal morphine (150–500 μg) has emerged as an alternative to epidural anaesthesia. Recent reviews have confirmed improved patient outcomes with decreased individual opiate requirements, and improvement in pain scores. This is often combined with local or regional neural block in major abdominal surgery.

Systemic lidocaine

The intravenous infusion of lidocaine has been used as an opiate-sparing analgesic. It is a potent anti-inflammatory, suppressing the operative stress response. It also increases peristalsis of the GIT, allowing early oral intake and provides effective analgesia lasting for up to 24 hours following surgery; this improves mobility and recovery times.

Other options

Other analgesic strategies suggested include the use of low-dose ketamine (a dissociative anaesthetic) infusion and dexmedetomidine (a centrally acting alpha-2 adrenergic agonist) given in titrated doses. These agents have intraoperative analgesic effects and reduce postoperative opiate requirements.

Perioperative analgesia requires a multidisciplinary approach with the aim of providing adequate safe analgesia. The strategies and techniques adopted usually reflect the expertise of the institution.

Surgical techniques

Drains

The insertion of surgical drains should be kept to a minimum and they should be removed as early as possible. Prolonged abdominal drainage is associated with an increase in intra-abdominal complications and increased recovery times.

Laparoscopic surgery

There is little data on the impact of minimal invasive surgery within an ERAS protocol setting, Information on pain scores, complications, LOS and overall costs are variable and may reflect the case load and expertise of the institution. In general, major laparoscopic abdominal surgery is associated with improved pain scores, decreased complication rates (wound sites, pulmonary) and increased operating times. Conflicting data exists on its effects on major abdominal complications, hospital LOS and hospital costs. More data is required before definitive conclusions can be reached.

Fluid administration

Excessive fluid administration has been shown to increase inflammatory responses and is associated with increased external lung interstitial water. This may lead to multi-organ dysfunction with increased complication rates and prolonged recovery times. Optimization of IV fluid administration is thus essential in modifying the risk according to the incidence of perioperative complications.

Restricted fluid regimens have been traditionally recommended to overcome adverse effects of excessive fluid administration. Several trials have shown conflicting results in respect of the benefits of restrictive fluid regimens. A large multicentre randomized study demonstrated that a restricted fluid regimen conferred no advantage over a liberal fluid regime. The restrictive group had a higher incidence of renal dysfunction and an equivalent complication rate (wound sepsis) to the liberal group. Most clinical trials investigating the relationship between the amount of IV fluid and perioperative complications use a fixed protocol approach for intraoperative fluid intervention.

Fluid directed goal therapy has been shown to decrease perioperative complications and shorten the recovery period when compared to other traditional fluid regimes. This concept uses a flexible and dynamic response to the amount and type of fluid administered and the need of vasoactive agents to maintain organ perfusion. It utilizes the concept of continuous monitoring of parameters including cardiac output, stroke volume variation, pulse pressure variation and mean arterial pressure to determine fluid requirements. Traditional assessment of fluid requirements using central venous pressure (CVP), urine output and pulse rate are not sufficiently sensitive and should no longer be used as a guide to fluid requirements and administration.

Hypothermia

Avoiding intraoperative hypothermia is essential (a core temperature below 36°C). It is associated with cardiac arrythmias, coagulopathies, prolonged anaesthetic recovery times and a higher complication rate. Normal temperatures are usually achieved using a variety of warming devices.

Prophylactic antibiotics

These should be considered for major abdominal surgery as they reduce the rate of septic complications with a consequent prolonged recovery time. A single dose (usually a cephalosporin) is given less than 60 minutes before beginning the skin incision but generally no postoperative antibiotics are necessary. If positive cultures are available preoperatively (bile, wound sites) an appropriate antibiotic should be given as a full therapeutic course.

Nasogastric tubes

Tubes are associated with increased patient discomfort, delayed GI function and increased aspiration rates. A selective approach with early removal is recommended. Prophylactic or routine insertion should be avoided.

POSTOPERATIVE PHASE

Principles of management in the postoperative phase include adequate pain relief using no, or minimal, opiate analgesia, early mobilization and oral feeding, maintaining a normal volume fluid status and addressing issues of nausea and vomiting (6). Early removal of NG tubes, wound drains and urinary catheters should be undertaken when appropriate and thromboembolic prophylaxis should be maintained. All these measures are associated with improved patient outcomes.

Postoperative nausea and vomiting (PONV)

Several factors contribute to nausea and vomiting in the postoperative period and these should be addressed. These include avoiding the use of volatile anaesthetic agents and opiate analgesia, early removal of NG tubes and the correction of dehydration. Patient risk scores have been defined to allow the prophylactic use of anti-emetic medication for the high-risk patient. Four predictive risk factors have been identified. These include being female, previous history of postoperative nausea and vomiting (PONV), non-smoking status and the use of opiate analgesia. The risks of PONV are 10% for no risk factors, 20% for two risk factors, 40% for three risk factors and 60% for four risk factors. The number and nature of anti-emetics administered is dependent on the risk score and physician preference.

The administration of dexamethasone on induction should also be considered for the high-risk patient.

Hyperglycaemic control

Hyperglycaemia, during and immediately following major abdominal surgery is associated with increased complication and mortality rates. This is due to insulin resistance with impaired uptake of peripheral glucose and accelerated hepatic glucose release. Therapeutic aims are to lower the blood glucose to base line levels without compromising patient safety. There is however currently no high-level evidence to support the premise that correction of hyperglycaemia leads to improved patient outcomes.

Prevention of ileus

Adherence to ERAS principles of the use of non-narcotic analgesia alongside early postoperative oral feeding and decreased preoperative fasting promote early return of GI function. Other factors such as early ambulation and fluid optimization also contribute.

Chewing gum, oral magnesium and several prokinetic agents have been suggested as GI stimulants to prevent or decrease the incidence of ileus with mixed results.

ERAS AND MAJOR HEPATIC RESECTION

Major liver resections are associated with morbidity rates approaching 25–30% and mortality rates of 1–3% when performed for malignant disease. ERAS protocols specifically designed around major liver resection first appeared in 2008, mostly adopting principles of colorectal ERAS programs, with modified intervention for organ specific issues. The majority of studies have demonstrated that patients undergoing open liver resection within ERAS programs were associated with reduced LOSs and decreased complication rates. There was earlier recovery of both synthetic liver and GI bowel function although there was no difference in mortality rates. Patient satisfaction was significantly better in the ERAS group and patient reported outcomes (PRO) should be an integral part of any ERAS program (7).

A further suggested outcome measure of ERAS based protocols following liver resection is return to intended oncological treatment (RIOT). This parameter is a ratio between the number of patients initiating oncological treatment compared to the number of patients intended to have adjuvant chemotherapy. A recent study from the USA (MD Anderson Cancer Centre) demonstrated that patients treated within ERAS protocols increased RIOT to 95% at 21 days compared to 87% at 32 days for patients undergoing standard treatment which may have an impact on patient survival. All general principles of ERAS protocols apply to patients undergoing open liver surgery but there are additional specific issues related to hepatic resection and these include:

Haemorrhage

A significant complication of major liver resection is intraoperative haemorrhage predominantly from the hepatic veins during parenchymal dissection. This may lead to hypotension, multiorgan failure and death. A low CVP less than 5 mmHg has traditionally been recommended to lower hepatic venous outflow pressure and decrease bleeding, Studies have confirmed that a low CVP (2–5 mmHg) is associated with less intraoperative blood loss and transfusion requirements. This is generally achieved usings vasodilators, fluid restrictions or patient positioning.

CVP measurements appear to be an inaccurate guide to a patient's volume status or the degree of perfusion of other organs. It also varies with underlying cardiac disease and intraoperative mechanical factors. Stroke volume variation (SVV), pulse pressure variation (PPV) and mean arterial pressure (MAP) are alternative haemodynamic parameters to CVP measurements. They appear to be more accurate in assessing volume status and underlying organ perfusion then CVP. In addition, these indices provide information on intraoperative fluid requirements and the need for vasoactive agents using an individualized algorithm-based goal directed therapeutic approach.

A SSV above 15–20% is associated with decreased blood loss and transfusion requirements during major hepatectomy. It is equivalent to that achieved by a low CVP and is associated with comparable complication rates.

Surgical issues

Evidence regarding the routine use of prophylactic abdominal drains following hepatectomy remains controversial and the larger consensus view is that it confers no major advantage and should be avoided. Unless specifically indicated, 'Mercedes Benz' incision should be avoided as it is associated with a high rate of incisional hernias.

Minimally invasive surgery

Laparoscopic major liver resection has been found to be safe and feasible if performed by experienced HPB surgeons in high-volume centres. Evidence is inconclusive but suggests improvements in operative blood loss, improved pain scores and shortened hospital LOS. R0 resection margins appear comparable to open surgery and overall conversion rates approach 15–20%.

No randomized studies comparing laparoscopic versus open techniques for major liver resections in an ERAS setting exists. One small study compared major laparoscopic liver resection under standard hospital treatment to those having open major liver resection using ERAS protocols and no differences were found. A multicentre randomized study compared open and laparoscopic left lateral sectionectomy, both groups under ERAS protocols and again there was no significant difference in outcomes.

The status of multisystem inflammatory syndrome (MIS) in major liver resection remains inconclusive, although with a trend towards favourable outcomes more clinical trials under an ERAS setting are required (8).

ERAS AND PANCREAS SURGERY

ERAS protocols specific to the pancreas first appeared over a decade ago. Most data from clinical trials, reviews and several meta-analyses largely confirm the benefits of patients having major pancreatic surgery under ERAS protocols compared with similar patients receiving standard hospital care. These improvements include decreased complication rates, faster patient recovery times with decreased LOS and hospital costs. Readmission and mortality rates appear to be similar (9).

ERAS guidelines for major pancreatic surgery follow similar guidelines to those for abdominal surgery. Pancreatic specific issues related to pancreaticoduodenectomy (PD) include preoperative biliary drainage, delayed gastric emptying, the management of perianastomotic drains and pancreatic fistulae and the role of minimally invasive surgery.

Preoperative biliary decompression

Preoperative biliary decompression and drainage remains a controversial issue in the jaundiced patient with pancreatic malignancy. Several clinical trials and multiple reviews showed no benefits post-PD and were associated with increased postoperative complications predominantly related to sepsis. There is no effect on mortality and no difference in the complication rates between the endoscopic and percutaneous transhepatic approaches and no difference in complication rates between the use of plastic or metal endoscopic stents.

Specific indications for preoperative biliary drainage include patients with cholangitis. those having neoadjuvant therapy, those patients with severe malnutrition and patients with impending organ failure.

Delayed gastric emptying (DGE)

DGE occurs in 15–35% of patients following PD and is usually secondary to intra-abdominal bleeding, sepsis or fluid collections. Apart from eliminating abdominal causes, no pharmacotherapy such as prokinetic agents or variations in surgical techniques have proven effective in the prevention or treatment of this condition.

Postoperative pancreatic fistula (POPF)

POPF is the most frequent complication following PD occurring in 15–40% of patients and is a major cause of morbidity and mortality.

The association between POPF and the placement of perianastomotic drains at operation remains controversial and a number of clinical trials have resulted in conflicting evidence. One study demonstrated that the insertion of drains increased the risk of clinically-relevant POPF. A no-drain group in other studies showed an increased incidence of POPF and morbidity and mortality rates compared with the group having drainage. Using the fistula risk score (FRS), low-risk patients have increased complications with drain insertion while medium- to severe-risk patients have a lower incidence of complications.

Because of these controversies, a selective policy of early drain removal has been proposed. Data suggest that early elevation of drain tube amylase levels to greater than 5000 U/L on day 3 are highly predictive of POPF development. Comparative studies have shown in these low-risk patients, removal of drains on day 3 compared with day 5 (late removal) is associated with a decreased incidence of POPF and other related complications and a shortened LOS. The use of somatostatin analogues has been shown to have no prophylactic or therapeutic effect on POPF.

Selective, early removal of drain tubes on day 3 based on elevated drain tube amylase is currently the preferred option.

Laparoscopic pancreaticoduodenectomy (LPD)

Uncertainty remains regarding the feasibility, safety, and overall benefits of minimally invasive surgery for PD. At present LPD should only be performed in select cases by high-volume centres with the necessary clinical and training expertise. One report cited a 3.7% increase in mortality if LPD was performed in low-volume centres compared to high-volume centres.

Two recent studies could not reach any definitive conclusion regarding complications, but reported decreased operating blood loss, prolonged operating times and decreased LOS. A recent multicentre study compared LPD and open surgery within ERAS management protocols. No beneficial effects were evident and the study was terminated because of safety concerns although studies have shown no difference in mortality, morbidity and LOS.

SUMMARY

In any unit working within ERAS protocols, or considering implementing them, a continued assessment and formal audit is important. ERAS recommended protocols in liver and pancreatic surgery have demonstrated that there are substantial advantages, compared with standard hospital treatment. These include, decreased complication rates, shortened patient recovery times and hospital LOSs. Mortality rates appeared unchanged between the two groups. Monitoring of patient outcomes and compliance is an essential component in an ERAS protocol-based program.

REFERENCES

1. Kehlet H. Multimodal approach to control postoperative pathophysiology and rehabilitation. *Br J Anaesth* 1997;**78(5)**:606–17. doi: 10.1093/bja/78.5.606. PMID: 9175983.
2. Li C, Cheng Y, Li Z, Margaryan D, Perka C, Trampuz A. The pertinent literature of Enhanced Recovery After Surgery programs: A bibliometric approach. *Medicina* 2021;**57(2)**:172.
3. Hajibandeh S, Hajibandeh S, Bill V, Satyadas T. Meta-analysis of Enhanced Recovery After Surgery (ERAS®) protocols in emergency abdominal surgery. *World J Surg* 2020;**44**:1336–48.
4. Visioni A, Shah R, Gabriel E, Attwood K, Kukar M, Nurkin S. Enhanced Recovery After Surgery for noncolorectal surgery? A systematic review and meta-analysis of major abdominal surgery. *Annals Surg* 2018;**267(1)**:57–65.
5. Elhassan A, Elhassan I, Elhassan A, Sekar KD, Rubin RE, Urman RD, et al. Essential elements for Enhanced Recovery After intra-abdominal Surgery. *Curr Pain Headache Rep* 2019;**23**:1–4.
6. Tang JZJ, Weinberg L. A literature review of intrathecal morphine analgesia in patients undergoing major open hepato-pancreatic-biliary (HPB) surgery. *Anesth Pain Med* 2019;**9(6)**:e94441.
7. Melloul E, Hübner M, Scott M, Snowden C, Prentis J, Dejong CHC, et al. Guidelines for perioperative care for liver surgery: Enhanced Recovery After Surgery (ERAS®) Society recommendations. *World J Surg* 2016;**40**:2425–40.
8. HA Lillemoe, Aloia TA. Enhanced Recovery After Surgery: Hepatobiliary. *Surg Clin North Am* 2018;**98(6)**:1251–64.
9. Melloul E, Lassen K, Roulin D, Grass F, Perinel J, Adham M, et al. Guidelines for perioperative care for pancreatoduodenectomy: Enhanced Recovery After Surgery (ERAS®) recommendations. *World J Surg* 2020;**44**:2056–84.

Bailey & Love's Essential Operations Bailey & Love's Essential Operatio
Bailey & Love's Essential Operatic
Bailey & Love's Essential Operations Bailey & Love's Essential Operatio

SECTION 1 | BASIC PRINCIPLES

Chapter

8

Principles of Laparoscopic Surgery

Jenifer Barrie

INTRODUCTION

Physicians have always aimed to achieve the maximum benefit for their patients while causing the least harm. This is the basis for the Hippocratic oath where clinicians promised that they would 'first, do no harm' (or '*primum non nicer*' the Latin translation from the Ancient Greek). In situations where it is not possible to do no harm because access to a body cavity is required, then the corollary is to reduce the insult as far as possible. For hundreds of years, it has been realized that it should be possible to directly examine orifices and cavities minimally invasively.

Endoscopy is derived from the Ancient Greek '*endo*' and '*skopein*' meaning 'to view the inner spaces of the human body' suggesting that the concept was considered over 2000 years ago. Although the development of techniques to examine patients using illuminated hollow tubes is not well documented, it is known that Hippocrates (460–375 BCE) performed the first recorded proctoscopy in 370 BCE and examples of rectal specula were found in the ruins of Pompeii, Italy. The earliest gastrointestinal 'endoscopes' were hollow reeds or bamboo canes illuminated by candles and are believed to have been used by both the Egyptians and Ancient Greeks. Major technical advances were required to facilitate the modern era of laparoscopic surgery, but early advances and the advocates who utilized them met with considerable resistance.

Fortunately, early advocates and particularly Kurt Karl Stephan Semm were so convinced of the benefits of this new minimally invasive approach that they persisted, and within a remarkably short period of time laparoscopic surgery became the default approach for a rapidly expanding number of gynaecological, general surgical, urological and thoracic procedures.

The aim of this chapter is to describe the main principles of laparoscopic surgery, including the set-up, equipment used and their advantages and limitations.

THE EARLY HISTORY OF MINIMALLY INVASIVE AND LAPAROSCOPIC SURGERY

On 13th September 1980, Semm performed the first laparoscopic appendicectomy at the University of Kiel. Semm was a gynaecologist and trained toolmaker and the combination of skills enabled him to radically alter traditional surgical approaches. His demonstration unfortunately was not well received and he was universally condemned. The hostility from the medical profession was widespread and he was unable to get his work published until 1983. Following the appendicectomy, Semm was summoned from the operating theatre and in the words of his colleague Liselotte Mettler in her book (herself an internationally renowned gynaecologist) 'had to undergo a computed tomography (CT) investigation of his skull to prove that he was in good health'. Subsequently, in 1981, the President of the German Surgical Society wrote to the Board of Directors of the German Gynaecological Society suggesting that they revoke Semm's medical license and suspend him from medical practice for the offence of trying to show surgeons how to perform an appendicectomy.

Although the first record of a mirror being used to reflect light into an internal organ is credited to Albucasis (936–1013 CE), an Arabian physician, who used the device to inspect a cervix, modern laparoscopic surgery developed due to advances pioneered from the 16th century onwards summarized in *Table 8.1*.

THE MODERN ERA OF LAPAROSCOPIC HEPATOBILIARY AND PANCREATIC SURGERY

The first laparoscopic cholecystectomy heralded the beginning of a new era of laparoscopic abdominal surgery (1) and in the 40 years which followed the indications for the treatment of both benign and malignant conditions has expanded. Laparoscopic hepato-pancreatico-biliary (HPB) surgery is no longer restricted to cholecystectomy and diagnostic procedures. Complex benign pathologies and malignant disease are now routinely treated minimally invasively. The enthusiasm for these minimally invasive liver and pancreatic surgery procedures has grown exponentially worldwide since the 1990s and there is no doubt that this trend will continue. A number of technical advances facilitated the application of minimally invasive surgery (MIS) to more advanced HPB procedures (*Table 8.2*).

DOI: 10.1201/9781003080060-8

Table 8.1 The early history and development of modern laparoscopic techniques

~980 BCE	The first record of a mirror being used to reflect light into an internal organ is credited to Albucasis (936–1013), an Arabian physician who used the device to inspect a cervix.
1585	Tulio Caesare Aranzi focused light through a flask of water and documented the first examination of the nasal cavity. Giulio Cesare Aranzio (1530–1589) brought light to endoscopy in the true sense of the word when he used a camera obscura in Venice to examine the inside of the nasal cavity by focusing the light beam.
1694	Thomas Corneille was the first person to use the term 'trocar' from the French '*trocart*', from '*trois*' meaning 'three' and '*carre*' meaning 'side, or face of an instrument'. The term 'trocar' was first recorded in the *Dictionnaire des Arts et des Sciences*.
1806	Philipp Bozzini developed the 'Lichtleiter' (light conductor), for inspecting the ear, urethra, rectum, female bladder, cervix, mouth, nasal cavity or wounds. It used an aluminium tube with incorporated mirrors illuminated by a wax candle.
1853	Antoine Jean Desormeaux, a French surgeon, first introduced the 'Lichtleiter' of Bozzini to a patient. Desormeaux is considered the 'Father of Endoscopy'.
1869	Commander DC Pantaleoni of Ireland performed the first diagnostic and therapeutic hysteroscopy using a modified cystoscope to cauterize a haemorrhagic uterine tumour.
1877	Maximilian Nitze, the Berlin urologist, developed the first optical endoscope with an integrated light source with the help of the Viennese instrument maker, Josef Leiter. Nitze used this first illuminated cystoscope on a cadaver for the first time in October 1877 and successfully on a living patient a few months later.
1901	The German surgeon Georg Kelling performed the first experimental laparoscopy in Berlin using a cystoscope to examine the peritoneal cavity of a dog after air insufflation. Kelling proposed a high-pressure insufflation of the abdominal cavity which he called the 'Luft-tamponade'.
1910	Hans Christian Jacobaeus, a professor at the Karolinska Institutet in Stockholm, published a discussion of the inspection of the peritoneal, pleural and pericardial cavity.
1911	Bertram M Bernheim, from Johns Hopkins Hospital, introduced laparoscopic surgery to the United States. He named the procedure of minimal access surgery 'organoscopy' and he used a half-inch proctoscope with natural light for illumination.
1929	Kalk, a German physician, introduced the forward oblique 135°-view lens systems. He advocated the use of a separate puncture site for pneumoperitoneum. Goetze of Germany first developed a needle for insufflations.
1934	John C Ruddock, an American surgeon described laparoscopy as 'A good diagnostic method, many times, superior than laparotomy'. John C. Ruddock used the instrument for diagnostic laparoscopy which used forceps with electro-coagulation capacity.
1938	Jànos Veress worked at the St. Gellèrt Hotel in Budapest, Hungary and developed a specially designed spring-loaded needle for the induction of a pneumothorax not a pneumoperitoneum.
1944	Raoul Palmer, of Paris, performed gynaecological examinations using laparoscopy placing the patients in the Trendelenberg position (named after German surgeon Friedrich Trendelenburg), so air could fill the pelvis.
1952	Fourestier, Gladu, and Vulmière provided the first description of a *fiberoptic bronchoscope* that transmitted intense, but cool, light.
1960	Kurt Semm, a German gynaecologist invented the automatic insufflator and published his experience in 1966. Largely unrecognized in Germany but enthusiastically adopted by American physicians and instrument makers.
1960	British gynaecologist Patrick Steptoe adapted the techniques of sterilization by two puncture technique.
1961	British physicist Harold Hopkin's interest in medical endoscopy began when he had a chance encounter with Dr Hugh Gainsborough, a physician based at St George's Hospital, London. He developed an innovative rod-lens system which, although rigid, provided a fifty-fold increase in light transmission, a more panoramic, wider field of view and as a consequence a sharper, brighter image.
1963	Kurt Semm introduced an automatic insufflation device capable of monitoring intra-abdominal pressure to reduce the problems associated with over-insufflation.

(Continued)

Table 8.1 (*Continued*) The early history and development of modern laparoscopic techniques

1972	H Courtney Clarke devised a simplified technique for *laparoscopic suturing* using a knot pusher, which was rediscovered in 1992 by Harry Reich.
1978	Hasson suggested a new method of trocar placement employing a blunt mini-laparotomy to permit direct visualization of entry into the peritoneal cavity.
1980	In the United Kingdom, Patrick Steptoe started to perform laparoscopic procedures. He was the first in Britain to use laparoscopy for the routine diagnosis of gynaecological disorders, and the first in the world to use it as a standard technique for sterilization.
1980	Semm, a German gynaecologist, performed the first laparoscopic appendicectomy.
1985	The first documented laparoscopic cholecystectomy was performed by Erich Muhe in Germany in 1985.
1987	On March 17, 1987, Philippe Mouret performed the first video laparoscopic cholecystectomy, in Lyon, France. He is recognized as the pioneer of the modern laparoscopic surgery technique. He used two separate incisions in the abdomen, while other surgeons such as Palmer and Muhe only used one incision. This was a very important innovation and is often described as the 'Second French Revolution'.
1989	Reddick and Olsen reported that common bile duct (CBD) injury after laparoscopic cholecystectomy was five-times higher than with conventional cholecystectomy and the USA government announced that surgeons should be supervised for at least 15 laparoscopic cholecystectomies before being allowed to do this procedure independently.

Table 8.2 Technical advances that have facilitated the development of safe, major laparoscopic HPB surgery

Stapling devices	The first surgical stapler was invented in 1908, by Victor Fischer and Hümér Hültl. In the 1960s disposable devices were developed and in the 1990s these became available for use laparoscopically.
Gas humidification and warming	Permits longer procedures due to the prevention of hypothermia and reduced cytokine release. Improves postoperative pain.
High-definition (HD) 4K optics	Reduce surgical operating time and blood loss compared with normal HD technology and improve surgical comfort and accuracy due to more efficient movement by virtue of better depth perception. More rapid acquisition of basic MIS skills.
Laparoscopic ultrasound	First introduced by Fukuda et al. in 1981 and now very accurate and sensitive for the identification of liver lesions and CBD stones. Facilitates intraoperative planning for laparoscopic liver resection especially segmental resection when combined with indocyanine green clearance (ICG) infusion.
Hand access devices	Enabled the development of laparoscopic liver resection. Easier mobilization of the liver and control of bleeding.
Live teleconferencing capabilities	The use of telecommunication technology to provide remote guidance and assistance during surgical procedures.
Remote presence systems	Enable experienced surgeons to mentor and proctor less experienced colleagues in real-time during laparoscopic procedures. These systems often utilize HD video streaming, audio communication, and even telestration using a head mounted device.
Virtual reality (VR)	The use of proficiency-based VR training under supervision and the use of haptic feedback has proven to be an effective method for surgical training and is now incorporated into many training programmes.
3D cameras	3D-HD view confers great depth perception which makes laparoscopic surgery less tiring due to improved ability to see fine anatomical detail and the simplification of procedures such as knot tying and suturing.
Ablative techniques; radiofrequency ablation (RFA); microwave ablation (MWA)	Used in the treatment of both primary and metastatic tumours. Laparoscopic use overcomes some of the anatomical problems associated with a percutaneous approach. Can be used as a hybrid-technique together with laparoscopic liver resection. MWA provides higher intra-tumoural temperatures, a more predictable ablation zone, and is not susceptible to the 'heat sink' phenomenon.

(Continued)

Table 8.2 *(Continued)* Technical advances that have facilitated the development of safe, major laparoscopic HPB surgery

Augmented reality (AR)	Preoperative images are registered in a stationary format then superimposed on intraoperative images from the laparoscopic camera.
Advanced energy devices/hybrid energy-sealing devices	A number of energy devices are available for use during laparoscopic surgery including monopolar and bipolar electrosurgical, ultrasonic energy and hybrid vessel-sealing devices. They improve coagulation, facilitate parenchymal (liver and pancreas) transection and reduce blood loss.
Robotic surgery	The da Vinci® surgical system, was approved by the US Food and Drug Administration (FDA) in 2000 for use in urological and general surgical procedures in children and adults. It is now increasingly used to augment laparoscopic procedures and facilitate surgery in areas which are difficult to access. It improves the accuracy of anastomotic suturing (hepaticojejunostomy and pancreaticojejunostomy).
Training programmes	Simulation-based training enables trainees to develop skills in a safe, and controlled, environment and is now a compulsory component of a number of formal training programmes. A number of platforms are available ranging from basic box trainers to highly complex, virtual reality systems.
Near-infrared (NIR) fluorescence imaging with indocyanine green	Useful for the identification of liver lesions, surgical resection planning and margin evaluation, particularly in cirrhotic patients having segmental resections. A positive-method staining the tumour or negative-technique staining adjacent normal parenchyma can be used (*see* Chapters 9 and 43 for more details).
Qualifications and certification	Laparoscopic surgery is increasingly used in all specialities, and more advanced and complex procedures are becoming routine. The formal recognition of training will be essential to identify those procedures surgeons are capable of performing unsupervised. Organisations, such as the Society of American Gastrointestinal and Endoscopic Surgeons (SAGES) and the European Association for Endoscopic Surgery (EAES), have developed guidelines and certification programs to ensure that surgeons possess the necessary skills to perform laparoscopic procedures safely and effectively.

The laparoscopic approach to pancreatoduodenectomy was first described by Gagner and Pomp in 1994 (2) and demonstrated that even the most challenging HPB procedures could be performed using MIS. Internationally, laparoscopic surgery has now been extensively employed for both hepatic and pancreatic resections. Particularly for hepatic resections, indications are no longer limited to anterior tumours in segments 2, 3, 4b and 5. Virtually all the technically challenging resections, including formal right and left hepatectomies, caudate lobe resection, extended resections and associating liver partition and portal vein ligation for staged hepatectomy (ALPSS) procedures have now been successfully completed. *Table 8.3* describes the HPB procedure for which a laparoscopic approach is appropriate.

BASIC REQUIREMENTS FOR LAPAROSCOPIC SURGERY

The minimum equipment required to perform MIS is at least one high-resolution monitor, an automated insufflator to maintaining a pneumoperitoneum, an audiovisual stack, a camera and the necessary instruments (diathermy hook, graspers, scissors etc.). The surgeon may stand between the legs of the patient, in the 'French' position or on the right or left side depending on the operation being performed. Given that up to 70% of laparoscopic surgeons suffer from work-related musculoskeletal injuries (3) the set-up is important and time should be spent ensuring it is optimal, with the monitor positioned just below the surgeon's eye level to avoid strain due to prolonged neck extension (4). *Figure 8.1* demonstrates a basic set-up with the surgeon in the 'French' position and camera height at eye level.

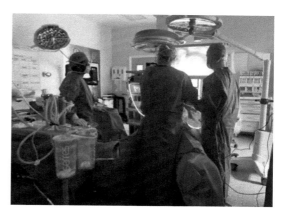

Figure 8.1 Typical set-up in the 'French' position for the performance of laparoscopic surgery.

Table 8.3 Examples of, and indications for, laparoscopic HPB surgery

Pathology	Procedure
Gallstone disease	• Laparoscopic cholecystectomy • Laparoscopic common bile duct exploration • Bile duct reconstruction following iatrogenic injury
Benign liver cysts	• Laparoscopic deroofing
Cancer staging	• Staging laparoscopy, intraoperative ultrasound +/− biopsies
Liver cancer	• Laparoscopic liver resection; major and minor
Benign pancreatic disease	• Spleen preserving distal pancreatectomy • Total pancreatectomy • Pancreatectomy and islet autotransplantation
Pancreatic cancer	• Distal pancreatectomy + splenectomy
Peri-ampullary cancer Duodenal cancer	• Whipple procedure
Choledochal cyst	• Roux-en-Y hepaticojejunostomy
Investigation of postoperative bleeding and bile leaks	• Washout, identify the source of bleeding or bile leak and address (energy device, clips)
Acute pancreatitis	• Treatment of refractory pseudocysts which have failed endoscopic treatment • Formal drainage or Roux-en-Y loop

Patient positioning

Meticulous patient positioning is essential for safe laparoscopic surgery. Major joints should be in a neutral position and any pressure points should be appropriately padded. Sliding of the patient during tilt can be prevented by air mattresses, shoulder supports and straps. During long operations it may be necessary to return to a neutral position for a break to avoid complications.

Imaging system

Imaging systems are composed of cameras, imaging consoles, light guides and a monitor(s). Standard cameras are 10 mm, but camera and lens technology allow for the use of 5 mm cameras. The camera is located at the tip of the scope with a fixed angle ranging from 0°–70°. There are two main types of laparoscopes; forward-oblique viewing laparoscope with a 30° or 45° view, or the more rarely used, flexible laparoscopes. Automatic focusing and charge-coupled devices (CCDs) are used to detect the degree of brightness and modify this for optimal image quality. Monitors are flat panel and mobile. Some recent systems include further advances such as touch screen panels and voice-activated systems.

Production of a pneumoperitoneum

The creation of a pneumoperitoneum can be achieved using an open or closed method. The closed method involves either puncture of the peritoneum using a Veress needle or entry to the peritoneum with a Visiport™. Optical port insertion in the left upper quadrant (with or without prior Veress needle pneumoperitoneum) may be safer for patients with a previous midline laparotomy or obesity (5). These methods are efficient and considered relatively safe. Morbid obesity may make pneumoperitoneum more challenging and standard instruments may be too short. Paradoxically, access may also prove more difficult in very thin patients, where increasing care needs to be taken to avoid visceral and vascular injuries, especially where there is a concomitant severe kyphosis. As a general rule, the lowest possible intra-abdominal pressure (IAP) should be maintained, and an IAP >15 mmHg is very rarely necessary (5).

INSTRUMENTATION AND BASIC TECHNIQUES

The standard laparoscopic instruments for tissue manipulation such as Maryland forceps, fenestrated graspers and diathermy hook will be familiar to hepatobiliary surgeons performing laparoscopic surgery. More advanced retractors such as fan retractors and articulated liver retractors have been developed to facilitate more complex procedures, many of them specifically tailored for use during laparoscopic liver resections. Technological progress continues as indications for surgery expand, and increasingly specialized devices such as laparoscopic intraoperative ultrasound, indocynanine green fluorescence and liver transection methods are discussed in **Chapters 9,14** and **43**.

Haemostasis

Laparoscopic vessel-sealing devices have greatly enhanced surgical capabilities in HPB surgery. There are two categories of devices, advanced bipolar and ultrasonic instruments which both efficiently seal vessels (≤7 mm and ≤5 mm in diameter, respectively, *see* **Chapter 10**), and the majority have a built-in tissue transection function (6). Conventional monopolar electrosurgery remains a popular laparoscopic modality because of its low cost, general availability, and diverse range of available tissue effects. Potential disadvantages include the need for a dispersive electrode, relatively high-power settings, and the inability to seal vessels larger than 1–2 mm diameter (6).

Haemostatic agents including surgical sealants, haemostatic clips and fibrin glue may be employed to control small bleeding vessels or bleeding from a raw surface during laparoscopic hepatobiliary surgery. These agents are useful particularly in areas where sutures or staplers are not feasible.

If there is a bleeding vessel which can be identified, a fine-tip grasper such as a Maryland, should be used to occlude it and then electrocautery, or a metal or locking plastic clip, applied depending on vessel size. When it isn't possible to identify an individual vessel and there is pooling of blood, compression should be immediately applied with a swab using a blunt instrument. Good suction irrigation is imperative. Once the area has been suctioned and cleared of clot and excess blood, pressure can be released gradually to pinpoint the source of the bleeding. Exposure and technical advantages can be improved by insertion of an extra port.

Due to the risks of major haemorrhage in advanced laparoscopic HPB surgery, and specifically liver resection, a laparoscopic vascular clamp should be available (7). With laparoscopic liver surgery, it is generally accepted today that the main factors contributing to reduced intraoperative blood loss are the positive pressure pneumoperitoneum, the development of new transection devices and the ability to achieve inflow and outflow control (8). In respect of the Pringle manoeuvre, Decailliot et al. (9) demonstrated in a nonrandomized comparative study that the use of the Pringle manoeuvre during laparoscopic liver resection reduces blood loss as effectively as it does during open surgery. Technically, this can be achieved using an intracorporeal or extracorporeal technique. Once the hepatoduodenal ligament has been exposed, the pars flaccida of the gastrohepatic ligament is opened. An umbilical tape is placed around the hepatoduodenal ligament with a laparoscopic dissector and then safely passed (from left or right depending on port placement) through

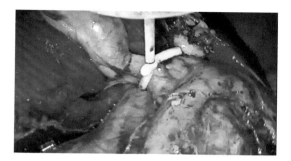

Figure 8.2 Intracorporeal inflow control using a Foley catheter.

the epiploic foramen behind the hepatoduodenal ligament. The umbilical tape is pulled to the halfway point with two laparoscopic graspers and both ends are exteriorized through the closest 5 mm port. The ends of the umbilical tape are threaded through a flexible plastic tourniquet that allows the internal end to remain intraperitoneally applied to the pedicle and the external end to remain outside of the patient, where it can be pushed into position and clamped (10). Alternative intracorporeal methods using a Foley catheter have also been described and *Figure 8.2* demonstrates the placement and use of this technique. Pro-coagulation of the liver is not a dissection or transection tool but rather an instrument that can be employed prior to the use of a transection device in order to decrease bleeding (8). This technique is not employed in many centres due to the incidence of bile duct injuries and strictures.

Laparoscopic suturing

Laparoscopic suturing, although cumbersome during the initial learning phase, is an essential technique to master, particularly for advanced laparoscopic HPB surgery. Selection of the correct needle size, length of the suture, suture material and proper handling of the needle at various angles are vital considerations for safe laparoscopic suturing. Certain practical considerations should be borne in mind, for example, a curved needle will not go through a 5 mm port whereas a ski-shaped needle will and curved needles can be lost intra-abdominally in an attempt to retrieve them through a 5 mm port. Visualizing the needle being retrieved is essential (5).

Stapling devices

Minimally invasive, linear-cutting, stapling devices apply two double-staggered or triple-staggered staple rows depending on the manufacture. These devices feature articulating joints for improved utility within a limited operating space and compression mechanisms to squeeze-out tissue oedema. Manual and powered stapling devices are available. A 'vascular' load, intended to be haemostatic, is available for these devices. There are a range of devices on the market and surgeons need to be familiar with the type of stapler they are using and have good working knowledge of different types of cartridges.

ADVANTAGES OF LAPAROSCOPIC RESECTION

It is well-recognized that laparoscopic surgery has the advantage of reducing tissue trauma and the risk of adhesion formation (11–13). Laparoscopic surgery results in a smaller scar which improves recovery time, shortens hospital stay and improves cosmesis (14). Most studies comparing laparoscopic surgery to the open approach have demonstrated reduced blood loss and postoperative pain, a shorter length of hospital stay, improved patient satisfaction and enhanced cost-effectiveness (15).

Advances in digital recording equipment allows surgeons to access the recorded laparoscopic procedure in full, which is valuable for training and to improve surgical technique. Video live streaming to any authorized remote viewer is now also facilitating remote mentoring and supervision, which is not possible with open surgery.

DISADVANTAGES OF LAPAROSCOPIC SURGERY

The advantages of laparoscopic surgery in terms of decreased rate of postoperative complications is well established (16). Nevertheless, there are technical, and surgeon-associated issues which are related to the use of a laparoscopic approach.

Technical drawbacks

Despite more advanced optical systems, visual limitations still hamper more difficult resections. Increased operative time and reduced economy of movement results when there are problems with any component of the imaging system resulting in a poor view. Issues occur with the camera view when there is fogging of the system which is a frequent problem in laparoscopy, particularly at the beginning of the procedure due to the temperature difference between cold scope and warm peritoneal cavity. This is avoided by pre-warming the camera with warm water, liquid scope warmer or an anti-fog solution. Intraoperative bleeding is problematic for the field of view as blood is very efficient at absorbing light and may significantly affect the quality of the image. This can lead to blind spots or an obscured view, making it challenging to ensure complete tumour removal, especially when they are located in deep-seated or complex anatomical regions. Reduced depth perception may influence decision-making and procedural

nuances, particularly in liver surgery. For example, the confined space in laparoscopic procedures can limit the movement of instruments, particularly when dealing with larger tumours. This can restrict the surgeon's ability to achieve optimal angles which is most apparent during difficult major liver resections where the liver parenchyma is stiff and fibrotic or friable and fragile following chemotherapy. In difficult cases these issues may require instruments to be repositioned frequently to gain adequate access, potentially prolonging the procedure due to the reduced economy of movement.

Unlike open surgery, laparoscopic procedures lack direct tactile feedback and surgeons must rely on visual cues and instruments to gauge tissue consistency and depth, which in some situations will be compromised due to altered depth perception. This lack of tactile feedback and altered depth perception can make it challenging to accurately gauge the pressure exerted on tissues, potentially leading to inadvertent tissue injury or incomplete resections. This is an area which has been extensively studied and presently the evidence from the literature regarding the importance of haptic feedback during laparoscopic surgery is unclear and contradictory (17–19). The most recent comprehensive systematic review on the role of haptic feedback in standard laparoscopic surgery, robot-assisted surgery, and virtual reality training concluded that, in the current literature, there is no clear consensus regarding the importance of haptic feedback in MIS (20). Hand-assisted laparoscopic surgery has been practiced since the development of major laparoscopic HPB surgery initially to aid mobilization and control any sudden significant bleeding. It involves the intra-abdominal placement of a hand or forearm through a mini-laparotomy incision whilst maintaining pneumoperitoneum and it allows for surgeons to examine tissue and potential pathologies as they would during open surgery.

The use of specialized instruments can also make the surgeon reliant on their consistent performance. The majority of minimally invasive surgeons have experienced laparoscopic linear stapler malfunction and 25% have had to significantly alter the planned operative procedure due to the malfunction (21). Strategies to mitigate against equipment failure are more challenging but necessary in a laparoscopic case. A number of reports have suggested that a hybrid approach is more economical than a totally laparoscopic approach, reducing the number of laparoscopic ports and instruments required. Some advocates of the technique claim that it is also easier to learn and perform than a totally laparoscopic approach.

Surgeon factors

Laparoscopic surgery results in a higher proportion of musculoskeletal complaints among surgeons compared with open or robotic surgery. This is one of the main purported advantages of robotic surgery and console operating. The learning curve associated with laparoscopic surgery demands dedicated training, potentially affecting the procedural duration and outcomes during the initial phases of adoption. There is heterogeneity in published learning curve data for each procedure, but using laparoscopic liver surgery as an example, the published cut-off for minor laparoscopic liver resection is defined as around 60 cases, with 15 cases for left lateral sectionectomy, and 60 minor livers needed before moving to major liver resection (22). Strategies to shorten learning curves, such as structured training and mentorship and simulation training have been proposed, but in order to gain experience in such cases, high volumes and long training durations will be required.

GENERAL COMPLICATIONS OF LAPAROSCOPIC SURGERY

The most routinely reported symptoms, in patients, after laparoscopic procedures are upper abdominal pain, nausea and referred shoulder pain from diaphragmatic irritation. A number of methods have been developed to reduce postoperative pain and improve recovery including local anaesthetic infiltration, which although used almost ubiquitously, has surprisingly not been convincingly proven to be effective (23). Shoulder-tip pain is usually maximal 24 hours after the operation, settles within 2–3 days and is relieved by simple analgesia.

In some cases a laparoscopic approach may involve longer operating times and the pneumoperitoneum may provoke cardiac arrhythmias. It has been demonstrated that increased intra-abdominal pressure, particularly when prolonged, produces changes in the cardiovascular and pulmonary dynamic which may be poorly tolerated when cardiopulmonary reserve is poor (24).

Most electrosurgical injuries which occur during laparoscopy follow the use of monopolar diathermy and are potentially serious. The overall incidence is 1–2 cases per 1000 operations but unfortunately, they are frequently unrecognized. Patients commonly present 3–7 days later with abdominal pain and pyrexia. Due to the delay, the reasons for their occurrence are largely speculative. Potential mechanisms of electrosurgical trauma include direct application of the electrosurgical probe from mistaken targeting or unintended activation; stray current arising from defective insulation; direct coupling when the active electrode is accidentally activated or in close proximity to another metal instrument and capacitive coupling, when the electric current is transferred from one conductor (the active electrode), through intact insulation, into adjacent conductive materials such as the bowel without the need for direct contact. Finally, alterative burn sites, usually the

Table 8.4 Reported causes of iatrogenic visceral injury at laparoscopy in a review of 273 instances (26).

Instrument	Number of injuries n (%)
Trocar or Veress needle	114 (41.8%)
Coagulator or laser	70 (25.6%)
Grasping forceps	3 (1.1%)
Scissors	2 (0.7%)
Other	84 (30.8%)

skin, can occur if the return electrode contact is poor due to placement or fluid leakage onto the plate preventing safe dispersal of the current over an adequate surface area. Under these circumstances, the exiting current may have a high enough density to produce an unintended burn (25).

Even with surgical experience, iatrogenic injuries do occur. In 2004, van der Voort et al. (26) conducted a comprehensive, systematic review of laparoscopy induced bowel injury. The incidence of laparoscopy-induced GI injury was 0.13% (430 of 329 935) and of bowel perforation 0.22% (66 of 29 532). The most frequently injured organ was the small intestine (55.8%) followed by the large intestine (38.6%) (26). The causes of injury are shown in *Table 8.4*.

The factors that contribute to these errors include surgeon technical error (due to inexperience, fatigue or inadequate view) and complex pathology resulting in inflamed tissue or obliteration of normal tissue planes, making the operation more technically difficult. Often it is difficult to attribute these injuries to one single factor, and it is often a combination of surgeon error and complex pathology (27).

It is important to stress that conversion due to complications that cannot be managed laparoscopically, pathology that requires an open approach, or uncontrolled bleeding, are not complications of laparoscopic surgery but sensible and safe decisions made by a competent surgeon.

SUMMARY

The emergence of laparoscopy brought about a fundamental change in the way surgical procedures were performed. Despite the technique now being over 100 years old significant technological progress was required to facilitate the dramatic expansion of its use since the end of the 20th century. This period witnessed the evolution of laparoscopy from an essentially diagnostic technique into an exciting new discipline which was appropriate for a rapidly expanding range of indications.

It is salutary to remember that laparoscopy was initially shunned, and its protagonists treated like pariahs for bringing the medical profession into disrepute. Due to the perseverance of a small number of dedicated enthusiasts, there has fortunately been a rapid change of heart and a widespread adoption of the new techniques. Today, benign and malignant pathologies can be safely treated, and major resections are becoming routine. Future developments will see the expansion of robot-assisted laparoscopic surgery, the inclusion of artificial intelligence (AI) systems and augmented reality. Improvements in training methods will be possible due to advances in simulators and virtual reality.

REFERENCES

1. Litwin D, Girotti M, Poulin E, Mamazza J, Nagy A. Laparoscopic cholecystectomy: Trans-Canada experience with 2201 cases. *Can J Surg* 1992;**35(3)**:291–6.
2. Gagner M, Pomp A. Laparoscopic pylorus-preserving pancreatoduodenectomy. *Surg Endosc* 1994;**8**:408–10.
3. Stomberg MW, Tronstad S-E, Hedberg K, Bengtsson J, Jonsson P, Johansen L, et al. Work-related musculoskeletal disorders when performing laparoscopic surgery. *Surg Laparosc Endos Percutan Tech* 2010;**20(1)**:49–53.
4. Seghers J, Jochem A, Spaepen A. Posture, muscle activity and muscle fatigue in prolonged VDT work at different screen height settings. *Ergonomics* 2003;**46(7)**:714–30.
5. Madhok B, Nanayakkara K, Mahawar K. Safety considerations in laparoscopic surgery: A narrative review. *World J Gastrointest Endosc* 2022;**14(1)**:1–16.
6. Lyons SD, Law KS. Laparoscopic vessel sealing technologies. *J Minim Invasive Gynecol* 2013;**20(3)**:301–7.
7. Ogiso S, Araki K, Gayet B, Conrad C. Optimal operating room set-up and equipment used in laparoscopic hepatopancreatobiliary surgery. In: Conrad C, Gayet B (eds). *Laparoscopic Liver, Pancreas, and Biliary Surgery*, Wiley, 2016, chapter 3, pp. 28–46.
8. Tranchart H, O'Rourke N, Van Dam R, Gaillard M, Lainas P, Sugioka A, et al. Bleeding control during laparoscopic liver resection: A review of literature. *J Hepatobiliary Pancreat Sci* 2015;**22(5)**:371–8.
9. Decailliot F, Streich B, Heurtematte Y, Duvaldestin P, Cherqui D, Stéphan F. An echocardiography prospective study of hemodynamic effects of portal triad clamping with and without pneumoperitoneum. *Anesth Analg* 2005;**100**:617–22.
10. Dua MM, Worhunsky DJ, Hwa K, Poultsides GA, Norton JA, Visser BC. Extracorporeal Pringle for laparoscopic liver resection. *Surg Endosc* 2015;**29**:1348–55.
11. Burns E, Currie A, Bottle A, Aylin P, Darzi A, Faiz O. Minimal-access colorectal surgery is associated with fewer adhesion-related admissions than open surgery. *Br J Surg* 2013;**100(1)**:152–9.
12. Yamada T, Okabayashi K, Hasegawa H, Tsuruta M, Yoo J, Seishima R, et al. Meta-analysis of the risk of small bowel obstruction following open or laparoscopic colorectal surgery. *Br J Surg* 2016;**103(5)**:493–503.
13. Aquina CT, Probst CP, Becerra AZ, Iannuzzi JC, Hensley BJ, Noyes K, et al. Missed opportunity: Laparoscopic colorectal resection is associated with lower incidence of small bowel obstruction compared to an open approach. *Ann Surg* 2016;**264(1)**:127–34.
14. Wang C-L, Qu G, Xu H-W. The short-and long-term outcomes of laparoscopic versus open surgery for colorectal cancer: A meta-analysis. *Int J Colorectal Dis* 2014;**29**:309–20.
15. Vanounou T, Steel JL, Nguyen KT, Tsung A, Marsh JW, Geller DA, et al. Comparing the clinical and economic impact of laparoscopic versus open liver resection. *Ann Surg Oncol* 2010;**17**:998–1009.
16. Kennedy GD, Heise C, Rajamanickam V, Harms B, Foley EF. Laparoscopy decreases postoperative complication rates after abdominal colectomy: Results from the National Surgical Quality Improvement Program. *Ann Surg* 2009;**249(4)**:596–601.
17. Morris D, Tan H, Barbagli F, Chang T, Salisbury K. Haptic feedback enhances force skill learning. *Second Joint EuroHaptics Conference and Symposium on Haptic Interfaces for Virtual Environment and Teleoperator Systems* (WHC'07); 2007: IEEE.
18. Panait L, Akkary E, Bell RL, Roberts KE, Dudrick SJ, Duffy AJ. The role of haptic feedback in laparoscopic simulation training. *J Surg Res* 2009;**156(2)**:312–16.
19. Reiley CE, Akinbiyi T, Burschka D, Chang DC, Okamura AM, Yuh DD. Effects of visual force feedback on robot-assisted surgical task performance. *J Thorac Cardiovasc Surg* 2008;**135(1)**:196–202.
20. Van der Meijden OA, Schijven MP. The value of haptic feedback in conventional and robot-assisted minimal invasive surgery and virtual reality training: A current review. *Surg Endosc* 2009;**23**:1180–90.
21. Kwazneski D, Six C, Stahlfeld K. The unacknowledged incidence of laparoscopic stapler malfunction. *Surg Endosc* 2013;**27**:86–9.
22. Guilbaud T, Birnbaum DJ, Berdah S, Farges O, Beyer Berjot L. Learning curve in laparoscopic liver resection, educational value of simulation and training programmes: A systematic review. *World J Surg* 2019;**43**:2710–19.
23. Suragul W, Tantawanit A, Rungsakulkij N, Muangkaew P, Tangtawee P, Mingphrudhi S, et al. Effect of local anaesthetic infiltration on postoperative pain after laparoscopic cholecystectomy: Randomized clinical trial. *BJS Open* 2022;**6(3)**:zrac066.
24. Ortenzi M, Montori G, Sartori A, Balla A, Botteri E, Piatto G, et al. Low-pressure versus standard-pressure pneumoperitoneum in laparoscopic cholecystectomy: A systematic review and meta-analysis of randomized controlled trials. *Surg Endosc* 2022;**36(10)**:7092–113.
25. Huang H-Y, Yen C-F, Wu M-P. Complications of electrosurgery in laparoscopy. *Gynecol Minim Invasive Ther* 2014;**3(2)**:39–42.
26. Van der Voort M, Heijnsdijk E, Gouma D. Bowel injury as a complication of laparoscopy. *J Br Surg* 2004;**91(10)**:1253–8.
27. Barrie J. Next generation of atraumatic laparoscopic instruments through analysis of the instrument-tissue interface. PhD thesis. University of Leeds; 2017.

Chapter 9

Principles of Robotic Surgery

Jian Zhou, Xiao-Ying Wang and Kai Zhu

INTRODUCTION

This chapter gives a general introduction to the application of robotic surgical systems in hepatobiliary and pancreatic (HPB) operations. Robotic surgery is minimally invasive surgery (MIS) performed with the help of a surgical robot. Instead of the surgeon directly holding the surgical instruments, surgery is done by the surgeon through a console. This has a joystick that controls the robot arm which holds specially designed surgical instruments (*Figure 9.1*).

HISTORY OF ROBOTIC SURGERY IN HPB OPERATIONS

Robotic surgery has been performed for over 30 years. The first documented operation performed with robotic assistance was in 1985, when a brain biopsy was performed using the PUMA surgical robot (Westinghouse Electric, Pittsburgh, USA). Since then, robotic surgery has evolved in leaps and bounds, leading to the first robotic cholecystectomy in 1987 (1). In 2000, the US Food and Drug Administration (FDA) approved

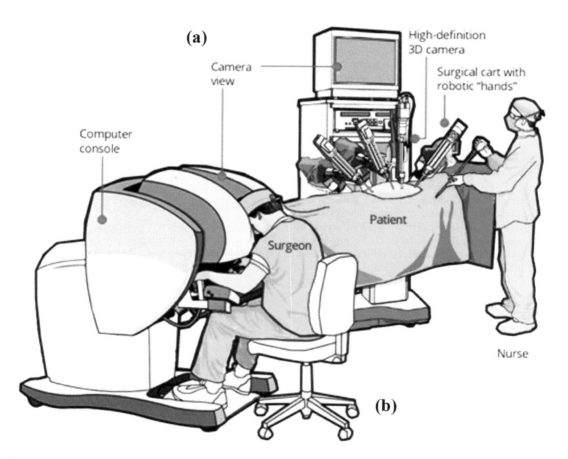

(a)

High-definition 3D camera

Camera view

Surgical cart with robotic "hands"

Computer console

Patient

Surgeon

Nurse

(b)

Figure 9.1 Diagrammatic representation of the setup in a robotic theatre (a) and (b) the surgeon is at a console using joysticks to control the robotic arms.

DOI: 10.1201/9781003080060-9

the da Vinci® surgical system as the first surgical robotic system for general laparoscopic surgery. Since then, robotic surgery has emerged as one of the most promising surgical advances. Currently, almost all surgical specialties have performed, or are performing, some level of robotic surgery, with urology leading the way (2). However, despite its worldwide acceptance in many different surgical specialties, the use of robotic assistance in the field of HBP surgery remains relatively low. This is almost certainly due to the complexity of the procedures performed and the difficult location and access to the liver, biliary tract and pancreas.

In 2002, Giulianotti et al. (3) reported the first robotic-assisted hepatectomy. Subsequently the United States, Europe and China have reported their own experiences with robotic hepatectomy. The initial experience and the potential applications in HPB surgery, together with the incumbent challenges, stimulated HPB surgeons around the world to look for ways to expand the applications in their fields. The earliest cases of robotic hepatectomy were understandably and sensibly confined to relatively straightforward procedures such as local excisions and wedge hepatectomy for lesions situated antero-inferiorly (segments 2, 3, 4b, 5 and 6). With increasing experience and confidence, hemihepatectomy and extended hemihepatectomy procedures were gradually performed. As the technique has matured, some surgeons also utilized robotic systems to perform segmental resection of posterosuperior segments, and the associating liver partition with portal vein ligation for staged hepatectomy (ALPPS) (4–6).

Advances in robotic liver surgery have also driven progress towards minimally invasive living-donor transplantation. In 2011, Giulianotti et al. (7) performed the world's first living-donor hepatectomy of the right lobe using the da Vinci robot. In 2014, Fan and Zhou from Zhongshan Hospital of Fudan University performed the first da Vinci robot-assisted adult-child liver transplant in Asia (8). In 2021, Kyung-Suk Suh et al. (9) developed a safe and reproducible method for total robotic living-donor liver transplantation, which consists of an explant hepatectomy and implantation of the graft. Although robotic living-donor hepatectomy is technically safe and feasible, it does not confer significant benefits in terms of postoperative morbidity compared to open and conventional laparoscopic approaches (10). Such procedures should only be performed by experienced surgeons, and the benefits of robotic donor hepatectomy need further investigation and research.

With advances in laparoscopic technology, laparoscopic biliary operations such as cholecystectomy, choledochotomy and congenital choledochal cyst removal have been performed routinely in a large number of centers around the world. However, for surgery of malignant biliary tract pathologies, such as gallbladder cancer and perihilar cholangiocarcinomas (Klatskin

tumours), due to the complexity of the surgical procedure, which involves lymph node dissection in the hilar region often combined with liver resection, and in some cases biliary reconstruction, these procedures are difficult to perform laparoscopically. The advent of robotic surgical systems with the ability to manoeuvre in confined spaces and EndoWrist instruments heralded the dawn of minimally invasive biliary surgery. There are now numerous reports in the literature describing robotic biliary surgery including choledochotomy for stone extraction, congenital choledochal cyst excision, gallbladder cancer, perihilar cholangiocarcinoma, extrahepatic bile duct cancer and other miscellaneous biliary procedures.

Since the first report of robotic distal pancreatectomy (RDP) in 2001 (3), pancreaticoduodenectomy, central pancreatectomy, total pancreatectomy, and pancreas tumour enucleation have been performed using robotic systems (11). There is clearly a range of pancreatic procedures which can be safely performed using these systems and oncological results appear to be broadly equivalent. Nevertheless, for the more complex operations such as pancreaticoduodenectomy there remain concerns about the attendant morbidity which appears to be high when these procedures are performed using an open approach. These concerns, together with the inevitable costs and the relatively long learning curve, may inhibit the widespread uptake and acceptance of robotic systems for pancreatic surgery for the foreseeable future despite an increasing number of centres reporting their experience.

ADVANTAGES AND DISADVANTAGES OF ROBOTIC SURGERY

Advantages

Robot-assisted laparoscopic surgical systems possess a number of clear advantages. The maneuverability of the multifunctional manipulators addresses the technical limitations inherent in the use of the traditional rigid instrument with conventional minimally invasive techniques (*Figure 9.2*).

The robot can filter physiological tremors, increase ergonomics, and offer a clear, stable, magnified, and unmatched 3D-view of the surgical field (12). Robotic arms allow an increased range of movement and robotic instruments offer extended freedom compared to laparoscopic instruments. As the surgeon remotely controls the operation from a console, has 3D-endoscopic sight, restored hand-eye coordination and with more recent systems force feedback, comfort is significantly improved and the common occupational problems suffered by the vast majority of surgeons (neck and shoulder ailments) may be abrogated. As a consequence the learning curve is shorter than for conventional laparoscopic surgery.

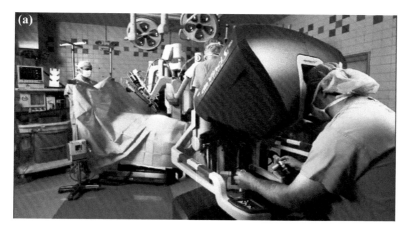

(b)

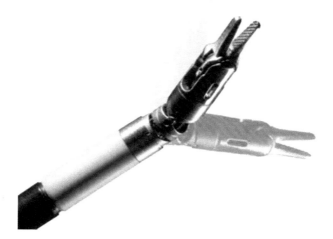

Figure 9.2 The range of movement of the most recent robotic instruments addresses the technical limitation with laparoscopic surgery and the early robotic systems.

For HBP surgery, there are certain specific advantages for robotic systems. Major HPB procedures are generally long and many HBP surgeons find laparoscopic HPB operations physically challenging (for both the surgeon and assistant). With robotic-assisted operations, the surgeon is seated while working at the console, the camera is held by the robot and even a very lengthy robotic procedure can be completed in comfort, in a pleasant environment with breaks if necessary and without surgeon or assistant fatigue. HPB surgery requires meticulous attention to detail particularly in respect of haemostasis, suturing, bile duct and digestive tract reconstruction, and access to some tumours is difficult, for example, the posterosuperior segments of the liver (segments 7 and 8) (13). Robotic surgery facilitates very delicate and intricate movement and can filter hand tremors which makes suturing more precise.

These are generally more effective in controlling bleeding, and make reconstruction of the biliary and digestive tracts much simpler when compared to laparoscopic surgery. In addition, the view obtained with the imaging systems is state of the art and particularly valuable when accessing difficult-to-reach tumours (14).

Disadvantages

The cost of robotic surgery is high, not only due to the initial cost of purchasing the system but also the annual servicing costs, expense of the instruments which are specifically designed for a single platform and finally the construction of special operating theatres. Also, in the early phase of implementation, the use of precious theatre time and consequent loss of productivity add to the cost. The longer operating times when using robotic systems persist even beyond the learning curve compared with laparoscopic, or open, approaches. Proponents argue that these can be offset if intensive care and hospital stays can be reduced.

With early systems there was no tactile feedback while operating through the consul which meant that excess force could be applied inadvertently. As a consequence, force feedback systems have been introduced on newer models. It can also be difficult to lose sight of additional robotic arms in the surgical field which can lead to accidental trauma from instruments outside the surgeon's field of view. Finally, current robotic systems do not offer cavitronic ultrasonic surgical aspirator (CUSA) equivalent parenchymal transection (*see* **Chapter 44**).

THERAPEUTIC EFFICACY

According to the findings from current studies, the effectiveness of robotic surgery is essentially identical to that of conventional laparoscopic and open surgery. However, the outcome from studies reporting on operative time, intraoperative bleeding, conversion rates, complications, length of stay in hospital, perioperative mortality, R0 resection rates, and oncological outcome remain inconclusive. Generally, robotic surgery is associated with longer operating times, increased intraoperative blood loss, and higher costs (15–18). However, much of this data is historical. Guan et al. published results in 2010 that demonstrated lower conversion rates and intraoperative blood loss and operation times that were equivalent to laparoscopic and open surgery (19).

The indications for robot-assisted and laparoscopic hepatectomy are similar and include primary tumours (hepatocellular carcinoma and intrahepatic cholangiocarcinoma), metastatic lesions from colorectal, neuroendocrine, breast and renal tumours, benign tumours (enlarging haemangiomas, adenomas, focal nodular hyperplasia) and miscellaneous symptomatic lesions including cysts and abscesses. Minimally invasive surgical approaches to liver pathologies, whether laparoscopic or robotic, are now equally safe and feasible with results equivalent to traditional open hepatectomy. However, for relatively simple procedures such as wedge hepatectomy, hemihepatectomy and extended hepatectomy, conventional laparoscopic hepatectomy has achieved good outcomes and is as effective as robotic surgery and consequently should be the preferred approach (20). Indeed, for some hepatectomies, such as a laparoscopic resection of the left lateral lobe, a laparoscopic approach is superior in terms of operative time and overall procedure costs. For complex procedures such as resection of tumours in caudate lobe, posterosuperior segments, and ALPPS, robotic surgery has clear advantages over conventional laparoscopic techniques. For skilled robotic surgeons, the site, size and number of liver lesions are no longer absolute

indications. This is, in part, due to the far superior image quality with robotic stacks and also the rapid response of industry who have produced new instruments to overcome early technical issues. Controversy has shifted instead to discussions regarding operative times (theatre utilization), procedure morbidity and cost. Robotic surgery is, however, still contraindicated in cases where the lesion is too large ($\geq 15\,\text{cm}$) as tumours of this size prevent proper visualization and mobilization is not possible safely.

Paradoxically for biliary operations, minor procedures such as cholecystectomy are so well established and straightforward to perform laparoscopically that there is no justification for the use of a robot. For more major biliary procedures including biliary resection/reconstruction, those where they are combined with a liver resection (gallbladder cancer) or where extensive lymph node dissection is required, robotic systems with their three-dimensional field of view and multifunctional instruments with seven degrees of motion; a range of movement greater than the human wrist, are superior (*Figure.9.3*).

The excellent field of view and the ever-expanding range of instruments now available (*Figure 9.4*) enables surgeons to perform more delicate dissection of important vessels and bile ducts, and to complete reconstruction more quickly and efficiently.

Robot-assisted pancreatic surgery is safe and feasible for almost all pancreatic surgical procedures, including pancreatic tumour enucleation, pancreaticoduodenectomy, distal, central and total pancreatectomies. The robotic instruments again dramatically reduce the difficulty of laparoscopic suturing, making even the most complex reconstructions such as the pancreaticojejunostomy possible, quick and safe. In addition, the feasibility of vascular anastomoses

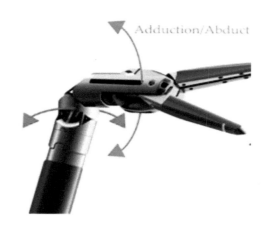

Figure 9.3 Seven degrees of motion with robotic instruments exceeds that of the human wrist.

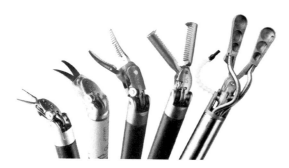

Figure 9.4 The number and range of available robotic instruments is expanding rapidly.

(which are extremely difficult to perform with conventional laparoscopy) means that radical and extensive resections which are normally only performed at open surgery can be considered (21,22). This is supported by some encouraging data regarding patients undergoing robotic pancreatic procedures which suggests faster recovery times, less blood loss and conversion rates are reduced. Negative margins are more frequently achieved and there is better lymph node dissection with a higher spleen preservation rate when compared to the laparoscopic approach (23–27).

FUTURE PERSPECTIVES

Robotic surgery is safe and feasible for most HPB operations. It is an exciting and challenging development which makes MIS possible and safe in otherwise very challenging cases. The high cost of robotic systems, their running costs and concerns regarding the use of theatre time have prevented wholesale approval and uptake in most countries around the world. In the future there is no doubt that indications will expand, surgical experience will improve and the robotic platforms will become less expensive. Together with more data demonstrating, unequivocally, the advantages of a robotic approach and economic data from different healthcare systems identifying those areas where the approach is cost-effective, it is inevitable that there will be an expansion of this exciting field. The technology underpinning the robot systems will also improve and if the rate of development mirrors that seen in the past 2 decades, then systems will quickly evolve with further miniaturization and the addition of 'intelligent' components and support with the use of artificial intelligence (AI).

REFERENCES

1. Lomanto D, Cheah WK, So JB, Goh PM. Robotically assisted laparoscopic cholecystectomy: A pilot study. *Arch Surg* 2001;**136(10)**:1106–8.

2. Laviana AA, Williams SB, King ED, Chuang RJ, Hu JC. Robot assisted radical prostatectomy: The new standard. *Minerva Urol Nefrol* 2015;**67(1)**:47–53.
3. Giulianotti PC, Coratti A, Angelini M, Sbrana F, Cecconi S, Balestracci T, et al. Robotics in general surgery: Personal experience in a large community hospital. *Arch Surg* 2003;**138(7)**:777–84.
4. Choi SB, Park JS, Kim JK, Hyung WJ, Kim KS, Yoon DS, et al. Early experiences of robotic-assisted laparoscopic liver resection. *Yonsei Med J* 2008;**49(4)**:632–8.
5. Croner RS, Perrakis A, Brunner M, Matzel KE, Hohenberger W. Pioneering robotic liver surgery in Germany: First experiences with liver malignancies. *Front Surg* 2015;**2**:18.
6. Vicente E, Quijano Y, Ielpo B, Fabra I. First APPS procedure using a total robotic approach. *Surg Oncol* 2016;**25(4)**:457.
7. Giulianotti PC, Tzvetanov I, Jeon H, Bianco F, Spaggiari M, Oberholzer J, et al. Robot-assisted right lobe donor hepatectomy. *Transpl Int* 2012;**25(1)**:e5–9.
8. Wang XY, Gao Q, Duan M. Outcomes of robot-assisted laparoscopic liver resection: A report of 142 cases. *Chin J Pract Surg* 2017;**37(05)**:548–51.
9. Suh KS, Hong SK, Lee S, Hong SY, Suh S, Han ES, et al. Pure laparoscopic living donor liver transplantation: Dreams come true. *Am J Transplant* 2022;**22(1)**:260–5.
10. Chen PD, Wu CY, Hu RH, Ho C-M, Lee P-H, Lai H-S, et al. Robotic liver donor right hepatectomy: A pure, minimally invasive approach. *Liver Transpl* 2016;**22(11)**:1509–18.
11. Zhao W, Liu C, Li S, Geng D, Feng Y, Sun M. Safety and efficacy for robot-assisted versus open pancreaticoduodenectomy and distal pancreatectomy: A systematic review and meta-analysis. *Surg Oncol* 2018;**27(3)**:468–78.
12. Ghezzi TL, Campos Corleta O. 30 years of robotic surgery. *World J Surg* 2016;**40(10)**:2550–7.
13. Kornaropoulos M, Moris D, Beal EW, Makris MC, Mitrousias A, Petrou A, et al. Total robotic pancreaticoduodenectomy: A systematic review of the literature. *Surg Endosc* 2017;**31(11)**:4382–92.
14. Giulianotti PC, Bianco FM, Daskalaki D, Gonzalez-Ciccarelli LF, Kim J, Benedetti E. Robotic liver surgery: Technical aspects and review of the literature. *Hepatobiliary Surg Nutr* 2016;**5(4)**:311–21.
15. King JC, Zeh HJ 3rd, Zureikat AH, Celebrezze J, Holtzman MP, Stang ML, et al. Safety in numbers: Progressive implementation of a robotics program in an academic surgical oncology practice. *Surg Innov* 2016;**23(4)**:407–14.
16. Nguyen KT, Gamblin TC, Geller DA. World review of laparoscopic liver resection 2,804 patients. *Ann Surg* 2009;**250(5)**:831–41.
17. Hu L, Yao L, Li X, Jin P, Yang K, Guo T. Effectiveness and safety of robotic-assisted versus laparoscopic hepatectomy for liver neoplasms: A meta-analysis of retrospective studies. *Asian J Surg* 2018;**41(5)**:401–16.
18. Tsilimigras DI, Moris D, Vagios S, Merath K, Pawlik TM. Safety and oncologic outcomes of robotic

liver resections: A systematic review. *J Surg Oncol* 2018;**117(7)**:1517–30.

19. Guan R, Chen Y, Yang K, Ma D, Gong X, Shen B, et al. Clinical efficacy of robot-assisted versus laparoscopic liver resection: A meta analysis. *Asian J Surg* 2019;**42(1)**:19–31.

20. Liu R, Wakabayashi G, Kim HJ, Choi G-H, Yiengpruksawan A, Fong Y, et al. International consensus statement on robotic hepatectomy surgery in 2018. *World J Gastroenterol* 2019;**25(12)**: 1432–44.

21. Kendrick ML, Cusati D. Total laparoscopic pancreaticoduodenectomy: Feasibility and outcome in an early experience. *Arch Surg* 2010;**145(1)**:19–23.

22. Kendrick ML, Sclabas GM. Major venous resection during total laparoscopic pancreaticoduodenectomy. *HPB (Oxford)* 2011;**13(7)**:454–8.

23. Marino MV, Shabat G, Potapov O, Gulotta G, Komorowski AL. Robotic pancreatic surgery: Old concerns, new perspectives. *Acta Chir Belg* 2019; **119(1)**:16–23.

24. Daouadi M, Zureikat AH, Zenati MS, Choudry H, Tsung A, Bartlett DL, et al. Robot-assisted minimally invasive distal pancreatectomy is superior to the laparoscopic technique. *Ann Surg* 2013;**257(1)**: 128–32.

25. Peng L, Lin S, Li Y, Xiao W. Systematic review and meta-analysis of robotic versus open pancreaticoduodenectomy. *Surg Endosc* 2017;**31(8)**:3085–97.

26. Briggs CD, Mann CD, Irving GR, Neal CP, Peterson M, Cameron IC, et al. Systematic review of minimally invasive pancreatic resection. *J Gastrointest Surg* 2009;**13(6)**:1129–37.

27. Duran H, Ielpo B, Caruso R, Ferri V, Quijano Y, Diaz E, et al. Does robotic distal pancreatectomy surgery offer similar results as laparoscopic and open approach? A comparative study from a single medical center. *Int J Med Robot* 2014;**10(3)**:280–5.

Chapter 10

Energy Devices

Harsh Kanhere

INTRODUCTION

The development of energy devices has revolutionized surgical practice and been responsible for extraordinary innovation. The result of this fertile period is a range of instruments which have, in turn, facilitated surgical progress in a number of fields, particularly minimally invasive surgery. These devices are now ubiquitous, but their initial introduction over a hundred years ago was controversial and they were initially felt to be an insult to surgeons and very long-standing and engrained medical traditions. Surgeons who were at the forefront of the development and attempted to integrate these devices into surgical practice were branded charlatans. Fortunately, through their persistence there is a panoply of instruments available today that would have been inconceivable even 40 years ago. Available devices, as well as using a number of different technologies, are frequently specifically designed or modified for use in different surgical specialities including neurosurgery, colorectal and hepato-pancreatico-biliary (HPB) surgery. Technological advances have enabled the performance of complex HPB surgical procedures with less blood loss, reduced operation times and the minimising of trauma with the consequence of significantly improved outcomes.

This chapter will outline the historical aspects of the original electrosurgical cauterizing machines and trace their development through to the highly-specialized devices available today.

The technologies covered will encompass electrosurgery (monopolar and bipolar), ultrasonic technology including ultrasonic shears and cavitron ultrasonic surgical aspiration (CUSA), vessel sealing technology and laser and argon beam coagulation. I will not address energy devices used for tissue and tumour ablation as these are discussed in **Chapter 49**. For each device the mechanism of action, advantages and disadvantages and indication and value during HPB surgical procedures will be described.

THE HISTORY AND DEVELOPMENT OF ENERGY DEVICES

Methods for cauterizing tissue date back further than written records. Evidence exists for the use of heated stones to stem bleeding and there is widespread evidence of the recognition of the usefulness and use of conducted heat which is described as early as 600 BCE.

In 1881, Morton demonstrated that an oscillating current (a frequency of 100 kHz) could pass through human tissue between two electrodes without apparent harm and was painless.

As surgical practice developed, by the end of the 19th century and into the early 20th century, major procedures were possible, but a remaining area of concern was intraoperative blood loss. Options available to achieve haemostasis were extremely limited and surgeons relied on electrocautery, which is the direct application of heat to tissue and not to be confused with electrosurgery. Descriptions of cautery to address bleeding and infection are available dating back over 3000 years. In ancient times, fire was considered an effective treatment for various diseases such as warts, wounds, infections, bleeding, fatigue, stress disorders, gastrointestinal (GI) diseases, musculoskeletal pain and skin cancer. First reference to cautery can be found in surgical papyrus (1550 BCE) in Egyptian society. Cautery was also considered a cure for religious beliefs.

Pioneering work by Harvey Cushing (1869–1939) popularized the use of electrosurgery in neurosurgery following the development in 1926 of the first commercial electrosurgical unit by the physicist William T Bovie (an eccentric inventor with a doctorate in plant physiology) whilst he was working at Harvard University (1). The same year that Bovie developed his device, Harvey Cushing used it on October the 1st for the first time at the Peter Bent Brigham Hospital in Boston Massachusetts to remove a tumour from a man's head. Cushing's demonstration radically changed the surgical landscape and ushered in a new era of surgery. Cushing went on to use the Bovie device in over 500 neurosurgical operations and it was enthusiastically adopted by other surgeons and became standard equipment in operating theatres around the world (2).

The Bovie device or 'Bovie' used the passage of an electrical current through tissues to control bleeding. The first electrosurgical unit employed a powerful and high-frequency generator. The generator produced a radiofrequency spark between a probe and the surgical site which caused localized heating and damage to the tissue (desiccation and blood coagulation), controlling bleeding and producing haemostasis.

Before the 'Bovie', electrocautery had been available in other forms. Karl Franz Nagelschmidt, a Berlin physician, coined the term 'diathermy' in 1909 (from Greek words '*dia*' and '*therma*' meaning 'heating

DOI: 10.1201/9781003080060-10

through') in the Münchener Medizinische Wochen-schrift. In 1907, at a congress in Budapest, Nagelschmidt had demonstrated a prototype diathermy apparatus he had designed whilst at Dresden. He demonstrated the 'heating through' of tissues by high-frequency currents and suggested that they be used in the treatment of diseases of the circulation and joints. In the 1890s, Nikola Tesla (1856–1943) and Jacques-Arsene aeronaval (1851–1940) had both studied the medical applications of high-frequency currents and shown them to be safe for use in humans.

Since the era of the 'Bovie', technological advances have produced a range of devices to assist today's surgeons to control bleeding during surgical procedures. Surgeons now have a choice of different technologies, different handpieces and more recently devices which are designed for laparoscopic use. Many of the more recent energy devices are multifunctional and able to divide tissue while simultaneously sealing vessels and producing haemostasis. The consequences are reduced blood loss, frequently avoiding blood transfusions, shorter operating times and a more rapid and safer recovery. The technology involved to produce the various devices is often quite different and surgeons must be aware of the mechanism of action, advantages, disadvantages, necessary safety precautions and indications to enable them to be used safely. Energy devices fall into four broad categories:

1 Monopolar electrosurgery
2 Bipolar electrosurgery
3 Ultrasonic generators. Vessel sealing devices can be bipolar, ultrasonic or a combination of both
4 Lasers and argon beam coagulators used in major HPB surgery

THE MONOPOLAR ELECTROSURGERICAL UNIT

The most commonly used device in both open, and minimal access surgery, is the monopolar electrosurgical unit (ESU). Frequently this is referred to as a 'cautery' or 'diathermy' (diathermy is any technique that uses electric currents, radio and sound waves to generate heat). 'Cauterize' is a Middle English word borrowed from the Old French 'cauteriser', itself from Late Latin 'cauterizes' meaning 'to burn or brand with a hot iron' which means direct application of heat to tissues, and is as such, a misnomer. The principle of a monopolar ESU is to pass an electric current though the tissues at high frequencies to generate heat and other pro-thrombotic effects resulting in the ability to cut and coagulate.

COMPONENTS

There are four basic components of a monopolar ESU: generator; active electrode; tissue medium and patient return electrode.

Generator

The generator is the basic unit of any ESU and virtually all modern generators work on the principal of raising the frequency of the electrical current passing through it from about 60 Hz to over 300 kHz. There is considerable variation of current frequencies used in diathermy machines. Surgical diathermy units operate at 1–3 MHz, ultrasonic diathermy at 800–1000 kHz, short wave diathermy at 27 MHz. This high-frequency current is then applied to the tissue medium with the active electrode. The current passes through the tissues to the return plate and back to the unit to complete the electrical circuit (*Figure 10.1a*).

The original generators worked on the principle of grounding (grounded referenced generators), where the current passed from the return plate to the ground through the generator to complete the circuit. This approach risked current dispersion with leakage via any electrode that was grounded (ECG electrodes, exposed parts of the operating table, fixed retraction posts or any metal object in contact with the patient). With these devices patients were therefore at risk of burns at the site of contact with these alternate electrodes.

The current state-of-the-art generators are isolated generators meaning that the circuit is completed only through the generator and does not pass to a ground plate. In addition, newer generators are equipped with return electrode monitoring technology where the system measures the impedance between two conductors and is able to detect when it falls outside the nominal range due to current leakage and immediately deactivates the generator to protect the patient from inadvertent burns.

Active electrode

The active electrode (*Figure 10.1b*) is usually a handheld, pencil-type instrument (sometimes with smoke extraction) with a metal-Teflon™ (polytetrafluoroethylene [PTFE]) coated tip. The generation of the current occurs as a button on the handpiece, or a foot-operated pedal when depressed.

Return electrode

The return electrode is usually an adhesive pad with a large surface contact area. This is applied to the patient's skin as close to the surgical field as possible, ensuring there are no metallic implants (hip prostheses, pacemakers etc.) between the operative field and the plate. The area needs to be clean, preferably with minimal hair (clipped) and a broad, flat surface to provide constant and reliable contact. The lateral aspect of the thigh fits these criteria during the majority of abdominal surgical procedures and is the therefore the preferred site. Extreme care must also be taken when patients have pacemakers. Whilst monopolar ESUs can be used with care (if the current path does not include the pacemaker location), bipolar units are preferred where appropriate.

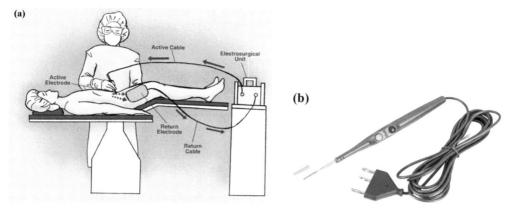

Figure 10.1 The basic layout of a monopolar ESU (a) and typical handpiece (b).

MODES OF OPERATION, WAVEFORMS AND TISSUE EFFECTS

Monopolar electrosurgery

All monopolar ESUs perform three basic functions: Cutting, coagulation and blend.

Mechanism of action

When activated, the cutting function produces a continuous waveform with a high-duty cycle, that is the 'on time' for the majority of the activated period. Cutting vaporizes or cuts tissues with very rapid production of heat. With the coagulation function, the waveform is intermittent and the duty cycle 'on time' is reduced. Less heat is generated over a longer period of time leading to the formation of a coagulum. A blended cycle is not as the name would suggest a mixture of cutting and coagulation, but a modification of the waveform with pulses providing differing degrees of cutting and coagulation effects. Further modes such as spray and fulguration are based on the current spread over a field. The waveforms are shown in *Figure 10.2*.

Advantages

Monopolar ESUs are simple to use, inexpensive, easy to set up and very effective for both cutting and coagulation of tissue.

Disadvantages

Transmission of current and heat can cause inadvertent tissue damage to any organ in the operative field and bowel injuries may go unnoticed at the time of surgery and lead to delayed perforations and major morbidity. It is not possible to seal vessels which are

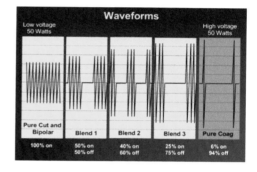

Figure 10.2 Different waveforms associated with the cut, coagulate and blend functions of a monopolar ESU.

larger than 1–2 mm in diameter and use in patients with pacemakers, defibrillators and other electromagnetic implants should be avoided, whenever possible, as the current may interfere with the correct working of these devices.

Use in HPB surgery

Monopolar ESUs are used for the majority of tissue dissection in pancreatic and biliary surgery, for marking the lines of transection for liver resections, coagulation of small vessels during liver transection and for performing minor liver biopsies. Considerable care needs to be taken whilst using monopolar ESUs in minimally invasive surgery. There is a risk of collateral damage due to restricted field of vision and transmission of current to adjacent organs due to the generation of electrostatic fields particularly when using mixed material ports (metal and plastic).

BIPOLAR ELECTROSURGERY

Bipolar ESUs work on similar principles as monopolar devices but there is no patient return electrode and the current flows between two closely placed electrodes to complete the circuit (*Figure 10.3*).

Mechanism of action

The electrodes are usually the opposing exposed tips of insulated forceps, one jaw acting as the working electrode and the second as the receiving electrode. Current will only pass through the tissues that are held in the jaws or tines of the forceps when the circuit is completed. The bipolar ESU consists of a generator (newly available generators can be used with monopolar and bipolar equipment), and as for a monopolar ESU, an active and passive electrode in the form of the jaws of the forceps with current passing through the tissue and returning to the generator via the second jaw of the forceps.

Advantages

Due to this very localized closed circuit the dissipation of the current is extremely limited with minimal risk of thermal injury to surrounding structures and tissues.

Disadvantages

Only limited tissue can be coagulated, and a bipolar ESU does not provide a cut function and hence tissues cannot be divided.

Use in HPB surgery

Many surgeons prefer to use bipolar diathermy forceps to coagulate and control bleeding from small vessels during dissection for pancreatic surgery especially during a Whipple procedure. Bipolar forceps can be utilized to coagulate small liver parenchymal vessels during a segmental or non-anatomical resection

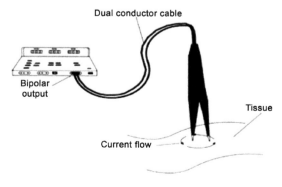

Figure 10.3 A bipolar device connected to tissue forceps.

although a small cohort of liver surgeons use bipolar diathermy for all resections.

VESSEL SEALING TECHNOLOGY

Vessel sealing technology is the term applied to any electrosurgical technology that combines pressure and energy to seal vessels. This technology utilizes a specialized generator and instrument combination to reliably grasp tissue and seal vessels that are larger than possible with ESU devices. The maximum diameter of the vessel that can be reliably sealed depends on the instrument used but some manufacturers claim that vessels up to 7 mm in diameter can be safely and reliably coagulated.

Mechanism of action

Optimal pressure is applied with the instrument (in shape of graspers with two jaws) to initially fuse the vessel wall together followed by application of a unique form of bipolar energy to create a permanent seal. The generator used is a bipolar device working at 180 V and a high 4 A current. The instruments are precisely calibrated, can apply high pressure and are suitable for use during open and laparoscopic procedures.

The bipolar output is controlled via a feedback mechanism which facilitates reliable tissue sealing in the minimal time independent of the type or amount of tissue in the jaws. The energy delivery cycle measures initial resistance of the tissue and chooses an energy setting that is appropriate. The energy is then delivered in a pulsed manner which adapts as the cycle progresses and the instrument provides feedback, indicating that the tissue has been completely sealed, and completes the cycle.

Advantages

As with the bipolar ESU, the thermal spread is significantly reduced. The sealed site is transparent and can be visualized prior to division if required. The manufacturers claim that seal strengths are comparable to mechanical ligation. Most of these devices are equipped with a small knife that can be activated with a trigger or a button on the grip of the instrument, thereby allowing the tissue to be cut after the seal has been completed.

Ligasure™ is the trade name of the original device (Medtronic, Minnesota, USA), and it is used in a variety of open, and minimal access, surgeries. New instruments using similar technologies are currently on the market. The array of instruments and generator is shown in *Figure 10.4* with lengths that vary for open, or laparoscopic use.

Disadvantages

The sealing cycle is slow compared with ultrasound technology and an additional action of activating the

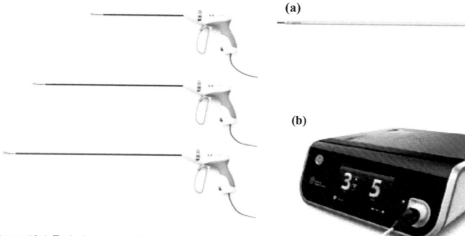

Figure 10.4 Typical vessel-sealing handpieces.

(a)

(b)

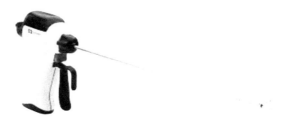

Figure 10.5 Harmonic™ scalpel (a) active blade and (b) generator.

knife is required to separate the tissue. The placement of the button/trigger for the knife is not always easily accessible or ergonomic.

Use in HPB surgery

A randomized trial examining the use of the Ligasure device, compared to stapling devices, during liver resection demonstrated a greater blood loss although with no difference in overall morbidity or complications (3). There are also a number of reports describing the use of bipolar vessel sealing devices which demonstrate their safety and effectiveness during open and laparoscopic liver transection (4) and they are widely used during pancreatic surgery for mobilization, dissection and division of the gland.

ULTRASONIC ENERGY DEVICES AND GENERATORS

The development of ultrasonically activated coagulating shears in the early 1990s provided an additional method of controlling blood vessels and the use of ultrasonic shears or devices is now virtually ubiquitous in open and laparoscopic surgery. These devices employ compression and friction to deliver mechanical energy to the tissues and produce coagulation, sealing and simultaneous division of tissues.

Mechanism of action

A high-frequency ultrasonic transducer transforms electrical energy from a generator into mechanical energy. The active blade delivers high-grade frictional force while the inactive upper arm holds tissue in apposition. Its main advantages include precise

Figure 10.6 Sonicision™ handpiece.

dissection, reliable haemostasis and less lateral thermal spread and charring. The mechanism of action is through the application of pressure and the subsequent sealing results from the ultrasonic vibration which denatures hydrogen bonds, forming a protein coagulum and haemostasis. The stability of the coagulum is achieved mechanically due to the tamponade and coaptation between the jaws (5). Division of tissue occurs through high-frequency (55 000 Hz) ultrasonic energy transmitted between the instrument blades. The active blade of the instrument such as a HARMONIC scalpel (ETHICON, J&J MedTech, New Jersey, USA) vibrates longitudinally against an inactive blade over an excursion of 50–100 μm (*Figure 10.5*).

A more recent instrument called the Sonicision has been introduced by Medtronic (Minnesota, USA) which uses similar technology, but has the advantage of being battery powered (*Figure 10.6*).

Advantages

Ultrasonic energy devices require no electrical current flow or patient return electrodes eliminating the risk of electrical burns to the skin. Coagulation and division of tissues occurs with activation of a single button instead of requiring two separate manoeuvres. The consensus among surgeons is that these devices complete the coagulation and cut cycle in less time than bipolar vessel sealing devices and they can be used in patients with electromagnetic devices, including defibrillators.

Disadvantages

Although the heat generated is claimed to be minimal, the active electrode remains hot for some time after inactivation of the cycle with the potential risk of thermal injury to the adjacent structures particularly when used during minimal access surgery. Indications for use in HPB surgery mirror those of the bipolar vessel-sealing technology devices.

CAVITRON ULTRASONIC SURGICAL ASPIRATOR (CUSA)

CUSA devices are specialized dissecting instruments that use ultrasonic frequencies to disrupt tissue. The main application for CUSA in HPB surgery is the liver parenchymal transection and it is still the device preferred by many surgeons (6).

The device employs a hollow titanium tip that vibrates along its long axis and the vibration occurs with a frequency of 23 kHz and with an adjustable stroke of 0–300 microns. It fragments tissues whilst simultaneously lavaging and aspirating the resulting fine residue from the surgical field. It is very effective in tissues with a high-water content such as the liver and glandular tissue and is consequently also used extensively in neurosurgery.

Advantages

Precise dissection is possible as biliary radicles and vessels are preserved while liver tissue is selectively removed. Safe identification of the portal-vein radicles and biliary ductules allows them to be safely ligated, clipped or diathermied if small and CUSA use minimizes blood loss.

Disadvantages

Dissection using CUSA devices is slow and prolongs the operation time (*Figure 10.7*).

HYBRID TECHNOLOGY

The THUNDERBEAT® (Olympus Medical Systems Corp., Tokyo, Japan) device integrates bipolar and

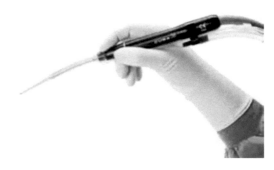

Figure 10.7 CUSA handpiece for transection of the liver parenchyma.

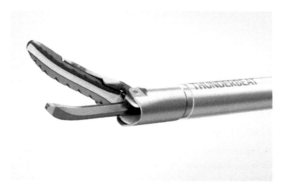

Figure 10.8 THUNDERBEAT hybrid energy device.

ultrasonic energy technologies into one instrument (*Figure 10.8*). The combination of technologies confer the ability to rapidly cut tissue with ultrasonic energy and create reliable vessel seals with bipolar energy.

Advantages

The main benefits include the rapid division of tissue, reliable 7 mm vessel sealing, precise dissection due to the jaw design and bipolar energy for haemostasis. There is also minimal thermal spread and reduced mist generation which produces a clear field of view at open, or laparoscopic, surgery.

Disadvantages

Heat generation and inadvertent thermal tissue injury issues are similar to those encountered with ultrasonic devices.

Use in HPB surgery

Use of the THUNDERBEAT device (Olympus Medical Systems, Hamburg, Germany) is increasing in the treatment of the same indications where bipolar and ultrasonic devices are used. There are similar caveats regarding the associated risks.

ARGON PLASMA-BEAM COAGULATION

Argon plasma-beam coagulation deserves a brief mention for the sake of completeness as it has been the mainstay for effective surface coagulation of the liver after transection for over 30 years. Argon is an inert gas that is non-combustible and easily ionized by radiofrequency energy. The principal on which the device is based, is the release of the ionization energy when the plasma comes in contact with tissue, which is earthed. In practice, argon gas flows through a tube containing an electrode and a discharge are generated between the active electrode and the tissue to be treated. This occurs due to the application of a high-frequency (HF) voltage difference between the wire and the tissue. The electrode may be a tungsten wire usually with a diameter of several tenths of a millimetre, or a needle- or spatula-shaped tip made of stainless steel. The distance between electrode and tissue is typically 2–10 mm. The argon flows through a tube which surrounds the electrode and an alternating current (AC) voltage with an amplitude of typically 4 kV and a frequency of typically 350 kHz is used to ignite the discharge (*Figure 10.9*). The HF current flows

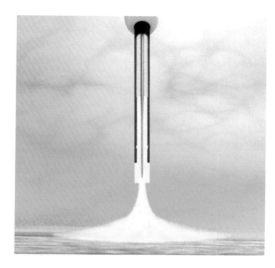

Figure 10.10 Diagrammatic representation of the surface coagulation resulting from the application of an argon plasma-beam device.

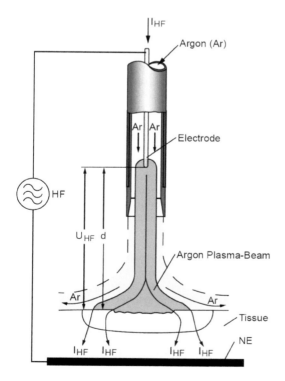

Figure 10.9 Schematic of an argon plasma-beam generator.

between the wire and the tissue causing a coagulation effect. It generates a flexible eschar over the raw, cut surface reducing blood loss and risk of re-bleeding. The current then flows back to the generator through the neutral electrode. It can be applied over large surface areas and the effect of coagulation remains superficial so that the underlying healthy liver tissue remains unaffected (*Figure 10.10*). The eschar is also undisturbed due to the non-contact nature of the process unlike any mechanism which has to deliver current through forceps which are holding the tissue.

LASER COAGULATION

In 1960, soon after Maiman discovered the first ruby-based working laser, the first experiments on medical laser application began. Only a couple of years after Maiman's discovery, ruby-laser use in ophthalmology was investigated leading eventually to its ubiquitous use. A number of different specialties now use lasers to cut, coagulate, and ablate tissue and the technology is attractive due to its minimally invasive, localized effect (7). Today, there are a number of types of lasers available for surgical and GI procedures and the wavelength and delivery system will depend on the planned application and the absorption chromophore (a chromophore is the part of a molecule responsible for its colour) of the tissue to be treated (*see Table 10.1*).

Percutaneous interstitial laser coagulation (ILC), has been used for the treatment of irresectable hepatocellular carcinoma (HCC) since 1983 and is reported to have very few side effects. Lasers have also been

Table 10.1 The various types of lasers used in surgery

Laser	Wavelength (nanometers)	Absorption chromophore
Er:YAG	2940	Water
Diode	630–980	Pigment, water
Argon	350–514	Pigment, haemaglobin
Nd:YAG	1064	Pigment, proteins
CO_2	10600	Water

Abbreviations: Er:YAG = erbium-doped yttrium aluminium garnet laser; Nd:YAG = neodymium-doped yttrium aluminium garnet.

investigated for the transection and coagulation of liver tissue in animal studies but the experience in the clinical setting is not yet available. Thulium lasers, characterized by the length of emission wave corresponding to a peak absorption of water, are a promising new method of cutting tissues efficiently and achieving haemostasis with minimal thermal damage. Over a decade ago, it was demonstrated that liver resections could be performed very rapidly with good haemostasis and minimal blood loss in animals using a diode-pumped, and continuous-wave Tm^{3+}-doped (Thulium) fibre-laser emitting 37.4 W of output power at ~1.94 µm wavelength (8). Samples collected intraoperatively demonstrated a superficial coagulated zone which was distinct and spared deeper tissues. Fourteen days following the resection, a zone of granulation tissue 765.35 µm deep was observed and again this was clearly separated from the healthy underlying tissue. In experimental animals, a thulium-doped fibre-laser was able to transect liver tissue rapidly. Doping refers to introducing small amounts of rare-earth elements such as erbium, ytterbium, neodymium, dysprosium, praseodymium, thulium and holmium to the laser fibres. Research is ongoing to develop devices for clinical use and although there is a limited experience of laser use in laparoscopic and robotic urological surgery (9), it is unlikely in the foreseeable future, that this technology will replace those presently available for HPB surgery.

RISKS OF ENERGY DEVICES

Adverse events and harm following the use of energy devices in medicine, endoscopy and surgery are surprisingly common and their frequency is increasing. Concern has been expressed as a root-cause-analysis and the investigation of serious untoward incidents (SUI) suggest that the vast majority of these events are avoidable. According to the Manufacturer and User Facility Device Experience (MAUDE) database set up by the US Food and Drug Administration (FDA), 178 deaths and 3553 injuries related to radiofrequency electrosurgical devices have been reported in the last two decades. Predictably, the usual injury is a burn (2353, 63%), followed by bleeding generally consequent upon an endoscopic therapeutic procedure (642, 17%), device failure (336, 9%), and fire (294, 8%). Burns were responsible for the most deaths (70, 39%). The rising incidence, possibly related to the rapid expansion of invasive endoscopic procedures, also has a significant impact on healthcare systems due to the medicolegal implications (10).

The picture is similar in Europe, and the French national database on adverse events in surgery (Evénements Porteurs de Risques [EPR]) maintained by the French Federation of Gastrointestinal and Digestive Surgery (Fédération de Chirurgie Viscérale et Digestive [FCVD]) contains over 7500 registered adverse events reported voluntarily by 900 surgeons between 2009–2014. Many of the reported events occurred in operating theatres (2345). Over the time period 648 (24%) involved the use of energy devices, including 51 operating room fires and 423 unintended skin or organ burns. Most injuries followed the use of monopolar diathermy and resulted in the need for a number of additional surgical procedures. There were also some deaths (10).

EDUCATIONAL ISSUES WITH ENERGY DEVICES

Education in the use of energy devices has historically been informal and to a large extent this is still the case today. Undergraduate and postgraduate training has no structured teaching regarding the use and risks of energy devices. The lack of formal teaching problem has been exacerbated by the proliferation of different technologies in addition to the fact that instruments cannot be visualized at all times in body cavities during inter-luminal and in minimally-invasive procedures. Problems are most acute for specialities that use advanced and potentially hazardous devices which included anaesthesia, cardiology, gastroenterology, urology, minimally invasive surgery (all specialities) and interventional radiology. There is also increasing 'technological crossover' with surgeons, physicians and radiologists using common pieces of equipment and frequently working together on a procedure. This relies on all team members having a full understanding of the technology and its appropriate use and hazards which is increasingly difficult with the burgeoning number of devices and applications. In the USA, these concerns resulted in the setting up of The Fundamental Use of Surgical Energy (FUSE) program by a multidisciplinary team under the auspices of the Society of American Gastrointestinal and Endoscopic Surgeons (SAGES) (10).

SUMMARY

The last three decades have seen the development in all areas of medicine and surgery advance at an incredible rate with the development of technology. Technologies have facilitated advances, such as minimally invasive surgery, which in turn has demanded further innovation to perform increasing complex procedures safely. The application of these technologies has benefitted HPB surgeons. Operating times have improved, blood loss has reduced, and tissue trauma lessened which ameliorated the inevitable morbidity associated with major liver and pancreatic surgery. The improvements are in no small part due to the energy devices that are now available, and it is likely that developments will continue at the same pace. The only note of caution relates to the cost burden on healthcare systems. If the new technologies can reduce lengths of stay, demands on intensive care and in-hospital costs while avoiding increasing the medicolegal burden, then those new technologies should be welcomed. If, however, the burgeoning costs and the negative aspects of new technologies, particularly when introduced without adequate scrutiny, outweigh the advantages then healthcare providers will be faced with a significant dilemma.

REFERENCES

1. Carter PL. The life and legacy of William T. Bovie. *Am J Surg* 2013;**205**(5):488–91.
2. Bovie WT, Cushing H. Electrosurgery as an aid to the removal of intracranial tumors with a preliminary note on a new surgical-current generator. *Surg Gynecol Obstet* 1928;**47**:51–84.
3. Fritzmann J, Kirchberg J, Sturm D, Ulrich AB, Knebel P, Mehrabi A, et al. Randomized clinical trial of stapler hepatectomy versus LigaSure™ transection in elective hepatic resection. *Br J Surg* 2018;**105**(9): 1119–27.
4. Huo YR, Shiraev T, Alzahrani N, Chu F. Reducing inflow occlusion, occlusion duration and blood loss during hepatic resections. *ANZ J Surg*, 2018;**88**(1–2): e25–e9.
5. Dutta DK, Dutta I. The Harmonic Scalpel. *J Obstet Gynaecol India* 2016;**66**(3):209–10.
6. Honda G, Ome Y, Yoshida N, Kawamoto Y. How to dissect the liver parenchyma: Excavation with cavitron ultrasonic surgical aspirator. *J Hepatobiliary Pancreat Sci* 2020;**27**(11):907–12.
7. Fuchshuber PR, Robinson TN, Feldman LS, Brunt LM, Madani A, Jones SB, et al. Fundamental Use of Surgical Energy (FUSE): Closing a gap in medical education. *Ann Surg* 2015;**262**(1):20–2. doi: 10.1097/SLA.0000000000001256. PMID: 26057558; PMCID: PMC4484398.
8. Khalkhal E, Rezaei-Tavirani M, Zali MR, Akbari Z. The evaluation of laser application in surgery: A review article. *J Lasers Med Sci* 2019;**10**(Suppl 1):S104–S11. doi: 10.15171/jlms.2019.S18. Epub 2019 Dec 1. PMID: 32021682; PMCID: PMC6983859.
9. Azadgoli B, Baker RY. Laser applications in surgery. *Ann Transl Med* 2016; **4**(23):452. doi: 10.21037/atm.2016.11.51. PMID: 28090508; PMCID: PMC5220034.
10. Theisen-Kunde D, Wolken H, Danicke V, Brinkmann R, H Bruch H, Kleemann, M. *In vivo* study of partial liver resection on pigs using a 1.9 μm Thulium fiber laser. Proceedings of SPIE-OSA Biomedical Optics (Optica Publishing Group, 2011), paper 809211.

Bailey & Love's Essential Operations Bailey & Love's Essential Operatio
Bailey & Love's Essential Operations Bailey & Love's Essential Operatio
Bailey & Love's Essential Operations Bailey & Love's Essential Operatio

SECTION 1 | BASIC PRINCIPLES

Chapter

11

Training of the HPB Surgeon

Greg M. Padmore and Elijah Dixon

INTRODUCTION

The subspecialty of hepato-pancreatico-biliary (HPB) surgery has evolved during the 20th century, from pioneers who were largely self-taught becoming familiar with the anatomy by practical experience, and synchronously developing various techniques through trial and error. The modern era continues to show maturation of the field as advances in pre-, intra- and postoperative care occur, along with the development of energy devices, and as more organized, high-volume fellowship institutions become available. This chapter discusses the historical development of this subspecialty and describes the various training paths that are available together with the geographical nuances involved for trainees wishing to become a HPB surgeon in the modern era.

HISTORY OF HPB SURGERY

Details and discussion around the essential requirements for the training of an HPB surgeon cannot be made without acknowledging the history of this amazing specialty which is now, thanks to pioneers who paved the way for us, an established and respected discipline. These giants in the field can be divided into first, second and modern generation HPB surgeons. Respectively, these timelines are prior to 1960, 1960–1970 and 1970-to-date although there are areas where there is inevitably some overlap.

Gallbladder followed by biliary tract operations were the first successful HPB surgical exploits. John Bobbs in Indiana in 1867 began the development of gallbladder surgery (1). He relieved a female patient with an enormous gallbladder filled with stones, performing a cholecystostomy with stone extraction and primary suture repair. In 1878, Marion Sims performed the first elective procedure for obstructive jaundice in Paris when he operated on a patient with obstructive jaundice. Following a cholecystostomy and extraction of 60 calculi the gallbladder was sutured to the abdominal wall and the jaundice resolved (2). Lawson Taitt, an English surgeon and the doyen of Swiss surgery, Theodore Kocher, almost simultaneously performed planned gallbladder operations which involved stone removal and suturing the gallbladder to the abdominal wall. Taitt was credited with the first cholecystostomy for cholelithiasis in 1885 but it was actually Carl Langenbuch in 1882 who performed the first cholecystectomy because he

had observed a high rate of stone recurrence with stone removal alone (2).

Following these early successes, the natural development saw surgeons begin to address the issues of stone disease in the common bile duct (CBD) developing methods to deal with this technically difficult problem. Hans Kehr in 1897 was the first to perform a CBD exploration leaving a rubber tube *in situ* through the cystic duct (3). In 1898, Thornton was the first to remove stones from the CBD, followed in 1899 by Courvoisier who successfully operated on another case of choledocholithiasis (4). Courvoisier published his observations which entered the literature and became known as Courvoisier's law which states that in patients with jaundice, if the gallbladder is not distended, the cause is more likely to be one of stones. Subsequently, following these very early pioneers, Hans Kehr was instrumental in advancing biliary surgery. In 1912, he was able to perform stone extractions via a tube he placed in the CBD via the cystic duct and he is credited with the development of the 'T' tube (5). In addition to this important development which is still in use today Hans Kerr was also the first person to perform a hepatico-enteric anastomosis.

These initial successful approaches stimulated the surgical community and demonstrated the feasibility of even technically difficult HPB procedures. As a consequence, the complexity of the procedures progressively increased with Halsted in Baltimore in 1900 performing a partial duodenectomy for a tumour which required reimplantation of the CBD and a cholecystectomy. Subsequently, Mayo in 1901 performed the first reported transduodenal ampullectomy where the periampullary tumour was removed following a duodenotomy and reconstruction by means of a choledochoduodenostomy (1).

The role of mentorship is undoubtably one of the main pillars of surgery without which surgical expertise could not be taught and disseminated. Roux trained under Kocher and in 1897 described the preparation of the jejunal loop used in gastric surgery which soon became almost ubiquitously used in biliary surgery (6). Couinaud in France in 1954 described the detailed liver anatomy, and Hepp and Couinaud and Soupault and Couinaud both in 1957, developed techniques for direct bilioenteric anastomosis, either to the left hepatic duct or to the segment III duct of the left liver (1).

Pancreatic surgery was in its infancy when war inflicted injuries became commonplace which in part

DOI: 10.1201/9781003080060-11

led to the development in 1881 of pancreatic cyst drainage procedures. The early 20th century witnessed the first attempts to perform pancreatic-enteric anastomoses, with Coffey in 1909 anastomosing the tail of the pancreas to the small bowel (7). Pancreatic neuroendocrine tumour surgery was first described by Wilder and colleagues in 1927 when they reported on the resection of an insulinoma (8). In 1935, Allen Oldfather Whipple began publishing his work on two staged cephalic duodenopancreatectomy for cancer of the ampulla of Vater (9) which eventually evolved into the one stage procedure which he initially performed in 1941. Surgery for pancreatitis was fraught and the morbidity and mortality was extremely high. The surgical management of chronic pancreatitis developed in a similar fashion through much trial, error and innovation. Surgeons such as Leger and Brehand in 1956 and von Puestow and Gillespy in 1958 opened the pancreatic duct along its length to decompress the gland and completed the procedures with a pancreatojejunostomy (1).

The infancy of liver surgery, similar to pancreatic surgery, developed against a background of war inflicted traumatic injuries. Important early developments included Langenbuch in Germany in 1888 who performed the first planned liver resection (10). A number of surgeons rapidly followed Langenbuch's example, and in 1890 Tiffany in the USA resected a liver tumour and, in 1891 Lucke also reported a liver resection for cancer (11). Rex in 1888 and Cantlie in 1897 contributed greatly to the art of controlled hepatic resections with their detailed anatomic studies and once the anatomical road map had been established, the next hurdle was to identify the optimal technique for parenchymal transection and haemostasis. Kousnetzoff and Pensky in 1896 wrote that 'these vessels were amenable to suture ligature once a sufficient margin of liver parenchyma is included', a principle that still holds today (11). Pringle in 1908 made another seminal contribution by describing the technique of portal inflow occlusion, which has stood the test of time and remains another key technique in the armamentarium of the modern liver surgeon. The next logical step was to attempt a formal major hepatectomy with hilar ligation, the first of which was achieved by Wendell in 1911. Further detailed anatomic studies by Hjortsjo 1951, Couinaud in 1952 and Healey and Schroy in 1953 led to the acceptance of the concept of segmental anatomy (11). In Japan in 1949, Honjo and Araki performed a right hepatectomy and in 1952, Lorat-Jacob and Robert performed the first true anatomical liver resection with preliminary vascular control.

The 1960s brought the drive and innovation of Thomas Starzl and Roy Calne who established the basis for orthotopic liver transplantation while at the same time pioneering immunosuppressive drug protocols. The work of these two pioneers and their mentorship which has produced generations of liver surgeons, clearly confirm them as the forefathers of liver transplantation. This era also introduced luminaries such as Blumgart, Bismuth, Langer, and Bengmark who started to develop specialist HPB centres in their countries (12). It is notable that during this period experience was gained by spending time with experts in the field as no formal training programmes existed. Subsequently there has also been much cross-fertilisation between transplant and HPB surgeons especially with regard to vascular techniques, patient selection, intraoperative and postoperative management, training and the skills and principles required by trainees.

Embarking on a career in HPB surgery requires at a minimum completion of a general surgery training programme. Although not mandatory it is also recommended that trainees spend time during their elective period in a prospective institution or institutions where recognized and established fellowship programmes exist. This exposure to the rigours and demands of HPB surgery, which may not be available in their own institution, will emphasize the skillset necessary for the speciality and provide an opportunity to develop relationships with the faculty and foster mentorship. This is particularly important today as the specialty continues to evolve and technological advances such as energy devices, intraoperative imaging, laparoscopic and robotic surgery and virtual training simulators challenge surgeons to advance the field in a safe and controlled manner. Finally, trainees will be encouraged to undertake a period of research (in some countries this is mandatory) to be competitive in applying for HPB fellowships, and developing relationships with recognized units with a proven track record for producing high quality research, will allow trainees to consider which areas interest them most.

Internationally, there are many training programmes where HPB subspecialization skills and training can be acquired with surprisingly different approaches, structures and duration. The route taken will depend heavily on your future career goals, long term aims, the time you are able to spend in the programme and whether you wish to get fully trained within that programme or spend a short time acquiring a specific skill (robotic procedures, oncological surgery). There are a variety of programmes available and their length and composition vary considerably depending largely on whether they are HPB alone, surgical oncology/HPB, transplant with HPB or HPB with gastrointestinal (GI) surgery.

In North America, HPB training is available through the American Society of Transplant Surgeons (ASTS), the Complex General Surgical Oncology Board (CGSO) and the Americas Hepato-Pancreato-Biliary Association (AHPBA) fellowships (13). In association with the Fellowship Council, the AHPBA offers 21 AHPBA-sponsored Fellowship Council accredited fellowship positions across the USA and Canada (13–15). These HPB-only programmes (11 one-year programmes and 10 two-year programmes) encompass all practice settings, including university, university-affiliated, and private hospitals (13).

Additionally, there are programmes which are dually accredited with CGSO (6 programmes) and ASTS (2 programmes), (13,16). In South America (Argentina and Brazil), there are 14 HPB fellowship programmes registered with the International Hepato-Pancreato-Biliary Association (IHPBA) (14) and in the Asia/Pacific region, there are a total of 15 fellowship programmes registered with the IHPBA and another 26 registered programmes in Europe, Africa and the Middle East (17).

The training curriculum for an HPB surgeon has core fundamentals and competencies which trainees are expected to have achieved upon completion. For example, the AHPBA/Fellowship Council curriculum includes core competencies in patient care, medical knowledge, practise-based learning and improvement, interpersonal and communication skills, professionalism, system-based practice and operative experience. After completion of the programme the fellow will be able to provide comprehensive, state-of-the-art medical and surgical care to patients with surgical diseases/disorders of the liver, pancreas, biliary tract and duodenum. This includes the ability to investigate, diagnose, recommend appropriate treatment options, perform operative procedures and provide pre-, peri- and late-postoperative care. Minimum clinical experience requirements for the AHPBA certification includes at least 100 cases which comprise a minimum of 20 major hepatectomies, 20 pancreaticoduodenectomies and 15 complex biliary surgical procedures with intraoperative diagnostic and guidance ultrasound competency (13). The fellow has to be acting as either the primary or teaching surgeon for at least 70 cases.

HPB ALONE

The programme length is usually 12–24 months and irrespective of the duration chosen the core structure is similar in terms of the minimum operative case requirements, knowledge and mastery of managing benign and malignant HPB conditions, participation in multidisciplinary conferences, outpatient and inpatient evaluations and management, research and scholarly activities. Some centres however will have unique opportunities, such as a higher volume of minimally invasive HPB cases, whether laparoscopic or robotic. Strengths of an HPB alone programme include the opportunity to be exposed to managing a wide variety of both benign and malignant HPB conditions. Depending on the programme, centre workload volume and the institutional practices, the fellow may also have a variable experience involving vascular resections in pancreatic and hepatic surgery.

CGSO HPB

These programmes fit together very well and the fellow's training will encompass surgical oncology including sarcoma, breast/melanoma and complex GI malignancies possibly including cytoreductive procedures and heated intraperitoneal chemotherapy. While the breadth of experience is valuable, particularly understanding that the core of surgical oncology is multidisciplinary care, the drawback of these programmes is the potential for a significantly reduced exposure to benign HPB pathology and procedures (laparoscopic bile duct exploration and acute and chronic pancreatitis including pancreatic necrosectomy). It is worth remembering however, that for the majority of HPB surgeons their substantive position will involve a workload which is not solely HPB, and the additional breadth of training will be of great benefit (18). The CGSO fellowship lasts 24 months and is arranged by disease-specific surgical rotations in addition to multidisciplinary non-surgical rotations such as medicine, radiation oncology and pathology (13). Currently there are 6 CGSO programmes that offer the possibility of a CGSO certification plus Fellowship Council HPB certification.

HPB/TRANSPLANT (ASTS PATHWAY) OR HPB/GI

In HPB/transplant, fellows are well trained in the nuances and science of organ failure, vascular techniques and transplantation. These accredited programmes must not only have an adequate volume of index HPB cases but also have a multidisciplinary approach towards the management of HPB malignancies. The IHPBA also has programmes which combined HPB with upper GI. Though these are not common fellowships, fellows have the benefit of having minimally invasive upper GI training, which will broaden the scope of their post fellowship practice and allow advanced MIS HPB surgery early in one's career.

GEOGRAPHICAL NUANCES

Globally, there are both similarities and differences when acquiring HPB subspecialization training. In Argentina, the HPB surgeons of the 1980s and 1990s were primarily trained in France and the US. Argentina now has 16 HPB fellowships through the IHPBA with 15 of the 16 incorporating transplant (some liver only and others liver and pancreas). A typical fellowship training in Argentina is 2 years after completing 5 years of general surgery residency. In Argentina however, following the completion of an HPB fellowship, there are employment issues relating to disparities between training numbers and trained job opportunities. Options include fellows who have completed the programme staying to work in transplant units or combining HPB with general surgery in a non-tertiary hospital. Similarly in France, HPB and transplant training are integrated and following 5 years of general and digestive surgery the requirement is for at least 2 years of HPB and transplant experience. Currently, post-fellowship positions match the number of HPB jobs with practices generally being pure HPB.

The structure in Ireland is also based on a programme comprising a combined 2-year HPB and transplant fellowship. There are differences however and Irish trainees who wish to pursue an HPB career are only required to complete 2 years of basic surgical training before entering the definitive HPB training programme which last a further 5 years. Many trainees also elect to take a year or two out to complete a higher degree meaning that the actual duration of training is 8–10 years. Even following a training programme of this length, job opportunities are limited but helped by the fact that most fellows are non-Irish EU citizens who return home post-fellowship.

In the Netherlands, there are a number of well-established training centres where 2-year fellowships are offered. The Dutch and Belgium training programmes can be either HPB oncology with transplantation or transplantation alone and generally obtaining pure HPB jobs is difficult and the number of posts very limited with some fellows ultimately having to work as general digestive surgeons performing only simple HPB procedures. Mixed practices remain common, and not unusually comprise a workload with 40% HPB, 40% surgical oncology and 20% general surgery.

In India, HPB and transplantation programmes are separate. India is unique in the volume of radical cholecystectomies performed due to their high incidence of gallbladder cancer. Training programme structures vary but generally include 3 years of general surgery followed by 3 years of surgical oncology or surgical gastroenterology, and an additional 2 years in a transplant fellowship is also an option. Most post-fellowship practices are mixed with at least 50–80% being HPB and the remainder GI surgery. Training options are far less than the demand in this country, which equates to most fellows being unable to acquire a position in their preferred HPB training programme.

In South Africa, pre-fellowship training requires the completion of a 5-year residency in general surgery. Subsequent fellowship programmes are separate with HPB training for 2 years and transplant experience, which includes kidney, for an additional 2 years. The HPB fellowship programmes are accredited unlike the transplant fellowship which is not formalized. The dual heathcare system allows those who cannot be accommodated in an academic HPB unit to continue to practice HPB surgery in private practice.

In Japan, board certification is obtained through the Japanese Society of HPB Surgery (IHPBA Japan chapter). HPB and transplant are integrated with over 200 designated training hospitals being recognized as appropriate institutions for HPB board certification. Pre-fellowship requirements include 2 years of junior residency, 3 years of general surgical residency, 2–5 years of GI surgery subspecialization and finally 3 years of HPB board certification potentially meaning 13 years before certification. Post-fellowship practices are usually pure HPB although some surgeons later in their careers become general GI surgeons.

The training pathway in Australia requires applicants to hold a general surgical fellowship of the Royal Australasian College of Surgeon. Fellowship training consists of 2 years of HPB and 3 years of transplant experience. Upon completion of the training, exit exams are completed, which include both written and oral components. The vast majority of graduates from fellowships are able to find rewarding jobs, whether in the public or private sector.

HPB training is evolving and there is no single optimal approach and debate continues regarding the ideal structure of a training programme particularly in terms of duration, the requirement for a research component and how structured they should be (19,20,15). All programmes have their advantages and disadvantages and the fellow needs to be genuinely eclectic to benefit maximally. One way to nurture a well-rounded fellow is to encourage exchange programmes between institutions spending a variable amount of time at each hospital depending on the training requirements (18). This would be particularly valuable where institutions have pure HPB training programmes and the fellow could be exposed to transplant, oncological or complex GI surgery at a different institution. The nature of the exchange should take into account the fellow's career goals and be sufficiently flexible. In some countries, there are potential issues with this sort of training relating to the licensing of a visiting fellow to ensure they are able to work clinically with no restrictions.

The specialty of HPB surgery is extremely fortunate having experts and educators who have a wide variety of backgrounds and training. For instance, the convergence of training streams can easily produce trainees who are transplant trained, pure HPB trained and HPB/surgical oncology trained. Presently the optimal pathway for training an HPB surgeon remains unclear but individual and national programmes are constantly being refined, aided by the input from international HPB societies. It is unlikely in the foreseeable future that there will be one template for the ideal programme but the goal should always be to ensure that the graduating fellows are well rounded and competent HPB surgeons. Our aim as experts and mentors should not only be to produce technically competent fellows well versed in HPB anatomy but fellows who also have a sound command of cancer biology, HPB diseases, research and multidisciplinary care. When experts from around the world were asked what are the core competencies of an HPB surgeon their answers were strikingly similar and include a thorough knowledge of oncologic principles, technical skills and precision, clinical experience in a high-volume centre, research, team work and empathy.

REFERENCES

1. Jarnagin WR (ed). *Blumgart's Surgery of the Liver, Biliary Tract and Pancreas*, 6th edn. London: Elsevier; 2016.
2. De U. Evolution of cholecystectomy: A tribute to Carl August Langenbuch. *Indian J Surg* 2004;**66(2)**:4.
3. Morgenstern L. Hans Kehr: Not first, but foremost. *Surg Endosc* 1993;**7(3)**:152–4.
4. Ahrendt SA. A history of the bilioenteric anastomosis. *Arch Surg* 1990;**125(11)**:1493.
5. Ioannis S, Petrou A, Christos C, Felekouras E. History of biliary surgery. *World J Surg* 2013;**37**:1006–12.
6. Deitel M. César Roux and his contribution. *Obes Surg* 2007;**17(10)**:1277–8.
7. Binkley JS. Telescopic pancreaticojejunostomy. *Cancer* 1951;**4(2)**:226–32.
8. Radhakrishnan N (ed). Neoplasms of the Endocrine Pancreas: Practice Essentials, Background, Pathophysiology. 2021. Available from: https://emedicine.medscape.com/article/276943-overview. (Accessed 28 August 2024).
9. Are C, Dhir M, Ravipati L. History of pancreaticoduodenectomy: Early misconceptions, initial milestones and the pioneers. *HPB* 2011;**13(6)**:377–84.
10. Bismuth H, Eshkenazy R, Arish A. Milestones in the evolution of hepatic surgery. *Rambam Maimonides Med* 2011;**2(1)**:e0021.
11. Blumgart LH. Resection of the liver. *J Am Coll Surg* 2005;**201(4)**:492–4.
12. Bengmark S. The early days of HPB: A personal reminiscence. *HPB* 2002;**4(3)**:117–21.
13. Jeyarajah DR, Abouljoud M, Alseidi A, Berman R, D'Angelica M, Hagopian E, et al. Training paradigms in hepato-pancreatico-biliary surgery: An overview of the different fellowship pathways. *J Gastrointest Surg* 2021;**25(8)**:2119–28.
14. de Santibañes M, de Santibañes E, Pekolj J. Training in hepato-pancreato-biliary surgery during residency: Past, present and future perspectives: training in hepato-pancreato-biliary surgery during residency: Past, present and future perspectives. *J Hepatobiliary-Pancreat Sci* 2016;**23(12)**:741–4.
15. Seshadri RM, Ali N, Warner S, Cochran A, Vrochides D, Iannitti D, et al. Training and practice of the next generation HPB surgeon: Analysis of the 2014 AHPBA residents' and fellows' symposium survey. *HPB* 2015;**17(12)**:1096–104.
16. Baker EH, Dowden JE, Cochran AR, Iannitti DA, Kimchi ET, Staveley-O'Carroll KF, et al. Qualities and characteristics of successfully matched North American HPB Surgery Fellowship candidates. *HPB* 2016;**18(5)**:479–84.
17. IHPBA. Available from: https://www.ihpba.org/fellowship/?group=Asia+%2F+Pacific (Accessed 30 August 2024).
18. D'Angelica MI, Chapman WC. HPB Surgery: The specialty is here to stay, but the training is in evolution. *Ann Surg Oncol* 2016;**23(7)**:2123–5.
19. Dixon E, Vollmer CM, Bathe O, Sutherland F. Training, practice, and referral patterns in hepatobiliary and pancreatic surgery: Survey of general surgeons. *J Gastrointest Surg Off J Soc Surg Aliment Tract* 2005;**9(1)**:109–14.
20. Edwards J, Bressan A, Dharampal N, Grondin S, Datta I, Dixon E, et al. Hepato-pancreato-biliary surgery workforce in Canada. *Can J Surg* 2015;**58(3)**:212–5.

APPENDIX

HPB-Certification-Requirements_-Incoming-Fellows-2019.pdf

Chapter 12

Hepatobiliary and Pancreatic Imaging

Louise I.T. Lee and Arumugam Rajesh

IMAGING OF THE GALLBLADDER AND BILIARY TRACT

The gallbladder and biliary tract can be evaluated using a variety of imaging modalities. The choice is guided by the patient's clinical presentation and the primary differential diagnosis suspected by the clinical team.

Ultrasound

In the acute setting, ultrasound (US) is the first-choice modality to investigate right upper quadrant pain and is ideal for evaluating gallbladder pathology and biliary obstruction. It is a rapid, reliable and dynamic imaging technique that avoids the use of ionizing radiation, making it an especially attractive option for the younger patient (1,2). Optimal imaging of the gallbladder requires patients to be fasted for 4–6 hours to allow adequate gallbladder distension and visualization of structure and contents.

US has the highest sensitivity and specificity, above 95%, for identifying cholelithiasis (3). Diagnosis of acute calculous cholecystitis is made by identifying cholelithiasis in combination with a positive sonographic Murphy sign, or gallbladder wall thickening, with high, positive predictive values of 92.2% and 95.2%, respectively (4) (*Figure 12.1*). Acute biliary diseases can be rapidly and definitively diagnosed, often with no further imaging required. Although able to detect biliary obstruction, US is somewhat limited in localizing the site and cause, such as in distal choledocholithiasis, where assessment is frequently inadequate due to overlying bowel gas (5). Magnetic resonance cholangiopancreatography (MRCP) is increasingly considered as the next-step imaging modality to localize, characterize and identify the extent of obstruction in such cases (6).

Despite the many recognized advantages of US, there are drawbacks limiting its use in certain clinical situations. These include patients with large body habitus, poor mobility or poor compliance as a result of their acute presentation or comorbidities, or overlying bowel gas degrading images of the biliary tract. Ultrasonography is also heavily operator-dependent, reliant on the training and skillset of the individual to identify and accurately characterize pathology in the context of the patient's clinical presentation.

Computed tomography

Contrast-enhanced computed tomography (CECT) is the most utilized imaging modality for patients presenting to an emergency department with acute abdominal pain. Being widely available and quick to perform (especially beneficial for patients in pain), timely assessment of acute conditions can be made to assist in clinical decision making (7). Superior spatial

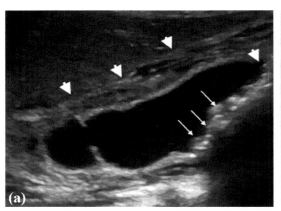
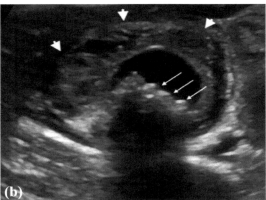

Figure 12.1 US images (a) and (b) show acute calculous cholecystitis. Hyperechogenic gallstones within the gallbladder causing posterior acoustic shadowing (arrows), thickening of the gallbladder wall and pericholecystic free fluid (arrowheads).

DOI: 10.1201/9781003080060-12

resolution delineates abdominal structures in fine detail, allowing for the assessment of acute pathology and complications that may arise with a high degree of accuracy (8). Despite this, CT is not generally regarded as the first-line modality for identifying cholelithiasis or acute biliary disease due to its lower sensitivity and specificity compared with US. Gallstones may not be radio-opaque due to varying composition from calcium to cholesterol, resulting in a sensitivity of 39–75% for the detection of gallstones (9) (*Figure 12.2*). CT is instead reserved for cases where wider differential diagnoses are being considered, such as patients presenting with generalized upper abdominal pain not confined to the right upper quadrant, or for the assessment of complications of gallbladder or biliary tract disease including perforation, gangrene, abscess formation or vascular complications (10).

In the postoperative setting, CT has great utility for complications such as fluid collections or biloma, bile

duct injury, abscess, or haematoma, the extent of which must be well defined to guide further interventional or surgical management (11).

In the non-acute setting when gallbladder or biliary tract malignancy is suspected, CT is preferred over US to identify the local, regional and distant extent of disease, allowing for tumour, node, metastasis (TNM) staging and to guide treatment and management options (12) (*Figure 12.3*).

Magnetic resonance cholangiopancreatography

MRCP is an accurate imaging technique for defining biliary tract anatomy. Patients are fasted for 4 hours to allow gallbladder distension, reduce secretions from the stomach and bowel peristalsis that may otherwise degrade image quality. Basic MRCP sequences vary across institutions, but at a minimum include a heavily

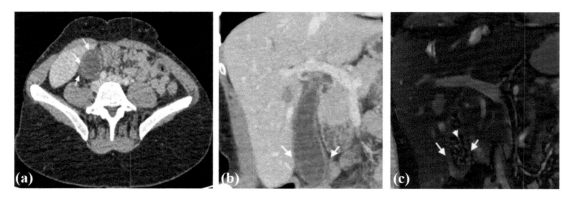

Figure 12.2 CT and MRI scans demonstrating acute cholecystitis. Axial (a) and coronal (b) CT scans show only mild mural-thickening of the gallbladder (arrows) but no radio-opaque gallstones. Coronal MRCP (c) of the same patient better demonstrates mural thickening of the gallbladder (arrows) containing numerous gallstones (arrowhead). This highlights the drawbacks of CT for acute gallbladder pathology, being less sensitive for gallstone detection compared to US and MRI.

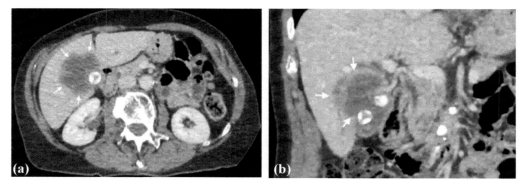

Figure 12.3 CT scans show gallbladder carcinoma. Axial (a) and coronal (b) CT of the upper abdomen shows a large gallbladder mass lesion with extension into the liver (arrows). This was pathologically proven stage T3 gallbladder carcinoma.

transverse relaxation time (T2)-weighted sequence, a T2-weighted maximum intensity projection (MIP) and 3D volume rendering to optimize visualization of the biliary tract (13).

MRCP is an attractive alternative for diagnosing biliary obstruction due to its non-invasive and non-ionising nature in comparison to endoscopic retrograde cholangio pancreatography (ERCP) (14). Characterization of suspected biliary obstruction based on clinical presentation and biochemical markers remains a key indication, especially when other imaging modalities have been exhausted but the cause not elucidated despite clinical suspicion. Both the presence and level of biliary obstruction can be identified with excellent sensitivity and specificity, both over 97% (*Figure 12.4*).

Detection of choledocholithiasis and differentiating benign from malignant biliary obstruction are amongst the strengths of the modality (15). Superior soft-tissue resolution and various sequences used in MRI and MRCP allows diagnosis of the extent of malignant biliary obstruction such as in cholangiocarcinoma (*Figure 12.5*). Tumour spread, biliary duct and blood vessel patency are all evaluated in a single examination, essential for determining surgical resectability, or guiding biliary drainage either through percutaneous routes or ERCP (16). A further benefit of MRCP lies in its ability to identify aberrant and variant biliary anatomy, which is particularly important in patients scheduled for cholecystectomy or hepaticobectomy/ segmentectomy (17).

Limitations of MRI include well-known contra-indications from certain metal work, patient claustrophobia and heavy reliance on patient compliance to 'breath hold' and lie still for relatively long periods of time, which may prove particularly challenging in the acutely unwell.

Hepatobiliary scintigraphy

Widely known as a hepatobiliary iminodiacetic acid (HIDA) scan, this functional imaging technique is most commonly performed using Tc-99m-IDA, a Technetium-99m radiotracer and hepatobiliary iminodiacetic acid agent, taken up by hepatocytes and excreted into the biliary system. Images are taken at intervals determined by the clinical indication. Although seldom used in the acute setting as the first imaging modality due to image acquisition time, patient preparation and relatively limited availability, the HIDA scan is a useful problem-solving tool in certain clinical scenarios when other imaging modalities have already been exhausted, yet findings remain equivocal. Main uses include diagnosis of acute cholecystitis or biliary obstruction. Postoperative

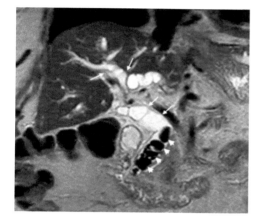

Figure 12.4 MRCP scan shows choledocholithiasis. Coronal T2-weighted image shows multiple common bile duct stones (arrowheads) causing gross intra- and extrahepatic biliary duct dilatation (arrows).

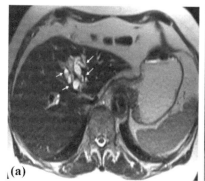 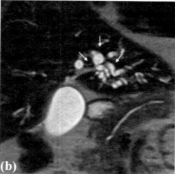 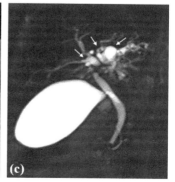

(a)   (b)   (c)

Figure 12.5 MRCP scan shows hilar cholangiocarcinoma causing intrahepatic biliary duct dilatation. Axial (a) and coronal (b) T2-weighted images demonstrate marked dilatation of the intrahepatic ducts (arrows), particularly the left ducts (arrows) due to a stricture proximal to the main biliary confluence. 3D MIP image (c) of the dilated intrahepatic ducts (arrows) and incidental distal common bile duct stone.

indications include assessment for bile leak or injury and biliary enteric anastomotic patency (18).

Percutaneous transhepatic cholangiography

Percutaneous transhepatic cholangiography (PTC) can be performed for diagnostic and/or therapeutic purposes through access to the biliary tract with a needle and catheter, followed by injection of contrast into the ducts under fluoroscopic guidance. Through direct injection of contrast into the proximal biliary ducts, proximal biliary pathology can be more readily identified in comparison to a retrograde approach such as ERCP. The mainstay of use is therapeutic drainage of obstructed biliary ducts caused by benign or malignant conditions. PTC may also be used to obtain histological specimens or direct stent insertion where ERCP attempts have been unsuccessful or technically impossible (19). *Table 12.1* provides a summary of the imaging modalities for the gallbladder and biliary tract.

IMAGING OF THE PANCREAS

Pancreatic imaging in the setting of acute pancreatitis is generally not indicated in patients with a mild, or uncomplicated, clinical course. The advantage of imaging lies in establishing the cause, assessing disease severity and evaluation of complications arising from pancreatic pathology that can guide therapeutic intervention or surgical options (20). On the other hand, imaging of pancreatic lesions requires a multimodality approach to evaluate the pancreatic parenchyma and neighbouring structures. The choice of modality is made considering clinical presentation, availability of local equipment and radiological expertise.

Ultrasound

US has limited ability in imaging the entirety of the pancreas. Imaging may be challenging due to a combination of variables including operator experience, large patient habitus and overlying bowel gas that may obscure clear views of the whole pancreas. Rather than confirming

Table 12.1 The main indications and pros and cons of each imaging modality for imaging of the gallbladder and biliary tract

Modality	Main indications	Pathology identified	Advantages	Disadvantages
US	• Ideal for gallbladder and biliary pathology • Identifies biliary obstruction	• Cholelithiasis • Cholecystitis • Choledocholithiasis • Gallbladder and biliary malignancy • Adenomyomatosis • Polyps	• Non-ionizing • Dynamic • Rapid • Widely available • Portable	• Operator and patient dependent • Limited in localizing distal biliary obstruction
CT	• Diagnosis of other causes of upper abdominal pain • Complications and extent of pathology	• Same as US • Complications: abscess/perforation/gangrene/vascular/etc.	• Widely available • High spatial resolution • Rapid • Other causes of abdominal pain	• Ionizing radiation • Lower sensitivity and specificity versus. US for gallbladder pathology
MRI/MRCP	• Cause and level of biliary obstruction • Aberrant and variant biliary anatomy for surgical planning • Local extent of disease	• Same as US/CT • Choledocholithiasis • Biliary strictures	• Non-ionizing • High soft-tissue contrast resolution • Best for biliary anatomy and cause of obstruction	• General MRI contraindications • Patient compliance • Acquisition time • Availability
HIDA	• Equivocal cases after other modalities exhausted	• Acute cholecystitis • Biliary leak/injury • Biliary obstruction • Biliary enteric anastomotic patency	• High sensitivity and specificity for acute cholecystitis • Physiological and functional assessment	• Ionizing radiation • Patient preparation • Acquisition time • Availability • Poor anatomical detail
PTC	• Therapeutic: relieves biliary obstruction/guides stent insertion • Diagnostic: histological sampling	• Biliary obstruction • Biliary strictures: benign/malignant	• Diagnostic and therapeutic • Ideal for proximal biliary tract • Can be useful when ERCP has failed	• Ionizing radiation • Invasive procedure: risk of sepsis/bile leak/haemorrhage/pneumothorax etc.

a diagnosis of acute pancreatitis, the role of US is reserved for identifying the causative factor, such as gallstones or biliary obstruction and is generally recommended in patients presenting with their first episode of acute pancreatitis (20,21). Due to limitations in imaging, the gland in its entirety and inability to definitively characterize lesions, other modalities such as CT, MRI or endoscopic US are often used in combination to image pancreatic lesions.

Computed tomography

CECT is widely accepted as the preferred imaging modality for evaluating a spectrum of pancreatic diseases. These include lesions such as pancreatic adenocarcinoma, neuroendocrine tumours and pancreatic cystic lesions, as well as determining severity and complications of inflammatory processes in acute and chronic pancreatitis.

The pancreas receives a rich blood supply from branches of the coeliac axis and the superior mesenteric artery. Optimal imaging of pancreatic mass lesions

should therefore involve at least dual-phase acquisition to maximize contrast between the lesion and normal pancreatic parenchyma. This is typically achieved by imaging in late arterial phase (35–40 seconds) and portal venous phase (65–70 seconds) (22).

CT has high-sensitivity, specificity and diagnostic accuracy of 90%, 87% and 89%, respectively, for pancreatic adenocarcinoma (23). Pancreatic adenocarcinoma is most commonly a hypovascular mass, with greatest conspicuity in the late arterial phase (pancreatic phase), where normal pancreatic tissue enhances maximally in comparison to the hypoattenuating lesion. As arterial vasculature is opacified, assessment for tumour invasion or encasement is ideal in this phase. The portal venous phase is important for venous and hepatic enhancement, allowing for assessment of venous thrombus, locoregional tumour spread and distant metastasis. Pancreatic adenocarcinoma carries a particularly poor prognosis so CT has great use in identifying the relatively few candidates suitable for surgical resection (22) (*Figure 12.6*). It is well-recognized that smaller pancreatic lesions less than 2 cm, or isoattenuating lesions, may remain occult

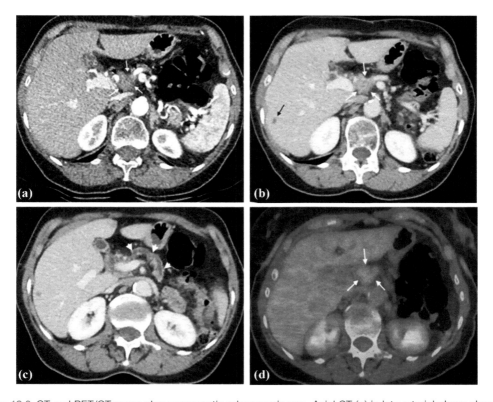

Figure 12.6 CT and PET/CT scans show pancreatic adenocarcinoma. Axial CT (a) in late arterial phase showing a hypoenhancing head of pancreas mass lesion (arrows) with involvement of the hepatic and splenic arteries (black arrowheads). Axial CT (b and c) images in portal venous phase showing the head of pancreas lesion (arrows), which appears less conspicuous compared to late arterial phase, and distal main pancreatic duct dilatation as a result (white arrowheads). Incidental hepatic cyst (black arrow) which was not FDG avid (b). Axial PET/CT (d) shows the FDG avid mass lesion (arrows). Whilst CT is the mainstay for staging pancreatic cancer, PET/CT may sometimes be used to assess for small distant metastasis not identified on CT in potential surgical candidates.

on CT, with only indirect signs present such as the double duct sign, interrupted duct sign or distal pancreatic atrophy. In such cases, endoscopic ultrasound (EUS) remains the 'gold standard' for investigation and diagnosis, enabling histological sampling at the same time. Smaller hepatic metastases may also remain occult on CT, requiring magnetic resonance imaging (MRI) for complete assessment (24).

Pancreatic neuroendocrine tumours (NETs) often present asymptomatically or with vague symptoms. Radiologically, they are usually well-defined, hypervascular tumours that may undergo cystic or necrotic change. Initial detection and staging are performed with CT, utilizing both arterial and portal venous phases, with the hypervascular NET primary and metastases appearing most conspicuous on arterial phase. Nuclear medicine studies such as indium-labelled octreotide and gallium-DOTATE scans play a central role in the diagnosis and staging of pancreatic NETs through improved detection of the primary lesion, distant disease and assessment of disease recurrence (25).

In the acute setting, CT is not indicated in those with mild or uncomplicated acute pancreatitis. Imaging is generally reserved for cases of diagnostic uncertainty, to confirm severity of disease and identify complications in those with a severe clinical course, or when conservative management has failed in clinically deteriorating patients (*Figure 12.7*). ERCP imaging aids in decision-making and guidance of interventional or surgical management. Timing of the initial CT is usually suggested after at least 72–96 hours following symptom onset, as early imaging may otherwise underestimate the final severity of the disease (26). Complications including necrotizing pancreatitis, acute peripancreatic fluid collections, acute necrotic collections, pseudocyst formation, walled-off necrosis or infected necrosis can be identified and may require close follow-up or drainage under image

guidance (*Figure 12.8*). Important vascular complications which can be identified include portal vein or splenic vein thrombosis, splenic artery pseudoaneurysm and/or haemorrhagic pancreatitis. CT is the imaging modality of choice for chronic pancreatitis as it detects both pathognomonic features and complications. Pathognomonic features include duct dilatation, coarse parenchymal and/or intraductal calcifications and atrophy of the parenchyma (27) (*Figure 12.9*).

Magnetic resonance imaging

MRI/MRCP are reliable methods of pancreatic assessment, serving as problem-solving tools when features are indeterminate on CT, due to excellent soft-tissue contrast resolution and the ability to assess pancreatic parenchyma, ductal integrity and neighbouring vascular structures in a single examination. MRI can be utilized in a range of pancreatic diseases including acute and chronic pancreatitis or characterization of solid or cystic pancreatic lesions and is often the next step following either US or CT.

Although at least as effective as CT in assessment of acute pancreatitis, MRI is rarely used in the acute setting in clinical practice generally due to limited accessibility and cost. Patients are often too unwell to co-operate with the 'breath holding' required to obtain satisfactorily diagnostic images. Nevertheless, MRI is useful in characterizing and classifying complex peripancreatic collections arising as a result of pancreatitis and for diagnosis and follow-up of chronic pancreatitis (28).

The principal use of MRI in pancreatic adenocarcinoma is to detect smaller or non-contour deforming lesions, characterize hepatic lesions that are indeterminate on CT and to identify hepatic or peritoneal metastases that remain occult on CT (29).

With cystic pancreatic lesions, MRCP better defines lesional communication with the pancreatic duct

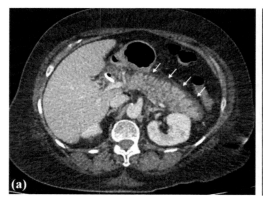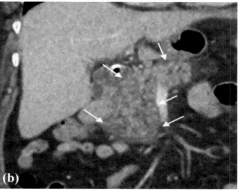

Figure 12.7 CT scan shows acute interstitial oedematous pancreatitis, which in this case occurred post ERCP. Axial (a) and coronal (b) images show pancreatic oedema, inflammatory stranding and free fluid (arrows).

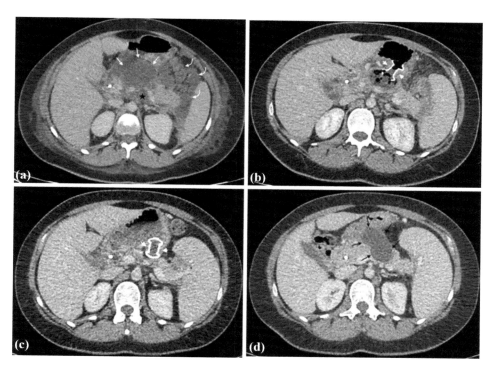

Figure 12.8 CT scans showing acute necrotizing pancreatitis with complications. Axial CT (a) shows marked pancreatic inflammation with an acute necrotic collection (arrows), hypoenhancing pancreatic body consistent with necrosis (star) and peripancreatic free fluid (curved arrows). Insertion of a gastrocystostomy (arrowheads) (b) to drain the pancreatic collection. Successful drainage of the pancreatic collection (c). Interval removal of the gastrocystostomy (d). The patient was reimaged on day 40 due to sepsis and the pancreatic collection had reaccumulated (black arrows), later drained again (not shown here), and found to contain necrotic debris, consistent with walled-off-necrosis.

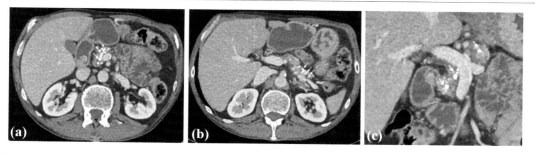

Figure 12.9 CT scans showing features of chronic pancreatitis (arrows). Axial (a,b), and coronal (c) images demonstrate course flecks of pancreatic calcification, atrophic parenchyma and mild duct dilatation.

(*Figure 12.10*). Studies have found similar overall accuracy between MRI and CT in characterizing cystic pancreatic lesions into benign or malignant categories. Either modality may be used for follow-up of cystic lesions (30).

Positron emission tomography/ computed tomography

18-Fluorodexoxyglucose (FDG) is the most commonly used radiotracer in positron emission tomography/ computed tomography PET/CT imaging. PET/CT is not routinely used in pancreatic cancer, but is useful for staging in patients who have localized pancreatic cancer identified on CT, where identification of metastatic disease would otherwise preclude operative management (*see Figure 12.6*). PET/CT may also be useful in selected cases of suspected recurrence where other imaging modalities remain equivocal or negative, despite elevated biochemical markers and persistent clinical suspicion (31).

Table 12.2 provides a summary of the imaging modalities for the pancreas.

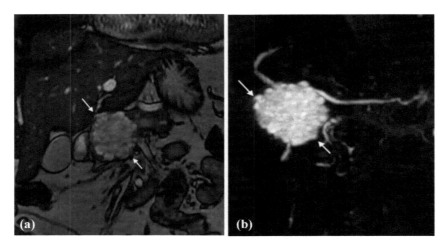

Figure 12.10 MRCP scans showing serous cystadenoma of the pancreas. Coronal T2 (a) and 3D MIP images (b) of a multicystic lesion at the head of pancreas in a 'bunch of grapes' morphology (arrows) with no connection to the main pancreatic duct.

Table 12.2 The main indications and advantages and disadvantages of each imaging modality for imaging of the pancreas

Modality	Main uses/Indications	Pathology identified	Advantages	Disadvantages
US	• Biliary cause of pancreatitis	• Gallstone pancreatitis • Biliary obstruction • May depict pancreatitis complications/ pancreatic lesions	• Non-ionizing • Dynamic • Rapid • Widely available • Portable	• May not visualize whole pancreas • Cannot definitively assess for pancreatic disease
CT	• Pancreatic cancer staging and assessment of surgical resectability • Guides management in complicated pancreatitis • Lesion follow-up	• Acute and chronic pancreatitis • Pancreatitis complications • Pancreatic adenocarcinoma • Cystic pancreatic lesions • Pancreatic NET	• Widely available • High spatial resolution • Rapid • Best modality for calcification	• Ionizing radiation • Small pancreatic lesions may be occult • May not identify small hepatic or peritoneal metastases
MR/MRCP	• Same as CT • Problem solving tool for indeterminate findings (e.g. hepatic lesions on CT)	• Same as CT	• Assesses parenchyma, ducts and vessels all at once • Superior soft-tissue contrast resolution to better characterize lesions	• Poor detection of calcification • Patient compliance in acute setting • Acquisition time • Availability • General MR contraindications
PET/CT	• Staging of localized pancreatic cancer identified on CT	• Pancreatic mass lesion • Distant sites of metastasis	• Identifies metastatic disease occult on other imaging modalities	• Ionizing radiation • Inflammatory or infective processes may be PET avid
Nuclear medicine scans: octreotide and gallium-DOTATE	• Diagnosis, staging and detection of NET recurrence	• Pancreatic NET • Distant sites of metastasis	• Identifies smaller lesions occult on other imaging modalities	• Ionizing radiation • Availability • Acquisition time • Patient preparation

IMAGING OF THE LIVER

Segmental anatomy

The Couinaud classification divides the liver into eight functional segments. Each segment contains dual vascular inflow and biliary drainage via the portal vein, hepatic artery and bile duct, allowing for surgical resection of selected segments without compromising the remainder (32).

The hepatic veins radiate from the inferior vena cava (IVC) and divide the liver into four sections in the vertical plane. In cross-sectional imaging, the middle hepatic vein runs in a plane from the IVC to the gallbladder fossa, known as Cantlie's line, separating the right and left lobes. The right hepatic vein further divides the right lobes into right medial and right lateral segments. The left hepatic vein divides the left lobes into the left medial and left lateral segments.

The bifurcation of the main portal vein (MPV) further divides the liver into upper and lower sections in the horizontal plane. Describing the segments located above and below the portal vein, respectively, the left lateral section contains segments 2 and 3, left medial section contains segments 4a and 4b, right medial section contains segments 8 and 5 and right lateral section contains segments 7 and 6.

Vascular supply

The liver receives dual blood supply, deriving 70–80% of nutrient rich blood from the portal vein and 20–30% of oxygen rich blood from the hepatic artery. Venous drainage occurs through the right, middle and left hepatic veins into the IVC. The caudate lobe (segment 1) is the exception draining directly into the IVC.

Overview of liver imaging

Imaging of the liver involves a multimodality approach directed by the clinical question, availability of imaging and radiological expertise. A variety of modalities including US, CT and MRI are used often in combination to characterize lesions that are indeterminate on one modality alone, to follow up lesions and to guide interventional and surgical procedures.

Ultrasound

Located in the right upper quadrant and close to the abdominal wall, the liver is situated in an ideal location to allow effective hepatic imaging in most patients. A multitude of pathologies can be assessed ranging from diffuse parenchymal disease such as hepatic steatosis or cirrhosis and focal hepatic lesions, for which size, number, morphology, location, echotexture and blood flow can be assessed (33). US is also often employed to direct percutaneous interventional procedures such as biopsies, drains or radiofrequency ablation therapy.

Relative drawbacks include the broad overlap of sonographic features between benign and malignant lesions, thus most focal lesions cannot be definitively characterized by standard B-mode US alone. Small lesions may also be missed, as US is highly dependent on both operator and patient factors.

Contrast-enhanced ultrasound

Contrast-enhanced (CEUS) allows real-time, dynamic assessment of focal hepatic lesions through a combination of a contrast agent, traditional B-mode and Doppler US. Microbubbles are injected into a peripheral vein, which circulate in the bloodstream and persist in the vascular compartment for 4–6 minutes depending on the agent. Dynamic visualization and quantification of blood flow and perfusion characteristics of lesions in the arterial, portal venous and delayed phases can be made, providing crucial information regarding wash-in and wash-out characteristics of benign and malignant hepatic lesions (34).

Over recent years, CEUS has emerged as a valuable imaging technique that has gained popularity around the world, with studies highlighting its accuracy, non-invasive nature, favourable safety profile and positive economic impact for characterizing hepatic lesions. CEUS may be used to complement findings on CT and MRI or as a first-line alternative in patients with renal failure, contrast allergy or claustrophobia. The use of CEUS for hepatic lesions remains highly variable between centres around the world, with a vast majority of the reported experience originating from Asia, Canada and Europe. Limitations include the relatively short transition time between imaging phases, precluding the ability to assess and characterize multiple lesions at once following a single injection of contrast, as well as the general limitations of standard B-mode US imaging (35).

Doppler ultrasound

Doppler US consists of standard grey-scale (B-mode) US with either colour Doppler or both colour Doppler and spectral Doppler superimposed. The haemodynamics of the portal vein, hepatic artery and hepatic veins can be assessed through the presence of blood flow, direction of blood flow, waveform morphology and velocity. Conditions resulting in alteration of normal hepatic blood flow such as cirrhosis and portal hypertension and hepatic veno-occlusive disease can be readily evaluated through this technique. Another use is for evaluation of transjugular intrahepatic portosystemic (TIPS) patency postintervention in those with portal hypertension (36,37).

Computed tomography

The single most-used protocol for general imaging of the abdomen is performed in single portal venous phase, most suited to cases where abdominal imaging is required, but not specifically to assess a hepatic lesion. The diverse nature of hepatic conditions means not one single CT protocol is suitable in all clinical scenarios. A protocol, tailored to the clinical question, must be selected to yield appropriate and beneficial information to the individual patient. The use of contrast and specific imaging phases serve to maximize conspicuity between the hepatic lesion in question and the background parenchyma.

Before selection of the appropriate protocol, it is important to consider the hepatic blood supply and type of lesion to be assessed across different imaging phases. The liver receives dual blood supply from the portal vein and hepatic artery, 70–80% of which arrives through the portal vein. The background parenchyma is therefore at maximal enhancement during the portal venous phase (65–70 seconds after injection).

Primary tumours, such as hepatocellular carcinoma (HCC), originating from the liver receive blood supply from the hepatic artery, are hypervascular tumours and best depicted on the late arterial (35–40 seconds) phase. In contradistinction, secondary tumours that metastasize to the liver, such as colorectal metastases, are hypovascular lesions, most conspicuous on the portal venous phase when the hepatic parenchyma is at maximal enhancement. The exceptions are hypervascular metastases of renal, thyroid, neuroendocrine, breast or melanoma origin, all best demonstrated in the arterial phase (38). Imaging in cases of intrahepatic cholangiocarcinoma benefit from an additional delayed phase as there may be areas of fibrosis that demonstrate persistent enhancement after normal contrast wash-out from the background liver parenchyma (39). A delayed phase is also required in cases of benign haemangioma, where there is usually homogenous contrast retention in the lesion on delayed blood pool images (*Figure 12.11*) (40).

Taking the above into account, general imaging of hepatic lesions requires at least dual-phase imaging (late arterial and portal venous), especially when screening patients with cirrhosis or HCC, or when there is a hypervascular primary tumour originating outside the liver, with suspected hepatic metastases. Depending on the institution and hepatic lesion to be interrogated, triple-phase (non-contrast, arterial and portal venous) or even quadruple-phase (triple-phase with addition delayed-phase) imaging may be utilized for benign and malignant lesions, in order to assess wash-in and wash-out characteristics and to assess contrast retention.

Magnetic resonance imaging

MRI provides the most comprehensive evaluation of hepatic pathology of all the imaging modalities. The range of imaging sequences allows characterization of diffuse parenchymal abnormalities and focal lesions beyond that possible with US or CT. Basic

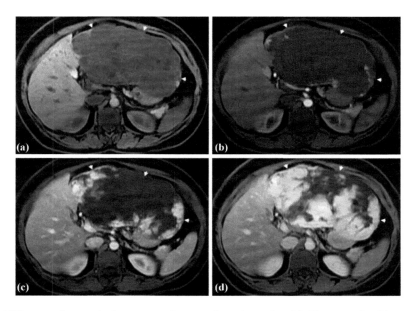

Figure 12.11 MRI scans show a giant cavernous haemangioma (arrowheads). T1 pre-contrast image (a) showing a large haemangioma centred in the left lobe of the liver. T1 post-contrast arterial (b), portal venous (c) and 10-minute delay (d), respectively. There is progressive, peripheral nodular enhancement and centripetal fill into near total by 10-minute delay. No contrast wash-out.

imaging protocols vary between institutions, but broadly encompass a combination of T2-weighted fast-spin-echo, gradient-echo T1-weighted in and opposed-phase, fat-saturated T2-weighted, dynamic pre- and post-contrast T1-weighted imaging and diffusion-weighted imaging. Contrast agents consist of extracellular agents and hepatocyte-specific agents, the selection depending on the clinical scenario. Extracellular agents equilibrate within the extracellular space and are excreted by the kidneys, allowing for enhancement patterns to be studied through arterial, portal venous and equilibration phases (41). Hepatocyte-specific agents are taken up by both the extracellular space and hepatocytes and excreted through the kidney and the biliary system, thus also allowing enhancement patterns to be studied in the hepatobiliary phase (42).

Application in hepatic imaging can broadly be split into two categories, either cases that require problem-solving or for surgical work-up. MRI is a great problem-solving tool when findings are equivocal on other modalities, such as clinically suspected lesions that have not been identified despite rising tumour markers or for characterizing indeterminate lesions. Smaller malignant lesions, which were not visualized on other modalities may be identified, as well as relationship with important neighbouring vasculature and biliary structures. Overall sensitivity and specificity for the detection of small hepatic metastases, especially with colorectal metastases (*Figure 12.12*) and identifying small HCC in cirrhotic patients (*Figure 12.13*) is higher compared with CT (43,44). MRI therefore plays an important role in the surgical workup of patients being assessed for hepatic resection, transplantation or chemoembolization/ablation therapy.

Table 12.3 provides a summary of the imaging modalities for the liver and *Table 12.4* the typical imaging characteristics of common benign and malignant hepatic lesions.

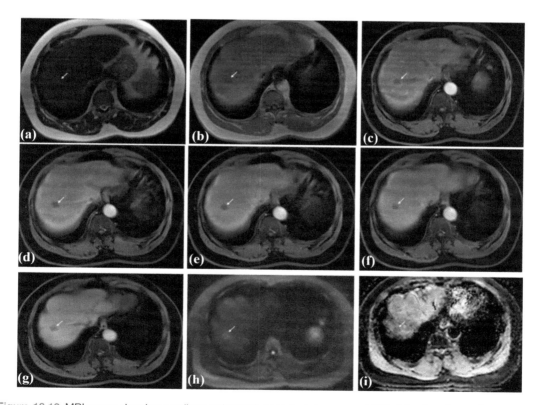

Figure 12.12 MRI scans showing a solitary colorectal metastasis in segment 7/8 of the liver (arrows), which was less conspicuous on CT (not shown). Slightly hyperintense on T2 (a). T1 pre-contrast (b). T1 post-contrast arterial phase demonstrating perilesional enhancement (c). T1 post-contrast portal venous phase demonstrating rapid wash-out (d). T1 post-contrast 90 seconds (e), 2 minutes (f) and 20 minutes delay (g) demonstrating no retention of contrast. Diffusion images, diffusion weight imaging (DWI) (h) and apparent diffusion coefficient (ADC) (i) demonstrating diffusion restriction. Colorectal hepatic metastases tend to show rapid lesional/perilesional enhancement and wash-out with no retention of contrast and demonstrates diffusion restriction.

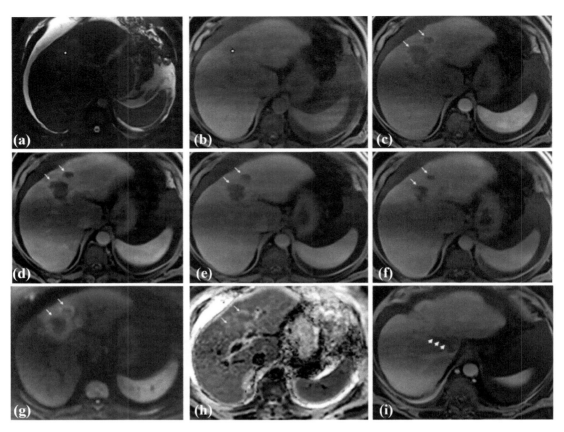

Figure 12.13 MRI scans showing multifocal hepatocellular carcinoma in a cirrhotic liver with ascites. Lesions are slightly hyperintense on T2 (star) (a). T1 pre-contrast appears rather inconspicuous (star) (b). T1 post-contrast arterial (c) and portal venous phases (d), both demonstrating perilesional enhancement (arrows). T1 post-contrast 2-minute (e) and 10-minute delay (f) demonstrating perilesional wash-out with no retention of contrast (arrows). Diffusion images DWI (g), and ADC (h), respectively, demonstrating diffusion restriction (arrows). Showing hepatic vein thrombosis (arrowheads) (i).

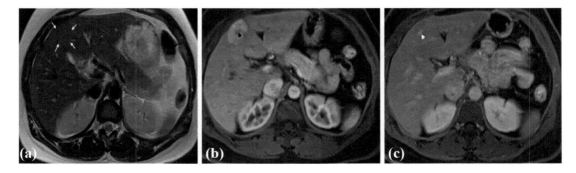

Figure 12.14 MRI scans showing focal nodular hyperplasia. T2 image showing FNH in segment 4 (a), appearing isointense to surrounding liver parenchyma (arrows). Post-contrast portal venous phase image (b) showing enhancement of most of the lesion and a centrally hypoenhancing scar (black arrowhead). 20-minute delay image (c) shows lesion wash-out with a centrally enhancing scar (white arrowhead).

Table 12.3 The main indications and advantages and disadvantages of each imaging modality for imaging the liver

Modality	Main uses/Indications	Pathology identified	Advantages	Disadvantages
US	• Often first line to assess the liver	• Diffuse liver disease • Focal lesions: benign and malignant	• Non-ionizing • Dynamic • Rapid • Widely available • Portable • Guides IR procedures: biopsy/drainage/treatment	• Operator and patient dependent • May miss smaller lesions • Cannot definitively characterize lesions (except simple cysts)
CT	• Staging of malignancy • Assessment of surgical resectability • Guides IR/surgical management	• Same as US • Features of decompensated liver disease: cirrhosis, portal hypertension (HTN), ascites, splenomegaly	• Widely available • High spatial resolution • Rapid • Allows TNM staging	• Ionizing radiation • Lesions may remain indeterminate • May not identify smaller lesions
MRI	• Characterization of lesions • Same as CT	• Same as US/CT	• Non-ionizing • High soft-tissue contrast resolution • Most comprehensive modality to evaluate liver pathology	• General MRI contraindications • Patient compliance • Acquisition time • Availability

Table 12.4 The typical imaging characteristics of common benign and malignant hepatic lesions (non-exhaustive list)

BENIGN LESIONS

	US (Non contrast)	CT	MRI
Simple cyst	• Anechoic • Well defined • Thin/imperceptible wall • No colour Doppler flow	• Fluid/water attenuation • Thin/imperceptible wall • No soft-tissue component	• T1 hypointense • T2 hyperintesnse • No diffusion restriction • No enhancement
Haemangioma	• Well defined • Hyperechoic • Peripheral feeding vessel	• Low attenuation • Arterial phase: peripheral, nodular enhancement • Portal venous (PV) phase: progressive peripheral enhancement + centripetal fill-in • Delayed phase: contrast retention	• T2 shine through • Same enhancement characteristics as CT
Focal nodular hyperplasia (FNH)	• Variable, may be isoechogenic • May have central scar which displaces peripheral vessels on colour Doppler flow	• Arterial phase: homogenous enhancement, except central scar • PV phase: hypo/isodense • Delayed phase: fibrotic central scar may enhance	• T1 isointense/hypointense with hypointense central scar • T2 isointense/hyperintense with hyperintense central scar • Post-contrast: avid arterial enhancement, isointense PV, central scar retains contrast on delayed phase (*Figure 12.14*) • Hepatocyte specific contrast: enhancement on hepatobiliary phase

(Continued)

Table 12.4 (*Continued*) The typical imaging characteristics of common benign and malignant hepatic lesions (non-exhaustive list)

BENIGN LESIONS

	US (Non contrast)	CT	MRI
Adenoma	• Well-defined, heterogeneous mass • Variable echotexture	• Variable: hyperattenuating if haemorrhagic/hypoattenuating if fat-containing • Post-contrast: arterial enhancement, isodense on PV and delayed	• T1 hyperintense if fat-containing • Signal drop-out between T1, in-and-out phases, if fat-containing • Heterogenous signal if haemorrhagic • Same enhancement characteristics as CT

MALIGNANT LESIONS

	US (Non contrast)	CT	MRI
HCC	• Hypoechoic if small • Mixed echogenicity if large – may contain fibrosis, fat, necrosis, calcification	• Background cirrhotic liver • Post-contrast: avid arterial enhancement and non-peripheral rapid wash-out, becoming indistinct on PV and delayed • May have persistently enhancing pseudocapsule, perfusion abnormality: arterioportal shunt or enhancing portal vein tumour thrombus	• Same enhancement characteristics as CT • Diffusion restriction
Intrahepatic Cholangiocarcinoma	• Well-defined, irregular mass • May have capsular retraction, dilated distal bile ducts, peripheral hypoechoic halo of compressed liver parenchyma	• Well-defined, irregular mass • Post-contrast: incomplete, minimal rim enhancement during arterial and PV Centrally may retain contrast on delayed phase • Dilated distal bile ducts • Capsular retraction • Rarely causes tumour thrombus in vessels (versus HCC)	• Same enhancement characteristics as CT • Diffusion restriction
Hypovascular metastases (e.g. colorectal)	• Most are hypoechoic • May have hypoechoic halo • Mass effect, distorts vessels	• Hypoattenuating versus normal liver parenchyma on PV phase • Typically, perilesional enhancement with wash-out on delayed phase	• T1 hypointense • T2 mildly hyperintense • Enhancement: lesional or perilesional with wash-out • Diffusion restriction
Hypervascular metastases (e.g. RCC/NET)	• Mostly hyperechoic	• Hyperenhancement on arterial phase • Rapid wash-out on PV and delayed phases	• Same enhancement characteristics as CT • Diffusion restriction

REFERENCES

1. Yarmish GM, Smith MP, Rosen MP, Baker ME, Blake MA, Cash BD, et al. ACR appropriateness criteria right upper quadrant pain. *J Am Coll Radiol* 2014;**11**(**3**):316–22.
2. Harvey RT, Miller WT. Acute biliary disease: Initial CT and follow-up US versus initial US and follow-up CT. *Radiology* 1999;**213**(**3**):831–6.
3. Shea JA. Revised estimates of diagnostic test sensitivity and specificity in suspected biliary tract disease. *Arch Intern Med* 1994;**154**(**22**):2573.
4. Ralls PW, Colletti PM, Lapin SA, Chandrasoma P, Boswell WD, Ngo C, et al. Real-time sonography in suspected acute cholecystitis. Prospective evaluation of primary and secondary signs. *Radiology* 1985;**155**(**3**):767–71.

5. Laing FC, Jeffrey RB, Wing VW, Nyberg DA. Biliary dilatation: Defining the level and cause by real-time US. *Radiology* 1986;**160**(**1**):39–42.

6. Mandelia A. The value of magnetic resonance chol-angio-pancreatography (MRCP) in the detection of choledocholithiasis. *J Clin Diagn Res* 2013;**7**(**9**):1941–5.

7. Lameris W, van Randen A, van Es HW, van Hee-sewijk JPM, van Ramshorst B, Bouma WH, et al. Imaging strategies for detection of urgent conditions in patients with acute abdominal pain: Diagnostic accuracy study. *BMJ* 2009;**338**:b2431.

8. Wang J, Fleischmann D. Improving spatial resolution at CT: Development, benefits, and pitfalls. *Radiology* 2018;**289**(**1**):261–2.

9. Benarroch-Gampel J, Boyd CA, Sheffield KM, Townsend CM, Riall TS. Overuse of CT in patients with complicated gallstone disease. *J Am Coll Surg* 2011;**213**(**4**):524–30.

10. Shakespear JS, Shaaban AM, Rezvani M. CT Find-ings of acute cholecystitis and its complications. *Am J Roentgenol* 2010;**194**(**6**):1523–9.

11. Thurley PD, Dhingsa R. Laparoscopic cholecys-tectomy: Postoperative imaging. *Am J Roentgenol* 2008;**191**(**3**):794–801.

12. Kalra N, Suri S, Gupta R, Natarajan SK, Khandelwal N, Wig JD, et al. MDCT in the staging of gallbladder carcinoma. *Am J Roentgenol* 2006;**186**(**3**):758–62.

13. Griffin N, Charles-Edwards G, Grant LA. Magnetic resonance cholangiopancreatography: The ABC of MRCP. *Insights Imaging* 2012;**3**(**1**):11–21.

14. Chen W, Mo J-J, Lin L, Li C-Q, Zhang J-F. Diag-nostic value of magnetic resonance cholangiopan-creatography in choledocholithiasis. *World J Gastro-enterol* 2015;**21**(**11**):3351–60.

15. Romagnuolo J, Bardou M, Rahme E, Joseph L, Reinhold C, Barkun AN. Magnetic resonance chol-angiopancreatography: A meta-analysis of test per-formance in suspected biliary disease. *Ann Intern Med* 2003;**139**(**7**):547.

16. Vanderveen KA. Magnetic resonance imaging of cholangiocarcinoma. *Cancer Imaging* 2004;**4**(**2**):104–15.

17. Mortelé KJ, Ros PR. Anatomic variants of the bili-ary tree: MR cholangiographic findings and clinical applications. *Am J Roentgenol* 2001;**177**(**2**):389–94.

18. Ziessman HA. Nuclear medicine hepatobiliary im-aging. *Clin Gastroenterol Hepatol* 2010;**8**(**2**):111–16.

19. van der Gaag NA, Kloek JJ, de Castro SMM, Bus-ch ORC, van Gulik TM, Gouma DJ. Preoperative biliary drainage in patients with obstructive jaun-dice: History and current status. *J Gastrointest Surg* 2009;**13**(**4**):814–20.

20. Baker ME, Nelson RC, Rosen MP, Blake MA, Cash BD, Hindman NM, et al. ACR Appropri-ateness Criteria® Acute Pancreatitis. *Ultrasound Q* 2014;**30**(**4**):267–73.

21. Koo BC, Chinogureyi A, Shaw AS. Imaging acute pancreatitis. *Br J Radiol* 2010;**83**(**986**):104–12.

22. Ichikawa T, Erturk SM, Sou H, Nakajima H, Tsu-kamoto T, Motosugi U, et al. MDCT of pancreat-ic adenocarcinoma: Optimal imaging phases and multiplanar reformatted imaging. *Am J Roentgenol* 2006;**187**(**6**):1513–20.

23. Toft J, Hadden WJ, Laurence JM, Lam V, Yuen L, Janssen A, et al. Imaging modalities in the diagnosis of pancreatic adenocarcinoma: A systematic review and meta-analysis of sensitivity, specificity and diag-nostic accuracy. *Eur J Radiol* 2017;**92**:17–23.

24. Müller MF, Meyenberger C, Bertschinger P, Schaer R, Marincek B. Pancreatic tumors: Evaluation with endoscopic US, CT, and MR imaging. *Radiology* 1994;**190**(**3**):745–51.

25. Sundin A. Radiological and nuclear medicine imaging of gastroenteropancreatic neuroendocrine tumours. *Best Pract Res Clin Gastroenterol* 2012;**26**(**6**):803–18.

26. IAP/APA evidence-based guidelines for the man-agement of acute pancreatitis. *Pancreatology* 2013;**13**(**4**):e1–15.

27. Thoeni RF. The Revised Atlanta Classification of Acute Pancreatitis: Its importance for the ra-diologist and its effect on treatment. *Radiology* 2012;**262**(**3**):751–64.

28. Robinson PJA, Sheridan MB. Pancreatitis: Comput-ed tomography and magnetic resonance imaging. *Eur Radiol* 2000;**10**(**3**):401–8.

29. Miller FH, Rini NJ, Keppke AL. MRI of Ad-enocarcinoma of the pancreas. *Am J Roentgenol* 2006;**187**(**4**):W365–74.

30. Visser BC, Yeh BM, Qayyum A, Way LW, Mc-Culloch CE, Coakley FV. Characterization of cys-tic pncreatic masses: Relative accuracy of CT and MRI. *Am J Roentgenol* 2007;**189**(**3**):648–56.

31. The Royal College of Radiologists, Royal College of Physicians of London, Royal College of Physi-cians and Surgeons of Glasgow, Royal College of Physicians of Edinburgh, British Nuclear Medicine Society, Administration of Radioactive Substances Advisory Committee. Evidence-based indications for the use of PET-CT in the United Kingdom 2016. *Clin Radiol* 2016;**71**(**7**):e171–88.

32. Couinaud C. *Le foie. Etudes anatomiques et chirurgi-cales*. Paris: Masson; 1957.

33. Harvey CJ, Albrecht T. Ultrasound of focal liver le-sions. *Eur Radiol* 2001;**11**(**9**):1578–93.

34. Claudon M, Dietrich C, Choi B, Cosgrove D, Kudo M, Nolsøe C, et al. Guidelines and Good Clinical Practice Recommendations for Contrast Enhanced Ultrasound (CEUS) in the Liver – Update 2012. *Ul-traschall Med Eur J Ultrasound* 2012;**34**(**01**):11–29.

35. D'Onofrio M, Crosara S, De Robertis R, Canestrini S, Mucelli RP. Contrast-enhanced ultrasound of focal liver lesions. *Am J Roentgenol* 2015;**205**(**1**):W56–66.

36. Kok EJ van der Jagt, EB Haag Th. The value of doppler ultrasound in cirrhosis and portal hyperten-sion. *Scand J Gastroenterol* 1999;**34**(**230**):82–8.

37. McNaughton DA, Abu-Yousef MM. Dop-pler US of the liver made simple. *RadioGraphics* 2011;**31**(**1**):161–88.

38. Oliver JH, Baron RL. Helical biphasic contrast-enhanced CT of the liver: Technique, indications, in-terpretation, and pitfalls. *Radiology* 1996;**201**(**1**):1–14.

39. Lacomis JM, Baron RL, Oliver JH, Nalesnik MA, Federle MP. Cholangiocarcinoma: Delayed CT con-trast enhancement patterns. *Radiology* 1997;**203**(**1**):98–104.

40. Oto A, Kulkarni K, Nishikawa R, Baron RL. Contrast enhancement of hepatic hemangiomas on multiphase MDCT: Can we diagnose hepatic hemangiomas by comparing enhancement with blood pool? *Am J Roentgenol* 2010;**195**(2):381–6.

41. Morcos SK. Extracellular gadolinium contrast agents: Differences in stability. *Eur J Radiol* 2008;**66**(2):175–9.

42. Thian YL, Riddell AM, Koh D-M. Liver-specific agents for contrast-enhanced MRI: Role in oncological imaging. *Cancer Imaging Off Publ Int Cancer Imaging Soc* 2013;**13**(4):567–79.

43. Floriani I, Torri V, Rulli E, Garavaglia D, Compagnoni A, Salvolini L, et al. Performance of imaging modalities in diagnosis of liver metastases from colorectal cancer: A systematic review and meta-analysis. *J Magn Reson Imaging* 2010;**31**(1): 19–31.

44. Wang G, Zhu S, Li X. Comparison of values of CT and MRI imaging in the diagnosis of hepatocellular carcinoma and analysis of prognostic factors. *Oncol Lett* 2019;**17**(1):1184–8.

Chapter

13

Tissue and Molecular Diagnosis

Trisha Kanani and Wen-Ning Cong

INTRODUCTION

Hepato-pancreatico-biliary (HPB) surgery requires precise diagnostic approaches to optimize treatment planning and improve patient outcomes. The management of complex HPB disease necessitates a multidisciplinary approach to ensure accurate preoperative diagnosis and the implementation of targeted and efficient treatment strategies. Given the intricate and complex nature of these pathologies which often manifest non-specific symptoms, a solid interspecialty understanding of the histopathological features and molecular characteristics of HPB lesions is increasingly important for HPB surgeons. This is particularly crucial in a time of rapid technological advancements and the integration of artificial intelligence (AI).

This chapter aims to provide a comprehensive overview of the value of tissue and molecular diagnostic techniques in HPB surgery. It emphasizes the significance of these approaches in enhancing precision, guiding treatment decisions, and improving patient outcomes. The chapter will examine the principles and applications of tissue diagnosis, including histopathological examination, margin assessment, and immunohistochemistry. Additionally, molecular diagnostic techniques such as next-generation sequencing, *in situ* hybridization, and polymerase chain reaction (PCR) will be discussed. We emphasize the role of these techniques in tumour classification, therapeutic targeting, and the detection of minimal residual disease. Furthermore, novel approaches with targeted treatment strategies and immunotherapies based on specific molecular abnormalities is a promising tool for improving outcomes in HPB disease.

BENEFITS OF TISSUE AND MOLECULAR DIAGNOSIS

HPB surgery is complex and the range of pathologies mandates the consideration of radiological imaging, surgical findings and postoperative histopathology in the context of a multidisciplinary team (MDT) in order to plan management strategies that are targeted and efficient. These pathologies vary considerably, and not infrequently present a diagnostic conundrum with non-specific symptoms. A sound interspeciality professional understanding of the histopathological features

Table 13.1 Benefits of tissue and molecular diagnosis

- Establishing a definitive diagnosis
- Differential diagnosis and subtyping
- Predicting prognosis and patient outcomes
- Aiding risk stratification
- Guiding treatment decisions
- Monitoring treatment response
- Detecting recurrence

and molecular characteristics of HPB lesions is of increasing importance for the HPB surgeon, particularly in an era of rapidly evolving technology and advances in precision medicine based on sophisticated technologies. Not only do these diagnostic techniques allow effective evaluation and characterization of hepatic and pancreatic lesions, but they also have a fundamental role in guiding treatment strategies, predicting outcomes and facilitating comparisons between series. The benefits of precision from tissue and molecular diagnosis are outlined in *Table 13.1*.

TISSUE DIAGNOSIS IN HPB SURGERY

Biopsy techniques

The precise identification and characterization of HPB lesions is imperative to provide a foundation for surgical planning and predicting potential outcomes of disease. Tissue diagnostic techniques involve the analysis of specimens retrieved following a biopsy, which is a representative sample of tissue or cells. This critical diagnostic tool allows assessment and evaluation of histopathological, cytological or molecular characteristics and *Table 13.2* summarizes the various presently available biopsy techniques.

Percutaneous biopsies are often needle biopsies obtained under radiological guidance, whereas endoscopic biopsies are retrieved during gastroscopy, endoscopic ultrasound (EUS) or endoscopic retrograde cholangiopancreatography (ERCP). Surgical biopsies can be taken intraoperatively and if required sent for real-time frozen section analysis. The specimen is routinely fixed in formalin and processed using

DOI: 10.1201/9781003080060-13

Table 13.2 Presently available biopsy techniques and their advantages and limitations

	Percutaneous	Endoscopic	Surgical	Frozen section
Principle	• Needle biopsy under image guidance	• Tissue obtained using an endoscope (ERCP or EUS)	• Direct tissue excision during surgical procedure	• Frozen section analysis of samples taken intraoperatively
Indication	• Commonly used to diagnose and stage liver lesions	• Commonly used to diagnose and stage pancreatic lesions	• Performed during open or minimally invasive surgical procedures	• Margin assessment and facilitate decision-making intraoperatively
Advantages	• Minimally invasive • Cost-effective • Access to deep-seated lesions	• Direct visualization • Precision • Simultaneous therapeutic intervention (e.g. stenting)	• Macroscopic assessment of lesion • Simultaneous resection	• Real-time assessment • Guides surgical management
Limitations	• Risk of sampling error • Risk of injury to adjacent structures and bleeding	• Risk of complications such as bleeding or perforation • Size and location of lesion may affect sampling	• Invasive • Complications such as bleeding, infection and anaesthetic risks	• Sampling error • Inter-observer variability • Prolongs surgery

haematoxylin and eosin (H&E) staining. Highly skilled histopathologists have a pivotal role in defining these lesions by examining distinct cellular aberrations, tissue architecture and the presence, or absence of specific molecular biomarkers.

Immunohistochemistry

Immunohistochemistry (IHC) facilitates the detection of specific proteins or antigens expressed in tissue samples. Selected primary antibodies are used and bind to a target antigen in the tissue section and subsequently antigen-antibody complexes can be visualized after signal amplification with a secondary antibody (indirect IHC). This allows the differentiation of various malignancies, subtyping of tumours, and the identification of specific biomarkers that have prognostic significance. For example, the detection of Ki-67 as a marker of the proliferative activity of tumour cells is frequently used to predict aggressive malignant potential and poor prognosis. It is also valuable in differentiating benign lesions (such as focal nodular hyperplasia and hepatocellular adenoma) from hepatocellular carcinoma (HCC). Ki-67 is also frequently used to assess the response to neoadjuvant chemotherapy in patients with pancreatic ductal adenocarcinoma (PDAC) and to predict prognosis, with a lower Ki-67 index being favourable.

Another crucial role of IHC is the ability to identify primary cell types from metastatic lesions in the liver and pancreas. Hepatocyte-specific antigen (also known as HepPar-1) is a reliable marker for HCC as it is highly expressed in hepatocytes and so can be used in IHC staining to differentiate primary HCC from a secondary metastasis. Furthermore, cytokeratins are proteins expressed in epithelial cells and have also proved valuable in differentiating HCC from metastatic adenocarcinomas. The protein cytokeratin-7 (CK7) is another marker which is often positive in primary HCCs as it is expressed by biliary epithelial cells, whereas CK20 positivity would be more associated with colorectal adenocarcinoma. Lung metastases to the liver are usually positive for thyroid transcription factor 1 (TTF-1). This differentiation is vital to allow appropriate management.

Key histopathological features

Tissue diagnosis provides key details pertaining to the nature of these lesions and their malignant potential, as well as identifying specific molecular alterations which may influence treatment strategies. As clinical signs and symptoms are usually vague and non-specific and radiological features are frequently initially similar for a number of HPB pathologies especially with liver lesions, the ability to achieve a definitive diagnosis as quickly as possible is crucial. As well as confirming malignant transformation, tissue diagnosis can also detect benign conditions such as hepatitis or cirrhosis. *Table 13.3* outlines the characteristic histopathological features of common HPB lesions, including HCC, cholangiocarcinoma, and PDAC.

Margin assessment

Histopathological evaluation of resection margins is an important tool in HPB surgery to confirm adequate tumour resection margins and indicate the potential for residual disease or the risk of recurrence, which helps

Table 13.3 The characteristic histopathological features of common HPB lesions

Common HPB lesions	Characteristic histopathological features	IHC markers
Hepatocellular carcinoma	• Trabecular or pseudoglandular growth pattern • Nuclear atypia, including enlarged and hyperchromatic nuclei • Mallory bodies • Fibrous stroma • Mitotic figures • Sinusoidal invasion	• HepPar1 • Glypican 3 • Alpha-fetoprotein • Hepatocyte-specific antigen
Cholangiocarcinoma	• Tubular or glandular growth patterns • Desmoplastic stromal reaction around tumour glands • Nuclear atypia, including enlarged and hyperchromatic nuclei • Mucin production • Perineural invasion • Ductal differentiation	• Cytokeratin 7 • Cytokeratin 19 • MUC1
Pancreatic ductal adenocarcinoma	• Infiltrating glands composed of cuboidal or columnar epithelium • Dense desmoplastic stromal reaction • Nuclear atypia, with enlarged nuclei, irregular nuclear contours, prominent nucleoli • Intra- or extra-cellular mucin production, identified with mucin stains such as mucicarmine or alcian blue	• Cytokeratin 19 • Carcinoembryonic antigen • Ca 19-9
Pancreatic neuroendocrine tumours	• Nests or cords of uniform cells with round nuclei and stippled chromatin • Mitotic figures • Cytoplasmic granules • Nuclear pseudoinclusions • Vascular invasion	• Chromogranin A • Synaptophysin • Insulin

to establish the need for further operative intervention, adjuvant therapy, or closer surveillance. Frozen section analysis of tissue samples taken intraoperatively allows for the rapid assessment of margins during surgery and is able to guide the surgeon, in real time, to ensure an adequate, potentially curative resection. This technique, although valuable, is limited by the risk of freezing artefacts and inadequate sampling which may compromise diagnostic accuracy.

A resected specimen with no malignant cells at the resected margin (R0 resection) is associated with optimal oncological outcomes. Positive resection margins (R1 and R2 resections) suggest that there are malignant cells at the margin of the surgical specimen, and this is associated with a higher risk of recurrence and reduced survival. R1 resections may require further operative intervention or adjuvant systemic chemotherapy to achieve local tumour control and the best possible outcome.

Staging and grading

The accurate staging and grading of HPB tumours within standardized frameworks is essential to predict prognosis, guide clinical decision-making, and determine treatment strategies. The tumour, node, metastasis (TNM) system stages tumours based on the size of the primary tumour (T), involvement of lymph nodes (N) and the presence or absence of metastases (M). This system can be used to stage HCC, cholangiocarcinoma and PDAC. Examples of other staging systems include the Barcelona clinic liver cancer staging system for HCC (1) and the Bismuth–Corlette classification for hilar cholangiocarcinoma (2). Tumour differentiation is assessed with grading systems such as the Edmondson–Steiner classification for HCC (3) and the World Health Organization grading system.

Despite the benefits, inter-observer variability and subjectivity in interpreting histopathological characteristics can affect the reliability of these staging and grading systems. Achieving a precise tissue diagnosis with tumour stage and grade is crucial in facilitating multidisciplinary and interspeciality decision-making in HPB surgery. Histopathological features serve as the foundation for further molecular analyses and patient-specific approaches to management.

MOLECULAR DIAGNOSIS IN HPB SURGERY

Advances in molecular diagnostic techniques have revolutionized the diagnosis and management of HPB cancers, which are characterized by a range of genetic mutations and alterations. These biological assays detect markers of a disease and due to the sensitivity of the assays, sample acquisition is far less invasive than traditional techniques such as biopsies. The identification of specific genetic alterations can guide targeted therapies and predict response to treatment.

These techniques involve DNA/RNA analysis, gene expression profiling and the detection of mutations. DNA sequencing and genotyping allows specific genetic alterations to be identified, such as point mutations, insertions, and deletions. The ability to profile tumours based on DNA analysis allows them to be differentiated into subtypes with different potential therapeutic targets. RNA analysis with gene expression profiling allows the molecular pathways driving tumour growth to be understood, further assisting tumour classification and prediction of treatment response rates. Molecular diagnostic techniques also allow genetic mutations associated with HPB tumours to be detected which is fundamental to the development of targeted therapies and personalized treatment strategies.

GENETIC AND EPIGENETIC ALTERATIONS IN HPB TUMOURS

Genetic alterations refer to changes in DNA sequences as a result of copy number alterations or mutations in tumour suppressor genes and oncogenes. Epigenetic alterations, however, involve changes to DNA and proteins without modification of the DNA sequence.

Mutations in tumour suppressor genes and oncogenes

Mutations in tumour suppressor genes and oncogenes play a critical role in the development and progression of HPB tumours. Tumour suppressor gene mutations, such as in *TP53* and *CDKN2A*, can lead to the loss of normal cell function, allowing uncontrolled cell growth and tumour formation. More than half of pancreatic cancers have the TP53 mutation which impairs the detection of abnormal DNA and allows cells to avoid apoptotic signals (4). Activating mutations in oncogenes drive uncontrolled cell proliferation and survival. Approximately 90% of PDACs have the Kirsten rat sarcoma virus (*KRAS*) oncogene mutation which inhibits intrinsic GTPase activity, with mutations in the aspartic acid, valine and cysteine amino acids being the most common (5). *TP53* and *KRAS* mutations are also frequently observed in HCC and cholangiocarcinoma. Detection of genetic alterations in oncogenes and tumour suppressor genes provides valuable information for tumour characterisation, prognosis and targeted therapies.

Copy number alterations

Copy number alterations refer to changes in the number of copies of specific genes or genomic regions.

These alterations can occur as amplifications or deletions and are commonly observed in HPB tumours. Gene amplifications, such as in the human epidermal growth factor receptor 2 (*HER2*) gene, can result in overexpression of the protein, making it a potential therapeutic target in PDAC and a predictor of aggressive tumour potential in pancreatic neuroendocrine tumours. Deletions of tumour suppressor genes, such as *CDKN2A* in cholangiocarcinoma, can lead to loss of their tumour-inhibiting functions and are associated with a poor prognosis. Furthermore, *SMAD4* deletion results in loss of SMAD4-dependent inhibition of TGF-β, accelerating tumorigenesis in PDAC (5).

DNA methylation

DNA methylation is an epigenetic alteration that involves the addition of a methyl group to the DNA molecule, by the enzyme DNA methyltransferase. This process alters gene regulation and genomic stability. Abnormal DNA methylation patterns have been detected in HPB tumours and are associated with altered gene expression. Hypermethylation of promoter regions can result in the silencing of tumour suppressor genes such as *CDKN2A*, while global hypomethylation may contribute to genomic instability and oncogene activation. DNA methylation profiles have been found to be distinctive, allowing tumour subtyping in PDAC and these patterns can serve as diagnostic, prognostic, and predictive biomarkers in HPB tumours.

Histone modifications

Histone modifications are the chemical alterations which occur to key components of chromatin, which makes up the structure of chromosomes. They play a crucial role in the regulation of gene expression by modifying the structure and accessibility of chromatin. Alterations in histone modifications, such as acetylation, methylation, and phosphorylation, can affect gene expression patterns and contribute to tumour development. These alterations may affect various amino acids of the histone protein. Dysregulation of histone modifications has been implicated in HPB tumours and can provide insights into tumour biology and potential therapeutic targets. Alterations in acetylation and methylation have been observed in HCC, cholangiocarcinoma, PDAC, and neuroendocrine tumours. The specific histone modifications vary based on tumour subtype and have differing impacts on gene expression.

Microsatellite instability and DNA mismatch repair deficiency

Microsatellites are repetitive sequences of DNA distributed throughout the genome. Microsatellite instability (MSI) refers to mutations or variations in the length of repetitive DNA sequences due to a defective DNA mismatch repair (MMR) system. The DNA MMR system usually recognizes and corrects errors in DNA replication and maintains genomic stability. HPB tumours with MSI and DNA mismatch repair deficiency have distinctive clinical and pathological features and have implications for predicting prognosis and response to treatment. The ability to diagnose MSI and DNA MMR deficiency has a novel role in helping to identify patients who may benefit from immunotherapy or have an increased risk of hereditary cancer syndromes, such as Lynch syndrome.

TECHNIQUES FOR MOLECULAR ANALYSIS

Polymerase chain reaction

PCR is a well-known molecular technique allowing the amplification of specific DNA sequences. Targeted mutation analysis is a PCR-based method which allows the detection of specific DNA mutations by amplifying specific regions of interest that are known to result in HPB malignancy or have an association with treatment resistance. Furthermore, gene expression profiling can be performed by quantifying mRNA of specific genes to allow deeper understanding of tumour biology and facilitate patient specific treatment strategies.

In situ hybridization

In situ hybridization (ISH) is a molecular technique used to detect and localize specific nucleic acid sequences within cells and tissue sections. It is particularly useful for evaluating gene expression patterns and identifying specific genetic alterations in HPB tumours. Fluorescent *in situ* hybridization (FISH) is a variant that uses fluorescently labelled probes to visualize genetic abnormalities, such as gene amplifications or rearrangements. ISH and FISH techniques have proved valuable in diagnosing certain types of cholangiocarcinoma with rearrangements involving the fibroblast growth factor receptor 2 (*FGFR2*) gene. This technique is also valuable in the detection of amplifications of the *HER2* gene in some subsets of PDAC, identifying patients who may benefit from HER2-targeted therapies. This technique can also detect hepatitis B or C viruses in HCC, allowing a deeper understanding of the tumour aetiology and guide further treatment strategies.

Next generation sequencing

Next generation sequencing (NGS) technologies allow simultaneous analysis of multiple RNA or DNA fragments, allowing comprehensive profiling of genetic and genomic alterations. One application of this technique in HPB surgery is for molecular subtyping to improve the accuracy of diagnosis, such as the HCC subgroups with distinctive characteristics and clinical outcomes. Mutations in *TP53*, *KRAS* and proto-oncogene B-Raf (*BRAF*) are frequently observed in HCC, cholangiocarcinoma and PDAC and are associated with variable treatment responses and prognosis. Chromosomal alterations can also be detected,

such as the amplification of *HER2* gene in PDAC, and are a potential therapeutic target. NGS-based assays studying mutations and methylation abnormalities in bile are a promising development in the diagnosis of pancreatic and biliary malignancy with higher sensitivity and specificity than 'gold standard' methods (6).

Circulating tumour DNA analysis

Circulating tumour DNA (ctDNA) and circulating tumour cell (CTC) analysis involves the detection and analysis of circulating tumour cells or DNA fragments in peripheral blood. This technique is non-invasive and often referred to as a liquid biopsy. Liquid biopsy is promising as a minimally invasive diagnostic tool, providing real-time information about tumour genetic alterations, monitoring treatment response, and predicting recurrence. By analysing ctDNA and CTCs, it is possible to detect specific mutations, monitor tumour heterogeneity, and identify resistance mechanisms. Liquid biopsy has the potential to revolutionize the field of HPB surgery by providing dynamic and personalized information for guiding treatment decisions, although there is a requirement for the development of assay technology. Combined with tissue histopathological evaluation, molecular profiling increases diagnostic precision and accuracy and also guides treatment strategies. This novel strategy allows a more personalized approach to diagnosis, treatment selection and patient management.

SUMMARY

Tissue and molecular diagnosis play a pivotal role in HPB surgery, providing a definitive diagnosis and facilitating diagnostic precision, tumour classification, predicting outcomes, guiding treatment strategies, monitoring response and detecting recurrence. Histopathological evaluation, immunohistochemistry, *in situ* hybridization, molecular profiling, and liquid biopsy are essential techniques that are complementary to one another and aid deeper understanding of tumour biology allowing personalized treatment strategies.

Future directions involve the integration of genomics, transcriptomics and proteomics to gain a further comprehensive understanding of tumour molecular biology. AI and machine-learning algorithms can support diagnosis with data analysis, pattern recognition and prediction of treatment response. Novel approaches with targeted treatment strategies and immunotherapies based on specific molecular abnormalities is a promising tool for improving outcomes in HPB disease.

REFERENCES

1. Reig M, Forner A, Rimola J, Ferrer-Fabrega J, Burrel M. Garcia-Criado A, et al. BCLC strategy for prognosis prediction and treatment recommendation: the 2022 update. *J Hepatol* 2022;**76(3)**:681–93. doi:10.1016/j.jhep.2021.11.018

2. Passeri MJ, Baimas-George MR, Sulzer JK, Iannitti DA, Martinie JB, Baker EH, et al. Prognostic impact of the Bismuth-Corlette classification: higher rates of local unresectability in stage IIIb hilar cholangiocarcinoma. *Hepatobiliary Pancreat Dis Int* 2020;**19(2)**:157c62. doi:10.1016/j.hbpd.2020.02.001

3. Zhou L, Rui JA, Zhou WX, Wang SB, Chen SG, Qu Q. Edmondson-Steiner grade: a crucial predictor of recurrence and survival in hepatocellular carcinoma without microvascular invasio. *Pathol Res Pract* 2017;**213(7)**:824–30. doi:10.1016/j.prp.2017.03.002

4. Mizrahi JD, Surana R, Valle JW, Shroff RT. Pancreatic cancer. *Lancet* 2020;**395(10242)**:2008–20. doi:10.1016/S0140-6736(20)30974-0

5. Wang S, Zheng Y, Yang F, Zhu L, Zhu XQ, Wang ZF, et al. The molecular biology of pancreatic adenocarcinoma: translational challenges and clinical perspectives. *Signal Transduct Target Ther* 2021;**6(1)**:249. doi:10.1038/s41392-021-00659-4

6. He S, Zeng F, Yin H, Wang P, Bai Y, Song Q. Molecular diagnosis of pancreatobiliary tract cancer by detecting mutations and methylation changes in bile samples. *EClinicalMedicine* 2023;**55**:101736. doi:10.1016/j.eclinm.2022.101736

Chapter
14

History of Intraoperative Ultrasound during Open and Laparoscopic Liver Surgery

Masatoshi Makuuchi and Yoshihiro Sakamoto

INTRODUCTION

Intraoperative ultrasound (IOUS) is indispensable in liver surgery, not only for the diagnosis of tumour spread in the liver, but also as a direct guide in hepatectomy. Real-time B-mode IOUS was introduced in Japan in the 1970s as the first means of detecting small hepatocellular carcinomas (HCCs). In liver surgery for HCC, IOUS showed a higher sensitivity for detecting intrahepatic metastasis or tumour thrombus compared with other preoperative diagnostic modalities. In the 1980s, we developed systematic subsegmentectomy of the liver for HCC with staining of tumour-harbouring liver subsegments under the guidance of IOUS, and this technique has become the standard procedure for treatment of HCC. Colour Doppler IOUS, enabled estimation of hepatic arterial, portal, and venous flow during hepatectomy and has become indispensable for confirming blood flow in liver grafts during transplantation. Compared with conventional IOUS, contrast-enhanced IOUS (CE-IOUS) achieved even more accurate diagnosis of HCC and metastatic tumours. The introduction of fluorescence imaging using indocyanine green (ICG) enabled clear visualization of the stained hepatic segments as well as intraoperative identification of some malignant tumours. With advances in preoperative simulation systems for liver surgery made from 3D-computed tomography (CT) images (3D-CT), real-time virtual sonography (RVS) has been utilized in liver surgery. New technologies such as CE-IOUS, fluorescent ICG images and RVS have been introduced for laparoscopic hepatectomy where it is more difficult to identify tumour location and hepatic segment boundaries compared with open hepatectomy.

IOUS IN LIVER SURGERY

First experience of IOUS in liver surgery

IOUS was first employed in surgery for renal calculi, biliary calculi and cerebral lesions in the 1960s, providing images that were one-dimensional and of limited clinical use (1,2). In 1979, the first author of this chapter, Masatoshi Makuuchi and colleagues described their experience using IOUS with real-time B-mode imaging. They made a small side-viewing probe designed specifically for IOUS scanning of the liver, which consisted of electronic linear-array transducers. The probe quickly became popular in Japan, and is now commonly used during liver surgery (*Figure 14.1*).

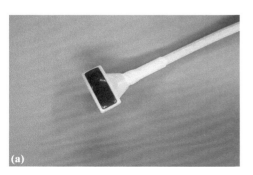
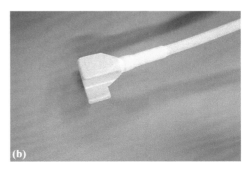

Figure 14.1 Intraoperative C42T probe (miniconvex) (7.5 MHz, Hitachi Aloka Medical). The scanner is aligned in a lateral line (a). The back of the probe can be grasped by the fingers (b).

DOI: 10.1201/9781003080060-14

Diagnosis of cancer spread of HCC using IOUS

The need for IOUS for liver surgery became critical in far eastern countries in the 1970s, due to the increasing incidence of liver cirrhosis and visible and non-visible hepatocellular carcinomas (HCCs). In the 8 years following our first introduction of IOUS in liver surgery in October 1979, 386 patients underwent laparotomy and 347 underwent hepatectomy using IOUS with 5–7.5 MHz linear-array transducers in either I-shaped or T-shaped configurations (3). Of these, 245 patients had HCC and 152 tumours were ≤5 cm in diameter. These smaller tumours included intrahepatic metastases and daughter nodules around the main tumours. The sensitivity of IOUS for the detection of these tumours was 99%, whereas that of angiography and CT scans was 84.1% and 89.6%, respectively. IOUS detected 23/33 (70%) of tumour thrombus that were detected in only 7/33 (21%) by preoperative US and angiography. These results demonstrate the higher diagnostic accuracy of IOUS compared with CT.

Development of systematic subsegmentectomy

In the 1970s, the conventional anatomical hepatectomy procedure was resection of some of Healey's four segments of the liver. As the boundary of Couinaud's segments are unclear on the liver surface, it was considered difficult to remove these subsegments. We introduced systematic subsegmentectomy that enabled anatomically precise resection of Couinaud's segments which are smaller than Healey's segments (4). It is known that HCC sometimes involves the portal venous branches and that cancer cells can spread via the portal vein in the hepatic segments harbouring the tumour. In patients with impaired hepatic function, massive hepatectomy can easily evoke post-hepatectomy liver failure and complete resection limited to the unit containing the tumour is the only practical solution. As there are no hepatic segmental landmarks on the liver surface, systematic subsegmentectomy guided by IOUS was developed to enable rational hepatectomy following visualization of subsegments containing tumours.

The operative procedure for systematic subsegmentectomy is shown in *Figure 14.2*. To identify the portal unit, the portal venous branches are punctured, indigo carmine solution (ICS) is injected, and the stained area is then marked by electrocautery. Arterio-portal shunt is not rare in patients with HCC, and the injected dye sometimes washes out rapidly. To maintain staining with the blue dye, either arterial occlusion or arterial injection is performed. The parenchyma of the liver is tattooed to enable identification of the ligation point of each vessel. Hepatic transection is performed after

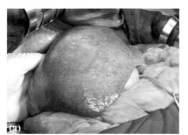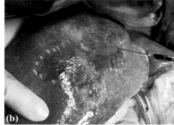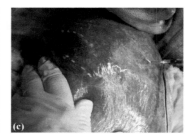
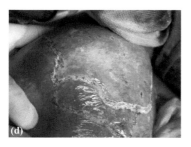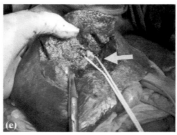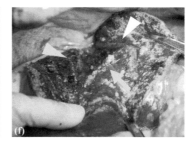

Figure 14.2 Systematic subsegmentectomy for a hepatocellular carcinoma in segment 8. No boundary of segment 8 can be seen on the liver surface (a). Dye (indigo carmine solution) was injected into the ventral portal branch in segment 8 under the guidance of intraoperative ultrasonography, stains the area harbouring the tumour (b). Segment 8 dorsal area is stained (c). The transection line was marked with electrocautery (d). Liver transection is performed under Pringle's manoeuvre using the clamp-crushing method. The Glissonean branch of segment 8 ventral is taped (e). After resection of segment 8, the middle hepatic vein (white arrowhead), right hepatic vein (yellow arrowhead), and Glissonean pedicle of segment 8 (yellow arrow) are exposed on the raw surface of the liver (f).

occlusion of inflow blood to the liver by hemihepatic blood occlusion technique or under Pringle's total inflow occlusion method. After complete removal of the right anterior superior area (right anterior section), the main trunks of the middle and right hepatic veins are exposed on the raw surface of the liver.

We performed 96 systematic subsegmentectomies in the 8 years following introduction in September 1980, which comprised systematic resection of S8 (n = 34), S7 (n = 13), S6 (n = 12), S8 + 4 (n = 8), S5 (n = 5), S5 + 6 (n = 5), S4 or extended S4 (n = 7) (3).

More than 40 years have passed since the introduction of systematic segmentectomy of the liver for HCC. The oncological advantage of anatomical resection including systematic subsegmentectomy using IOUS have been recognized in terms of decreasing the risk of local recurrence and death compared with non-anatomical limited resection (5,6).

Inferior right-hepatic vein-preserving hepatectomies

Other than the three principal major hepatic veins, the broad, short-hepatic vein located on the caudal side of the right hepatic vein is termed the inferior right-hepatic vein (IRHV) in accordance with Couinaud's nomenclature, and was found in 27/269 (10%) of patients studied in 1983 (7). The diameter of the IRHV was less than 4mm in 9/269 patients, and wider than the right hepatic vein in 8/269. IOUS is essential for identifying the draining area of the IRHV and thus preserving the corresponding segments. In patients with Budd–Chiari syndrome, the IRHV is the main draining vein of the right lobe.

Since July 1981, we have performed IRHV-preserving hepatectomies sacrificing the right-hepatic veins in six patients and proposed the concept of four new IRHV-preserving hepatectomies including left trisectionectomy (3,8). Left trisectionectomy, severing all major hepatic veins preserving segment 6 and IRHV (9), was finally performed 20 years after our proposition.

Counterstaining technique

Identification of the hepatic segments to be removed is not always successful using injection of ICS into the portal branches harbouring HCC if the dye solution washes out due to arterial-portal shunting or decreased portal flow in the corresponding segments. To reveal the boundary between segments to be removed and preserved, it is useful to inject dye into the surrounding segments to be preserved. Takayama et al. termed this method the counterstaining technique (10), and it was utilized in a recent study that employed ICG fluorescence imaging to visualize the corresponding hepatic segments (11).

Our IOUS-guided subsegmentectomy technique was soon adopted by French as well as Japanese surgeons. Bismuth (12,13) and Belghiti (14) followed our work and introduced IOUS and our techniques for liver surgery. These French surgeons spread the concept of IOUS-guided subsegmentectomy widely within Europe, and by the mid-1980s, IOUS became an indispensable component in conducting surgical treatment for HCC in patients with cirrhosis (15).

Use of IOUS in resection of colorectal liver metastasis

The use of IOUS for the detection of and screening for liver metastases from colorectal cancer has been investigated extensively. Machi et al. compared the accuracy of diagnosing liver metastasis between IOUS and other modalities and reported a sensitivity of 93.3% for IOUS, which was significantly higher than that for preoperative US (41.3%), CT (47.1%) and surgical exploration (66.3%) (16). IOUS has become essential in the management of colorectal liver metastasis (CRLM), because it can identify small metastatic lesions that are undetectable by other preoperative imaging studies (17).

Using IOUS, hepatectomy for bilobar multiple CRLM can be performed with preservation of as much of the hepatic parenchyma as possible, which increases the chance of being able to perform second or third resectional procedures for recurrent CRLM. This parenchyma-sparing strategy is very important in the treatment of CRLM because of the greater than 70% chance of recurrence of multiple CRLM. Kokudo et al. demonstrated the advantage of non-anatomical, parenchyma-preserving resections compared with anatomical resections in patients with CRLM (18). Torzilli et al. advocated the importance of parenchyma-sparing radical but conservative resection of CRLM that permits R1 resection of adjacent vital hepatic veins or Glissonean pedicles (19,20). Mise et al. demonstrated the advantage of a parenchyma-sparing strategy rather than anatomical resection on survival in patients with CRLM (21). Thus, limited non-anatomical liver resection using IOUS has become a standard hepatectomy for bilobar CRLM in Japan.

Colour or power Doppler imaging

Intraoperative colour Doppler imaging was first performed during cardiovascular surgery because of its ability to provide blood flow information (22). In liver transplantation, IOUS is indispensable (23,24). In living-donor operations, IOUS is used to estimate the transection line of the liver and in recipient operations, Doppler IOUS is indispensable for evaluating reconstructed hepatic, portal and arterial flow to avoid vascular complications. When the size of a partial liver graft is smaller than the recipient liver, adequate positioning of the graft in the abdominal cavity must be arranged using Doppler IOUS to maintain blood flow in the graft. Doppler IOUS can also be used to evaluate hepatopetal and hepatofugal flow in the portal vein to determine the indication for ligation of the collateral veins forming a porto-systemic shunt in cirrhotic patients undergoing liver transplantation.

We have proposed a method for evaluating liver congestion using Doppler IOUS (25). The state of venous congestion in the right liver graft for living-donor liver transplantation (LDLT) can be estimated after temporary clamping of the hepatic artery, and assessed using Doppler IOUS. Criteria for reconstruction of the middle hepatic vein of the donor graft can be determined based on the extent of the congested area in the graft.

Extended, directional power Doppler ultrasonography (e-Flow) is an advanced imaging mode that has high axial- and lateral-spatial resolution as well as flow sensitivity, which is useful for differentiating arterial and portal flows in a Glissonean sheath (26).

INTRODUCTION OF CONTRAST-ENHANCED IOUS AND ICG FLUORESCENCE IMAGING IN LIVER SURGERY

Contrast-enhanced US

Patients with cirrhosis develop new liver lesions other than HCC, including regenerative and dysplastic nodules, which can be easily located using conventional IOUS (27). Contrast-enhanced IOUS (CE-IOUS) is useful for the differential diagnosis of these small liver lesions in cirrhotic liver. Gaseous perflutren and gaseous sulfur hexafluoride have been widely used as agents for ultrasonographic enhancement. In addition to acting as intravascular contrast agents, they accumulate in the Kupffer cells of the liver, enabling Kupffer imaging in a similar manner to superparamagnetic iron oxide (SPIO)-enhanced MRI. In CE-US, the vascularity of each tumour can be estimated in the vascular phase at 1 min after injection and at the Kupffer phase at approximately 15 min after injection of Sonazoid®. CE-IOUS may be superior to extracorporeal CEUS, because IOUS has better spatial resolution and can avoid artifacts by dead angle or breathing motion associated with extracorporeal CEUS.

Torzilli et al. introduced CE-IOUS in 2002 and investigated whether CE-IOUS could provide additional information to that of conventional IOUS (28). They also reported that 6/16 (37.5%) nodules detected in cirrhotic liver by IOUS were identified accurately as HCC by CE-IOUS examination (29). Arita et al. screened 72 new focal liver lesions detected by conventional IOUS, in which the diagnosis of the lesions was HCC in 17 (22%). The accuracy of CE-IOUS in these 17 lesions was 87% (30). They also showed a strong correlation between dynamic CT and CE-IOUS using Sonazoidâ in estimating the histological grade of HCC (31). Takahashi et al. further revealed that CE-IOUS increased the accuracy of identification of hepatic metastases from colorectal cancer in comparison with conventional IOUS. They found that CE-IOUS was also useful for visualizing the spatial relationship between tumours and vascular structures (32). CE-IOUS has recently

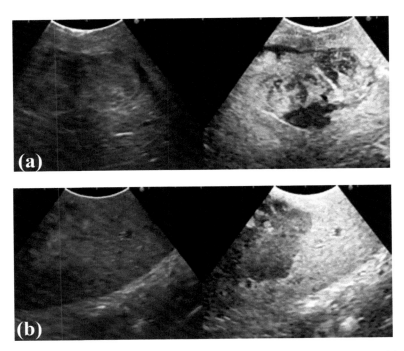

Figure 14.3 CE-IOUS of ruptured hepatocellular carcinoma. Vascular phase image (a) obtained immediately after systemic injection of Sonazoid (right side) shows more intensive vascularity within the tumour compared with an image obtained in conventional mode (left side). Kupffer phase image (b) obtained at 15 minutes after injection of Sonazoid (right side) shows greater hypo-echogenicity within the tumour compared with conventional mode (left side).

become indispensable in the differential diagnosis of liver tumours (*Figure 14.3*).

Fluorescence images on IOUS

Identification of hepatic segments to be removed by injection of ICS into the portal branches harbouring HCC is sometimes difficult, as mentioned above. During repeat resection where extensive adhesions are present, the liver surface is often too irregular to enable visualization of stained hepatic segments even with the counterstaining identification technique. A new technique using fluorescence with IOUS can clearly elucidate the hepatic (sub)segments, and can also be used during laparoscopic liver surgery.

A fluorescent imaging technique using ICG was first introduced to assess coronary artery bypass graft patency. It was subsequently used to identify sentinel lymph nodes in breast and gastric cancer and was subsequently introduced for use in hepatobiliary surgery, enabling highly sensitive identification of liver cancers (33) and extrahepatic bile ducts (34).

Aoki et al. was the first to apply a fluorescence navigation system that used ICG for anatomical segmentectomy (35). Injection of ICG and observation of the liver surface with a near-infrared camera system can clearly visualize the anatomical boundary of each hepatic segment. This technique is useful even in patients with poor expression of ICS on the liver surface. In addition, Ishizawa and Kokudo applied ICG fluorescent imaging to liver surgery for the identification of the boundary of each segment to detect ICG deposits in the liver cancer (33,36). Thus, fluorescence imaging has significantly improved the identification of the demarcation area during anatomical liver resection (*Figure 14.4*) (37).

IOUS WITH A SIMULATION AND NAVIGATION SYSTEM BEFORE, AND DURING, OPEN AND LAPAROSCOPIC LIVER SURGERY

Preoperative simulation in liver surgery

Recent advances with 3D-simulation systems in liver surgery have enabled the precise preoperative localization of tumours, hepatic segments and virtual hepatectomy by 3D-CT analysis (38). Virtual hepatectomy can be performed using surgical planning software (*Figure 14.5*). Mise et al. have performed 1194 virtual hepatectomies before LDLT and hepatectomy for HCC and colorectal liver metastasis. The need for, and type of, venous reconstruction during LDLT was determined based on the congestive volume of sacrificed major hepatic veins. Thus, virtual hepatectomy in LDLT optimized decision-making regarding graft selection and venous reconstruction (39). Further utilization of

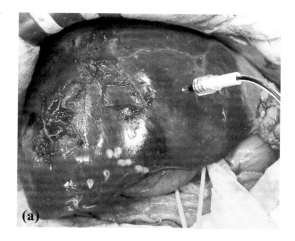

(a)

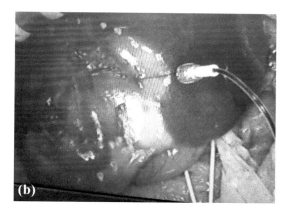

(b)

Figure 14.4 Identification of segment 5 during anatomical sectionectomy of segments 5 and 6 for a ruptured hepatocellular carcinoma (HCC). A volume of 2.5 mL of mixed indigo-carmine (5 mL) and ICG solution (0.1 mL) was injected into the portal branch in segment 5 (a). Indigo carmine solution shows the boundary of segment 5; however, the outer part is unclear because of intrahepatic haemorrhage from the ruptured HCC. Near-infrared light camera image (b) more clearly visualizes the boundary of segment 5 stained by ICG in the mixed solution, even on the irregular surface of the liver.

these images is being planned for navigation during liver surgery.

Real-time virtual sonography

In real-time virtual sonography (RVS), virtual sonographic images reconstructed from CT or MRI images are adjusted according to the position and direction of the IOUS probe (*Figure 14.6*). Satou et al. first reported the use of RVS to visualize 26 tumours in 16 patients undergoing hepatectomy and confirmed the feasibility and safety of this navigation system (40). As the virtual RVS images are reconstructed with reference to the CT or MRI images and the real IOUS images at the initial setting point, there

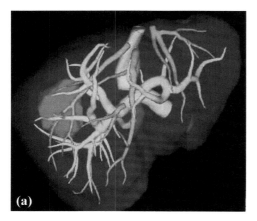

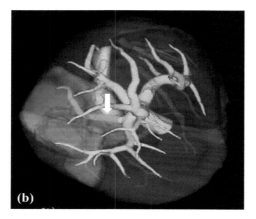

Figure 14.5 Preoperative simulation image using the Vincent system. The tumour located in segment 7 is involving the peripheral branches of the right hepatic vein (a). Anatomical resection of segment 7 was conducted, with planned division of the Glissonean branch of segment 7 at its root (arrow) (b).

is potential for misalignment between RVS and the real IOUS images. Miyata et al. evaluated the median degree of misalignment in 33 patients as 9.8 mm (41) and the adjustment time as 105 sec (range, 51–245 sec) using an ultrasonography system (HI VISION Ascendus, Hitachi-Ltd, Tokyo, Japan). Further investigation is needed to reduce the frequency of adjustment failure.

Laparoscopic IOUS

Laparoscopic IOUS rapidly became popular among surgeons performing minimally invasive surgery. Laparoscopic intracorporeal ultrasound was first performed by Japanese investigators using A-mode imaging (42). In the early- to mid-1980s, prototype laparoscopic ultrasound was performed using high-frequency real-time B-mode instruments developed for direct placement on the surface of organs (43). Laparoscopic IOUS was used initially for intraoperative diagnosis (44) but with the development of laparoscopic liver resection, it was incorporated into the intraoperative assessment during liver surgery. Laparoscopic hepatectomy must be performed without tumour palpitation or inspection and consequently, laparoscopic-IOUS has an essential role. Kawaguchi et al. reported that most near misses during laparoscopic hepatectomy were caused by a lack of understanding of both the laparoscopic view of the liver and the anatomical aspects unique to laparoscopic hepatectomy. In their review of 408 consecutive patients at a single institution who had undergone laparoscopic hepatectomy, they investigated technically important principles and advocated the need to identify the thick hepatic branches of major hepatic veins using laparoscopic IOUS (45). The limitations of laparoscopic IOUS include the difficulty of use within the limited space in the abdominal cavity, issues related to angulation and positioning of the probe, and difficulty in hand-eye coordination when the probe can be seen on the screen but there is no tactile feedback.

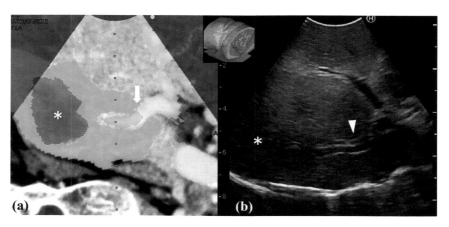

Figure 14.6 Real-time virtual sonography (RVS). Image (a) shows the root of segment 7 to be divided branching from the right Glissonean pedicle (arrow). Real intraoperative ultrasonography image (b) coincided with the RVS image. The Glissonean pedicle in segment 7 was planned to be divided at its root (arrowhead).

During laparoscopic anatomical liver resection, it is difficult (although not impossible) to puncture the corresponding portal branches in the abdomen to identify the boundary of each segment (46). As an alternative to portal branch puncture, hilar dissection and subsequent clamping of the corresponding Glissonean branches and injection of dye into the systemic circulation can be performed. This method of negative staining of the liver (47) is already utilized in anatomical liver resection as a variation of the Glissonean approach first described by Takasaki et al. (48). Positive and negative staining of hepatic segments is well-utilized during laparoscopic hepatectomy for resection of CRLM as well as HCC. When intraoperative positive or negative staining appears difficult, preoperative percutaneous staining under general anaesthesia using a thick needle would be an option although the difficulty in puncturing multiple or thin portal branches is a limitation of this technique (49).

Another strategy that could be used to overcome the technical issues relating to laparoscopic IOUS is virtual IOUS, which has been described in the section on RVS. Aoki et al. introduced a virtual real-time CT-guided volume navigation (VRCT) system during laparoscopic hepatectomy. They successfully removed 26 of 27 hepatic tumours with a mean diameter of 11 mm under VRCT guidance, and all surgical resection margins were negative with a mean margin to tumour distance of 9 mm. This system uses prerecorded 3D data of CT data and displays the calculated position of the instrument tip on a virtual IOUS image on the monitor screen (50).

SUMMARY

IOUS was first introduced in the 1970s and has become indispensable during open and laparoscopic liver surgery. In addition to conventional B-mode IOUS, colour Doppler IOUS and CE-IOUS have made huge contributions to successful anatomical and non-anatomical hepatectomy for hepatocellular carcinoma and colorectal liver metastasis and during liver transplantation. Recent advances in simulation and navigation systems for liver surgery and the use of ICG fluorescent imaging have enabled RVS. These techniques will be increasingly applied in the era of laparoscopic liver surgery.

REFERENCES

1. Makuuchi M, Torzilli G, Machi J. History of intraoperative ultrasound. *Ultrasound Med* 1998;**24**:1229–42.
2. Makuuchi M, Machi J, Torzilli G. Intraoperative procedures. *Ultrasound Med Biol* 2000;**26(Suppl S1)**:40–3.
3. Makuuchi M, Hasegawa H, Yamazaki S, Takayasu K, Moriyama N. The use of operative ultrasound as an aid to liver resection in patients with hepatocellular carcinoma. *World J Surg* 1987;**11**:615–21.
4. Makuuchi M, Hasegawa H, Yamazaki S. Ultrasonically guided subsegmentectomy. *Surg Gynecol Obstet* 1985;**161**:346–50.
5. Hasegawa K, Kokudo N, Imamura H, Matsuyama Y, Aoki T, Minagawa M, et al. Prognostic impact of anatomic resection for hepatocellular carcinoma. *Ann Surg* 2005;**242**:252–9.
6. Shindoh J, Makuuchi M, Matsuyama Y, Mise Y, Arita J, Sakamoto Y, et al. Complete removal of the tumor-bearing portal territory decreased local tumor recurrence and improves disease-specific survival of patients with hepatocellular carcinoma. *J Hepatol* 2016;**64**:594–600.
7. Makuuchi M, Hasegawa H, Yamazaki S, Bandai Y, Watanabe G, Ito T, et al. The inferior right hepatic vein: Ultrasonic demonstration. *Radiology* 1983;**148**:213–7.
8. Makuuchi M, Hasegawa H, Yamazaki S, Takayasu K. Four new hepatectomy procedures for resection of the right hepatic vein and preservation of the inferior right hepatic vein. *Surg Gynecol Obstet* 1987;**164**:69–72.
9. Machado MA, Bacchella T, Makdissi FF, Surjan RT, Machado MC. Extended left trisectionectomy severing all hepatic veins preserving segment 6 and inferior right hepatic vein. *Eur J Surg Oncol* 2008;**34**:247–51.
10. Takayama T, Makuuchi M, Watanabe K, Kosuge T, Takayasu K, Yamazaki S, et al. A new method for mapping hepatic segment: Counterstaining identification technique. *Surgery* 1991;**109**:226–9.
11. Kobayashi Y, Kawaguchi Y, Kobayashi K, Mori K, Arita J, Sakamoto Y, et al. Portal vein territory identification using indocyanine green fluorescence imaging: Technical details and short-term outcomes. *J Surg Oncol* 2017;**116**:921–31.
12. Bismuth H, Cnastaing D, Kunstlinger F. Preoperative echography in hepatobiliary surgery. *Presse Med* 1984;**13**:1819–22.
13. Castaing D, Emond J, Kunstinger F, Bismuth H. Utility of operative ultrasound in the surgical management of liver tumors. *Ann Surg* 1986;**204**:600–5.
14. Belghiti J, Menu Y, Cherqui D, Nahm H, Fekete F. Surgical treatment of hepatocellular carcinoma in cirrhosis. Value of intraoperative ultrasonography. *Gastroenterol Clin Biol* 1984;**13**:1819–22.
15. Bonnet P, Bernard JL, Delmout J, Huguet C. Intraoperative echography: An indispensable element in surgery of small hepatocarcinomas in cirrhotic patients. *Ann Chir* 1986;**40**:648–50.
16. Machi J, Osomoto H, Kurohji T, et al. Accuracy of intraoperative ultrasonography in diagnosing liver metastasis from colorectal cancer: Evaluation with postoperative follow-up results. *World J Surg* 1991;**15**:551–6.
17. Cervone A, Sardi A, Conaway GL. Intraoperative ultrasound (IOUS) is essential in the management of metastatic colorectal liver lesions. *Ann Surg* 2000;**66**:611–15.
18. Kokudo N, Tada K, Seki M, Ohta H, Azekura K, Ueno M, et al. Anatomical major resection versus nonanatomical limited resection for liver metastases from colorectal carcinoma. *Am J Surg* 2001;**181**:153–9.
19. Torzilli G, Montorsi M, Donandon M, Palmisano A, Del Fabbro D, Gambetti A, et al. "Radical but conservative" is the main goal for ultrasonography-guided liver resection: Prospective validation of this approach. *J Am Coll Surg* 2005;**201**:517–28.
20. Vigano L, Procopio F, Cimino MM, Donadon M, Gatti A, Costa G, et al. Is tumor detachment from

vascular structures equivalent to R0 resection in surgery for colorectal liver metastases? An observational cohort. *Ann Surg Oncol* 2016;**23**:1352–60.

21. Mise Y, Aloia TA, Brudvik KW, Schwarz L, Vauthey J-N, Conrad C, et al. Parenchymal-sparing hepatectomy in colorectal liver metastases improves salvageability and survival. *Ann Surg* 2016;**263**:146–52.

22. Takamoto S, Kyo S, Adachi H, Matsumura M, Yokote Y, Omoto R, et al. Intraoperative color flow mapping, by real-time two-dimensional Doppler echocardiography for evaluation of vascular and congenital heart disease and vascular disease. *J Thorac Cardiovasc Surg* 1985;**90**:802–12.

23. Kasai H, Makuuchi M, Kawasaki S, Ishizone S, Kitahara S, Matsunami H, et al. Intraoperative color Doppler ultrasonography for a partial-liver transplantation from the living donor in pediatric patients. *Transplantation* 1992;**54**:173–4.

24. Makuuchi M, Kawarazaki H, Iwanaka T, Kamada N, Takayama T, Kumon M. Living related liver transplantation. *Surg Today* 1992;**22**:297–300.

25. Sano K, Makuuchi M, Miki K, Maema A, Sugawara, Imamura H, et al. Evaluation of hepatic venous congestion: Proposed indication criteria for hepatic vein reconstruction. *Ann Surg* 2002;**236**:241–7.

26. Kaneko J, Sugawara Y, Yanhong Q, Makuuchi M. *J Gastroenterol Hepatol* 2007;**22**:1345.

27. Kokudo N, Bandai Y, Imanishi H, Minagawa M, Uedera Y, Harihara Y, et al. Management of new hepatic nodules detected by intraoperative ultrasonography during hepatic resection for hepatocellular carcinoma. *Surgery* 1996;**119**:634–40.

28. Torzilli G, Fabbro DD, Olivari N, Calliada F, Montorsi M, Makuuchi M, et al. Contrast-enhanced ultrasonography during liver surgery. *Br J Surg* 2004;**91**:1165–7.

29. Tozlilli G, Olivari N, Moroni E, Del Fabbro D, Gambetti A, Leoni P, et al. Contrast-enhanced intraoperative ultrasonography in surgery for hepatocellular carcinoma in cirrhosis. *Liver Transpl* 2004;**10**:S34–8.

30. Arita J, Takahashi M, Hata S, Shindoh J, Beck Y, Sugawara Y, et al. Usefulness of contrast-enhanced intraoperative ultrasound using Sonazoid in patients with hepatocellular carcinoma. *Ann Surg* 2011;**254**:992–9.

31. Arita J, Hasegawa K, Takahashi M, Hata S, Shindoh J, Sugawara Y, et al. Correlation between contrast-enhanced intraoperative ultrasound using Sonazoid and histologic grade of resected hepatocellular carcinoma. *Am J Roentgenol* 2011;**196**:1314–21.

32. Takahashi M, Hasegawa K, Arita J, Hata S, Aoki T, Sakamoto Y, et al. Contrast-enhanced intraoperative ultrasonography using perfluorobutane microbubbles for the enumeration of colorectal liver metastases. *Br J Surg* 2012;**99**:1271–7.

33. Ishizawa T, Fukushia N, Shibahara J, Masuda K, Tamura S, Aoki T, et al. Real-time identification of liver cancers by using indocyanine green-fluorescent imaging. *Cancer* 2000;**115**:2491–504.

34. Ishizawa T, Bandai Y, Kokudo N. Fluorescent cholangiography using indocyanine green for laparoscopic cholecystectomy: An initial experience. *Arch Surg* 2009;**115**:2491–504.

35. Aoki T, Yasuda D, Shimizu Y, Odaira M, Niiya T, Kusano T, et al. Image-guided liver mapping using fluorescence navigation system with indocyanine green for anatomical hepatic resection. *World J Surg* 2008;**32**:1763–7.

36. Kokudo N, Ishizawa T. Clinical application of fluorescence imaging of liver cancer using indocyanine green. *Liver Cancer* 2012;**1**:15–21.

37. Inoue Y, Arita J, Sakamoto T, Ono Y, Takahashi M, Takahashi Y, et al. Anatomical liver resections guided by 3-dimensional parenchyma staining using fusion indocyanine green fluorescence imaging. *Ann Surg* 2015;**262**:105–11.

38. Takamoto T, Hashimoto T, Ogata S, Inoue K, Maruyama Y, Miyazaki A, et al. Planning of anatomical liver segmentectomy and subsegmentectomy with 3-dimensional simulation software. *Am J Surg* 2013;**206**:530–8.

39. Mise Y, Hasegawa K, Satou S, Shindoh J, Miki K, Akamatsu N, et al. How has virtual hepatectomy changed the practice of liver surgery? Experience of 1194 virtual hepatectomy before liver resection and living donor liver transplantation. *Ann Surg* 2018;**268**:127–33.

40. Satou A, Aoki T, Kaneko J, Sakamoto Y, Hasegawa K, Sugawara Y, et al. Initial experience of intraoperative three-dimensional navigation for liver resection using real-time virtual sonography. *Surgery* 2014;**155**:255–62.

41. Miyata A, Arita J, Shirata C, Abe S, Akamatsu N, Kaneko J, et al. Quantitative assessment of the accuracy of real-time virtual sonography for liver surgery. *Surg Innov* 2020;**27**:60–7.

42. Yamakawa K, Naito S, Azuma K, et al. Laparoscopic diagnosis of intraabdominal organs: Ultrasound diagnosis through laparoscopy. *Jpn J Gastroenterol* 1958;**55**:741.

43. Machi J, Schwartz JH, Zaren HA, Noritomi T, Sigel B. Technique of laparoscopic ultrasound examination of the liver and pancreas. *Surg Endosc* 1996;**10**:684–9.

44. Ohta Y, Fujiwara K, Sato Y, Niwa H, Oka H. New ultrasound laparoscope for diagnosis for intraabdominal diseases. *Gastrointest Endosc* 1983;**29**:289–94.

45. Kawaguchi Y, Velayutham V, Fuks D, Mal F, Kokudo N, Gayet B, et al. Operative techniques to avoid near misses during laparoscopic hepatectomy. *Surgery* 2017;**161**:341–6.

46. Ito D, Ishizawa T, Hasegawa K. Laparoscopic positive staining of hepatic segments using indocyanine green-fluorescence imaging. *J Hepatobiliary Pancreat Sci* 2020;**22**:441–3.

47. Ishizawa T, Zuker NB, Kokudo N, Gayet B. Positive and negative staining of hepatic segments by use of fluorescent imaging techniques during laparoscopic hepatectomy. *Arch Surg* 2012;**147**:393–4.

48. Morimoto M, Tomassini F, Berardi G, Mori Y, Shirata C, Hilal MA, et al. Glissonean approach for hepatic inflow control in minimally invasive anatomic liver resection: A systematic review. *J Hepatobiliary Pancreat Sci* 2022;**29(1)**:51–65.

49. Aoki T, Koizumi T, Mansour DA, Fujimori A, Kusano T, Matsuda K, et al. Percutaneous indocyanine green fluorescence staining for laparoscopic anatomical liver resection. *J Am Coll Surg* 2020;**230**:e7–12.

50. Aoki T, Mansour DA, Koizumi T, Wada Y, Enami Y, Fujimori A, et al. Laparoscopic liver surgery guided by virtual real-time CT guided volume navigation. *J Gastrointest Surg* 2021;**25(7)**:1779–86.

Chapter

15

Intraoperative Anaesthesia for Liver and Pancreas Surgery

Rachel Wong and Dave Patel

INTRODUCTION

Hepato-pancreatico-biliary (HPB) surgery presents unique challenges to the anaesthetist on account of the significant associated morbidity, mortality and potentially high-risk patient population (1). The delicate balance between minimizing surgical blood loss, while maintaining optimal perfusion targets, demands meticulous attention to detail and open communication between surgeon and anaesthetist. This chapter will focus on the salient intraoperative anaesthetic measures required for common HPB procedures.

MONITORING

Standard electrocardiogram (ECG), non-invasive blood pressure and oxygen saturation monitoring is established prior to the induction of anaesthesia. In addition, intra-arterial cannulation facilitates continuous blood pressure monitoring and repeated blood sampling. Pre-induction placement should be considered in those patients with significant cardiorespiratory comorbidity or hepatic impairment (2). Continuous arterial pressure monitoring helps to provide information regarding the patient's volume and perfusion status, allows serial arterial blood gas sampling and monitoring of intraoperative of glucose, electrolytes, lactate and coagulation (3).

Central venous pressure (CVP) monitoring is recommended with the placement of a central venous catheter, which also provides central access for vasopressor administration (4). This should not replace peripheral intravenous (IV) access and in procedures where large volume blood loss can be predicted, widebore venous cannulae are inserted to enable rapid volume resuscitation (5). Rapid infuser devices should be readily available and cell salvage considered in such cases. All but minor cases, should have cross-matched blood available.

Cardiac output monitoring varies across individual centres. 'Non-invasive' cardiac output monitoring using Doppler *(Figure 15.1)* or arterial-waveform analysis *(Figure 15.2)* and their derived parameters is preferred as the documented use of pulmonary artery catheters is deemed too invasive by most units (3,4,6).

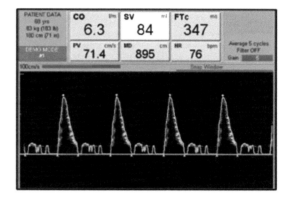

Figure 15.1 Oesophageal Doppler cardiac output monitoring screen demonstrating the following haemodynamic parameters: Cardiac output (CO); stroke volume (SV); corrected (systolic) flow-time (FTc), indicating preload; peak velocity (PV) indicating contractility; and heart rate (HR).

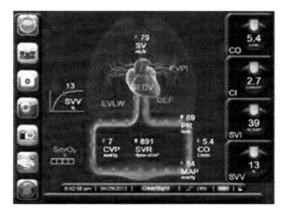

Figure 15.2 Edward Lifesciences FloTrac™ cardiac output monitoring using arterial waveform analysis to calculate: Cardiac output (CO); cardiac index (CI); stroke volume (SV); stroke volume index (SVI); stroke volume variation (SVV) and systemic vascular resistance (SVR).

DOI: 10.1201/9781003080060-15

There may be a role for transoesophageal echocardiography (TOE), particularly in larger resection surgery, however, the presence of varices and requirement for specialist interpretation, may preclude TOE or even the use of oesophageal Doppler-based 'non-invasive' cardiac output monitoring (3). In liver resection surgery, in particular, the maintenance of a low CVP to minimize blood loss and frequent haemodynamic changes due to surgical liver manipulation make the information garnered intraoperatively unreliable at best.

A urinary catheter is inserted to monitor urine output and allow targeted fluid resuscitation. This is of particular importance in patients with associated renal dysfunction, and during procedures where large volume shifts may occur.

As thermoregulation is impaired under the influence of anaesthesia and prolonged surgical times, temperature should be closely monitored and actively controlled through the use of fluid warmers and active warming devices. This is important to avoid the exacerbation of coagulation disorders and impaired wound healing. A peripheral nerve stimulator should always be used to monitor neuromuscular blockade when muscle relaxants are used.

CHOICE OF ANAESTHETIC TECHNIQUE

Anaesthetic technique will vary between individual anaesthetists but should focus on an awareness of the effects of anaesthesia on liver function. Particular attention must be paid to changes in the pharmacodynamics and pharmacokinetics in patients with associated organ dysfunction, where altered protein binding and drug metabolism may lead to residual effects of drugs being prolonged (2).

A standard approach would be an IV co-induction using propofol or thiopentone, along with a short-acting opioid such as alfentanil or fentanyl. Propofol elimination is not significantly impaired in liver disease, whereas the fraction of unbound thiopentone may increase, leading to prolonged effects (2). Opioids act by sparing the amount of induction agent required, reducing the resultant vasodilation and thereby cardiovascular instability. Dose adjustments should be made in the presence of liver disease as altered absorption, distribution, metabolism and excretion often leads to prolonged drug half-lives and duration of action (3,4). Benzodiazepines are avoided as these may precipitate encephalopathy in the recovery phase.

Muscle relaxants are used to facilitate endotracheal intubation (ET) and provide optimal operating conditions, ensuring the abdominal wall muscles are relaxed during surgery. Operative duration and patient comorbidity should be considered when selecting the appropriate agent for use. Suxamethonium (which acts by mimicking acetylcholine at the neuromuscular junction) may be useful for ET, however its short

duration of action is unlikely to benefit surgical access, even if this is prolonged through a reduction in pseudocholinesterase concentrations in liver disease (2,3). Rocuronium provides the prolonged neuromuscular blockade required, however its dependence on hepatic elimination can lead to an extremely prolonged duration of action in severe liver disease. Therefore atracurium, exclusive in its ability to undergo spontaneous degradation, (Hofmann elimination is where an amine is degraded to form alkenes) is the superior agent. Furthermore, a continuous intraoperative infusion of atracurium (0.3–0.6 mg/kg/hr) may be considered to achieve a high degree of muscle relaxation. Rapid sequence induction should be considered when there is a risk of gastric-outlet obstruction with pancreatic or biliary masses. A nasogastric tube is placed during the induction phase of anaesthesia in these cases or where prolonged surgery or multiple bowel anastomoses are likely to result in a postoperative ileus.

Intraoperative anaesthesia is maintained through the delivery of volatile agents such as sevoflurane, isoflurane or desflurane which undergo minimal hepatic metabolism (7). Desflurane offers the quickest emergence, has minimal effect on the hepatic arterial buffer response and relatively preserves hepatic blood flow (3), however, with 20 times the environmental impact of other less harmful greenhouse gases (8), units are moving away from its use. Nitrous oxide is also avoided as it causes bowel distension (5). There is a role for total IV anaesthesia as we work to reduce the carbon footprint from anaesthetic practices, using target-controlled infusions of propofol and remifentanil, in combination with depth of anaesthesia monitoring. The clinical application of processed electroencephalogram (EEG) in modern depth of anaesthesia monitors has permitted better titration of IV agents to mitigate the haemodynamic instability often seen with large doses of propofol and offer a rapid emergence from prolonged anaesthesia. All anaesthetic agents may contribute to vasodilation and a reduction in cardiac output and thus organ perfusion (9). This should be anticipated and treated judiciously with the use of vasopressors such as metaraminol, phenylephrine or noradrenaline.

In association with strict asepsis, antibiotic prophylaxis should be considered in accordance with local guidelines and discussion with the surgical team, with the first dose administered within 30–60 minutes of the surgical incision. This may be of particular importance in large resections, where disruption to Kupffer cells may increase susceptibility to bacterial infections (4).

ANALGESIA

Effective analgesia is essential, both during the intraoperative and postoperative phases, as inadequate pain relief is associated with an increased risk of postoperative complications and length of stay in hospital (10).

The different approaches to pain relief will be fully explored in **Chapter 16**. Patient compliance with physiotherapy, mobilization and breathing exercises, is only achieved with good analgesia.

The use of patient-controlled analgesia containing opiates in patients with pre-existing liver or renal failure may result in the prolonged elimination of the opioids (11). Morphine, and its active metabolite morphine-6-glucuronide, can accumulate leading to increased side effects, drowsiness, respiratory depression and a risk of encephalopathy (3). Fentanyl, in large doses can also accumulate. Remifentanil can be used intraoperatively as its metabolism by plasma esterases is independent of organ function, however, its short duration of action makes it unsuitable for use in the postoperative period.

The placement of a thoracic epidural as part of the anaesthetic technique minimizes the requirement for opioid-based analgesia. A combination infusion of low dose (0.1%) levobupivacaine and fentanyl (2 µg/mL) is associated with relative haemodynamic stability, superior postoperative analgesia, a reduced stress response, decreased incidence of pulmonary or cardiac morbidity, earlier return of intestinal function and reduced thromboembolic complications (1,4,9,12). The vasodilatation and reduced sympathetic activity can aid in the production of a low CVP which is pivotal during liver resection surgery. Studies have suggested that it is the lowered sympathetic activity that plays a crucial role in reducing stress-induced hepatic injury and insulin resistance and improving immune function by reducing the release of corticosteroids and catecholamines (11,13). Epidurals have also been reported to reduce the rate of cancer recurrence following surgical resection (1).

An intraoperative epidural may be sufficient to relax the abdomen, reducing the requirement for further muscle relaxant doses. This infusion can continue in the postoperative period for up to 5 days. In the event of hepatic decompensation or concerns over the cumulative effects of epidural fentanyl, the infusion can be switched to plain levobupivacaine or ropivacaine.

Opinion is divided regarding the use of epidural analgesia in procedures carrying an increased potential for major blood loss and coagulation deficits, such as extensive liver resection or liver resection in the presence of liver impairment (14,15). The relative hypotension, along with a low CVP state and haemodilution because of its treatment with fluid, is thought to explain why epidural anaesthesia is independently associated with an increased risk of blood transfusions (6). Post-resection impairment of coagulation raises the concern of the development of an epidural haematoma. Transfusion of clotting factors or fresh frozen plasma may be required to safely remove the epidural catheter. There is growing evidence for the utilization of other regional techniques to mitigate these concerns (16,17).

LIVER SURGERY

Hepatic blood flow may decrease by as much as 40% following induction of anaesthesia (11). Lack of perfusion and hepatocyte apoptosis can precipitate liver failure and the subsequent development of ascites, oedema and other postoperative complications (6). Haemodynamic goals in liver resection include the maintenance of organ perfusion and oxygen delivery while minimizing surgical bleeding by maintaining a low CVP (18). Low CVP may also help to improve portal venous flow through the liver by providing a better portal perfusion pressure gradient across the acini. In particular, it may offer some protection to hepatic acinus zone 3, which has the lowest partial pressure of oxygen. As the liver is a highly vascular organ, various blood loss limiting anaesthetic and surgical methods are utilized during surgery.

Massive blood loss has been reported following hepatic resection, with transfusions being an independent risk factor for postoperative morbidity and mortality (5). Associated postoperative morbidity includes coagulopathy, infection and cancer recurrence. A multidisciplinary approach is thereby needed to reduce perioperative blood loss, with modern techniques reducing mean blood loss to 300–900 mL (5,15,19,20). Intraoperative cell salvage may be beneficial, however its use in malignancy is controversial. Tranexamic acid also has a role in reducing blood transfusion requirements (19,21).

Anaesthetic methods

General anaesthesia can facilitate a reduction in CVP by vasodilatation and direct cardiac depression (22). It is common practice to restrict IV fluid resuscitation and maintain a low CVP until the liver specimen has been resected. Maintenance of mean arterial blood pressure is achieved using vasopressors such as metaraminol, phenylephrine or noradrenaline and judicious fluid administration. Clinical judgement, often gained through experience, is required to walk the tightrope between hypoperfusion of tissues from hypovolaemia and maintaining a low CVP to minimize blood loss. Non-invasive cardiac monitoring derived parameters are limited in these circumstances, but cardiac output and systemic vascular resistance parameter trends produced by these instruments may aid clinical awareness. Careful monitoring of lactate and urine output to determine adequate organ perfusion is needed to avoid the risk of exacerbating hepatocellular injury. The requirement for frequent use of vasoconstrictors, a rising lactate and significantly reduced urine output indicates the patient is too 'dry'.

Whilst a low CVP will reduce bleeding during liver resection, it results from a decreased venous return from a lower circulating volume, and thus a decreased cardiac output. Sudden hypovolaemia as a result of bleeding or transient surgical compression of the inferior vena cava (retractors, packs, pneumoperitoneum), can therefore potentiate extreme cardiovascular instability and anaesthetists must remain vigilant to this (4,5,18). Patients with associated impaired left or right ventricular function may require a higher CVP to maintain organ perfusion. In these instances, close communication with the surgeon is key to achieving the best patient outcome. In situations with elevated right-heart pressures and high CVPs, despite low volume resuscitation, diuretics or nitrates can be used (4,5). These patients can often be highlighted early in the preoperative phase and the team should be aware that these pose a high degree of likelihood of large intraoperative bleeding.

Positive pressure ventilation may impair hepatic blood flow and venous return to the heart due to increased intrathoracic pressure. Intraoperative ventilation strategies should aim to target normal oxygen and carbon dioxide levels to ensure adequate organ perfusion and oxygenation. A temporary reduction in positive end-expiratory pressure (PEEP) or no PEEP may be warranted to minimize bleeding during the resection phase (4), however this should be restored once the resection is complete. Some anaesthetists may choose to 'recruit' the lung with some vital capacity breaths at the end of the procedure to reduce lung atelectasis and risk of pulmonary complications (4).

Surgical methods

Blood loss is reduced by the Pringle manoeuvre which produces hepatic artery and portal vein occlusion, in a continuous or more usually an intermittent technique (6). The route for blood loss then becomes backflow through the valveless hepatic veins. It is for this reason that a low central venous, and thus hepatic, pressure is preferential, ideally below 5 cm H_2O to reduce blood loss. Application of the Pringle manoeuvre is associated with a 10% reduction in the cardiac index as a result of the reduced venous return, and a 40% increase in systemic vascular resistance (SVR) from a hepatic neuro-humoral reflex and an increase in mean arterial pressure (6). Profound haemodynamic instability may also occur on release of the clamp as a result of reperfusion. Other vascular occlusions techniques exist, such as total hepatic vascular exclusion, which may be associated with profound reductions in cardiac output requiring pre-emptive volume loading. Close communication with the anaesthetist is paramount when planning surgical occlusion technique, and at points during parenchymal resection where profound haemodynamic fluctuations may occur.

Prolonged clamping can cause warm ischaemia of the liver, and this should be restricted with breaks for reperfusion to allow the liver to recover. Periods of intermittent clamping of up to 1 hour are often well-tolerated in non-cirrhotic livers, when compared to the consequences of major blood loss, therefore most centres advocate the use of the Pringle manoeuvre (4,6). Despite intermittent clamping allowing hepatic blood

flow to be restored, sinusoidal epithelial cell death occurs due to paradoxical reduced blood flow from microcirculatory change following reperfusion (5,23). There is some evidence that N-acetylcysteine works to reduce the resulting hepatic dysfunction during clamping, and reperfusion, although its use is often isolated to hepatic transplants or in those with fulminant hepatic failure (5,14). It may improve oxygen delivery and consumption and reduce base deficit. Regular glucose monitoring is necessary, and a dextrose infusion may be required during clamping and resection, as hypoglycaemia may occur as a result of the depletion of glycogen stores.

There is an associated risk of venous air embolism during liver resection, as air can easily be entrained into the low CVP venous system (4–6). A high index of suspicion is required when the hepatic vein is opened and during episodes of rapid blood loss. Communication between the anaesthetist and surgeon is vital to coordinate a rapid response to such an event. The surgeon must be made aware if infusions of large volumes of fluid occur to restore circulating volume, and they may need to flood the surgical field with fluid to stop the entrainment of air. The patient should be placed in the Trendelenburg position and the central venous catheter aspirated.

Post-resection fluid resuscitation should be initiated as the risk of bleeding is reduced at this point. Factors such as patient size, blood loss and insensible losses should be taken into account when restoring circulating volume. This will enable identification of bleeding points as circulating volume is restored. The patient should also be monitored for coagulopathy with real-time thromboelastography and coagulation studies, correcting any deficits with specific clotting components such as fresh frozen plasma or platelets.

SPECIAL CIRCUMSTANCES

Liver failure

Patients with liver disease can be extremely unwell with deranged physiology and have a high perioperative morbidity and mortality. A thorough preoperative assessment should highlight any pre-existing coagulopathy, portal hypertension, ascites, varices and encephalopathy. These conditions should be optimized where possible as these patients are extremely susceptible to hepatic decompensation in the perioperative phase. Associated cardiovascular disease can be unmasked during anaesthesia and surgery, and the anaesthetist should be prepared for this.

Importantly, knowledge of the altered metabolism of drugs in liver failure is required during the delivery of anaesthesia. Established liver dysfunction can lead to prolonged effects of anaesthesia and an increased likelihood of hepatic decompensation in the postoperative phase. Massive ascites impairs ventilation from raised intra-abdominal pressure and splinting of the diaphragm and impairs the function of other intra-abdominal organs. This includes adverse effects on renal function, exacerbating the unpredictability of anaesthetic drug pharmacokinetics in these patients. Tense ascites may need to be drained preoperatively but leads to massive fluid shifts and potentially a large loss of protein. The ascitic patient may require intravascular volume resuscitation with human albumin solution as crystalloids are less effective in these circumstances (2,5). Early commencement of a dextrose infusion to prevent hypoglycaemia should be considered.

Regional anaesthesia can be useful as it avoids many of the systemic side effects of commonly used analgesics although concurrent coagulopathy may preclude its use. Portal hypertension can also be associated with epidural varices which may pose additional risks when considering the use of regional anaesthesia (14).

Most liver resection patients, irrespective of aetiology, can be safely extubated at the end of surgery, once particular attention is made to the restoration of circulating volume, normothermia, pH, glucose, lactate, electrolytes and ensuring the effects of drugs, particularly neuromuscular blockade, have worn off. These patients are best monitored in high-dependency environments.

Microwave liver ablation

Radiofrequency ablation has the potential to cause large areas of tissue destruction and places patients at risk of a systemic inflammatory response syndrome (SIRS)-like response (4). This may precipitate intraoperative instability.

PANCREATIC SURGERY

Pancreatic surgery is a technically challenging intra-abdominal surgery. Patients are often elderly with significant major comorbidities. Furthermore, pancreatic surgery is often associated with a higher degree of postoperative complications, morbidity and mortality due to the complexity and complications related to some of the operations (1,10). Intraoperative anaesthesia follows measures similar to that required for liver surgery, with specific preparation for major fluid shifts, including blood loss, and large-volume fluid replacement.

Pancreaticoduodenectomy

Multiple studies highlight the impact of fluid resuscitation on adverse events following pancreaticoduodenectomy (24). Large, volume fluid resuscitation has previously been used during major abdominal surgery to account for losses from an abdominal incision, prolonged surgery, during the formation of anastomoses and into the gut. The volume of fluids received is believed to often exceed actual fluid losses, leading to worsening postoperative outcome. Complications arising from salt and water overload include impaired

wound healing, dehiscence, anastomotic leak and ileus (1,13,24).

The judicious administration of balanced crystalloids, with a goal-directed approach, is therefore needed to maintain a near neutral fluid balance. CVP measurements should be used in conjunction with mixed venous saturations, lactate, haematocrit, and urine output monitoring when calculating individual fluid requirements. The use of non-invasive cardiac output monitoring and its derived parameters is useful to establish baseline and ongoing volume status and can alert the anaesthetist to any acute changes in stroke volume and cardiac output. Care should be taken not to mistake epidural-induced hypotension for excessive fluid depletion as in this instance the use of a vasopressor is preferred.

Octreotide, a synthetic analogue of somatostatin, may be used to reduce pancreatic exocrine secretions although its evidence remains controversial (10,13). A recent meta-analysis concluded that whilst octreotide reduced the crude rate of pancreatic fistulas, the rate of clinically significant fistulas as well as the overall major morbidity and mortality remain unchanged (25). Its use is largely dependent upon institutional and surgical preference.

Endocrine resection

The principle of anaesthesia in hormone-secreting tumours of the pancreas (*see Table 15.1*) is in the prevention and treatment of the effects of the excreted hormone (10). In carcinoid tumours, octreotide infusions are often commenced preoperatively and continued into the postoperative period for symptom control. A close watch on blood glucose levels should be maintained during operations for insulinomas and glucagonomas and derangements appropriately treated. Diabetes may occur, particularly after total pancreatectomy, therefore tight glucose monitoring should be observed in all these cases. Patients are often more sensitive to exogenous insulin and caution should be taken when prescribing insulin regimes. Surgery for phaeochromocytomas and VIPomas may result in severe haemodynamic instability as vasoactive compounds are released and result in associated morbidity. During surgical manipulation of the pancreas, patients may develop a SIRS-like response, requiring the use of vasopressors to maintain mean arterial pressure.

Table 15.1 Principles of anaesthesia for hormone-secreting tumours

- Insulinoma
- Glucagonoma
- Gastrinoma
- VIPoma
- Phaeochromocytoma
- Carcinoid

Autologous islet cell infusion

Total pancreatectomy and autologous islet cell transplantation has become the final common pathway for patients with life-altering pain from chronic pancreatitis. The total pancreatectomy is effective in treating the pain from chronic pancreatitis and the islet cell transplant mitigates or prevents the brittle diabetes which results from complete removal of the endocrine function. Organ preservation during the potentially long warm ischaemic time of the resection relies on both surgical and anaesthetic input. Careful surgical dissection, maintaining blood supply to the pancreas for as long as possible and a metabolically stress-free anaesthetic with tight blood sugar control to keep the pancreas metabolically quiescent is key to preserving the islets. A combined regional and balanced general anaesthetic technique is the currently preferred approach with invasive arterial and CVP monitoring. Goal-directed fluid therapy using non-invasive cardiac output monitoring helps maintain tissue perfusion throughout the extremely long procedure. As the patients are anticoagulated prior to islet cell infusion, scrupulous haemostasis helps reduce the requirement for blood transfusion. Techniques of islet cell infusion vary between centres, but most commonly the islets are infused into the portal circulation of the liver. Monitoring of portal venous pressure is important during the islet infusion as the islets embolize and occlude the tributaries of the portal circulation and give rise to a steadily increasing portal venous pressure. Post-transplant transient portal hypertension which usually resolves within 96 hours potentially leads to significant postoperative morbidity including both liver dysfunction upstream and bowel congestion (occasionally ischaemia) and prolonged ileus downstream. Postoperative monitoring of coagulation is recommended before removal of epidural catheters. Pain management in patients with chronic pancreatitis is often difficult and requires a multidisciplinary approach in the pre- and postoperative periods with chronic pain team and psychological support and multimodal analgesia in the perioperative phase. Weaning from long-term opiate usage must be undertaken slowly and monitored carefully often over weeks and months and sometimes years following surgery.

CARCINOID: LIVER OR PANCREAS

Carcinoid is associated with significant morbidity and mortality, exhibiting many unpredictable physiological symptoms due to the release of vasoactive hormones (26). The aim of anaesthesia is to maintain patient stability and avoid any stressors which could potentiate a carcinoid crisis. Association particularly with right-sided heart disease, warrants a thorough cardiovascular assessment when planning anaesthesia and surgery (18). Pulmonary hypertension and right heart failure are associated with extremely high mortality and should be excluded with ECG, echocardiogram and, if indicated, CT chest and right heart catheterization.

The literature supports the avoidance of histamine-releasing drugs such as morphine and atracurium, and the peptide-releasing agent suxamethonium (26), as these may trigger a crisis. The anaesthetist should be familiar with the clinical features of carcinoid syndrome, in order to anticipate and treat life-threatening features such as bronchospasm and severe haemodynamic instability.

A perioperative octreotide infusion should commence, at least 12 hours prior to surgery to help reduce tumour hormonal activity (18). Intraoperative instability, as a result of vasoactive hormone release, can be treated with further boluses of octreotide. This should then be continued IV or subcutaneously in the postoperative period.

A thoracic epidural should be sited prior to anaesthetic induction to attenuate the surgical stress response. Epidural drug loading should be titrated cautiously as accompanying hypotension may respond erratically to vasopressors, with unpredictable fluctuations in blood pressure. Phenylephrine is the vasopressor of choice and should be titrated to effect. Adrenaline and noradrenaline can lead to exaggerated haemodynamic responses. Noradrenaline and similarly metaraminol, through noradrenaline liberation from the pre-synaptic storage vesicles, may result in paradoxical hypotension due to kallikrein activation and bradykinin release (26). Vasopressin may be useful if prolonged vasoconstriction is required.

Where a patient is undergoing hepatic resection for carcinoid metastases, it may not be possible to maintain a low CVP as hypotension may be exaggerated during the Pringle manoeuvre. Suggested mechanisms for the exaggerated haemodynamic effects include the disruption of the hepatic metabolism of carcinoid vasoactive metabolites during the liver ischaemia and then release of the accumulated metabolites when the Pringle inflow occlusion is released. The severe nature of the haemodynamic effects may completely preclude the use of inflow control. Blood loss and the effects of epidural anaesthesia should also always be considered when treating haemodynamic instability in carcinoid. Conversely, in episodes of extreme hypertension, labetalol or alpha blockade agents may be used.

SUMMARY

This chapter, whilst not exhaustive, highlights the key features of anaesthesia which are unique to hepatopancreatico-biliary surgery. The combination of a highly complex patient cohort and surgical technique demands focus and understanding of the individual roles of the surgeon and anaesthetist. Close communication throughout will facilitate pre-emptive actions and lead to improved patient outcomes.

REFERENCES

1. Pietri LD, Montalti R, Begliomini B. Anaesthetic perioperative management of patients with pancreatic cancer. *World J Gastroenterol* 2014;**20(9)**: 2304–20. doi: 10.3748/wjg.v20.i9.2304.

2. Vaja R, McNicol L, Sisley I. Anaesthesia for patients with liver disease. *BJA Education* 2010;**10(1)**:15–19.

3. Drury N. *Anaesthesia and Liver Disease – Part 2 Tutorial 272.* WFSA. 2012. Available from: https://resources.wfsahq.org/atotw/anaesthesia-and-liver-disease-part-2-anaesthesia-tutorial-of-the-week-272/ (Accessed 19 August 2024).

4. Mills GH. Anaesthesia and the perioperative management of hepatic resection. *Trends Anaesth CritCare* 2011;**1(3)**:147–52.

5. Hartog A, Mills GH. Anaesthesia for hepatic resection surgery. *BJA Education* 2009;**9(1)**:1–5.

6. Page AJ, Kooby, DA. Perioperative management of hepatic resection. *J Gastrointest Oncol* 2012;**3(1)**:19–27.

7. Zaleski L, Abello D, Gold MI. Desflurane versus isoflurane in patients with chronic hepatic and renal disease. *Anesth Analg* 1993;**76(2)**:353–6.

8. Greener NHS. Putting anaesthetic-generated emissions to bed. Available from: https://www.england. nhs.uk/greenernhs/whats-already-happening/putting-anaesthetic-generated-emissions-to-bed/ (Accessed 28 August 2024).

9. Rahimzadeh P, Safari S, Faiz SHR, Alavian SM. Anesthesia for patients with liver disease. *Hepatitis Monthly.* 2014;**14(7)**: 1–7.

10. Pai S, Hughes T. *Perioperative Management and Anaesthetic Considerations for Pancreatic Resection Surgery Tutorial 391.* WFSA. 2018. Available from: https://resources.wfsahq.org/wp-content/uploads/391_english.pdf (Accessed 28 August 2024).

11. Popping DM, Elia N, Van Aken HK, et al. Impact of epidural analgesia on mortality and morbidity after surgery: Systematic review and meta-analysis of randomized controlled trials. *Ann Surg* 2014;**259**:1056–67.

12. Ginsburg R. *Anaesthesia and Liver Disease. Update in Anaesthesia.* 2007. Available from: https://resources.wfsahq.org/wp-content/uploads/uia-16-ANAESTHESIAAND-LIVER-DISEASE.pdf (Accessed 28 August 2024).

13. Redai I, Emond J, Brentjens T. Anesthetic considerations during liver surgery. *Surg Oncol Clin N Am* 2004;**84**:401–11.

14. Mungroop T, Veelo D, Besselink M, van Dieren S, van Gulik TM, Karsten TM, et al. Continuous wound infiltration versus epidural analgesia after hepato-pancreato-biliary surgery (POP-UP): A randomised controlled, open-label, non-inferiority trial. *Lancet Gastroenterol Hepatol* 2016;**1**:105–13.

15. Kasivisvanathan R, Abbassi-Ghadi N, Mallett S, Prout J, Clevenger B, Fusai GK, Mallett SV, et al. A prospective cohort study of intrathecal versus epidural analgesia for patients undergoing hepatic resection. *HPB (Oxford)* 2014;**16(8)**:768–75.

16. Prout J, Jones T, Martin D (eds). *Advanced Training in Anaesthesia: the essential curriculum.* Oxford: Oxford University Press; 2014.

17. Wu CC, Ho WM, Cheng SB, Yeh D-C, Wen M-C, Liu T-J, et al. Perioperative parenteral tranexamic acid in liver tumor resection. A prospective randomized trial toward a 'blood transfusion' free hepatectomy. *Ann Surg* 2006;**243**:173–80.

18. Simmonds PC, Primrose JN, Colquitt JL, Garden OJ, Poston GJ, Rees M, et al. Surgical resection of hepatic metastases from colorectal cancer: A systematic review of published studies. *Br J Cancer* 2006;**94(7)**:982–99.

19. Henry DA, Carless P, Moxey A, , O'Connell D, Stokes BJ, Fergusson DA, et al. Anti-fibrinolytic use for minimising perioperative allogeneic blood transfusion. *Cochrane Database Syst Rev* 2007;**(4)**:CD001886.

20. Nishiyama T, Yokoyama T, Hanaoka K. Effects of sevoflurane and isoflurane anesthesia on arterial ketone body ratio and liver function. *Acta Anaesthesiol Scand* 1999;**43**:347–51.

21. Selzner N, Rudiger H, Graf R, Clavien P-A, et al. Protective strategies against ischemic injury of the liver. *Gastroenterology* 2003;**125**:917–36.

22. Behman R, Hanna S, Coburn N, Law C, Cyr DP, Truong J, et al. Impact of fluid resuscitation on major adverse events following pancreaticoduodenectomy. *Am J Surg* 2015;**210(5)**:896–903.

23. Koti RS, Gurusamy KS, Fusai G, Davidson BR, et al. Meta-analysis of randomized controlled trials on the effectiveness of somatostatin analogues for pancreatic surgery: A Cochrane review. *HPB (Oxford)* 2010;**12**:155–65.

24. Powell B, Mukhtar AA, Mills GH. Carcinoid: The disease and its implications for anaesthesia. *BJA Education* 2011;**11(1)**:9–13.

25. Veall GR, Peacock JE, Bax ND, Reilly CS, et al. Review of the anaesthetic management of 21 patients undergoing laparotomy for carcinoid syndrome. *Br J Anaesth* 1994;**72**:335–34.

Bailey & Love's Essential Operations Bailey & Love's Essential Operatio
Bailey & Love's Essential Operations Bailey & Love's Essential Operatio
Bailey & Love's Essential Operations Bailey & Love's Essential Operatio

SECTION 3 | PREOPERATIVE CARE

Chapter

16

Pain Relief

Pankaj Kundra and Stalin Vinayagam

INTRODUCTION

Pain management plays an important part in the perioperative care of patients undergoing hepato-pancreatico-biliary (HPB) surgery. Inadequate pain relief leads to unpleasant patient experiences, increases complication rates, affects the stress response and prolongs the hospital stay. Pain relief is inadequate in up to 50% of patients undergoing major HPB surgery (1). Perioperative pain is a well-recognized hurdle on the road to rapid recovery following an HPB surgical procedure, and successful pain control continues to be a challenge. Moreover, perioperative pain varies depending upon the specific hepatic, pancreatic and biliary procedure performed and differs between patients undergoing the same procedure. Optimal perioperative pain management requires a multidisciplinary and multimodal approach and should include a combination of regional anaesthetic techniques and parenteral drugs. This chapter will review the standard and evidence-based pain relief strategies for providing optimal pain relief for patients undergoing HPB surgery.

INNERVATION OF THE ABDOMEN

The leading cause for pain after open HPB surgery is trauma to the abdominal wall (somatic pain) and abdominal organs (visceral pain). In laparoscopic procedures, pneumoperitoneum induced abdominal wall distension leads to pain.

The abdominal skin, muscles and peritoneum receive their sensory nerve supply from the T7–T12 intercostal nerves, originating from the ventral rami of the thoracic nerve root (*Figure 16.1*). The abdominal viscera receive autonomic innervation from the splanchnic (sympathetic) nerves and the vagus (parasympathetic) nerve. The hepatic capsule is innervated by branches of the lower intercostal nerves that are stimulated when the capsule is stretched although the liver *per se* does not have any sensory innervation. The bile ducts and the gallbladder sense pain when the surrounding thin layer of tissue is stretched. The pancreas has a dual afferent nerve supply, from branches of the abdominal vagus nerve and the splanchnic nerves, which are responsible for visceral pain (2).

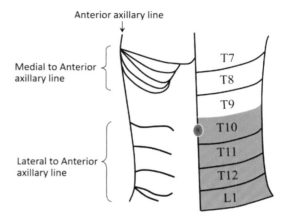

Figure 16.1 Illustration showing the intercostal and subcostal nerve supply of the anterior abdominal wall.

MULTIMODAL ANALGESIA

Multimodal analgesia is a pharmacological method of pain management that combines different groups of medications for pain relief. These drugs act at different levels of pain pathways starting from the generation of painful stimuli at the periphery to blocking the transmission of such impulses to the central nervous system (3). The effectiveness of this analgesic technique in major abdominal surgery has been long established (4) and in HPB surgeries it is advisable to avoid intense, single modality analgesic treatment. The multimodal analgesic technique will reduce the dose of individual drugs and their associated side effects. Studies have shown that by lowering systemic opioid requirements, multimodal analgesia can facilitate early enteral feeding and postoperative mobilization in patients undergoing HPB surgery (5). Such multimodal analgesia techniques should be specific to a particular HPB procedure and include regional anaesthetic techniques and parenteral analgesics.

VARIOUS ANALGESIC MODALITIES

Regional: Epidural anaesthesia; spinal anaesthesia; transverse abdominis plane (TAP) block and wound infiltration.

Parenteral: Opioids; lidocaine; non-steroidal anti-inflammatory drugs (NSAIDs) and paracetamol.

DOI: 10.1201/9781003080060-16

Regional

Regional anaesthesia plays an important role in the perioperative management of pain in patients undergoing HPB surgery. Besides providing improved pain relief, regional anaesthesia has anti-inflammatory effects, facilitates early mobilization and decreases postoperative ileus and pulmonary complications. Various regional anaesthetic techniques have been used, but the most commonly employed methods include: epidural anaesthesia; spinal anaesthesia; transverse abdominis plane block and wound infiltration catheters.

Epidural anaesthesia

Epidural analgesia, an important tool in the anaesthesiologist's armamentarium is widely used in HPB surgery because it provides superior analgesia compared with systemic opioids (6). Most commonly, epidural anaesthesia is combined with general anaesthesia, with the catheter being placed before induction and continued for 3–5 days postoperatively. Epidural placement is performed either sitting or in a lateral position, and the epidural space is approached via a midline or paramedian approach. Recently, ultrasound (US) has been used to facilitate epidural insertion, particularly in obese patients and a longitudinal paramedian scan is the preferred approach for the visualization of the epidural space. Epidural analgesia produces a segmental block over many spinal levels on either side of the insertion point and the point of epidural placement is important as it determines the final segmental block. Usually, a thoracic epidural is preferred for HPB operations due to the high placement of the surgical incision.

Local anaesthetics (LA) are the most commonly used analgesic drugs in epidural anaesthesia and together with a sensory block, they also produce motor blockade, which is dependent on the concentration and dose of LA used. The addition of opioids to the LA improves the quality of analgesia, minimizes the motor block, and decreases the incidence of hypotension by reducing the dose of LA required. In the postoperative period, patients receive either a continuous epidural infusion or variable rate via a patient-controlled analgesia (PCA) pump. The type of infusion and dosing of analgesia depends on the individual anaesthetist's preference. Epidural anaesthesia has been demonstrated to substantially reduce the risk of postoperative pulmonary complications, deep vein thrombosis, ileus, blood loss and renal dysfunction (7).

Epidural analgesia causes sympathetic blockade which may result in hypotension, potentially requiring increased intravenous (IV) fluid administration in patients undergoing HPB surgery (8). Clinical experience over several decades has demonstrated the safety of epidural catheter insertion in hepatic surgery, however following major liver resections elevations in international normalized ratio (INR) can delay epidural catheter removal due to the increased risk of epidural haematoma formation particularly in patients with an INR of more than 1.5 (6). Epidural analgesia is also commonly used in pancreatic surgery. It is an integral and important component of ERAS® pathways and has been shown to improve outcomes (9).

Spinal anaesthesia

Spinal anaesthesia is a simple, and safe, technique where local anaesthesia is administered into the intrathecal space. When combined with general anaesthesia, it has several benefits in HPB surgery, including better pain control, early mobility and decreased postoperative opioid consumption. Compared with epidural anaesthesia, the need for postoperative IV fluids and vasopressors is significantly less (10). Bupivacaine is the most commonly used LA for spinal anaesthesia, either with or without opioids. The addition of opioids has the advantage of prolonging analgesia, but it also increases the risk of respiratory depression in the postoperative period.

Spinal analgesia has not been extensively studied in HPB surgery despite it being one of the most commonly employed anaesthetic techniques for open abdominal surgery. Those studies, which have been performed, have shown that spinal anaesthesia facilitates early mobilization and decreases the hospital stay in patients undergoing hepatic resection compared with epidural anaesthesia (11). Moreover, single-shot spinal anaesthesia nullifies the complications associated with any coagulopathy and has consequently been proposed as an alternative to epidural anaesthesia (12).

Transverse abdominis plane (TAP) block

TAP block is a peripheral nerve-block technique, and its efficacy is well demonstrated in a number of HPB scenarios. It is performed either through a median or paramedian incision and LA such as bupivacaine is deposited in the plane between the internal oblique and transverse abdominis muscles. It provides excellent analgesia for pain originating from the anterior and lateral abdominal wall by blocking somatic nerves but does not provide analgesia for visceral pain. The absence of a motor block with this technique enables early mobilization and speedy recovery in the postoperative period. As the procedure is easy to perform, it can be safely utilized in patients who are anticoagulated, where epidural anaesthesia is contraindicated. The procedure can be performed either as a landmark-based technique or using US after induction of general anaesthesia (*Figure 16.2*). The three main techniques involved are lateral, subcostal, and posterior approaches and TAP blocks can also be performed by surgeons at the end of an operation prior to closure of the abdomen. Studies have shown that preoperative administration of TAP block is found to have an improved analgesic effect when compared with a postoperative block (13). Continuous infusion catheters can also be placed under US-guidance allowing analgesia to be extended for significantly longer in the postoperative period. Bilateral TAP blocks can be considered when epidural analgesia is contraindicated and have the added advantage of decreasing respiratory and cardiovascular complications in the postoperative period. TAP blocks are also frequently used for

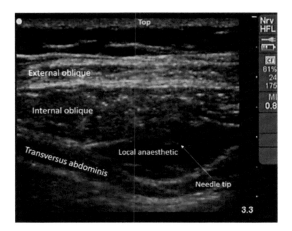

Figure 16.2 US image showing deposition of local anaesthetic by US-guided TAP block.

minimally invasive and laparoscopic HPB procedures. In centres not equipped with US in the operating theatre laparoscopy-assisted TAP blocks, which are as effective as USG-guided blocks should be considered (14). The incidence of hypotension and urinary retention in the postoperative period is less with TAP blocks than epidural anaesthesia (15) and they also lower the total opioid requirement in the first 24 h after surgery which was confirmed in 2010 by a Cochrane Review (16).

Wound infiltration

Wound infiltration is a technique of administering LA directly to the surgical incision in the immediate postoperative period and this technique has been shown to have significant analgesic effects. This is a very simple technique which is performed under direct vision without the need for any specialized equipment such as US which reduces the possibility of iatrogenic injury. In this technique, a sterile multi-orifice catheter is usually placed in the pre-peritoneal space and secured using sutures. The catheter is brought out through the skin using a separate port created with a Tuohy's needle (*Figure 16.3a*). The proximal end of the

catheter is connected to a filter and an adapter with an injection port, which is fixed to the skin using adhesive tape (*Figure 3.16b*). Studies have shown that subfascial placement of the catheter is more effective in terms of analgesic effect compared to subcutaneous placement (17,18). These catheters can also be connected to elastomeric pumps, designed to deliver a constant infusion of LA at a fixed rate for 24–48 h, thereby extending the analgesic benefit in the postoperative period. The most commonly used drugs are 0.25% bupivacaine, 0.25% levobupivacaine or 0.2% ropivacaine at a flow rate of around 10 mL/h for good spread along the desired plane (19).

As a part of a multimodal analgesic regimen, catheter wound infiltration is generally considered safe and can facilitate early recovery following HPB surgery (20). Although experience with wound catheters is relatively limited in HPB surgery they have been shown to produce fewer complications, shorter critical care unit stays, earlier mobilization, and more rapid discharge when compared with epidural analgesia (21). In addition, there is a potential role for this technique in patients in whom epidural anaesthesia is contraindicated and wound infiltration can also be considered as a rescue technique in patients who have undergone laparoscopic HPB procedures which have been converted to an open approach.

Parenteral drugs

Opioids

Opioids are among the most commonly used drugs for treating surgical pain and are extensively prescribed in the postoperative period as rescue analgesic. Opioids are usually administered parenterally via the IV, intramuscular and subcutaneous routes. Commonly used medications include fentanyl, sufentanil, remifentanil, and morphine, typically administered either intermittently or as a continuous infusion (22). Opioid use is associated with various side effects which increase the risk of poor surgical outcomes following HPB surgery. The most common opioid-related side effects are respiratory depression, nausea and postoperative ileus (23). Opioids directly suppress the central ventilatory drive resulting in a respiratory impairment

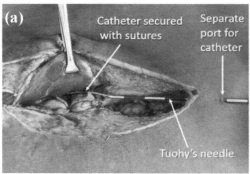
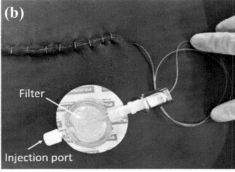

Figure 16.3 Patient images showing wound infiltration catheter placement (a) and fixation (b).

exacerbated by various other factors, including but not limited to, patient comorbidities, obstructive sleep apnoea and the use of additional sedatives (24). Acute and chronic opioid use can directly affect bowel function and lead to postoperative ileus (25) and in HPB surgery, the prime objective of selecting a drug is to minimize the effect of the opioid particularly on the sphincter of Oddi (26). Drugs such as meperidine should be selected instead of other opioids as it has a negligible effect on sphincter of Oddi function. The clearance and metabolism of opioids in the context of hepatic dysfunction are altered, leading to more significant variations in plasma concentrations and frequently a decreased dose requirement. Therefore, the dosing of opioids needs to be carefully monitored in patients with compromised liver function.

Novel formulations and routes of delivery have been developed to reduce the incidence of opioid-induced side effects and improve patients' long-term outcomes after HPB surgery. Administration of opioids through the transdermal route is a simple and painless technique that provides a more prolonged duration of action (*Figure 16.4*) and the commonly used drugs for this route are fentanyl and buprenorphine. Transdermal fentanyl patches are found to have fewer side effects compared with oral morphine (27). In addition, respiratory complications in the postoperative period can be significantly reduced by administering lower doses through transdermal patches. One of the novel patient-controlled analgesia systems, the fentanyl iontophoretic transdermal system (fentanyl ITS), has been found to produce analgesic effects which are as effective as an IV morphine patient-controlled analgesia (PCA). It has the advantage of a rapid rate of absorption with no skin depot effect compared to the classical passive diffusion of transdermal fentanyl (28,29).

Intravenous lidocaine

IV lidocaine, a potent anti-inflammatory and anti-hyperalgesic drug, has been used as an analgesic adjunct to treat postoperative pain following a range of surgical procedures. Level 1 evidence from gastrointestinal (GI) surgery demonstrates decreased pain scores, reduced opioid consumption and fewer side effects in the postoperative period (30). Though lidocaine infusion is yet to be explicitly evaluated in HPB surgery, ERAS guidelines recommend the perioperative use of IV lidocaine as an analgesic whenever epidural anaesthesia is contraindicated (31). The usual recommended dose is a bolus of 100 mg before the start of the surgery followed by a continuous infusion of 1–2 mg/kg/hour to maintain a plasma concentration under 5.0 mg/mL (32). The liver plays an essential role in the metabolism of lidocaine through the cytochrome p450 system, resulting in the formation of various key active metabolites which are then excreted by the kidneys. Thus, plasma concentrations of free lidocaine are significantly affected by diminished hepatic and renal function. One of the major advantages of IV lidocaine is that when a continuous infusion is stopped it has been shown that plasma-levels decrease rapidly (33).

Non-steroidal anti-inflammatory drugs

Non-steroidal anti-inflammatory drugs (NSAIDs) are potent analgesic and anti-inflammatory agents that provide pain relief and attenuate the inflammatory response caused by surgical trauma. Several NSAIDs have been used to treat perioperative pain at different doses and within variable regimens. NSAIDs act on cyclooxygenase-1 and cyclooxygenase-2 and inhibit the synthesis of prostaglandins and thromboxanes, leading to beneficial analgesic and anti-inflammatory effects in the postoperative patient and meta-analyses demonstrate the advantage of NSAIDs in reducing opioid-related side effects (34). Nevertheless, they should only be used for short intervals as there is an increased risk of severe GI bleeding and anastomotic leak after GI surgery (35,36).

Paracetamol

Paracetamol has both analgesic and antipyretic properties and is commonly used for postoperative pain management, as part of multimodal analgesic regimens. Paracetamol can be administered orally, IV, and rectally, and the route chosen influences the bioavailability of the drug. IV paracetamol has a better analgesic effect than the oral route due to higher plasma concentrations and greater CNS penetration (30). Paracetamol is metabolized in the liver by cytochrome p450 and gets conjugated by glutathione. Liver toxicity is a well-documented complication of paracetamol overdose, so the dose should be limited to 4 g over 24 h. Extensive liver resections affect

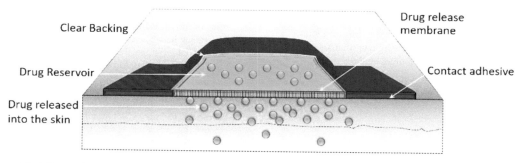

Figure 16.4 Illustration demonstrating the drug dispersal system of a transdermal patch.

paracetamol metabolism, but no deficiency in glutathione is observed (37). Paracetamol should be avoided in patients with acute hepatitis or liver failure.

Enhanced Recovery After Surgery

Enhanced Recovery After Surgery (ERAS) is a multimodality treatment regimen implemented in various surgeries for improved clinical outcomes (*see* Chapter 7) and decreased length of stay, necessitating multidisciplinary management (38). One of the key aims of ERAS programmes is to suppress the physiological stress response following surgery, thereby reducing the morbidity and mortality. Respiratory pre-habilitation by incentive spirometry (39) and optimal analgesia techniques (40) plays vital roles as components of ERAS programmes which improve outcomes in patients undergoing laparotomy. Recent guidelines by the ERAS Society no longer recommends routine thoracic epidural analgesia for open liver surgery and supports the use of intrathecal opioids or wound infusion catheters for optimal postoperative pain management (41). Moreover, there is also a risk of renal failure secondary to epidural induced hypotension and potential delay in catheter removal due to elevated coagulation abnormalities (elevated INR or prothrombin time). There are a large number of trials comparing epidural analgesia with continuous wound infiltration after open liver resection and no differences between the two techniques in respect of complications, length of stay and mobilization have been demonstrated (20,21). This contrasts with ERAS pathways developed for pancreatic surgery where epidural anaesthesia is the recommended approach as it is found to provide superior analgesia with fewer respiratory complications (42).

Pain relief plays a vital role in the perioperative management of patients undergoing HPB surgery. Optimal perioperative pain management requires a multidisciplinary and multimodal approach and should include a combination of regional anaesthetic techniques and parenteral drugs. Most commonly employed regional techniques include epidural, spinal, transverse abdominis plane blocks and wound infiltration, and their selection should be based on potential merits and disadvantages of the individual techniques. Among parenteral drugs, opioids remain the mainstay despite a number of well-documented shortcomings. Other drugs such as NSAIDs and paracetamol should also be considered to avoid or reduce opioid-related side effects. As an analgesic adjuvant, IV lidocaine has been employed in HPB surgery in recent years and found to be effective. The aim of a successful pain management strategy should be to achieve optimal analgesia while minimizing the side effects of a particular technique and achieving the goals of Enhanced Recovery After Surgery.

SUMMARY

Epidural analgesia remains an essential part of perioperative pain management, but recent evidence shows that other techniques such as TAP blocks and wound infiltration catheters are equally effective. Parenteral drugs like lidocaine and paracetamol can decrease the adverse events associated with opioids and improve overall patient outcomes. The available evidence for approaches designed to achieve optimal pain relief in HPB surgery is mixed and often contradictory and the key is to minimize the potential side effects of a particular technique while achieving ERAS goals.

REFERENCES

1. Weinbroum AA. Non-opioid IV adjuvants in the perioperative period: Pharmacological and clinical aspects of ketamine and gabapentinoids. *Pharmacol Res* 2012;**65(4)**:411–29.
2. Jensen KJ, Alpini G, Glaser S. Hepatic nervous system and neurobiology of the liver. *Compr Physiol* 2013;**3(2)**:655–65.
3. Gritsenko K, Khelemsky Y, Kaye AD, Vadivelu N, Urman RD, et al. Multimodal therapy in perioperative analgesia. *Best PractRes Clin Anaesthesiol* 2014; **28(1)**:59–79.
4. Kehlet H, Dahl JB. The value of 'multimodal' or 'balanced analgesia' in postoperative pain treatment. *Anesth Analg* 1993;**77**:1048–56.
5. Wheeler M, Oderda GM, Ashburn MA, Lipman AG, et al. Adverse events associated with postoperative opioid analgesia: A systematic review. *J Pain* 2002;**3(3)**:159–80.
6. Tzimas P, Prout J, Papadopoulos G, Mallett SV, et al. Epidural anaesthesia and analgesia for liver resection. Anaesthesia 2013;68(6):628–35.
7. Moraca RJ, Sheldon DG, Thirlby RC. The role of epidural anesthesia and analgesia in surgical practice. *Ann Surg* 2003;**238(5)**:663–73.
8. Popping DM, Elia N, Van Aken HK, Schug SA, Kranke P, Wenk M, et al. Impact of epidural analgesia on mortality and morbidity after surgery: Systematic review and meta-analysis of randomized controlled trials. *Ann Surg* 2014;**259(6)**:1056–67.
9. Bruns H, Rahbari NN, Löffler T, Diener MK, Seiler CM, Glanemann M, et al. Perioperative management in distal pancreatectomy: Results of a survey in 23 European participating centres of the DISPACT trial and a review of literature. *Trials* 2009;**10**:58.
10. Levy BF, Scott MJ, Fawcett W, Fry C, Rockall TA, et al. Randomized clinical trial of epidural, spinal or patient-controlled analgesia for patients undergoing laparoscopic colorectal surgery. *Br J Surg* 2011; **98(8)**:1068–78.
11. Kasivisvanathan R, Abbassi-Ghadi N, Prout J, Clevenger B, Fusai GK, Mallett SV, et al. A prospective cohort study of intrathecal versus epidural analgesia for patients undergoing hepatic resection. *HPB* 2014;**16(8)**:768–75.
12. De Pietri L, Siniscalchi A, Reggiani A, Masetti M, Begliomini B, Gazzi M, et al. The use of intrathecal morphine for postoperative pain relief after liver resection: A comparison with epidural analgesia. *Anesth Analg* 2006;**102(4)**:1157–63.
13. Favuzza J, Delaney CP. Outcomes of discharge after elective laparoscopic colorectal surgery with trans-versus abdominis plane blocks and enhanced recovery pathway. *J Am Coll Surg* 2013;**217**:503–6.
14. Ravichandran NT, Sistla SC, Kundra P, Ali SM, Dhanapal B, GalidevaraI, et al. Laparoscopic-assisted tranversus abdominis plane (TAP) block

versus ultrasonography-guided transversus abdominis plane block in postlaparoscopic cholecystectomy pain relief: Randomized controlled trial. *Surg Laparosc Endosc Percutan Tech* 2017;**27**(**4**):28–32.

15. Rao Kadam V, Van Wijk RM, Moran JI, Miller D, et al. Epidural versus continuous transversus abdominis plane catheter technique for postoperative analgesia after abdominal surgery. *Anesth Intensive Care* 2013;**41**(**4**):476–81.

16. Keir A, Rhodes L, Kayal A, Khan OA, et al. Does a transversus abdominis plane (TAP) local anaesthetic block improve pain control in patients undergoing laparoscopic cholecystectomy? A best evidence topic. *Int J Surg* 2013;**11**(**9**):792–4.

17. Forastiere E, Sofra M, Giannarelli D, Fabrizi L, Simone G, et al. Effectiveness of continuous wound infusion of 0.5% ropivacaine by On-Q pain relief system for postoperative pain management after open nephrectomy. *Br J Anaesth* 2008;**101**:841–7.

18. Yndgaard S, Holst P, Bjerre-Jepsen K, Thomsen CB, Struckmann J, Mogensen T, et al. Subcutaneously versus subfascially administered lidocaine in pain treatment after inguinal herniotomy. *Anesth Analg* 1994;**79**:324–7.

19. Beaussier M, El'Ayoubi H, Schiffer E, Rollin M, Parc Y, Mazoit J-X, et al. Continuous pre-peritoneal infusion of ropivacaine provides effective analgesia and accelerates recovery after colorectal surgery. *Anesthesiology* 2007;**107**:461–8.

20. Hughes MJ, Harrison EM, Peel NJ, Stutchfield B, McNally S, Beattie C, et al. Randomized clinical trial of perioperative nerve block and continuous local anaesthetic infiltration via wound catheter versus epidural analgesia in open liver resection (LIVER 2 trial). *Br J Surg* 2015;**102**(**13**):1619–28.

21. Revie EJ, McKeown DW, Wilson JA, Garden OJ, Wigmore SJ, et al. Randomized clinical trial of local infiltration plus patient-controlled opiate analgesia vs. epidural analgesia following liver resection surgery. *HPB (Oxford)* 2012;**14**:611–8.

22. Derrode N, Lebrun F, Levron JC, Chauvin M, Debaene B, et al. Influence of peroperative opioid on postoperative pain after major abdominal surgery: Sufentanil TCI versus remifentanil TCI. A randomized, controlled study. Br J Anaesth 2003;91(6):842–9.

23. Erstad BL, Puntillo K, Gilbert HC, Grap MJ, Li D, Medina J, et al. Pain management principles in the critically ill. *Chest* 2009;**135**(**4**):1075–86.

24. Barletta JF. Clinical and economic burden of opioid use for postsurgical pain: Focus on ventilatory impairment and ileus. *Pharmacotherapy* 2012;**32**(**9**):3–9.

25. Barletta JF, Senagore AJ. Reducing the burden of postoperative ileus: Evaluating and implementing an evidence-based strategy. *World J Surg* 2014;**38**(**8**):1966–77.

26. Thompson DR. Narcotic analgesic effects on the sphincter of Oddi: A review of the data and therapeutic implications in treating pancreatitis. *Am J Gastroenterol* 2001;**96**(**4**):1266–72.

27. Radbruch L, Sabatowski R, Loick G, Kulbe C, Kasper M, Grond S, et al. Constipation and the use of laxatives: A comparison between transdermal fentanyl and oral morphine. *Palliat Med* 2000;**14**(**2**):111–19.

28. Rawal N, Langford RM. Current practices for postoperative pain management in Europe and the potential role of the fentanyl HCl iontophoretic transdermal system. *Eur J Anaesthesiol* 2007;**24**(**4**):299–308.

29. Mattia C, Coluzzi F, Sonnino D, Anker-Møller E, et al. Efficacy and safety of fentanyl HCl iontophoretic transdermal system compared with morphine intravenous patient-controlled analgesia for postoperative pain management for patient subgroups. *Eur J Anaesthesiol* 2010;**27**(**5**):433–40.

30. Tan M, Law LS-C, Gan TJ. Optimizing pain management to facilitate Enhanced Recovery After Surgery pathways. *Can J Anaesth* 2014;**62**(**2**):203–18.

31. Fearon KC, Liunggvist O, Von Meyenfeldt M, Revhaug A, Dejong CHC, Lassen K, et al. Enhanced Recovery After Surgery: A consensus review of clinical care for patients undergoing colonic resection. *Clin Nutr* 2005;**24**:466–77.

32. Daykin H. The efficacy and safety of intravenous lidocaine for analgesia in the older adult: A literature review. Br J Pain 2017;11:23–31.

33. Kundra P, Vinayagam S. Perioperative intravenous lidocaine: Crossing local boundaries and reaching systemic horizons. *Indian J Anaesth* 2020;**64**:363–5.

34. Marret E, Kurdi O, Zufferey P, Bonnet F. Effects of nonsteroidal antiinflammatory drugs on patient-controlled analgesia morphine side effects: Meta-analysis of randomized controlled trials. Anesthesiology 2005;102(6):1249–60.

35. Rushfeldt CF, Sveinbjørnsson B, Søreide K, Vonen B. Risk of anastomotic leakage with use of NSAIDs after gastrointestinal surgery. *Int J Color Dis* 2011;**26**(**12**): 1501–9.

36. Kagedan DJ, Ahmed M, Devitt KS, Wei AC. Enhanced recovery after pancreatic surgery: A systematic review of the evidence. *HPB* 2015;**17**(**1**):11–16.

37. Hughes MJ, Harrison EM, Jin Y, Homer N, Wigmore SJ. Acetaminophen metabolism after liver resection: A prospective case-control study. *Dig Liver Dis* 2015;**47**(**12**):1039–46.

38. Hughes MJ, McNally S, Wigmore SJ. Enhanced recovery following liver surgery: A systematic review and meta-analysis. *HPB (Oxford)* 2014;**16**(**8**):699–706.

39. Swaminathan N, Kundra P, Ravi R, Kate V. ERAS protocol with respiratory prehabilitation versus conventional perioperative protocol in elective gastrectomy: A randomized controlled trial. *Int J Surg* 2020;**81**:149–57.

40. Khuri SF, Henderson WG, DePalma RG, Mosca C, Healy NA, Kumbhani DJ, et al. Determinants of long-term survival after major surgery and the adverse effect of postoperative complications. *Ann Surg* 2005;**242**:326–41.

41. Melloul E, Hübner M, Scott M, Snowden C, Prentis J, Dejong CHC, et al. Guidelines for perioperative care for liver surgery: Enhanced Recovery After Surgery (ERAS®) Society recommendations. *World J Surg* 2016;**40**(**10**):2425–40.

42. Lassen K, Coolsen MM, Slim K, Carli F, de Aguilar-Nascimento JE, Schäfer M, et al. ERAS® Society; European Society for Clinical Nutrition and Metabolism; International Association for Surgical Metabolism and Nutrition. Guidelines for perioperative care for pancreaticoduodenectomy: Enhanced Recovery After Surgery (ERAS®) Society recommendations. *Clin Nutr* 2012;**31**:817–30.

Bailey & Love's Essential Operations Bailey & Love's Essential Operations
Bailey & Love's Essential Operations Bailey & Love's Essential Operations
Bailey & Love's Essential Operations Bailey & Love's Essential Operations

SECTION 3 | PREOPERATIVE CARE

Chapter

17

Day Case Surgery

Thomas MacCabe and Andrew Strickland

INTRODUCTION

This chapter discusses the current practices of day case surgery in the wider field of hepato-pancreatico-biliary (HPB) surgery. It introduces the concept of selection criteria that permit successful day case surgery which can improve the patient experience, in addition to offering significant financial incentives to healthcare providers. The recent advances in anaesthesia which have facilitated the evolution of day case surgery are reviewed, including the prevention of common problems such as postoperative nausea and vomiting and pain control. Measures for successful day case surgery are explored, including methods to reduce unplanned admissions, whilst maintaining the safety and welfare of each patient. Since this is a rapidly progressing field of surgery, this chapter describes the current variations in practice and recent developments that may guide hepatobiliary surgery in day case surgery going forward.

The provision of surgical intervention, without requiring hospital admission has been a significant development in modern medical practice. The avoidance of an overnight stay has a substantial impact for both patients and healthcare providers, allowing for a quicker recovery for patients, less disruption to an individual's daily routine and reduces the risk of hospital-acquired infections. Additionally, day case surgery reduces the demand on inpatient bed pressures and has considerable financial incentives, with estimated average savings of between 11–70% compared with the same procedure when performed as an inpatient (1). The success of day case surgery has resulted in a wider range of procedures being offered in the day case setting with ever-increasing complexity (*Figure 17.1*). The main drivers facilitating this change have resulted from improvements in anaesthesia, surgical technique and technology including minimally invasive surgery. In the UK, day case surgery is defined as the intended admission, operation and discharge of a patient within the same day. Most other healthcare systems, including the United States, use a '23-hour stay' to describe patients who require an overnight admission postoperatively.

PATIENT SELECTION CRITERIA

The Academy of Medical Royal Colleges recommend that 'day surgery should be considered as the default for most surgical procedures' and that the majority of patients are suitable. The success of day case surgery is dependent on three key factors: Medical, surgical and social.

Medical factors

The assessment of an individual's fitness and suitability for day case surgery should be determined by functional and physiological capacity, rather than a single parameter such as age or body mass index (BMI). Historical limits

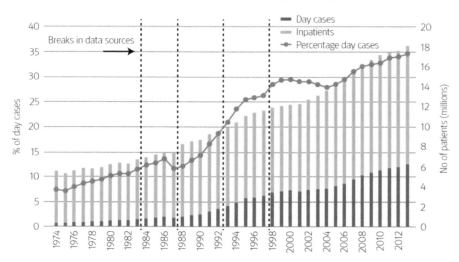

Figure 17.1 Proportion of all patient activity carried out as day cases: England: 1974–2013. Adapted from (14).

DOI: 10.1201/9781003080060-17

to a patient's age, American Society of Anaesthesiology (ASA) grade or BMI, when considering day case surgery, are no longer applicable with more elderly, obese and comorbid individuals safely undergoing day case surgery. Elderly patients can safely be operated on in the day case surgery environment, preventing admissions which interfere with normal routines which are well recognized triggers of acute confusion. The physiological stress from starvation, anaesthesia and surgery may prompt hypoglycaemia and dehydration and therefore needs consideration in selected individuals before undergoing surgery. Obese patients with a BMI >35 should not be excluded from day case surgery as evidence demonstrates no increase in re-admission or complication rates in this group if they are selected appropriately. Obese patients, however, are more likely to be comorbid, with poorly controlled chronic health conditions and therefore most centres would recommend formal preoperative assessment by an experienced anaesthetist. In general, a thorough assessment by preoperative assessment nurses or anaesthetists can successfully determine suitability for day case surgery and identify comorbidities that need optimizing prior to surgery.

Patients with a stable chronic disease such as diabetes, asthma or epilepsy are often better managed when a procedure's disruption to their normal routine is minimized. Additionally, unstable conditions such as poorly controlled diabetes or unstable angina can be optimized prior to surgery. The use of anticoagulants and antiplatelet therapy is increasingly commonplace among the general population and is not *per se* considered an absolute contraindication for day surgery. Local guidelines concerning anticoagulants should be followed with clear communication to patients and clinicians regarding the timing of the cessation of anticoagulants preoperatively and subsequent recommencement postoperatively. Additionally, and if appropriate, communications should include information pertaining to the use of bridging plans and therapies such as low-molecular weight heparin until adequate anticoagulation is restored.

Surgical factors

Several advances in technology and surgical technique have allowed more complex surgical procedures to be performed as day cases. There are several key principles to consider when determining whether a procedure is suitable for day surgery. These include the duration of the procedure, the risk of major complications that may require urgent intervention, and the speed at which patients are likely to return to their baseline function postoperatively. Successful discharge after day case surgery requires patients to be able to mobilize safely, resume oral intake and have pain controlled through a combination of oral medications and local anaesthetic techniques. Therefore, when considering the surgical technique, minimal access approaches should always be used when possible and the surgeon should limit any tissue trauma and ensure meticulous haemostasis.

Social factors

A prerequisite for safe, same day discharge, is that a responsible adult escorts the patient home and supports them at home for the following 24 hours. This 24-hour rule is true for any procedure under general anaesthetic or sedation, however frailer patients and more invasive procedures may necessitate a longer recuperation time and so management should be tailored on an individual basis. Whoever is providing care should be designated prior to the day of surgery and appropriate transport arrangements made to minimize failed discharge on the day of surgery due to inadequate social preparations.

An additional factor that must be considered is the distance from the patient's home to the hospital. In the event of a complication requiring urgent intervention, patients living in rural areas, in particular, could be a considerable distance or travel time from hospital facilities, and it is generally recommended that the journey time from home to hospital should be an hour or less. Many self-contained day surgery units are freestanding and as a result often located closer to patient's homes than hospitals with inpatient beds. An alternative for individuals who live far from hospital is limited care accommodation or medi-motels, where non-professional staff act as replacements for carers and relatives. These have reduced cost implications than inpatient beds and allow patients to recover safely when social factors precluded day surgery.

OUTPATIENT AND PREOPERATIVE ASSESSMENT CLINIC

Once a decision for day surgery has been made, it should be communicated to the patient as soon as possible. Introducing the concept of day surgery, at an early stage, allows patients to develop realistic expectations, make appropriate postoperative arrangements and become motivated to recover promptly following their procedure. All patients should be considered for day case surgery until it is demonstrated they cannot meet the day case criteria. This decision may be straightforward for many individuals, but all require a formal anaesthetic assessment by trained preoperative assessment nursing staff or anaesthetists. This assessment can also help identify social problems that might preclude day surgery, for example, individuals without relatives or relations to provide postoperative care. At the same time, it offers an opportunity to optimize comorbidities and provide prehabilitation advice regarding weight loss, exercise regimes and smoking cessation.

ANAESTHESIA IN DAY SURGERY

In recent years, advances in anaesthesia and the successful introduction of specific pathways for day case surgery have contributed to the increasing volume and complexity of surgical procedures being performed globally. Total intravenous anaesthesia (TIVA) where anaesthesia is induced and maintained using intravenous propofol and short-acting opiates is a practice that has revolutionized day case surgery. TIVA has allowed clinicians to avoid inhalational agents such as nitrous oxide or fluorinated ethers, which commonly cause postoperative nausea and vomiting (PONV). In addition to reducing the rates of PONV in day case surgery, TIVA has also been shown to reduce recovery times and length of hospital stay, without affecting unplanned re-admission rates.

There is a cost implication for the use of TIVA, which in the UK is estimated to be £5–8 more expensive, per patient anaesthetic episode, when compared to inhaled agents (2). Irrespective of which anaesthetic methods is used, it is well-recognized that the success of day case surgery relies on prompt management of pain and PONV to facilitate discharge and prevent avoidable admissions.

Postoperative nausea and vomiting (PONV)

The pathophysiology of nausea and vomiting is complex and involves multiple organs and pathways including the chemoreceptor trigger zone (CTZ), a vagal mucosal pathway in the gastrointestinal system, neuronal pathways from the vestibular system, a reflex afferent pathway from the cerebral cortex and midbrain afferents. Despite the complexity of PONV, there are several well-recognized risk factors which have been incorporated into predictive scoring systems, the most recognized being the Apfel et al. (3) and Koivuranta et al. scoring systems (4) (*Table 17.1*). These validated scoring systems can help to identify those at risk, though there is limited evidence supporting specific anti-emetic regimens. Clinical practice, however, would commonly include multiple agents such as ondansetron, dexamethasone and dopamine receptor antagonists such as metoclopramide, haloperidol and chlorpromazine.

Table 17.1 Postoperative nausea and vomiting (PONV)-risk scoring systems

Risk factor included in scoring system	Apfel et al. (3)	Koivuranta et al. (4)
Female	✓	✓
Non-smoker	✓	✓
History of PONV		✓
History of motion sickness		✓
Combined history of PONV/motion sickness	✓	
Surgical duration >1 h		✓
Postoperative opiates	✓	
Total score	/4	/5

Analgesia

Multimodal oral analgesia and limiting opiate use, to give adequate pain control without initiating PONV, is essential for successful day case surgery (5). When opiates are required, it is recommended that very short-acting opiates such as remifentanil are used instead of longer-acting compounds. Preoperative loading with paracetamol and non-steroidal anti-inflammatories, unless contra-indicated, should be given to all patients and when possible, long-acting local anaesthetic agents should be used as an adjunct. Whether given as a local infiltration or regional nerve block, local anaesthetics provide excellent pain relief in the day case surgery setting.

Venous thromboembolism prophylaxis

The risk of venous thromboembolism (VTE) must be assessed preoperatively on an individual basis. Although early mobilization reduces VTE risk, patient and surgical factors frequently increase this risk, necessitating a clinical decision to use mechanical prophylaxis such as thromboembolic deterrent stockings (TEDS), intermittent pneumatic compression or chemical prophylaxis with low-molecular weight heparin.

POSTOPERATIVE RECOVERY

Postoperative recovery is divided into two phases. The first phase being defined as the time from the end of anaesthesia until the return of protective reflexes and motor function, and the second phase encompassing the ongoing recovery until the patient meets pre-defined discharge dependant criteria. The exact criteria vary between institutes and operations, but generally include stable observations, controlled symptoms, ability to understand postoperative instructions and receipt of appropriate safety-netting information. Clear verbal and written instructions with the healthcare unit's contact details are of paramount importance in day case surgery. This ensures that patients who do experience complications return promptly to an appropriate place for assessment and intervention.

POSTOPERATIVE COMPLICATIONS

Major morbidity and mortality following day case surgery is extremely rare. Minor complications, however, are more common and a cause for failed discharges or readmission. As such, it has become increasingly important for patients to not only understand the risks of surgery, but are also aware of the common signs and symptoms and what to do when they occur. The most common causes for reattendance are pain, PONV, bleeding and infections. Following hepatobiliary surgery, additional complications such as bile duct injury, bile leaks and retained stones are encountered albeit infrequently, particularly after laparoscopic cholecystectomy with reported incidence rates of around 0.5%, 0.3% and 1.8%, respectively (6,7).

UNPLANNED ADMISSIONS

The success of a day case surgery unit is commonly defined as the proportion of patients who undergo the proposed surgery and are safely discharged, without requiring overnight admission. The rate of unplanned overnight admission due to surgical, medical, anaesthetic or social complications after any day case surgery averages 1% in most units (5), with bleeding being the most common surgery-related cause. Although this is clearly a testament to the success of day case surgery protocols, admission rates vary significantly depending on the operative procedure undertaken and also between centres. For example, unplanned admission rates after laparoscopic cholecystectomy have been reported in one retrospective study as 4.5% (8), compared with 24.2% from another unit (9). In order to measure the standard of care, provide quality assurance and ensure patient safety, the International Association for Ambulatory Surgery has developed a set of clinical indicators (*Table 17.2*). These parameters can be used to help structure regular audits that are essential for each unit to identify shortcomings, help improve practice and facilitate comparative studies.

SOCIAL OUTCOMES

Patient reported outcome measures are now recognized as a fundamental assessment of the quality of care being delivered by healthcare professionals. Patient

Table 17.2 Clinical indicators set by the International Association for Ambulatory Surgery (IAAS)

Indicator	Details
1	Cancellation of booked procedures
1.1	Failure to attend the day surgery centre/unit
1.2	Cancellation of the booked procedure after arrival at the day surgery centre/unit
2	Unplanned return to the operation room on the same day
3	Unplanned overnight admission
4	Unplanned return of the patient to an ambulatory surgery unit or hospital
5	Unplanned readmission of the patient to an ambulatory surgery unit or hospital

Additional clinical indicators considered inappropriate

Mortality rate

Infection

Table 17.3 Factors associated with improved patient satisfaction

- Good postoperative pain control
- No postoperative nausea and vomiting
- Good pre- and postoperative information
- Increased surgery availability and short waiting time before surgery
- Avoiding longer operating room and post-anaesthetic care unit times
- Courtesy of staff and friendly environment
- Privacy within the day surgery facility
- Avoidance of patients feeling that they are being discharged too early or rushed
- Telephone follow-up contact on the next day

satisfaction is often positive following day case surgery with high satisfaction occurring when events match a patient's expectations. This highlights the importance of clear information and education pre- and postoperatively to manage these expectations, but several other variables have been shown to be linked with improved satisfaction (*Table 17.3*). Additionally, a prompt uninterrupted return to baseline function is important not only for patient's physical and psychological wellbeing, but also economically as any delay in recovery can affect an individual's return to work and potentially cause economic hardship.

CURRENT PRACTICE

Since the first reports of day case laparoscopic cholecystectomies in 1990 (10), it has rapidly been adopted as standard practice. Conversion and complication rates have fallen, but the rates of successful same day discharge vary significantly from 40% to 83% (11). Based upon a UK-wide audit, the cholecystectomy-as-a-day-case (CAAD) scoring system has been developed to help predict patients who are less likely to be successfully discharged on the same day (*Table 17.4*). Patients with CAAD scores of ≤5 were associated with an 80% chance of a successful day case cholecystectomy compared to those with scores >5 where the rate was 20%.

Bile duct exploration could feasibly be performed as day case surgery, if undertaken as the first case on an operating list, particularly if percutaneous drains are placed. This allows the surgeon to assess for evidence of a bile leak once the patient has recovered and determine if the drain can be removed prior to discharge. When considering the technique to be used for exploration, a trans-cystic approach will have a significantly lower bile leak rate than transductal, but has limitations including the cystic duct diameter, duct length, stone size and location.

In current practice, day case surgery for malignant hepatobiliary disease is limited. Laparoscopy with adjuncts such as ultrasound (US) for staging of

Table 17.4 Cholecystectomy-as-a-day-case (CAAD) score. Predicting successful same-day discharge after laparoscopic cholecystectomy

Patient and preoperative factors	
<30	0
30–60	1
61–70	2
71+	3
Gender	
Female	0
Male	1
ASA	
ASA1	0
ASA2	1
ASA3+	3
Previous admission to hospital[1]	1
Primary indication for surgery	
Biliary colic	0
Cholecystitis	1
Pancreatitis	1
CBD stone	2
Other	0
Preoperative investigations[2]	
US only	0
Radiological	1
Endoscopic	2
US findings	
Thick-walled gallbladder	1
Dilated CBD	1

Abbreviation: ASA: American Society of Anesthesiologists (Physical-status classification score); *CBD:* common bile duct.
[1]Previous gallstone-related emergency admission to hospital.
[2]Preoperative investigations: Radiological: CT and MR cholangiopancreatography (MRCP); endoscopic: ERCP and EUS.

hepatobiliary cancers are ideally suited for day case surgery. Additionally, laparoscopy can be used to facilitate radiofrequency or microwave ablation for liver tumours in close proximity to organs that preclude percutaneous access.

Interventional endoscopic techniques have advanced significantly in the last decade allowing more complex and invasive procedures to be performed. Endoscopic retrograde cholangiopancreatography (ERCP) to access the common bile duct and more recently Spyglass® cholangioscopy to visualize intra-hepatic bile ducts has transformed the investigation of and intervention for biliary disease. Endoscopic ultrasound (EUS),

performed by experienced clinicians, can add valuable anatomical, cytological and biochemical information when assessing upper gastrointestinal tract pathology and additionally be used to perform minimally invasive interventional procedures. However, these longer and more complex procedures are often not tolerated well by the patients, and frequently require deeper sedation or general anaesthesia, to ensure adequate views and allow the procedure to be performed safely.

FUTURE PROSPECTS

In parallel with other surgical specialties, more complex hepatobiliary procedures are being undertaken as day cases and although these are still in their infancy, the results are promising. Two small prospective studies have reported two series of 23 and 20 patients who have undergone laparoscopic liver surgery with the aim of discharge on the same day (12,13). Both studies included single segment or left lateral sectionectomy for liver metastases, benign lesions, hepatocellular carcinomas (12) and fenestration of liver cysts (13). Both studies adopted strict inclusion criteria and arranged early postoperative follow-up with a nurse-led telephone call on day one and with the operating surgeon on days 3 and 4. Same day discharge, without readmission was successful in 83% and 100% of patients, respectively, with neither study reporting any major complications of Clavien-Dindo 3 or above.

REFERENCES

1. Castoro C, Bertinato L, Baccaglini U, Drace CA, McKee M. 2007. *Day surgery: Making it happen. Policy brief, 12.* Available from: https://iris.who.int/handle/10665/107831 (Accessed March, 2024).
2. Kumar G, Stendall C, Mistry R, Gurusamy J, Walker DA. Comparison of total intravenous anaesthesia using propofol with sevoflurane or desflurane in ambulatory surgery: Systematic review and meta-analysis. *Anaesthesia* 2014;**69**:1138–50.
3. Apfel CC, Korttila K, Abdalla M, Kerger H, Turan A, Vedder I, et al. A factorial trial of six interventions for the prevention of postoperative nausea and vomiting. *N Engl J Med* 2004;**350**:2441–51.
4. Koivuranta M, Laara E, Snare L, Alahuhta S. A survey of postoperative nausea and vomiting. *Anaesthesia* 1997;**52**:443–9.
5. Deutsch N, Wu CL. Patient outcomes following ambulatory anesthesia. *Anesthesiol Clin North Am* 2003;**21**:403–15.
6. Vecchio R, MacFayden BV, Latteri S. Laparoscopic cholecystectomy: An analysis on 114,005 cases of United States series. *Int Surg* 1998;**83(3)**:215–19.
7. Lee DH, Ahn YJ, Lee HW, Chung JK, Jung IM. Prevalence and characteristics of clinically significant retained common bile duct stones after laparoscopic cholecystectomy for symptomatic cholelithiasis. *Ann Surg Treat Res* 2016;**91(5)**:239–46. doi:10.4174/astr.2016.91.5.239

8. Lau H, Brookes DC. Contemporary outcomes of ambulatory laparoscopic cholecystectomy in a major teaching hospital. *World J Surg* 2002;**26**:1117–21.

9. Solodkyy A, Hakeem AR, Oswald N, Di Franco F, Gergely S, Harris AM. 'True Day Case' laparoscopic cholecystectomy in a high-volume specialist unit and review of factors contributing to unexpected overnight stay. *Minim Invasive Surg* 2018;1260358.

10. Reddick EJ, Olsen DO. Outpatient laparoscopic laser cholecystectomy. *Am J Surg* 1990;**160(5)**:485–7. doi: 10.1016/s0002-9610(05)81009-8. PMID: 2146896.

11. El-Sharkawy AM, Tewari N, Vohra R, CholeS Study Group, West Midlands Research Collaborative. The cholecystectomy as a day case (CAAD) Score: A validated score of preoperative predictors of successful day-case cholecystectomy using the CholeS Data Set. *World J Surg* 2019;**43**:192–3.

12. Rebibo L, Leourier P, Badaoui R, Le Roux F, Lorne E, Regimbeau J. Minor laparoscopic liver resection as day-case surgery (without overnight hospitalisation): A pilot study. *Surg Endosc* 2019;**33**:261–71.

13. Gaillart M, Tranchart H, Lainas P, Tzanis D, Franco D, Dagher I. Ambulatory laparoscopic minor hepatic surgery: Retrospective observational study. *J Visceral Surg* 2015;**152**:292–6.

14. Appleby J. Day case surgery: A good news story for the NHS. *BMJ* 2015;**351**:h4060. doi:10.1136/bmj.h4060

FURTHER READING

Bailey CR, Ahuja M, Bartholomew K, Bew S, Forbes L, Lipp A, et al. Guidelines for day-case surgery 2019: Guidelines from the Association of Anaesthetists and the British Association of Day Surgery. *Anaesthesia* 2019;**74(6)**:778–92. doi: 10.1111/anae.14639. Epub 2019 Apr 8. PMID: 30963557.

Lemos P, Jarrett P, Phillip B. 2006. *Day Surgery, Development and Practice International Association for Ambulatory Surgery.* Available from: https://theiaas.net/wp-content/uploads/2022/06/DaySurgery.pdf (Accessed March, 2024).

Russon K, Stocker M, Montgomery J, Ahuja M. 2020. *Guidelines for the Provision of Anaesthesia Services for Day Surgery.* Royal College of Anaesthetists. Available from: https://rcoa.ac.uk/gpas/chapter-6 (Accessed March, 2024).

Bailey & Love's Essential Operations Bailey & Love's Essential Operatio
Bailey & Love's Essential Operations Bailey & Love's Essential Operatic
Bailey & Love's Essential Operations Bailey & Love's Essential Operatic

SECTION 3 | PREOPERATIVE CARE

Chapter 18
Cirrhosis and Portal Hypertension

Hossamaldin Nawara, Xiao-Ping Chen and Zhen Yang

INTRODUCTION

Cirrhosis is the transformation of liver parenchyma into multiple nodules of regenerating hepatocytes surrounded by fibrous septa. This occurs as a consequence of chronic liver damage which can be due to a number of conditions and leads to increased portal venous pressure and a decline in liver function.

The most common cause of cirrhosis in the UK is alcohol-induced liver disease (ALD), followed by non-alcoholic steatohepatitis (NASH), and chronic infection with viral hepatitis B and C. Together these account for more than 90% of patients with liver cirrhosis (1) and other causes of cirrhosis are listed in *Table 18.1*. These figures vary in different regions of the world, where viral hepatitis remains the leading cause of liver disease in Africa, most of Asia and the Middle East.

Over the last few decades, death rates from major diseases have plummeted secondary to improvements and investment in healthcare. The mortality from liver disease contrasts with this and has increased significantly owing to the rising prevalence of obesity and increased alcohol consumption.

Since 2001, according to the Office for National Statistics (ONS), there has been a progressive rise in the incidence of liver disease and liver cancer-related mortality among individuals below the age of 75 in England. In 2020, the rate of such fatalities reached a record of 20.6 per 100 000 population, compared with 15.4 per 100 000 population in 2001 (2).

PATHOPHYSIOLOGY

Cirrhosis is the ultimate pathological sequela of hepatic parenchymal destruction and inflammation and is characterized by replacement of normal liver parenchyma with nodules of regenerating hepatocytes, with loss of the normal histological architecture. The destruction and loss of hepatocytes incites an inflammatory process with activation of fibrogenesis and deposition of fibrous tissue in place of the damaged cells. Fibrogenesis is a dynamic process and is mediated by hepatic stellate cells, and portal myofibroblasts which, when activated, respond to stimuli from cytokines and inflammatory mediators, primarily transforming growth factor-α (TGF-α), resulting in deposition of collagen and other extracellular matrix proteins (3). Collagen deposition leads to loss of fenestrations in the sinusoid wall and obliteration of the space of Disse, impairing the contact and exchange between the blood and hepatocytes, and restricting the normal blood flow from the portal tract through the sinusoids to the central vein leading to portal hypertension. The direct shunting of blood with compromised exchange with the hepatocytes and the loss of liver cell mass result in impaired liver function. The fibrotic nodules are formed of hepatocytes surrounded by fibrous tissue and lack a central vein (*Figure 18.1*) (4,5).

This process may take years and can be classified into two dynamic and progressive phases. The compensated phase where patients don't exhibit any clinical symptoms or signs, and the late decompensated phase, where patients present with the complications of liver dysfunction and portal hypertension.

Portal hypertension leads to formation of collateral portosystemic shunts in different anatomical sites, with shunting of blood through to the systemic circulation. This contributes to hepatic encephalopathy as the bacterial products and ammonia escape trapping and metabolism by the liver (6). Oesophageal and gastric varices result from dilated collateral veins in the walls of lower oesophagus and stomach.

The development of ascites in portal hypertension can be explained by the so-called peripheral arterial vasodilatation hypothesis (7). Portal hypertension stimulates the production of endogenous vasodilators such as nitric oxide (NO), which act on the systemic vascular beds especially the splanchnic circulation. This results in splanchnic arteriolar dilatation and effective hypovolaemia. This leads to stimulation of the renin-angiotensin-aldosterone axis as well as antidiuretic hormone (ADH) and sympathetic stimulation and subsequent increase in cardiac output, renal vasoconstriction and salt and water

Table 18.1 Causes of cirrhosis

- Alcoholic liver disease
- Hepatitis B & C
- Non-alcoholic fatty liver disease (NAFLD)
- Primary biliary cholangitis
- Haemochromatosis
- Wilson's disease
- Autoimmune hepatitis

DOI: 10.1201/9781003080060-18

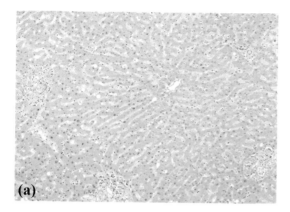

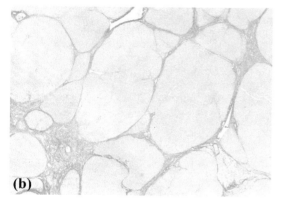

Figure 18.1 Liver lobule histology. Normal histology (a), histology of liver cirrhosis showing multiple nodules of hepatocytes surrounded by fibrous tissue (b). (Reproduced with permission from ref 46.)

retention. In the long term, these mechanisms lead to impaired cardiac function, and predispose patients to renal failure (hepatorenal syndrome) especially when exposed to hypovolaemia, haemorrhage, infection, or surgical stress, with a high risk of mortality (8).

Liver cirrhosis is the most common aetiology of portal hypertension, however, there are other causes which can be classified according to the anatomical location of blood flow resistance into prehepatic, intrahepatic (presinusoidal, sinusoidal and post-sinusoidal), and post-hepatic (*Table 18.2*) (9).

Prehepatic causes result from obstruction of the main portal vein secondary to thrombosis, where liver cirrhosis forms the most common risk factor and can lead to worsening of portal hypertension, or compression from malignancy or inflammatory conditions as in pancreas cancer or pancreatitis (10).

Left-sided (sinistral) portal hypertension results from splenic vein thrombosis, usually secondary to pancreatitis, and leads to the development of collateral veins draining the spleen and stomach, which may lead to the formation of gastric varices, and recurrent bleeding (11).

Sinusoidal obstruction syndrome (previously called veno-occlusive disease) can result from chemotherapeutic agents, leading to damage of the sinusoidal endothelial cells, which are shed into the lumen to cause obstruction and congestion, with activation of stellate cells and fibrosis. These effects in combination with direct cytotoxic effect from the chemotherapeutic drugs are the cause of hepatocyte necrosis and hepatic impairment in these patients (12). This is relevant to surgeons when planning hepatic resection for colorectal and other cancer metastases in patients who had chemotherapy.

DIAGNOSIS OF CIRRHOSIS AND PORTAL HYPERTENSION

Patients in the early compensated stage of liver cirrhosis are usually asymptomatic, but risk for cirrhosis can be suggested from the history, and some patients may exhibit clinical symptoms and signs related to the aetiology of the disease (alcohol-related pancreatitis, or a previous history of acute alcoholic or viral hepatitis).

In the decompensated phase, patients may present with a wide range of symptoms including muscle cramps, muscle wasting, insomnia, fatigue, pruritis, erectile dysfunction, anxiety and depression (13). Additionally, they may develop complications related to end-stage liver disease or portal hypertension, such as encephalopathy, ascites, variceal bleeding, hepatorenal syndrome, spontaneous bacterial peritonitis and development of hepatocellular carcinoma.

Several grading systems exist for the severity of cirrhosis. Child-Pugh score which was originally designed

Table 18.2 Causes of portal hypertension

Prehepatic	Intrahepatic, presinusoidal	Intrahepatic, sinusoidal	Intrahepatic, post-sinusoidal	Post-hepatic

• Portal vein thrombosis
• Splenic vein thrombosis (left-sided portal hypertension)
	• Schistosomiasis
	• Sarcoidosis
	• Congenital hepatic fibrosis
		• Cirrhosis
		• Non-cirrhotic:
		  ○ Acute hepatitis (Drug-induced, Alcoholic etc.)
			• Veno-occlusive disease
			  ○ Sinusoidal obstruction syndrome (SOS)
				• Budd–Chiari syndrome

Table 18.3 Child-Pugh scoring system and contributory factors

Factor	1 point	2 points	3 points
Total Bilirubin (µmol/L)	<34	34–50	>50
Serum Albumin (g/L)	>35	28–35	<28
INR	<1.7	1.7–2.3	>2.3
Ascites	Absent	Mild	Moderate
Encephalopathy	No encephalopathy	Grade 1–2	Grade 3–4

Class A: 5–6 points, **Class B**: 7–9 points, **Class C**: 10–15 points

for risk stratification in patients undergoing shunt surgery for portal hypertension, is still the most frequently used tool for grading and prediction of morbidity and mortality in cirrhosis (*Table 18.3*). Similarly, the model for end-stage liver disease (MELD) score was initially developed to predict survival in patients having trans-jugular intrahepatic portosystemic shunt (TIPS). Including objective parameters of bilirubin, INR, creatinine, and sodium, MELD is now a widely-used tool to list patients for liver transplantation, according to their predicted mortality (14).

Laboratory tests help in reaching the diagnosis and may be evident in the early stage of the disease. Thrombocytopenia is common due to impaired synthesis secondary to decreased thrombopoietin from the diseased liver, or increased sequestration in the spleen in portal hypertension (15). Impaired synthetic function will manifest as reduced serum albumin level, and prolonged prothrombin and thromboplastin times. Elevated serum bilirubin level result from impaired bilirubin conjugation and excretion.

Liver biopsy has traditionally been considered the gold standard for the diagnosis of cirrhosis, however, there are several limitations including sampling error, quantity of tissue, subjectivity and invasiveness. The development of accurate non-invasive techniques, such as transient elastography (an ultrasound [US] exam that uses pulse-echo US acquisitions to measure liver stiffness) and imaging with US, CT, and MRI has made biopsy unnecessary (16). Endoscopy is indicated for diagnosis and follow-up of patients with portal hypertension and varices.

The 'gold standard' for the diagnosis of portal hypertension is the measurement of hepatic venous pressure gradient (HVPG), which is the difference between the portal pressure and the hepatic venous pressure. It can be measured with the help of interventional radiology techniques using a round-tipped catheter to measure the free hepatic venous pressure in the hepatic vein (FHVP) and then wedged into the hepatic vein branch to measure the sinusoidal pressure which is reflective of portal venous pressure in portal hypertension (WHVP) (17). The normal HVPG is 2–5 mmHg and a value of 6 mmHg or more defines portal hypertension, and

a value over 10 indicates clinically significant/severe portal hypertension (CSPH) with high risk of development of complications such as ascites and variceal bleeding. Direct measurement of the portal venous pressure using a transhepatic approach is now rarely done due to risk of intraperitoneal bleeding. Similarly, with the improved accuracy of the above-mentioned techniques, measurement of HVPG is not necessary in most clinical settings.

Transient elastography (Fibroscan)

Transient elastography (TE) is a technique that utilizes US waves to measure stiffness of the liver. A wave of external vibration is applied, and the US detects the transmission of the shear wave through the liver parenchyma to measure liver stiffness in kilopascals (kPa) (18). In a large meta-analysis, TE had 83% sensitivity and 89% specificity for diagnosing cirrhosis, with mean cut-off value of 15 kPa (range: 9–26.5). TE can also predict the development of complications of cirrhosis, such as portal hypertension and varices. In a large meta-analysis, TE had a 90% sensitivity and 79% specificity for the diagnosis of significant portal hypertension (cut-off values: 13.6–34.9) (19).

Imaging

US is one of the most commonly used non-invasive tools to diagnose cirrhosis. Morphological changes associated with cirrhosis such as coarse or nodular liver parenchyma, hepatomegaly, portal vein diameter, splenomegaly or caudate lobe hypertrophy can be detected using US. Doppler mode can detect portal vein flow velocity and direction. Hepatopetal forward portal flow (FPF) and hepatofugal non-forward portal flow (NFPF) refer to the direction of portal vein blood flow towards or away from the liver, respectively. Reversal of blood flow is associated with increased severity of portal hypertension and reduced survival (20).

Computed tomography (CT) is also used to diagnose cirrhosis, through identification of morphological changes, in the same way as US. CT can also detect the presence of varices, and collateral vessels indicating severe portal hypertension (*Figures 18.2*

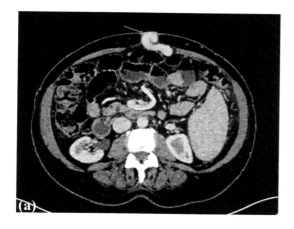

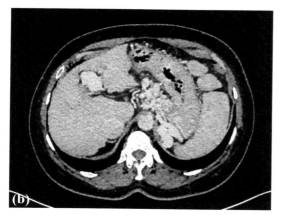

Figure 18.2 CT scan of patient with liver cirrhosis and portal hypertension (a). Note extensive collateral vessels near the gastroesophageal junction, and recanalized umbilical vein (b).

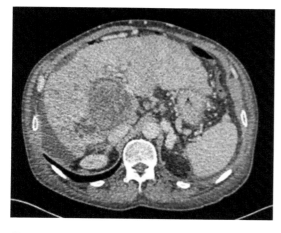

Figure 18.3 CT scan of patient with end-stage liver cirrhosis, showing irregular liver, ascites, collaterals and HCC.

and *18.3*). More recently, dynamically enhanced CT using measurement of multiphase contrast images has shown more accurate estimate of the severity of liver cirrhosis, correlating well with the Child-Pugh score (*Table 18.3*), however, this modality is still experimental, and has not yet been applied in clinical practice (21).

Endoscopy

All patients with liver cirrhosis should have an upper gastrointestinal (GI) endoscopy for the diagnosis and follow-up of oesophageal varices.

MANAGEMENT

Management of patients with liver cirrhosis is of necessity, multifactorial and requires input from different clinical teams. Supportive and symptomatic treatment, control of the aetiological factor, treatment of complications, and referral for consideration of transplantation if appropriate are all important aspects of management. Regular follow-up and surveillance for oesophageal varices and hepatocellular carcinoma (HCC) is required for most patients.

In early compensated cirrhosis, management is mainly aimed at slowing the progression or reversal of cirrhosis, prevention of decompensation by avoiding risk factors, symptomatic treatment and surveillance for varices and HCC. In addition to symptomatic treatment, addressing causative factors by the use of antiviral agents in hepatitis B and C, and the cessation of alcohol intake, prevent the progression of cirrhosis and may produce partial reversal. Patients should have 6-monthly follow-ups with liver US scanning and alpha fetoprotein (AFP) tests for HCC surveillance, and upper-GI endoscopy at regular intervals according to the initial findings at diagnosis.

Control of the Aetiology

Studies have shown that treatment of hepatitis B and C with antiviral agents not only slows the progression of cirrhosis, but also in some patients leads to regression to a lower fibrosis stage or no cirrhosis (22,23).

Behavioural and/or pharmacotherapy-based treatment for alcohol use disorder in patients with liver cirrhosis has been shown, in a retrospective cohort study, to reduce the incidence of decompensation and long-term all-cause mortality (24).

Weight reduction is the key treatment in non-alcoholic fatty liver disease. In the early phase of NAFLD, histological improvement may be achieved, and steatosis may be reversed. The effect of bariatric surgery on NAFLD was studied in a systematic review and a meta-analysis of 15 studies. Histological examination revealed improvement or complete resolution of steatosis, steatohepatitis, and fibrosis, in the majority of patients included in the studies (25). Similar findings were shown in a recent randomized controlled trial, where bariatric surgery achieved a statistically significant higher rate of NASH resolution than lifestyle modification after follow-up for a year (26).

The long-term clinical outcomes of bariatric surgery on NAFLD patients were studied in a retrospective cohort study by Aminian et al. in 1158 patients with biopsy-proven steatohepatitis without cirrhosis. Bariatric surgery was performed in 650 patients (no surgical treatment in 508) and after 10-year follow-up, major adverse liver outcomes (varices, ascites, encephalopathy, HCC, liver transplantation, histological cirrhosis and liver-related mortality) were higher in the control than the surgical group (9.6% versus 2.3%, respectively) (27).

Patients with established cirrhosis and decompensated liver disease have a high risk of morbidity and mortality and require appropriate resources and expertise to manage liver-related complications. These figures support the use of weight reduction surgery in patients with NAFLD including those with early fibrosis, but the available evidence to allow dogmatic conclusions is not presently available. Further studies of larger cohorts with matched controls and longer follow-up will be required to clarify the place of weight-reduction surgery in this complex cohort (28).

Table 18.4 Summary of BASL care bundle for decompensated cirrhosis

Treatment	Details
Laboratory investigations	• Full blood count (FBC) • Urea and electrolyte (U&E) • Liver function tests (LFTs) • Coagulation test • Glucose test • Blood cultures
Acitic tap	In all patients
Alcohol-related	• IV pabrinex • Clinical institute withdrawal assessment for alcohol (CIWA) in alcohol withdrawal
IV antibiotics	In suspected sepsis
Management of acute kidney injury (AKI)	–
Upper GI bleeding	Resuscitation with fluids and blood, aim for Hb >8 g/L
Encephalopathy	Lactulose, look for precipitant
Venous thromboembolism (VTE) prophylaxis	–

MANAGEMENT OF COMPLICATIONS OF CIRRHOSIS

Decompensation

The British Association for the Study of the Liver has published a care bundle for the acute management of decompensated cirrhosis in the first 24 hours of admission (*Table 18.4*). This aims to standardize and optimize treatment for decompensated cirrhosis and is composed of a checklist of necessary investigations and treatments to be done in all patients presenting with advanced liver disease and provides clinicians with clear guidance on the initial management of alcohol withdrawal, infection, AKI, GI bleeding and encephalopathy (29). It has shown in subsequent reviews to improve the care provided to these patients (30).

Ascites

First line therapies for ascites include dietary salt restriction, and diuretics such as spironolactone. Paracentesis may be indicated in symptomatic ascites, and albumin should be given if large volume paracentesis is performed. Patients with refractory ascites are considered for a transjugular intrahepatic portosystemic shunt (TIPS), which has a lower recurrence rate than paracentesis, but at the expense of higher rates of encephalopathy (31). Diagnostic paracentesis should be performed for all patients admitted with GI bleeding, shock, fever, worsening liver and renal function tests, and if spontaneous bacterial peritonitis is suspected (32). As with other complications of cirrhosis, liver transplantation represents the only definitive curative treatment for ascites.

Variceal bleeding

Routine screening endoscopy was previously indicated for all patients with diagnosis of cirrhosis, however the most recent Baveno guidelines recommended a more selective approach based on TE and platelet count. Patients with liver stiffness measurement (LSM) ≤ 15 kPa by TE, and platelet count $\geq 150 \times 10^9$/L rules out clinically significant portal hypertension (CSPH). This approach has a sensitivity and negative predictive value of 90%, and screening endoscopy can be avoided. Otherwise, screening is indicated for patients with higher LSM and/or thrombocytopenia <150 (33).

Nonselective beta-blockers (NSBB) are indicated in patients with diagnosis of cirrhosis and CSPH defined as HVPG ≥ 10, or with an endoscopic diagnosis of varices, or previous bleeding. These agents induce splanchnic vasodilatation and reduce the HVPG, which translates clinically into a significant decreased risk of bleeding and decompensation (33).

Acute variceal bleeding (AVB) requires prompt resuscitation with fluids and blood products. Unconscious patients and those at risk of aspiration require

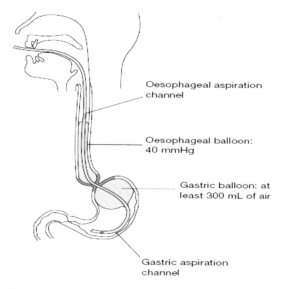

Figure 18.4 Illustration of a Sengstaken-Blakemore or Minnesota tube demonstrating the oesophageal and gastric balloon tamponade. The tube must be carefully managed.

intubation. Following resuscitation, urgent endoscopy is indicated and band ligation is recommended as the first line treatment for bleeding varices.

Terlipressin is a synthetic vasopressin analogue used in acutely bleeding varices and it activates V1 receptors in arterial smooth muscles to cause vasoconstriction which reduces splanchnic blood flow and portal pressure. Several studies have shown a significant improvement in the control of bleeding and reduction in mortality with the use of Terlipressin (34). Antibiotic prophylaxis is indicated in all patients with AVB to reduce the risk of bacterial infections (35), and lactulose should be given to reduce ameliorate the risk of encephalopathy (36).

Balloon tamponade using a Sangestaken-Blakemore or Minnesota tube, is a temporary method that can be used to control bleeding, in cases where endoscopic measures are unavailable or have been unsuccessful. The Sangestaken-Blakemore tube has three lumens (*Figure 18.4*), one for the gastric balloon, one for the oesophageal balloon and a gastric aspiration port. After insertion into the stomach (50 cm marking), the gastric balloon is inflated with 50 mL of air, and the position confirmed radiologically before further inflation with an additional 200 mL. The balloon is then pulled up against the GOJ, and a traction of 1 kg is applied, following this, the oesophageal balloon is inflated to a pressure of 40 mmHG (37). Deflation of the oesophageal balloon should be performed every 12 hours to avoid necrosis. Balloon tubes shouldn't be used for longer than 24–48 hours, following which definitive treatment with endoscopy or TIPS should be instituted.

TRANSJUGULAR INTRAHEPATIC PORTOSYSTEMIC SHUNT (TIPS)

TIPS is an interventional radiological procedure where a shunt is created between a hepatic vein and a portal vein branch, aiming to reduce portal hypertension and its complications (*Figure 18.5*). This was first performed on a human in 1988 by Richter et al. in Germany (38). Early TIPS (within 72 hours) is now considered the first line treatment of choice for patients who have persistent bleeding or rebleed within 5 days of combined pharmacologic and endoscopic therapy.

In a study by García-Pagán et al., 63 patients with Child C (10–13) or B (7–9) with active bleeding, were randomized to the standard pharmacological and endoscopic treatment with or without TIPS. Rebleeding or failure to control bleeding occurred in 14 patients in the standard group and only one patient in the TIPS group (39). The most recent Baveno consensus guidelines recommend pre-emptive TIPS for Child C <14, and actively bleeding Child B, or patients with HVPG > 20, as these patients have a high risk of recurrent bleeding. In patients with Child C ≥14, TIPS is considered futile, and is not indicated.

Expanded polytetrafluoroethylene coated stents are now the most widely used type of stents in TIPS, as they have longer patency rates than the previously used bare metal stents. TIPS has a success rate of 93–100% after initial placement although rebleeding may occur

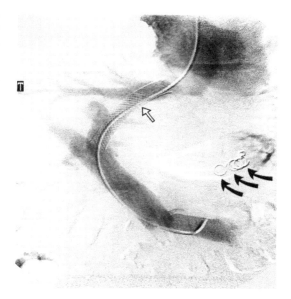

Figure 18.5 A check angiogram following insertion of a TIPS (open arrow). Injection of contrast into the portal vein flows through the metallic stent and outlines the right hepatic vein. Pressure measurements are taken from within the portal vein before and after insertion. Solid arrows indicate coils placed at the site of previous embolization.

in 20% of patients as a consequence of the long-term risk of occlusion or stenosis which occurs in about 75% of patients. With adequate surveillance using Doppler US, this can be diagnosed early, and patency can be re-established in most cases using interventional radiology (IR) techniques (40).

TIPS is also the method of choice for patients who are intolerant of standard secondary prophylaxis and is also recommended and effective therapy for patients with Budd–Chiari syndrome (41).

SURGICAL TREATMENT OF PORTAL HYPERTENSION

Surgical shunts have traditionally been used in the past to treat patients with complications of portal hypertension. They work by diverting blood from the portal to the systemic circulation which reduces portal pressure and thus the risk of variceal bleeding, and ascites (42).

However, with the development of the less invasive radiological shunt, e.g. TIPS, surgical shunts are used much less frequently, and fewer surgeons are familiar with these procedures. Surgical shunts can be classified into total, partial and selective shunts (*Figure 18.6*). Total shunts can be an end-to-side (portal vein ligated at its bifurcation and anastomosed to the vena cava), or side-to-side (portal vein or a tributary

>10 mm anastomosed to the vena cava). They are associated with high risk of encephalopathy and are no longer performed. Partial portosystemic shunting is achieved with a prosthesis lumen of 8 mm in diameter, which reduces the portal pressure, while maintaining hepato-petal flow in the majority of patients. Selective shunting aims to decompress the gastroesophageal varices while maintaining portal hypertension which can be achieved by the construction of a distal lienorenal shunt. To achieve long-term patency a side-to-side splenic to left renal vein anastomosis is performed. Portal azygous disconnection should also be performed as part of this procedure through ligation of right and left gastric veins and gastroepiploic disconnection (43).

The indications for surgical shunts are limited to patients with portal hypertension complications and preserved liver function Child A, B, and patients with non-cirrhotic portal hypertension, or patients with failed TIPS (44,45).

SUMMARY

The main cause of complications in cirrhosis prior to the onset of decompensated liver disease is portal hypertension. Some of the aetiological factors can be addressed with alcohol cessation and the use of antiviral drugs and there are now clear guidelines for the management of patients presenting with cirrhosis and portal

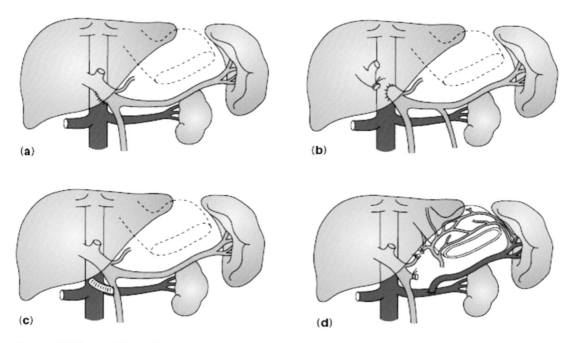

Figure 18.6 Surgical shunts. Surgical shunts for portal hypertension involve shunting portal blood into the systemic veins. This commonly involves a side-to-side portocaval anastomosis (a) or end-to-side portocaval (b), mesocaval 'H graft' (c) or splenorenal (d) anastomoses.

hypertension which have improved the outlook for these patients. HVPG is the most accurate method of assessing the degree of portal hypertension and has replaced older methods. There is good concordance with functional and histological changes and predictions of the mortality risk are accurate. Traditionally the treatment of portal hypertension relied on the construction of a surgical shunt. This has been replaced by the radiological insertion of TIPS which is used to treat the complications of portal hypertension in patients with advanced cirrhosis. TIPS has a significantly lower morbidity than surgery and is effective for the control of refractory ascites or recurrent variceal bleeding but is associated with the development of hepatic encephalopathy.

REFERENCES

1. Verne J. 2014. *Liver disease: A preventable killer of young adults. Public Health England.* Available from: https://publichealthmatters.blog.gov.uk/2014/09/29/liver-disease-a-preventable-killerof-young-adults. (Accessed March, 2024).

2. ONS. 2022. Liver disease: Applying All Our Health. Office for National Statistics. Available at https://www.gov.uk/government/publications/liver-disease-applying-all-our-health/liver-disease-applying-all-our-health. (Accessed 28 August, 2024).

3. Friedman SL. Mechanisms of hepatic fibrogenesis. *Gastroenterology* 2008;**134**:1655–69.

4. Schuppan D, Afdhal NH. Liver cirrhosis. *Lancet* 2008;**371(9615)**:838–51.

5. Tapper EB, Parikh ND. Diagnosis and management of cirrhosis and its complications: A review. *JAMA* 2023;**329(18)**:1589–602.

6. Haj M, Rockey DC. Ammonia levels do not guide clinical management of patients with hepatic encephalopathy caused by cirrhosis. *Am J Gastroenterol* 2020;**115(4)**:723–28.

7. Schrier RW, Arroyo V, Bernardi M, Epstein M, Henriksen JH, Rodés J. Peripheral arterial vasodilation hypothesis: A proposal for the initiation of renal sodium and water retention in cirrhosis. *Hepatology* 1988;**8(5)**:1151–7.

8. Zaccherini G, Tufoni M, Iannone G, Caraceni P. Management of ascites in patients with cirrhosis: An update. *J Clin Med* 2021;**10(22)**:5226.

9. Gioia S, Nardelli S, Ridola L, Riggio O. Causes and management of non-cirrhotic portal hypertension. *Curr Gastroenterol Rep* 2020;**22(12)**:56.

10. Acuna-Villaorduna A, Tran V, Gonzalez-Lugo JD, Azimi-Nekoo E, Billett HH. Natural history and clinical outcomes in patients with portal vein thrombosis by etiology: A retrospective cohort study. *Thromb Res* 2019;**174**:137–40.

11. Thompson RJ, Taylor MA, McKie LD, Diamond T. Sinistral portal hypertension. *Ulster Med J* 2006;**75(3)**:175–7.

12. Zhang Y, Jiang HT, Wei Y, Song B. Sinusoidal obstruction syndrome: A systematic review of etiologies, clinical symptoms, and magnetic resonance imaging features. *World J Clin Cases* 2019;**7(18)**:2746–59.

13. Peng J-K, Hepgul N, Higginson IJ, Gao W. Symptom prevalence and quality of life of patients with end-stage liver disease: A systematic review and meta-analysis. *Palliat Med* 2019;**33(1)**:24–36.

14. Pugh RNH, Murray-Lyon IM, Dawson JL, Pietroni MC, Williams R. Transection of the oesophagus for bleeding oesophageal varices. *Br J Surg* 1973;**60(8)**:646–9.

15. Mitchell O, Feldman DM, Diakow M, Sigal SH. The pathophysiology of thrombocytopenia in chronic liver disease. *Hepat Med* 2016;**8**:39–50.

16. Yeom SK, Lee CH, Cha SH, Park CM. Prediction of liver cirrhosis, using diagnostic imaging tools. *World J Hepatol* 2015;**7(17)**:2069–79.

17. Sanyal AJ, Bosch J, Blei A, Arroyo V. Portal hypertension and its complications. *Gastroenterology* 2008;**134(6)**:1715–28.

18. Moavenzadeh S, Palmeri ML, Ferraioli G, Barr RG. Liver stiffness measurement techniques: Basics. In: Barr RG and Ferraioli G (eds). *Multiparametric Ultrasound for the Assessment of Diffuse Liver Disease*, Elsevier, 2024, Chapter 3, pp. 25–34.

19. Sharma S, Khalili K, Nguyen GC. Non-invasive diagnosis of advanced fibrosis and cirrhosis. *World J Gastroenterol* 2014;**20(45)**:16820–30.

20. Kondo T, Maruyama H, Sekimoto T, Shimada T, Takahashi M, Yokosuka O. Reversed portal flow: Clinical influence on the long-term outcomes in cirrhosis. *World J Gastroenterol* 2015;**21(20)**:8894–902.

21. Van Beers BE, Leconte I, Materne R, Smith AM, Jamart J, Horsmans Y. Hepatic perfusion parameters in chronic liver disease: Dynamic CT measurements correlated with disease severity. *AJR Am J Roentgenol* 2001;**176(3)**:667–73.

22. Mauro E, Crespo G, Montironi C, Londoño MC, Hernández-Gea V, Ruiz P, et al. Portal pressure and liver stiffness measurements in the prediction of fibrosis regression after sustained virological response in recurrent hepatitis C. *Hepatology* 2018;**67(5)**:1683–94.

23. Marcellin P, Gane E, Buti M, Afdhal N, Sievert W, Jacobson IM, et al. Regression of cirrhosis during treatment with tenofovir disoproxil fumarate for chronic hepatitis B: A 5-year open-label follow-up study. *Lancet* 2013;**381(9865)**:468–75.

24. Rogal S, Youk A, Zhang H, Gellad WF, Fine MJ, Good CG, et al. Impact of alcohol use disorder treatment on clinical outcomes among patients with cirrhosis. *Hepatology* 2020;**71(6)**:2080–92.

25. Mummadi RR, Kasturi KS, Chennareddygari S, Sood GK. Effect of bariatric surgery on nonalcoholic fatty liver disease: Systematic review and meta-analysis. *Clin Gastroenterol Hepatol* 2008;**6(12)**:1396–402.

26. Verrastro O, Panunzi S, Castagneto-Gissey L, De Gaetano A, Lembo E, et al. Bariatric-metabolic surgery versus lifestyle intervention plus best medical care in non-alcoholic steatohepatitis (BRAVES): a multicentre, open-label, randomised trial. *Lancet* 2023;**401(10390)**:1786–97.

27. Aminian A, Al-Kurd A, Wilson R, Bena J, Fayazzadeh H, Singh T, et al. Association of bariatric

surgery with major adverse Liver and cardiovascular outcomes in patients with biopsy-proven nonalcoholic steatohepatitis. *JAMA* 2021;**326(20)**:2031–42.

28. Patton H, Heimbach J, McCullough A. AGA Clinical practice update on bariatric surgery in cirrhosis: Expert review. *Clin Gastroenterol Hepatol* 2021;**19(3)**:436–45.

29. McPherson S, Dyson J, Austin A, Hudson M. Response to the NCEPOD report: Development of a care bundle for patients admitted with decompensated cirrhosis–the first 24 h. *Frontline Gastroenterol* 2016;**7(1)**:16–23.

30. Smethurst K, Gallacher J, Jopson L, Majiyagbe T, Johnson A, Copeman P, et al. Improved outcomes following the implementation of a decompensated cirrhosis discharge bundle. *Frontline Gastroenterol* 2021;**13(5)**:409–15.

31. Will V, Rodrigues SG, Berzigotti A. Current treatment options of refractory ascites in liver cirrhosis: A systematic review and meta-analysis. *Dig Liver Dis 2022*;**54(8)**:1007–14.

32. Aithal GP, Palaniyappan N, China L, Härmälä S, Macken L, Ryan JM, et al. Guidelines on the management of ascites in cirrhosis. *Gut* 2021;**70(1)**:9–29.

33. de Franchis R, Bosch J, Garcia-Tsao G, Reiberger T, Ripoll C. Baveno VII Faculty. Baveno VII: Renewing consensus in portal hypertension. *J Hepatol* 2022;**76(4)**:959–74.

34. Zhou X, Tripathi D, Song T, Shao L, Han B, Zhu J, et al. Terlipressin for the treatment of acute variceal bleeding: A systematic review and meta-analysis of randomized controlled trials. *Medicine (Baltimore)* 2018;**97(48)**:e13437.

35. Lee YY, Tee HP, Mahadeva S. Role of prophylactic antibiotics in cirrhotic patients with variceal bleeding. *World J Gastroenterol* 2014;**20(7)**:1790–6.

36. Sharma P, Agrawal A, Sharma BC, Sarin SK. Prophylaxis of hepatic encephalopathy in acute variceal bleed: A randomized controlled trial of lactulose versus no lactulose. *J Gastroenterol Hepatol* 2011;**26(6)**:996–1003.

37. Powell M, Journey JD. *Sengstaken-Blakemore tube.* StatPearls Publishing; 2024.

38. Richter GM, Palmaz JC, Nöldge G, Rössle M, Siegerstetter V, Franke M, et al. The transjugular intrahepatic portosystemic stent-shunt. A new nonsurgical percutaneous method. *Radiologe* 1989;**29(8)**:406–11.

39. García-Pagán JC, Caca K, Bureau C, Laleman W, Appenrodt B, Luca A, et al. Early TIPS (Transjugular Intrahepatic Portosystemic Shunt) Cooperative Study Group. Early use of TIPS in patients with cirrhosis and variceal bleeding. *N Engl J Med* 2010;**362(25)**:2370–9.

40. Luo X, Zhao M, Wang X, Jiang M, Yu J, Li X, et al. Long-term patency and clinical outcome of the transjugular intrahepatic portosystemic shunt using the expanded polytetrafluoroethylene stent-graft. *PLoS One* 2019;**14(2)**:e0212658.

41. Inchingolo R, Posa A, Mariappan M, Tibana TK, Nunes TF, Spiliopoulos S, et al. Transjugular intrahepatic portosystemic shunt for Budd–Chiari syndrome: A comprehensive review. *World J Gastroenterol* 2020;**26(34)**:5060–73.

42. Henderson JM, Anderson CD. The surgical treatment of portal hypertension. *Clin Liver Dis (Hoboken)* 2020;**15(Suppl 1)**:S52–S63.

43. Li JC, Henderson JM. Portal hypertension. In: Holzheimer RG, Mannick JA (eds). *Surgical Treatment: Evidence-Based and Problem-Oriented.* Zuckschwerdt, 2001, pp. 313–24.

44. Koh C, Heller T. Approach to the diagnosis of portal hypertension. *Clin Liver Dis (Hoboken)* 2012;**1(5)**:133–5.

45. Kamath PS, Shah VH. Portal hypertension related to bleeding. In: Boyer TD, Lindor KD, Sanyal, AJ, Terrault NA (eds). *Zakim and Boyer's Hepatology: A Textbook of Liver Disease*, Elsevier, 2018, pp. 233–61.

46. Leonard N,Evason JK, Chan AWH, et al. Available from: from https://www.pathologyoutlines.com/ (Accessed 30 August 2024).

Chapter 19
Surgery in the High-Risk Patient

Andrew Packham and Philippa Graff-Baker

INTRODUCTION

This chapter will discuss the physiological challenges presented by the perioperative period, the preoperative impact of liver or pancreatic disease, and the postoperative complications that can occur. Priorities for preoperative evaluation include the assessment and management of comorbidities, geriatric appraisal and shared decision-making. The assessment of physical fitness is discussed in detail including questionnaires, simple fitness tests and cardiopulmonary exercise testing (CPET). Prehabilitation with exercise, nutrition and psychological support is outlined.

THE CHALLENGE OF SURGERY

Major surgery results in pain stimulus and release of pro-inflammatory mediators that result in sympathetic activation and a hormonal stress response with release of cortisol, growth hormone and vasopressin.

These changes lead to salt and water retention, an increased metabolic rate and hence increased cardio-respiratory demand, altered energy metabolism and immune system modulation.

The surgical stress response leads to greater muscle catabolism compared to starvation due to steroid and cytokine effects.

Perioperative period

The perioperative period carries the risk of:

- Surgical complications and return to theatre
- Infections of surgical site, lines, lungs, urinary system, etc.
- Thromboembolic disease
- Disruption of therapy for pre-existing diseases such as Parkinson's disease medication due to fasting and/or poor absorption
- Exacerbation of pre-existing conditions including chronic kidney disease, coronary or cerebrovascular disease
- Postoperative delirium, deconditioning and loss of function
- Organ failure and perioperative death

The risks of complications in the individual patient may relate to their disease process or underlying medical comorbidity.

Additional considerations

Patients for liver resection may have:

- Had recent major surgery including a bowel resection for surgical treatment of the primary disease
- Had recent chemotherapy
- Underlying liver disease
- Carcinoid syndrome

Patients for pancreatic resection may have:

- Upper gastrointestinal (GI) symptoms due to the disease process
- Acute, significant weight-loss and sarcopenia
- Obstructive jaundice with malabsorption of fats, fat-soluble vitamins (A, D, E and K) and calcium, malaise and general GI symptoms that may further reduce food intake, chronic dehydration and associated renal dysfunction
- Pancreatic insufficiency with the malabsorption of carbohydrate, fat and protein

Table 19.1 Factors addressed during the preoperative preparation process

Physical activity	Educational	Nutritional	Psychological	Clinical
Aerobic exercise	Lifestyle modification	Treat causes (e.g. biliary obstruction)	Self-care strategies	Optimizing medication and comorbidities
Strength training	Perioperative care process	Alleviate symptoms	Anxiety reducing interventions	Diabetes/blood glucose control
Avoidance of sedentary behaviours	Sources of support	Nutritional supplementation	Any cognitive or behavioural intervention	Treating anaemia

DOI: 10.1201/9781003080060-19

Summary

The hepatobiliary patient may approach major surgery with a poor physiological reserve due to their disease process, recent treatment, comorbidities and lifestyle factors. *Table 19.1* summarizes the factors which are addressed in the preparation process.

MEDICAL PREOPERATIVE ASSESSMENT

A full medical history including functional status should be taken. Consideration should be given to all aspects of the patient's general health and assessment of the control of any medical conditions. Where appropriate, other specialities should be involved to optimize comorbidities and plan postoperative support as necessary, for example, drug bridging plans, organ specific physiotherapy support or long-term renal support. It may be necessary for patients to have urgent cardiovascular intervention preoperatively for occult, or worsening conditions, such as valvular or ischaemic heart disease.

Some liver resection patients present with metastatic disease in other systems, such as pulmonary disease, that may require surgical diagnosis and/or treatment and it is important that a multidisciplinary approach is adopted for treatment planning.

Chronic liver disease

The presence of liver cirrhosis is a significant independent risk factor for poor outcomes after major surgery, with the risk related to the degree of derangement in baseline liver function. There are various scoring systems available to predict outcomes in non-liver surgery.

Child-Pugh scoring matrix

The Child-Pugh, or Child-Turcotte-Pugh (CTP), scoring matrix is based on the assessment of bilirubin, albumin, coagulation international normalized ratio (INR) or prothrombin time and the presence of hepatic encephalopathy (*Table 19.2*).

MELD score

Model for end-stage liver disease (MELD) is a scoring system used to assess the severity of liver disease. It is primarily used to stratify patients ≥12-years-old on liver transplant waiting lists and predicts mortality in the following situations: 1) Following transjugular intrahepatic portosystemic shunt (TIPS); 2) Cirrhotic patients undergoing surgical procedures other than liver transplantation; 3) Patients with acute alcoholic hepatitis; 4) Following acute variceal haemorrhage.

VOCAL-Penn cirrhosis surgical-risk score

The Veterans' Outcomes and Costs Associated with Liver Disease (VOCAL) cohort contains granular data on patients with cirrhosis from 128 US medical centres which was merged with the Veterans' Affairs Surgical Quality Improvement Program (VASQIP) to identify surgical procedures. This scoring system was introduced in early 2021 by Mahmud et al. from Pennsylvania. Early studies suggest that for the prediction of mortality following surgery in patients with cirrhosis, it may outperform previously used systems.

Histological scoring systems

Histological scoring systems for chronic liver disease are used to characterize and predict disease progression, determine prognosis, guide treatment strategies and allow comparison in clinical trials. Although histology is frequently not available preoperatively, many cirrhotic patients will have had a percutaneous or laparoscopic biopsy to clarify the aetiology of their disease. A number of predictive systems are available. The clinical variability with different aetiopathological factors mandates multiple models that incorporate morbidity, mortality and histological systems which are often multiparametric and include a combination of liver indices (*Figure 19.1*).

However, despite the availability of the various scoring systems, it is generally accepted that severe liver impairment remains a relative contraindication to major elective surgery. Clinical decision-making for patients with cirrhotic liver disease should be cautious and multidisciplinary.

Factor	1 point	2 points	3 points
Table 19.2 Child-Pugh scoring matrix			
Hepatic encephalopathy	None	Grade I–II	Grade III–IV
Ascites	None	Mild	Moderate to severe
Total bilirubin (mg/dL)	<2	2–3	>3
Serum albumin (g/L)	>35	28–35	<28
PT INR	<1.7	1.71–2.30	>2.30

Child-Pugh A: 5–6 points indicate the least severe liver disease with 1–5-year survival, 95%

Child-Pugh B: 7–9 points indicate moderately severe liver disease, 1–5-year survival, 75%

Child-Pugh C: 10–15 points indicate most severe liver disease 1–5-year survival, 50%

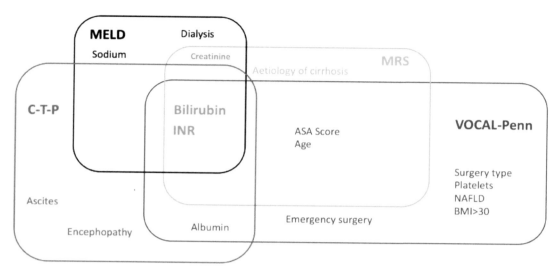

Figure 19.1 Scoring systems for the preoperative assessment of patients with cirrhosis, demonstrating the important factors used for assessment, and the overlap.

Frailty

Frailty is an independent risk-factor for perioperative morbidity and failure of the patient to return to their preoperative functional baseline. With increasing longevity, general frailty, without other specific diseases, can be present. It is also important to note that acute severe illness or major surgery can result in the presence of significant frailty and this may preclude further major surgery being in the patient's best interests.

The geriatric patient

Comprehensive assessment and care planning by a geriatrician may be particularly helpful in older patients with:

- Cognitive impairment
- Parkinson's disease
- Multimorbidity and/or polypharmacy
- Frailty syndromes such as falls or incontinence

The aims are to:

- Optimize diagnosis and rationalize management of comorbidities
- Produce care plans for the inpatient stay
- Reduce inpatient complications such as delirium
- Reduce the level of dependency and new care requirements post-discharge
- Pre-optimization, with the early involvement of other specialities, is essential for the high-risk patient

Risk-prediction tools

There have been multiple attempts over the years to develop risk-prediction scoring systems to quantify risk. In 1941, the American Society of Anesthetists (ASA)

developed the ASA scoring system. This classification was designed to allow for the collection and analysis of important statistical data relevant to anaesthesia. The ASA score evaluates the patient's condition preoperatively and calculates a score based on information from the patient's past medical history and current physical examination. The score ranges from 1–6 and correlates with the risk of complications and mortality with higher scores indicating increased risk.

Nevertheless it remains a challenge, even to experienced clinicians, to reliably quantify the overall risk of perioperative morbidity and mortality, and of failure to return to preoperative baseline function (1). The ASA scoring system is still in use but is not particularly helpful for complex hepato-pancreatico-biliary (HPB) patients. A number of other tools are available:

- *P-POSSUM:* This scoring system can be useful to estimate relative risk for 30-day morbidity and mortality for a patient with chronic cardiorespiratory disease. It is less helpful for patients with other organ disease such as chronic renal disease, neurological disorders, diabetes or generalized frailty. More recent evaluations of its usefulness in predicting absolute risk suggest that it overestimates morbidity and mortality.
- *SORT:* This is an easy tool to use, however, it is less helpful for higher-risk patients and it does again only evaluate up to 30 days.
- *ACS NSQIP:* This is a very comprehensive scoring system that, in addition to 30-day morbidity and mortality, also estimates long-term reduction in functional status. Its limitations relate to the fact that the data has been collated only from private healthcare patients in the United States.

ASSESSING PHYSICAL FITNESS

A range of tools are available to assess physical fitness. Caution should be exercised in interpretation when patients are, or have recently been, acutely unwell. 1 MET (metabolic equivalent) is the energy required when sleeping and equals a $\dot{V}O_2$ of approximately 3.5 mL/kg/min. Four METs therefore approximates to a $\dot{V}O_2$ of 14 mL/kg/min. Guidelines for the assessment of cardiac risk in non-cardiac surgery suggest that an exercise capacity of less than 4 METs is associated with increased cardiac risk after surgery (2,3).

Questionnaires

The Duke Activity Status Index (DASI) was developed as a self-reported questionnaire to estimate peak $\dot{V}O_2$ in cardiac patients. The 12-question tool gives a weighted score from 0 (2.74 METs) to 58.2 (9.89 METs). A score of 13.45 points equates to 4.4 METs.

The exercise tolerance before surgery (METS) study showed a small, but statistically significant, correlation between the DASI score and cardiac events after major surgery (adjusted odds ratio [OR] 0.96, 95% CI = 0.83–0.99; p = 0.03); however, the correlation between DASI score and peak $\dot{V}O_2$ measured on CPET was of limited clinical utility (Spearman correlation coefficient between DASI scores and peak oxygen consumption was 0.41 [p <0.0001]) (4). The DASI questionnaire may be best placed as a screening tool to identify patients requiring formal evaluation of physical fitness.

Consulting room tests

These tests are quick and simple to perform in the consulting room and can serve as simple screening-tools for general fitness, muscle strength and stability. They are not of sufficient duration to test aerobic capacity.

Sit-to-stand in 60 seconds (STS-60)

The patient stands up from a chair, without using their hands, as many times as possible in 60 seconds. Patients presenting to our multi-speciality cancer prehabilitation service have an average initial STS-60 of 25 repetitions with an average improvement of 4–5 repetitions during the programme.

Timed up-and-go

The patient stands from a chair, walks 3 m, turns, returns to the chair and sits down. A performance within 10–12 seconds indicates normal mobility.

Field exercise tests

These tests provide a more formal measure of aerobic fitness and can be useful for assessing the effect of exercise programmes. They require a 10 m straight walking course. Simple monitoring such as heart rate and oxygen saturations can be added. Either test must

be performed twice to account for learning effect with a minimum 30 minutes rest in between.

6-minute walk distance (6-MWD)

The patient walks as many lengths of the course as they can in 6 minutes.

Incremental shuttle walk test (ISWT)

The patient walks lengths of a course in a specific time with recorded beeps. The time intervals shorten each minute and the test ends when the patient can no longer complete the course length in the allowed time. The result, stated in metres walked, can be used to estimate $\dot{V}O_2$ max with 410 m approximating to a treadmill measured $\dot{V}O_2$ max of 15 mL/kg/min (5). The ISWT is reported to give a better demonstration of peak exercise capacity than the 6-MWD test (6).

Cardiopulmonary exercise tests

A Cardiopulmonary Exercise Test (CPET or CPX) also known as cardiopulmonary exercise (CPEX) testing, provides a non-invasive integrative assessment of cardiorespiratory function. It is usually provided with support from a clinical physiology department (respiratory or cardiac). As well as global fitness measures, the test provides diagnostic information about cardiorespiratory performance which refines the risk assessment, guides preoperative optimization and informs postoperative care (*Table 19.3*).

Clinical testing is usually performed on a cycle ergometer and the available perioperative literature is based on cycle testing. The patient pedals unloaded for 3

Table 19.3 Normal cardiopulmonary test variables

Variables	Normal value
Peak oxygen uptake ($\dot{V}O_2$ peak)	>84% predicted
Anaerobic threshold (AT)	>40% of predicted $\dot{V}O_2$ peak
Maximum heart rate (HR$_{max}$)	>90% age predicted
Heart rate reserve (HRR)	<15 beats/min
Blood pressure (BP)	<220/90 mmHg
O2 pulse ($\dot{V}O_2$/HR)	>80% predicted
Ventilatory reserve (VR)	MVV-VE$_{max}$ >11 L or VE$_{max}$/MVV x 100 <85%
Respiratory rate (RR)	<60 breaths/min
Minute ventilation/ carbon dioxide output ratio (VE/ $\dot{V}CO_2$) at AT	<34

Abbreviations: MVV: maximal voluntary ventilation; VE: expired ventilation.

Adapted from ATS/ACCP statement on cardiopulmonary exercise testing.

minutes, and then work-rate increases continuously on a pre-programmed ramp until the patient reaches volitional exhaustion. Continuous respiratory measurements are obtained via a facemask along with exercise electro-cardiogram (ECG), heart rate, blood pressure and oxygen saturation measurements. Pre-test spirometry is also recorded, with testing of reversibility where indicated.

The test provides measures of physiological capacity and efficiency with direct measurement of Peak Oxygen Uptake ($\dot{V}O_{2peak}$) and estimation of Anaerobic Threshold (AT) and ventilatory efficiency (VE/VCO_2 at AT). It also provides a range of diagnostic information concerning respiratory mechanics, pulmonary gas exchange and cardiovascular performance. Anaerobic threshold is the level of oxygen consumption for metabolic work, at which anaerobic metabolism starts to supplement aerobic metabolism resulting in a rise in blood lactate. It is normally quoted as mL of oxygen consumed per kg of actual body weight per minute.

The METS study demonstrated that $\dot{V}O_{2peak}$ measured on CPET is a better predictor of moderate or severe in-hospital complications after major surgery than DASI or NT-proBNP, noting that most complications are pulmonary complications, surgical site infections, unexpected critical care unit admissions, and re-operations rather than cardiac complications (4). A systematic review of eight studies of CPET in liver or pancreas cancer surgery concluded that:

'The CPET variable most reported and relevant to morbidity in both liver and pancreas cancer surgery appeared to be anaerobic threshold (AT). A preoperative AT of less than ~10.5 mL/min/kg seems to be associated with a worse postoperative convalescence'(7).

A study of CPET in liver transplant surgery showed that a reduced AT was associated with a prolonged postoperative hospitalization and reduced survival (8).

CPET, and other maximal exercise tests, are contra-indicated in patients with unstable cardiac syndromes, severe aortic stenosis or hypertrophic obstructive cardio-myopathy (HOCM), severe hypoxaemia or untreated thromboembolic disease. Many patients with restricted walking ability are able to undertake a cycle-based test, however some patients with limited or painful knee flexion, or lower limb amputation without a prosthesis will be unable to pedal on a cycle ergometer.

In patients who are unable to undertake exercise testing, static lung-function tests should be requested as undiagnosed chronic obstructive pulmonary disease (COPD) is common. Stress echocardiogram (ECHO) and stress MRI will demonstrate any cardiac structural abnormalities, and disorders of contractility occurring within the range of heart rates tested.

IMPROVING FITNESS BEFORE SURGERY

Alongside medical optimization, multimodal prehabilitation aims to improve physical fitness, nutrition, psychological wellbeing and lifestyle factors such as smoking and alcohol intake (9).

Exercise

The UK Chief Medical Officers' physical activity guidelines recommend that adults should accumulate 150 minutes of moderate intensity activity, or 75 minutes of vigorous intensity activity per week, and carry out muscle-strengthening activities on at least 2 days a week. Older adults, defined as age 65 and over, should undertake activities to improve balance and flexibility in addition to the above (10). Dedicated prehabilitation programmes should provide rapid access to specialist assessment and exercise support, suited to the complexities of patients approaching major HPB surgery.

Nutrition

All patients should be screened for malnutrition with a suitable tool such as the Malnutrition Universal Screening Tool (MUST) or short-form Patient-Generated Subjective Global Assessment (PG-SGA©).

Specialist assessment will often follow the PG-SGA. Intervention should treat specific causes of malabsorption, such as biliary obstruction or pancreatic insufficiency, treat other symptoms impeding food intake such as nausea or bloating, and provide nutritional supplementation where necessary.

Psychological wellbeing

Patients should be screened for psychological distress, for example using the Hospital Anxiety and Depression Scale (HADS), also taking note of active or past psychiatric diagnoses. Patients will often derive significant psychological benefit from their general prehabilitation interventions such as group exercise classes but specific psychological support should be utilized when indicated.

SHARED DECISION-MAKING

The decision for an individual to have major surgery is very challenging. A diagnosis of cancer and the fear of what that diagnosis engenders, combined with the hope that surgery can be curative, means that patients will often see a complex major operation as the easiest, or only option. Sometimes surgery is not the best choice of treatment in terms of the best long-term outcome. Quantity and quality of life may be optimized for some individuals if they choose not to have surgery which is particularly so for the elderly patient, those with significant comorbidity or when assessment indicates a high likelihood of complications. In these situations, it is possible that the risks of surgery outweigh the benefits and a full and frank discussion with the patient is essential.

Shared decision-making is a collaborative process that brings together the clinician's expertise, with information about treatment options, evidence, risks and benefits, and the patient's priorities around their preferences, personal circumstances, goals values and beliefs. This enables the clinician to support the patient to make decisions that are right for them (11).

SUMMARY

Preparation of the high-risk patient for HPB surgery should include:

- Individualized assessment of the risks and benefits of surgery versus other treatment options including doing nothing
- Shared decision-making between clinician and patient about the decision to proceed to surgery
- Identification and optimization of significant comorbidities, and perioperative care planning
- Improvement of modifiable risk factors including smoking, reduced physical activity, excess alcohol and poor nutrition, and improvement of psychological preparedness (12)

REFERENCES

1. Nag DS. Assessing the risk: Scoring systems for outcome prediction in emergency laparotomies. *Biomedicine (Taipei)* 2015;**5(4)**:20. doi: 10.7603/s40681-015-0020-y. Epub 2015 Nov 28. PMID: 26615537; PMCID: PMC4662940.
2. Fleisher LA, Fleischmann KE, Auerbach AD, Barnason SA, Beckman JA, Bozkurt B, et al. 2014 ACC/AHA Guideline on perioperative cardiovascular evaluation and management of patients undergoing noncardiac surgery. *Circulation* 2014;**130**:e278–e333.
3. Kristensen SD, Knuuti J, Saraste A, Anker S, Bøtker HE, De Hert S, et al. 2014 ESC/ESA Guidelines on non-cardiac surgery: Cardiovascular assessment and management. *Eur Heart J* 2014;**35(35)**:2383–431.
4. Wijeysundera DN, Pearse RM, Shulman MA, Abbott TEF, Torres E, Ambosta A, et al. Assessment of functional capacity before major non-cardiac surgery: An international, prospective cohort study. *Lancet* 2018;**391**:2631–40.
5. Singh SJ, Morgan MDL, Hardman AE, Rowe C, Bardsley PA. Comparison of oxygen uptake during a conventional treadmill test and the shuttle walking test in chronic airflow limitation. *Eur Respir J* 1994;**7**:2016–20.
6. Singh SJ, Morgan MDL, Scott S, Walters D, Hardman AE. Development of a shuttle walking test of disability in patients with chronic airways obstruction. *Thorax* 1992;**47**:1019–24.
7. Kumar R, Garcea G. Cardiopulmonary exercise testing in hepato-biliary & pancreas cancer surgery – A systematic review: Are we any further than walking up a flight of stairs? *Int J Surg* 2018;**52**:201–7.
8. Bernal W, Martin-Mateos R, Lipcsey M, Tallis C, Woodsford K, CmPhail MJ, et al. Aerobic capacity during cardiopulmonary exercise testing and survival with and without liver transplantation for patients with chronic liver disease. *Liver Transpl* 2014;**20**:54–62.
9. Macmillan Cancer Support. *Prehabilitation for people with cancer. Principles and guidance for prehabilitation within the management and support of people with cancer.* Available from: https://cdn.macmillan.org.uk/dfsmedia/1a6f23537f7f4519bb0cf14c45b2a629/1532-source/prehabilitation-for-people-with-cancer-tcm9-353994, (Accessed August, 2024).
10. Department of Health & Social Care. 2019. *UK Chief Medical Officers' Physical Activity Guidelines.* Available from: assets.publishing.service.gov.uk/media/5d839543ed915d52428dc134/uk-chief-medical-officers-physical-activity-guidelines.pdf (Accessed March, 2024).
11. NHS England. *Shared decision-making.* Available from: www.england.nhs.uk/personalisedcare/shared-decision-making. NHS England. (Accessed August, 2024).
12. Centre for Perioperative Care. 2021. *Preoperative Assessment and Optimisation for Adult Surgery.* Available from: https://www.cpoc.org.uk/preoperative-assessment-and-optimisation-adult-surgery. (Accessed August, 2024).

Chapter
20

Post-Hepatectomy Liver Failure

John W. Chen and S. George Barreto

INTRODUCTION

Post-hepatectomy liver failure (PHLF) is a serious and often life-threatening complication which manifests with progressive jaundice, coagulopathy, frequent renal failure, ascites and encephalopathy. Historically, PHLF has been a poorly defined entity but there have been recent attempts to produce a definition incorporating the timing, degree of jaundice and coagulopathy. In this chapter, we will discuss the clinical issues and provide the reader with a comprehensive understanding of PHLF, and its management (including mitigating preoperative, operative and postoperative risk factors) based on the current evidence in the literature.

Mortality following liver resection has significantly improved in the last three decades and the risk of mortality following a liver resection for colorectal liver metastases is <2% in most series. The mortality risk, however, increases with the complexity of the surgery including procedures such as resection and reconstruction for a hilar cholangiocarcinoma (Klatskin's tumour), or surgery for hepatocellular carcinoma (HCC) in a patient with parenchymal disease. While transient liver dysfunction after liver resection is not uncommon and usually resolves within 1–2 weeks, the most serious form of this complication is PHLF occurring as a result of inadequate future liver remnant (FLR) volume 'small for size' or with postoperative infectious or vascular complications in a patient with a borderline remnant. The pathophysiology of PHLF is multifactorial and it is associated with impaired hepatic synthetic and secretory function presenting as progressive jaundice, coagulopathy, a rising serum ammonia level and, eventually, the development of encephalopathy that persists beyond the first week. The incidence of PHLF is estimated to be between 8–12% (the wide range is likely to be due to the lack of an internationally accepted definition) and the subsequent morbidity and mortality are substantial.

DEFINITION OF PHLF

Clinically acute liver failure due to any cause, presents with a derangement of liver function (elevated bilirubin, hypoalbuminaemia) and a coagulopathy often associated with clinical signs such as the development of jaundice, ascites, ecchymosis and encephalopathy. With increasing severity, patients will also develop hypoglycaemia and elevated levels of serum ammonia and lactate. The term PHLF has been used in more recent times to describe the occurrence of acute liver failure following liver resection. The existing definitions of PHLF incorporate clinical and biochemical parameters of liver function which are indicative of synthetic function, including albumin and the international normalized ratio (INR), and markers of excretory and detoxification functions, namely, serum bilirubin and ammonia levels (*Table 20.1*). Clinical parameters such as the presence of encephalopathy and the need for clinical and/or invasive management have been used to predict the outcome of PHLF.

Table 20.1 Evolution of PHLF definitions

Author or reference	Publication year	Criteria
Balzan et al. (1)	2005	Prothrombin <50% of normal (INR >1.7) and serum bilirubin of >50 μmol/L on postoperative day 5
Mullen et al. (2)	2007	Peak post-hepatectomy bilirubin of >7 mg/dL
ISGLS (3)	2011	An increased INR and concomitant hyperbilirubinemia on, or after, postoperative day 5 *Severity grading:* • Grade A: no clinical intervention required • Grade B: clinical, no invasive intervention • Grade C: invasive intervention required

Abbreviations: INR: International normalized ratio; ISGLS: International Study Group of Liver Surgery.

DOI: 10.1201/9781003080060-20

One of the earliest attempts to define PHLF was made by Balzan et al. (1) in 2005. The authors noted that patients who fulfilled their '50–50 criteria' had a 59% risk of early (60–day) postoperative mortality. On applying these criteria to a cohort of non-cirrhotic patients who underwent liver resection, Mullen et al. (2) noted a low sensitivity of 50% and the authors noted that a peak post-hepatectomy serum bilirubin of >70 mg/L was more accurate in predicting PHLF-related mortality.

The most-widely accepted definition of PHLF is the one proposed by the International Study Group of Liver Surgery (ISGLS) in 2011 (3). Based on a comprehensive review of the published literature, this international consortium of liver surgeons proposed a relatively simple definition of PHLF. As per the ISGLS, PHF is characterized by 'the impaired ability of the liver to maintain its synthetic, excretory, and detoxifying functions, which are characterized by an increased INR and concomitant hyperbilirubinemia (according to the normal limits of the local laboratory) on, or after, postoperative day 5'. They defined PHLF as an increasing serum bilirubin concentration and increasing INR on, or after, postoperative day 5 compared with the values of the previous day. A downward trend in the abnormal levels of serum bilirubin or the INR on, or after, day 5 post-resection would not be deemed to be PHLF. They further proposed a severity grading system based on the need for clinical and/or invasive intervention. This severity grading system has been used as an outcome measure for predicting PHLF complications.

FACTORS CONTRIBUTING TO PHLF

Numerous factors contribute to the development of PHLF (*Figure 20.1*) and some of these factors can be mitigated before, during and after, surgery. They can be broadly divided into the following.

Inadequately functioning FLR

In younger patients with normal liver parenchyma, resection of up to 75–80% of the liver volume, representing a FLR of 20–25% can be performed without significant risk of PHLF. PHLF occurs when the post-resection liver remnant is inadequate. The volume of liver that needs to be preserved, the FLR depends on a number of factors including age, pre-existing parenchymal disease, the presence of portal hypertension, extent of jaundice, previous locoregional or systemic chemotherapy, and the location of the tumours requiring resection. There are strategies to produce liver remodelling that can assist in increasing FLR volume to reduce the risk of PHLF.

Liver parenchymal disease

Liver parenchymal disease reduces functional capacity. In patients with steatosis, liver fibrosis and cirrhosis, or in those with a history of systemic, or local-regional therapy for tumours, the FLR needs to be proportionately larger and not the 25% volume acceptable in those with normal liver parenchyma. Liver resection in patients with Child-Pugh B- or C-score for cirrhosis is associated with a significantly increased risk of complications and death.

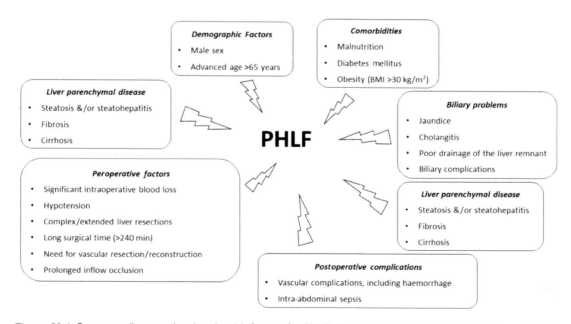

Figure 20.1 Summary diagram showing the risk factors for PHLF. *Abbreviations:* BMI: body mass index; NAFLD: non-alcoholic fatty liver disease.

Biliary obstruction and cholestasis

Liver resection in the presence of cholestasis is associated with a higher incidence of PHLF. If the FLR has a partial or complete biliary occlusion, resection is associated with high risk of PHLF. In this setting, the FLR needs to be adequately drained preoperatively for days and not infrequently weeks prior to undertaking liver resection. Classically this is the issue with resections for hilar cholangiocarcinoma (Klatskin's tumour) where patients have frequently been deeply jaundiced for a number of weeks and where attempts to relieve the jaundice have only been partially successful. Of particular importance in these patients is to ensure that the FLR has been adequately drained as opposed to the liver which is to be re-sected. Cholangitis with or without prior biliary intervention is also a significant contributing factor for the development of PHLF.

OPERATIVE COMPLICATIONS

Truant et al. (4) highlighted the significance of concomitant perioperative factors, especially severe vascular events, in increasing the risk of mortality from PHLF. They noted that the death of only 4 of 22 patients could be unequivocally attributed to PHLF and in the remaining 18 patients, additional perioperative factors contributed to which severe vascular events were the most common.

Vascular inflow and outflow injuries

During complex resectional liver surgery, such as for Klatskin's tumour or extended right and left hepatic resections, arterial and venous inflow and outflow injuries may occur and if left untreated, PHLF can occur. Prolonged hepatic arterial and portal venous occlusion can result in ischaemic hepatitis and increase the risk of PHLF. Hepatic arterial and portal vein resection and reconstruction are associated with periods of vascular clamping which can increase the risk of thrombosis and inflow occlusion. Resection of tumours close to the hepatic venous outflow can result in hepatic vein injuries with narrowing and consequent hepatic outflow restriction, or occlusion.

Intraoperative haemorrhage and blood transfusion

Bleeding during liver surgery is not uncommon and the risk increases with the magnitude and complexity of the resection. Significant haemorrhage in excess of 1200 mL and perioperative blood transfusion increases the risk of post-hepatectomy complications, including PHLF and the risk is exacerbated by intraoperative hypotension.

Complex liver resections in the setting of cholangiocarcinoma and hepatocellular carcinoma

Hepatectomy for hilar cholangiocarcinoma and hepatocellular carcinoma is associated with a greater incidence of PHLF. The pathophysiology responsible is probably the underlying liver disease causing large duct cholestasis or cholangitis in addition to the presence of fibrosis, or cirrhosis. Similarly, complex resections with associated biliary and vascular resections and reconstruction also have a higher incidence of PHLF.

STRATEGIES TO MITIGATE PHLF

Preoperative

PHLF will occur if the post-hepatectomy FLR is anatomically or functionally inadequate. In liver transplantation, a 'small for size' graft is one that provides insufficient functional capacity for the recipient resulting in post-transplant liver failure manifesting as a congested graft which fails to regenerate. For hepatectomy in a normal liver, the minimum FLR required is two contiguous segments representing at least 20–25% of the liver volume or 0.5% of the patient's weight. For a liver with parenchymal disease, the required FLR is expected to be higher approaching 40% (5) to reduce the possibility of remnant congestion and PHLF.

Liver remodelling to increase FLR volume

Computed tomography (CT) volumetric analysis is a standard 3D measure of FLR volume. In patient's undergoing major hepatectomies, if the FLR volume is predicted to be less than required for postoperative regeneration and recovery, a two or three-stage intervention can be performed to attain the desired volume.

Portal vein embolization or portal vein ligation and staged resection

For extended right hemihepatectomy where the FLR of segment II and III is predicted to be inadequate, embolization of the right portal vein with, or without, segment IVa and IVb portal vein branches can be performed. This renders the embolized right lobe ischaemic, (and segment IV if the portal inflow to this segment has been embolized or ligated), resulting in hypertrophy of the left lateral segments. It usually takes 3–8 weeks to achieve maximal hypertrophy of the proposed FLR. Right portal vein ligation as an operative approach can also be combined synchronously with non-anatomical resections of small tumours within the FLR.

Hepatic vein occlusion

In some instances, portal vein embolization is inadequate and transjugular right hepatic vein occlusion may be performed to achieve further contralateral liver hypertrophy.

Associating liver partition and portal-vein ligation for staged hepatectomy

The associating liver partition and portal vein ligation for staged hepatectomy (ALPPS) was developed to promote rapid expansion of segments II and III through ligation of right portal vein and all of the inflow to segments IVa and IVb (arterial, portal venous and biliary branches). Segment IV ischaemia often results in rapid hypertrophy of the future segments II and III. The second stage of extended completion right hemihepatectomy, is usually performed within 2 weeks of the initial surgery. The proponents of ALPPS have highlighted its use in patients requiring complex liver resections such as trisectionectomies for multiple bilateral liver metastases or intrahepatic cholangiocarcinoma. The shorter period before the second-stage operation, where possible, has the additional advantage of reducing the risk of disease progression. Recent studies have confirmed that this staged modality is associated with a higher rate of resection compared with right portal vein and segment IV portal vein embolization but it also has a higher rate of complications and an increased mortality.

Assessment of liver parenchymal disease

Gross changes of steatosis, fibrosis and cirrhosis may not be obvious on routine imaging. In patients in whom the suspicion of possible parenchymal liver disease has been raised due to abnormal preoperative clinical, biochemical and/or radiological parameters, a biopsy of the non-tumour bearing portion of the liver must be performed. This will help guide the estimations of the minimum-required FLR volume for that individual. Non-invasive measurement of liver stiffness using Fibroscan® may be useful prior to performing a liver biopsy.

Assessment of portal hypertension

CT features of portal hypertension such as an enlarged spleen, a dilated portal vein, the presence of collateral vessels and recanalization of the ligamentum teres are considered a contraindication to resection. In cases where cross-sectional imaging raises the suspicion of portal hypertension, a transjugular hepatic-vein wedge pressure measurement must be performed. A portal-hepatic vein gradient of greater than 10 mmHg is an absolute contraindication to major liver resection.

Drainage of biliary obstruction and the treatment of cholangitis

In the setting of biliary obstruction secondary to a cholangiocarcinoma, it is vital to ensure that the FLR is sufficiently drained, and the jaundice has resolved prior to undertaking a major liver resection. The presence of cholangitis can usually be adequately treated with drainage and antibiotics prior to surgery.

PERIOPERATIVE

A low central venous pressure and the avoidance of excessive bleeding

This is important especially with predicted borderline FLRs. Parenchyma transection in the presence of a high central venous pressure (CVP) is associated with significantly increased bleeding. A CVP of 1–5 mmHg is ideal during the parenchymal transection phase.

Avoidance of prolonged portal inflow occlusion (Pringle's manoeuvre)

Intermittent portal inflow clamping (10 minutes clamping followed by 5-minute revascularization) can reduce blood loss during parenchymal transection but prolonged inflow clamping is associated with FLR ischaemia and a risk of PHLF.

Vascular injuries and thrombosis

Excessive and prolonged clamping of vascular structures, as well as vascular resection and reconstruction contribute to the risk of PHLF. Due care should be taken to avoid vascular compromise.

N-acetyl cysteine infusion

N-acetyl cysteine (NAC) infusion is routinely used for paracetamol overdose to reduce hepatotoxicity-related liver failure. It has been used as a liver protective agent in high-risk cases although clinical trials have been inconclusive.

POSTOPERATIVE

The early recognition and treatment of post-hepatectomy complications and in particular haemorrhage, biliary obstruction, and intra-abdominal sepsis is crucial. As noted previously, attendant complications increase the risk of mortality should the patient additionally develop PHLF.

Management of PHLF

Once a patient fulfils the criteria for PHLF (listed in *Table 20.1*), the patient must be managed aggressively to avoid further deterioration. The initial management of PHLF is similar to acute liver failure from other causes including viral, drug or ischaemia-induced fulminant hepatitis. Progressive cholestasis and coagulopathy on, or after, postoperative day 5 (as defined by the ISGLS) indicates the failure of hepatic regeneration. The vast majority of patients with PHLF succumb due to associated complications such as bleeding, sepsis and other organ failure. Hence, central to the supportive management is the correction of coagulopathy, early recognition and treatment of surgical complications (vascular and biliary), treatment of hepatic encephalopathy, and the establishment of nutritional support, whilst avoiding complications, including sepsis.

Cross-sectional imaging should be performed to identify any undrained collections and to rule out vascular complications. Drainage of any collections is essential especially if there is evidence or suspicion that they are infected. Patients may require ascitic drainage with corresponding infusions of concentrated albumin. Judicious use of prophylactic antibiotics as well as antifungals is warranted in consultation with the microbiology team. The use of 'liver dialysis' circuits,

or liver support systems, which use either plasma exchange (PE) or a molecular adsorbent recirculating system (MARS) have been trialled. The main purpose of using a liver dialysis circuit is mainly to dialyze out and bind toxic metabolites to allow time for the liver remnant to regenerate. In a recent systematic review (6), the use of liver support systems for the treatment of PHLF was not supported by the existing literature. However, if liver failure becomes unresponsive to the traditional supportive treatments, and if there are no contraindications, patients should be referred for consideration of liver transplantation before the onset of septic complications. In the event that the patient has an identifiable source of sepsis, appropriate treatment with antibiotics and antifungals (guided by the microbiology team) along with drainage of collections if applicable should be pursued. Liver transplantation can be considered if the sepsis can be cleared and confirmed by negative cultures (*Figure 20.2*). The high risk-benefit ratio, high attendant costs and the global shortage of donor organs must be considered and this can only be done in the setting of a multidisciplinary team.

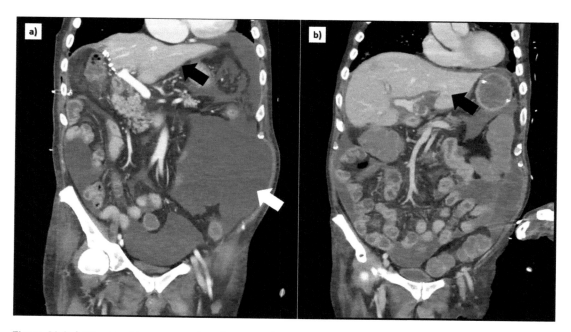

Figure 20.2 A 63-year-old man was referred to our unit with PHLF following a right hemi-hepatectomy and extra-hepatic biliary resection for presumed hilar cholangiocarcinoma. The main risk for PHLF was that the resection was performed while he still had significant jaundice. His course was complicated by pleural effusion, acute kidney injury, coagulopathy, fungal and systemic sepsis. Surgical pathology of the resected right liver and extrahepatic bile duct confirmed Immunoglobulin G4 disease. This was deemed not to represent a contraindication to liver transplant at the multidisciplinary team meeting. After negative bacterial and fungal cultures were confirmed, he underwent a successful orthotopic deceased donor liver transplantation 10 weeks after his initial resection. Images show contrast-enhanced computed tomography (CECT) scan sections of the abdomen. Pre-transplant, sagittal section (a) of the abdomen in portal venous phase demonstrating large volume ascites (white arrow) with his remnant left liver (black arrow). Post-transplant, sagittal section (b) of the abdomen in portal venous phase, demonstrating a full orthotopic liver graft (black arrow).

SUMMARY

PHLF is a serious complication associated with a significantly increased morbidity and mortality. The range of presentations varies from a mild derangement of liver function (transient hyperbilirubinaemia and coagulopathy) to features consistent with acute liver failure with the downstream effects on other organ systems necessitating support in an intensive care setting. While an anatomically and functionally inadequate FLR is the most likely cause, especially following complex liver resections, the development of PHLF in individuals with a seemingly adequate FLR is often the result of underlying unrecognized parenchymal liver disease (steatosis, fibrosis or cirrhosis) and/or the effects of risk factors including diabetes, obesity, chemotherapy, significant intraoperative blood loss, vascular and biliary complications and sepsis. Accurate preoperative planning with estimation of the required FLR, taking into consideration the influence of the aforementioned factors on the function of the remnant are essential to avoid PHLF. Management of PHLF involves supportive therapy that includes the correction of any coagulopathy, early recognition and treatment of surgical complications (vascular and biliary), treatment of hepatic encephalopathy, and the establishment of nutritional support, while avoiding potential complications, including sepsis. In patients with progressive deterioration despite maximal supportive therapy, consideration should be given to liver transplantation which must be discussed within a multidisciplinary forum.

REFERENCES

1. Balzan S, Belghiti J, Farges O, Ogata S, Sauvanet A, Delefosse D, et al. The '50-50 criteria' on postoperative day 5: An accurate predictor of liver failure and death after hepatectomy. *Ann Surg* 2005;**242(6)**:824–8.
2. Mullen JT, Ribero D, Reddy SK, Donadon M, Zorzi D, Gautam S, et al. Hepatic insufficiency and mortality in 1,059 noncirrhotic patients undergoing major hepatectomy. *J Am Coll Surg* 2007;**204(5)**:854–62.
3. Rahbari NN, Garden OJ, Padbury R, Brooke-Smith M, Crawford M, Adam R, et al. Posthepatectomy liver failure: A definition and grading by the International Study Group of Liver Surgery (ISGLS). *Surgery* 2011;**149(5)**:713–24.
4. Truant S, El Amrani M, Skrzypczyk C, Boleslawski E, Sergent G, Hebbar M, et al. Factors associated with fatal liver failure after extended hepatectomy. *HPB (Oxford)* 2017;**19(8)**:682–7.
5. Ribero D, Chun YS, Vauthey JN. Standardized liver volumetry for portal vein embolization. *Semin Intervent Radiol* 2008;**25(2)**:104–9.
6. Pufal K, Lawson A, Hodson J, Bangash M, Patel J, Weston C, et al. Role of liver support systems in the management of post hepatectomy liver failure: A systematic review of the literature. *Ann Hepatobiliary Pancreat Surg* 2021;**25(2)**:171–8.

Chapter

21

Diagnostic and Therapeutic Endoscopy

Richard J. Robinson and John J. McGoran

INTRODUCTION

This chapter addresses the endoscopic evaluation and management of patients with oesophageal and gastric varices. The elective management of non-bleeding oesophageal varices will be reviewed including screening and surveillance and the technique of applying variceal bands will be outlined. The initial assessment, management and specific endoscopic techniques for controlling active variceal haemorrhage is also discussed. Specific techniques for managing gastric varices will be considered. Salvage techniques when endoscopic therapy fails will also be reviewed including the role of balloon tamponade, transjugular intrahepatic porto-systemic shunts (TIPS) and self-expanding metal stents (SEMS).

The endoscopic management of duodenal polyps will be discussed, including lesion recognition, detailed endoscopic assessment for features of malignancy and the importance of photo documentation. The endoscopic techniques required to safely manage pedunculated and sessile duodenal polyps will be considered with reference to endoscopic mucosal resection and endoscopic submucosal dissection.

ENDOSCOPIC MANAGEMENT OF GASTRO-OESOPHAGEAL VARICES

Elective management of non-bleeding varices

Variceal screening, surveillance and bleeding prophylaxis is established practice for those with cirrhotic liver disease and individuals with clinical or radiological portal hypertension. The recognition of oesophageal varices is a simple but essential examination skill in upper gastrointestinal (GI) endoscopy. The modified Paquet classification is a common approach to grading varices, with Grade I disappearing on air insufflation and Grade III occluding the lumen (1).

On detection of oesophageal varices, the endoscopist may consider primary prophylaxis of bleeding using variceal band ligation (VBL), prescribing agents such as beta-blockers, or a combination of these. This will depend on the characteristics of the varices (Grade 0–III), and patient factors, including the patient's tolerance of beta-blockers. Early involvement of a hepatologist or gastroenterologist is advised to initiate appropriate prophylaxis, manage other features of decompensated liver disease that may arise and consider referral for transplantation at an appropriate stage for those who may require it.

Patients with a new diagnosis of cirrhotic liver disease satisfying agreed criteria for risk of varices and those with significant decompensated change, should undergo upper GI endoscopy for variceal screening and surveillance using Baveno criteria as an additional reference (2). One-year endoscopic follow-up of Grade I varices is to ensure no progression in the interim period. Generally, if electing to conduct VBL, the clinician should schedule endoscopic assessment every 2–4 weeks until complete eradication, with a follow-up upper GI endoscopy 3 months, thereafter, then at 6 months and yearly (*Figure 21.1*) (1).

When performing VBL (procedural details) it is recommended to begin band application at the level of the gastro-oesophageal junction and apply bands to the columns of varices in a helical fashion on withdrawal of the scope. Banding can cease when varices have collapsed, signifying cessation of blood flow (*Figures 21.1* and *21.2*).

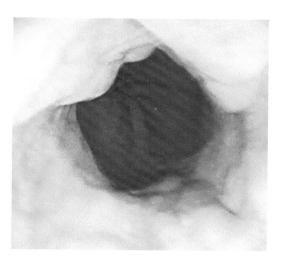

Figure 21.1 Grade I oesophageal varices.

DOI: 10.1201/9781003080060-21

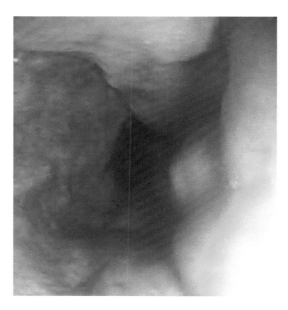

Figure 21.2 Grade II oesophageal varices.

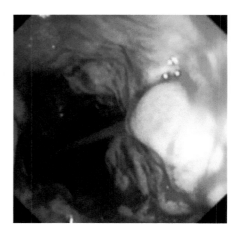

Figure 21.3 Bleeding oesophageal varices.

Oesophageal variceal bleeding

Variceal bleeding is a major contributor to death from liver disease, conferring a mortality rate of 33% for those who recover, with outcomes worse in Child-Pugh Class-C disease. Timely intervention can significantly reduce re-bleeding rates, however the impact on longer term prognosis is dependent on the severity of the underlying liver disease (3).

This medical emergency requires vigilant initial resuscitation and early intervention primarily through endoscopic means. Serious consideration should be given to airway protection through tracheal intubation, however, the risks of concomitant encephalopathy and infection must be considered and early discussion with a senior anaesthetist is advised. The aim of endoscopic intervention is to arrest bleeding at the source.

Following initial resuscitation and prior to endoscopic intervention, broad-spectrum antibiotic prophylaxis and vasoconstrictors such as terlipressin or somatostatin, should be administered.

VBL is the preferred method of endoscopic haemostasis in oesophageal variceal (OV) bleeding. This is achieved by initial examination of the upper GI tract, followed by forward-view identification of the bleeding source and band application along the length of the involved varix up to the bleeding point. Bands are applied by suction of the varix segment into the endoscopic cap until 'red-out' and deployment of the band before releasing suction. This practice should be completed progressively up the variceal columns to approximately 6 cm aboral to the gastro-oesophageal junction if significant congestion remains and performed on all other visible significant varices until they collapse.

Patients should receive non-selective beta blockade and follow-up endoscopies approximately every 4 weeks with repeat variceal banding until complete obliteration is achieved. For OV bleeding, VBL has largely replaced variceal sclerotherapy, which carries a higher risk of complications (4) (*Figure 21.3*).

Gastric varices

Bleeding of gastric varices (GVs) is less common than oesophageal variceal bleeding and achieving haemostasis can prove more challenging. Except in select cases (bleeding from type 1 gastro-oesophageal varices) where there is effectively extension of oesophageal varices to the lesser curve of the stomach, the preferred haemostatic approach is injection of either cyanoacrylate glue or thrombin directly to the bleeding varix (4).

Endoscopic ultrasound guided treatment, in the form of sclerotherapy, coil insertion, or a combination of the two, is an emerging safe and effective modality for treating gastric varices (5).

When endoscopic efforts fail

When initial endoscopic efforts fail to achieve haemostasis or significant variceal bleeding recurs, alternative methods of controlling blood loss must be considered. Balloon tamponade using for example, a Sengstaken-Blakemore or Minnesota tube can make a lifesaving, if temporary contribution until definitive treatment is available (*Figure 21.4*).

Generally, patients having balloon tamponade tube insertion should be intubated as a conscious patient will find it extremely difficult to tolerate. The device should be inserted by an experienced operator and inflated through the gastric port with 250 mL of air. Placement confirmation by initial inflation of 50 mL air followed by X-ray, is recommended. Gastric balloon inflation with traction applied to tamponade the varices at the gastro-oesophageal junction is usually enough to

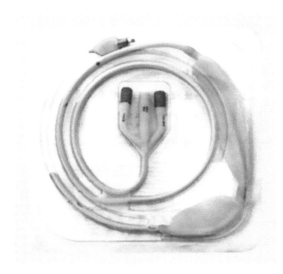

Figure 21.4 A Sengstaken-Blakemore tube with oesophageal and gastric balloons.

achieve haemostasis. If bleeding continues the oesophageal balloon may require inflation with 60–70 mL air, until intra-balloon pressure reaches 30 mmHg. Haemostatic powders such as Hemospray® may have a place in the emergency management of variceal bleeding and have been shown to be safe (7).

SEMS are an emerging alternative to balloon tamponade for control of oesophageal variceal bleeding prior to more definitive intervention such as TIPS and liver transplantation. The clinical success rate where haemostasis is achieved is 96% at 24 hours in suitably skilled hands (8).

In recent decades interventional radiology has become a central component in the management of variceal bleeding. TIPS insertion may be undertaken in cases of refractory or recurrent variceal bleeding. While this can be a useful way of reducing the portal pressure gradient and controlling bleeding, consideration must be made to co-existing factors like hepatic encephalopathy, heart failure and uncontrolled sepsis, which may serve as relative or absolute contraindications.

DUODENAL POLYPS

Duodenal polyps are uncommon, found in up to 1.5% of upper GI endoscopies and most commonly represent benign conditions for which no intervention is warranted (8). High-quality endoscopic assessment is fundamental to the diagnosis and onward management of duodenal polyps. The endoscopist must be mindful of obtaining a comprehensive luminal view of the lesion and ensure slow withdrawal with reinsertion if the endoscope retracts into the stomach before full assessment can be made. Air bubbles should be cleared with the help of an anti-foaming agent such as simethicone. Full assessment

of the ampulla is best performed with a side-viewing duodenoscope, which will require an operator skilled in its use. This is not required in the vast majority of diagnostic endoscopies.

Documented assessment and description of a polyp is an essential requirement of planning onward management. Location (including relationship to the ampulla and pylorus), diameter, morphology and surface characteristics are all vital pieces of information in making a judgement regarding therapy (10). Photographic or video documentation are extremely useful tools for this. Lesion surface characteristics can be assessed using enhanced methods such as narrow-band imaging or chromoendoscopy however high-quality white light endoscopy is the mainstay of assessment and interpretation. Distal attachment caps also have utility in close-up visualization of luminal lesions.

Lipomas and Brunner's gland hamartomas are benign growths that do not usually require resection, unless in rare circumstances, they lead to symptoms such as obstruction or bleeding.

For lesions with malignant potential, endoscopic resection may be considered. Solitary Peutz-Jegher (SPJ) polyps, adenomas, carcinoids and gastrointestinal stromal tumours (GISTs) are all in this category.

SPJ polyps are uncommon hamartomas that have the potential for malignant transformation and as such, resection is advised. The typical appearance is of a lobular pedunculated lesion with white surface markings. The characteristic clinical features of Peutz–Jegher's syndrome (mucocutaneous pigmentation) help to point towards this diagnosis. Genetic testing, colonoscopy and small bowel imaging should follow this.

Duodenal adenomas are usually found in the second or third part of the duodenum and can arise sporadically or in association with polyposis syndromes like familial adenomatous polyposis (FAP). In patients with FAP, where they occur in up to 90% of cases the lifetime risk of duodenal adenocarcinoma is estimated to be up to 5% for that entire patient population. Most duodenal polyps are sessile, with a characteristic hypo-pigmented surface. Careful surface examination should be performed to evaluate the lesion for dysplastic or malignant features. A loss of pit pattern, depression, ulceration or 'non-lifting' of an adenoma may suggest advanced dysplasia or invasive carcinoma, with larger adenomas conferring greater malignant potential. Significant caution should be exercised prior to planning resection of lesions exceeding 20 mm in diameter (*Figures 21.5–21.7*).

The Spigelman classification was devised to predict the risk of developing cancer with a polyp burden in FAP, guiding surveillance and intervention (*Tables 21.1 and 21.2*) (11).

When planning endoscopic resection of duodenal polyps, consideration must be given to the likelihood of safe and complete endoscopic removal. This is influenced by patient factors such as comorbidity

Table 21.1 Spigelman classification for guiding surveillance

Spigelman score	Spigelman stage	Recommendation
0	0	Re-scope in 5 years
1–4	I	Re-scope in 3–5 years
5–6	II	Re-scope in 3 years
7–8	III	Re-scope in 1 year
9–12	IV	Consider duodenectomy versus re-scope in 6 months

Table 21.2 Spigelman classification for duodenal polyps in FAP

Criteria	Points		
	1	2	3
Polyp number	1–4	5–20	>20
Polyp size (mm)	1–4	5–10	>10
Histology	Tubular	Tubulovillous	Villous
Dysplasia	Mild	Moderate	Severe

Note: Stage 0 = 0 points; Stage I = 1–4 points; Stage II = 5–6 points; Stage III = 7–8 points; Stage IV = 9–12 points.

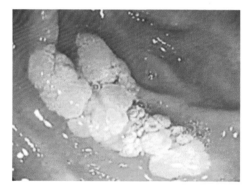

Figure 21.5 Adenoma within the second part of the duodenum, with characteristic pale surface and lobular morphology.

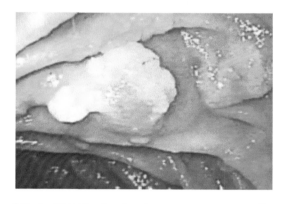

Figure 21.7 Duodenal adenoma appearance after submucosal lifting with agent containing adrenaline.

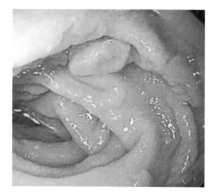

Figure 21.6 Multiple adenomatous polyps in the context of FAP.

and tolerance, operator factors such as skill set and resources, and the position and morphology of the polyp itself. The histological diagnosis, size and possibility of ampullary involvement are a few such factors.

Pedunculated polyps

European guidelines pertaining to colorectal pedunculated lesions advise that pre-injection of the stalk with adrenaline containing solution or placement of a clip before resection of thick-stalked lesions can be helpful in reducing the incidence of major bleeding. The evidence supporting this has prompted a similar approach in resecting pedunculated duodenal lesions (*Figure 21.8*) (12).

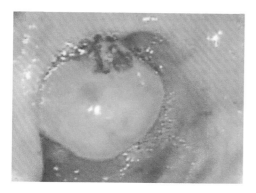

Figure 21.8 Pedunculated polyp situated between the first and second parts of the duodenum. Note the limitations on the calibre of the lumen, making attempts at resection more difficult.

Sessile polyps

As with colorectal intervention, endoscopic mucosal resection (EMR) can be performed using snare polypectomy. Adenomas are often sessile and the duodenal wall is thin. Submucosal injection separates the mucosa from the muscularis propria, creating a 'cushion' to decrease the risk of perforation and haemorrhage while also examining for 'non-lifting' sign indicative of invasive neoplastic tissue (13).

Commonly, snare polypectomy is then conducted, either *en-bloc* or piecemeal. Careful evaluation of the endoscopic margins is essential post-resection to ensure completeness of excision. Retrieval of polyp tissue can be achieved with aspiration via the suction channel and trap or with a net. After EMR, careful inspection of the base is vital and a low threshold for prophylactic deployment of endoscopic clips when significant concerns exist over perforation or post-procedural bleeding risk may be beneficial, with some evidence pointing to a lower complication rate with this practice (*Figure 21.9*) (14).

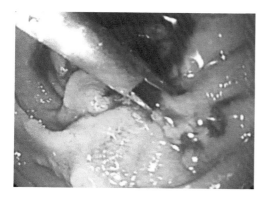

Figure 21.9 Prophylactic endoclip deployment to site of duodenal EMR.

Ampullary adenomas have traditionally been subject to surgical approaches for removal, however, endoscopic techniques have evolved and it is now possible to offer a less invasive management strategy in many cases. Endoscopic papillectomy is usually performed with a side-viewing duodenoscope, with hot snare polypectomy and insertion of a pancreatic duct stent to prevent post-procedure pancreatitis. As with standard endoscopic retrograde cholangiopancreatography (ERCP), rectal non-steroidal anti-inflammatory medication is advised to further reduce pancreatitis risk (15).

Sub-epithelial lesions such as sizeable carcinoids and GISTs were once the sole preserve of surgery for complete resection, however, endoscopic submucosal dissection (ESD) has progressed to the stage that it can now be offered as a safe alternative technique. Although ESD is associated with higher perforation rates and procedure duration than EMR in addition to the breadth of lesions amenable to this approach, ESD confers higher rates of complete extirpation of adenomas with an *en-bloc* resection. It should only be performed in high-volume centres by skilled operators. Adverse effects are often more common with ESD but this is balanced against improved therapeutic outcomes for larger lesions (16).

REFERENCES

1. Tripathi D, Stanley AJ, Hayes PC, Patch D, Milson C, Mehrzad H, et al. UK Guidelines on the management of variceal haemorrhage in cirrhotic patients. *Gut* 2015;**64(11)**:1–25. Doi10.1136/gutjnl–2015309262.
2. de Franchis R, Bosch J, Garcia-Tsao G, Reiberger T, Ripoll C, Faculty B VII. Baveno VII: Renewing consensus in portal hypertension. *J Hepatol* 2022;**76(4)**:959–74.
3. Puente A, Hernández-Gea V, Graupera I, Roque M, Colomo A, Poca M, et al. Drugs plus ligation to prevent rebleeding in cirrhosis: An updated systematic review. *Liver Int* 2014;**34(6)**:823–33.
4. Poza Cordon J, Froilan Torres C, Burgos García A, Gea Rodriguez FG, Manuel J, de Parga S. Endoscopic management of esophageal varices. *World J Gastrointest Endosc* 2012;**4(7)**:312–22.
5. Sarin SK, Lahoti D, Saxena SP, Murthy NS, Makwana UK. Prevalence, classification and natural history of gastric varices: A long-term follow-up study in 568 portal hypertension patients. *Hepatology* 1992;**16(6)**:1343–9.
6. McCarty TR, Bazarbashi AN, Hathorn KE, Thompson CC, Ryou M. Combination therapy *versus* monotherapy for EUS-guided management of gastric varices: A systematic review and meta-analysis. *Endosc Ultrasound* 2020;**9(1)**:6–15. doi: 10.4103/eus.eus_37_19. PMID: 31417066; PMCID: PMC7038733.
7. Ibrahim M, El-Mikkawy A, Abdel Hamid M, Abdalla H, Lemmers A, Mostafa I, et al. Early application of haemostatic powder added to standard management

for oesophagogastric variceal bleeding: A randomised trial. *Gut* 2019;**68**:844–53.

8. McCarty TR, Njei B. Self-expanding metal stents for acute refractory esophageal variceal bleeding: A systematic review and meta-analysis. *Digestive Endoscopy* 2016;**28**:539–47.

9. Jepsen JM, Persson M, Jakobsen NO, Christiansen T, Skoubo-Kristensen E, Funch-Jensen P, et al. Prospective study of prevalence and endoscopic and histopathologic characteristics of duodenal polyps in patients submitted to upper endoscopy. *Scand J Gastroenterol* 1994;**29**(6):483–7. doi: 10.3109/00365529409092458. PMID: 8079103.

10. Axon, A, Diebold MD, Fujino M, Fujita R, Genta RM, Gonvers JJ, et al. Update on the Paris classification of superficial neoplastic lesions in the digestive tract. *Endoscopy* 2005;**37**(6):570–78.

11. Spigelman AD, Williams CB, Talbot IC, Domizio P, Phillips RK. Upper gastrointestinal cancer in patients with familial adenomatous polyposis. *Lancet* 1989;**2**(**8666**):783–5.

12. Ferlitsch M, Moss A, Hassan C, Bhandari P, Dinis-Ribeiro M, Risio M, et al. Colorectal polypectomy and endoscopic mucosal resection (EMR): European Society of Gastrointestinal Endoscopy (ESGE) clinical guideline. *Endoscopy* 2017;**49**(3):270–97.

13. Castro R, Libânio D, Pita I, Dinis-Ribeiro M. Solutions for submucosal injection: What to choose and how to do it. *World J Gastroenterol* 2019;**25**(7):777–88.

14. An JY, Kim BW, Park JM, Park J-M, Kim TH, Lee J. Prophylactic clipping for the prevention of delayed complication after endoscopic resection for superficial non-ampullary duodenal tumor. *Endoscopy* 2019;**51**:S118.

15. Vanbiervliet G, Strijker M, Arvanitakis M, Aelvoet A, Arnelo U, Benya T, et al. Endoscopic management of ampullary tumors: European Society of Gastrointestinal Endoscopy (ESGE) guideline. *Endoscopy* 2021;**53**(4):429–48.

16. Gaspar JP, Stelow EB, Wang AY. Approach to the endoscopic resection of duodenal lesions. *World J Gastroenterol* 2016;**22**(2):600–17.

Chapter 22

Endoscopic Retrograde Cholangiopancreatography

Alexander Ney and Stephen P. Pereira

INTRODUCTION

The first endoscopic visualization of Vater's papilla dates back to the late 1960s but it required the development of long side-viewing endoscopes from Olympus Medical Systems (Hamburg, Germany) before it was routinely possible. The new side-viewing endoscopes formed the basis for the establishment of endoscopic retrograde cholangiopancreatography (ERCP) as a 'gold standard' diagnostic and therapeutic tool for the work-up of biliary and pancreatic pathologies. ERCP allows high-quality visualization of the pancreatic-biliary ductal system and localization of obstructing lesions. With the parallel developments in non-invasive imaging such as ultrasound (US), computed tomography (CT), magnetic resonance imaging (MRI) and magnetic resonance cholangiopancreatography (MRCP), the diagnostic utility of ERCP has declined, and it is now mostly used as a minimally invasive therapeutic modality. ERCP is commonly used for biliary and pancreatic duct (PD) stone retrieval and the relief of biliary obstruction in cases of benign and malignant biliary strictures. There is also still a role for diagnostic ERCP in cases of inconclusive imaging and for the purpose of tissue acquisition.

INDICATIONS FOR ERCP

ERCP is commonly indicated for both diagnostic (obtaining tissue biopsies for confirmation or exclusion of malignancy) and therapeutic purposes, in a variety of benign and malignant conditions of the pancreas and biliary tree (*Table 22.1*).

ERCP in gallstone disease

The relief of mechanical biliary obstruction due to biliary lithiasis is the most common indication for therapeutic ERCP. When acute biliary pancreatitis is suspected, US or MRCP evidence of gallbladder stones or CBD dilatation or stones should be sought ideally within 24 hours. Cholangitis secondary to a CBD stone is associated with upper abdominal pain, deranged liver function tests and clinical signs of biliary sepsis (Charcot's triad, Reynold's pentad). Concomitant CBD dilatation, which is often identified using abdominal ultrasound (USS) or MRCP, requires urgent intervention within 24 hours in a septic patient who does not respond to initial resuscitation and antibiotic treatment

Table 22.1 Indications for ERCP (1,86,123)

The jaundiced patient

- Common bile duct (CBD) stones, with or without cholangitis
- Evaluation of suspected malignant biliary strictures in the presence of equivocal or normal imaging, CT, MRI and endoscopic ultrasound (EUS)

Pancreatitis

- Stenting of pancreatic duct leaks
- Obstructing pancreatic duct stones
- Balloon dilatation/stenting of pancreatic duct strictures

Clinical or radiological findings suggestive of biliary or pancreatic duct disease in the non-jaundiced patient

- Evaluation and tissue sampling of biliary and pancreatic ducts

Endoscopic sphincterotomy

- Choledocholithiasis
- Papillary dilatation
- Choledochocele
- Sump syndrome

Stenting/balloon dilatation in benign biliary strictures

- Bile duct injury, fistulae
- Non-surgical biliary drainage in large obstructing stones
- Primary sclerosing cholangitis (PSC) with dominant stricture

Malignant biliary strictures

- Tissue sampling/brush cytology
- Cholangioscopy/pancreatoscopy
- Stenting
- Ampullary resection

(1). Prior to stone extraction, sphincterotomy with, or without, balloon sphincteroplasty is performed to enable the passage of instruments, stones or debris.

Sphincterotomy performed at the 11–12-o'clock position when viewing the duodenal papilla will usually allow extraction of CBD stones which are less than 1 cm in size. Best practice is to ensure duct clearance at the time of ERCP in order to prevent potential complications such as stone impaction with subsequent cholangitis or pancreatitis. Bile duct stones

DOI: 10.1201/9781003080060-22

can be retrieved using a balloon catheter, by basket extraction, or fragmented using a mechanical lithotripter in cases of stones which are larger than 1 cm or impacted. Balloon sphincteroplasty and single operator cholangioscopy-guided lithotripsy have particular roles. Where such approaches fail or are incomplete, placement of naso-biliary drains or removable plastic or metal mesh stents ensure duct drainage until definitive management in the form of repeat endoscopy or surgery is possible.

The British Society of Gastroenterology (BSG) recommends 'interval cholecystectomy' within 2 weeks of an admission with acute, mild gallstone pancreatitis (2). However, evidence from the PONCHO trial showed that same admission cholecystectomy is associated with reduced rates of complications and recurrence of symptoms compared with interval cholecystectomy (3). Patients undergoing laparoscopic cholecystectomy can be further assessed intraoperatively using 'on-table cholangiography'. In the hands of an experienced surgeon, laparoscopic common bile duct exploration can be safely performed with comparable stone clearance rates, and favourable patient outcomes equivalent to those seen with postoperative ERCP (4). Retrieval of retained stones, as well as the management of complications such as bile duct injuries can also be managed postoperatively using ERCP. Biliary leaks are treated with decompression by sphincterotomy and/or stenting (typically for 4–6 weeks) or by placement of naso-biliary drains (5).

In the non-surgical patient, ERCP-guided stone removal or endoscopic biliary stenting alone in patients with large, impacted stones, facilitates bile drainage. Several studies however, favour complete stone clearance due to high adverse-event rates observed with stenting alone (6).

Acute pancreatitis

A diagnosis of acute pancreatitis (AP) is made based on the clinical presentation, usually with characteristic abdominal pain and laboratory parameters including elevated serum pancreatic enzymes and typical findings on non-invasive imaging (USS/CT/MRI) of the pancreas and biliary tree. In the case of gallstone pancreatitis which is complicated by cholangitis, early intervention with ERCP should be considered during the first 24 hours of admission (7).

Recurrent and chronic pancreatitis

Causes of recurrent acute pancreatitis include gallstones, microlithiasis, benign biliary strictures (BBS), obstructing neoplasms and anatomical and physiological anomalies such as pancreas divisum and sphincter of Oddi dysfunction (SOD) (8–10). When non-invasive imaging (CT or MRI/MRCP) are equivocal, an endoscopic (EUS or ERCP) approach can be performed to establish a diagnosis or with therapeutic intent. Parenchymal, ductal injury and fibrosis in chronic pancreatitis (CP) result in stricturing and stenoses of the PD, with consequent obstruction to pancreatic outflow. Other complications include pseudocyst formation, duct leakage, the development of ascites and peri-pancreatic collections, all of which can result in chronic abdominal pain (8,9). ERCP is rarely used in the diagnosis of mild CP due to its low sensitivity, generally less than 65%, compared with MRCP or EUS (10,11). Therapeutic ERCP can be used for PD evaluation and drainage in patients with PD strictures and obstructing stones, however (10). Benign PD strictures can be stented or balloon-dilated following pancreatic sphincterotomy. Symptomatic or evolving peripancreatic collections and pseudocysts complicated by infection, bleeding, gastric/duodenal outlet or biliary obstruction should be drained (10,11). Endoscopic drainage offers comparable pain control, albeit with lower morbidity and reduced hospital stay and costs compared to surgical drainage (12,13). In cases of so-called type II and III SOD, biliary and pancreatic-sphincter manometry guided sphincterotomy were previously used and the actual role of manometry in these patients has been a subject of considerable debate

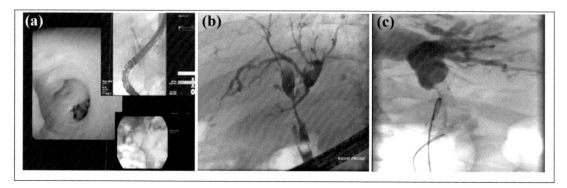

Figure 22.1 Benign biliary hilar stricture secondary to IgG4 disease (a) visualized using single operator cholangioscopy (spyglass image with left hepatic duct stones) and ERCP. Bilateral hilar benign biliary strictures (b) managed with balloon dilatation or stenting (c) under fluoroscopy-guided ERCP.

(14–16). The largest randomized controlled trial, the EPISOD study (Evaluating Predictors and Interventions in Sphincter of Oddi Dysfunction) demonstrated that outcomes following endoscopic sphincterotomy in patients with suspected SOD III were comparable or worse than sham intervention, and manometry is no longer recommended (17).

Benign and malignant bile duct strictures

Benign ductal strictures are usually iatrogenic and in the surgical patient can be seen following hepatic or pancreato-biliary surgery including cholecystectomy and at the site of biliary anastomoses (18,19). Other causes include inflammation (chronic pancreatitis), autoimmune (primary sclerosing cholangitis [PSC]) or IgG4-related disease), infectious (liver fluke), vascular and post-radiotherapy duct sclerosis (*Figure 22.1*) (20,21). Postoperative anastomotic strictures and iatrogenic injuries during cholecystectomy, can be managed with balloon dilatation or stenting using ERCP. In unresolving cases, surgical reconstruction of the bile duct is generally required (22,23).

Primary sclerosing cholangitis

In primary sclerosing cholangitis (PSC), the British Society of Gastroenterology (BSG), UK-PSC and European Society for Gastrointestinal Endoscopy (ESGE) guidelines do not recommend ERCP for the initial evaluation or follow-up, with ERCP reserved for cases following discussion by a multidisciplinary team (24,25). Where ERCP is advised, dominant strictures can be balloon-dilated or stented with comparable recurrence free survival (25). In patients with an intact duodenal papilla, balloon dilatation should be the first choice (24,25), as procedure-related adverse events (pancreatitis and cholangitis) are more frequently observed with stenting (45% versus 26% with dilatation) (26).

Indeterminate and malignant biliary strictures

Indeterminate strictures where laboratory findings, imaging or histology are inconclusive, are an indication for diagnostic ERCP, coupled with biliary brush cytology (ERCP–BC). Inadequate tissue sampling, cellular atypia or a well-differentiated phenotype in certain carcinomas, however, limit the predictive value of ERCP–BC (sensitivity 6–64% and 98–100% specificity) (27). Other sampling techniques include endobiliary biopsies and EUS-guided fine needle aspiration (FNA) are often used together, and can significantly increase diagnostic accuracy (28,29).

Certain morphological features, which can be identified with cholangioscopy (surface irregularity, nodularity or neovascularization), or detection of specific chromosomal aberrations (aneuploidy or polysomy in chromosomes 3, 7, 14 or 21, respectively) using fluorescence *in situ* hybridisation (FISH), enhance the diagnostic accuracy of BC (30–34). High-definition, optical enhancement of the visualized mucosa using chromoendoscopy, biliary narrow band imaging or probe-based confocal laser endomicroscopy (pCLE), can also be used in the assessment of biliary strictures although these relatively novel techniques still lack prospective validation in larger cohorts (35–37). Nevertheless, the addition of pCLE to ERCP–BC has shown to increase the former's sensitivity by over 30% (38). Real-time pCLE (intra-ductal fluorescein dye injection, or intravenous for pancreatic indications) enables high resolution visualization of the biliary epithelium, with diagnostic sensitivity of 98% compared with ERCP alone (45%), in the diagnosis of malignant biliary strictures (39,40).

Malignancy of non-biliary origin

Malignant biliary strictures (MBS) can be of biliary origin (cholangiocarcinoma), or secondary to cancers of the liver, pancreas, ampulla and gallbladder as well as of more distal origin (*Figure 22.2*). Where a

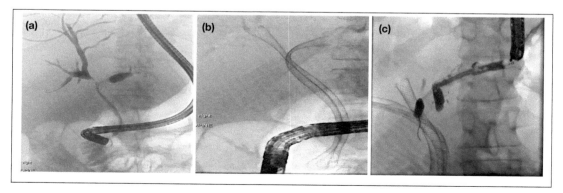

Figure 22.2 Metastatic malignant hilar stricture (a) (colorectal adenocarcinoma), stented (b) with uncovered self-expanding metallic stents. Left hepatico-gastrostomy (c) for malignancy hilar stricture with endoscopically inaccessible left hepatic duct.

pancreatic mass is identified on non-invasive imaging, preoperative biliary decompression with ERCP is not recommended unless neoadjuvant therapy is indicated, as it may in fact complicate or even preclude surgical intervention (41,42). In non-operable cancers, palliation of malignant biliary obstruction (MBO) can be achieved using ERCP or EUS-guided stenting (*Figure 22.2b*), as well as by surgical bypass with comparable technical success (43–45). Unresectable, obstructing ampullary tumours can be stented, while low-grade, well-differentiated exophytic tumours less than 3 cm, in the absence of duodenal or pancreatic invasion and PD dilatation, can be curatively resected endoscopically (46). Endoscopic *en-bloc* snare papillectomy has largely replaced radical surgical resections by Whipple's procedure in the management of ampullary adenomas which have a high rate of malignant transformation (47,48).

ADVANCED TECHNIQUES IN PALLIATION OF MALIGNANCY

Photodynamic therapy (PDT) is a locoregional therapeutic modality approved by the US Food and Drug Administration (FDA) for the treatment of oesophageal and bronchial cancers, that has shown limited efficacy in small patient cohorts with locally advanced pancreatic cancer (LAPC) and non-operable hilar cerebral amyloid angiopathy (CCA) (49–53). Similarly, ablation of intra/extrahepatic biliary tract lesions with intraductal radiofrequency ablation (RFA) has been shown to improve strictures or stent patency in patients with obstructing biliary cancers, albeit with increased procedure-related morbidity (54,55). Considering their invasive nature, costs and associated risk (photosensitivity in PDT, pain, cholangitis, pancreatitis or haemobilia with RFA), these techniques together with high intensity focused ultrasound remain largely unvalidated beyond small cohort studies (56,57).

The technique

Patients undergoing ERCP should be well informed of the indications, the procedure and potential complications and risks. In the anti-coagulated patient, specific considerations are recommended (*Table 22.2*) (58). Informed consent should be obtained by professionals with relevant training and experience, who are familiar with the procedure and its risks. Under conscious or deep propofol sedation (59) or general anaesthesia with cardiovascular monitoring, the endoscopist intubates the oesophagus and passes the endoscope through the pylorus into the duodenum. Visualization and cannulation of the major papilla on the medial wall of the second part of the duodenum requires the use of a side-viewing endoscope, which allows 90–120° up/down angulation, 90–110° right–left angulation and manipulation of the angle at which accessories leave the endoscope. A side-viewing duodenoscope enables selective cannulation of both the biliary tree and the pancreatic duct, using a sphincterotome and guidewire or contrast injection (cholangiopancreatography). ERCP is mainly indicated for therapeutic purposes, and modern endoscopes have a large 4.2 mm working channel which enables the passage of catheters, balloon dilators for sphincteroplasty, plastic or self-expanding metallic stents and mechanical lithotripters for biliary stone crushing and removal. Biliary interventions require deep cannulation of the CBD with either a standard catheter or a sphincterotome, to which an electrosurgical cutting wire is attached for the purpose of sphincterotomy or tissue dissection.

COMPLICATIONS OF ERCP AND THEIR MANAGEMENT

Compared to other endoscopic procedures, ERCP has a higher risk profile with procedure-related complication rates of around 5% (60,61) although ERCP associated mortality is relatively low at 1:500 for diagnostic procedures but approaches 1:200 for therapeutic interventions (61,62). The main complications associated with ERCP include post-ERCP pancreatitis and sphincterotomy-related issues. Other complications which are seen in less than 1% of cases include haemorrhage, cholangitis, intestinal perforation and cardiopulmonary events including myocardial ischaemia, arrhythmias and deep vein/pulmonary thrombosis (61,62).

Post-ERCP pancreatitis

Post-procedural hyper-amylasemia is seen in up to 75% of patients undergoing ERCP and is most often transient (63). Post-ERCP pancreatitis (PEP) complicates around 3% (up to 20% in certain high-risk cases) of ERCPs and is diagnosed in the presence of post-procedural abdominal pain with a 3-fold elevation in pancreatic enzymes within 24-hours of ERCP (11,63). Severe PEP may be complicated by pancreatic necrosis and sepsis, leading to multiorgan failure and death in <0.5% of cases (63,64). Risk factors include patient (younger age, sex, previous PEP), procedural (sphincterotomy, pancreatic injection, difficult cannulation) and operator (skills and experience) related factors (63,65,66). The risk of PEP is reduced with intra-procedural administration of rectal non-steroidal anti-inflammatory drugs (NSAIDS) (indomethacin or diclofenac) and pancreatic stenting in high-risk cases (67–70).

Haemorrhage

Severe intraprocedural haemorrhage during ERCP occurs in <1% of patients (61,71–73) but the risk is significantly increased (up to 9%) when sphincterotomy is performed (odds ratio [OR] 4.7), especially in the hands of less experienced endoscopists (72). Significant intra-procedural haemorrhage often follows an uncontrolled and long incision which may result in a retroduodenal artery injury. Other predictors of post-ERCP bleeding include the presence of a bleeding diatheses (cirrhosis or renal dysfunction), anti-coagulation, concomitant cholangitis and significant intra-procedural bleeding. During the procedure, haemostasis may be achieved using balloon tamponade, electro-cautery or argon plasma coagulation, clipping or local epinephrine injection (74). Short-term stenting using self-expanding metallic stents offers a safe alternative (74,75). Percutaneous arterial embolization or surgical

haemostasis are reserved for cases where endoscopic manoeuvres have failed (74). In the case of bile duct stones, the use of endoscopic balloon dilatation rather than sphincterotomy, significantly reduces the risk of post-procedural bleeding (76). Specific guidelines provided by the American Society for Gastrointestinal Endoscopy (ASGE), BSG or ESGE for the management of the anticoagulated patient, exist to guide clinicians (*Table 22.2*), and patients at moderate to high risk for cardiovascular complications and thrombosis. These

Table 22.2 ESGE and BSG guidelines for management of the anti coagulated patient undergoing endoscopy (58,77)

Anticoagulant	Indication/risk procedure	Action
Antiplatelet Therapy Aspirin (Acetylsalicylic acid) (dual or single agent)	● Low-risk (diagnostic +/− biopsy, biliary/pancreatic stenting, device-assisted enteroscopy)	● Continue
	● High-risk (sphincterotomy, stricture dilatation EUS-FNA)	● Continue
	● High-risk (ampullectomy, polypectomy, endoscopic mucosal resection/sub-mucosal dissection)	● Consider discontinuation (risk of haemorrhage vs. thrombosis) on individual basis
Antiplatelet Therapy **P2Y12 Receptor Antagonist** (Clopidogrel, prasugrel, ticagrelor)	● Low-risk (diagnostic +/− biopsy, biliary/pancreatic stenting, device-assisted enteroscopy without polypectomy)	● Continue
	● High-risk (sphincterotomy, polypectomy, stricture dilatation, ampullectomy, endoscopic mucosal resection/sub-mucosal dissection, EUS-FNA)	● Low thromboembolic risk (IHD without coronary stenting, CVD, PVD) – Discontinue 7 days prior to endoscopy ● High thromboembolic risk (stented coronary artery) – Discuss with cardiologist; consider discontinuation 5 days prior to endoscopy if: ○ Drug-eluting stent inserted 6–12 months or ○ Metal stent inserted >1 month prior to endoscopy
Warfarin/ Coumadin	● Low (diagnostic +/−biopsy, biliary/pancreatic stenting, device-assisted enteroscopy without polypectomy)	Check INR the week prior to endoscopy: ● If within therapeutic range: continue daily dose ● If above therapeutic range (but <5): adjust dose until INR within therapeutic range
	● High-risk (sphincterotomy, polypectomy, stricture dilatation, ampullectomy, endoscopic mucosal resection/sub-mucosal dissection, EUS-FNA)	● Low thromboembolic risk: metallic aortic valve, xenograft valve, AF without valve disease (>3 months following VTE), thrombophilia: ○ Ensure pre-procedural INR<1.5 ○ Restart warfarin evening of endoscopy ○ Follow-up INR in 1 week to ensure adequate anti-coagulation ● High thromboembolic risk: ○ Metallic mitral valve, prosthetic valve+AF, AF with MS, <3 months following VTE ○ Discontinue warfarin 5 days prior to endoscopy and: □ Commence LMWH 2 days following warfarin discontinuation □ Last LMWH dose should be given ≥24 h prior to endoscopy □ Restart usual warfarin dose evening of endoscopy □ Bridge with LMWH until INR within therapeutic range

(Continued)

Table 22.2 *(Continued)* ESGE and BSG guidelines for management of the anti coagulated patient undergoing endoscopy (58,77)

Anticoagulant	Indication/risk procedure	Action
Direct Oral Anticoagulants (DOAC) (dabigatran, apixaban, rivaroxaban)	• Low (diagnostic +/– biopsy, biliary/pancreatic stenting, device-assisted enteroscopy without polypectomy) • High-risk (sphincterotomy, polypectomy, stricture dilatation, ampullectomy, endoscopic mucosal resection/sub-mucosal dissection, EUS-FNA)	• Omit daily dose on morning of endoscopy Withhold agent 3 days prior to endoscopy: • If eGFR 30–50 mL/min, last dabigatran dose should be given 5 days prior to endoscopy • Cases of severe renal dysfunction should be consulted with a haematologist

Abbreviations: AF: atrial fibrillation; CVD: cerebrovascular disease; eGFR: estimated glomerular filtration rate; IHD: ischaemic heart disease; INR: international normalized ratio; LMWH: low molecular weight heparin; MS: mitral stenosis; PVD: peripheral vascular disease; VTE: venous thromboembolism.

guidelines are frequently discussed with a cardiologist prior to ERCP (58,77). The relative risks for bleeding versus thrombosis should be considered, and the ASGE guidelines offer a systematic approach for their assessment (77). Furthermore, electronic clinical decision support tools such as ENDOAID are currently being developed to aid clinicians apply evidence-based practice (78–80).

Perforation

ERCP-related visceral perforations are rare (0.08–0.6%) but associated with a high mortality rate (61,81). Increased risk for perforation is observed in cases of surgically altered anatomy (Billroth-II or bariatric surgery), sphincterotomies (periampullary perforation), intramural contrast injection, prolonged procedures, biliary dilatations or SOD (82). Luminal (including biliary/pancreatic duct) perforations may be scope or accessory induced following the use of sphincterotomy pre-cut devices and guidewires, or a later complication following stent migration. Post-ERCP surgical emphysema may be a manifestation of retroperitoneal air due to an over-extended sphincterotomy or pancreatic or bile duct injury, and should be suspected in the presence of worsening abdominal pain where serum amylase levels are normal. While subclinical perforations may be conservatively managed, worsening clinical signs such as peritonism or the development of sepsis, or radiological findings on abdominal or chest radiographs or a CT scan may require surgical intervention (62,83).

Infection

ERCP-related infections are uncommon occurring in less than 1% of procedures (60,61,84). An increased risk is seen in liver transplant patients, those with hilar or intrahepatic strictures due to PSC or perihilar CCA, in the presence of inadequate biliary drainage, or intra-peritoneal biliary leakage following contrast injection during stent insertion following a bile duct

injury. Although not routinely indicated prior to ERCP, the selective administration of prophylactic antibiotics reduces the risk of ascending cholangitis as well as cholecystitis and bacteraemia in such patients (84–87). High-level disinfection, instrument sterilization with ethylene oxide or peracetic acid or the use of single-use endoscopes reduces the risk of carbapenem-resistant entero-bacterial sepsis (81).

ERCP IN THE SURGICALLY ALTERED GASTROINTESTINAL ANATOMY

ERCP is the standard intervention for the management of biliary disease, with technical success rates of over 90% in patients with normal gastrointestinal (GI) anatomy. Gastric or proximal intestinal reconstructions during gastrectomy (Billroth-II gastrojejunostomy, Roux-en-Y bypass), pancreatic resections such as Whipple's procedure or hepaticojejunostomy formation in liver transplantation, challenge later endoscopic access for postoperative biliary and pancreatic indications (choledocholithiasis, SOD, biliary strictures). Postoperative adhesions can further complicate endoscopic procedures due to difficulty advancing the instruments through a narrow gastric lumen or a long and acutely angled surgical afferent limb. Medical rather than surgical treatment of benign gastric ulcers (proton pump inhibitors) has largely replaced Billroth-II procedures but there has been a dramatic increase in the number of patients having bariatric procedures due to the global rise in the incidence of obesity.

ERCP in the bariatric patient

Bariatric surgery is indicated in the morbidly obese (body mass index [BMI] over 40 kg/m^2) and it is recommended for the management of comorbidities such as diabetes mellitus type 2 and hypertension. In those with a BMI over 35 kg/m^2 BMI sleeve gastrectomy and Roux-en-Y gastric bypasses are the most commonly performed procedures (88–90). Gallstone disease is a late complication of bariatric surgery which occurs in over half of bariatric cases, with CBD stones seen in 10% (90,91). Following sleeve gastrectomy, the postoperative narrow gastric lumen can be safely traversed with an endoscope. In the case of Roux-en-Y bypasses, however, alternative access is required for biliary or pancreatic duct cannulation. Approaches can be sought trans-gastrically, by trans-enteric or percutaneous routes.

Trans-gastric ERCP

In laparoscopic assisted ERCP (LAP-ERCP) the surgeon will form a gastrostomy with a 15–18 mm port after securing the gastric remnant to the abdominal wall (*Figure 22.3a*) (92). The endoscope is then passed into the duodenum to facilitate papillary access for ERCP. Alternatively, under EUS guidance (endoscopic ultrasound-directed trans-gastric ERCP [EDGE]), apposition of the gastric pouch (or proximal Roux-limb in a trans-enteric approach [EDEE], *see Figure 22.3b*) and the bypassed gastric portion with a lumen-apposing metallic stent (LAMS), facilitates peroral duodenal access. Following completion, the LAMS can be removed and the defect is closed endoscopically (using sutures or clips) or left to heal by secondary intention.

Trans-enteric ERCP

Trans-enteric approaches require surgical formation of a jejunostomy in the biliopancreatic limb. Double balloon enteroscopy (DBE) allows the operator to advance a video endoscope (up to 200 cm working length) through the small intestinal lumen using a push-and-pull technique which is facilitated by inflating and deflating a latex balloon attached to the tip of the endoscope (*Figure 22.3c*) (93,94). Visualization of both large and small bowel is possible with DBE, and a relatively large working channel of 22 mm enables simultaneous tissue acquisition as well as the application of other endoscopic interventions including polypectomy, therapeutic injections or tattooing (94,95). In single balloon endoscopy (SBE), the role of the over-tube balloon is replaced by an angled, or sucking, endoscope tip for the purpose of bowel advancement with reduced complexity of instrumentation compared with DBE. Despite differences in the extent of bowel visualization, DBE and SBE have a similar therapeutic success rate and comparable risks (96,97). Spiral over-tube-assisted endoscopy (SAE) eschews the use of balloons and relies on rotational energy for linear advancement along the intestinal lumen. In the hands of an experienced endoscopist, SAE may be used as an alternative with success rates comparable to balloon-driven techniques (97,98).

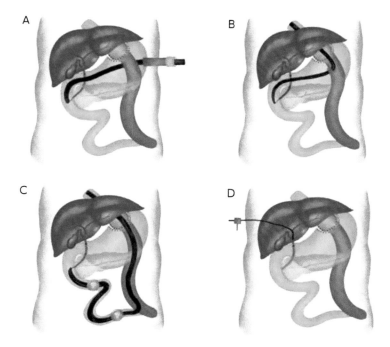

Figure 22.3 Biliary access after bariatric surgery (A) with LAP-ERCP. EU-directed trans-gastric ERCP (B). Enteroscopy-assisted ERCP (C). Percutaneous transhepatic drainage (D). Reproduced with permission, Martin H et al. (92).

ALTERNATIVE APPROACHES TO ERCP – EUS AND PERCUTANEOUS TRANSHEPATIC CHOLANGIOGRAPHY

Antegrade biliary access in the presence of altered GI anatomy (surgically, by significant stricturing or by obstructing malignancies) can be safely gained under EUS guidance (92,99,100). EUS is superior to non-invasive imaging such as CT or positron emission tomography (PET) and MRI in the detection of small pancreatic and ampullary tumours less than 3 cm in size (101–104), and is extremely useful for the evaluation or surveillance of pancreatic cysts with a high risk of transformation (105–107). EUS-guided fine needle aspiration tissue biopsy outperforms cross-sectional imaging guided biopsies in the diagnosis of both benign (BBS, CP) and malignant pancreaticobiliary conditions (pancreatic/ampullary neoplasms, MBS, CCA) where CT or ERCP-guided tissue sampling is equivocal or negative (108–112). With an accuracy of over 90% for the detection of CBD calculi less than 4 mm in size, EUS is recommended by the BSG and ESGE as the first-line investigation which when positive avoids exposing patients to the risks of ERCP (59,113–115). EUS-guided drainage of MBO (hepatico/duodeno-gastrostomy or stenting), offers a safer alternative to surgical, percutaneous transhepatic cholangiography (PTC) and endoscopic approaches, with similarly high technical success rates (99,116–120). Although PTC is associated with considerable morbidity compared to endoscopic approaches (121), the preference of one, over the other, in complex hilar lesions remains controversial (*Figure 22.3d*). Endoscopic preoperative biliary drainage using self-expanding metallic stents is recommended by the ESGE in cases of severe jaundice, cholangitis, or if resection with a curative intent is delayed (122). In non-operable patients, percutaneous transhepatic access to the biliary tree under sonographic or fluoroscopic guidance is therefore reserved for cases where endoscopic access is anatomically impossible, clinically perilous, or not available (123).

SUMMARY

Coupled with radiography, ERCP allows high-quality visualization of the pancreaticobiliary ductal system and localization of obstructing lesions. With the evolution of non-invasive imaging such as US, CT, MRI and MRCP, the diagnostic utility of ERCP has declined. It is currently used almost exclusively as a minimally invasive therapeutic modality. ERCP is commonly used for biliary- and pancreatic-duct stone retrieval and relief of biliary obstruction in cases of benign and malignant biliary strictures. There is also still a role for diagnostic ERCP in cases of inconclusive imaging, as well as for the purpose of tissue acquisition.

REFERENCES

1. Buxbaum JL, Abbas Fehmi SM, Sultan S, Fishman DS, Qumseya BJ, Cortessis VK, et al. ASGE guideline on the role of endoscopy in the evaluation and management of choledocholithiasis. *Gastrointest Endosc* 2019;**89(6)**:1075–105.e15.
2. UK guidelines for the management of acute pancreatitis. *Gut* 2005;**54(suppl 3)**:1–9.
3. da Costa DW, Bouwense SA, Schepers NJ, Besselink MG, van Santvoort HC, van Brunschot S, et al. Same-admission versus interval cholecystectomy for mild gallstone pancreatitis (PONCHO): A multicentre randomised controlled trial. *Lancet* 2015;**386(10000)**:1261–8.
4. Rhodes M, Sussman L, Cohen L, Lewis M. Randomised trial of laparoscopic exploration of common bile duct versus postoperative endoscopic retrograde cholangiography for common bile duct stones. *Lancet* 1998;**351(9097)**:159–61.
5. Mergener K, Strobel JC, Suhocki P, Jowell PS, Enns RA, Branch MS, et al. The role of ERCP in diagnosis and management of accessory bile duct leaks after cholecystectomy. *Gastrointest Endosc* 1999;**50(4)**:527–31.
6. Kaw M, Al-Antably Y, Kaw P. Management of gallstone pancreatitis: Cholecystectomy or ERCP and endoscopic sphincterotomy. *Gastrointest Endosc* 2002;**56(1)**:61–5.
7. Kuo VC, Tarnasky PR. Endoscopic management of acute biliary pancreatitis. *Gastrointest Endosc Clin N Am* 2013;**23(4)**:749–68.
8. Etemad B, Whitcomb DC. Chronic pancreatitis: Diagnosis, classification, and new genetic developments. *Gastroenterology* 2001;**120(3)**:682–707.
9. Witt H, Apte MV, Keim V, Wilson JS. Chronic pancreatitis: Challenges and advances in pathogenesis, genetics, diagnosis, and therapy. *Gastroenterology* 2007;**132(4)**:1557–73.
10. Löhr JM, Dominguez-Munoz E, Rosendahl J, Besselink M, Mayerle J, Lerch MM, et al. United European Gastroenterology evidence-based guidelines for the diagnosis and therapy of chronic pancreatitis (HaPanEU). *United Eur Gastroenterol J* 2017;**5(2)**:153–99.
11. Tenner S, Baillie J, DeWitt J, Vege SS. American College of Gastroenterology guideline: Management of acute pancreatitis. *Am J Gastroenterol* 2013;**108(9)**:1400–15.
12. Smits ME, Rauws EAJ, Tytgat GNJ, Huibregtse K. The efficacy of endoscopic treatment of pancreatic pseudocysts. *Gastrointest Endosc* 1995;**42(3)**:202–7.
13. Mark DH, Flamm CR, Aronson N. Evidence-based assessment of diagnostic modalities for common bile duct stones. *Gastrointest Endosc* 2002;**56(6)**:S190–4.
14. Geenen JE, Hogan WJ, Dodds WJ, Toouli J, Venu RP. The efficacy of endoscopic sphincterotomy after cholecystectomy in patients with sphincter-of-Oddi dysfunction. *N Engl J Med* 1989;**320(2)**:82–7.

15. Pfau PR, Banerjee S, Barth BA, Desilets DJ, Kaul V, Kethu SR, et al. Sphincter of Oddi manometry. *Gastrointest Endosc* 2011;**74(6)**:1175–80.

16. Cotton PB, Durkalski V, Romagnuolo J, Pauls Q, Fogel E, Tarnasky P, et al. Effect of endoscopic sphincterotomy for suspected sphincter of Oddi dysfunction on pain-related disability following cholecystectomy. *JAMA* 2014;**311(20)**:2101.

17. Cotton PB, Pauls Q , Keith J, Thornhill A, Drossman D, Williams A, et al. The EPISOD study: Long-term outcomes. *Gastrointest Endosc* 2018;**87(1)**: 205–10.

18. Bowlus CL, Olson KA, Gershwin ME. Evaluation of indeterminate biliary strictures. *Nat Rev Gastroenterol Hepatol* 2016;**13(1)**:28–37.

19. Greif F, Bronsther OL, Van Thiel DH, Casavilla A, Iwatsuki S, Tzakis A, et al. The incidence, timing, and management of biliary tract complications after orthotopic liver transplantation. *Ann Surg* 1994;**219(1)**:40–5.

20. Zepeda-Gómez S, Baron TH. Benign biliary strictures: Current endoscopic management. *Nat Rev Gastroenterol Hepatol* 2011;**8(10)**:573–81.

21. Costamagna G, Boškoski I, Familiari P. Benign Biliary Strictures. In: *ERCP*. London: Elsevier; 2019, pp. 417–21.e2.

22. Davids PHP, Tanka AKF, Rauws EAJ, van Gulik TM, van Leeuwen DJ, de Wit LT, et al. Benign biliary strictures surgery or endoscopy? *Ann Surg* 1993;**217(3)**:237–43.

23. Tocchi A. Management of benign biliary strictures. *Arch Surg* 2000;**135(2)**:153.

24. Schramm C, Eaton J, Ringe KI, Venkatesh S, Yamamura J. Recommendations on the use of magnetic resonance imaging in PSC-A position statement from the International PSC Study Group. *Hepatology* 2017;**66(5)**:1675–88.

25. Chapman MH, Thorburn D, Hirschfield GM, Webster GGJ, Rushbrook SM, Alexander G, et al. British Society of Gastroenterology and UK-PSC guidelines for the diagnosis and management of primary sclerosing cholangitis. *Gut* 2019;**68(8)**:1356–78.

26. Ponsioen CY, Arnelo U, Bergquist A, Rauws EA, Paulsen V, Cantú P, et al. No superiority of stents vs balloon dilatation for dominant strictures in patients with primary sclerosing cholangitis. *Gastroenterology* 2018;**155(3)**:752–9.

27. Avadhani V, Hacihasanoglu E, Memis B, Pehlivanoglu B, Hanley KZ, Krishnamurti U, et al. Cytologic predictors of malignancy in bile duct brushings: A multi-reviewer analysis of 60 cases. *Mod Pathol* 2017;**30(9)**:1273–86.

28. Khan SA, Davidson BR, Goldin R, Pereira SP, Rosenberg WMC, Taylor-Robinson SD, et al. Guidelines for the diagnosis and treatment of cholangiocarcinoma: Consensus document. *Gut* 2002; **51(Suppl 6)**:vi1–9.

29. Jailwala J, Fogel EL, Sherman S, Gottlieb K, Flueckiger J, Bucksot LG, et al. Triple-tissue sampling at ERCP in malignant biliary obstruction. *Gastrointest Endosc* 2000;**51(4)**:383–90.

30. Kipp BR, Stadheim LM, Halling SA, Pochron NL, Harmsen S, Nagorney DM, et al. A comparison of routine cytology and fluorescence in situ hybridization for the detection of malignant bile duct strictures. *Am J Gastroenterol* 2004;**99(9)**:1675–81.

31. Brooks C, Gausman V, Kokoy-Mondragon C, Munot K, Amin SP, Desai A, et al. Role of fluorescent in situ hybridization, cholangioscopic biopsies, and EUS-FNA in the evaluation of biliary strictures. *Dig Dis Sci* 2018;**63(3)**:636–44.

32. Kim H-J, Kim M-H, Lee S-K, Yoo K-S, Seo D-W, Min Y-I. Tumor vessel: A valuable cholangioscopic clue of malignant biliary stricture. *Gastrointest Endosc* 2000;**52(5)**:635–8.

33. Parsa N, Khashab MA. The role of peroral cholangioscopy in evaluating indeterminate biliary strictures. *Clin Endosc* 2019;**52(6)**:556–64.

34. Badshah MB, Vanar V, Kandula M, Kalva N, Badshah MB, Revenur V, et al. Peroral cholangioscopy with cholangioscopy-directed biopsies in the diagnosis of biliary malignancies: A systemic review and meta-analysis. *Eur J Gastroenterol Hepatol* 2019;**31(8)**:935–40.

35. Shieh FK, Drumm H, Nathanson MH, Jamidar PA. High-definition confocal endomicroscopy of the common bile duct. *J Clin Gastroenterol* 2012;**46(5)**:401–6.

36. Choi HJ, Moon JH, Lee YN. Advanced imaging technology in biliary tract diseases: Narrow-band imaging of the bile duct. *Clin Endosc* 2015;**48(6)**: 498–502.

37. Fugazza A, Gaiani F, Carra MC, Brunetti F, Lévy M, Sobhani I, et al. Confocal laser endomicroscopy in gastrointestinal and pancreatobiliary diseases: A systematic review and meta-analysis. *Biomed Res Int* 2016;**2016**:4638683.

38. Slivka A, Gan I, Jamidar P, Costamagna G, Cesaro P, Giovannini M, et al. Validation of the diagnostic accuracy of probe-based confocal laser endomicroscopy for the characterization of indeterminate biliary strictures: Results of a prospective multicenter international study. *Gastrointest Endosc* 2015;**81(2)**:282–90.

39. Meining A, Chen YK, Pleskow D, Stevens P, Shah RJ, Chuttani R, et al. Direct visualization of indeterminate pancreaticobiliary strictures with probe based confocal laser endomicroscopy: A multicenter experience. *Gastrointest Endosc* 2011;**74(5)**:961–8.

40. Chauhan SS, Abu Dayyeh BK, Bhat YM, Gottlieb KT, Hwang JH, Komanduri S, et al. Confocal laser endomicroscopy. *Gastrointest Endosc* 2014;**80(6)**:928–38.

41. van der Gaag NA, Rauws EAJ, van Eijck CHJ, Bruno MJ, van der Harst E, Kubben FJGM, et al. Preoperative biliary drainage for cancer of the head of the pancreas. *N Engl J Med* 2010;**362(2)**:129–37.

42. Eshuis WJ, van der Gaag NA, Rauws EAJ, van Eijck CHJ, Bruno MJ, Kuipers EJ, et al. Therapeutic delay and survival after surgery for cancer of the pancreatic head with or without preoperative biliary drainage. *Ann Surg* 2010;**252(5)**:840–9.

43. Han SY, Kim S-O, So H, Shin E, Kim DU, Park DH. EUS-guided biliary drainage versus ERCP for first-line palliation of malignant distal biliary obstruction: A systematic review and meta-analysis. *Sci Rep* 2019;**9(1)**:16551.

44. Artifon ELA, Sakai P, Cunha JEM, Dupont A, Filho FM, Hondo FY, et al. Surgery or endoscopy for palliation of biliary obstruction due to metastatic pancreatic cancer. *Am J Gastroenterol* 2006;**101(9)**:2031–7.

45. Paik WH, Lee TH, Park DH, Choi J-H, Kim S-O, Jang S, et al. EUS-guided biliary drainage versus ERCP for the primary palliation of malignant biliary obstruction: A multicenter randomized clinical trial. *Am J Gastroenterol* 2018;**113(7)**:987–97.

46. Anderson MA, Appalaneni V, Ben-Menachem T, Decker GA, Early DS, Evans JA, et al. The role of endoscopy in the evaluation and treatment of patients with biliary neoplasia. *Gastrointest Endosc* 2013;**77(2)**:167–74.

47. Jung MK, Cho CM, Park SY, Jeon SW, Tak WY, Kweon YO, et al. Endoscopic resection of ampullary neoplasms: a single-center experience. *Surg Endosc* 2009;**23(11)**:2568–74.

48. Catalano MF, Linder JD, Chak A, Sivak M V, Raijman I, Geenen JE, et al. Endoscopic management of adenoma of the major duodenal papilla. *Gastrointest Endosc* 2004;**59(2)**:225–32.

49. Dumoulin FL, Gerhardt T, Fuchs S, Scheurlen C, Neubrand M, Layer G, et al. Phase II study of photodynamic therapy and metal stent as palliative treatment for nonresectable hilar cholangiocarcinoma. *Gastrointest Endosc* 2003;**57(7)**:860–7.

50. Rumalla A, Baron TH, Wang KK, Gores GJ, Stadheim LM, de Groen PC. Endoscopic application of photodynamic therapy for cholangiocarcinoma. *Gastrointest Endosc* 2001;**53(4)**:500–4.

51. Cheon YK, Lee TY, Lee SM, Yoon JY, Shim CS. Longterm outcome of photodynamic therapy compared with biliary stenting alone in patients with advanced hilar cholangiocarcinoma. *HPB (Oxford)* 2012;**14(3)**:185–93.

52. DeWitt JM, Sandrasegaran K, O'Neil B, House MG, Zyromski NJ, Sehdev A, et al. Phase 1 study of EUS-guided photodynamic therapy for locally advanced pancreatic cancer. *Gastrointest Endosc* 2019;**89(2)**:390–8.

53. Hanada Y, Pereira SP, Pogue B, Maytin EV, Hasan T, Linn B, et al. EUS-guided verteporfin photodynamic therapy for pancreatic cancer. *Gastrointest Endosc* 2021;**94(1)**:179–86.

54. Sofi AA, Khan MA, Das A, Sachdev M, Khuder S, Nawras A, et al. Radiofrequency ablation combined with biliary stent placement versus stent placement alone for malignant biliary strictures: A systematic review and meta-analysis. *Gastrointest Endosc* 2018;**87(4)**:944–51.

55. Tal AO. Intraductal endoscopic radiofrequency ablation for the treatment of hilar non-resectable malignant bile duct obstruction. *World J Gastrointest Endosc* 2014;**6(1)**:13.

56. Prat F, Lafon C, Theillière J-Y, Fritsch J, Choury A-D, Lorand I, et al. Destruction of a bile duct carcinoma by intraductal high intensity ultra sound during ERCP. *Gastrointest Endosc* 2001;**53(7)**:797–800.

57. Prat F, Lafon C, de Lima DM, Theilliere Y, Fritsch J, Pelletier G, et al. Endoscopic treatment of cholangiocarcinoma and carcinoma of the duodenal papilla by intraductal high-intensity US: Results of a pilot study. *Gastrointest Endosc* 2002;**56(6)**:909–15.

58. Veitch AM, Radaelli F, Alikhan R, Dumonceau JM, Eaton D, Jerrome J, et al. Endoscopy in patients on antiplatelet or anticoagulant therapy: British Society of Gastroenterology (BSG) and European Society of Gastrointestinal Endoscopy (ESGE) guideline update. *Gut* 2021;**70(9)**:1611–28.

59. Williams E, Beckingham I, El Sayed G, Gurusamy K, Sturgess R, Webster G, et al. Updated guideline on the management of common bile duct stones (CBDS). *Gut* 2017;**66(5)**:765–82.

60. Loperfido S, Angelini G, Benedetti G, Chilovi F, Costan F, De Berardinis F, et al. Major early complications from diagnostic and therapeutic ERCP: A prospective multicenter study. *Gastrointest Endosc* 1998;**48(1)**:1–10.

61. Masci E. Complications of diagnostic and therapeutic ERCP: A prospective multicenter study. *Am J Gastroenterol* 2001;**96(2)**:417–23.

62. Anderson MA, Fisher L, Jain R, Evans JA, Appalaneni V, Ben-Menachem T, et al. Complications of ERCP. *Gastrointest Endosc* 2012;**75(3)**:467–73.

63. Freeman ML, Guda NM. Prevention of post-ERCP pancreatitis: A comprehensive review. *Gastrointest Endosc* 2004;**59(7)**:845–64.

64. Kochar B, Akshintala VS, Afghani E, Elmunzer BJ, Kim KJ, Lennon AM, et al. Incidence, severity, and mortality of post-ERCP pancreatitis: A systematic review by using randomized, controlled trials. *Gastrointest Endosc* 2015;**81(1)**:143–9.

65. Cheng CL, Sherman S, Watkins JL, Barnett J, Freeman M, Geenen J, et al. Risk factors for post-ERCP pancreatitis: A prospective multicenter study. *Am J Gastroenterol* 2006;**101(1)**:139–47.

66. Bailey AA, Bourke MJ, Kaffes AJ, Byth K, Lee EY, Williams SJ. Needle-knife sphincterotomy: Factors predicting its use and the relationship with post-ERCP pancreatitis (with video). *Gastrointest Endosc* 2010;**71(2)**:266–71.

67. Elmunzer BJ, Waljee AK, Elta GH, Taylor JR, Fehmi SMA, Higgins PDR. A meta-analysis of rectal NSAIDs in the prevention of post-ERCP pancreatitis. *Gut* 2008;**57(9)**:1262–7.

68. Elmunzer BJ, Scheiman JM, Lehman GA, Chak A, Mosler P, Higgins PDR, et al. A randomized trial of rectal indomethacin to prevent post-ERCP pancreatitis. *N Engl J Med* 2012;**366(15)**:1414–22.

69. Fazel A, Quadri A, Catalano MF, Meyerson SM, Geenen JE. Does a pancreatic duct stent prevent post-ERCP pancreatitis? A prospective randomized study. *Gastrointest Endosc* 2003;**57(3)**:291–4.

70. Choudhary A, Bechtold ML, Arif M, Szary NM, Puli SR, Othman MO, et al. Pancreatic stents for prophylaxis against post-ERCP pancreatitis: A meta-

analysis and systematic review. *Gastrointest Endosc* 2011;**73(2)**:275–82.

71. Vandervoort J, Soetikno RM, Tham TCK, Wong RCK, Ferrari AP, Montes H, et al. Risk factors for complications after performance of ERCP. *Gastrointest Endosc* 2002;**56(5)**:652–6.

72. Cotton PB, Garrow DA, Gallagher J, Romagnuolo J. Risk factors for complications after ERCP: A multivariate analysis of 11,497 procedures over 12 years. *Gastrointest Endosc* 2009;**70(1)**:80–8.

73. Navaneethan U, Parsi MA, Lourdusamy D, Grove D, Sanaka MR, Hammel JP, et al. Volatile organic compounds in urine for noninvasive diagnosis of malignant biliary strictures: A pilot study. *Dig Dis Sci* 2015;**60(7)**:2150–7.

74. Valats J-C, Funakoshi N, Bauret P, Hanslik B, Dorandeu A, Christophorou D, et al. Covered self-expandable biliary stents for the treatment of bleeding after ERCP. *Gastrointest Endosc* 2013;**78(1)**:183–7.

75. Bilal M, Chandnani M, McDonald NM, Miller CS, Saperia J, Wadhwa V, et al. Use of fully covered self-expanding metal biliary stents for managing endoscopic biliary sphincterotomy related bleeding. *Endosc Int Open* 2021;**9(05)**:E667–73.

76. Baron TH, Harewood GC. Endoscopic balloon dilation of the biliary sphincter compared to endoscopic biliary sphincterotomy for removal of common bile duct stones during ERCP: A metaanalysis of randomized, controlled trials. *Am J Gastroenterol* 2004;**99(8)**:1455–60.

77. Acosta RD, Abraham NS, Chandrasekhara V, Chathadi KV, Early DS, Eloubeidi MA, et al. The management of antithrombotic agents for patients undergoing GI endoscopy. *Gastrointest Endosc* 2016;**83(1)**:3–16.

78. Nutalapati V, Tokala KT, Desai M, Kanakadandi V, Olyaee M, Parasa S, et al. Development and validation of a web-based electronic application in managing antithrombotic agents in patients undergoing GI endoscopy. *Gastrointest Endosc* 2019;**90(6)**:906–12.

79. Hatta W, Tsuji Y, Yoshio T, Kakushima N, Hoteya S, Doyama H, et al. Prediction model of bleeding after endoscopic submucosal dissection for early gastric cancer: BEST-J score. *Gut* 2020;**70(3)**:476–84.

80. James TW, Baron TH. Algorithmic anticoagulation: Streamlining the decision to hold and restart blood thinners in the periendoscopy period. *Gastrointest Endosc* 2019;**90(6)**:913–14.

81. Chandrasekhara V, Khashab MA, Muthusamy VR, Acosta RD, Agrawal D, Bruining DH, et al. Adverse events associated with ERCP. *Gastrointest Endosc* 2017;**85(1)**:32–47.

82. Anderson MA, Fisher L, Jain R, Evans JA, Appalaneni V, Ben-Menachem T, et al. Complications of ERCP. *Gastrointest Endosc* 2012;**75(3)**:467–73.

83. Kumbhari V, Sinha A, Reddy A, Afghani E, Cotsalas D, Patel YA, et al. Algorithm for the management of ERCP-related perforations. *Gastrointest Endosc* 2016;**83(5)**:934–43.

84. Cotton PB, Connor P, Rawls E, Romagnuolo J. Infection after ERCP, and antibiotic prophylaxis: A sequential quality-improvement approach over 11 years. *Gastrointest Endosc* 2008;**67(3)**:471–5.

85. Dumonceau J-M, Kapral C, Aabakken L, Papanikolaou IS, Tringali A, Vanbiervliet G, et al. ERCP-related adverse events: European Society of Gastrointestinal Endoscopy (ESGE) Guideline. Endoscopy 2020;52(02):127–49.

86. Adler DG, Baron TH, Davila RE, Egan J, Hirota WK, Leighton JA, et al. ASGE guideline: The role of ERCP in diseases of the biliary tract and the pancreas. *Gastrointest Endosc* 2005;**62(1)**:1–8.

87. Brand M, Bizos D, O'Farrell PJ. Antibiotic prophylaxis for patients undergoing elective endoscopic retrograde cholangiopancreatography. *Cochrane Database Syst Rev* 2010;**(10)**CD007345.

88. Buchwald H, Avidor Y, Braunwald E, Jensen MD, Pories W, Fahrbach K, et al. Bariatric surgery. *JAMA* 2004;**292(14)**:1724.

89. Buchwald H, Oien DM. Metabolic/Bariatric Surgery Worldwide 2011. *Obes Surg* 2013;**23(4)**:427–36.

90. Dixon JB, le Roux CW, Rubino F, Zimmet P. Bariatric surgery for type 2 diabetes. *Lancet* 2012;**379(9833)**:2300–11.

91. Li VKM, Pulido N, Fajnwaks P, Szomstein S, Rosenthal R. Predictors of gallstone formation after bariatric surgery: A multivariate analysis of risk factors comparing gastric bypass, gastric banding, and sleeve gastrectomy. *Surg Endosc* 2009;**23(7)**:1640–4.

92. Martin H, El Menabawey T, Webster O, Parisinos C, Chapman M, Pereira SP, et al. Endoscopic biliary therapy in the era of bariatric surgery. *Frontline Gastroenterol* 2021;**13(2)**:133–9.

93. May A, Nachbar L, Ell C. Double-balloon enteroscopy (push-and-pull enteroscopy) of the small bowel: Feasibility and diagnostic and therapeutic yield in patients with suspected small bowel disease. *Gastrointest Endosc* 2005;**62(1)**:62–70.

94. Yamamoto H, Sekine Y, Sato Y, Higashizawa T, Miyata T, Iino S, et al. Total enteroscopy with a nonsurgical steerable double-balloon method. *Gastrointest Endosc* 2001;**53(2)**:216–20.

95. Yamamoto H, Kita H, Sunada K, Hayashi Y, Sato H, Yano T, et al. Clinical outcomes of double-balloon endoscopy for the diagnosis and treatment of small-intestinal diseases. *Clin Gastroenterol Hepatol* 2004;**2(11)**:1010–16.

96. Wadhwa V, Sethi S, Tewani S, Garg SK, Pleskow DK, Chuttani R, et al. A meta-analysis on efficacy and safety: Single-balloon vs. double-balloon enteroscopy. *Gastroenterol Rep* 2015;**3(2)**:148–55.

97. Skinner M, Popa D, Neumann H, Wilcox C, Mönkemüller K. ERCP with the overtube-assisted enteroscopy technique: A systematic review. *Endoscopy* 2014;**46(07)**:560–72.

98. Khashab MA, Lennon AM, Dunbar KB, Singh VK, Chandrasekhara V, Giday S, et al. A comparative evaluation of single-balloon enteroscopy and spiral enteroscopy for patients with mid-gut disorders. *Gastrointest Endosc* 2010;**72(4)**:766–72.

99. Holt BA, Hawes R, Hasan M, Canipe A, Tharian B, Navaneethan U, et al. Biliary drainage: Role of EUS guidance. *Gastrointest Endosc* 2016;**83(1)**:160–5.

100. Shah JN, Marson F, Weilert F, Bhat YM, Nguyen-Tang T, Shaw RE, et al. Single-operator, single-session EUS-guided anterograde cholangiopancreatography in failed ERCP or inaccessible papilla. *Gastrointest Endosc* 2012;**75(1)**:56–64.

101. DeWitt J, Devereaux BM, Lehman GA, Sherman S, Imperiale TF. Comparison of endoscopic ultrasound and computed tomography for the preoperative evaluation of pancreatic cancer: A systematic review. *Clin Gastroenterol Hepatol* 2006;**4(6)**:717–25.

102. Müller MF, Meyenberger C, Bertschinger P, Schaer R, Marincek B. Pancreatic tumors: Evaluation with endoscopic US, CT, and MR imaging. *Radiology* 1994;**190(3)**:745–51.

103. Tang S, Huang G, Liu J, Liu T, Treven L, Song S, et al. Usefulness of 18F-FDG PET, combined FDG-PET/CT and EUS in diagnosing primary pancreatic carcinoma: A meta-analysis. *Eur J Radiol* 2011;**78(1)**:142–50.

104. Ishikawa T, Itoh A, Kawashima H, Ohno E, Matsubara H, Itoh Y, et al. Usefulness of EUS combined with contrast-enhancement in the differentia diagnosis of malignant versus benign and preoperative localization of pancreatic endocrine tumors. *Gastrointest Endosc* 2010;**71(6)**:951–9.

105. Vege SS, Ziring B, Jain R, Moayyedi P, Adams MA, Dorn SD, et al. American Gastroenterological Association Institute Guideline on the Diagnosis and Management of Asymptomatic Neoplastic Pancreatic Cysts. *Gastroenterology* 2015;**148(4)**:819–22.

106. Pereira SP, Oldfield L, Ney A, Hart PA, Keane MG, Pandol SJ, et al. Early detection of pancreatic cancer. Lancet Gastroenterol Hepatol 2020;5(7):698–710.

107. Bhandari P, Longcroft-Wheaton G, Libanio D, Pimentel-Nunes P, Albeniz E, Pioche M, et al. Revising the European Society of Gastrointestinal Endoscopy (ESGE) research priorities: A research progress update. *Endoscopy* 2021;**53(05)**:535–54.

108. Fritscher-Ravens A, Broering DC, Knoefel WT, Rogiers X, Swain P, Thonke F, et al. EUS-Guided Fine-Needle Aspiration of suspected hilar cholangiocarcinoma in potentially operable patients with negative brush cytology. *Am J Gastroenterol* 2004;**99(1)**:45–51.

109. Eloubeidi MA, Chen VK, Jhala NC, Eltoum IE, Jhala D, Chhieng DC, et al. Endoscopic ultrasound-guided fine needle aspiration biopsy of suspected cholangiocarcinoma. *Clin Gastroenterol Hepatol* 2004;**2(3)**:209–13.

110. Rösch T, Meining A, Frühmorgen S, Zillinger C, Schusdziarra V, Hellerhoff K, et al. A prospective comparison of the diagnostic accuracy of ERCP, MRCP, CT, and EUS in biliary strictures. *Gastrointest Endosc* 2002;**55(7)**:870–6.

111. DeWitt J, Misra VL, LeBlanc JK, McHenry L, Sherman S. EUS-guided FNA of proximal biliary strictures after negative ERCP brush cytology results. *Gastrointest Endosc* 2006;**64(3)**:325–33.

112. Horwhat JD, Paulson EK, McGrath K, Stanley Branch M, Baillie J, Tyler D, et al. A randomized comparison of EUS-guided FNA versus CT or US-guided FNA for the evaluation of pancreatic mass lesions. *Gastrointest Endosc* 2006;**63(7)**:966–75.

113. Lachter J, Rubin A, Shiller M, Lavy A, Yasin K, Suissa A, et al. Linear EUS for bile duct stones. *Gastrointest Endosc* 2000;**51(1)**:51–4.

114. Karakan T, Cindoruk M, Alagozlu H, Ergun M, Dumlu S, Unal S. EUS versus endoscopic retrograde cholangiography for patients with intermediate probability of bile duct stones: A prospective randomized trial. *Gastrointest Endosc* 2009;**69(2)**:244–52.

115. Manes G, Paspatis G, Aabakken L, Anderloni A, Arvanitakis M, Ah-Soune P, et al. Endoscopic management of common bile duct stones: European Society of Gastrointestinal Endoscopy (ESGE) guideline. *Endoscopy* 2019;**51(5)**:472–91.

116. Hara K, Yamao K, Niwa Y, Sawaki A, Mizuno N, Hijioka S, et al. Prospective clinical study of EUS-guided choledochoduodenostomy for malignant lower biliary tract obstruction. *Am J Gastroenterol* 2011;**106(7)**:1239–45.

117. Paik WH, Lee TH, Park DH, Choi J-H, Kim S-O, Jang S, et al. EUS-guided biliary drainage versus ERCP for the primary palliation of malignant biliary obstruction: A multicenter randomized clinical trial. *Am J Gastroenterol* 2018;**113(7)**: 987–97.

118. Park JK, Woo YS, Noh DH, Yang J-I, Bae SY, Yun HS, et al. Efficacy of EUS-guided and ERCP-guided biliary drainage for malignant biliary obstruction: Prospective randomized controlled study. *Gastrointest Endosc* 2018;**88(2)**:277–82.

119. Anderloni A, Fugazza A, Troncone E, Auriemma F, Carrara S, Semeraro R, et al. Single-stage EUS-guided choledochoduodenostomy using a lumen-apposing metal stent for malignant distal biliary obstruction. *Gastrointest Endosc* 2019;**89(1)**:69–76.

120. Sharaiha RZ, Khan MA, Kamal F, Tyberg A, Tombazzi CR, Ali B, et al. Efficacy and safety of EUS-guided biliary drainage in comparison with percutaneous biliary drainage when ERCP fails: A systematic review and meta-analysis. *Gastrointest Endosc* 2017;**85(5)**:904–14.

121. Nennstiel S, Weber A, Frick G, Haller B, Meining A, Schmid RM, et al. Drainage-related complications in percutaneous transhepatic biliary drainage. *J Clin Gastroenterol* 2015;**49(9)**:764–70.

122. Dumonceau J-M, Tringali A, Papanikolaou I, Blero D, Mangiavillano B, Schmidt A, et al. Endoscopic biliary stenting: indications, choice of stents, and results: European Society of Gastrointestinal Endoscopy (ESGE) Clinical Guideline – Updated October 2017. *Endoscopy* 2018;**50(9)**:910–30.

123. Bukhari M, Kowalski T, Nieto J, Kunda R, Ahuja NK, Irani S, et al. An international, multicenter, comparative trial of EUS-guided gastrogastrostomy-assisted ERCP versus enteroscopy-assisted ERCP in patients with Roux-en-Y gastric bypass anatomy. *Gastrointest Endosc* 2018;**88(3)**: 486–94.

Chapter

23

Endoscopic Ultrasound in Pancreatic and Biliary Diseases

Laurent Palazzo and Maxime Palazzo

INTRODUCTION

Endoscopic ultrasound (EUS) is an endoscopic technique that combines ultrasonography and endoscopy with a dedicated endoscope at the end of which is placed a miniaturized ultrasound probe. The endoscope is linked to both an endoscopic processor and an ultrasound processor. Despite the routine use of high-definition cross-sectional imaging; computed tomography (CT) and magnetic resonance imaging (MRI), EUS remains invaluable in the management of pancreatic and biliary diseases because of its unrivalled spatial resolution. Indeed, the distance between the transducer and the target is reduced to a few millimeters allowing the use of high frequencies with no disturbance due to peri-digestive fat and luminal air, regardless of the morphology of the patient.

Presently, and for the foreseeable future, the use of EUS-guided fine needle biopsy (EUS-FNB) and the development of therapeutic EUS will be key elements for the management of pancreatic and biliary diseases.

EUS is performed under intravenous sedation or general anaesthesia because the procedure can be prolonged and requires the patient to remain still. For examination of the pancreatic and biliary systems a left lateral decubitus position, tilted forward by 30° is the preferred position (1).

DIAGNOSTIC ENDOSCOPIC ULTRASOUND

Pancreatic diseases

EUS can be used to examine the whole of the pancreas from the uncinate process to the tail in almost all patients (*Figure 23.1*). The head cannot be completely seen in patients with impassable duodenal strictures or a previous gastrectomy with a Billroth-2 anastomosis. Previous endoscopic biliary sphincterotomy, or the presence of an uncovered metal stent, may also hinder visualization of part of the pancreatic head. EUS should ideally be performed prior to the insertion of a stent in the common bile duct.

Solid pancreatic masses

The sensitivity of EUS for the diagnosis of pancreatic cancer is greater than 95% even in small cancers with a diameter of 2 cm or less. These small cancers are not detectable by external imaging (CT and MRI) in 30% of cases and EUS remains the reference examination. A normal EUS examination essentially excludes a diagnosis of pancreatic cancer.

EUS-FNB is a technique that uses a specific needle through the operator channel to obtain histopathological samples. The second-generation FNB needles (called cutting needles) are disposable and designed for single use. The available gauge diameters are 25G, 22G, 20G and 19G. They have a specifically designed tip that allows the needle to obtain core tissue from the tumour. Core samples facilitate immunohistochemistry and molecular biology for personalized oncological therapy. Twenty-two-gauge cutting needles and flexible 20G cutting needles are an excellent compromise and are more suitable than 25G cutting needles as they obtain a larger tissue sample. Nineteen-gauge cutting needles obtain large tissue samples but are associated with more complications.

The diagnostic accuracy of EUS-FNB for solid pancreatic masses exceeds 90% with a specificity close to 100% (2). The main complications of EUS-FNB are bleeding, pancreatitis, perforation and superinfection of cystic lesion. Complications occurs in 2–6% of cases.

EUS-FNB indications are:

1   Histopathological diagnosis of a solid pancreatic mass is important to distinguish between adenocarcinoma, other types of cancer (neuroendocrine tumours), pancreatic metastasis and an inflammatory mass. New methods of tissue characterization such as contrast harmonic EUS (CH-EUS) and elastography (3,4) are helpful for the aetiological diagnosis of solid pancreatic masses but their accuracy is still insufficient to replace EUS-FNB

2   Assessment of locoregional involvement in pancreatic cancer. The sensitivity of EUS for the diagnosis of moderate involvement of the mesenteric-portal vein confluence in patients with pancreatic cancer smaller than 3 cm is close to 100%. EUS is able to detect, and confirm by FNB, small subcapsular liver metastases of segment II and I that are invisible on CT and MRI. EUS is the most sensitive method for the diagnosis of early low-volume ascites suggestive of peritoneal carcinomatosis

DOI: 10.1201/9781003080060-23

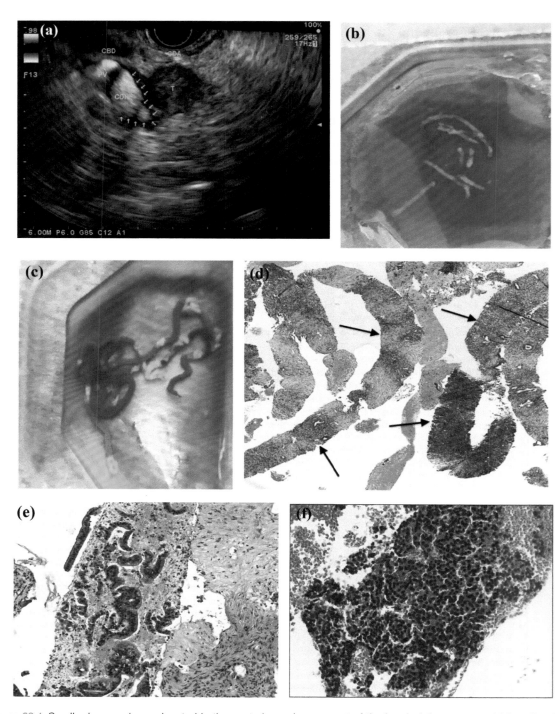

Figure 23.1 Small adenocarcinoma located in the posterior and upper part of the head of the pancreas (a) invading (white arrows) more than 200° of the mesenteric-portal confluence. Fine needle biopsy sample (b) (macroscopic on-site evaluation) with second generation 22G cutting needle. Fine needle biopsy sample (c) (macroscopic on-site evaluation) with 20G cutting needle. Histological aspect (d) (low magnification) of pancreatic adenocarcinoma (black arrows). Histological aspect (e) (high magnification) of pancreatic adenocarcinoma demonstrating thickened stroma infiltrated by malignant glands. Histological aspect (f) (high magnification) of pancreatic neuroendocrine tumour. The quality of the sample is sufficient for a satisfactory assessment of the proliferation index (Ki 67). *Abbreviations*: GDA: gastroduodenal artery; CBD: common bile duct; PV: portal vein; CONF: confluence; T: tumour.

Pancreatic cysts

Pancreatic cysts are very common and the prevalence in the general population is high. The prevalence increases with age and they are present in 5% of the population aged 50, at least 15% of the population aged 70, and in excess of 25% after 80. Pancreatic cysts result from a number of different pathologies with variable behaviour and will have a different specific risk of malignancy. For example, serous cystadenoma (SCA) has almost no risk of malignant transformation in contrast with mucinous cystadenoma (MCA) or main-duct intraductal papillary mucinous neoplasms (IPMN). Obtaining an accurate diagnosis of the precise nature of the cyst is the key element for guiding management and EUS is very useful for cystic lesions when their nature cannot be clarified by a combination of CT and MRI scanning.

There are key EUS features used to classify cysts. A microcystic appearance is suggestive of SCA while a clearly visible communication between the cyst and the main pancreatic duct is suggestive of a branch-duct IPMN. The presence of wall thickening, mural nodule and droplets of mucus is suggestive of a mucinous cyst (MCA, branch-duct IPMN). When diagnostic uncertainty remains, EUS-guided fine needle aspiration (EUS-FNA) is mandatory to allow evaluation of the intra-cystic fluid. The evaluation includes an assessment of the macroscopic appearance of the fluid. A milky appearance suggests a cystic lymphangioma, a positive string-test suggests a mucinous lesion, and a chocolate-brown appearance suggests a necrotic pseudocyst. Biochemical analysis including for amylase, carcinoembryonic antigen (CEA) and glucose are mandatory (5). An amylase level of <250 rules out a pseudocyst. A glucose level below 50 ng/dL is in favour of a mucinous cyst whilst a (CEA) level greater than 200 ng/dL is in favour of a mucinous lesion. Cytology, despite a very high specificity, is disappointing with a sensitivity of around 50%. Molecular biology analysis of the fluid is promising but not presently routinely available in clinical practice.

Through-the-needle techniques are available where additional devices are introduced via a 19G needle. These are needle-based confocal laser endomicroscopy (nCLE) devices which consists of an *in vivo* histology of the cyst wall after IV injection of fluorescein. Diagnostic accuracy is greater than 90% and morbidity is less than 5% (6). When a superficial vascular network is observed, the specificity for the diagnosis of SCA is close to 100%. When papillae are observed, the specificity for the diagnosis of mucinous lesions, mainly branch-duct IPMN, is also close to 100%. The other option is endocystic wall microbiopsy, with microforceps (7) that are introduced through the 19G needle. Diagnostic accuracy is slightly lower than nCLE and morbidity is higher at around 10% including intra-cystic bleeding and acute pancreatitis. Though-the-needle techniques are indicated when the multidisciplinary team of gastroenterologist, surgeon and radiologist are considering surgery for a cystic lesion with a mucinous appearance at risk of rapid progression to malignancy (>3–4 cm in diameter), or when discontinuing surveillance (macrocystic or mixed-type SCA) is proposed. In both these scenarios, it is absolutely essential to have an unequivocal diagnosis. In the absence of a clear communication between the cystic lesion and the main pancreatic duct that confirms the diagnosis of branch-duct IPMN, or positive cytology, having a diagnostic test that ensures a specificity approaching 100% is essential and extremely reassuring.

Acute pancreatitis of unknown cause

EUS has clearly been established as the most accurate technique for identifying an unrecognized biliary cause for acute pancreatitis; responsible for almost half of the acute cases of pancreatitis of indeterminate origin at initial presentation. The sensitivity for the diagnosis of gallbladder microlithiasis exceeds 90% when abdominal ultrasound has suggested no abnormality (8). EUS is also the 'gold standard' method for the diagnosis of common bile duct stones which are known to be present in 20% of cases of acute biliary pancreatitis. EUS is also very sensitive for the diagnosis of early non-calcifying chronic pancreatitis, which is the second most common cause of acute pancreatitis of indeterminate origin. EUS remains the most sensitive technique for the diagnosis of small solid tumours causing an obstructive acute pancreatitis and, as described earlier, is also very accurate for the diagnosis of IPMN.

Chronic pancreatitis including autoimmune pancreatitis

EUS is useful in the setting of early, non-calcifying chronic pancreatitis (9) and the diagnostic criteria are known as the 'Rosemont criteria' (hyperechoic foci with shadowing and main pancreatic duct calculi (Major A) and lobularity with honeycombing (Major B). When chronic pancreatitis is advanced with calcifications, EUS is poor because of the shadowing due to the ultrasound beam being unable to pass through the calcified areas. In cases of duodenal stricture in the setting of excess alcohol consumption, EUS is the gold standard for the diagnosis of cystic dystrophy of the duodenal wall arising from an aberrant pancreas (paraduodenal pancreatitis, groove pancreatitis). EUS is also able to sample a pancreatic mass in the setting of chronic pancreatitis using EUS-FNB in order to rule out a pancreatic malignancy.

EUS is the imaging modality of choice when a diagnosis of autoimmune pancreatitis (AIP) is suspected. There will be diffuse hypertrophy with a 'sausage-shaped' gland, peripheral rim enhancement and a main pancreatic duct, which cannot be seen. In cases of a localized mass-forming pancreatitis, irregular narrowing of the main pancreatic duct with thickening of the wall is highly suggestive and specific. EUS-FNB sensitivity, using second-generation cutting needles for the diagnosis of type 1 AIP (IgG4-related pancreatitis), is 60% (10).

Biliary diseases

Stones

EUS is the 'gold standard' technique and superior to magnetic resonance cholangiopancreatography (MRCP), endoscopic retrograde cholangiopancreatography (ERCP), abdominal ultrasound (US) and CT scanning for the diagnosis of common bile duct stones with a diagnostic accuracy of 95% (11) (*Figure 23.2*). EUS is also the 'gold standard' technique, again superior to MRCP, ERCP, abdominal US and CT scanning for the diagnosis of gallbladder stones with a diagnostic accuracy of 95% (including microlithiasis). In patients who have had a cholecystectomy with biliary pain and liver function test abnormalities, EUS is the ideal examination for confirming or ruling out a residual stone, the absence of which suggests sphincter of Oddi dysfunction.

Tumours

The sensitivity of EUS for the diagnosis of cholangiocarcinoma of the subhilar biliary tract and arising from the ampulla is close to 100%. EUS is comfortably the most accurate examination for the assessment of the locoregional (vascular and lymph node) involvement from these cancers. If necessary, histopathological assessment is possible with EUS-FNB but tumour seeding is a concern when targeting proximal lesions. As a consequence, EUS-FNB of extra pancreatic cholangiocarcinoma is not recommended in potentially resectable cases and is contraindicated when liver transplantation is considered. Conversely, it can be performed safely in cases of distal cholangiocarcinoma and non-resectable proximal cholangiocarcinoma or when sampling lymph nodes (12).

In patients with ampullary tumours, EUS is essential for selecting patients with usT1N0 tumours, since they may benefit from curative ampullectomy.

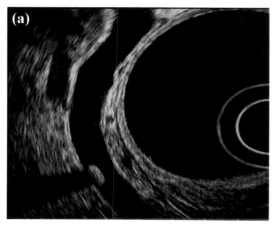

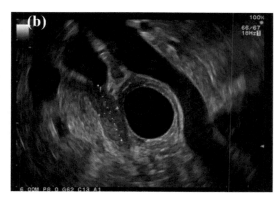

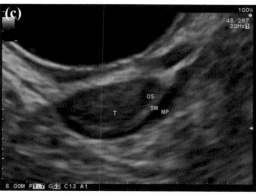

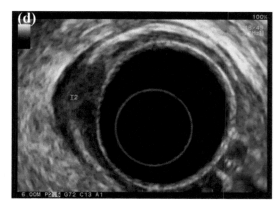

Figure 23.2 A stone (3 mm) (a) in the lower part of a normal CBD. Distal (b) cholangiocarcinoma. Small (10 mm) intra-ampullary tumour (T) (c) sparing the SM and MP, suitable for an ampullectomy. Small (12 mm) (d) intra-ampullary tumour invading the submucosa and the muscularis propria justifying pancreaticoduodenectomy. *Abbreviations*: SM: submucosa; MP: muscularis propria; OS: sphincter of Oddi.

THERAPEUTIC ENDOSCOPIC ULTRASOUND

EUS-guided drainage of pancreatic pseudocysts and walled-off necrosis

Pancreatic fluid collections are classified as, early acute peripancreatic fluid collections, pseudocysts and walled-off necrosis. Acute pancreatic fluid collections should not be drained during the early phase of their development because of the high rate of spontaneous resolution. Pseudocysts and walled-off necrosis should only be drained if symptomatic or complications occur. EUS-guided drainage should always be preferred if the collection is close to a digestive wall, usually the stomach or duodenum. EUS-guided drainage is an internal drainage technique which obviates the need for a percutaneous drain or catheter and the associated complications and morbidity.

EUS-guided drainage is done under radiological (X-ray) guidance in a dedicated interventional (usually ERCP) suite. Prior to the procedure, EUS and MRI are the best modalities to evaluate the amount of solid tissue in the pancreatic fluid collections. EUS-guided drainage can be performed with plastic, double-pigtail stents or a fully covered dedicated metallic stent called a 'lumen apposing metallic stent' (LAMS). Drainage by plastic double-pigtail stents is preferable when a rupture of the main pancreatic duct (MPD) is suspected and a disconnected pancreatic duct syndrome (DPDS) is likely. LAMS facilitates an endoscopic necrosectomy which is performed by introducing the endoscope into the cavity for the debridement of necrotic tissue. The efficacy of EUS-guided drainage of pancreatic collection is very high with a very low rate of adverse events (13).

EUS-guided drainage of pancreatic collections with double-pigtail plastic stents requires a number of stages. The EUS scope is positioned so the collection can be visualized and Doppler mode analysis of the wall is performed prior to puncturing the collection to avoid traversing a blood vessel. Puncture of the cyst is performed with a 19G needle or directly with the cystotome using a pure cutting current. Aspiration of the fluid for bacteriological analysis is mandatory. An 0.035 inch hydrophilic guidewire (GLIDEWIRE®) is inserted into the cyst and a tract produced with a 10 F cystotome or a 4 mm balloon. A second guidewire is then introduced, and the two plastic double-pigtail stents are placed under radiological and endoscopic control. In case of suspicion of DPDS the plastic stents should be left in place as long as possible to avoid pseudocyst recurrence.

EUS-guided drainage (mainly for abscesses or walled-off necrosis) with LAMS is easier because of the 'all-in-one concept'. Direct puncture of the cyst is performed with the integrated cystotome. Release of the distal flange uses EUS guidance and the catheter is then retrieved in order to oppose the two lumens. The proximal flange is then released under EUS or endoscopic guidance. LAMS should be removed ideally 2–3 weeks later to minimize the risk of secondary complications, particularly haemorrhage.

EUS-guided biliary drainage

Endoscopic retrograde cholangiography (ERC) is the 'gold standard' for the drainage of pancreatic or biliary malignancies involving the distal end of the common bile duct. It is also very useful in cases of malignant obstruction at the hilum. In cases where ERC is unsuccessful, however, the next step usually involves percutaneous drainage. More recently, EUS-guided biliary drainage has emerged as an alternative approach. The procedure involves constructing an anastomosis between the digestive tract (stomach or duodenum) and the biliary tree (14) *(Figures 23.3* and *23.4)*.

Two types of anastomoses can be performed, either a hepaticogastrostomy or choledocoduodenostomy. Dedicated, and specially developed, equipment and stents are required to facilitate this technique and ensure that the rate of adverse events is acceptable. For hepaticogastrostomy, bile ducts within segments 2 or 3 are identified and targeted with a 19G needle. Aspiration of bile and subsequent cholangiography are performed to confirm placement and clarify the anatomy. A 0.025 inch or 0.035 inch hydrophilic guidewire is then inserted into the selected bile duct and a tract formed with a 6 F cystotome or a 4 mm balloon. A fully

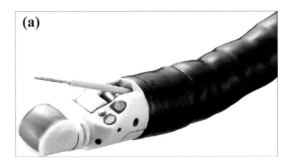

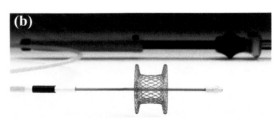

Figure 23.3 Curved array echoendoscope (a) which allows EUS-guided FNB and EUS-guided therapy. Lumen-apposing metallic stent (LAMS) (b) is useful in case of EUS-guided drainage of pancreatic collection and choledocoduodenostomy. It is mandatory in the cases of EUS-guided gallbladder drainage, gastroenterostomy and gastrogastrostomy.

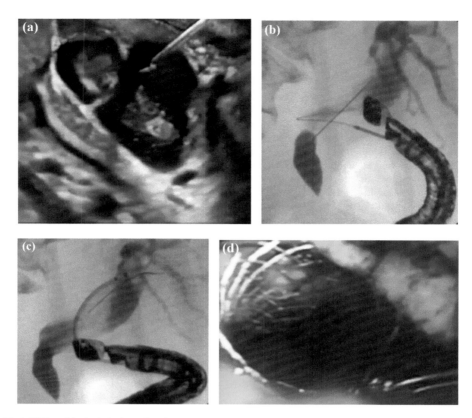

Figure 23.4 EUS-guided choledocoduodenostomy. Puncture of the dilated common bile duct (a) using a 19G needle. Introduction of the 6-French cystotome (b) on the guidewire previously set up through the 19G needle. Introduction (c) of the self-expanding covered metal stent. Endoscopic view (d) of the fully deployed stent.

covered or specific partially covered stent is introduced and released under EUS, radiological and endoscopic guidance.

Choledocoduodenostomy can be performed using the same technique through the duodenal bulb or second part of the duodenum. Small LAMS are very useful for choledocoduodenostomy formation with a very high success rate, and low risk of adverse events. EUS-guided gallbladder drainage is another very efficient technique in case of acute cholecystitis in patients unfit for surgery (15) and should be preferred to transhepatic percutaneous gallbladder drainage. The use of LAMS in this indication is mandatory.

EUS-guided coeliac neurolysis

The coeliac plexus is composed of two groups of ganglia, located anterior and lateral to the aorta at the level of the coeliac trunk. Coeliac plexus neurolysis (CPN) refers to the permanent ablation of the coeliac plexus and is usually performed with phenol or alcohol in patients with malignant disease. Coeliac plexus block (CPB) refers to the temporary inhibition of pain using corticosteroids and long-acting anaesthetics and is

usually performed in patients with chronic pancreatitis. Coeliac ganglia neurolysis (CGN) and coeliac ganglia block are a more recent development. They refer to the direct injection of alcohol or corticosteroid into the ganglia. CPN/CPB and CGN/CGB rarely relieve pain completely but reduce opioid requirements and side effects (16).

EUS-guided radiofrequency ablation

Radiofrequency ablation is a thermal ablative therapy which has been in use for over two decades traditionally employing a percutaneous approach. It facilitates the delivery of a controlled thermal insult in order to destroy tumours such as hepatic metastases. Specific needles have been developed which can be used through the operating channel of an EUS endoscope. Results are very promising with an efficacy of 90% and adverse events recorded in less than 10% of cases during the treatment of pancreatic neuroendocrine tumours of less than 2 cm (17). This technique is also ideal for the treatment of pancreatic insulinomas due to their benign behaviour, small size and the difficulty in managing, often very difficult, symptoms in functioning

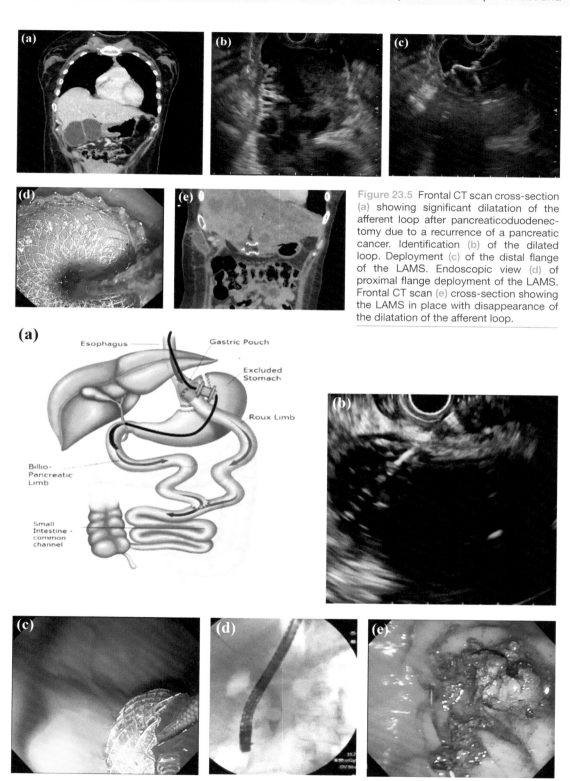

Figure 23.5 Frontal CT scan cross-section (a) showing significant dilatation of the afferent loop after pancreaticoduodenectomy due to a recurrence of a pancreatic cancer. Identification (b) of the dilated loop. Deployment (c) of the distal flange of the LAMS. Endoscopic view (d) of proximal flange deployment of the LAMS. Frontal CT scan (e) cross-section showing the LAMS in place with disappearance of the dilatation of the afferent loop.

Figure 23.6 Endoscopic ultrasound-directed trans-gastric ERCP (EDGE). Labelled anatomical diagram (a) of the procedure. Deep introduction (b) of the guidewire slipped through the 19G needle. Endoscopic view (c) of proximal flange deployment of the LAMS. Opacification of the bile duct (d) with the presence of a stone (>1 cm). Endoscopic view (e) of stone fragments after mechanical lithotripsy.

lesions. Small pancreatic metastases less than 2 cm in size from renal cancers and branch-duct IPMN with mural nodules, in patients unfit for surgery are also suitable candidates for this technique.

EUS-guided gastroenterostomy and gastrogastrostomy

EUS-guided gastroenterostomy is a new technique for the treatment of malignant gastric outlet obstruction. As for EUS-guided biliary drainage, the use of LAMS is mandatory (18). EUS-guided gastrogastrostomy with a LAMS, where a previous Roux-en-Y gastric bypass has been performed, allows reconnection of the pouch and the excluded stomach in order to access the remnant stomach and duodenum. Endoscopic diagnosis or treatment (EDGE) of the biliary tract and pancreas can then be done in a classical fashion using the LAMS technique (19) (*Figures 23.5* and *23.6*).

REFERENCES

1. Palazzo L, Lennon AM, Penman I. Endosonography. In: Canard JM, Letard C, Palazzo L, Penman I, Lennon AM (eds). *Gastrointestinal Endoscopy in Practice*, Churchill Livingstone Elsevier; 2011, Chapter 9, pp. 274–369.
2. Renelus BD, Jamorabo DS, Boston I, Briggs WM, Poneros JM, et al. Endoscopic ultrasound-guided fine needle biopsy needles provide higher diagnostic yield compared to endoscopic ultrasound-guided fine needle aspiration needles when sampling solid pancreatic lesions: a meta-analysis. *Clin Endosc* 2021; **54(2)**:261–8.
3. Yamashita Y, Shimokawa T, Napoleon B, Fusaroli P, Gincul R, Kudo M, et al. Value of contrast-enhanced harmonic endoscopic ultrasonography with enhancement pattern for diagnosis of pancreatic cancer: A meta-analysis. *Diag Endosc* 2019;**31(2)**:125–33.
4. Ignee A, Jenssen C, Arcidiacono PG, Hocke M, , Möller K, Saftoiu, et al. Endoscopic ultrasound elastography of small solid pancreatic lesion: a multicenter study. *Endoscopy* 2018;**50**:1071–9.
5. Faias S, Cravo M, Chaves P, Pereira L. Comparative analysis of glucose and carcinoembryonic antigen in the diagnosis of pancreatic mucinous cysts: A systematic review and meta-analysis. Gastrointest Endosc 2021;**94(2)**:235–47.
6. Napoleon B, Palazzo M, Lemaistre AI, Caillol F, Palazzo L, Aubert A, et al. Needle-based confocal laser endomicroscopy of pancreatic cystic lesions: A prospective multicenter validation study in patients with definite diagnosis. *Endoscopy* 2019;**51(9)**:825–35.
7. Yang D, Trindade AJ, Yachimski P, Benias P, Nieto J, Manvar A, et al. Histologic analysis of endoscopic ultrasound-guided through the needle microforceps biopsies accurately identifies mucinous pancreatic cysts. *Clin Gastroenterol Hepatol* 2019;**17(8)**:1587–96.
8. Dahan P, Andant C, Levy PH, Amouyal P, Amouyal G, Dumont M, et al. Prospective evaluation of endoscopic ultrasonography and microscopic examination of duodenal bile in the diagnosis of chole-

cystolithiasis in 45 patients with normal conventional ultrasonography. *Gut* 1996;**38(2)**:277–81.
9. Mayerle J, Hoffmeister A. Chronic pancreatitis (German, Austrian and Swiss guideline). Ârzteb Int 2013;110(22):387–93 (in English).
10. Ishikawa T, Kawashima H, Ohno E, Suhara H, Hayashi D, Hiramatsu Y, et al. Usefulness of endoscopic ultrasound-guided fine-needle biopsy for the diagnosis of autoimmune pancreatitis using a 22G Franseen needle: A prospective multi-center study. *Endoscopy* 2020;**52**:978–85.
11. Meeralam Y, Al-Shammari K, Yaghoobi M. Diagnostic accuracy of EUS compared with MRCP in detecting choledocholithiasis: A meta-analysis of diagnostic test accuracy in head-to-head studies. *Gastrointest Endosc* 2017;**86(6)**:986–93.
12. El Chafic AH, Dewitt J, Leblanc JK, El Hajj II, Cote G, House MG, et al. Impact of preoperative endoscopic ultrasound-guided fine needle aspiration on postoperative recurrence and survival in cholangiocarcinoma patients. *Endoscopy* 2013;**45**:883–9.
13. Guzmán-Calderón E, Chacaltana A, Díaz R, Li B, Martinez-Moreno B, Aparicio JR, et al. Head-to-head comparison between endoscopic ultrasound guided lumen apposing metal stent and plastic stents for the treatment of pancreatic fluid collections: A systematic review and meta-analysis. *J Hepatobiliary Pancreat Sci* 2022;**29(2)**:198–211.
14. Paik WH, Lee TH, Park DH, Choi J-H, Kim S-O, Jang S, et al. EUS-guided biliary drainage versus ERCP for the primary palliation of malignant biliary obstruction: A multicenter randomized clinical trial. *Am J Gastroenterol* 2018;**113(7)**:987–97.
15. Teoh AYB, Kitano M, Itoi T, Pérez-Miranda M, Ogura T, Chan SM, et al. Endosonography-guided gallbladder drainage versus percutaneous cholecystostomy in very high-risk surgical patients with acute cholecystitis: An international randomized multicentre controlled superiority trial. *Gut* 2020;**69(6)**:1085–91.
16. Doi S, Yasuda I, Kawakami H, Hayashi T, Hisai H, Irisawa A, et al. Endoscopic ultrasound-guided celiac ganglia neurolysis vs. celiac plexus neurolysis: A randomized multicenter trial. *Endoscopy* 2013;**45(5)**:362–9.
17. Barthet M, Giovannini M, Lesavre N, Boustiere C, Napoeon B, Koch S, et al. Endoscopic ultrasound guided radiofrequency ablation for pancreatic neuroendocrine tumors and pancreatic cystic neoplasms: A prospective multicenter study. *Endoscopy* 2019;**51**:836–42.
18. Khashab MA, Bukhari M, Baron TH, Nieto J, El Zein M, Chen Y-I, et al. International multicenter comparative trial of endoscopic ultrasonography-guided gastroenterostomy versus surgical gastrojejunostomy for the treatment of malignant gastric outlet obstruction. *Endosc Int Open* 2017;**05(04)**: E275–E281.
19. Kedia P, Tarnasky PR, Nieto J, Steele SL, Siddiqui A, Xu M-M, et al. EUS-directed transgastric ERCP (EDGE) versus laparoscopy-assisted ERCP (LA-ERCP) for Roux-en-Y gastric bypass (RYGB) anatomy: A multicenter early comparative experience of clinical outcomes. *J Clin Gastroenterol* 2019;**53(4)**:304–8.

Chapter 24

Liver Trauma

Eduard Jonas and Jake Krige

INTRODUCTION

The liver is the most commonly injured intra-abdominal organ following trauma (1). Occupying the space between the anterior- and posterior-upper abdominal wall on the right- and lower-right thoracic wall, it is at risk for injury from blunt trauma either due to direct impact or compression. Partial attachment superiorly to the diaphragm, and posterior to the inferior vena cava (IVC) and retroperitoneum, also makes it susceptible to shear forces especially from vertical deceleration injuries. In addition, its relatively large size and anterior location make it vulnerable to penetrating trauma from stab or gunshot wounds (GSW). Associated injuries to other intra-abdominal organs which are reported in up to 80% of patients, occur more frequently in penetrating than blunt trauma (2,3). Mechanisms of injury vary amongst different regions but blunt trauma dominates in most high-income countries and penetrating causes are more common in middle and low-income countries (3,4).

ANATOMICAL CONSIDERATIONS

The liver is anatomically and functionally divided into eight segments and morphologically into left and right hemi-livers, defined by the plane connecting the gallbladder fossa and the IVC in which the middle hepatic vein runs. The hepatic blood supply is via the common hepatic artery and portal vein, dividing into left and right branches supplying the respective hemi-livers. The liver receives approximately 25% (1500–1900 mL/min) of the cardiac output with 75% delivered through the portal vein and 25% through the hepatic artery. Anatomical variations in terms of aberrant and accessory arteries may need to be considered in extrahepatic control of the arterial supply in a trauma situation (5). Whereas the hepatic parenchyma receives both arterial and portal venous blood, the vascular supply of the bile ducts is exclusively arterial. Venous drainage into the IVC is through the right, middle and left hepatic veins and a varying number of smaller inferior veins. The relatively high blood flow of the liver, three possible anatomical sources of bleeding, and intimate relation of the IVC makes control of bleeding especially with major liver injuries extremely challenging.

DIAGNOSIS AND SPECIAL INVESTIGATIONS

The possibility of a liver injury should be considered in any patient with a history of blunt abdominal or lower thoracic trauma, or a penetrating entry wound to the upper abdomen. Focused assessment with sonography in trauma (FAST) is useful for the assessment of abdomino-thoracic trauma in general but lacks accuracy for diagnosing liver injuries. Contrast-enhanced computed tomography with arterial, porto-venous and delayed sequences is the preferred modality for the diagnosis and grading of liver injuries, assessment of ongoing bleeding and identification of associated abdominal and chest injuries. Magnetic resonance imaging (MRI) is of limited value in the immediate assessment of liver trauma but is helpful in the subsequent assessment of biliary injuries. Functional contrast-enhanced MRI (CE-MRI) using hepatocyte specific contrast is useful for the detection and characterization of bile leaks (6). CT angiography has to a large extent replaced diagnostic arteriography in liver trauma which is now generally reserved for angioembolization to control bleeding (7).

CLASSIFICATION OF LIVER INJURIES

The American Association for the Surgery of Trauma (AAST) Organ Injury Scale (OIS) for liver injury was first published in 1989 as an anatomical description of injuries as assessed at open exploration, and ranked severity from 1–5. It was mainly used for clinical research and risk stratification (8) but has undergone several revisions based on emerging evidence and the development of better preoperative diagnostic modalities. These changes were responsible for the evolution in the treatment of liver injuries and especially the introduction of non-operative management (NOM). The most recent update consists of three sets of criteria for grading, namely imaging, operative and pathology which allows for grading regardless of treatment modality (*Table 24.1*) (9). In patients where more than one set is applicable, the highest of the three criteria is used to calculate the final AAST grade. As initial treatment decisions for patients with liver injuries are exclusively based on clinical parameters, it does not aid in early decision-making. The classification has been used for predicting outcome and may be useful in guiding subsequent management, specifically the use of angioembolization.

DOI: 10.1201/9781003080060-24

Table 24.1 The American Association for the Surgery of Trauma (AAST) Organ Injury Scale (OIS) for liver injury, 2018 update

AAST grade[#]	Imaging criteria	Operative criteria	Pathologic criteria
I	• Subcapsular haematomas <10% surface area • Parenchymal laceration <1 cm in depth	• Subcapsular haematomas <10% surface area • Parenchymal laceration <1 cm in depth • Capsular tear	• Subcapsular haematomas <10% surface area • Parenchymal laceration <1 cm in depth • Capsular tear
II	• Subcapsular haematomas 10–50% surface area; intraparenchymal haematomas <10 cm in diameter • Laceration 1–3 cm in depth and ≤10 cm in length	• Subcapsular hematomas 10–50% surface area; intraparenchymal haematomas <10 cm in diameter • Laceration 1–3 cm in depth and ≤10 cm in length	• Subcapsular haematomas 10–50% surface area; intraparenchymal haematomas <10 cm in diameter • Laceration 1–3 cm in depth and ≤10 cm in length
III	• Subcapsular haematomas >50% surface area; ruptured subcapsular or parenchymal haematomas • Intraparenchymal haematomas >10 cm • Laceration >3 cm in depth • Any injury in the presence of a liver vascular injury* or active bleeding^ contained within liver parenchyma	• Subcapsular haematomas >50% surface area or expanding; ruptured subcapsular or parenchymal haematomas • Intraparenchymal haematomas >10 cm • Laceration >3 cm in depth	• Subcapsular haematomas >50% surface area; ruptured subcapsular or intraparenchymal haematomas • Intraparenchymal haematomas >10 cm • Laceration >3 cm in depth
IV	• Parenchymal disruption involving 25–75% of a hepatic lobe • Active bleeding extending beyond the liver parenchyma into the peritoneum	• Parenchymal disruption involving 25–75% of a hepatic lobe	• Parenchymal disruption involving 25–75% of a hepatic lobe
V	• Parenchymal disruption >75% of hepatic lobe • Juxtahepatic venous injury to include retrohepatic vena cava and central major hepatic veins	• Parenchymal disruption >75% of hepatic lobe • Juxtahepatic venous injury to include retrohepatic vena cava and central major hepatic veins	• Parenchymal disruption >75% of hepatic lobe • Juxtahepatic venous injury to include retrohepatic vena cava and central major hepatic veins

[#] Grade based on highest grade assessment made on imaging, at operation or on pathological specimen. More than one grade of liver injury may be present and should be classified by the higher grade of injury. Advance one grade for multiple injuries up to a grade III.

* Vascular injury is defined as a pseudoaneurysm or arteriovenous fistula and appears as a focal collection of vascular contrast that decreases in attenuation with delayed imaging.

^ Active bleeding from a vascular injury presents as vascular contrast, focal or diffuse, that increases in size or attenuation in delayed phase. Vascular thrombosis can lead to organ infarction.

¶ Table content adapted from Kozer at al. 2018 (9).

MANAGEMENT

Improvements in the understanding of trauma management in general, with focus on trauma pathophysiology, the importance of correction of trauma-related physiological impairment, readily available diagnostic imaging and advances in interventional radiology and endoscopy have revolutionized the treatment of liver trauma over the past three decades.

Initial management

Initial management principles in patients with thoraco-abdominal trauma are applicable to patients with suspected liver injury. Primary management should follow Advanced Trauma Life Support (ATLS©) principles (10). After initial priority airway management, vascular access is established for volume resuscitation and rapid blood analyses are performed to measure the haemoglobin concentration, white cell count, urea, creatinine, electrolytes and blood gases and to establish the patient's blood group. A more detailed history regarding time and mechanism of injury is obtained and a comprehensive clinical examination is performed during ongoing resuscitation. Guidelines such as the Definitive Surgical Trauma Care (DSTC©) guidelines facilitate further management (11). In patients with haemodynamic instability and a suspicion of ongoing bleeding, goal-directed fluid replacement using massive haemorrhage protocols should be employed, following damage control resuscitation (DCR) principles (12,13). Based on clinical findings, the response to resuscitation and blood results, a decision is made whether immediate surgical exploration is indicated or if a CECT scan should be performed. Imaging results, interpreted in the context of the evolving clinical picture, will confirm whether operative or non-operative treatment is indicated. Special investigations, including imaging, should not delay transfer to the operating theatre for a trauma laparotomy if major intraperitoneal bleeding is suspected.

Non-operative management

Despite a NOM approach in the context of blunt liver trauma being suggested as early as 1929, operation was the preferred treatment for all liver trauma until the 1980s with reported mortality rates of between 9 and 19% (14–16). Following several case series of NOM in paediatric patients with success rates of up to 90%, NOM was applied to adults with blunt trauma (17–19). Indications were subsequently extended to penetrating trauma, including GSW with comparable mortality and complication rates (3,20,21). Patients who are haemodynamically stable at initial assessment without clinical suspicion of associated injuries that require operation should be considered for NOM (22). Patients are best managed in dedicated trauma units with resources for continuous monitoring of vital parameters (blood pressure, pulse and respiratory rates and oxygen saturation), serial clinical evaluations, 2–4 hourly haemoglobin measurements, operating facilities available for urgent laparotomy and access to multimodality interventions, applying institutionally tailored protocols and algorithms. CECT for grading of the injury, detection of ongoing bleeding and assessment of extrahepatic injuries should be performed routinely (23). For optimal outcomes, failure of NOM should be recognized promptly, and laparotomy, laparoscopy or radiological intervention performed as appropriate (3).

Selective NOM has become the treatment of choice for patients with liver injuries regardless of aetiology (3,4) and advances in interventional radiology and endoscopy as adjuncts to NOM have further increased the proportion of patients who can now be managed non-operatively. Fewer patients with penetrating injuries, especially GSW fulfil the criteria for NOM, compared with blunt injury (21). Successful NOM has resulted in lower transfusion requirements, shorter hospital and intensive care unit (ICU) stays, lower complication rates and improved survival, compared with patients who are treated surgically (2). Numerous studies have reported success rates of NOM in blunt liver trauma in excess of 90%, including patients with severe (AAST grade IV and V) injuries (22,24). Levels of evidence regarding factors predicting failure of NOM are low but shock on admission, the need for volume resuscitation, the number of blood transfusions, peritoneal signs, severity of the liver injury and evidence of other intra-abdominal injuries have been associated with failure (25).

Operative management

The need for operative management of patients with liver injuries may be immediate (haemodynamic instability not responsive to resuscitation), urgent (non-liver-related indication for operation or failed NOM) or elective (management of late complications). In haemodynamically unstable patients with suspected ongoing bleeding, immediate laparotomy is mandatory and should not be delayed. In keeping with trauma laparotomy principles, a midline laparotomy is performed with draping allowing an incision from symphysis pubis to the sternal notch and intrathoracic extension if needed. An early intraoperative judgement should be made as to whether a damage control procedure or definitive surgery should be performed, based on the severity of injuries, the condition of the patient, metabolic parameters and the estimated time required for definitive management (*Table 24.2*).

Damage control surgery (DCS) involves an abbreviated procedure to firstly control bleeding and luminal contamination with definitive management deferred to a subsequent procedure. Manual compression of the liver as a first manoeuvre, approximating the raw edges of fractures or lacerations, is usually effective in controlling low-pressure venous but not arterial bleeding. Reduction in bleeding following occlusion of the hepatic artery and portal vein *en masse* (Pringle manoeuvre) with placement of a non-crushing vascular clamp across the porta hepatis indicates bleeding from these vessels. Continued bleeding despite a Pringle manoeuvre indicates bleeding from outflow vessels (IVC and hepatic veins). A Pringle manoeuvre is a temporizing measure and should be released every 20–30 minutes to allow intermittent liver perfusion. If bleeding is controlled by manual compression, therapeutic packing is performed as the definitive damage control intervention. Major arterial bleeding is not well controlled by packing and if bleeding arteries are visible in fractures and can be dealt with swiftly, ligation or suture ligation should be performed. If interventional radiology expertise is available in a hybrid theatre facility, deep arterial bleeds are best managed by immediate angioembolization as an adjunct to packing (26). In facilities where radiological intervention is not available, surgical arterial ligation may be the only option for controlling major life-threatening arterial bleeding. If arterial bleeding is localized to a hemi-liver, selective ligation of the right or left hepatic artery distal to the hepatic artery bifurcation is preferred. With extensive bilateral injuries or an inability to separately identify the right or left hepatic arteries, non-selective ligation of the common hepatic artery may be indicated. With intact portal vein inflow hepatic ischaemia is unlikely, but there is a risk of eventual ischaemic biliopathy.

When performing definitive therapeutic packing, extensive mobilization of the liver should be avoided. Dry large gauze packs, usually 6–8, are packed around the superior, anterior, lateral, and inferior surfaces of the liver to restore the shape and anatomical contour and keep raw parenchymal surfaces reapproximated. Packs should not be inserted into fractures and excessive packing, especially too many packs between the diaphragm, should be avoided as it may cause IVC compression, compromising venous outflow and aggravating bleeding from parenchymal veins. Following definitive packing and temporary abdominal wall closure, patients should be sedated and ventilated, and intravenous (IV) antibiotics administered. Re-laparotomy for removal of packs and definitive management of injuries is performed when the deranged physiology of the patient, including acidosis, hypothermia, and coagulopathy have been corrected, usually 24–48 hours following the initial DCS procedure. In severe liver injuries delaying re-laparotomy for 48 hours has been shown to reduce re-bleeding rates with no increase in septic complications or bile leaks (27). If no bleeding occurs after pack removal no further treatment is required and the abdomen is definitively closed following drain placement. Closed suction drains are preferred to address the potential for bile leaks.

The definitive management of liver injuries, where there are exposed raw surfaces of fractures or lacerations, is principally a careful examination to identify bleeding vessels and bile leaks which should be controlled with suture ligation or clips. Thermal coagulation devices such as monopolar or bipolar electrocautery, and argon beam coagulation and topical haemostatic agents are useful adjuncts. In AAST grade I–III injuries reapproximating fractures can be facilitated and maintained by placement of 1.0 absorbable sutures, if needed with Teflon or rectus sheath pledgets. Plugging an injury tract using an inflated urine catheter balloon or a Sengstaken-Blakemore oesophageal balloon may control venous bleeding where the source is not accessible and avoids extensive exploration. Drains, preferably with closed suction, should be used selectively in patients with increased risk of bile leaks.

Liver resection at initial laparotomy is seldom indicated and should be limited to ligating the remaining attachments of a partially avulsed portion of the liver. Following initial DCS, definitive management at re-laparotomy may require removal of ischaemic or necrotic liver tissue which usually entails resectional debridement of devitalized liver tissue along non-anatomical planes (*Figure 24.1*). Previously, mortality rates of over 50% have been reported for major liver resections for trauma (28,29) but more recent studies have shown

improved results especially when involving experienced liver surgeons (30,31).

A substantial proportion of patients with AAST grades IV and V liver injuries still require surgery, either primarily or following failed NOM and overall mortality rates exceed 50% (*Figure 24.2*) (4,32).

Table 24.2 Criteria for damage control surgery

Absolute indications
Transfusion requirements: >10 units packed red cells
Hypothermia: temperature <35 °C
Acidosis: pH <7.2; base deficit >8 mEq/L; lactate <5 mmol/L
Clinical onset of coagulopathy
Relative indications
Complex pattern of injuries
Expected operating time for definitive management of injuries >60–90 min

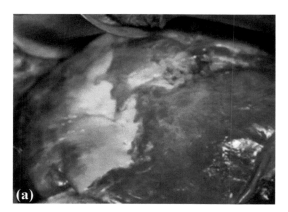

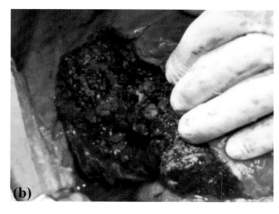

Figure 24.1 Following initial damage (a) control surgery resectional debridement of a devitalized right hemi-liver is performed (b) as definitive treatment at re-laparotomy.

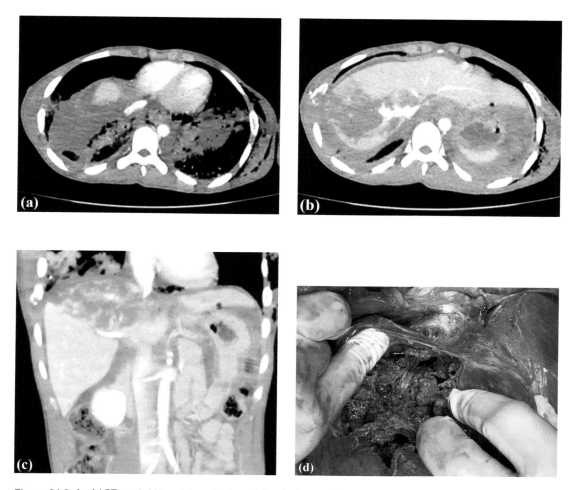

Figure 24.2 An AAST grade V liver injury due to a high velocity gunshot with entrance wound in the mid-axillary line in the 6th intercostal space and exit wound anterolateral on the right fracturing the 6th rib **(a)**. Contrast-enhanced CT shows a complex injury of the IVC/hepatic vein junction **(b)** with contained contrast extravasation and preserved retrohepatic IVC flow **(c)**. The patient was treated non-operatively but became haemodynamically unstable 24 hours later. At laparotomy profuse bleeding from a non-reconstructable IVC/hepatic vein junction was found and the patient demised **(d)**.

Interruption of perihepatic caval flow may be required for injuries of the retrohepatic IVC or central hepatic veins. Total vascular exclusion can be achieved by a Pringle manoeuvre and infra- and suprahepatic control of the IVC. However, the reduced venous return may be poorly tolerated and require veno-venous bypass (33). The use of atrio-caval shunts has been abandoned.

Interventional management

In the pre-DCS and -NOM era, radiological and endoscopic interventions were mostly used for the management of late complications following primary surgical management. In the modern multidisciplinary management of liver trauma, radiological intervention has a central role in the initial treatment of liver trauma (34). In DCS situations where hybrid theatre facilities are available, intraoperative angioembolization can be used for immediate control of arterial bleeding as an adjunct to packing (26). Angioembolization is also the treatment of choice for arterial bleeding following DCS and in patients treated non-operatively with clinical signs of bleeding or contrast extravasation on CECT scans (35–37). Endoscopic treatment for the definitive management of associated biliary injuries in the initial management period has been described, thereby avoiding the need for surgical reconstruction (*Figure 24.3*) (38).

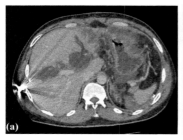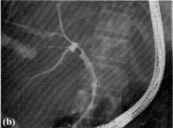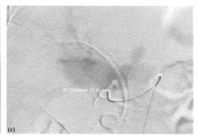

Figure 24.3 An injury of the common hepatic duct with 25 mm substance loss complicated by a porto-biliary fistula following a gunshot injury of the liver initially managed with a damage control laparotomy (a), managed definitively with a bridging fully covered self-expanding metal stent (b). The patient developed haemobilia 48 hours later. Angiography showed a bleeding right hepatic artery false aneurysm, which was managed with placement of a bridging endovascular stent endovascular stent (c).

MANAGEMENT OF COMPLICATIONS

Complications following the treatment of liver injuries occurs in up to 50% of patients and the incidence and severity are directly related to the grade of liver injury (3,39). Between 4% and 23% of patients will have bile leaks following liver trauma (29). Complications related to biliary injuries present as intraperitoneal bile leaks or biliary fistulae although the majority of bile leaks are minor and usually settle with conservative management. Major leaks may require intervention (40). Trans-papillary stenting at endoscopic retrograde cholangiography (ERC) is successful in controlling leaks in most patients, including complicated fistulation such as bilio-portal and thoraco-biliary fistulae (38,41). Bile leaks with large volumes of free bile in the abdomen or signs of peritonitis will require open or laparoscopic drainage and washout of the peritoneum. Localized bile collections and other fluid collections including infected haematomas and abscesses can usually be managed with antibiotics and ultrasound (US)- or CT-guided percutaneous drainage. Bile leaks refractory to conservative or interventional treatment, usually due to disconnected ducts, may require elective liver resection.

Hepatic necrosis may occur in liver segments, devascularized by the actual trauma or as a complication of treatment, including total or selective hepatic artery ligation and angioembolization which may cause necrosis in 15% of patients (42). Whereas limited necrosis can be treated expectantly, resection is indicated with infection or extensive necrosis. Resection is usually performed as non-anatomical debridement of devitalized or necrotic tissue with the planes dictated by the injury. Formal anatomical resections may be indicated in selected patients where the necrosis follows anatomical segmental borders or where repeated debridement procedures are anticipated (43). Delayed bleeding following liver injury is usually due to hepatic artery pseudoaneurysms with the incidence increasing with higher grade liver injures, ranging from 1.8% in AAST grade III to 17.3% in AAST grade V injuries (44). Surveillance for hepatic pseudoaneurysm in high-risk patients with interval CECT scan has been proposed.

PROGNOSIS AND FOLLOW-UP

The prognosis of liver injuries is related to the severity of the injury and associated organ involvement. Over the last three decades there has been a dramatic improvement in survival rates with individualized multimodality treatment of patients in dedicated multidisciplinary units. Treatment has been revolutionized by the refinement of indications based on evolving classifications and procedural improvements in NOM and DCS. Nevertheless, the management of major liver injuries remains challenging with high mortality rates seen in AAST grades IV and V injuries requiring surgery. Long-term follow up of patients for late complications should be individualized and is warranted where there is a risk of late hepatic artery aneurysm formation and in patients at risk of ischaemic biliopathy following arterial angioembolization or ligation.

SUMMARY

The liver is the most commonly injured intra-abdominal organ following trauma. Emphasis on trauma pathophysiology and correction of physiological impairment, better and readily available diagnostic imaging and advances in interventional radiology and endoscopy have revolutionized the treatment of liver trauma over the past three decades. Survival has improved significantly with individualized multimodal treatment of patients in dedicated multidisciplinary units. Selective non-operative management has become the treatment of choice for patients with liver injuries regardless of aetiology. DCS with abbreviated index procedures to control bleeding and definitive management deferred to a subsequent procedure has significantly improved outcomes in severely injured patients with severely deranged physiology. The management of major liver injuries remains challenging with high mortality rates seen in severe injuries requiring surgery.

REFERENCES

1. Clancy TV, Maxwell JG, Covington DL, Brinker CC, Blackman D. A statewide analysis of level I and II trauma centers for patients with major injuries. *J Trauma* 2001;**51(2)**:346–51.
2. Hommes M, Navsaria PH, Schipper IB, Krige JE, Kahn D, Nicol AJ. Management of blunt liver trauma in 134 severely injured patients. *Injury* 2015;**46(5)**:837–42.
3. Keizer AA, Arkenbosch JHC, Kong VY, Hoen camp R, Bruce JL, Smith MTD, et al. Blunt and penetrating liver trauma have similar outcomes in the modern era. *Scand J Surg* 2021;**110(2)**:208–13.
4. Gaski IA, Skattum J, Brooks A, Koyama T, Eken T, Naess PA, et al. Decreased mortality, laparotomy, and embolization rates for liver injuries during a 13-year period in a major Scandinavian trauma center. *Trauma Surg Acute Care Open* 2018;**3(1)**:e000205.
5. Michels NA. Newer anatomy of the liver and its variant blood supply and collateral circulation. *Am J Surg* 1966;**112(3)**:337–47.
6. Wong YC, Wang LJ, Wu CH, Chen HW, Fu CJ, Yuan KC, et al. Detection and characterization of traumatic bile leaks using Gd-EOB-DTPA enhanced magnetic resonance cholangiography. *Sci Rep* 2018;**8(1)**:14612.
7. Lacobellis F, Scaglione M, Brillantino A, Scuderi MG, Giurazza F, Grassi R, et al. The additional value of the arterial phase in the CT assessment of liver vascular injuries after high-energy blunt trauma. *Emerg Radiol* 2019;**26(6)**:647–54.
8. Moore EE, Shackford SR, Pachter HL, McAninch JW, Browner BD, Champion HR, et al. Organ injury scaling: Spleen, liver, and kidney. *J Trauma* 1989;**29(12)**:1664–6.
9. Kozar RA, Crandall M, Shanmuganathan K, Zarzaur BL, Coburn M, Cribari C, et al. Organ injury scaling 2018 update: Spleen, liver, and kidney. *J Trauma Acute Care Surg* 2018;**85(6)**:1119–22.
10. Trauma ACoSCo. *Advanced Trauma Life Support: Student Course Manual*, 10th edition. Chicago, IL: American College of Surgeons; 2018.
11. Boffard KD (ed). *Manual of Definitive Surgical Trauma Care: Incorporating Definitive Anaesthetic Trauma Care*, 10th edition, CRC Press; 2019.
12. Holcomb JB, Tilley BC, Baraniuk S, Fox EE, Wade CE, Podbielski JM, et al. Transfusion of plasma, platelets, and red blood cells in a 1:1:1 vs a 1:1:2 ratio and mortality in patients with severe trauma: The PROPPR randomized clinical trial. *JAMA* 2015;**313(5)**:471–82.
13. Moore EE, Moore HB, Chapman MP, Gonzalez E, Sauaia A. Goal-directed hemostatic resuscitation for trauma induced coagulopathy: Maintaining homeostasis. J Trauma Acute Care Surg 2018;84(6S Suppl 1):S35–S40.
14. Hinton JW. Injuries to the abdominal viscera: Their relative frequency and their management. *Ann Surg* 1929;**90(3)**:351–6.
15. Hasselgren PO, Almersjo O, Gustavsson B, Seeman T. Trauma to the liver during a ten-year period. With special reference to morbidity and mortality after blunt trauma and stab wounds. *Acta Chir Scand* 1981;**147(6)**:387–93.
16. Carmona RH, Lim RC Jr., Clark GC. Morbidity and mortality in hepatic trauma. A 5-year study. *Am J Surg* 1982;**144(1)**:88–94.
17. Cywes S, Rode H, Millar AJ. Blunt liver trauma in children: Nonoperative management. *J Pediatr Surg* 1985;**20(1)**:14–18.
18. Oldham KT, Guice KS, Ryckman F, Kaufman RA, Martin LW, Noseworthy J. Blunt liver injury in childhood: Evolution of therapy and current perspective. *Surgery* 1986;**100(3)**:542–9.
19. Farnell MB, Spencer MP, Thompson E, Williams HJ, Jr., Mucha P, Jr., Ilstrup DM. Nonoperative management of blunt hepatic trauma in adults. *Surgery* 1988;**104(4)**:748–56.
20. MacGoey P, Navarro A, Beckingham IJ, Cameron IC, Brooks AJ. Selective non-operative management of penetrating liver injuries at a UK tertiary referral centre. *Ann R Coll Surg Engl* 2014;**96(6)**:423–6.
21. Navsaria P, Nicol A, Krige J, Edu S, Chowdhury S. Selective nonoperative management of liver gunshot injuries. *Eur J Trauma Emerg Surg* 2019;**45(2)**:323–8.
22. Brooks A, Reilly JJ, Hope C, Navarro A, Naess PA, Gaarder C. Evolution of non-operative management of liver trauma. *Trauma Surg Acute Care Open* 2020;**5(1)**:e000551.
23. Yoong S, Kothari R, Brooks A. Assessment of sensitivity of whole body CT for major trauma. *Eur J Trauma Emerg Surg* 2019;**45(3)**:489–92.
24. Melloul E, Denys A, Demartines N. Management of severe blunt hepatic injury in the era of computed tomography and transarterial embolization: A systematic review and critical appraisal of the literature. *J Trauma Acute Care Surg* 2015;**79(3)**:468–74.
25. Boese CK, Hackl M, Muller LP, Ruchholtz S, Frink M, Lechler P. Nonoperative management of blunt hepatic trauma: A systematic review. *J Trauma Acute Care Surg* 2015;**79(4)**:654–60.
26. Johnson JW, Gracias VH, Gupta R, Guillamondegui O, Reilly PM, Shapiro MB, et al. Hepatic angiography in patients undergoing damage control laparotomy. *J Trauma* 2002;**52(6)**:1102–6.
27. Nicol AJ, Hommes M, Primrose R, Navsaria PH, Krige JE. Packing for control of hemorrhage in major liver trauma. *World J Surg* 2007;**31(3)**:569–74.
28. Beal SL. Fatal hepatic hemorrhage: An unresolved problem in the management of complex liver injuries. *J Trauma* 1990;**30(2)**:163–9.
29. Cogbill TH, Moore EE, Jurkovich GJ, Feliciano DV, Morris JA, Mucha P. Severe hepatic trauma: A multi-center experience with 1,335 liver injuries. *J Trauma* 1988;**28(10)**:1433–8.

30. Strong RW, Lynch SV, Wall DR, Liu CL. Anatomic resection for severe liver trauma. *Surgery* 1998;**123**(3):251–7.

31. Tsugawa K, Koyanagi N, Hashizume M, Ayukawa K, Wada H, Tomikawa M, et al. Anatomic resection for severe blunt liver trauma in 100 patients: Significant differences between young and elderly. *World J Surg* 2002;**26**(5):544–9; discussion 9.

32. van der Wilden GM, Velmahos GC, Emhoff T, Brancato S, Adams C, Georgakis G, et al. Successful nonoperative management of the most severe blunt liver injuries: A multicenter study of the research consortium of new England centers for trauma. *Arch Surg* 2012;**147**(5):423–8.

33. Baumgartner F, Scudamore C, Nair C, Karusseit O, Hemming A. Venovenous bypass for major hepatic and caval trauma. *J Trauma* 1995;**39**(4):671–3.

34. Cadili A, Gates J. The role of angioembolization in hepatic trauma. *Am Surg* 2021;**87**(11):1793–801.

35. Asensio JA, Roldan G, Petrone P, Rojo E, Tillou A, Kuncir E, et al. Operative management and outcomes in 103 AAST-OIS grades IV and V complex hepatic injuries: Trauma surgeons still need to operate, but angioembolization helps. *J Trauma* 2003;**54**(4):647–53;discussion 53–4.

36. Matsushima K, Hogen R, Piccinini A, Biswas S, Khor D, Delapena S, et al. Adjunctive use of hepatic angioembolization following hemorrhage control laparotomy. *J Trauma Acute Care Surg* 2020;**88**(5):636–43.

37. Virdis F, Reccia I, Di Saverio S, Tugnoli G, Kwan SH, Kumar J, et al. Clinical outcomes of primary arterial embolization in severe hepatic trauma: A systematic review. *Diagn Interv Imaging* 2019;**100**(2):65–75.

38. Lindemann J, Kloppers C, Burmeister S, Bernon M, Jonas E. Mind the gap! Extraluminal percutaneous-endoscopic rendezvous with a self-expanding metal stent for restoring continuity in major bile duct injury: A case series. *Int J Surg Case Rep* 2019;**60**:340–4.

39. Kozar RA, Moore FA, Cothren CC, Moore EE, Sena M, Bulger EM, et al. Risk factors for hepatic morbidity following nonoperative management: Multicenter study. *Arch Surg* 2006;**141**(5):451–8; discussion 8–9.

40. Hommes M, Kazemier G, Schep NW, Kuipers EJ, Schipper IB. Management of biliary complications following damage control surgery for liver trauma. *Eur J Trauma Emerg Surg* 2013;**39**(5):511–16.

41. Burmeister S, Krige JE, Bornman PC, Nicol AJ, Navsaria P. Endoscopic treatment of persistent thoracobiliary fistulae after penetrating liver trauma. *HPB (Oxford)* 2009;**11**(2):171–5.

42. Green CS, Bulger EM, Kwan SW. Outcomes and complications of angioembolization for hepatic trauma: A systematic review of the literature. *J Trauma Acute Care Surg* 2016;**80**(3):529–37.

43. Dabbs DN, Stein DM, Philosophe B, Scalea TM. Treatment of major hepatic necrosis: Lobectomy versus serial debridement. *J Trauma* 2010;**69**(3):562–7.

44. Wagner ML, Streit S, Makley AT, Pritts TA, Goodman MD. Hepatic Pseudoaneurysm incidence after liver trauma. *J Surg Res* 2020;**256**:623–8.

Chapter 25

Pancreas Trauma

Martin D. Smith and John W. S. Devar

INTRODUCTION

Trauma is an international public health issue. It represents a significant financial and resource burden on healthcare systems and is one of the leading causes of injury, disability and death. Global deaths from trauma far exceed all other causes in working age individuals. Annually, almost 6 million people die from accidental and violent injuries, 40 million people are permanently injured and almost 100 million suffer an injury from which they recover. In 2022 there were 67.1 million deaths worldwide with trauma responsible for about 8–9% exceeding those from infectious diseases including malaria (619 000), tuberculosis (1.6 million), HIV/AIDS (630 000) and COVID-19 (up to 3 million over the period of the pandemic).

The injury severity score (ISS) is an anatomical system that provides an overall score for patients with multiple injuries. Each injury is assigned an abbreviated injury code (AIS) score and is allocated to one of six body regions. The highest AIS score in each body region is used and major trauma is defined as an ISS of 15 or greater (*Table 25.1*).

Following major trauma, serious injuries to the liver, spleen, pancreas, biliary tract and duodenum are responsible for significant morbidity and mortality. With blunt abdominal trauma, injuries are more likely to affect solid organs (liver and spleen being the most common) and pancreatic involvement is unusual. However, when pancreatic injuries are present, due to its relatively protected retroperitoneal position, injury to other organs is likely. In a Scottish population study the incidence of pancreatic trauma was recorded at 0.21% of over 52 000 trauma patients (1–3) and injury to the pancreas occurs in less than 10% of all abdominal injuries. Penetrating injuries are more common in regions with a high prevalence of gunshot wounds, such as North America and South Africa, but in most other regions blunt abdominal trauma is the predominant aetiology. Immediate and early mortality from pancreatic trauma is usually related to major concomitant vascular involvement and injury to other abdominal organs, whereas late morbidity and mortality follow complications of pancreatic parenchymal and ductal injuries. The management of a pancreatic injury depends on the status of the main pancreatic duct, the degree of parenchymal damage, and the anatomical location of the injury.

Selecting the appropriate management strategy requires a detailed understanding of pancreatic anatomy, the nature of the injury (blunt or penetrating) and any associated damage to other organs. This chapter will describe the present evidence relating to pancreas trauma, guidelines and selection of non-operative and surgical approaches.

SURGICAL ANATOMY

The pancreas lies behind the lesser sac and posterior and inferior to the stomach (*Figure 25.1*). The first three parts of the duodenum are inseparable from the head of the pancreas (HOP) and share a common blood supply via the superior and inferior pancreaticoduodenal arteries. The distal end of the common bile duct (CBD) courses through the HOP and appreciating its involvement in an injury to the HOP is essential when planning a surgical approach. The tail of the pancreas is intimately related to the hilum of the spleen and posteriorly to the left kidney.

The pancreas can be divided anatomically into three distinct 'zones' based on intrinsic and extrinsic landmarks – head, body and tail. The appreciation of these zones is important to enable use of the available grading systems and decide on management of injuries based on their location. The main pancreatic duct runs the length of the pancreas and joins with the CBD at the ampulla of Vater (the papilla duodeni or ampulla 'of Vater', or papilla 'of Santorini' is named after Abraham Vater [1684–1751] a botanist and professor of medicine in Wittenberg who was responsible for an important collection of anatomical preparations). Its position in the pancreas is variable, and while it often lies more posteriorly, this is not consistent. The parenchyma of the pancreas is soft with the main duct usually being less than 3 mm. The ductal system has a 'fish bone' appearance with multiple small side branch ducts. Injuries to the main pancreatic duct do not usually

Table 25.1 Abbreviated injury score

AIS Score	Injury	AIS % probability of death
1	Minor	0
2	Moderate	1–2
3	Serious	8–10
4	Severe	5–50
5	Critical	3–50
6	Maximum	100
9	Not specified	

DOI: 10.1201/9781003080060-25

settle spontaneously and will require an intervention, but damage to side branch ducts often heal spontaneously. Understanding the ductal anatomy and the different approaches needed allows interpretation of the various grading systems and facilitates logical operative decisions.

The inferior border of the pancreas gives rise to the mesentery of the transverse colon and contains the middle colic veins that enter the superior mesenteric vein (SMV) below the entry of the splenic vein. Inferiorly the body on the pancreas is very close to the duodeno-jejunal junction at the ligament of Trietz (Václav Treitz, 1819–1872, was born in Hostomice, Bohemia and in 1851 accepted an appointment as a Prosector at the Jagellonian University in Krakow, publishing his first major paper in which he described the suspensory duodenal ligament that still bears his name almost 200 years later). The 4th part of the duodenum travels slightly superiorly at this point and is in close proximity to the junction of the neck and body of the pancreas.

Posteriorly, the head and neck of the pancreas are closely related to the inferior vena cava (IVC) and the aorta. Retroperitoneal haematomas, particularly in penetrating injuries, may be associated with concomitant vascular injuries including the IVC and the aorta. Together with the rest of the complex vascular anatomy of the pancreas, this explains why there is such a high mortality rate when the pancreatic injury involves adjacent structures (*Figure 25.1*).

The blood supply to the pancreas is complex and arises predominantly from the coeliac axis via the hepatic artery. The two main branches are the gastroduodenal artery (GDA), and the splenic artery which has multiple pancreatic branches. The superior mesenteric artery (SMA) gives rise to the inferior pancreaticoduodenal (PD) artery. An accessory right hepatic artery (HA) may arise from the SMA and usually runs behind to the HOP towards the right lateral aspect of the porta hepatis. This complex vascular arrangement means that pancreatic ischaemia is only rarely a significant issue following a pancreatic injury but that controlling bleeding from the pancreas can be challenging.

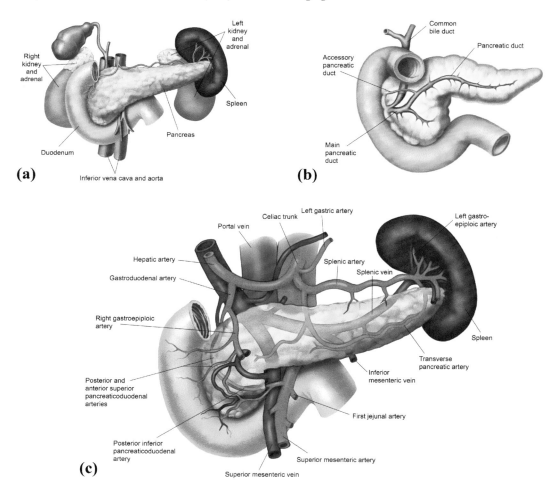

Figure 25.1 Anatomical illustrations showing the location of the pancreas and its relationship to other organs (a). Pancreatic and bile duct anatomy (b) and relevant vascular structures (c).

INCIDENCE AND MECHANISM OF PANCREATIC TRAUMA

Pancreatic injuries are rare, occurring in approximately 0.4% of trauma patients, but can be devastating. The pancreas is more likely to be involved with blunt abdominal trauma, occurring in 5–12% of such injuries compared with 2% of penetrating injuries.

Penetrating traumas, caused by stab or gunshot wounds are usually associated with other injuries which determine the presentation (*Table 25.2*) (4,5).

Blunt trauma to the pancreas occurs following road traffic, bicycle and pedestrian accidents and direct blows to the epigastrium during assaults. The mechanism is a consequence of the anatomical relationship to the spine as the soft pancreas is crushed against unyielding bony vertebrae.

PRESENTATION AND DIAGNOSIS

With penetrating trauma, the presentation is generally due to the consequence of an injury to another organ or from pancreatic bleeding. Following blunt trauma, the nature and extent are much more difficult to diagnose.

Table 25.2 Associated abdominal and extra-abdominal injuries after Petrone et al. (4)

Abdominal injuries	n	%
Liver	1899	20.9
Stomach	1564	17.2
Major vascular injury	1305	14.3
Spleen	1094	12
Urological	803	8.8
Colon	791	8.7
Duodenum	773	8.5
Small bowel	553	6
Gallbladder and biliary tract	165	1.8
Diaphragm	163	1.8
Total	**9110**	**100**
Extra-abdominal injuries	**n**	**%**
Thorax	234	44.5
Musculoskeletal	138	26.2
Head	92	17.5
Neck and spinal column	57	10.8
Heart	5	1
Total 4559 injuries	**526**	**100**

Often patients, with isolated pancreas injuries from blunt trauma, will present late with the sequelae of a duct injury resulting in fluid collection which becomes symptomatic or causes complications.

In patients who have evidence of peritonitis due to an associated organ injury the diagnosis of a pancreatic injury is frequently only made intraoperatively and 95% of pancreatic injuries can be diagnosed by careful inspection following adequate exposure. The remaining 5% of injuries may require more elaborate intraoperative investigative techniques to identify a ductal injury (6). This can include intraoperative US or endoscopy to identify the injury to the duct although the applicability and accuracy of these approaches has not been validated (6,7).

The next important consideration that determines management is the haemodynamic stability of the patient. Unstable patients, following appropriate resuscitation, will require urgent laparotomy. The stable patient allows time for further investigations and in this group, there remains controversy about the value of the different modalities and the timing and sequence for their use.

Radiological investigations

US or focused assessment with sonography in trauma (FAST), can reveal the presence of free abdominal fluid and provide supportive, albeit indirect evidence, in cases of suspected pancreatic injury. The assessment of the pancreas *per se* is difficult on US due to its retroperitoneal position and the presence of overlying transverse colonic producing a gas fluid interface (8).

Contrast-enhanced computed tomography (CECT) remains the 'gold standard' for radiological investigation in the stable patient with an overall accuracy of >80%. However, in the initial phases of investigations, CECT may miss or underestimate the severity of the injury and normal findings do not exclude an isolated pancreatic injury. CECT findings, associated with pancreatic trauma, include soft signs such as extraperitoneal fluid, fluid in the lesser sac or between the splenic vein and the pancreatic parenchymal space, and hard signs which include pancreatic oedema, peripancreatic haematomas, spinal fracture and thickening of the anterior renal fascia (*Table 25.3*) (9,10).

Morbidity and mortality rates for isolated pancreatic trauma are directly related to the injury to the pancreatic duct and it has been shown that delayed detection of pancreatic duct disruption is related to increased rates of morbidity and mortality. Magnetic resonance cholangiopancreatography (MRCP) and endoscopic retrograde cholangiopancreatography (ERCP) have higher sensitivities (approaching 100%) and are indicated when pancreatic injury with ductal disruption is suspected. MRCP has the advantage

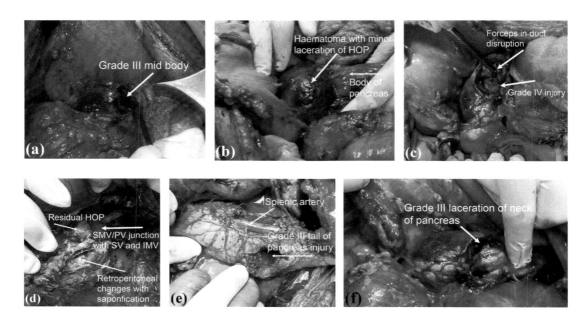

Figure 25.2 Images showing pancreatic trauma injuries with AAST organ injury score where relevant. Gunshot wound to the mid-body, Grade III (a). Haematoma with minor laceration of the HOP (b). Grade IV injury to the HOP (c). Appearance of the retroperitoneum at re-look, 72 hours following a distal pancreatectomy (d). Gunshot to the tail of the pancreas, Grade III injury. Splenic artery exposed (e). Grade III laceration of the neck of the pancreas from a stab wound (f).

Table 25.3 CECT signs of pancreatic trauma

Direct (hard) signs	Indirect (soft) signs	Delayed signs
Fracture of the pancreas	Fluid separating the splenic vein from posterior aspect	Pancreatic ductal dilatation
Pancreatic laceration	Fluid surrounding the superior mesenteric vessels	Pseudocyst formation/ peripancreatic fluid collection
Focal or diffuse pancreatic enlargement/oedema	Fluid in the anterior and posterior pararenal spaces	
Pancreatic haematoma	Fluid in transverse mesocolon and lesser sac	
Active bleeding/extravasation of intravenous contrast	Inflammatory changes in peripancreatic fat and mesentery	
	Thickening of the left anterior renal fascia	

of being non-invasive and is the first choice in a stable patient when trying to confirm an injury to the main pancreatic duct. Intra-parenchymal haematoma may cause duct compression showing as loss of duct on imaging and can be difficult to differentiate from ductal loss or disruption. Confirmation of a true duct disruption may require ERCP which will reveal contrast extravasation from the injury site if there is a significant side- or main-duct injury (*Table 25.4*).

Historically, peritoneal lavage (DPL) was the diagnostic method of choice but several cases of complete transection with normal lavage findings have been

described and recent evidence confirmed that it is not a reliable method and should no longer be used (11,12). The elevation of amylase in either serum or DPL fluid is not sufficiently sensitive or specific in the diagnosis of pancreatic injury (13,14) and it is also important to note that raised serum amylase is not a reliable indicator of pancreatic injury when associated with a head injury as elevations of both *serum amylase* and *lipase* have been observed in trauma patients with *intracranial* bleeding (15). Nevertheless, an elevated amylase in serum or peritoneal lavage fluid in the setting of blunt abdominal trauma does mandate further investigation. People

Table 25.4 Frey and Wardell classification of pancreatic injuries

Grade and location of injury	Description of the injury
Pancreas	
Class I (P_1)	Capsular damage, minor parenchymal damage
Class II (P_2)	Partial/complete duct transection in the body/tail
Class III (P_3)	Major duct injury involving the head of pancreas or the intrapancreatic common bile duct
Duodenum	
Class I (D_1)	Contusion, haematoma or partial thickness injury
Class II (D_2)	Full thickness duodenal injury
Class III (D_3)	Full thickness injury with >75% circumference injury or injury to the extrahepatic common bile duct
Combined pancreas and duodenum	
Type 1	P_1D_1, P_2D_1, D_2P_1
Type 2	D_2P_2
Type 3	D_3P_{1-2}, P_3D_{1-2}
Type 4	D_3P_3

by addressing the key issues of parenchymal disruption and major pancreatic duct status in more severe injuries through focusing on anatomical location, see *Figure 25.2a–f*. There are similarities between these three scoring systems, but their differences create problems when attempting to compare outcomes of studies that use differing systems. In clinical practice, the AAST remains the most commonly used system (*Tables 25.4–25.6*) (17).

LOCATING THE PANCREATIC INJURY

When a laparotomy is required, a midline incision is the optimal approach providing adequate exposure to all the abdominal viscera, including the pancreas. Once the bleeding and the ongoing contamination are controlled, and if the patient is physiologically stable, the surgeon proceeds to open the lesser sac to identify signs suggesting a pancreatic injury (*Table 25.3*). There are a number of findings which will indicate a significant injury including a fluid collection in the lesser sac,

Table 25.5 Lucas classification of pancreatic injuries

Grade	Description of injury
1	Superficial contusion with minimal damage
2	Deep laceration or transection of the left portion of the pancreas
3	Injury of the pancreatic head

with a reliable history, lack of significant clinical signs and elevated serum amylase should be observed and undergo repeated amylase measurements. Persistent elevation or the development of abdominal signs necessitate further evaluation by other methods such as abdominal CECT, ERCP or surgical exploration (16).

Patients with hyperamylasaemia, persistent abdominal pain and questionable CECT findings, who are being considered for non-operative management, should have the integrity of the duct system demonstrated. MRCP remains the investigation of choice in these patients and ERCP may be of value in cases with delayed presentation or injuries missed by CECT. ERCP has a very high-sensitivity and can also be therapeutic when duct disruption is demonstrated enabling the insertion of a pancreatic stent to facilitate drainage.

GRADING OF PANCREATIC INJURIES

The Frey and Wardell, the Lucas Score and American Association for the Surgery of Trauma Committee on Organ Injury Scale (AAST), are grading systems used in pancreatic trauma. All three systems guide management

Table 25.6 AAST organ injury scoring for pancreatic trauma

Grade		Description of the Injury
I	Haematoma	Major contusion without ductal injury or tissue loss
	Laceration	Major laceration without ductal injury or tissue loss
II	Haematoma	Contusion involving >1 portion of the pancreas
	Laceration	Disruption <50% of circumference
III	Laceration	Parenchymal injury with major pancreatic duct injury or distal transection
IV	Laceration	Major pancreatic duct injury right of SMV (proximal pancreatic transection)
V	Laceration	Massive disruption of the pancreatic head

Abbreviations: AAST: Association for the Surgery of Trauma; SMV: superior mesenteric vein.

Table 25.7 Suggested ERCP grading of pancreatic trauma after Takishima et al. (14)

Classification	Description of ERCP findings
1	Normal ERCP finding
2a	Contrast leak from side branch but is contained within the pancreas parenchyma
2b	Contrast leak from side branch to retroperitoneal space
3a	Main pancreatic duct injury in pancreas body or tail
3b	Main pancreatic duct injury in the pancreas head

bile staining of retroperitoneal tissues, the presence of fat necrosis involving the omentum or in the retroperitoneum, or a haematoma overlying the pancreas (18). In penetrating trauma, the surgeon should attempt to predict and follow the trajectory of the injury throughout its length. Contusions and lacerations constitute the majority of pancreatic injuries, and should be treated with haemostasis and drainage.

The most important factor predicting outcome is the presence, or absence of a main pancreatic duct (MPD) injury. ERCP can define and grade ductal injuries very precisely, but in the acute situation and especially with penetrating trauma, there is no place for the evaluation of the injury radiologically or by ERCP (*Table 25.7*).

Intraoperative observation is the main method used to detect ductal damage, and is based on the intraoperative criteria described in 1976 by Heitsch et al. and which remain valuable today (19). These include, direct visualization of duct damage, complete transection of the pancreas, laceration of more than half the diameter of the pancreas, central perforation and severe maceration of the gland. To identify these criteria, the injured area must be fully mobilized and more recent techniques using intraductal US have been reported but there is limited evidence supporting its routine use (7).

MOBILIZATION OF THE HEAD OF THE PANCREAS

Intraoperative evaluation of the head of pancreas must include an assessment of the integrity of the MPD, the presence of a devitalized pancreatic head or duodenum, the extent of any associated duodenal injury, the integrity of the ampulla and bile duct and whether there is a concomitant vascular injury.

Exposure of the head of the pancreas is achieved by mobilizing the hepatic flexure of the colon. The assistant retracts the colic flexure and the proximal

colon caudally thereby visualizing the second part of the duodenum and gentle left and upward traction of the duodenal loop allows a Kocher manoeuvre to be performed. Full mobilization using electrocautery or an energy device separates the duodenum from Gerota's fascia and the dissection is extended medially until the infra-hepatic IVC and the left renal vein are exposed. The dissection continues until the SMV is seen crossing the third part of the duodenum. Care must be taken during this manoeuvre as excessive upward traction of the duodenum and pancreas may tear the superior mesenteric vein. The cranial extent of the mobilization ends when the foramen of Winslow is identified and/or when the lateral aspect of the common bile duct is identified. Following this Kocherization it should be possible to palpate the aorta behind the pancreas and visualize the anterior and posterior aspects of the second and third part of the duodenum, as well as the head and uncinate process of the pancreas (20).

MOBILIZATION OF THE BODY AND TAIL OF THE PANCREAS

The entire lesser sac should be opened, including the inferior short gastric vessels. This is achieved by detaching the greater omentum from the transverse colon along the bloodless plane (this is also described as a ligament, veil, or the bloodless fold of Treves after the English surgeon Sir Frederick Treves who is also credited with performing the first appendicectomy in Britain). Despite the bloodless plane moniker, the ileocecal fold often contains a number of small vessels and when the greater omentum and the transverse mesocolon are adherent, it can be difficult to separate them without risking injury to the transverse colon and its mesentery. In this case, lift the stomach by grasping the anterior surface with the right hand and break the lesser omentum with a finger fracture using the left hand, making sure that the vasculature of the lesser curvature of the stomach is preserved. Then the whole left hand is inserted along the back of the stomach, fingers pointing caudally, and by moving the whole palm in a transverse and caudal plane one will open the left-lateral lesser sac by separating the greater omentum from the transverse mesocolon. The lesser sac can also be entered by using an energy device or serially applied artery forceps outside the vascular arcade of the greater curvature of the stomach (20).

Mobilization is continued to the left and laterally if there is any suspicion of a distal tail injury near the hilum of the spleen. The phrenocolic, splenocolic, splenorenal and gastrosplenic ligaments are incised and the spleen mobilized by rotating it medially and lifting it upwards into the incision, being careful not to damage the short gastric arteries. This will allow inspection of the anterior, as well as the posterior, aspects of the tail of the pancreas. The same manoeuvre can be used to visualize the body and the tail, but because it requires significant mobilization of the spleen and the pancreas from the retroperitoneal space, it can lead to bleeding, especially in the coagulopathic patient.

An alternative approach to visualizing the body of the pancreas is by incising the avascular peritoneal attachment of the transverse mesocolon to the pancreas and exposing the inferior border of the pancreas. This is done by sharp dissection and as the peritoneum is divided, a few millimetres of retroperitoneal fat will bulge at the line of division between the lower border of the pancreas and incised mesocolon. The incision is extended as far laterally as possible towards the spleen. The pancreas should be mobilized anteriorly by inserting the right index and middle finger, in the retroperitoneal space behind the pancreas until they reach the superior border of the pancreas and the peritoneum exposed along the superior border of the pancreas is then incised. This plane, posterior to the body of the pancreas and tail, is avascular and limited bleeding occurs. The splenic artery, however, runs along the superior border of the pancreas and when the peritoneum along the superior border of the pancreas is divided, care should be taken not to inadvertently injure it. The pancreas will now be sufficiently mobilized to be allow cephalad rotation, inspection of the posterior surface and bimanual palpation.

DISTAL PANCREATECTOMY

The indication to perform a distal pancreatectomy is guided by the grading system (*Tables 25.4–25.6*). If the injury requires a distal pancreatectomy, the first step should be to ligate the splenic artery and vein to decrease the possibility of extensive bleeding during the resection. Ligation of both vessels, about 2 cm to the right of the injury site, is performed so that they are not damaged during the transection of the parenchyma. Mobilization of the proximal pancreas should also be performed to 2 cm to the right of the site of the proposed transection. Most surgeons use electrocautery for parenchymal transection but a soft bowel clamp can be applied to the proximal pancreas and the gland divided with a scalpel or a stapler can be used. The superior and inferior pancreatic arteries are under-run with an absorbable monofilament 5-0 suture with care being taken to ensure that the stitch is applied as close as possible to the vessel and care is taken to apply just sufficient tension to ensure that the parenchyma of the pancreas is not damaged.

Identification of a small main pancreatic duct can be difficult, but it is usually possible. Historically, a number of authors preferred transecting the pancreas with a blade as the use of electrocautery was believed to make identification of the opening of the duct against the background of the cauterized, coagulated pancreatic parenchyma difficult. Practice has changed over the last decade and the majority of surgeons now transect the pancreas with an energy device. The cut-surface is

closed using a non-absorbable 5-0 suture using a figure-of-eight suture. Different techniques described to achieve closure of the pancreatic stump all aim to control bleeding and reduce the incidence of leaks from pancreatic ducts by compressing them within the pancreatic tissue. Applying a figure-of-eight suture, separately to the main pancreatic duct, can lessen the risk of fistula formation. The pancreatic stump should be closed by inserting overlapping interrupted mattress sutures of polypropylene or silk (20).

Linear stapling devices when available may be used with graded closure and tension slowly applied to thin down the parenchyma, prior to stapling. Care should be taken not to fracture the parenchyma and lacerate the duct. There is no difference in pancreatic leak rates between stapled and handsewn methods (21).

The use of drains after a distal pancreatectomy remains controversial, but in the trauma scenario and particularly if damage control surgery is not implemented, we recommend their use.

The distal pancreas should be removed together with the spleen if the patient is haemodynamically unstable. If the patient is physiologically stable, which is often the case with isolated pancreatic injuries, an attempt can be made to preserve the spleen. This does mean additional time to identify and dissect the small perforating vessels originating from splenic vasculature on the posterior surface of the pancreas. As a rule, we do not attempt splenic preservation when performing a distal pancreatectomy for trauma in adults.

PANCREATICODUODENECTOMY

Pancreaticoduodenectomy (PD) is rarely done as the initial procedure in trauma patients, however, where there is massive tissue destruction with injuries involving the pancreas, duodenum and common bile duct it can be unavoidable and in fact much of the dissection will have effectively already been done by the forces applied when the injury occurred. The overall physiological status of the patient and the extent of damage will be the determining factors when deciding whether this is the appropriate management. Generally, however, more patients are salvaged by drainage, total parenteral nutrition and meticulous overall care than by an emergency pancreaticoduodenectomy in a desperately unwell and unstable patient.

If a PD is inevitable it should, where possible, be performed as a two-stage procedure (22–25). The initial damage-control operation should aim to achieve haemostasis, control or repair gastric and jejunum perforations, oversew or staple off the pancreatic stump and ligate or drain the bile duct. The anastomoses are completed at reoperation within the next 48 hours, when the patient is stable and the damage has had time to fully mature and can be properly assessed (26).

When performing a PD for trauma it is not necessary to remove the uncinate process which simplifies the procedure, as the surgeon can operate away from the SMV. It is also not necessary to remove the gallbladder and it can be used as a component of a biliary-enteric reconstruction when the common bile duct is compromised (26). There is controversy regarding the management of the pancreatic stump after PD largely because a soft, normal pancreas with a small pancreatic duct is found in the vast majority of trauma cases. This combination is recognized to increase the technical difficulty and consequently the incidence of complications. In an attempt to abrogate this increased rate of complications, a number of different approaches have been suggested including ligation of the pancreatic duct and a pancreaticoenteric or pancreaticogastric anastomosis. Although ligation of the pancreatic duct in the non-trauma situation has been associated with a significantly higher fistula rate when compared with performing an anastomosis, the mortality rate is the same (27,28). The experience and data following trauma is limited, and pancreatic duct ligation following a trauma PD has been advocated as a valuable technique when faced with an unstable patient unable to tolerate more complex or lengthy surgery (29). The theoretical long-term risks of beta-cell depletion and eventual insufficiency among young trauma patients are disputed (29). A comparison of pancreaticoenteric and pancreaticogastric anastomosis however, has suggested that the latter is associated with fewer complications (30), but it has not been compared with other more recent conventional techniques which have demonstrated a reducing incidence of pancreatic fistula and related mortality following elective pancreaticojejunostomy (27,28). Total pancreatectomy has also been advocated to remove any potential complications related to a pancreatic anastomosis but can result in unstable diabetes and hypoglycaemic unawareness.

COMPLICATIONS

Sepsis and multiple organ failure, usually due to complications from concomitant abdominal injuries, cause 30% of deaths following pancreatic trauma (31). The most common complication after surgical treatment for pancreatic trauma is a pancreatic fistula (32). Most fistulae resolve spontaneously within 1–2 weeks after injury, provided adequate external drainage and nutritional support have been established. Fistulae secondary to major disruption of the pancreatic duct can generally be treated endoscopically (stenting or sealing of the damaged portion of the duct) and when this is not successful a distal pancreatectomy is recommended for fistulae of the neck, body and tail, and a Roux-en-Y loop to the head of the pancreas for fistulae of the head of the gland.

The incidence of abscess formation after pancreatic trauma ranges from 10–25% depending on the number and nature of any associated injuries (17). Endoscopic US or percutaneous drainage should be performed as early as possible and subhepatic/subphrenic fluid collections dealt with by percutaneous drainage under US or CECT guidance.

Secondary haemorrhage is often from the pancreatic bed or the surrounding vessels as a result of an infected retroperitoneal collection. First-line management is angiographic embolization. Laparotomy is only considered if this fails or the patient becomes rapidly and irreversibly unstable. A laparotomy, when the bleeding vessel is identified, should be under-run or suture-ligated but if this is not possible, due to the condition of the vessel or the presence of a significant coagulopathy, temporary control with abdominal packs may be necessary until the patient is again stable (25).

Pseudocyst formation resulting from pancreatic trauma can present weeks or months following the original injury (33). The major determinant of outcome and indicator of preferred treatment is the status of the pancreatic duct. If the pancreatic duct is intact and this has been confirmed by ERCP or MRCP, percutaneous aspiration or pigtail drainage is sufficient in the majority of cases (32,34,35). If investigations show disruption of the duct, this can lead to a chronic fistula and endoscopic drainage with an apposing wall stent, endoscopic stenting, internal surgical drainage or, in selected cases, a central or distal pancreatectomy will be required (36,37).

Mild pancreatitis presenting with transient abdominal pain and raised serum amylase occurs in up to 18% of people who have undergone surgery for pancreatic trauma (38–40) but resolves spontaneously with conservative management.

Endocrine and exocrine insufficiencies are very unusual after resections for pancreatic trauma (41) and the remaining pancreatic tissue is generally sufficient, as in the great majority of cases it was healthy prior to the injury. It must however be remembered that patients undergoing splenectomy are at risk of developing overwhelming post-splenectomy sepsis syndrome and need to be vaccinated against encapsulated bacterial pathogens, pneumococcal, meningococcal and *Haemophilus influenzae* (type b). This should be administered at least 2 weeks following surgery.

SUMMARY

Pancreatic trauma is uncommon and usually associated with other intra-abdominal injuries. It can occur following either blunt or penetrating trauma. The well-known resident's mantra, 'Eat when you can, sleep when you can, and don't mess with the pancreas' certainly holds true for pancreatic trauma. The evaluation of the patient requires a good knowledge of the mechanism of injury. The initial management focuses on the haemodynamic status of the patient. In unstable patients or those with clear indications for surgery, no further investigations are needed. In the stable patient with equivocal clinical signs, further investigations are required usually with US and CECT scan. In penetrating trauma, the approach to diagnosis and treatment is usually obvious but following blunt trauma, especially with the increased use of conservative management, diagnosis or exclusion of a pancreatic injury in the stable patient is essential.

A knowledge of the anatomy of the pancreas and its surrounding structures is important to guide operative management following trauma and enable the interpretation of established guidelines. Intraoperatively, identifying a main duct injury requires mobilization of the pancreas and the approach and technical aspects vary for the different anatomical regions of the pancreas. Injury to the body and tail usually requires a distal resection with splenectomy, but injuries of the head are best managed by drainage. When resection is necessary it is best performed by experienced pancreatic surgeons, particularly the reconstruction. The outcome is usually determined by concomitant injuries to other organs but postoperative complications require the input of a multidisciplinary team including interventional radiologists and endoscopists. Pancreatic injuries occur as part of a complex scenario but modern approaches to imaging and surgery have significantly improved the outcome for these patients.

REFERENCES

1. Scollay JM, Yip VS, Garden OJ, Parks RW. A population-based study of pancreatic trauma in Scotland. *World J Surg* 2006;**30(12)**:2136–41.
2. World Health Organization. 2010. *Injuries and violence: the facts*. Available from: https://www.who.int/news-room/fact-sheets/detail/injuries-and-violence (Accessed March, 2024).
3. Kuza CM, Hirji SA, Englum BR, Ganapathi AM, Speicher PJ, Scarborough JE. Pancreatic injuries in abdominal trauma in US adults: Analysis of the National Trauma Data Bank on Management, Outcomes, and Predictors of Mortality. *Scand J Surg* 2020;**109(3)**:193–204.
4. Petrone P, Álvarez SM, González Pérez M, Ceballos Esparragón J, Marini CP. Management of pancreatic trauma: A literature review *Science Direct* 2017;**95(3)**;123–30.
5. Krige JE. Pancreatic trauma. In: Nicol AJ, Steyn E (eds). *Handbook of Trauma*, 2nd edition, Oxford University Press, 2004, pp. 250–7.
6. Jurkovich GJ, Carrico CJ. Pancreatic trauma. *Surg Oncol Clin N* 1990;**70(3)**:575–93.
7. Hofmann LJ, Learn PA, Cannon JW. Intraoperative ultrasound to assess for pancreatic duct injuries. *J Trauma Acute Care Surg* 2015;**78(4)**:888–91.
8. McKenney KL. Ultrasound of blunt abdominal trauma. *Radiol Clin North Am* 1999;**37(5)**:879–93.
9. Mullinix AJ, Foley WD. Multidetector computed tomography and blunt thoracoabdominal trauma. *J Comput Assist Tomogr* 2004;**28(Suppl 1)**:S20–7.
10. Patton JH Jr, Fabian TC. Complex pancreatic injuries. *Surg Oncol Clin N* 1996;**76(4)**:783–95.
11. Jones RC. Management of pancreatic trauma. *Ann Surg* 1978;**187(5)**:555–64. Epub 1978/05/01. doi: 10.1097/00000658-197805000-00015. PMID: 646495; PubMed Central PMCID: PMCPMC1396562.
12. Wisner DH, Wold RL, Frey CF. Diagnosis and treatment of pancreatic injuries: An analysis of management principles. *Arch Surg* 1990;**125(9)**:1109–13.
13. Bradley EL 3rd, Young PR Jr, Chang MC, Allen JE, Baker CC, Meredith W, et al. Diagnosis and initial management of blunt pancreatic trauma: Guidelines from a multiinstitutional review. *Ann Surg* 1998;**227(6)**:861–9. Epub 1998/06/24. doi: 10.1097/00000658-199806000-00009. PMID: 9637549; PubMed Central PMCID: PMCPMC1191392.
14. Takishima T, Sugimoto K, Hirata M, Asari Y, Ohwada T, Kakita A. Serum amylase level on admission in the diagnosis of blunt injury to the pancreas: Its significance and limitations. *Ann Surg* 1997;**226(1)**:70–6. Epub 1997/07/01. doi: 10.1097/00000658-199707000-00010. PMID: 9242340; PubMed Central PMCID: PMCPMC1190909.
15. Liu KJ, Atten MJ, Lichtor T, Cho MJ, Hawkins D, Panizales E, et al. Serum amylase and lipase elevation is associated with intracranial events. *Am Surg* 2001;**67(3)**:215–19; discussion 9–20. Epub 2001/03/29. PMID: 11270877.
16. Jurkovich GJ. Duodenum and pancreas. In: Mattox KL, Feliciano DV (eds). *Trauma*. Appleton and Lange, 2005, pp. 573–94.
17. Ho VP, Patel NJ, Bokhari F, Madbak FG, Hambley JE, Yon JR, et al. Management of adult pancreatic injuries: A practice management guideline from the Eastern Association for the Surgery of Trauma. *J Trauma Acute Care Surg* 2017;**82(1)**:185–99.
18. Oláh A, Issekutz A, Haulik L, Makay R. Pancreatic transection from blunt abdominal trauma: Early versus delayed diagnosis and surgical management. *Dig Surg* 2003;**20(5)**:408–14.
19. Heitsch RC, Knutson CO, Fulton RL, Jones CE. Delineation of critical factors in the treatment of pancreatic trauma. *Surgery* 1976;**80(4)**:523–9.
20. Yilmaz TH, Hauer TJ, Smith MD, Degiannis E, Doll D. Operative techniques in pancreatic trauma – A heuristic approach. *Injury* 2013;**44(1)**:153–5.
21. Degiannis E, Glapa M, Loukogeorgakis SP, Smith MD. Management of pancreatic trauma. *Injury* 2008;**39(1)**:21–9.
22. Asensio JA, Petrone P, Roldán G, Kuncir E, Demetriades D. Pancreaticoduodenectomy: A rare procedure for the management of complex pancreaticoduodenal injuries. *J Am Coll Surg* 2003;**197(6)**:937–42.
23. Koniaris LG, Mandal AK, Genuit T, Cameron JL. Two-stage trauma pancreaticoduodenectomy: Delay facilitates anastomotic reconstruction. *J Gastrointest Surg* 2000;**4(4)**:366–9.
24. Krige J, Bornman PC, Terblanche J (eds). *The Role of Pancreatoduodenectomy in the Management of Complex Pancreatic Trauma*. Springer; 1997.

25. Krige JE, Nicol AJ, Navsaria PH, Jones O, Bornman PC. Emergency pancreaticoduodenectomy for complex pancreatic trauma. *HPB Surg* 2005;**7**:104.

26. Hirshberg A, Mattox KL. *Top Knife: The Art and Craft of Trauma Surgery. The Wounded Surgical Soul.* TSM publishing; 2005.

27. Patton JH Jr, Lyden SP, Croce MA, Pritchard FE, Minard G, Kudsk KA, et al. Pancreatic trauma: A simplified management guideline. *J Trauma* 1997;**43**(2): 234–9.

28. Sikora SS, Posner MC. Management of the pancreatic stump following pancreaticoduodenectomy. *Br J Surg* 1995;**82**(12):1590–7.

29. Gentilello LM, Cortes V, Buechter KJ, Gomez GA, Castro M, Zeppa R. Whipple procedure for trauma: Is duct ligation a safe alternative to pancreaticojejunostomy? *J Trauma* 1991;**31**(5):661–7.

30. Morris DM, Ford RS. Pancreaticogastrostomy: Preferred reconstruction for Whipple resection. *J Surg Res* 1993;**54**(2):122–5. Epub 1993/02/01. doi: 10.1006/jsre.1993.1018. PMID: 8479169.

31. Jurkovich GJ. Duodenum and Pancreas. In: Mattox KL, Feliciano DV (eds). *Trauma.* Appleton and Lange, 2005, pp. 709–34.

32. Lin BC, Chen RJ, Fang JF, Hsu YP, Kao YC, Kao JL. Management of blunt major pancreatic injury. *J Trauma* 2004;**56**(4):774–8. Epub 2004/06/10. doi: 10.1097/01.ta.0000087644.90727.df. PMID: 15187740.

33. Bornman PC, Krige JE. *Management Strategies in Pancreatic Trauma. Surgical Emergencies and New Technologies.* University of the Witwatersrand Press Johannesburg; 2006.

34. Jones RC. Management of pancreatic trauma. *Am J Surg* 1985;**150**(6):698–704.

35. Lewis G, Krige JE, Bornman PC, Terblanche J. Traumatic pancreatic pseudocysts. *Br J Surg* 1993;**80**(1): 89–93.

36. Beckingham IJ, Krige JE, Bornman PC, Terblanche J. Endoscopic management of pancreatic pseudocysts. *Br J Surg* 1997;**84**(12):1638–45.

37. Beckingham IJ, Krige JE, Bornman PC, Terblanche J. Long term outcome of endoscopic drainage of pancreatic pseudocysts. *Am J Gastroenterol* 1999;**94**(1): 71–4.

38. Cogbill TH, Moore EE, Morris JA Jr, Hoyt DB, Jurkovich GJ, Mucha P Jr, et al. Distal pancreatectomy for trauma: A multicenter experience. *J Trauma* 1991;**31**(12):1600–6.

39. Moore JB, Moore EE. Changing trends in the management of combined pancreatoduodenal injuries. *World J Surg* 1984;**8**(5):791–7.

40. Stone HH, Fabian TC, Satiani B, Turkleson ML. Experiences in the management of pancreatic trauma. *J Trauma* 1981;**21**(4):257–62. Epub 1981/04/01. doi: 10.1097/00005373-198104000-00001. PMID: 7218391.

41. Degiannis E, Levy RD, Potokar T, Lennox H, Rowse A, Saadia R. Distal pancreatectomy for gunshot injuries of the distal pancreas. *Br J Surg* 1995; **82**(9):1240–2.

Chapter
26
Duodenal Trauma

Leo Lin, Steven C. Stain and Ali Salim

INTRODUCTION

Traumatic duodenal injury is rare but can result in significant morbidity and mortality if not diagnosed and treated promptly. This chapter will review the anatomy and physiology of the duodenum and provide a comprehensive overview of the epidemiology, mechanism, evaluation, and management of traumatic duodenal injuries, including an in-depth discussion of operative and nonoperative approaches. It showcases classic surgical techniques and highlights the recent 'less is more' trend, advocating primary repair with nasogastric tube decompression for even extensive and high-grade injuries. The chapter also aims to clarify the complex decision-making process in managing duodenal trauma based on recent data and societal guidelines and outline the diagnostic algorithm, including operative and nonoperative approaches, and potential complications and long-term outcomes.

Lastly, by examining other management aspects, such as nutrition and associated complications, the chapter intends to demonstrate the importance of a multidisciplinary approach in improving patient outcomes.

ANATOMY AND PHYSIOLOGY

The duodenum is the first portion of the small intestine and is a peritoneal and retroperitoneal organ. Its name is derived from the Latin word *duodeni* or 'twelve each,' referencing its length measuring approximately 12 'fingerbreadths' (20 cm) (1). The duodenum has four anatomical segments. The first portion is superior and primarily intraperitoneal. The second portion runs vertically downward and is entirely retroperitoneal. The bile and pancreatic duct drain into the duodenum at this level via the ampulla of Vater. It is also the most common site for injury (2,3). The third portion runs transversely and posterior to the superior mesenteric vessels. The last portion runs vertically upwards and connects to the jejunum.

The duodenum has a robust arterial circulation, receiving blood from the coeliac trunk and the superior mesenteric artery. The gastroduodenal artery and the superior pancreaticoduodenal artery supply the duodenal bulb, and the inferior pancreaticoduodenal artery supplies the second portion. The superior mesenteric artery supplies the third and fourth portions. Venous drainage is through the superior mesenteric vein, draining into the portal vein.

On average, the duodenum sees about five litres of combined salivary (800 mL), gastric (2500 mL), biliary (1000 mL), and pancreatic (1000 mL) secretion per day (1). Such massive efflux highlights the importance of maintaining duodenal integrity and the challenges in managing traumatic duodenal injuries.

EPIDEMIOLOGY, MECHANISM AND ASSOCIATED INJURIES

Duodenal trauma is infrequent and constitutes only 1–4.7% of all abdominal trauma injuries, with an overall incidence of 0.2–0.6% of all trauma patients (4). Seventy percent of duodenal injuries occur in individuals between 16 and 30 years of age (2). Penetrating mechanisms are the most common cause of duodenal trauma, accounting for 77.7% of cases, whereas blunt mechanisms account for only 22.3%. Most blunt injuries are due to high-speed motor vehicle collisions (85%). Within the category of penetrating injuries, gunshot wounds account for 81%, while stabbings account for the remaining 19% (2).

Duodenal injuries are rarely isolated and are often associated with injuries to adjacent organs, including the liver, pancreas, small bowel, colon and stomach. The liver is the most injured organ, accounting for 17% of associated injuries (2–5). Associated major vascular injuries can also occur, leading to life-threatening exsanguination. Prominent abdominal veins were injured in 10% of patients, mostly involving the inferior vena cava, and major arteries were injured in 7% of patients, mostly involving the aorta (5,6).

EVALUATION

Trauma patients' initial resuscitation and evaluation should follow the Advanced Trauma Life Support (ATLS) algorithm with an efficient primary and secondary survey. The history and physical examination are non-specific in the context of duodenal injury. Focused assessment with sonography for trauma (FAST) has replaced Diagnostic Peritoneal Lavage (DPL) as a diagnostic adjunct to identify the presence of free peritoneal fluid (7). As a part of routine trauma assessment, laboratory studies typically include serum amylase or lipase although these tests are not specific enough to confirm or exclude the diagnosis (8,9).

DOI: 10.1201/9781003080060-26

Based on the mechanism and FAST evaluation, haemodynamically unstable patients with high suspicion of the abdomen being the source of instability should undergo immediate laparotomy. Typically, most duodenal perforations are apparent during the initial inspection but instilling methylene blue via a nasogastric tube can further aid in identifying subtle full-thickness injuries by looking for duodenal subserosal staining (10).

Diagnosing blunt duodenal injury in haemodynamically stable patients relies primarily on imaging as history, physical and laboratory findings are non-specific. The most efficient imaging modality is a contrast-enhanced CT (CECT) scan, which has a sensitivity and specificity of 86% and 88%, respectively, for diagnosing blunt hollow-viscus injury (11–13). However, it has been reported that up to 27% of injuries can be missed on initial imaging (14). Furthermore, no substantial evidence suggests oral contrast enhances the ability to identify bowel injuries compared to scanning using IV contrast alone at the initial evaluation (4).

Table 26.1 AAST duodenum injury grade with associated OIS scale

Grade	Type of Injury	Description of Injury	OIS-90
I	Haematoma	Involving single portion of duodenum	2
	Laceration	Partial thickness, no perforation	3
II	Haematoma	Involving more than one portion	2
	Laceration	Disruption <50% of circumference	4
III	Laceration	Disruption 50–75% of the circumference of D2	4
		Disruption 50–100% of D1, D3 or D4	4
IV	Laceration	Disruption >75% of circumference of D2	5
		Involving ampullar or distal common bile duct	5
V	Laceration	Massive disruption of duodenopancreatic complex	5
	Vascular	Devascularization of duodenum	5

Abbreviations: D1: first portion of duodenum; D2: second portion of duodenum; D3: third portion of duodenum; D4: fourth portion of duodenum.

Source: Reprinted with permission from Moore EE, et al. Organ Injury Scaling, 11: Pancreas, Duodenum, Small Bowel, Colon, and Rectum. *J Trauma Acute Care Surg* 1990;*30(11)*:1427.

The American Association for the Surgery for Trauma (AAST) Organ Injury Scale (OIS) (*Table 26.1*) is an anatomically based classification system commonly used to grade the extent and severity of duodenal injuries. It is an effective tool to help guide management by standardizing the approach to specific anatomical injury in the ideal situation. For example, injuries designated Grades I–II are straightforward and amenable to primary repair. On the other hand, AAST Grades III, IV and V indicate more complex trauma potentially requiring reconstruction.

OPERATIVE MANAGEMENT

An injured patient's presenting physiology should always govern the initial operative decision-making. In haemodynamically unstable patients, the principal tenet is damage control surgery aiming to stop haemorrhage and contain any gastrointestinal (GI) contamination by closing the affected section with suturing, stapling, or complete resection if feasible leaving the GI tract in discontinuity (15). In cases of severe tissue destruction resulting in difficult-to-control contamination, placing multiple closed suction drains is crucial to mitigate risks associated with uncontrolled bile and pancreatic leaks. After damage control surgery, temporary abdominal closure followed by expedient transfer to the intensive care unit for fluid resuscitation, rewarming, and correction of coagulopathy and acidosis should be the next goal. Restoration of GI continuity with definitive reconstruction can be planned after the patient demonstrates improved physiology.

For haemodynamically stable patients, the principles guiding surgical management should encompass debridement of non-viable tissue, restoration of GI continuity, and gastric and pancreaticobiliary diversions if necessary (15). Nevertheless, it is worth emphasizing that the objectives can be achieved in a staged approach. It is essential to avoid complex repair and reconstruction during the initial encounter, allowing time to optimize the patient's physiology and mobilize the necessary resources and expertise to tackle the challenge more methodically. As mentioned above, the AAST-OIS can provide a scaffold to guide surgical planning accordingly (*Figure 26.1*).

Grade I lacerations can be repaired by suturing the serosa in a Lembert style (named after Antoine Lembert, who carried out his operations in France in the early 1800s and was the beginning of attempts to overcome some of the problems faced during suturing the intestine. He stated that 'the quality of muco-mucosal sutures is low and sero-serous sutures should be preferred over this type of suture'). Grade II lacerations are treated with tension-free primary closure in one or two layers after debriding to a healthy wound edge. It is vital to perform the repair in a transverse orientation to reduce the risk of luminal narrowing. Periduodenal drain placement post-repair is controversial, and there is no substantial evidence to guide its routine use (15). Nasogastric tube decompression should be placed for proximal decompression to reduce gastric effluent through the repair. Periduodenal haematomas

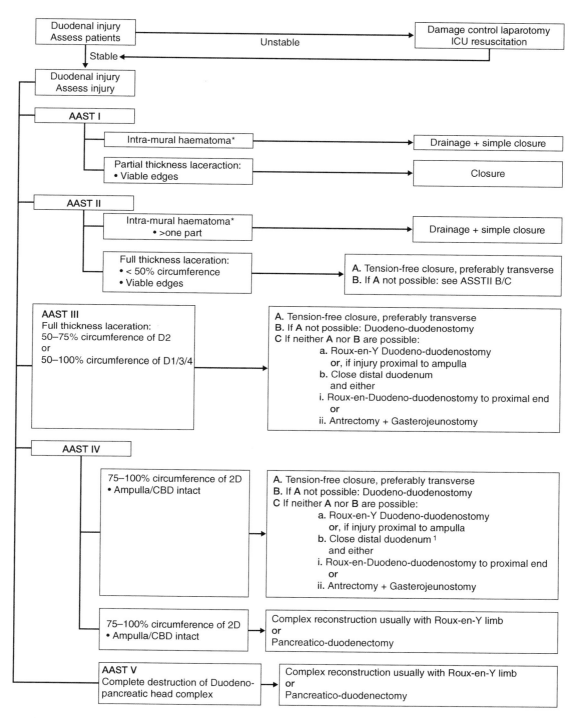

*If detected by CT and there is no other indication to operate observe with gastric decopression. If does not resolve during observation then operate and manage as **AAST I** above.

Figure 26.1 Proposed algorithm for the management of duodenal injuries. Reprinted with permission from (36).

encountered during exploration should lead to a thorough inspection of the duodenum to exclude perforation. However, only obstructing haematomas involving more than 50% of the duodenal diameter should be considered for evacuation (4).

Operative management of AAST Grades III and IV injuries without ampullary involvement has been controversial. There has been an evolution towards primary repair with nasogastric tube decompression and external drain placement, even for extensive and high-grade injuries. More recent studies demonstrate improved morbidity and mortality with primary repairs compared with more complex reconstructive and drainage procedures (16,17). If tension-free primary repair is not feasible or may result in luminal narrowing, a jejunal serosal patch sewn to the edges of the duodenal injury can be considered (18). A pedicled mucosal flap from the jejunum has also been described as an alternative (19). Segmental resection with primary duodeno-duodenostomy is another option if the two ends are mobile enough for tension-free anastomosis in an end-to-end or side-to-side fashion (*Figure 26.2*).

If neither primary repair nor resection with primary anastomosis is possible due to the extent of the injury, more complex reconstruction may be necessary. In such cases, the location of the injury to the ampulla will dictate the reconstruction. Antrectomy incorporating injured proximal duodenum followed by distal duodenum closure is an option for injuries occurring at the first or proximal second portion of the duodenum (4). Billroth II or Roux-en-Y gastrojejunostomy are both viable methods of reconstruction and the Roux-en-Y approach has less risk for bile reflux (*Figure 26.3*). For injuries located distal to the ampulla, reconstruction with primary duodeno-duodenostomy is often feasible if the bowel is adequately mobilized to allow for tension-free anastomosis (*Figure 26.4*).

Grade IV injuries involving the distal common bile duct will require both biliary and enteric tract reconstruction. The biliary continuity can be restored with the common bile duct reimplantation via choledochoduodenostomy or reconstruction via a Roux-en-Y choledochojejunostomy. Placing a biliary stent is recommended during the reconstruction, given the high risk of biliary stenosis (15). Conversely, Roux-en-Y gastrojejunostomy

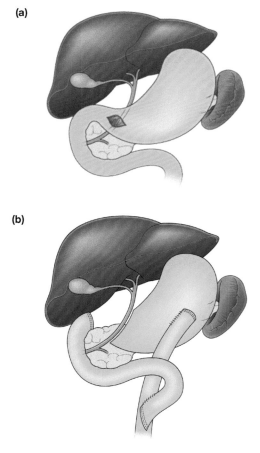

Figure 26.3 AAST Grades III and IV injuries without ampullary involvement that are not amenable for primary repair or anastomosis. Injury is proximal to the ampulla (a), the injured segment is resected (b), and enteric continuity is restored via a Roux-en-Y gastrojejunostomy reconstruction.

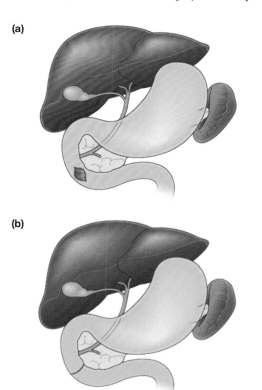

Figure 26.2 AAST Grade III injury managed with debridement (a) and a primary end-to-end anastomosis (b).

(a)

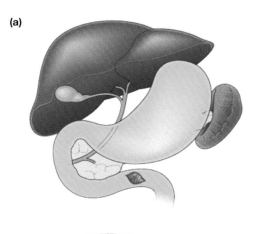

(b)

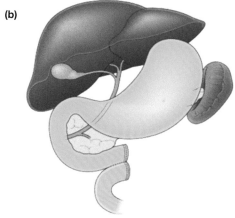

Figure 26.4 AAST Grades III and IV injuries without ampullary involvement. Injury is distal to the ampulla (a), the injured segment is resected (b), and enteric continuity is restored via a side-to-side reconstruction.

is the favoured option for enteric restoration, especially when biliary reconstruction is required. Finally, the pancreaticoduodenectomy (Whipple's procedure) is the procedure of choice for extensive injury involving the pancreaticoduodenal complex and ampulla of Vater. Different from patients with pathological pancreas from malignancy or chronic inflammation, creating a pancreaticojejunal anastomosis in otherwise healthy trauma patients can be difficult due to the small size of the pancreatic duct and the soft texture of the pancreatic tissue. To reduce the risk of anastomotic dehiscence, the 'dunking the pancreas' manoeuvre may be performed by suturing the pancreatic capsule to the bowel (15).

ANCILLARY SURGICAL TECHNIQUES

Duodenal exposure

The Kocher manoeuvre, first published in 1903 by Theodor Kocher, is a fundamental surgical technique to expose the duodenum's first and second portions by

dissecting its lateral peritoneal attachments (20). The posterior aspect of the first portion and the medial aspect of the second portion can be inspected by dividing the gastrocolic ligament to enter the lesser sac. The third and fourth portions can be revealed via a right medial visceral rotation (Cattell–Braasch manoeuvre) by extending the incision from the Kocher manoeuvre along the right white line of Toldt and incising the posterior mesenteric attachments towards the ligament of Treitz followed by releasing the ligament itself.

Diverticulization

In 1968, Berne and colleagues described duodenal diverticulization in 16 patients (21). The technique consisted of primary duodenal wound closure, antrectomy, truncal vagotomy, end-to-side gastrojejunostomy, insertion of biliary T-tube, and tube duodenostomy to achieve complete diversion of gastric and biliary flow away from newly repaired duodenum (21). However, due to its intricate and time-consuming nature, it has fallen out of favour.

Triple tube ostomy

The triple tube ostomy was initially introduced in 1954 for the closure of the duodenal stump after gastrectomy and was later applied in trauma management by Stone and Fabian in 1979 (22). It incorporates antegrade decompression via a gastrostomy tube, retrograde biliary drainage via a jejunostomy tube, and distal feeding access via another separate jejunostomy. However, its effectiveness in reducing the incidence of suture line dehiscence has not been clearly demonstrated.

Pyloric exclusion

Vaughan devised the concept in 1977 to exclude gastric efflux from entering the duodenum by closing the pylorus and diverting gastric outflow with a loop gastrojejunostomy (23). The pylorus can be closed with staples or sutures. The suturing technique requires a longitudinal gastrostomy incision on the antrum proximal to the pylorus, which can be used as the site for gastrojejunostomy. The exposed pyloric muscle is then approximated using partial-thickness absorbable sutures to close the outflow tract. The stapling technique employs a non-cutting linear stapler applied transversely just distal to the pylorus. Although the technique is still used as an adjunct to protect a distal repair, several studies have demonstrated little benefit compared with primary repair with nasogastric tube decompression but with a higher overall complication rate (71% vs. 33%) (17,24,25).

NON-OPERATIVE MANAGEMENT

Most duodenal injuries are diagnosed and managed operatively because the penetrating mechanism is the most common cause (2). However, nonoperative management is a safe option for haemodynamically stable patients with blunt trauma without any associated injuries requiring operative interventions. The decision of nonoperative management in these patients is based on the combination of the patient's physical examination and CECT scan findings. For example, diffuse peritonitis or evidence of full-thickness laceration on the CT scan, such as extravasation of enteral contrast or free air, would necessitate immediate operative exploration. On the other hand, Grades I or II duodenal haematomas diagnosed on the CT scan can be safely observed (4,26,27).

The principles of nonoperative management are proximal decompression, continuous assessment of progressive symptoms and nutritional support. A nasogastric tube should be placed in patients with symptoms of proximal bowel obstruction due to duodenal haematoma or swelling. Imaging studies, either an upper GI series or a CT scan with oral contrast, should be repeated when the nasogastric tube shows decreasing output to evaluate for duodenal patency. It is safe to resume an oral diet if the obstruction is no longer present. In most cases, obstruction caused by duodenal haematoma will resolve within 14 days (28) but surgical intervention may be necessary if it persists for longer than this (4). Laparoscopic evacuation is a safe alternative to the more common open approach (29).

According to a multicentre retrospective study on the nonoperative management of blunt pancreaticoduodenal injury, the failure rate is about 10.3% (30). Hence, close monitoring of patients managed nonoperatively with serial abdominal exams and laboratory studies is critical. Worsening abdominal pain, peritonitis on physical examination, intolerance of oral intake, or emerging sepsis can be clinical clues alerting clinicians to the failure of nonoperative management. Further investigations with repeat imaging, diagnostic laparoscopy, or exploratory laparotomy are necessary depending on the patient's haemodynamics and the clinician's index of suspicions.

NUTRITION

Nutritional optimization should always be a cornerstone in managing any trauma patient and early enteral nutrition is preferred to the parenteral route (31,32). Operative management of duodenal injuries should integrate surgical planning for enteral access. A post-pyloric nasoenteric feeding tube extending beyond the injury is preferred but can be challenging to place and a surgical jejunostomy is an alternative approach. Jejunostomy placement however should be thoroughly evaluated in individual cases as jejunostomy-related complications, including soft-tissue infection, leak, enteric fistula and bowel obstruction occurs in approximately 4% of patients (33). On the other hand, establishing and maintaining enteral access can be problematic for patients with blunt duodenal injury managed non-operatively and when enteral feeding is not feasible for more than seven days, parenteral nutrition should be considered (4).

OUTCOMES AND COMPLICATIONS

Based on the recent case series review, the overall mortality rate for duodenal injuries ranges from 5.3–30%.

Exsanguination from associated vascular injuries is typically responsible for early mortality, while later deaths often result from sepsis leading to multiorgan failure (34). The mortality rate also correlates with the duodenal injury grade according to the AAST classification: Grade I (8.3%), Grade II (18.7%), Grade III (27.6%), Grade IV (30.8%) and Grade V (58.8%) (2). Most importantly, delay in diagnosis or intervention significantly increases mortality by almost 50% (35).

The morbidity rate associated with duodenal trauma is reported to be 22% (36). The complication observed most frequently is intra-abdominal abscesses, accounting for 68% of all morbidities (5). Two primary factors leading to significant retroperitoneal abscess formation are delayed surgical intervention and dehiscence of the duodenal wound. Antibiotics and percutaneous drainage can achieve source control in most cases without reoperation.

Duodenal fistula, commonly resulting from suture line dehiscence, is the second most common complication, accounting for up to 28% of morbidities associated with traumatic duodenal injury (5) and it can be the most life-threatening complication if not managed well. The management paradigm revolves around controlling output, treating sepsis, optimizing nutrition, and wound care. Given its complexity, a multidisciplinary approach incorporating nutritionists and wound care is highly desirable in managing duodenal fistula.

SUMMARY

Traumatic duodenal injury is a rare but severe entity that requires careful evaluation and prompt treatment to minimize associated morbidity and mortality. The diagnosis of duodenal injury can be incredibly challenging with blunt mechanisms. Penetrating injuries require operative management, with damage control surgery necessary for haemodynamically unstable patients or patients with extensive damage at the initial presentation. For complex injuries, there has been a significant shift towards a 'less is more' approach, with recent data advocating primary repair with nasogastric tube decompression for even extensive and high-grade injuries. Non-operative management can be safe and effective for selected patients. Given its complexity, it is vital to have a thoughtful and multidisciplinary approach to treating duodenal trauma and its complications to improve patient outcomes.

REFERENCES

1. Lopez PP, Gogna S, Khorasani-Zadeh A. *Anatomy, Abdomen and Pelvis: Duodenum*, In StatPearls. 2023, Treasure Island, FL: StatPearls Publishing.
2. Garcia Santos E, Soto Sánchez A, Verde JM, Marini CP, Asensio JA, Petrone P. et al. Duodenal injuries due to trauma: Review of the literature. *Cir Esp* 2015;**93(2)**:68–74.
3. Pandey S, Niranjan A, Mishra S, Agrawal T, Singhal BM, Prakash A, et al. Retrospective analysis of duodenal injuries: A comprehensive overview. *Saudi J Gastroenterol* 2011;**17(2)**:142–4.

4. Coccolini F, Kobayashi L, Kluger Y, Moore EE, Ansaloni L, Biffl W, et al. Duodeno-pancreatic and extrahepatic biliary tree trauma: WSES-AAST guidelines. *World J Emerg Surg* 2019;**14**:56.

5. Asensio JA, Feliciano DV, Britt LD, Kerstein MD. Management of duodenal injuries. *Curr Probl Surg* 1993;**30(11)**:1023–93.

6. Chen C, Schuster K, Bhattacharya B. Motor vehicle collision patient with simultaneous duodenal transection and thoracic aorta injury: a case report and review of the literature. *Case Rep Surg* 2015;**2015**:519836.

7. Rinta-Kiikka I. FAST ultrasonography *Duodecim* 2016;**132(8)**:791–5.

8. Takishima T, Sugimoto K, Hirata M, Asari Y, Ohwada T, Kakita A. Serum amylase level on admission in the diagnosis of blunt injury to the pancreas: Its significance and limitations. *Ann Surg* 1997;**226(1)**:70–6.

9. Buechter KJ, Arnold M, Steele B, Martin L, Byers P, Gomez G, et al. The use of serum amylase and lipase in evaluating and managing blunt abdominal trauma. *Am Surg* 1990;**56(4)**:204–8.

10. Brotman S, Cisternino S, Myers RA, Cowley RA. A test to help diagnosis of rupture in the injured duodenum. *Injury* 1981;**12(6)**:464–5.

11. Choi AY, Bodanapally UK, Shapiro B, Patlas MN, Katz DS. Recent advances in abdominal trauma computed tomography. *Semin Roentgenol* 2018;**53(2)**:178–86.

12. Joseph DK, Kunac A, Kinler RL, Staff I, Butler KL. Diagnosing blunt hollow viscus injury: is computed tomography the answer? *Am J Surg* 2013;**205(4)**:414–8.

13. Rodriguez C, Barone JE, Wilbanks TO, Rha C-K, Miller K. Isolated free fluid on computed tomographic scan in blunt abdominal trauma: A systematic review of incidence and management. *J Trauma* 2002;**53(1)**:79–85.

14. Ballard RB, Badellino MM, Eynon CA, Spott MA, Staz CF, Buckman RF Jr. Blunt duodenal rupture: a 6-year statewide experience. *J Trauma* 1997;**43(2)**:229–32; discussion 233.

15. Bolaji T, Ratnasekera A, Ferrada P. Management of the complex duodenal injury. *Am J Surg* 2023;**225(4)**:639–44.

16. Aiolfi A, Matsushina K, Chang G, Bardes J, Strumwasser A, Lam L, et al. Surgical trends in the management of duodenal injury. *J Gastrointest Surg* 2019;**23(2)**:264–9.

17. Ordoñez C, García A, Parra MW, Scavo D, Pino LF Millán M, et al. Complex penetrating duodenal injuries: less is better. *J Trauma Acute Care Surg* 2014;**76(5)**:1177–83.

18. Ivatury RR, Gaudino J, Ascer E, Nallathambi M, Ramirez-Schon G, Stahl WM. Treatment of penetrating duodenal injuries: primary repair vs. repair with decompressive enterostomy/serosal patch. *J Trauma* 1985;**25(4)**:337–41.

19. Takei R, Hashimoto M, Zaimoku R, Terakawa H, Terada I, Tsukioka Y, et al. Pedicled jejunal flap reconstruction for partial duodenectomy: a report of two cases. *J Surg Case Rep* 2020;**2020(10)**:rjaa296.

20. Livani A, Angelis S, Skandalakis PN, Filippou D, et al. The story retold: The Kocher manoeuvre. *Cureus* 2022;**14(9)**:e29409.

21. Berne CJ, Donovan AJ, White EJ, Yellin AE. Duodenal "diverticulization" for duodenal and pancreatic injury. *Am J Surg* 1974;**127(5)**:503–7.

22. Stone HH, Fabian, TC. Management of duodenal wounds. *J Trauma* 1979;**19(5)**:334–9.

23. Vaughan GD, 3rd, Frazier OH, Graham DY, Mattox KL, Petmecky FF, Jordan GL Jr, et al. The use of pyloric exclusion in the management of severe duodenal injuries. *Am J Surg* 1977;**134(6)**:785–90.

24. DuBose JJ, Inaba K, Teixeira PGR, Shiflett A, Putty B, Green JD, et al. Pyloric exclusion in the treatment of severe duodenal injuries: results from the National Trauma Data Bank. *Am Surg* 2008;**74(10)**:925–9.

25. Seamon MJ, Pieri PG, Fisher CA, Gaughan J, Santora TA, Pathak AS, et al. A ten-year retrospective review: Does pyloric exclusion improve clinical outcome after penetrating duodenal and combined pancreaticoduodenal injuries? *J Trauma* 2007;**62(4)**:829–33.

26. Cogbill TH, Moore EE, Feliciano DV, Hoyt DB, Jurkovich GJ, Morris JA, et al. Conservative management of duodenal trauma: A multicenter perspective. *J Trauma* 1990;**30(12)**:1469–75.

27. Jewett TC, Jr, Caldarola V, Karp MP, Allen JE, Cooney DR. Intramural hematoma of the duodenum. *Arch Surg* 1988;**123(1)**:54–8.

28. Czyrko C, Weltz CR, Markowitz RI, O'Neill JA. Blunt abdominal trauma resulting in intestinal obstruction: when to operate? *J Trauma* 1990;**30(12)**:1567–71.

29. Nolan GJ, Bendinelli C, Gani J. Laparoscopic drainage of an intramural duodenal haematoma: a novel technique and review of the literature. *World J Emerg Surg* 2011;**6(1)**:42.

30. Velmahos GC, Tabbara M, Gross R, Willette P, Hirsch E, Burke P, et al. Blunt pancreatoduodenal injury: A multicenter study of the Research Consortium of New England Centers for Trauma (ReCONECT). *Arch Surg* 2009;**144(5)**:413–9; discussion 419–20.

31. McClave SA, et al. Guidelines for the Provision and Assessment of Nutrition Support Therapy in the Adult Critically Ill Patient: Society of Critical Care Medicine (SCCM) and American Society for Parenteral and Enteral Nutrition (A.S.P.E.N.). *JPEN J Parenter Enteral Nutr* 2009;**33(3)**:277–316.

32. Dissanaike S, Pham T, Shalhub S, Aarner K, Hennessy L, Moore EE, et al. Effect of immediate enteral feeding on trauma patients with an open abdomen: protection from nosocomial infections. *J Am Coll Surg* 2008;**207(5)**:690–7.

33. Holmes JH, Brundage SI, Yeun P, Hall RA, Maier RV, Jurkovich GJ. Complications of surgical feeding jejunostomy in trauma patients. *J Trauma* 1999;**47(6)**:1009–12.

34. Phillips B, Turco L, McDonald D, Mause A, Walters RW. Penetrating injuries to the duodenum: An analysis of 879 patients from the National Trauma Data Bank, 2010 to 2014. *J Trauma Acute Care Surg* 2017;**83(5)**:810–17.

35. Snyder WH, 3rd, Weigelt JA, Watkins WL, Beitz DS. The surgical management of duodenal trauma. Precepts based on a review of 247 cases. *Arch Surg* 1980;**115(4)**:422–9.

36. Malhotra A, et al. Western Trauma Association Critical Decisions in Trauma: Diagnosis and management of duodenal injuries. *J Trauma Acute Care Surg* 2015; **79(6)**: 1096–1101.

Bailey & Love's Essential Operations Bailey & Love's Essential Operatic
Bailey & Love's Essential Operatic Bailey & Love's Essential Operatic
Bailey & Love's Essential Operatic Bailey & Love's Essential Operatic

SECTION 5 | HEPATOBILIARY TRAUMA AND CONTROL OF BLEEDING

Chapter 27

Biliary Trauma

Rahul Deshpande and Jenifer Barrie

INTRODUCTION

Injuries to the biliary tract are extremely rare. They can result from both blunt and penetrating abdominal trauma or be iatrogenic. The nature and extent of injury and modes of presentation vary widely depending on the mechanism of trauma and whether there are any associated injuries. The type of injury and the initial and definitive management are generally different for blunt as compared to penetrating trauma. Iatrogenic injuries are mostly related to complications of laparoscopic and open cholecystectomy but may also infrequently result from other upper gastrointestinal (GI) operations and interventional biliary procedures. This chapter deals specifically with trauma to the extrahepatic biliary system unrelated to gallbladder surgery.

INCIDENCE AND EPIDEMIOLOGY

Injuries of the extrahepatic biliary tree are extremely rare and account for about 0.1% of all adult and paediatric trauma admissions (1–3). The male to female ratio varies significantly between 5:1–25:1 depending on the reporting geographical area, the latter related to the higher incidence of penetrating trauma in that series (4,5). The vast majority of injuries of the extrahepatic biliary tree, particularly in relation to blunt trauma are associated with other abdominal injuries, specifically, liver and pancreatoduodenal. Extrahepatic biliary trauma will be encountered in about 4–5% of all cases of liver trauma (6), regardless of aetiology and in up to 2–3% of all cases of abdominal trauma (1). Isolated extrahepatic bile duct injuries are rare with only a very small number reported in the setting of blunt trauma (7,8). However, in a recently reported large series, isolated bile duct injury, after blunt abdominal trauma, without concomitant liver or pancreatic injury, was recorded in 11.3% of patients (9). Significantly, the injury severity score and grade of liver injury after blunt trauma also tends to be higher when there is associated biliary trauma (9). Penetrating injuries account for most gallbladder injuries whereas the bile ducts are more frequently injured with blunt trauma. Conversely, in another relatively recent series, all gallbladder injuries were encountered secondary to blunt trauma (2) and importantly, a significant proportion of patients with biliary trauma present with haemodynamic instability (10).

The site of biliary trauma varies with the mechanism of injury. Penetrating trauma to the lower liver accounts for almost all traumatic gallbladder perforations. Similar injuries to the portal area are frequently fatal due to injury to portal vein and hepatic artery. Blunt trauma tends to spare these vessels due to their tortuosity whereas the relative stiffness of the bile duct lends itself to disruptive trauma. With blunt trauma, the predominant gallbladder injury is either contusion or avulsion with perforation being relatively uncommon whereas perforation is the predominant feature of penetrating trauma (11). When both blunt and penetrating trauma is taken into account, the most common site of injury to the extrahepatic biliary tree is actually the common bile duct (CBD) and/or the common hepatic duct (CHD) and involves either a laceration or complete transection in nearly 70% of cases while similar injuries to either the right or the left main ducts are much less frequent (2). In a historical report of a large series of blunt biliary trauma, partial or complete transection of the CBD or CHD accounted for nearly 60% of all biliary injuries (12). In the paediatric population, however, the incidence of complete CBD transection is relatively rare (3).

Most iatrogenic biliary injuries result from complications of cholecystectomy and are discussed in **Chapter 62**. Gastric and pancreatic operations are often complex and especially if there has been previous surgery or inflammation (pancreatitis, cholangitis) may rarely cause iatrogenic biliary injuries. Any procedure for biliary intervention has the potential for causing biliary trauma and perforations occur in about 0.6% of all endoscopic retrograde cholangiopancreatographys (ERCP) (13) but the majority are duodenal or ampullary rather than of the extrahepatic biliary tree.

CLASSIFICATION OF BILIARY TRAUMA

Biliary trauma can be broadly classified anatomically into injury to the intrahepatic or extrahepatic biliary tract and intrahepatic injuries can be further classified arbitrarily into central and peripheral (6). Central injuries involve the main right- or left-ducts and intrahepatic or sectoral ducts within 5 cm of the biliary confluence whereas peripheral injuries are

DOI: 10.1201/9781003080060-27

those within the parenchyma more than 5 cm beyond the confluence.

Extrahepatic biliary injuries specifically associated with abdominal trauma are classified according to the organ injury scale (OIS) adopted by the American Association for the Surgery of Trauma (AAST) (14). They are graded from 1–5 with increasing severity and are listed in *Table 27.1*. The World Society of Emergency Surgery (WSES) recently published comprehensive guidelines for duodenopancreatic and extrahepatic biliary tree injuries (15). The WSES classifies these injuries into four classes based both on the AAST grading and haemodynamic status of the patient. These are then graded as: Minor (WSES Class I), Moderate (WSES Class II) and Severe (WSES Class III and IV). A combined AAST-OIS and WSES grading and classification system for the biliary tree is listed in *Table 27.2*. Although many biliary injuries are technically in the minor or moderate categories, a significant number of these patients present with haemodynamic instability due to associated organ trauma and consequently will be classified in the severe category.

Table 27.1 AAST-OIS grading of biliary tract injuries (15)

Grade of injury*	Description of injury
I	Gallbladder contusion
	Portal triad contusion
II	Partial gallbladder avulsion from liver bed with intact cystic duct
	Laceration or perforation of gallbladder
III	Complete gallbladder avulsion from liver bed
	Laceration or disruption of cystic duct
IV	Partial or complete right duct laceration
	Partial or complete left duct laceration
	Partial common hepatic or common bile duct laceration (<50%)
V	>50% laceration of common hepatic or common bile duct
	Combined right and left hepatic duct injuries
	Intraduodenal or intrapancreatic bile duct injury

*Advance one grade for multiple injuries up to Grade III.

Table 27.2 Combined WSES and AAST-OIS grading of injury to biliary tree

Grade	WSES Class	AAST	Description of injury
Minor	Class I	I-II-III	Gallbladder contusion
			Portal triad contusion
			Partial gallbladder avulsion from liver bed with intact cystic duct
			Laceration or perforation of gallbladder
			Complete gallbladder avulsion from liver bed
Moderate	Class II	IV	Laceration or disruption of cystic duct
			Partial or complete right duct laceration
			Partial or complete left duct laceration
			Partial common hepatic or common bile duct laceration (<50%)
Severe	Class III	V	>50% laceration of common hepatic or common bile duct
			Combined right and left hepatic duct injuries
			Intraduodenal or intrapancreatic bile duct injury
Severe	Class IV	Any	Any degree of injury with haemodymanic instability

Adapted from Coccolini et al., 2019 (15).

IATROGENIC EXTRAHEPATIC BILE DUCT INJURIES

Non-traumatic iatrogenic bile duct injuries outside of the setting of gallbladder surgery are incredibly rare. They can be associated with diagnostic and therapeutic procedures such as an ERCP (*Figure 27.1*) or percutaneous transhepatic cholangiography (PTC). They have also been described in setting of upper abdominal surgery, particularly radical gastric surgery (16).

ERCP-related bile duct injuries often go unreported and the exact site is sometimes unclear. Perforations, in general, occur in about 0.6% of all ERCPs but are related to a mortality of about 8% (17). Guidewire perforations are often unrecognized, and hence not reported, but if recognized and dealt with, rarely cause a significant bile leak due to the minor nature of the injury (*Figure 27.1*). The majority of ERCP-related perforations are lateral duodenal wall injuries or a consequence of a sphincterotomy. True distal biliary injuries, the Stapfer Type 3 (Stapfer described four types of perforations; Type 1 is a lateral or medial wall duodenal perforation; Type 2 are periampullary injuries; Type 3 are bile or pancreatic duct injuries and Type 4 describe retroperitoneal air with no other identifiable injury) account for less than 25% of all perforations (17).

More recently, endoscopic ultrasound (US)-guided trans-duodenal direct side-puncture of the bile duct has been introduced for the relief of biliary obstruction where the ampulla is inaccessible. Both, standard and lumen-apposing metal stents can be deployed using this technique. Although considered a relatively safe procedure the rates of perforation appear to be higher (18) and due to the dimensions of the stents used, maldeployment can lead to a significant defect in the side wall of the bile duct requiring urgent surgery or further intervention. *Figure 27.2* demonstrates the effects of a maldeployed biliary stent resulting in a side-perforation (*Figure 27.2a*), needing urgent PTC (*Figure 27.2b*) and rescue by deployment of a covered self-expanding metal stent. *Figure 27.3a,b* demonstrates a malpositioned distal end of a direct-puncture biliary stent lying free in the peritoneal cavity and needing urgent corrective surgery.

PTC-related extrahepatic bile duct injuries are rarely reported and injury to the extrahepatic ducts usually results from guidewire perforations with or without stent deployment. With many of these injuries there is a pre-existing biliary pathology of the main CBD, most commonly, a stricture.

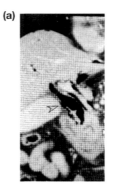
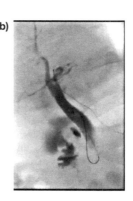

Figure 27.2 CT of a patient with a maldeployed Axios stent (a) (stent accidentally withdrawn during the procedure) showing a lateral wall-loss of the CBD (arrow) and portal free gas. PTC image of the same patient (b) demonstrating contrast extravasation from the biliary perforation locally and into peri-duodenal space.

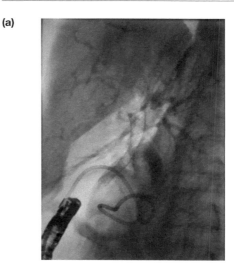

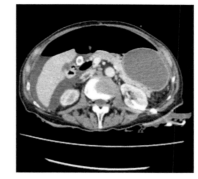

Figure 27.3 ERCP picture of an US-guided bile duct stent insertion (a) demonstrating the distal end lying free in the abdominal cavity (nephrostomy tube in the background). CT scan of the same patient (b) showing the position of the stent outside the CBD and massive pneumoperitoneum.

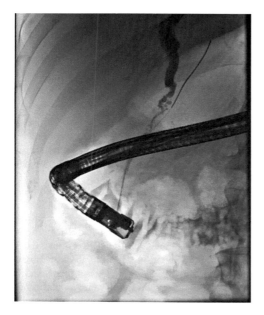

Figure 27.1 ERCP guidewire perforation of the CBD.

CLINICAL PRESENTATION AND DIAGNOSIS

In general, the timing of presentation of biliary trauma can broadly be considered as immediate, delayed or late. In the immediate setting, biliary trauma is encountered at laparotomy performed for trauma, typically in an unstable patient or in a haemodynamically stable patient with a clear indication for a laparotomy. Intraoperative findings that indicate extrahepatic biliary trauma include contusion or laceration to the gallbladder, haematoma or distortion of the porta hepatis or a frank bile leak from the portal or supraduodenal area. In a stable patient with a suspected injury which can't be identified after a thorough exploration, an on-table cholangiogram can be diagnostic (19). Avulsion or major damage to the head of the pancreas or duodenum or a major liver parenchymal injury close to the hilum should lead to a suspicion of bile duct trauma.

With the increasing trend towards conservative management, biliary injuries now commonly present in the delayed phase of a hospital admission. Moreover, with damage-control surgery being commonplace, intraoperative recognition of biliary trauma is often not possible or can be missed. These patients then present with a whole range of symptoms of bile leaks and biliary peritonitis, often concomitant with manifestations of other abdominal injuries. In patients who have had a damage-control laparotomy with abdominal drain placement, the presentation is usually that of a postoperative bile leak (6). In patients treated conservatively after blunt trauma, biliary ascites or bilomas can occur in up to 20% of patients, indicating an unrecognized injury (20). Delay in diagnosis leads to a longer in-hospital stay with early diagnosis resulting in better outcomes.

Finally, a subset of patients will present late due solely to the biliary injury. They have delayed bile leaks, or more typically symptoms related to biliary strictures such as recurrent cholangitis, failure to thrive and obstructive jaundice. This is a result of ischaemic damage to the ducts in a mechanism similar to that encountered with injuries related to cholecystectomy.

INVESTIGATIONS

Unless traumatic biliary injuries are recognized and fully defined intraoperatively on initial and immediate laparotomy, radiological and interventional investigations are key to the definitive diagnosis and management of biliary trauma.

Abdominal ultrasound

In the context of acute trauma, an abdominal US in the form of a focused assessment with sonography in trauma (FAST) scan merely detects free fluid. Even in the absence of a solid organ injury, free fluid in the upper abdomen is rarely diagnostic of biliary or even associated pancreatoduodenal trauma (21). However abdominal US does play some role in monitoring patients with trauma-related collections and bilomas.

Computed tomography

A contrast-enhanced CT (CECT) scan is the most rapid and comprehensive investigation in general for a trauma patient. However, signs and appearances, specifically of biliary trauma, can be quite subtle and non-specific. Gallbladder injuries may present as a collapsed gallbladder with pericholecystic fluid, wall thickening or differential enhancement although occasionally a clear discontinuity of the wall can be seen (19). Displacement of the gallbladder or intraluminal haemorrhage may be seen with, or without, associated local liver laceration, indicative of an avulsion (22).

CT findings of bile duct injury proper are even more non-specific and fluid or haematoma around the porta may be the only initial sign. Injury to the portal blood vessels, if seen, may suggest the likelihood of associated bile duct trauma. A central liver laceration or a major pancreaticoduodenal injury may similarly suggest that a biliary injury is likely. However, a significant number of the latter injuries can be missed on the initial CT (23) and serial scans depending on the clinical indication are useful and may provide an evolving picture of any bile duct injury in the form of an increasing local collection, compression of the duct leading to proximal dilatation or signs of biliary peritonitis. Drip-infusion cholangiographic CT (DIC-CT) enables high-resolution and three-dimensional visualization of even small bile ducts. It provides, in effect, a dynamic image of the biliary tree with the potential to diagnose and localize injuries better than standard CT (24). However, its use is very limited, and it carries a higher risk of contrast allergy.

Iatrogenic injuries resulting from complications of procedures such as an ERCP may be incredibly difficult to see, given the relatively small puncture wound. Gas in the porta and around the bile duct may be demonstrated on the CT and a wall defect or damage can be identified in some cases (*Figure 27.2a*).

Hepatobiliary scintigraphy

Unlike other radiological modalities, scintigraphy such as a hepatobiliary iminodiacetic acid (HIDA) scan will demonstrate physiological real-time biliary excretion, which can be traced and tracked over the study period. Slow leaks can be diagnosed with delayed images although it is poor at determining the precise site of the leak and has poor spatial imaging quality (25). The sensitivity and precision of scintigraphy can be further enhanced by the addition of single-photon emission computed tomography (SPECT-CT) which enhances the resolution of the images, providing a much more specific anatomical definition of the injury (26). Scintigraphy can differentiate between free abdominal leaks and slow contained ones which can help determine treatment options, the latter being predominantly managed conservatively (26). However, scintigraphy can be a cumbersome and prolonged diagnostic test and many aspects of it have largely been superseded by magnetic resonance cholangiopancreatography (MRCP).

Magnetic resonance cholangio-pancreatography

MRCP is a non-invasive investigation which obviates radiation exposure and facilitates mapping of the biliary tree with a high level of precision. Gadolinium-based contrast agents now permit dynamic biliary imaging during the hepatobiliary phase and have been shown to improve diagnostic accuracy and anatomical localization of a leak or injury compared with standard T2-weighted images (27). As with scintigraphy, it is possible to differentiate between a free abdominal and a contained leak. Significant free fluid in the upper abdomen, particularly around the biliary tree can reduce the diagnostic yield of an MRCP as can reduced filling of the bile ducts due to compromised liver function (24). Often, a combination of these non-invasive modalities is necessary for the precise delineation of a biliary injury.

Endoscopic retrograde cholangio-pancreatography

ERCP is rarely the first investigation of choice for suspected biliary trauma and is almost invariably preceded by one or more of the cross-sectional imaging modalities described previously. However, ERCP provides excellent detailed images of the biliary tree and, with the ability to instil contrast with balloon occlusion, will identify the site and the extent of injury in virtually all cases. It can be performed after a trauma laparotomy where a definitive repair to a suspected injury has not been possible. It may however not be feasible or safe to perform an ERCP in the event of an associated high-grade duodenal trauma and there are well-known complications associated with the ERCP procedure *per se* including pancreatitis and duodenal perforation. Nevertheless, complications are relatively uncommon and ERCP is an acceptable procedure in the context of a trauma setting. There are no available studies examining different modalities following biliary trauma which compare the diagnostic accuracy of ERCP with MRCP or scintigraphy.

The major advantage of ERCP, over non-invasive investigations, is its potential therapeutic value. A significant number of biliary injuries are now managed conservatively with ERCP playing a major role in the overall management of biliary trauma. Sphincterotomy performed at ERCP enables and maintains decompression of the biliary tree and this, in itself, can either be a definitive management or an adjunct to definitive repair. Upon identification of the injury, if a stent can be placed across the site of leak, it can be controlled to a substantial extent and in many cases, is the only treatment necessary in both the short- and long-term (28).

Percutaneous transhepatic cholangiography

PTC has a very limited role in the diagnosis and acute management of biliary trauma. It could potentially be used in the event of a failed cannulation at ERCP, but non-invasive cross-sectional imaging is much safer. Moreover, in the event of a major ductal injury or free abdominal bile leak, the intrahepatic ducts are usually collapsed rendering safe access to the biliary tract difficult.

MANAGEMENT

Management of traumatic biliary injuries differs considerably from the treatment of those which are iatrogenic. The initial management of biliary trauma largely follows the general principles of trauma management and is dictated by the general condition of the patient and associated organ injuries. The definitive management is then further determined by the injury severity scale. Patients with any WSES Class IV severity trauma need an emergency laparotomy which is then performed with the usual principles of damage-control surgery. Even when biliary injuries are recognized, definitive repair is often not possible (technically or due to the patient's condition) or not advised in presence of shock due to suboptimal short- and long-term results (29).

Gallbladder injury

In the setting of a laparotomy, conservative management could potentially be tried for a minor contusion (AAST Grade I). Although cholecystography was tried historically, a cholecystectomy is the safest, simplest and most expeditious treatment and can be performed either at the initial laparotomy or during definitive surgery (10,15). In a non-operative setting, patients with gallbladder contusions or haematomas without perforation can be managed conservatively.

Common bile duct and common hepatic duct injuries

Major CBD and CHD injuries (AAST Grade IV and V) are most frequently encountered in the setting of major abdominal trauma with haemodynamic instability (WSES Class IV). The optimum initial management in such situations is controlled drainage with large drains in the subhepatic area. A T-tube may be used as the definitive treatment if the initial tangential wall loss is <50% but delayed biliary strictures occur and often present at a later stage (2,30). The definitive management for a complete transection or major wall loss of the CBD/CHD is a Roux-en-Y hepaticojejunostomy. If there is an associated, major hepatic artery injury, a high repair such as a Hepp–Couinaud repair offers the best chance of long-term anastomotic patency (1,2,9).

Patients with biliary trauma initially managed non-operatively and in whom the trauma has gone unrecognized despite a laparotomy, typically present with bile leaks, bilomas or even biliary peritonitis. Suspected bilomas and leaks should be diagnosed on a CT scan and initially drained percutaneously. In many patients with low-volume or self-resolving bile leaks, no further procedures or interventions are needed and up to one third of injuries can be treated expectantly (6,9,15). In patients with persistent and high-volume leaks, ERCP is the investigation and treatment of choice in combination, as needed, with other investigations such as an MRCP or rarely these days, biliary scintigraphy. Endoscopic sphincterotomy alone usually settles some of these leaks but particularly when there is tangential wall loss, stenting may be necessary.

Failure of non-operative management needs surgical reconstruction at the appropriate time. A formal biliary disconnection and a Roux-en-Y hepaticojejunostomy is the treatment of choice and in patients with complete transection of the bile duct initially managed conservatively, a formal reconstruction is necessary. End-to-end primary anastomosis may be attempted in selected cases with minimal length and circumferential loss and good vascularity (31) although, in the majority, a Roux-en-Y hepaticojejunostomy is the treatment of choice.

Segmental ductal injuries

These injuries are fortunately even rarer as they can be difficult to manage. The basic principles are similar to the management of CBD/CHD injuries. Definitive surgery is rarely possible at the initial damage-control laparotomy and a significant number of these are associated with major central liver injury. At definitive surgery, minor leaks can be managed by suture repair over a stent or T-tube, if feasible. Occasionally, a formal ductal hepaticojejunostomy may be possible. In difficult situations, ligation of the sectoral duct may be the safest option, although this not infrequently leads to delayed complications such as segmental liver atrophy with or without recurrent biliary sepsis (3,28).

FOLLOW-UP AND MANAGEMENT OF DELAYED COMPLICATIONS

Follow-up after any biliary injury is usually symptom directed. Injuries managed conservatively alone with no luminal loss rarely have long-term complications. Luminal compromise associated with primary closure, T-tube repairs or endoscopic stenting can lead to delayed stricture formation similar to that seen with post cholecystectomy bile duct injuries and their management follows similar principles. Non-operative interventional management with ERCP and stricture dilatation is successful in a significant number of patients. In others where endoscopic management has not been successful,

a formal hepaticojejunostomy is the treatment of choice. Likewise, patients who have already undergone a definitive hepaticojejunostomy may present with recurrent cholangitis and anastomotic strictures which can be treated initially with PTC dilatations or revision of the anastomosis after failed non-operative management (32,33). In some instances, recurrent episodes of sepsis and biliary obstruction lead to secondary biliary cirrhosis and liver failure. In general, long-term outcomes are predominantly related to the primary success of repair and maintenance of patency (32).

SUMMARY

Traumatic biliary injuries are quite rare and make up only about 0.1% of all trauma cases. The vast majority of biliary trauma is associated with other abdominal organ injuries, particularly, the liver and pancreaticoduodenal complex.

Biliary trauma is classified according to the AAST and WSES scoring systems. The main bile duct is the most frequently injured part, followed by the gallbladder and then segmental extrahepatic ducts. Patients may present immediately, shortly following the injury or at a later stage due to insidious complications and the mode of presentation will vary widely. Diagnosis and precise delineation of the extent and morphology of biliary trauma is frequently challenging. Signs and symptoms may be subtle, and diagnosis relies on a variety of radiological investigations and interventional procedures.

Management is usually dictated by associated injuries and the mode of presentation. Early diagnosis, control of other injuries and definitive repair at the optimum time are important to achieve optimal outcomes. Conservative or non-operative management is usually very successful in Grade I–III injuries whereas Grade IV–V injuries and patients with failed non-operative treatment need surgical repair, or more commonly biliary diversion. Patients suffering from biliary trauma need ongoing follow-up and often experience significant delayed complications and long-term morbidity.

REFERENCES

1. Sawaya DE, Johnson LW, Sittig K, et al. Iatrogenic and noniatrogenic extrahepatic biliary tract injuries: A multi-institutional review. *Am Surg* 2001;**67(5)**:473–7.
2. Thomson BNJ, Nardino B, Gumm K, et al. Management of blunt and penetrating biliary tract trauma. *J Trauma Acute Care Surg* 2012;**72(6)**:1620–5.
3. Soukup ES, Russell KW, Metzger R, et al. Treatment and outcome of traumatic biliary injuries in children. *J Pediatr Surg* 2014;**49(2)**:345–8.
4. Parks RW, Diamond T. Non-surgical trauma to the extrahepatic biliary tract. *Br J Surg* 1995;**82(10)**:1303–10.
5. Bade PG, Thomson SR, Hirshberg A, Robbs JV. Surgical options in traumatic injury to the extrahepatic biliary tract. *Br J Surg* 1989;**76(3)**:256–8.

6. Hommes M, Nicol AJ, Navsaria PH, et al. Management of biliary complications in 412 patients with liver injuries. *J Trauma Acute Care Surg* 2014;**77(3)**:448–51.

7. Mishra PK, Saluja SS, Nag HH, et al. Isolated extrahepatic bile duct injury after blunt trauma abdomen. *Am Surg* 2012;**78(9)**:1014–6.

8. Balzarotti R, Cimbanassi S, Chiara O et al. Isolated extrahepatic bile duct rupture: A rare consequence of blunt abdominal trauma. Case report and review of the literature. *World J Emerg Surg WJES* 2012;**7(1)**:16.

9. Zakaria HM, Oteem A, Gaballa NK, et al. Risk factors and management of different types of biliary injuries in blunt abdominal trauma: Single-center retrospective cohort study. *Ann Med Surg* 2020;**52**:36–43.

10. Ball CG, Dixon E, Kirkpatrick AW, et al. A decade of experience with injuries to the gallbladder. *J Trauma Manag Outcomes* 2010;**4**:3.

11. Sharma O. Blunt gallbladder injuries: Presentation of twenty-two cases with review of the literature. *J Trauma* 1995;**39(3)**:576–80.

12. Rydell WB. Complete transection of the common bile duct due to blunt abdominal trauma. *Arch Surg* 1970;**100(6)**:724–8.

13. Andriulli A, Loperfido S, Napolitano G, et al. Incidence rates of post-ERCP complications: A systematic survey of prospective studies. *Am J Gastroenterol* 2007;**102(8)**:1781–8.

14. Moore EE, Jurkovich GJ, Knudson MM, et al. Organ injury scaling. VI: Extrahepatic biliary, esophagus, stomach, vulva, vagina, uterus (nonpregnant), uterus (pregnant), fallopian tube, and ovary. *J Trauma* 1995;**39(6)**:1069–70.

15. Coccolini F, Kobayashi L, Kluger Y, et al. Duodeno-pancreatic and extrahepatic biliary tree trauma: WSES-AAST guidelines. *World J Emerg Surg WJES* 2019;**14**:56.

16. Dadoukis J, Prousalidis J, Botsios D, et al. External biliary fistula. *HPB Surg* 1998;**10(6)**:375–7.

17. Vezakis A, Fragulidis G, Polydorou A. Endoscopic retrograde cholangiopancreatography-related perforations: Diagnosis and management. *World J Gastrointest Endosc* 2015;**7(14)**:1135–41.

18. Mohan BP, Shakhatreh M, Garg R, et al. Efficacy and safety of endoscopic ultrasound-guided choledochoduodenostomy: A systematic review and meta-analysis. *J Clin Gastroenterol* 2019;**53(4)**:243–50.

19. Gupta A, Stuhlfaut JW, Fleming KW, et al. Blunt trauma of the pancreas and biliary tract: A multimodality imaging approach to diagnosis. *Radiogr Rev Publ Radiol Soc N Am Inc* 2004;**24(5)**:1381–95.

20. Wahl WL, Brandt M-M, Hemmila MR, Arbabi S. Diagnosis and management of bile leaks after blunt liver injury. *Surgery* 2005;**138(4)**:742–7.

21. Körner M, Krötz MM, Degenhart C, et al. Current role of emergency US in patients with major trauma *Radiographics* 2008;**28(1)**:225–42.

22. Wittenberg A, Minotti AJ. CT diagnosis of traumatic gallbladder injury. *AJR Am J Roentgenol* 2005;**185(6)**:1573–4.

23. Elbanna KY, Mohammed MF, Huang S-C, Mak D, et al. Delayed manifestations of abdominal trauma: Follow-up abdominopelvic CT in posttraumatic patients. *Abdom Radiol N Y* 2018;**43(7)**:1642–55.

24. Hyodo T, Kumano S, Kushihata F, et al. CT and MR cholangiography: Advantages and pitfalls in perioperative evaluation of biliary tree. *Br J Radiol* 2012;**85(1015)**:887–96.

25. Melamud K, LeBedis CA, Anderson SW, Soto JA. Biliary imaging: Multimodality approach to imaging of biliary injuries and their complications. *Radiographics* 2014;**34(3)**:613–23.

26. Kousik V, Bhattacharya A, Yadav TD, Mittal BR. Hepatobiliary scintigraphy-role in preliminary diagnosis and management of biliary tract injuries. *Clin Nucl Med* 2020;**45(1)**:e1–7.

27. Kantarcı M, Pirimoglu B, Karabulut N, et al. Non-invasive detection of biliary leaks using Gd-EOB-DTPA-enhanced MR cholangiography: Comparison with T2-weighted MR cholangiography. *Eur Radiol* 2013;**23(10)**:2713–22.

28. Jaik NP, Hoey BA, Stawicki SP. Evolving role of endoscopic retrograde cholangiopancreatography in management of extrahepatic hepatic ductal injuries due to blunt trauma: Diagnostic and treatment algorithms. *HPB Surg* 2008;**2008**:259141.

29. Thomson BNJ, Parks RW, Madhavan KK, et al. Early specialist repair of biliary injury. *Br J Surg* 2006;**93(2)**:216–20.

30. Feliciano DV. Biliary injuries as a result of blunt and penetrating trauma. *Surg Clin North Am* 1994;**74(4)**:897–907.

31. Jabłonska B. End-to-end ductal anastomosis in biliary reconstruction: Indications and limitations. *Can J Surg* 2014;**57(4)**:271–7.

32. Cho JY, Baron TH, Carr-Locke DL, et al. Proposed standards for reporting outcomes of treating biliary injuries. *HPB* 2018;**20(4)**:370–8.

33. Booij KAC, Coelen RJ, de Reuver PR, et al. Long-term follow-up and risk factors for strictures after hepaticojejunostomy for bile duct injury: An analysis of surgical and percutaneous treatment in a tertiary center. *Surgery* 2018;**163(5)**:1121–7.

Chapter 28

Aneurysms and Arterio-Venous Fistulae

Balaji Mahendran and Colin Wilson

INTRODUCTION

Abdominal aneurysms were previously considered uncommon but are increasingly diagnosed due to an ageing population and the availability of cross-sectional imaging. The presentation of such lesions is often incidental. In this chapter we will consider both true aneurysms (involving all vascular layers) and pseudoaneurysms, defined as disruptions in arterial wall continuity with patent flow in a defined space beyond the vessel walls. These conditions are associated with significant mortality rates, especially upon rupture.

The true incidence of such aneurysms is unknown but they have been reported to be between 0.01–2% (1). The most commonly reported site for a visceral aneurysm is the splenic artery (60–80%), followed by the hepatic artery (14–20%), and the superior mesenteric artery (5–7%) (1–3). The prevalence of the different locations of aneurysms are shown in *Table 28.1*. The aetiology of these aneurysms is not fully understood, but there are several known risk factors that can influence their formation. Cardiovascular risk factors (atherosclerosis, smoking history, previous myocardial infarctions) are always important to elicit in the patient's history, as they play an important role in the pathophysiology of these cases.

Complications of aneurysms are typically haemorrhagic and dramatic, although occlusion secondary to thrombosis or dissection can also occur leading to distal ischaemia. 'Herald' bleeds with pain and hypotension followed by a period of stability can portend more devastating sequelae. In most cases of arterial rupture, permissive hypotensive resuscitation is the most advisable immediate management. Definitive repair, in the current and future era of complex interventional radiological facilities, is often provided by an expedient and accurate endovascular approach, although there are notable exceptions. In all cases, contrast angiography and close communication between radiologists, vascular and hepatobiliary surgeons are essential to plan successful management.

RISK FACTORS

Numerically most aneurysms and arterio-venous (AV) malformations related to the pancreas and spleen are the consequence of pancreatitis and represent the result of chronic active inflammation degrading the integrity of the arterial wall. In the older population, atherosclerotic damage to the vessel wall is a common cause. However, there are rare inherited syndromes that can lead to multiple true aneurysms and in addition, peripheral vascular disease can also manifest with true aneurysms that require surgical attention. Causal factors of these aneurysms are listed in *Table 28.2*. Concomitant aneurysms are subsequently discovered in 33–46% of diagnosed aneurysms, including the thoraco-abdominal aorta, iliac and intracranial arteries (4,5).

Table 28.1 Relative prevalence of visceral artery aneurysms

Aneurysm location	Relative prevalence
Splenic artery	60–80%
Hepatic artery	14–20%
Superior mesenteric artery	5–7%
Gastric artery	4%
Coeliac artery	3–4%
Pancreaticoduodenal artery	2%
Gastroduodenal artery	1.5%
Inferior mesenteric artery	<1%
Renal artery	<0.1%

Table 28.2 Risk factors leading to the formation of aneurysms

- Atherosclerosis
- Cigarette use
- Diabetes mellitus
- Infection/chronic inflammation
- Chronic pancreatitis
- Abdominal trauma
- Connective tissue disorders and congenital diseases (Marfan syndrome, Ehlers–Danlos syndrome, von Recklinghausen disease, Behçet disease)
- Conditions causing increased flow through vessels (pregnancy, portal hypertension)
- Pregnancy
- Segmental arterial mediolysis (SAM)
- Coeliac axis stenosis

DOI: 10.1201/9781003080060-28

Segmental arterial mediolysis (SAM) is a rare, non-atherosclerotic, non-inflammatory arteriopathy, commonly found in the middle-aged and elderly population. It is characterized by lysis of the smooth muscle of the outer media of the arterial wall. This commonly affects the medium-sized branches of the superior mesenteric artery and there is some histological similarity to fibromuscular dysplasia, but the lesion distribution and clinical features are characteristic.

There are no gender, or age differences, in the distribution of these aneurysms. Whilst there is no recognized age distribution in the incidence, the pathophysiology of aneurysms differs according to the age of the patient. Younger patients are more likely to have connective tissue disorders while older patients are more likely to have a disease process driven by underlying endothelial damage due to atherosclerotic disease.

A further subgroup of patients has an established link between coeliac axis stenosis and pancreaticoduodenal (PDA) aneurysms, with 50–80% of PDA aneurysms associated with coeliac axis stenosis (6). This is likely due to the hyperkinetic flow through the pancreaticoduodenal arcade due to the shift of blood from the coeliac axis to the superior mesenteric artery branches in the presence of stenosis (6). This subset of aneurysms differs slightly in that there seems to be a lower risk of rupture compared with other types (7).

Pregnancy

A significant number of aneurysms are seen in multiparous, young pregnant women, likely due to the effect of oestrogen, progestogen and relaxin on the vessel wall (8,9). Histology may reveal sub-endothelial thickening, medial fibrodysplasia and glycosaminoglycan accumulation in the subintimal and medial layers (10,11). These aneurysms are more likely to rupture, and the risk of rupture not only poses a threat to the patient but to the unborn child as well. Maternal mortality can be between 70–75%, whilst the fetal mortality rate can be up to 95% (9). These aneurysms are normally diagnosed at the point of rupture however, some are diagnosed on routine ultrasound scans, which can then be confirmed through further cross-sectional imaging. Given the high-mortality risk, the decision to operate should be made expediently in consultation with the obstetric, neonatology and vascular/general surgical teams.

Liver biopsy and other hepatic procedures

Iatrogenic injury to the liver either by direct puncture for biopsy, portal venous embolization (*Figure 28.1*) or more commonly cholangiography can lead to arterial complications demanding immediate re-intervention. Mortality risks associated with these procedures are almost directly related to the risks of arterial injury and delayed diagnosis. Often the initial clinical picture is subtle and elusive, but signs such as hypotension and capsular pain if inappropriate should suggest further investigation. Capsular rupture leads to the loss of tamponade and a large volume haemoperitoneum which demands immediate management.

Liver and pancreas transplant-related false aneurysms

Transplantation of the liver and pancreas is associated with an almost unique subset of aneurysmal complications, the mycotic visceral aneurysm. Fungi are by far the most common cause, although technical suture failure can also rarely be responsible (*Figure 28.2*). Graft pancreatitis, either secondary to ischaemia or rejection, has also been a leading pathogenic mechanism. A recent review in solid organ pancreatic transplantation cited an incidence of 8% (12). Graft biopsy to assess for allograft rejection can lead to arterio-venous (AV) malformations but this is relatively rare. This is one area of vascular surgery where definitive surgical management, rather than interventional radiology, is often the key to success. Whilst endovascular stent placement may seem the most straightforward solution in the short-term, long-term this can lead to complicated problems with infected stent grafts eroding through compromised native vessels. Endovascular stent placement is often still considered in these patients, to avoid the morbidity of another major operation, however, there remains a significant risk of stent erosion through compromised native vessels (13).

ARTERIO-VENOUS FISTULAE

Arterio-venous fistulae (AVF) in the abdomen are generally caused by trauma to the related region but can also be due to iatrogenic trauma following biopsy or embolization. Hepato-portal fistulae (HPF) have also been

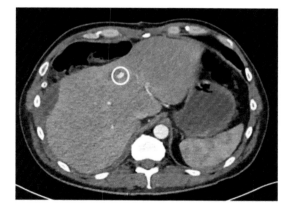

Figure 28.1 Intrahepatic aneurysm (white circle) diagnosed following a diagnostic procedure to biopsy the liver.

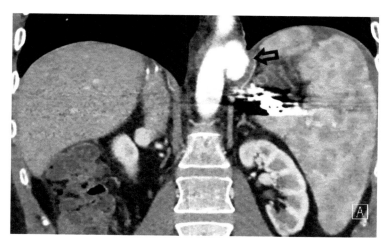

Figure 28.2 A transplant-related aneurysm (black arrow). This is likely a mycotic aneurysm – the transplanted liver has multiple hypoattenuating areas within the parenchyma which are probably abscesses from the translocation of the fungi.

reported following hepatic-artery aneurysm ruptures (14). Pancreatic AVFs are rare, and generally congenital, with pancreatitis being a rare causal pathology (15). The work-up of such cases would require the same investigations as discussed below, with intervention options including the same endovascular procedures, and in some cases, open resection of the affected segment.

Liver transplant false aneurysms are associated with conduits used to restore continuity between the aorta and the graft either in the supra-renal or infra-renal configuration. Specific risk factors associated with their development are biliary complications particularly bile leak, contamination of the transport preservation solution, requirement for augmented immunosuppression, for instance ABO incompatible or antibody-mediated rejection necessitating anti-thymocyte globulin utilization. Presentation can be dramatic or insidious with swinging pyrexia. Often re-transplant is required but removal of all infected material and sterilization of the operative field can prove impossible. In up to 20%, the re-graft will be affected by the same process and pragmatic decisions will need to be made in the context of organ demand and supply.

The situation is no less straightforward in pancreas transplantation, even though the pancreas graft can be explanted and the patient returned to insulin therapy with comparatively little short-term consequence. Most cases are due to fungal infection on the background of graft pancreatitis and pancreatectomy is the surgical option of choice with careful assessment of the arteriotomy and patch closure with biological patches, preferably autologous.

CLINICAL PRESENTATION

Hepatico-pancreatico-biliary (HPB) aneurysms of the abdomen are usually silent, but in the context of infection, pancreatic necrosis can be anticipated. Where symptoms are present, generalized abdominal pain with a peritonitic abdomen, including signs of shock and/or sepsis are all possible. The specific symptoms are directed by the function of the organ supplied by the aneurysmal vessel. Symptoms might be mistaken for other conditions, commonly an acute flare of pancreatitis, thereby making diagnosis based on history and examination alone difficult. Thrombotic occlusion of aneurysmal vessels or peripheral embolization of thrombi can cause end-organ ischaemia. This can lead to symptoms of post-prandial abdominal pain, or generalized abdominal pain. Ischaemic injury to the liver or ischaemic hepatitis may not classically present with abdominal pain, but with other symptoms including weakness, fatigue, oliguria and jaundice. Large coeliac artery aneurysms may cause compression of neighbouring structures, such as the stomach, duodenum and bile ducts (1). This may cause symptoms such as early satiety, post-prandial vomiting and episodes of jaundice.

Initial blood tests may reveal an element of inflammation and ischaemia including an elevation of C-reactive protein (CRP), the platelet count and lactate with a neutrophilia. However, none of these markers on their own would indicate the presence of an aneurysm, or a rupture.

In today's age of high-resolution cross-sectional imaging, a patient with undifferentiated abdominal pain requires expedient access to such imaging. Basic modalities such as abdominal X-ray or routine ultrasounds do not have a role in the diagnosis of aneurysms, however an ultrasound scan may incidentally notice an aneurysm or AVF. Computed tomography (CT) scans play a vital role in establishing the diagnosis in these cases.

IMAGING OF VASCULAR PATHOLOGY

The advent of CT scans has allowed for the planning of an aneurysm repair even in an emergency situation. An appropriate arterial phase is required to fully assess the aneurysm and plan surgery. Planning should take place in the presence of an interventional radiologist who is able to consider more minimally invasive options for repair. Routine 2D-CT imaging can be used to measure aneurysmal sizes, with more sophisticated 3D-reconstructed images allowing for better visualization of the aneurysm (*Figure 28.3a*).

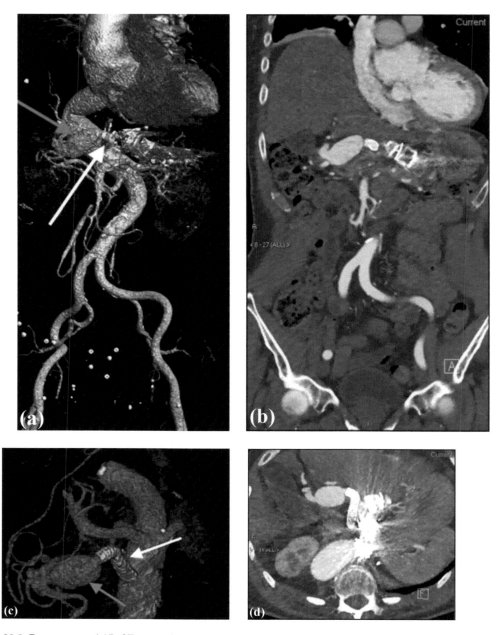

Figure 28.3 Reconstructed 3D-CT scan of a patient (a) with a previously stented (white arrow) common hepatic artery, who had presented with a subsequent distal aneurysmal segment (red arrow). CT angiogram (b) showing a common hepatic artery aneurysm that has been previously stented. A reconstructed 3D image is shown (c) and CT angiogram (d).

CT angiography

This is now the 'gold standard' imaging modality in most institutions. A routine CT scan with contrast is commonly performed in the porto-venous phase but this in itself is inadequate to appropriately diagnose aneurysms. If the clinical suspicion is high, a CT angiogram should be requested and even if not performed in the first instance, a CT angiogram should be done as part of the complete work up of the patient (*Figure 28.3b*).

MR angiography

Magnetic resonance angiography (MRA) scans can be preferred in certain situations. MRAs can reveal mild atherosclerotic disease better than CT angiograms, and do not routinely require intravenous contrast. Although MRAs take significantly longer to perform they have their role for patients where a CT scan is contraindicated, such as in pregnant women, or patients with an allergy or contraindication to the contrast medium used.

INDICATIONS FOR TREATMENT

Whilst most aneurysms are only diagnosed upon rupture and with the patient *in extremis*, incidental aneurysms should be carefully evaluated for repair. The current literature suggests a maximum aneurysmal diameter of 2–2.5 cm as the cut-off for elective intervention, with a more aggressive approach suggested for symptomatic true aneurysms, and for aneurysms with a higher risk of rupture (pancreaticoduodenal, gastroduodenal and branches of the hepatic artery) (5). Current guidelines suggest interval imaging at 2–3 years for aneurysms less than 2.5 cm may be considered although 6% of patients with asymptomatic aneurysms will require an intervention within 2 years and false or mycotic aneurysms should almost always be repaired (5). However, the authors would recommend a more nuanced approach, allowing for closer follow-up of such patients. Asymptomatic patients in whom such aneurysms have been fortuitously picked up should be kept under closer follow-up, with their first follow-up scan performed at 1 year. Aneurysms over 1.5 cm would have yearly cross-sectional imaging in the authors' unit. Recipients of abdominal organ transplants are more likely to benefit from treatment of aneurysms at any diameter. There is no evidence that aneurysm calcification is a protective factor that reduces the risk of rupture.

MINIMALLY INVASIVE PROCEDURES

Endovascular therapy options offer major benefits to high-risk patients, including those with multiple comorbidities and previous abdominal surgery. Other patients might opt for an endovascular treatment option for their aneurysms, after a thorough consent process. Endovascular options include embolization or stenting

of the target vessel (*Figure 28.3c,d*). The technique to be selected depends on the necessity of preserving the parent artery, and anatomical considerations including the shape and type of the aneurysm (with regards to the neck) and the tortuosity of the vessel. There is a reported high success rate with such treatment options, with up to 95.2% of cases treated endovascularly being considered a technical success and only 1.8% of such cases requiring conversion to an open surgical approach (16).

Various techniques have been described and used successfully, including deployment of coils and vascular plugs, injection of liquid embolic agents, placement of covered or flow-limiting stents, and percutaneous injection of thrombin. Successful embolization requires occlusion of all inflow and outflow arteries, which may happen in the form of occlusion of the distal and proximal arteries along with coil packing of the aneurysmal segment. Embolization using liquid agents, whilst a feasible technique, poses an increased risk of distal ischaemia making the procedure more technically challenging and potentially hazardous.

Another common endovascular option is the use of self-expanding stents within the aneurysm, which have provided good results with up to 96% success rate in elective cases and an 84% success rate in emergency cases (17). Covered stents are also a useful option for iatrogenic pseudoaneurysms of the hepatic arteries, splenic artery, or gastroduodenal artery, as there is a significant risk of liver failure secondary to ischaemia upon coil embolization of these vessels. There are nevertheless limitations to this technique, especially as current delivery systems for these stents are not small or flexible enough to negotiate the complex arterial anatomy commonly found in this region. Covered stents also require a straight landing-zone with reduced tortuosity as with the renal arteries. In the future, novel devices with smaller delivery systems and more flexible stent grafts are likely to make this technique appropriate for more patients.

The decision to perform an endovascular procedure to treat an aneurysm should take into account the need for arterial reconstruction (either primary or delayed). The spleen receives an abundant collateral supply from the short gastric arteries and a pure coil embolization of a splenic artery aneurysm would be a feasible option. However, aneurysms of the proper hepatic artery, or left or right hepatic artery which are distal to the gastroduodenal artery are unlikely to be amenable to an endovascular repair due to the lack of collateral supply to the liver. In such cases, a surgical repair with reconstruction or a bypass of the aneurysmal segment should be considered.

SURGICAL INTERVENTION

Prior to the advent of evidence-based interventional radiology, open repair was considered the standard treatment option. Open procedures allow for clear visualization of the condition of the end organ prior to deciding upon the best course of action and avoids more serious postoperative sequelae. There are several options available to the operating surgeon when faced with an aneurysm, the advantages and disadvantages of which will be discussed here.

The most common indication for an operative approach to these aneurysms is a rupture. Whilst more of these cases can still be managed using an endovascular approach, the unstable patient will require an operation. In a truly unstable patient who is hypotensive and tachycardic with a significant hypovolaemia response, damage control laparotomy principles apply. Gaining proximal and distal control is of utmost importance. Subsequently restoring arterial continuity can be considered, especially in the case of a distal hepatic-artery aneurysm. The common hepatic artery (CHA) can be ligated if there is adequate collateral circulation from the pancreaticoduodenal and gastroduodenal arteries (*Figure 28.4*). Splenic artery aneurysms can generally be ligated, with the additional option of a splenectomy in an emergency. Splenectomy should certainly be considered when the aneurysm is found in the branches close to the splenic hilum, and this can be performed laparoscopically in the elective situation. It should be

mentioned that the majority of aneurysms that are operated on are true aneurysms. False aneurysms, commonly occurring after trauma or inflammatory conditions, will require tying off if not amenable to endovascular techniques in the first instance.

The reconstruction of the artery can be achieved either by performing a bypass procedure, or an aneurysmectomy with an end-to-end anastomosis which is technically feasible when the artery is of sufficient length. Aneurysmectomy can also be followed by an interposition graft, either with a vein or prosthetic material. Prosthetic interposition grafts have a higher risk of infection and therefore are normally only considered in the elective setting and vein grafts are preferred. Bypassing the aneurysm will reduce the risk of rupture by reducing the flow through the aneurysmal segment. Hepatic artery aneurysms requiring continuity of flow are amenable to bypass procedures, using whichever conduit is available. The proximal anastomosis can be performed on a number of arteries, including the aorta, iliac, splenic and renal arteries. A reno-hepatic bypass, from the right renal artery is technically simple and offers the highest chance of success, due to the diameters of the vessels involved, and the short distance from the right renal artery to the hepatic artery (18). When the right or left extra-hepatic arteries are involved, the omental artery can be used to form an end-to-end anastomosis without complicating the supply to the omentum (3).

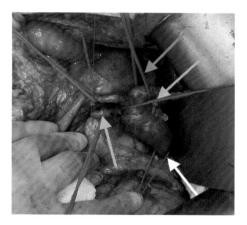

Figure 28.4 Intraoperative image of an open CHA aneurysm repair. This is the same patient from the scans shown in *Figure 28.3*. There are rubber slings placed around important landmarks; including the neck of the aneurysm beyond the previously stented segment (white arrow), below the bifurcation of the CHA into the hepatic artery proper and right gastric artery (orange arrow), hepatic artery proper (blue arrow), right gastric artery (pink arrow) and the gastroduodenal artery (green arrow). After careful assessment of the retrograde supply to the branches through the gastroduodenal artery, the decision was made to ligate the aneurysmal segment. The patient required a re-look laparotomy the following day for persistent hypotension, which revealed no further bleeding or ischaemic segments. The patient was then subsequently discharged at day 7, and kept on follow-up.

SUMMARY

Aneurysms and fistulae of the visceral arteries around the liver and pancreas are a rare phenomenon with the majority of cases due to complications following an inflammatory process such as pancreatitis. However, other aetiologies also contribute to the pathophysiology of these aneurysms, including iatrogenic injury, trauma, and underlying soft-tissue disorders but irrespective of the aetiology they have devastating sequelae if not treated appropriately. The relative rarity of this condition may render clinicians oblivious to their presence and a high index of suspicion is required to avoid overlooking them. A large proportion of these cases present as an emergency after rupture, requiring urgent intervention. Some patients (pregnant women) require intervention regardless of the presence of symptoms, as do aneurysms over 2–2.5 cm in diameter. The availability of advanced cross-sectional imaging facilitates the diagnosis, and multidisciplinary care with vascular and HPB surgeons and radiologists is key. Minimally invasive options including embolization and stenting, enabled by advances in interventional radiology has allowed more patients to be afforded treatment, with open surgery as a viable alternative in a carefully selected patient population. Careful follow-up is also required to prevent further propagation of aneurysms and to enable early intervention where appropriate.

REFERENCES

1. Juntermanns B, Bernheim J, Karaindros K, Walensi M, Hoffmann J. Visceral artery aneurysms. *Gefässchirurgie* 2018;**23(Suppl 1)**:19–22.
2. Sousa J, Costa D, Mansilha A. Visceral artery aneurysms: review on indications and current treatment strategies. *Int Angio* 2019;**38(5)**:381–94.
3. Obara H, Kentaro M, Inoue M, Kitagawa Y. Current management strategies for visceral artery aneurysms: an overview. *Surg Today* 2020;**50(1)**:38–49.
4. Erben Y, Brownstein AJ, Rajaee S, Li Y, Rizzo JA. Natural history and management of splanchnic artery aneurysms in a single tertiary referral center. *J Vasc Surg* 2018;**68(4)**:1079–87.
5. Björck M, Koelemay M, Acosta S, Goncalves FB, Kölbel T, Kolkman JJ, et al. Management of the diseases of mesenteric arteries and veins clinical practice guidelines of the European Society of Vascular Surgery (ESVS). *Eur J Vasc Endovasc Surg* 2017;**53(4)**:460–510.
6. Mano Y, Takehara Y, Sakaguchi T, Alley MT, Isoda H, Shimizu T, et al. Hemodynamic assessment of celiaco-mesenteric anastomosis in patients with pancreaticoduodenal artery aneurysm concomitant with celiac artery occlusion using flow-sensitive four-dimensional magnetic resonance imaging. *Eur J Vasc Endovasc Surg* 2013;**46(3)**:321–8.
7. Suzuki K, Kashimura H, Sato M, Hassan M, Yokota H, Nakahara A. Pancreaticoduodenal artery aneurysms associated with celiac axis stenosis due to compression by median arcuate ligament and celiac plexus. *J Gastroenterol* 1998;**33**:434–8.
8. Mattar SG, Lumsden AB. The of splenic artery aneurysms: Experience with 23 Cases. *Am J Surg* 1995;**169(6)**:580–4.
9. Sadat U, Dar O, Walsh S, Varty K. Splenic artery aneurysms in pregnancy: A systematic review. *Int J Surg* 2008;**6**:261–5.
10. Selo-Ojeme D, Welch C. Review: Spontaneous rupture of splenic artery aneurysm in pregnancy. *Eur J Obstet Gynaecol Reprod Biol* 2003;**109(2)**:124–7.
11. Abbas M, Stone W, Fowl R, Gloviczki P, Oldenburg WA, Pariolero P, et al. Splenic artery aneurysms: Two decades experience at Mayo clinic. *Ann Vasc Surg* 2002;**16(4)**:442–9.
12. Lubezky N, Goykhman Y, Nakache R, Kessler A. Early and late presentations of graft arterial pseudoaneurysm following pancreatic transplantation. *World J Surg* 2013;**37**:1430–7.
13. Gao X, de Jonge J, Verhagen H, Dinkelaar W, ten Raa S, van Rijn MJ. Unsuccessful stent graft repair of a hepatic artery aneurysm presenting with haemobilia: Case report and comprehensive literature review. *EJVES VF* 2021;**52**:30–6.
14. Fagot H, Guieu M, Zemour J, Pierre S. Intra-hepatic arterio-venous fistula after penetrating liver injury. *J Visc Surg* 2020;**157**:453–4.
15. Holsbeeck A Van, Dalle I, Geldof K, Verhaeghe L, Ramboer K. Acquired pancreatic arteriovenous malformation. *J Belgian Soc Radiol* 2015;**99(1)**:37–41.
16. Hogendoorn W, Lavida A, Hunink MGM. Open repair, endovascular repair, and conservative management of true splenic artery aneurysms. *J Vasc Surg* 2014;**60(6)**:1667–76.e1.
17. Venturini M, Marra P, Colombo M, Panzeri M, Agostini G, Balzano G, et al. Endovascular repair of 40 visceral artery aneurysms and pseudoaneurysms with the viabahn stent-graft: Technical Aspects, clinical outcome and mid-term patency. *Cardiovasc Intervent Radiol* 2018;**41(3)**:385–97.
18. Bowens NM, Woo EY, Fairman RM. Reno-hepatic artery bypass for an inferior pancreaticoduodenal artery aneurysm with associated celiac occlusion. *J Vasc Surg* 2011;**53(6)**:1696–8.

Chapter 29

Control of Iatrogenic Bleeding in Hepatobiliary Surgery

Jaekeun Kim, Steven C. Stain and Mohamed E. Akoad

INTRODUCTION

Significant bleeding during hepato-biliary surgery (HBS) is associated with increased morbidity and mortality, and successful control of iatrogenic bleeding is essential for a successful procedure. Although there is no way to guarantee that unexpected bleeding will not occur, several steps can be taken to reduce the risk. Preoperative planning and intraoperative prevention are fundamental, and early detection and control are essential steps for a good outcome.

The mechanisms of bleeding in HBS are complex and include the patients' pre-existing comorbidities, use of anticoagulation or antiplatelet agents, the type of procedure, and coagulopathy related to the hepatic function that affects the ability to maintain normal haemostasis (1). A multidisciplinary approach including preoperative risk stratification, surgical planning, appropriate consultations and perioperative management is critical (2). During the operation, the surgical field needs to be optimized and meticulous dissection and atraumatic tissue handling are mandatory to prevent iatrogenic bleeding.

Despite adherence to these principles, unexpected bleeding may occur, and the surgical team must be ready to control bleeding and minimize blood loss.

This chapter reviews the general principles and steps needed to manage iatrogenic bleeding in HBS.

GENERAL PRINCIPLES OF BLEEDING CONTROL

Preoperative considerations

Preparation and prevention are the keys to the management of bleeding. Preoperatively, a detailed history should be obtained, the use of anticoagulants or antiplatelet preparations should be evaluated, and comorbidities that will impact operative and postoperative course should be elucidated. Previous operative reports for surgical procedures in the upper abdomen should be reviewed. Consultation with cardiology and pulmonary services might be required to stratify operative risk, and this should be discussed with the anaesthetic team before the operation. Imaging studies should be thoroughly reviewed and compared to previous studies if available. Abnormal and variant anatomy or proximity of the planned surgical resection to major blood vessels should be clearly delineated. If major vascular resection or reconstruction is anticipated, it is advised to consult with vascular surgeons. The surgical plan should be clearly shared with the anaesthetic team, operating room staff and surgical assistants. The surgeon should request operating room staff have the specific instruments and devices that may be needed for the procedure available. Communication with the blood bank is essential to ensure blood products are available.

Operative general consideration

Invasive monitoring with an arterial line and central-venous catheter is often required and allows for continuous assessment of volume status and rapid resuscitation when needed. Relevant images should be displayed for quick access during surgery. Equipment should be checked, and the availability of blood products confirmed. During the surgical pause or timeout, a final check of the surgical plan should be outlined with the team. The surgical field needs to be exposed under appropriate lighting. Meticulous dissection and atraumatic tissue handling are mandatory to prevent and minimize bleeding. Awareness of vascular anomalies is essential to avoid iatrogenic injury and bleeding. Intraoperative ultrasound might be required to map vasculature and define resection planes. The use of table mounting retractors such as the Omni®, Thompson®, or Bookwalter® retractors are crucial in gaining adequate exposure in open cases. The use of headlights is a helpful adjunct in hepato-pancreatico-biliary (HPB) surgical cases.

Initial complete mobilization of structures is important to properly control and manage unexpected bleeding. In cases of partial hepatectomies, complete mobilization of the lobe or segment to be resected should be performed prior to starting the parenchymal transection. If bleeding is encountered, applying pressure to the mobilized lobe may temporarily control the bleeding allowing preparation for more definitive repair. Similarly, Kocherization of the duodenum allows the surgeon to place the hand behind the portal vein (PV), which is helpful in temporarily controlling PV bleeding.

Suturing and knot tying need to be atraumatic. The needle should penetrate the tissues at 90° and rotate along the needle's curvature whenever placing sutures. The knot-tying should be square to avoid tissue injuries by excess pulling or contact with adjacent tissue when pushing down the knot. Each tightening thread needs to be parallel to the cut surface to avoid unnecessary tissue avulsion, especially when tying small venous branches during partial hepatectomy.

VARIANT ANATOMY

Familiarity with variant arterial and venous anatomy is essential to avoid inadvertent injury to these structures that can have catastrophic consequences.

Arterial anatomy and variants

The anatomy of the coeliac, superior mesenteric artery (SMA), and hepatic arteries can be quite variable. An accessory or replaced right hepatic-artery is reported in 10–30% in the general population. It originates from the SMA and is the first large branching artery from the SMA. When there is a replaced right hepatic artery (HA), the main or accessory cystic artery usually is a branch of that vessel (3,4) (*Figure 29.1*).

The accessory, or left replaced, HA is found in about 10–20% of the general population and usually originates from the left gastric artery. When the left replaced HA is present, 70% of the cases are accompanied by another arterial variant, such as the right replaced HA and middle HA. In most cases, variant hepatic vasculature can be easily identified preoperatively in contrast-enhanced cross-sectional imaging studies and intraoperatively these vessels can be identified by palpation. An accessory or replaced right HA can be easily identified by palpating around the hepatoduodenal ligament with index fingers and thumb and feeling for the pulsation posterior to the common bile duct. The accessory or replaced left HA can be found running along with the lesser omentum. In laparoscopic or robotic cases, these vessels may be visualized with the scope.

PORTAL VEIN AND THE VARIANTS

In standard or conventional anatomy, the PV originates at the confluence of the superior mesenteric vein (SMV) and the splenic vein at the level of the neck of the pancreas. PV variants have been reported in 20–35% of the patients and the most common variants are the anterior and posterior right portal vein branches originating directly from the main PV (PV trifurcation) (5). Rarely, the segment IV, PV-branch originates from the right anterior PV (*Figure 29.2*).

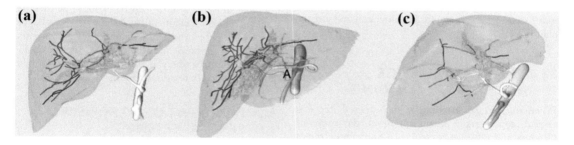

Figure 29.1 Illustration of standard anatomy of the hepatic artery (a). Variations include right replace HA from SMA (b) and left accessory HA from left gastric artery (c).

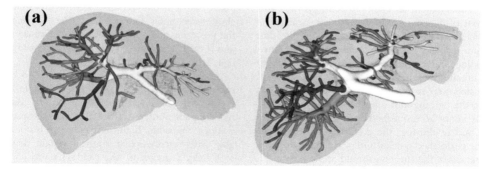

Figure 29.2 Illustration of standard portal vein anatomy (a). Note how the main portal bifurcates the right- and left-PV. Variation of trifurcation of the PV in (b). Note the main portal trifurcates the right-anterior- and right-posterior-, and left-PV.

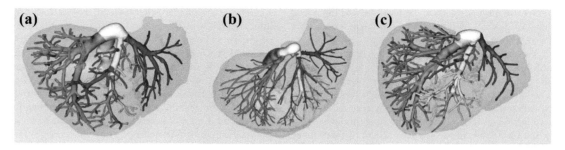

Figure 29.3 Illustration of standard HV anatomy (a). Variations include (b), where the right fissural vein drains to left- and middle-HV and (c) where the left- and middle-HV drains to the IVC separately.

Hepatic vein variations

The liver has three major draining hepatic veins (HV), the right, middle and left. A single right HV is present in 90% of cases on computed tomography (CT) evaluations (6). However, the presence of an accessory right-HV or inferior right-HV was previously under-reported in imaging studies and these veins have been found in about 25% of surgical patients (7) (*Figure 29.3*).

The left- and middle-HV join together for a common trunk in 70–73.5%, and 26.5% of the left-HV drained into inferior vena cava (IVC) (8, 9). These veins that drain extrahepatically into the IVC are less than 1 cm in length and most of the portion of the left-HV runs within the liver. Intraoperative ultrasound with, or without, marking on the surface of the liver helps more accurate assessment for HV direction and surgical planning (10).

STRATEGIES TO MANAGE INTRAOPERATIVE BLEEDING

When unexpected bleeding is encountered, the first critical step is rapid identification of the cause of bleeding and effective control (11). Sometimes, minor haemorrhage can progress to a significant bleeding diathesis. Therefore, indiscriminate and blind suturing should be avoided as it may cause more profound and complicated problems.

The management strategies depend on the cause and extent of bleeding (minor or major, arterial, or venous, localized or diffuse). Whenever major bleeding is encountered, the surgeon must temporarily control the bleeding and communicate with the anaesthetic team to initiate resuscitation.

The first step is to optimize the surgical field by adjusting the lighting and improving exposure. Sometimes this can be accomplished by simply extending the incision and readjusting the retractors. If the repair cannot be performed quickly and safely in laparoscopic or robotic cases, the surgeon should apply pressure to the bleeding area and temporarily control the bleeding before converting to an open approach.

The exposure of IVC, PV, SMA and infrarenal aorta is sometimes required to address iatrogenic bleeding not controlled by simple measures. It can be achieved by performing a right to medial visceral rotation (Cattell–Braasch manoeuvre) of the right colon with associated extended mobilization of the duodenum (Kocher). Exposing the retrohepatic IVC requires mobilization of the right hepatic lobe. The suprahepatic IVC can then be exposed by mobilizing the left lateral segment and being cleared above the HVs. The infrahepatic IVC can be exposed after mobilizing the right hepatic lobe and mobilization of the duodenum. Revealing the suprahepatic and infrahepatic IVC might be necessary in cases where total hepatic occlusion is required to control the bleeding.

The suprarenal aorta can be exposed by dividing the gastrohepatic ligament, mobilizing the esophagus, and dividing the crus of the diaphragm. Exposing the supracoeliac aorta or infrarenal aorta is necessary for the rare instances where an interposition graft from the aorta is needed to revascularize the HA or the SMA.

MANAGEMENT OF IATROGENIC ARTERIAL BLEEDING

Most of the iatrogenic arterial bleeding occurs from smaller arterial branches that can easily be controlled by ligating the vessel. Bleeding from injuries to the HA or its branches can be encountered during complex hilar resections but can also infrequently occur during cholecystectomies. During cholecystectomies, injury to the posterior cystic artery branch can cause bleeding and is easily controlled with the placement of a clip or ligation.

The right HA usually runs posterior to the common bile duct, but in 8.3%, it crosses anteriorly, where it can be mistaken for the cystic artery (12). Significant bleeding encountered from the HA requires repair whenever possible. If the surgical team is not comfortable with microvascular surgical repair, they should seek help. Ligation of the right HA will control the bleeding but might be complicated by bile duct strictures and the development of bilomas and intrahepatic abscesses. Bleeding from the coeliac artery can also be encountered during pancreatectomies. Repair with non-absorbable monofilament sutures should be used to control the bleeding while maintaining the continuity of the vessel, as ligation or narrowing of the coeliac artery can result in hepatic ischaemia. Bleeding from the SMA can occur during pancreaticoduodenectomy and should be repaired with monofilament sutures. Restoring the continuity of these vessels might require an end-to-end anastomosis and should be performed by experienced surgeons. Rarely interposition grafts from the supra-coeliac or infrarenal aorta will be needed.

MANAGEMENT OF IATROGENIC VENOUS BLEEDING

While most of the iatrogenic venous bleeding can be controlled with digital pressure and ligation or placement of sutures, iatrogenic injuries to major venous branches can be difficult to control. Intraoperative strategies to minimize bleeding during major parenchymal transection include a low CVP below 5 mmHg, fluid restriction, and permissive hypotension (13).

Hepatic venous bleeding can be encountered during liver mobilization or during parenchymal transection. Most of the bleeding from the hepatic parenchyma can simply be controlled with electrocautery or the argon beam coagulator and the application of topical haemostatic agents. Various haemostatic agents are available in the market and include oxidized regenerated cellulose, microporous polysaccharide spheres, and biological agents such as thrombin and fibrin. These are helpful to control bleeding with local compression during HPB surgery.

Bleeding from larger venous branches can be controlled with simple ligation or sutured with non-absorbable monofilament sutures. Excessive traction and pulling should be avoided while placing sutures on the cut surface of the liver as it can easily crack, resulting in more severe bleeding.

It is essential to dissect the lateral border of the IVC prior to dividing the short inferior HVs while mobilizing the liver. Clearing an adequate segment of the retrohepatic IVC is important for major hepatic resection and especially during the hanging manoeuver (14).

The retrocaval, short inferior-HVs, including the right, inferior-HV, caudate vein (draining from Spiegel's lobe), and short-HVs should be carefully dissected, and both sides of the short-HV to the vena cava and liver should be ligated or clipped, and the vessel divided. Sizable (larger than 3 mm) veins can be safely closed with transfixion and suture ligation. Dissection of the retrohepatic IVC can be treacherous, especially in patients with cirrhosis or in patients who have significant adhesions from prior operations, which may obscure plains and lead to injury. Sometimes attempts at controlling the bleeding from the IVC or its branches can make a tear worse, resulting in significant blood loss in a very

short time. If a large tear in the IVC is encountered, the patient should immediately be placed in Trendelenburg position to prevent a potentially fatal air embolism. Manual compression and placement of vascular clamps on the IVC below the injury can control the bleeding allowing for repair of the injury. If these manoeuvres fail, vascular occlusion should be attempted and is achieved by occlusion of the inflow (HA and PV) using a vascular clamp or Penrose drain and placing a clamp on the suprahepatic IVC and on the infrahepatic IVC above the renal veins. This can be accomplished rapidly and, in most instances, will control the bleeding and allow for resuscitation by the anaesthetic team and definitive repair.

The Pringle manoeuvre (temporal occlusion of the portal triad) provides total hepatic inflow occlusion (HA and PV) and can be helpful during parenchymal transection. A surgeon can perform the Pringle manoeuvre with the hand, vascular clamps, or a Penrose drain after opening the lesser sac. However, this method does not control bleeding from outflow vessels (hepatovenous back perfusion).

Intermittent Pringle manoeuvre for 15 mins and 5 mins off-clamp interval can be performed safely if the accumulated total ischaemic time is less than 120 mins. In a study by Man K et al., the intermittent Pringle manoeuvre group showed less blood loss than the no Pringle group, with no significant difference in postoperative complications (15). The clamping time has been reported from different authors with suggesting clamping times varying between 10–30 mins however, most reports allowing a reperfusion time of 5 mins or longer (16,17). The surgeon needs to be cautious as prolonged inflow occlusion can result in hepatic ischaemia and splanchnic congestion. Selective or hemi-hepatic vascular occlusion has been introduced to minimize ischaemia-reperfusion injury from total inflow occlusion as hemi-hepatic occlusion allows blood inflow to the contralateral hemi-liver. This technique was reported to be as effective as total hepatic inflow occlusion in terms of blood loss, but its impact on preserving hepatic function remains controversial (18).

Total hepatic vascular occlusion can be applied, as discussed above, to allow for control of bleeding from the IVC and it is also occasionally applied during resection of a large hepatic tumour or during a complex hepatectomy. In a report by Li et al., total vascular exclusion was associated with less blood loss and fewer complications than Pringle manoeuvre alone, with no difference in postoperative liver functions or hospital stay (19).

PV bleeding can result in exsanguinating haemorrhage and be difficult to control. Placing the index and middle fingers behind the PV is helpful in applying pressure to temporarily control the bleeding and allow for immediate repair of an unexpected injury. Most small bleeds from the PV are a result of avulsion of small PV tributaries and can be managed by carefully placing figure-of-eight or U stitches using non-absorbable monofilament sutures. Because the PV wall is often thin, too much traction can worsen the bleeding. If the tear is large and bleeding cannot be controlled with digital compression, either a side-biting clamp or proximal and distal clamps on the PV may be required. If bleeding is encountered from the confluence of the splenic and SMV during pancreaticoduodenectomies after transection of the pancreatic neck, clamps on both the SMV and splenic veins are needed to control the inflow. Once the bleeding is controlled, repair of the injury should be done. If it is noticed that the repair has narrowed the diameter of the PV to less than 50%, then PV reconstruction should be considered. Up to 2 cm of PV can be re-sected, and end-to-end anastomosis carried out without tension. When completing this type of repair, the sutures should be tied with an air knot to allow for expansion of the anastomosis (growth factor). A major PV injury has been reported to be associated with a mean blood loss of 5.6 L and 28% intraoperative mortality (20).

PV ligation to control bleeding should be avoided whenever possible. It is rarely required, has generally only been reported following significant injuries from trauma, and is associated with 60% in-hospital mortality (21).

MAJOR VASCULAR REPAIRS

Basic surgical principles include proximal and distal vascular control, including all branches. The fully exposed vessel can be isolated with vascular clamps, vessel loops, or umbilical tapes. Heparin (100 units/kg) should be considered unless contraindicated before clamping any blood vessel. When suturing, the needle should enter the tissue at 90° and include all the layers.

Non-absorbable monofilament sutures should be used, adjusting the size for vessel diameter. Needle holes usually become haemostatic with topical haemostatic agents. In general, aortic repairs will require a 3/4-0, IVC-portal 4/5-0, and hepatic artery 6/8-0 sutures.

The anastomosis can be done in an end-to-end, end-to-side and side-to-side fashion, depending on the tension between vessels, diameter and length of exposure.

VENOUS GRAFT AND PROSTHETIC MATERIALS

In some instances, such as concerns for stenosis or tension, vascular reconstruction may require the placement of an interposition graft using an autologous, homologous or prosthetic graft. The autologous vein (internal jugular, saphenous, iliac, inferior mesenteric, or renal veins) can be harvested from the patient and are the preferred conduits (*Figure 29.4*). Allograft vessels with cryopreserved iliac veins, iliac arteries and the aorta can be used if available. Prosthetic grafts, including Dacron®, GORE-TEX® and polytetrafluoroethylene (PTFE) can be used as an alternative, but are avoided in cases with extensive contamination.

Reconstruction of the PV or SMV may be required in cases where iatrogenic injury and repair resulted in significant narrowing of the vessels. A patch venoplasty or primary end-to-end anastomosis is the most common option for PV-SMV reconstruction. The end-to-end graft anastomosis can be performed using running 5-0 or 6-0 monofilament, non-absorbable sutures. Before completing the anastomosis, a graft should be irrigated with heparinized saline and flushed by unclamping the PV. Prosthetic graft reconstruction in pancreaticoduodenectomy has been reported to have patency rates of 76% during 14-month follow-up (22) and is reported

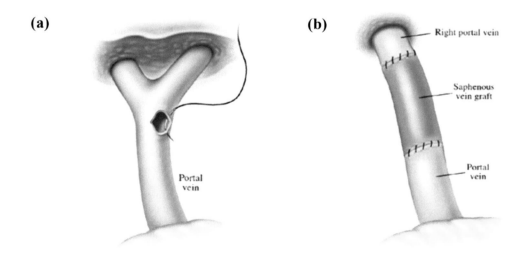

(a)

Portal vein

(b)

Right portal vein

Saphenous vein graft

Portal vein

Figure 29.4 Simple primary PV repair (a) and (b) using a saphenous interposition graft.

to be comparable to autologous grafts in a recent meta-analysis (23).

DAMAGE-CONTROL RESUSCITATION

When a patient develops uncorrectable coagulopathy, hypothermia and acidosis as a result of ongoing haemorrhage, applying damage-control resuscitation is a viable option when other methods fail. The surgical field should be carefully inspected and all obvious bleeding vessels controlled. When it is clear that the bleeding is a result of coagulopathy, laparotomy packs are placed on applying pressure to the oozing surfaces. Care should be taken not to apply too much pressure that would obstruct major vessels. Once reasonable control is achieved, the abdomen should be temporarily closed, and the patient sent to the intensive care unit (ICU) for resuscitation and restoration of physiologic stability. If available, viscoelastic assays such as rotational thromboelastometry (ROTEM) and thrombelastography (TEG) are useful in guiding the correction of any coagulopathy (12). A planned second-look operation or staged operation can be performed once the patient is stabilized (usually in 1–3 days) where the laparotomy packs are removed, and the precise location of any persistent bleeding can be identified and repaired.

REFERENCES

1. Shah A, Palmer AJR, Klein AA. Strategies to minimize intraoperative blood loss during major surgery. *Br J Surg* 2020;**107**(2):e26–e38 doi:10.1002/bjs.11393.
2. Spahn DR, Bouillon B, Cerny V, et al. Management of bleeding and coagulopathy following major trauma: An updated European guideline. *Critical Care* 2013;**17**(2):R76 doi:10.1186/cc12685.
3. Song SY, Chung JW, Yin YH, et al. Celiac axis and common hepatic artery variations in 5002 patients: Systematic analysis with spiral CT and DSA. *Radiology* 2010;**255**(1):278–88 doi:10.1148/radiol.09090389.
4. Favelier S, Germain T, Genson PY, et al. Anatomy of liver arteries for interventional radiology. *Diagn Interv Imaging* 2015;**96**(6):537–46 doi:10.1016/j.diii.2013.12.001.
5. Carneiro C, Brito J, Bilreiro C, et al. All about portal vein: A pictorial display to anatomy, variants, and physiopathology. *Insights Imaging* 2019;**10**(1):1–18 doi:10.1186/s13244-019-0716-8.
6. Sureka B, Sharma N, Khera PS, Garg PK, Yadav T. Hepatic vein variations in 500 patients: Surgical and radiological significance. *Br J Radiol* 2019;(**1102**):20190487 doi:10.1259/bjr.20190487.
7. Bageacu S, Abdelaal A, Ficarelli S, Elmeteini M, Boillot O. Anatomy of the right liver lobe: A surgical analysis in 124 consecutive living donors. *Clin Transplant* 2011;**25**(4):E447–54.
8. Cheng YF, Huang TL, Chen CL, et al. Variations of the left and middle hepatic veins: Application in living related hepatic transplantation. *J Clin Ultrasound* 1996;**24**(1):11–16 doi:10.1002/jcu.1996.1870240103.
9. Cawich SO, Johnson P, Gardner MT, et al. Venous drainage of the left liver: An evaluation of anatomical variants and their clinical relevance. *Clin Radiol* 2020;**75**(12):964.e1–964.e6 doi:10.1016/j.crad.2020.07.039.
10. Kesimal U, Çeken K, Kabaalioğlu A, et al. The role of intraoperative ultrasonography in detection of hepatic vein variations in living donor liver transplantation. *J Ultrasound* 2022;**25**(1):19–25.
11. Dandekar U, Dandekar K, Chavan S. Right hepatic artery: A cadaver investigation and its clinical significance. *Anat Res Int* 2015;**2015**:412595.
12. Carvalho M, Rodrigues A, Gomes M, et al. Interventional algorithms for the control of coagulopathic bleeding in surgical, trauma, and postpartum settings: Recommendations from the Share Network Group. *Clin Appl Thromb Hemost* 2016;**22**(2):121–37 doi:10.1177/1076029614559773.
13. Hughes MJ, Ventham NT, Harrison EM, Wigmore SJ. Central venous pressure and liver resection: A systematic review and meta-analysis. *HPB (Oxford)* 2015;**17**(10):863–71 doi:10.1111/hpb.12462.
14. Hirai I, Murakami G, Kimura W, Kanamura T, Sato I. How should we treat short hepatic veins and paracaval branches in anterior hepatectomy using the hanging maneuver without mobilization of the liver? An anatomical and experimental study. *Clin Anat* 2003;**16**(3):224–32 doi:10.1002/ca.10092.
15. Man K, Fan ST, Ng IOL, et al. Tolerance of the liver to intermittent Pringle maneuver in hepatectomy for liver tumors. *Arch Surg* 1999;**134**(5):533–9. doi:10.1001/archsurg.134.5.533.
16. Kim YI, Fujita S, Hwang YJ, Chun JM, Song KE, Chun BY. Successful intermittent application of the Pringle maneuver for 30 minutes during human hepatectomy: A clinical randomized study with use of a protease inhibitor. *Hepatogastroenterology* 2007;**54**(70):2055–60.
17. Al-Saeedi M, Ghamarnejad O, Khajeh E, et al. Pringle Maneuver in Extended Liver Resection: A propensity score analysis. *Sci Rep* 2020;**10**(1):1–10 doi:10.1038/s41598-020-64596-y.
18. Li M, Zhang C, Zhang T, et al. Outcome using selective hemihepatic vascular occlusion and Pringle maneuver for hepatic resection of liver cavernous hemangioma. *World J Surg Oncol* 2015;**13**(1):267 doi:10.1186/s12957-015-0680-9.
19. He P, He K, Zhong F, et al. Meta-analysis of infrahepatic inferior vena cava clamping combined with the pringle maneuver during hepatectomy. *Asian J Surg* 2021;**44**(1):18–25 doi:10.1016/j.asjsur.2020.04.022.
20. Oderich GS, Panneton JM, Hofer J, et al. Iatrogenic operative injuries of abdominal and pelvic veins: a potentially lethal complication. *J Vasc Surg* 2004;**39**(5):931–6. doi:10.1016/j.jvs 2003.11.040.
21. Sabat J, Hsu CH, Chu Q, Tan TW. The mortality for surgical repair is similar to ligation in patients

with traumatic portal vein injury. *J Vasc Surg Venous and Lymphatic Disorders* 2019;**7(3)**:399–404.

22. Stone HH, Fabian TC, Turkleson ML. Wounds of the portal venous system. *World J Surg* 1982;**6(3)**:335–40.

23. Song W, Yang Q, Chen L, et al. Pancreato-duodenectomy combined with portal-superior mesenteric vein resection and reconstruction with interposition grafts for cancer: A meta-analysis. *Oncotarget* 2017;**8(46)**:81520–8.

Chapter

30

Bleeding Following Radiological and Endoscopic Procedures

Rajesh Panwar and Peush Sahni

INTRODUCTION

Endoscopic and image-guided interventions are minimally invasive procedures that have replaced surgery as the technique of choice for a wide range of indications. Variceal bleeding in patients with cirrhosis is primarily tackled endoscopically and if it fails, a transjugular intrahepatic portosystemic shunt (TIPS) is performed. Patients who require biliary drainage either undergo endoscopic retrograde cholangiopancreatography (ERCP) or percutaneous transhepatic biliary drainage (PTBD) depending on the site of obstruction. Endoscopic and percutaneous interventions have also become the first-choice treatments in the management of acute pancreatitis.

Endoscopic stenting was commonly used to palliate gastrointestinal (GI) obstruction and obstructive jaundice but more recently, endoscopic ultrasound (EUS)-guided gastrojejunostomy and hepaticogastrostomy have emerged as alternative, potentially superior, therapeutic options. These advances in a number of different specialities have undoubted benefits and have reduced procedure-related morbidity in many patients. Nevertheless, any procedure, endoscopic, radiological or surgical, is associated with an inherent risk of complications and the risk increases proportionately with the complexity of the procedure. The risk is even higher during the learning curve of a newly developed technique. Procedure-related bleeding is one such complication that encompasses minor self-limiting to life threatening haemorrhage. This chapter describes the risk of bleeding after endoscopic and radiological procedures used for managing hepato-pancreato-biliary (HPB) diseases, the strategies to mitigate the risk and the management when bleeding occurs.

ENDOSCOPIC INTERVENTIONS

Endoscopic treatment of variceal bleeding

Endoscopic therapy including endoscopic variceal ligation (EVL) and endoscopic sclerotherapy (EST) is used for the treatment of acute variceal bleeding. It is also indicated for primary, as well as secondary, prophylaxis in patients with high-risk varices due to cirrhosis of the liver. Endoscopic therapy successfully controls bleeding in 80–90% of patients. Failure of endoscopic therapy occurs either because of an inability to control the varices due to poor visualization or re-bleeding from a successfully treated lesion (EVL-induced ulcer) and is associated with a high risk of mortality. The majority of endoscopic therapy failures are further managed endoscopically, either by cyanoacrylate injection, re-trial of EVL or EST or argon plasma coagulation (APC). Some patients with ongoing bleeding require the insertion of a Sengstaken–Blakemore (SB) or Minneapolis tube (*Figure 30.1*) that temporarily arrests the bleeding and provides invaluable time for resuscitation. These patients require a subsequent definitive procedure as there is significant risk of re-bleeding once the balloon of the SB tube is deflated. In this setting, the management depends on the functional status of the liver. Patients with liver cirrhosis should be managed with an emergency TIPS procedure. TIPS is successful in around 90% of these patients although the risk of mortality is approximately 35% (1). Balloon-occluded retrograde transvenous obliteration (BRTO) is another option in patients with bleeding gastric varices, especially in those who have a poor hepatic reserve (2). Although Orloff et al. (3) have published their experience of a rescue portacaval shunt following failure of EST in patients

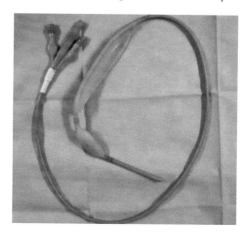

Figure 30.1 A Sengstaken–Blakemore tube.

DOI: 10.1201/9781003080060-30

with cirrhosis-related variceal bleeding, most centres do not favour this approach and surgery is only considered as a last option in this group of patients. Patients with non-cirrhotic portal hypertension do have the option of emergency shunt surgery employing a proximal lienorenal shunt in addition to TIPS or BRTO. The mortality of an emergency shunt procedure is naturally higher than procedures performed electively but is still acceptable given the clinical scenario (4). Some patients may require gastrotomy and suture ligation of the varices in order to directly control the bleeding varices. Splenectomy with esophagogastric devascularization is another option in patients in whom a shunt is not possible.

Endoscopic retrograde cholangiopancreatography

ERCP is a commonly performed endoscopic procedure for the treatment of choledocholithiasis and preoperative or palliative biliary drainage for distal bile duct obstruction. Other less common indications include acute biliary pancreatitis and chronic pancreatitis. ERCP is a relatively safe procedure in experienced hands with an overall complication rate of around 10% (5). Although, minor ooze and self-limiting bleeding are commonly seen, especially after endoscopic sphincterotomy (ES), the incidence of clinically significant bleeding is less than 2%. The risk factors for bleeding include anticoagulant usage, thrombocytopenia, coagulopathy, cirrhosis and acute cholangitis (6). The bleeding can be immediate, and visible during the procedure and delayed, occurring later after completion. Post-ERCP bleeding can usually be treated by a further endoscopic approach with norepinephrine injection, balloon tamponade, thermal coagulation or haemoclip application (*Figure 30.2*). Rarely, the bleeding is so severe that it obscures the endoscopic view and precludes endoscopic treatment and for these patients' angiographic embolization can be lifesaving. Surgery is usually not indicated unless the patient is haemodynamically unstable or has other associated complications such as a hollow viscus perforation that merits surgery *per se*. Recently, the placement of biliary self-expandable metallic stents has emerged as a primary modality for refractory post-ERCP bleeding (7).

Endoscopic ultrasound-guided fine needle aspiration

EUS-guided tissue acquisition is an important technique to differentiate between benign and malignant pancreatic, biliary and hepatic lesions. It is preferred over the percutaneous approach due to the lower risk of needle track seeding and is especially useful for confirming the diagnosis in malignant pancreato-biliary lesions that require neoadjuvant therapy. Overall, the rate of complications is approximately 2.5% with bleeding being the most common (8). The size of the needle does not appear to influence the risk of bleeding but patients on oral or injectable anticoagulants do have a higher risk of bleeding complications. Minor bleeding occurs in up to 2% of cases and is usually managed by endoscopy-guided local tamponade. Major bleeding that requires blood transfusion and/or angioembolization is rarely encountered with only a small number of reports of haemorrhage-related deaths following EUS-guided fine needle aspiration (FNA) (9).

Endoscopic procedures for complications of acute pancreatitis

Endoscopy provides a minimally invasive approach to the management of complicated acute pancreatitis. Endoscopic cysto-gastrostomy is commonly performed for persistent and symptomatic pseudocysts and walled-off necrosis (WON). Endoscopic necrosectomy has also become the first-line treatment in the management of infected pancreatic necrosis (10–12). The procedure used to be performed blind as the only guide available was the bulge in the gastric wall caused by a large lesser sac collection. Consequently, the procedure was only available to patients with large collections and the risk of complications, such as bleeding, infection and perforation, was high.

Bleeding used to be a common complication of these procedures due to the need to traverse a highly vascular gastric wall to reach the collection combined with the presence of branches of the coeliac and superior mesenteric artery. EUS guidance enables a short, straight path that avoids any major blood vessels to be selected which has led to a decrease in complications and

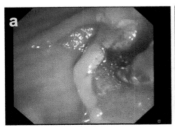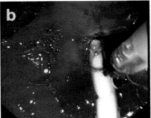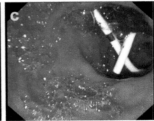

Figure 30.2 Endoscopic pictures showing (a) bleeding during ERCP. (b) Bleeding being controlled by using needle-knife. (c) Haemostasis achieved.

EUS-guided transmural drainage has become the standard of care for endoscopic management of complications of acute pancreatitis (13). Even though the safety of the procedure has improved with EUS-guidance, the risk of bleeding still ranges from 1–10% depending on the type of procedure (14). Necrosectomy is associated with additional risk when compared to drainage-alone procedures and bleeding may range from minor ooze from the puncture site to severe life-threatening haemorrhage from a ruptured pseudoaneurysm. The bleeding may occur during the procedure but is often delayed. Minor bleeding that is recognized during the procedure may be controlled endoscopically using electro-coagulation, clips or adrenaline injection. Placement of a fully covered self-expandable metallic stent (SEMS) may also help control the puncture-site bleeding by tamponade. Rarely, major arterial bleeding is encountered during the procedure, either from a ruptured pre-existing pseudoaneurysm in the cyst wall or cavity, or from a direct injury to a vessel. Delayed bleeding can occur a few days to weeks after the procedure and is usually from a ruptured pseudoaneurysm. Initial resuscitation followed by a digital subtraction angiography and embolization is the procedure of choice in these settings. Surgery is required if endoscopic and intervention radiological procedures fail to control the bleeding or if the haemodynamic instability precludes non-surgical approaches. In our experience, a trans-gastric surgical approach is the best option in this scenario (15) as it provides rapid access to the site of bleeding which is controlled by suture ligation. Failure to identify the bleeding source at surgery may require packing of the cyst cavity.

Other advanced endoscopic procedures

The armamentarium of endoscopic interventions is ever increasing and procedures that were once considered high risk or technically impossible are now being facilitated by technological developments and the evolution of related technical aspects. EUS-guided endoscopic hepaticogastrostomy and gastrojejunostomy are emerging as attractive options for the palliation of malignant obstructive jaundice and gastric outlet obstruction, respectively (16,17). As a consequence, advanced and often lengthy procedures are now possible and undertaken routinely, but the risk of complications is directly related to the complexity of a procedure. Bleeding is the most common complication of endoscopic hepaticogastrostomy, but usually settles with conservative management and blood transfusion. Inadvertent injury to the left hepatic artery or its branch may lead to formation of a pseudoaneurysm which can result in life-threatening haemorrhage.

RADIOLOGICAL INTERVENTIONS

Tissue/tumour biopsy

Percutaneous image, ultrasound (US)- or computed tomography (CT)-guided biopsy helps obtain tissue or tumour samples in a minimally invasive manner. It is a relatively safe procedure but may be associated with life-threatening haemorrhage. The risk of bleeding depends upon a number of factors including the size of the needle, the number of passes, the coagulation profile of the patient and vascularity of the target tissue. The overall rate of bleeding complications after percutaneous liver biopsy is 5.4%, but the rate of major bleeding is only 0.12% (18). Plugging the biopsy tract with gel-foam reduces the risk of bleeding especially in patients with coagulation disorders (19). Although delayed haemorrhage has also been reported, over 95% of the bleeding complications will occur within the first 24 hours. The majority are managed conservatively with embolization but surgery may sometimes be required (*Figure 30.3*).

Transjugular liver biopsy (TJLB) is an option in patients with coagulopathies who have a significant risk of bleeding with percutaneous biopsy (20,21). Although rare (<1%), TJLB itself may sometimes lead to intra-peritoneal haemorrhage due to inadvertent liver capsule perforation. The presence of liver dysfunction and coagulopathy as well as a difficult location of the bleeding site will further complicate matters in this scenario.

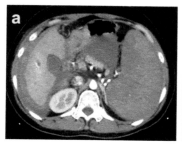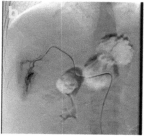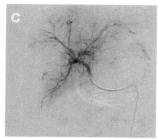

Figure 30.3 Post-percutaneous liver biopsy. CT scan shows contrast extravasation from the liver biopsy site (a). Digital subtraction angiography (DSA) image (b) shows contrast extravasation from a branch of right hepatic artery. Post-embolization DSA image (c) shows coils in the culprit vessel and no contrast extravasation.

Percutaneous drainage of abscesses, cysts or collections

US-, CT- and fluoroscopic-guided percutaneous drainage is the procedure of choice for the management of postoperative collections or abscesses. The step-up approach for pancreatitis places percutaneous drainage at the forefront in the management of acute pancreatitis and percutaneous drainage is also used in the management of hepatic cysts or abscesses. The procedure is usually safe as the image-guidance helps avoid any major vascular structures. However, aspiration of blood from the drainage catheter, which may result from pre-existing blood in the cavity or due to fresh bleeding during the procedure, is not uncommon. The latter may occur from a vascular injury as a result of the procedure or from a pre-existing pseudoaneurysm which is not uncommon in the setting of pancreatitis or a postoperative collection after a major HPB procedure. Minor bleeding is managed conservatively but severe bleeding may require embolization or even surgery (22) (*Figure 30.4*).

Percutaneous transhepatic procedures

Percutaneous transhepatic biliary drainage

Percutaneous transhepatic biliary drainage (PTBD) is a technically demanding procedure that is often required for preoperative or palliative drainage of the biliary tract especially in patients who are not candidates for endoscopic drainage. PTBD-guided stricture dilatation is also the treatment of choice for the management of anastomotic strictures. The proximity of bile ducts to the branches of the hepatic artery and portal vein endangers these structures during PTBD and bleeding is the most common complication with an incidence of 2–2.5% (23). Risk factors for bleeding include thrombocytopenia, coagulopathies, the use of anticoagulants, liver cirrhosis, larger access needles, multiple needle passes, central biliary access and a non-dilated biliary system. Bleeding may be acute, presenting either as blood in the drainage bag or haemobilia leading to melena or haematochezia depending on the severity. Delayed bleeding usually occurs due to a pseudoaneurysm consequent upon a vascular injury occurring during the performance of the PTBD.

Pulsatile bleeding which is bright-red in colour suggests damage to a branch of the hepatic artery and is often associated with a significant fall in haematocrit and haemodynamic instability and requires prompt diagnosis and management. The management depends on the size of the injured vessel and small, peripheral branches are treated by coil embolization while larger, central vessels may require the placement of a stent graft (*Figure 30.5*).

Bleeding from a portal vein branch is slow and intermittent and usually presents with dark blood in the drainage bag. Most often the culprit is a small peripheral branch which can be managed by up-sizing the drainage catheter and placing the side holes more centrally. Bleeding from a large central portal vein is rare and difficult to manage and endovascular options are preferred including coils and stent grafts. The placement of coils or a covered stent via the percutaneous track are other options but it is important to remember that placement in a central portal vein may lead to infarction of the hepatic segment or segments supplied by that branch.

Rarely, the source of bleeding may be outside the liver, suspected when the patient shows evidence of bleeding but the PTBD drainage bag contains only clear bile. Usually, an unrecognized anatomical variant involving a vessel such as the intercostal artery, makes it prone to injury during the percutaneous procedure but prompt angioembolization of the involved vessel is usually successful.

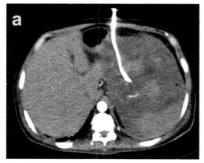 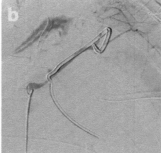 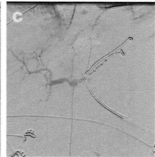

Figure 30.4 Post-percutaneous drainage of acute pancreatitis-related collection. CT scan (a) shows hyperdense contents (clots) in the lesser sac along with active contrast leak. DSA image (b) shows contrast leak from splenic artery. Post-embolization DSA image (c) shows coils in the splenic artery.

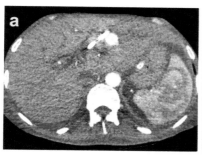
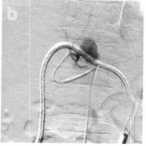
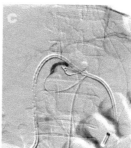

Figure 30.5 Post-percutaneous transhepatic biliary drainage. CT scan (a) shows a large pseudoaneurysm in the territory of left hepatic artery. DSA image (b) confirms the pseudoaneurysm arising from left hepatic artery. Post-embolization DSA image (c) shows no filling of contrast in the pseudoaneurysm.

Percutaneous transhepatic cholecystostomy

Percutaneous cholecystostomy (PC) is indicated for the treatment of acute cholecystitis in surgically unfit patients (24). With the availability of endoscopic drainage and PTBD, PC is no longer a preferred option for biliary drainage but may be required in some patients in whom endoscopic drainage and PTBD are not feasible. The procedure is usually less technically demanding compared with PTBD but may become difficult if the gall bladder is collapsed. Complications are infrequent and management is on similar lines to the complications of PTBD.

Portal vein embolization

Portal vein embolization (PVE) is a commonly performed procedure to increase the volume of a proposed future liver remnant (FLR) before a major hepatic resection. A percutaneous transhepatic approach is used to gain access into the portal vein followed by selective cannulation and embolization of the desired portal vein branches and the percutaneous tract is also embolized in order to reduce bleeding complications. Minor complications occur in up to 25% of patients while the incidence of major complications is less than 5% (25). Bleeding complications following PVE are similar to other transhepatic approaches and are managed along similar lines.

Endovascular procedures

TIPS is a non-selective shunt that connects the intrahepatic portions of a hepatic vein and a portal vein. TIPS is used as a bridge to transplantation and also to manage refractory variceal bleeding and ascites in patients with advanced liver cirrhosis. The initial access is usually gained through the right internal jugular vein and a cannula is passed over a guidewire into the intrahepatic portion of the right hepatic vein. The canula is then directed towards the right portal vein under transabdominal or intravascular ultrasound (IVUS)-guidance through the liver parenchyma. Subsequently, the track is dilated and a stent is placed to complete the procedure. Inadvertent liver capsule perforation or extrahepatic puncture of the portal vein may lead to severe intraperitoneal bleeding while injury to a hepatic artery branch may lead to pseudoaneurysm formation, arterio-venous fistula or arterio-biliary fistula. The rate of clinically significant bleeding after TIPS is 0.7–6% (25). Major intraperitoneal bleeding generally requires surgery while other vascular injuries may be tackled using an endovascular approach. The outcome depends not only on timely control of the bleeding but also on the functional status of the liver.

Balloon-occluded retrograde transvenous obliteration (BRTO) of gastric varices is another endovascular procedure with a risk profile similar to TIPS.

Bleeding is a common complication of endoscopic and radiological interventions. It is self-limiting in the majority of cases but may be life-threatening. A thorough understanding of the risk factors and careful patient selection will ensure complications are reduced as far as possible. Problems such as thrombocytopenia, coagulopathies, liver cirrhosis and use of anticoagulants identified pre-procedure must be appropriately addressed. A number of technical modifications such as a trans-jugular approach rather than percutaneous approach for liver biopsy and prophylactic embolization of the needle track or using a smaller size needle may be utilized in patients where despite the correction of problems the risk remains high and these procedures should be performed only if proper expertise is available. In the unfortunate event of significant bleeding the management will require a multidisciplinary team approach that includes endoscopists, interventional radiologists and surgeons.

SUMMARY

Endoscopic- and image-guided interventions have become the procedures of choice for a range of HPB pathologies. Although safe in experienced hands, these procedures are technically demanding and are associated with a risk of complications. Procedure-related haemorrhage is one such complication that can range from minor self-limiting to life-threatening bleeding. The risk of bleeding depends not only on the complexity of the procedure but also on patient-related factors such as coagulopathy, thrombocytopenia, anticoagulant use, etc. Pre-procedure optimization of the patients may help reduce the risk of bleeding. Minor bleeding may not need any treatment, but any major bleeding would require a prompt angio-embolization or endoscopic haemostasis. Surgery may be required if these interventions fail to achieve haemostasis or haemodynamic instability precludes any such intervention.

REFERENCES

1. Pandhi MB, Kuei AJ, Lipnik AJ, Gaba RC. Emergent transjugular intrahepatic portosystemic shunt creation in acute variceal bleeding. *Semin Interv Radiol* 2020;**37**:3–13.
2. Saad WEA, Darcy MD. Transjugular Intrahepatic Portosystemic Shunt (TIPS) versus Balloon-occluded Retrograde Transvenous Obliteration (BRTO) for the management of gastric varices. *Semin Interv Radiol* 2011;**28**:339–49.
3. Orloff MJ, Isenberg JI, Wheeler HO, Haynes KS, Jinich-Brook H, Rapier R, et al. Emergency portacaval shunt versus rescue portacaval shunt in a randomized controlled trial of emergency treatment of acutely bleeding esophageal varices in cirrhosis – Part 3. *J Gastrointest Surg* 2010;**14**:1782–95.
4. Prasad AS, Gupta S, Kohli V, Pande GK, Sahni P, Nundy S. Proximal splenorenal shunts for extrahepatic portal venous obstruction in children. *Ann Surg* 1994;**219**:193–6.
5. Glomsaker T, Hoff G, Kvaløy JT, Søreide K, Aabakken L, Søreide JA, et al. Patterns and predictive factors of complications after endoscopic retrograde cholangiopancreatography. *Br J Surg* 2013;**100**:373–80.
6. Johnson KD, Perisetti A, Tharian B, Thandassery R, Jamidar P, Goyal H, et al. Endoscopic retrograde cholangiopancreatography-related complications and their management strategies: A 'scoping' literature review. *Dig Dis Sci* 2020;**65**:361–75.
7. Moon SY, Heo J, Jung MK, Cho CM. Biliary self-expandable metal stent could be recommended as a first treatment modality for immediate refractory post-endoscopic retrograde cholangiopancreatography bleeding. *Clin Endosc* 2022;**55**:128–35.
8. Mizuide M, Ryozawa S, Fujita A, Ogawa T, Katsuda H, Suzuki M, et al. Complications of endoscopic ultrasound-guided fine needle aspiration: A narrative review. *Diagn Basel Switz* 2020;**10**:964.
9. Zhu H, Jiang F, Zhu J, Du Y, et al. Assessment of morbidity and mortality associated with endoscopic ultrasound-guided fine-needle aspiration for pancreatic cystic lesions: A systematic review and meta-analysis. *Dig Endosc* 2017;**29**:667–75.
10. Baron TH, DiMaio CJ, Wang AY, Morgan KA. American Gastroenterological Association Clinical Practice Update: Management of pancreatic necrosis. *Gastroenterology* 2020;**158**:67–75.e1.
11. Arvanitakis M, Dumonceau J-M, Albert J, Badaoui A, Bali MA, Barthet M, et al. Endoscopic management of acute necrotizing pancreatitis: European Society of Gastrointestinal Endoscopy (ESGE) evidence-based multidisciplinary guidelines. *Endoscopy* 2018;**50**:524–46.
12. Ramai D, McEntire DM, Tavakolian K, Heaton J, Chandan S, Dhindsa B, et al. Safety of endoscopic pancreatic necrosectomy compared with percutaneous and surgical necrosectomy: A nationwide inpatient study. *Endosc Int Open* 2023;**11**:E330–E9.
13. Guo J, Saftoiu A, Vilmann P, Fusaroli P, Giovannini M, Mishra G, et al. A multi-institutional consensus on how to perform endoscopic ultrasound-guided peri-pancreatic fluid collection drainage and endoscopic necrosectomy. *Endosc Ultrasound* 2017;**6**:285–91.
14. Rana SS, Shah J, Kang M, Gupta R. Complications of endoscopic ultrasound-guided transmural drainage of pancreatic fluid collections and their management. *Ann Gastroenterol* 2019;**32**:441–50.
15. George A, Panwar R, Pal S. Surgical management of life threatening bleeding after endoscopic cystogastrostomy. *J Investig Surg* 2018;**31**:503–8.
16. Cho JH, Park SW, Kim EJ, Park CH, et al. Long-term outcomes and predictors of adverse events of EUS-guided hepatico-gastrostomy for malignant biliary obstruction: Multicenter, retrospective study. *Surg Endosc* 2022;**36**:8950–8.
17. Vedantam S, Shah R, Bhalla S, Kumar S, Amin S. No difference in outcomes with 15 mm vs. 20 mm lumen-apposing metal stents for endoscopic ultrasound-guided gastroenterostomy for gastric outlet obstruction: A meta-analysis. *Clin Endosc* 2023;**56**:298–307.
18. Jing H, Yi Z, He E, Xu R, et al. Evaluation of risk factors for bleeding after ultrasound-guided liver biopsy. *Int J Gen Med* 2021;**14**:5563–71.
19. Singhal S, Pradeep MD, Inuganti S, Botcha S, et al. Percutaneous ultrasound-guided plugged liver biopsy: A single-centre experience. *Pol J Radiol* 2021;**86**:e239–e45.
20. Lavian JD, Thornton LM, Zybulewski A, Kim E, et al. Safety of percutaneous versus transjugular liver biopsy: A propensity score matched analysis. *Eur J Radiol* 2020;**133**:109399.
21. Sue MJ, Lee EW, Saab S, McWilliams JP, et al. Transjugular liver biopsy: Safe even in patients with severe coagulopathies and multiple biopsies. *Clin Transl Gastroenterol* 2019;**10**:e00063.
22. Lorenz J, Thomas JL. Complications of percutaneous fuid drainage. *Semin Interv Radiol* 2006;**23**:194–204.
23. Quencer KB, Tadros AS, Marashi KB, Cizman Z, et al. Bleeding after percutaneous transhepatic biliary drainage: Incidence, causes and treatments. *J Clin Med* 2018;**7**:94.
24. Gulaya K, Desai SS, Sato K. Percutaneous cholecystostomy: Evidence-based current clinical practice. *Semin Interv Radiol* 2016;**33**:291–6.
25. Madhusudhan KS, Sharma S, Srivastava DN. Percutaneous radiological interventions of the portal vein: A comprehensive review. *Acta Radiol Stockh Swed 1987* 2023;**64**:441–55.

Chapter 31 — Acute Pancreatitis

J. de Hondt, M. F. G. Francken, C. L. van Veldhuizen and Marc G. Besselink

INTRODUCTION

Acute pancreatitis is characterized by inflammation of the pancreas and elevated levels of pancreatic enzymes in the blood, clinically resulting in severe abdominal pain. It is diagnosed based on abdominal pain, elevated serum pancreas enzymes, and characteristic findings on imaging (1). The annual incidence of acute pancreatitis in the United States ranges from 4.9–35/100 000 people (2). The global incidence of acute pancreatitis is increasing, causing a further burden on healthcare systems (1,3). This may partly be explained by the evolving nature and extent of risk factors associated with acute pancreatitis, such as advancing age, biliary disease, alcohol abuse, obesity, metabolic syndrome, smoking and the use of pancreatitis-associated medications (3).

Acute pancreatitis has a broad aetiology, of which the most common is a biliary cause, such as a transient obstruction of the distal common bile duct secondary to oedema, choledocholithiasis or biliary sludge (2,4). Acute pancreatitis, with a biliary origin, accounts for half of all cases. The second most common cause, alcohol, accounts for 20% of cases. Other causes include post-endoscopic retrograde cholangiopancreatography (ERCP), viral infections trauma, iatrogenic related to the prescription of medications, hyperlipidaemia, hypercalcaemia and autoimmune pancreatitis. After extensive imaging and additional diagnostic work-up, as many as 25% of acute pancreatitis cases remain undiagnosed and are classified as idiopathic.

The clinical course and severity of acute pancreatitis varies widely. In 80% of patients, acute pancreatitis runs a mild course and is self-limiting. Most patients recover within days with a conservative approach, including analgesia and fluid resuscitation. However, 20% of patients develop a moderate-severe, or severe, pancreatitis with local, or systemic complications, or both, such as organ failure or peripancreatic necrosis. In these patients, a high mortality rate is seen of around 15–20% while mortality for mild pancreatitis is <1% (2,5). Identifying the aetiology and early detection of complications is the key to being able to offer effective treatment but the management of complications of acute pancreatitis remains challenging due to the heterogeneity of possible aetiologies (2).

Definitions and terminology

In 2012, a revision of the original Atlanta classification system was published. The goal was to enable medical specialists to introduce uniformity in diagnosis and definitions of acute pancreatitis and its complications; its severity and disease phases.

For the diagnosis of acute pancreatitis, the revised Atlanta classification is used which requires two of these three features: 1) abdominal pain consistent with acute pancreatitis, 2) serum lipase (or amylase) at least three times greater than the upper limit of normal and 3) characteristic findings of acute pancreatitis on contrast-enhanced computed tomography (CECT) or less commonly magnetic resonance imaging (MRI) or transabdominal ultrasonography (1). Imaging is not required for the diagnosis. The revised Atlanta classification has been included in best practice guidelines in Europe, Japan, Canada and Australia (1).

The severity of acute pancreatitis can be classified as a mild, moderate-severe, or severe. Mild pancreatitis is characterized by the absence of signs of organ failure and no local or systemic complications. Both moderate severe and severe pancreatitis may be accompanied by local or systemic complications and/or organ failure,

Table 31.1 Definition of severity according to the revised Atlanta classification with corresponding mortality rates (5)

	Mild	Moderate-severe	Severe
Organ failure	No	Transient (<48 h) or not present	Persistent (>48 h) Single or multiple organs
Local or systemic complications	No	Present	Present
Mortality (%)	0.1	2.1	52.2

DOI: 10.1201/9781003080060-31

with the difference that transient organ failure is classified as moderate-severe and persistent organ failure as severe acute pancreatitis. Persistent organ failure is defined as organ failure present for >48 hours, which is also considered the best predictor of mortality (1,5). See *Table 31.1* for summary.

IMAGING

Computed tomography

The 'gold standard' of imaging modality for acute pancreatitis, to determine the diagnosis and severity and to identify complications, is CECT. It is indicated for identifying pancreatic necrosis but is best performed >72 hours after onset of the disease. An early CECT could underestimate the extent of peripancreatic necrosis, due to the signs of necrosis evolving over several days. It is generally recommended that CECT should be performed after 6 days as some studies have reported that earlier CECT has no therapeutic benefit and prolongs hospital stay (1,5).

Magnetic resonance imaging

MRI in acute pancreatitis could be considered when CECT is suboptimal or contraindicated, such as allergy to contrast, young or pregnant patients, to avoid radiation exposure or patients with renal impairment. MRI can be helpful in detecting solid content in acute necrotic collections or acute peripancreatic fluid collections which may otherwise incorrectly be called 'pseudocysts' (1,6).

Endoscopic ultrasound and endoscopic retrograde cholangiopancreatography

Endoscopic ultrasound (EUS) and endoscopic retrograde cholangiopancreatography (ERCP) are two reliable diagnostic tools for the detection of biliary stones and sludge. ERCP should no longer be viewed as a diagnostic tool. It is not required in the first few days after presentation with biliary pancreatitis, except in patients with cholangitis (7). Additionally, some studies recommend performing EUS prior to therapeutic ERCP in suspected biliary pancreatitis due to the lower failure rate and reduced risk of complications (8). Also, EUS should be considered in cases of suspected idiopathic acute pancreatitis, since it has been shown to be an effective imaging tool to elucidate the aetiology (9).

INITIAL WORK-UP FOR DIAGNOSING ACUTE PANCREATITIS

Diagnosis of acute pancreatitis

The diagnosis of acute pancreatitis is made following the revised Atlanta classification. If the diagnosis of acute pancreatitis is established based on the first two criteria, the added value of CECT in the emergency room is relatively low, although it is still frequently performed. As a diagnostic tool, serum lipase is advised rather than serum amylase due to the lower specificity of the latter. If there is a strong suspicion of acute pancreatitis based on abdominal pain, but serum lipase is not more than three times the upper normal limit, imaging will be required to confirm the diagnosis (1,5).

Identifying aetiology of pancreatitis

After the diagnosis of acute pancreatitis is made, the main focus should be on initial treatment and identifying the aetiology. In approximately 75% of patients, an aetiology can be identified, leaving 25% categorized as idiopathic acute pancreatitis (IAP) (2). The initial evaluation should include an assessment of the medical history, laboratory evaluation and an abdominal ultrasound.

Key elements of the history are:

- Symptoms of gallstone disease (e.g. biliary colic) or documentation of cholelithiasis on imaging
- Amount and pattern of alcohol use
- Medication use (both unprescribed and prescribed) and changes in dose or usage
- Prior abdominal surgery, including ERCP within the last 24 hours
- Prior abdominal trauma
- History of hypertriglyceridaemia or hypercalcaemia
- Systemic symptoms, such as unexplained weight loss
- Direct family history of hereditary pancreatitis (2)

All acute pancreatitis patients should undergo routine laboratory tests, including triglyceride and serum calcium levels and liver function tests. Hypertriglyceridemia induced acute pancreatitis can be reliably diagnosed if levels are above 11.2 mmol/L. A 3-fold increase in alanine aminotransferase (ALT) levels within the first 48 hours, after onset, has a positive predictive value of more than 85% for acute biliary pancreatitis, but this diagnosis can only be made based on imaging. Hypercalcaemia can be challenging to diagnose, since calcium levels can decrease in cases of severe pancreatitis. Thus, levels should be re-evaluated some weeks after recovery. Hypercalcaemia is a rare cause of acute pancreatitis and can only be diagnosed after excluding other causes. All acute pancreatitis patients should undergo an abdominal ultrasound to evaluate the possibility of cholelithiasis or signs of biliary tract obstruction (2).

If an initial evaluation does not allow a conclusion to be reached regarding the aetiology, further evaluation should be performed. EUS is the recommended diagnostic tool to assess possible causes of the episode of acute pancreatitis, which has been shown to be a sensitive tool in detecting aetiology in presumed idiopathic cases as shown in the PICUS trial (7,9). In this case series of 105 patients, an aetiology could be detected in 32% of cases. During the EUS procedure, bile ducts and pancreas parenchyma should be evaluated for possible biliary sludge, microlithiasis, chronic pancreatitis or small pancreatic tumours. In case of a negative EUS, magnetic resonance cholangiopancreatography (MRCP) with secretin should be considered. ERCP is not recommended as a diagnostic test, due to the high-complication rate. Some studies have recommended performing a laparoscopic cholecystectomy in patients with IAP (4,10); although strong evidence regarding the benefit and safety of this treatment is still lacking.

MANAGEMENT OF ACUTE PANCREATITIS

Fluid resuscitation

Fluid resuscitation has been shown to have a beneficial effect on the clinical course of acute pancreatitis. Thus, controlled fluid therapy within the first 24 hours of presentation is highly recommended. Primary resuscitation should be performed with Ringer's lactate solution. Results from the WATERFALL trial showed that moderate fluid resuscitation (1.5 mL/kg/hour) was comparable to aggressive fluid resuscitation (bolus of 20 mL/kg and 3 mL/kg/hour) in respect of the occurrence of local complications, organ failure and severe or moderate-severe pancreatitis. Aggressive fluid resuscitation, however, resulted in a significantly higher risk of fluid overload and thus moderate fluid resuscitation of 1.5 mL/kg/hour with a bolus of 10 mL/kg over 2 hours, if hypovolemia present, is recommended (5,11).

Pain management

For pain management, opioids should be used. When patients require intensive care treatment, epidural anaesthesia can be considered (5,12).

Antibiotic therapy

Antibiotic prophylaxis to prevent infectious complications in predicted severe pancreatitis is not recommended. Recent meta-analyses of randomized trials showed no beneficial impact on mortality (5,13). Antibiotic treatment should however be considered for patients with a systemic inflammatory response (SIRS), infected necrosis, multi-organ failure or extrapancreatic infection.

Nutritional intervention

A prolonged catabolic illness and infectious complications are often seen in cases of acute pancreatitis, especially in those with moderate-severe or severe pancreatitis. Enteral nutrition will reduce or prevent catabolism, while also maintaining mucosal integrity. Commencing enteral nutrition very early, within 24 hours, if possible, reduces the occurrence of infected pancreatic necrosis, organ failure and mortality (14). Patients with mild acute pancreatitis can restart a normal oral diet within the first day of hospital admission. If oral food intake is not tolerated, enteral nutrition can be started after 72 hours, as shown by the PYTHON trial and nasojejunal or nasogastric feeding are both acceptable (5).

Management of acute biliary pancreatitis and biliary complications

In patients with mild biliary pancreatitis, cholecystectomy should be performed prior to discharge, as shown by the PONCHO trial (5,15). Early ERCP is not indicated for mild biliary pancreatitis and an early (within 24 hours) ERCP for patients with severe biliary pancreatitis without cholangitis does not reduce mortality, nor major complications in comparison to conservative treatment, as shown by the APEC trial (8). If concomitant cholangitis, choledocholithiasis and/or prolonged biliary obstruction is present, patients should undergo an ERCP with sphincterotomy.

Follow-up

A structured follow-up is recommended for the following patients: severe pancreatitis; alcohol-induced pancreatitis; idiopathic pancreatitis with an age >40 years and incomplete resolution of symptoms after discharge. Several cohort studies have shown an increased risk of pancreatic cancer after a first episode of acute pancreatitis compared to control populations, the adjusted hazard ratio is up to 19 : 28 (5). After 5–10 years, the risk returns to similar levels respective to the general population. Above the age of 40, there is a further increased risk of pancreatic cancer and these patients with idiopathic acute pancreatitis should undergo a CECT or EUS within 3 months after the end of symptoms to rule out an occult pancreatic cancer. Further follow-up after 1–2 years should also be considered (5).

COMPLICATIONS

Interstitial oedematous pancreatitis

Cases of acute pancreatitis can be divided into two subcategories based on imaging: interstitial oedematous pancreatitis (*Figure 31.1*) and necrotizing pancreatitis. Interstitial oedematous pancreatitis is the most common

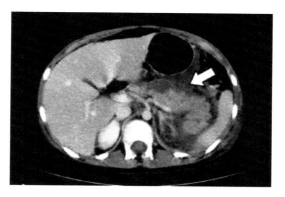

Figure 31.1 Imaging of patient with acute interstitial oedematous pancreatitis (arrow).

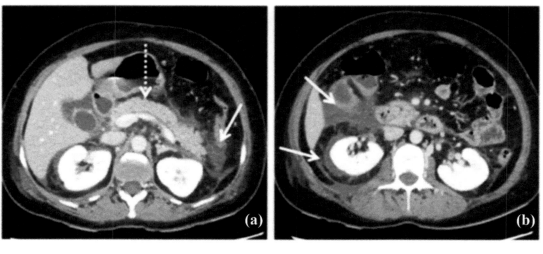

Figure 31.2 Imaging of patient with homogenous enhancement of the pancreas (dashed arrow) (a) and peripancreatic fluid collection (solid arrows) (a and b).

(80%) and is characterized by diffuse, or occasionally local, enlargement of the pancreas due to inflammation and oedema. Interstitial oedema can be seen on a CECT as a homogenous enhancement of the pancreas parenchyma (1).

Peripancreatic fluids collection

An early complication associated with acute pancreatitis is the incidence of acute peripancreatic fluid collection (APFC). The definition of APFC is a non-encapsulated homogeneous peripancreatic collection that develops within the first 4 weeks after disease onset (1). Approximately 25% of patients will develop APFC during the course of acute pancreatitis (*Figure 31.2*). In general, APFCs resolve spontaneously within a few weeks. If an APFC persists for more than 4 weeks, it is considered to be a pancreatic pseudocyst (1).

Pancreatic pseudocyst

Pancreatic pseudocysts are an unusual complication of acute pancreatitis occurring in 10–20% of patients and are more common in chronic pancreatitis (*Figure 31.3*). Pseudocysts are defined as encapsulated fluid collections and can be either asymptomatic or symptomatic, which can cause biliary or gastric obstruction, haemorrhage, or secondary infection but do not contain necrotic tissue. Pseudocysts will commonly present themselves in the lesser sac or anterior pararenal space, and often resolve spontaneously. However, in selected cases, treatment is needed, guided by the size and symptoms and includes endoscopic transluminal drainage. Secondary infections of the pseudocyst are rare but when they occur will usually require antibiotics and endoscopic or, rarely, surgical treatment (1,6).

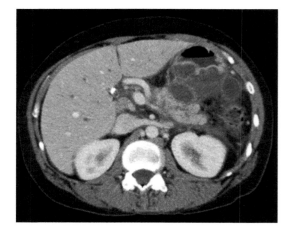

Figure 31.3 Imaging of patient with multiple pancreatic pseudocysts.

Necrotizing pancreatitis

The other subtype of acute pancreatitis is necrotizing pancreatitis. Necrotizing pancreatitis is less common with a prevalence of 5–10% and it is defined by necrosis of the pancreas parenchyma and peripancreatic tissue. Less commonly, only the peripancreatic tissue is affected, and even more rarely the pancreatic parenchyma alone. The impairment of pancreatic perfusion and signs of necrosis evolve over several days. An early CECT could therefore underestimate the extent of peripancreatic necrosis. After a week of acute pancreatitis, the full extent of the necrosis will be visible on a CECT (1) (*Figure 31.4*).

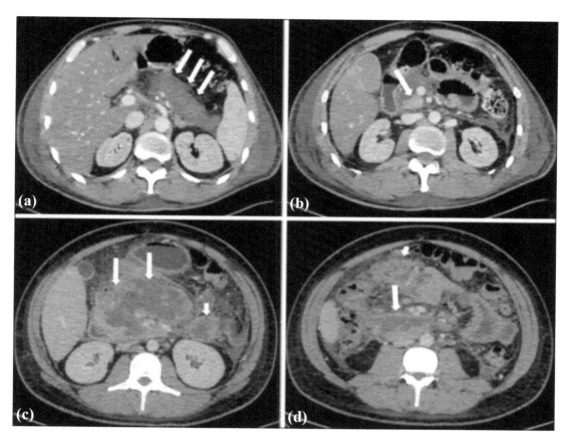

Figure 31.4 Imaging of patient (a–d) with pancreatic (long arrows) and peripancreatic (short arrows) necrosis (c and d).

Pancreatic necrosis can be seen as a hypodense region in the pancreas. In the initial stages of the disease patchy regions of necrosis may be observed on a CECT. In cases where only peripancreatic necrosis is present, the pancreas enhances normally, mimicking cases of interstitial oedematous pancreatitis (1).

Necrotizing collections are divided into two groups. In the first 4 weeks of necrotizing pancreatitis, the collections of necrotic material are referred to as acute necrotic collections (ANC). After 4 weeks and in case of persisting acute pancreatitis, ANCs mature and become walled-off necrosis (WON). Characteristic of WON is the fibrotic capsule surrounding the necrotic tissue. The walled-off collections can vary widely in size and may, or may not, be infected. The 4-week cut-off between both groups has been selected arbitrarily (1).

Sterile necrotizing pancreatitis can be managed conservatively; however, an infected necrosis remains an absolute indication for some form of invasive intervention. Intervention of infected necrotizing pancreatitis should be delayed as long as the situation of the patient permits it, or for at least 4 weeks, so a fibrotic capsule can be formed around the necrotic collection. Early debridement should only be considered if strong indications are present, and the necrotic collection is organized. The POINTER trial showed that delayed drainage of infected necrotizing pancreatitis was not inferior to immediate (within 24 hours) drainage in respect of occurrence of complications and even resulted in a lower rate of necrosectomy and reduced use of interventions (16) (*Figure 31.5*).

Infected necrosis

The diagnosis of infected ANC or WON can be made following the appearance of gas seen on CECT or the patient's clinical course. Half of all patients with infected necrotizing pancreatitis have gas in the collections and one third of patients with necrotizing pancreatitis will develop an infection. In cases of doubt, fine needle aspiration can be performed to culture the

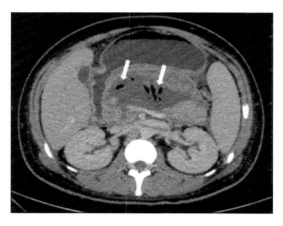

Figure 31.5 Imaging of patient with peripancreatic necrosis, as seen by the presence of gas (arrows).

content although this is not always necessary. Multiple treatment options are available for infected WON, such as image-guided percutaneous drainage and surgical or endoscopic procedures. Percutaneous and transmural drainage are both first-line nonsurgical approaches for managing patients with WON and can be considered in the acute phase (<4 weeks). Surgical procedures should be performed, if possible, minimally invasively as it has been shown to lower the risk of an inflammatory response and local sepsis (3,17).

Other local complications

Other, less common, complications following acute pancreatitis are colonic ischaemia, gastric outlet dysfunction, gastrointestinal perforation, bleeding and elevated intra-abdominal pressure.

Systemic complications

The course of acute pancreatitis can be complicated by systematic complications. These include organ failure and systemic inflammatory response syndrome (SIRS). SIRS commonly occurs in the early phase of severe acute pancreatitis and is associated with an increased risk of organ failure. The manifestation of organ failure is not limited to a specific part of the course of the disease and can occur at any stage. Transient organ failure (<48h) is associated with low mortality and complications. Persistent organ failure, which is present in severe pancreatitis, must always be treated in critical-care facilities.

SUMMARY

Acute pancreatitis is the acute inflammation of the pancreas, accompanied with abdominal pain, increased serum lipase (and amylase), and characteristic findings of acute pancreatitis on CT scan. The most common aetiology, in most countries, is biliary tract pathology,

followed by alcohol abuse and post-endoscopic retrograde cholangiopancreatography (ERCP). In about 25% of patients, no aetiology can be identified. In acute pancreatitis, 20% of patients develop moderate-severe, or severe, disease, which is associated with complications such as organ failure and pancreatic necrosis with a high rate of mortality.

Acute pancreatitis is diagnosed according to the revised Atlanta criteria based on the patient's history, laboratory results and, if necessary, a CECT scan. Other forms of imaging that could be performed, depending on the indication, are MRI, ERCP and a transabdominal ultrasound scan. The cornerstones of the management of acute pancreatitis are fluid resuscitation, pain management, and nutritional intervention. Prophylactic antibiotics are not recommended. Following the diagnosis of mild acute biliary pancreatitis an early (preferably index admission) cholecystectomy is recommended.

Based on imaging, acute pancreatitis may be divided into interstitial oedematous pancreatitis and necrotizing pancreatitis based on a delayed CECT after 3–4 days. Necrotizing pancreatitis, either pancreatic parenchyma or peripancreatic fat, can become infected, which is associated with a 15–20% risk of mortality with the majority of the deaths related to septic complications.

Key points

- Some 80% of episodes of acute pancreatitis are mild, although 20% of patients develop severe pancreatitis, which is associated with systemic complications and increased mortality.
- Acute pancreatitis and its complications are defined by the revised Atlanta classification.
- Management of acute pancreatitis consists of fluid resuscitation, pain management, nutrition, and if possible, to treat the specific cause of the pancreatitis (cholecystectomy in biliary pancreatitis).
- Acute pancreatitis can occur as a necrotizing pancreatitis or interstitial oedematous pancreatitis.
- Intervention in cases of infected necrotizing pancreatitis should be delayed for as long as possible, or for at least 4 weeks to lower the risk of mortality and complications.
- Systemic complications of acute pancreatitis are organ failure and SIRS, where SIRS occurs in the first stages of severe pancreatitis, and organ failure which can occur at any stage.

REFERENCES

1. Banks PA, Bollen TL, Dervenis C, Gooszen HG, Johnson CD, Sarr MG, et al. Classification of acute pancreatitis—2012: Revision of the Atlanta classification and definitions by international consensus. *Gut* 2013;**62**:102–11.
2. Vege SS. *Etiology of acute pancreatitis*. Whitcomb DC, Grover S, (eds). Waltham, MA: UpToDate Inc.

Available from: www-uptodate-com. (Accessed 3 September 2024).

3. Iannuzzi JP, King JA, Leong JH, Quan J, Windsor JW, Tanyingoh D, et al. Global incidence of acute pancreatitis is increasing over time: A systematic review and meta-analysis. *Gastroenterology* 2022;**162(1)**:122–34.

4. Umans DS, Hallensleben ND, Verdonk RC, Bouwense SAW, Fockens P, van Santvoort HC, et al. Recurrence of idiopathic acute pancreatitis after cholecystectomy: Systematic review and meta-analysis. *Br J Surg* 2020;**107(3)**:191–9.

5. Beyer G, Hoffmeister A, Lorenz P, Lynen P, Lerch MM, Mayerle J. Clinical practice guideline – Acute and chronic pancreatitis. *Dtsch Arztebl Int* 2022;**119(29–30)**:495–501.

6. Sandrasegaran K, Heller MT, Panda A, Shetty A, Menias CO. MRI in acute pancreatitis. Abdom Radiol 2020;**45**:1232–42.

7. Schepers NJ, Hollensleben NDL, Besselink MG, Anten M-PGF, Bollen TL, da Costa DW, et al. Urgent endoscopic retrograde cholangiopancreatography with sphincterotomy versus conservative treatment in predicted severe acute gallstone pancreatitis (APEC): A multicentre randomized controlled trial. *Lancet* 2020;**396(10245)**:167–76.

8. De Lisi S, Leandro G, Buscarini E. Endoscopic ultrasonography versus endoscopic retrograde cholangiopancreatography in acute biliary pancreatitis. *Eur J Gastroenterol Hepatol* 2011;**23(5)**:367–74.

9. Thevenot A, Bournet B, Otal P, Canevet G, Moreau J, Buscail L. Endoscopic ultrasound and magnetic resonance cholangiopancreatography in patients with idiopathic acute pancreatitis. *Dig Dis Sci* 2013;**58**:2361–68.

10. Raty S, Pulkkinen J, Nordback I, Sand J, Victorzon M, Gronroos J, et al. Can Laparoscopic cholecystectomy prevent recurrent idiopathic acute pancreatitis? A prospective randomized multicenter Trial. *Ann Surg* 2015;**262(5)**:736–41.

11. de-Madaria E, Buxbaum JL, Maisonneuve P, García García de Paredes A, Zapater P, Guilabert L, et al. Aggressive or moderate fluid resuscitation in acute pancreatitis. *New Engl J Med* 2022;**387(11)**:989–1000.

12. Basurto Ona X, Rigau Comas D, Urrútia G. Opioids for acute pancreatitis pain. *Cochrane Database Syst Rev* 2013:(**7**):CD009179

13. Ding N, Sun YH, Wen LM, et al. Assessment of prophylactic antibiotics administration for acute pancreatitis: A meta-analysis of randomized controlled trials. *Chin Med J (Engl)* 2020;**133**:212–20.

14. Bakker OJ, van Brunschot S, van Santvoort HC, Besselink MG, Bollen TL, Boermeester MA, et al. Early versus on-demand nasoenteric tube feeding in acute pancreatitis. *N Engl J Med* 2014;**371(21)**:1983–93.

15. da Costa DW, Bouwense SA, Schepers NJ, Besselink MG, van Santvoort HC, Brunschot S, et al. Same-admission versus interval cholecystectomy for mild gallstone pancreatitis (PONCHO): A multicentre randomized controlled trial. *Lancet* 2015;**386(10000)**:1261–8.

16. Boxhoorn L, van Dijk SM, van Grinsven J, Verdonk RC, Boermeester MA, Bollen TL, et al. Immediate versus postponed intervention for infected necrotizing pancreatitis. *New Engl J Med* 2021;**385(15)**:1372–81.

17. Besselink MG, van Santvoort HC, Nieuwenhuijs VB, Boermeester MA, Bollen TL, Buskens E, et al. Minimally invasive 'step-up approach' versus maximal necrosectomy in patients with acute necrotising pancreatitis (PANTER trial): Design and rationale of a randomized controlled multicenter trial [ISRCTN13975868]. *BMC Surg* 2006;**6**:6.

Bailey & Love's Essential Operations Bailey & Love's Essential Operations Bailey & Love's Essential Operatic
Bailey & Love's Essential Operations Bailey & Love's Essential Operatic
Bailey & Love's Essential Operations Bailey & Love's Essential Operatic

SECTION 6 | PANCREAS

Chapter 32

Chronic Pancreatitis

Ana Sather, Zachary Bergman and Greg Beilman

INTRODUCTION

Although surgery used to be the last choice of treatment for patients with chronic pancreatitis (CP), it is now being considered earlier in the disease process and may occasionally be indicated prior to endoscopic interventions. CP affects 25–98/100 000 people, with an incidence of approximately 5/100 000 per year (1). By far the most common symptom is pain (2). Other complications include pancreatic fluid collections, exocrine (steatorrhea, weight loss) and endocrine insufficiency (diabetes). This chapter will outline the primary aetiologies of CP, treatment, indications for surgery, and describe the operative choices based on pancreatic morphology.

An important first step is understanding the stages of pancreatitis. Acute pancreatitis is based on meeting criteria as per the revised Atlanta classification, discussed in detail in **Chapter 31**. Recurrent acute pancreatitis (RAP) is defined as two or more episodes of acute pancreatitis separated by 3, or more, disease-free months between episodes (3). In line with the complexity of CP, its definition has undergone multiple iterations with varying focus on symptoms, histology, function, and/or permanence. An appropriate definition, based on recent international consensus is a 'pathologic fibro-inflammatory syndrome of the pancreas in individuals with genetic, environmental and/or other risk factors who develop persistent pathologic responses to parenchymal injury or stress' (4). Morphological alterations that may be present include inflammation, fibrosis, atrophy, calcium deposits, and ductal changes (4,5).

AETIOLOGY

Part of the complexity of CP is the frequent multifactorial nature of the underlying aetiology. The TIGAR-O classification system lists risk factors associated with CP that include: toxic-metabolic; idiopathic; genetic; autoimmune; recurrent and severe acute pancreatitis, and obstructive (4). Alcohol remains the leading cause and is implicated in 40–70% of patients with CP (though less than 5% of heavy drinkers will develop CP) (6–8). Smoking is another lifestyle factor associated with CP, both independently, and in a synergistic fashion, with alcohol (7,9). Congenital anomalies, such as annular pancreas and pancreas divisum, are associated with increased risk but require a second risk factor, typically environmental or genetic (9). With the emergence of DNA sequencing, the rate of identifying hereditary pancreatitis has increased and cases deemed idiopathic have concurrently decreased. Genetic variations in *PRSS1*, *SPINK1*, *CFTR*, *CTRC*, and *CASR* are associated with CP (10). The majority of patients with recurrent acute, and chronic, pancreatitis have multiple variants in a gene, or epistatic interactions between multiple genes, coupled with environmental stressors (9).

Finally, autoimmune pancreatitis (AIP) represents a systemic autoimmune condition that has both pancreatic and extrapancreatic manifestations. AIP can be treated with steroids (although maintaining remission may be challenging) and does not generally require surgery (11). It is important to distinguish, since its characteristics may be similar to malignancy, and unnecessary pancreatic resection has been cited as high as 43% (12).

WORK-UP AND DECISION-MAKING PROCESS

In a patient with suspected CP (abdominal pain and/or symptoms of pancreatic exocrine insufficiency) (*Figure 32.1*), the diagnosis is made with a combination of imaging and laboratory testing. Functional testing includes the measurement of faecal fat and elastase levels, and pancreatic bicarbonate levels in response to intravenous secretin. In most patients, diagnosis is based on clinical symptoms but should be confirmed with a combination of endoscopic ultrasound (EUS), endoscopic retrograde cholangiopancreatography (ERCP), magnetic resonance cholangio pancreatography (MRCP) and/or computed tomography (CT) findings, focusing specifically on the presence of ductal dilation, pancreatic atrophy, and pancreatic calcification (13).

After the diagnosis of CP has been established, patients should be started on medical management. Steps in medical therapy include alcohol and smoking cessation, and analgesic agents starting with non-opioids such as nonsteroidal anti-inflammatory drugs. Opioids should be last line but are often required (14). Additional treatments for pain can include tricyclic antidepressants, neuromodulators such as gabapentin, and interventional procedures such as plexus nerve block or transcutaneous electrical nerve stimulation. Pancreatic enzymes can improve pain through a negative feedback mechanism (15). Finally, the detrimental effects on pancreatic endocrine function

DOI: 10.1201/9781003080060-32

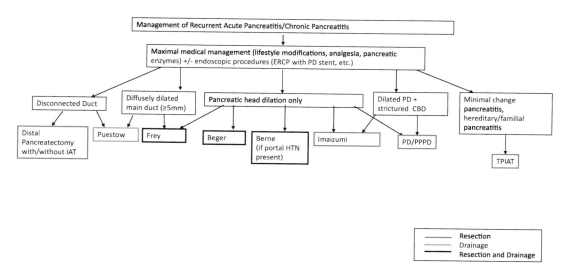

Figure 32.1 Decision tree to assist with surgical decision-making for chronic pancreatitis. *Abbreviations:* ERCP: endoscopic retrograde cholangiopancreatography; PD: pancreatic duct; IAT: islet autotransplant; HTN: hypertension; PD: pancreaticoduodenectomy; PPPD: pylorus preserving pancreaticoduodenectomy; TPIAT: total pancreatectomy with islet autotransplantation.

may require supplemental insulin and/or dietary changes, though this typically occurs later in the disease process (13,14).

Over the years, there has been a shift in the traditional paradigm of maximizing medical and endoscopic treatment prior to pursuing surgery for CP. A number of studies, including multiple randomized controlled trials (RCTs), have shown a greater improvement in overall pain relief with surgery rather than endoscopy (16–20). The 2020 International Consensus guidelines recommend that either endoscopy or surgery should be offered to a patient with severe pain due to CP, and that surgery should be offered after the first endoscopic attempt (21). Patients with pancreatic ductal obstruction due to stones and/or stricture may undergo ERCP with possible pancreatic ductal stenting, endoscopic drainage of pancreatic pseudocysts, extracorporeal shock wave lithotripsy (ESWL) of pancreatic stones, endoscopic celiac nerve block, or pancreatic sphincterotomy (21,22).

As mentioned previously, surgery is no longer the last resort once medical and endoscopic management have failed. The most common indication for surgery is intractable pain and operating early in the disease process prior to development of long-term side effects of chronic pain is recommended (23). Multiple studies have shown increased rates of partial, and complete, pain relief, decreased rates of exocrine insufficiency, and lower re-intervention rates when surgery is performed within 24–36 months of the initial diagnosis (17–19,23–26). Operating early in the disease process may prevent the ongoing inflammation and fibrosis leading to neuropathic pain, which is particularly difficult to treat, and pancreatic exocrine insufficiency

caused by ongoing destruction of acinar cells (27). Other indications for surgery include local complications, such as damage to surrounding vessels, pancreatic fistula, large pseudocysts, biliary or duodenal strictures, and suspicion of neoplasm (27).

Surgical decision making primarily depends on ductal dilation and inflammation of the pancreatic head. Drainage procedures (such as Puestow) focus on relieving ductal hypertension due to ductal obstruction, resection procedures (pancreaticoduodenectomy [PD] and distal pancreatectomy) are more historical in the context of CP and remove the inflammatory (or neoplastic) mass, and combination resection and drainage procedures (Frey and Beger with their associated modifications) address both of these issues (13,27–29). *Figure 32.1* demonstrates a decision tree for choosing the appropriate operations for a particular case. A number of small studies have been performed comparing various operations. In studies comparing PD and pylorus-preserving pancreaticoduodenectomy (PPPD) (*Figure 32.2a*) versus duodenum preserving pancreatic head resections (DPPHR) such as Beger or Frey (*Figure 32.2b,c*), pain relief is similar, but there is decreased operating time, intraoperative blood transfusion, hospital length of stay, delayed gastric emptying, morbidity, and improvement in quality of life in the DPPHR group (30–35). There is no significant difference when the Frey and Beger are compared, though Frey is generally preferred, as it also addresses the dilated pancreatic duct (35–37).

It is important to also note two further disease patterns. In minimal change CP (MCCP), total pancreatectomy with islet autotransplant (TPIAT) represents the best surgical option (38,39). For disconnected

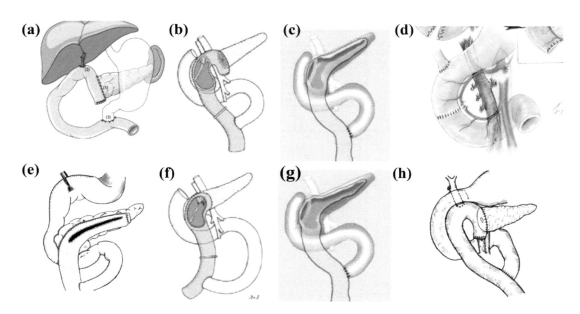

Figure 32.2 Illustrations of common procedures for chronic pancreatitis and their respective reconstructions: PPPD (a); Beger (b); Frey (c); TPIAT (d); Puestow (e); Berne (f); Hamburg (g); Imaizumi (h).

pancreatic duct, the surgical approach depends on the location of the duct disconnection, but often entails either distal pancreatectomy or Puestow (Fischer).

The following list is not comprehensive, as there are a number of historical operations and numerous modifications to the procedures that have been described. We are including the most common and well-followed operations (*Table 32.1*). The PD/PPPD and distal pancreatectomy have historically been used for CP, although as surgery has evolved and both drainage, as well as, resection and drainage procedures, have been developed, these operations are typically no longer done for CP. The incision utilized for the following procedures should be a bilateral subcostal incision, unless the patient has a narrow rib cage which may warrant an upper vertical midline incision. For all of these procedures we recommend leaving a single closed suction drain placed within the lesser sac (*Figure 32.2*).

OPERATION FOR DILATED MAIN PANCREATIC DUCT

Puestow procedure (lateral pancreaticojejunostomy)

Puestow and Gillesby originally described lateral pancreaticojejunostomy with distal pancreatectomy and splenectomy for CP in the late 1950s. This was modified in the 1960s by Partington and Rochelle to exclude distal

pancreatectomy and splenectomy. Although in theory safer and simpler than pancreatic head resections with drainage procedures, as it avoids dissection around the venous confluence, it does not address disease that involves the head of the pancreas. Long-term pain relief is also quite variable, from 40–90% (22,28,29,40,41).

Brief operative description

Upon entry into the abdomen, the gastrocolic ligament is divided to enter the lesser sac. The stomach and colon are retracted cephalad and caudally, respectively. Adhesions between the posterior wall of the stomach, and anterior surface of the pancreas, should be taken down carefully to avoid blood vessels and the vagus nerves along the lesser curvature. The anterior surface of the pancreas should be visible to within a few centimeters of the tail.

The anterior pancreas is palpated to locate the distended pancreatic duct and to identify ductal stones. The dilated pancreatic duct location is confirmed by using a small gauge needle to aspirate pancreatic fluid from the duct. If unable to identify the duct via aspiration, an intraoperative ultrasound can be used, or a vertical incision in the neck of the pancreas can be made, until the pancreatic duct is found. The duct is opened longitudinally from neck to tail using electrocautery. A 60 cm Roux-en-Y limb of small bowel is created and passed in a retrocolic fashion through the transverse mesocolon and positioned adjacent to the filleted open pancreatic duct. A side-to-side pancreaticojejunostomy is created

Table 32.1 Summary of operations for chronic pancreatitis

Procedure	Anastomosis	Resection	Drainage	Key manoeuvres
PD/PPPD (51) (Figure 32.2a)	End-to-side PJ to pancreatic body, end-to-side CDJ or HJ	Complete pancreatic head with duodenum, CBD	–	
Puestow (42) (Figure 32.2e)	Side-to-side PJ	–	Longitudinal opening of main pancreatic duct	
Beger (52) (Figure 32.2b)	End-to-side PJ to pancreatic body, side-to-side PJ to pancreatic head	Near complete resection pancreatic head	–	
Frey (45) (Figure 32.2c)	Side-to-side PJ	Partial resection pancreatic head	Longitudinal opening of main pancreatic duct	
Berne (53) (Figure 32.2f)	End-to-side PJ	Partial resection pancreatic head	Opening of CBD and main PD	
Hamburg (49) (Figure 32.2g)	V shaped side-to-side PJ	Partial resection pancreatic head	Wide opening of main pancreatic duct, secondary and tertiary ductal branches	
Imaizumi (47) (Figure 32.2h)	End-to-side PJ to pancreatic body, end-to-side CDD or CDJ	Complete pancreatic head, intrapancreatic CBD	–	
TPIAT (38) (Figure 32.2d)	End-to-side CDJ, end-to-side DJ	Entire pancreas with duodenum (w/wo pylorus), spleen	–	Transfusion of islet cells into portal system

Abbreviations: PD: pancreaticoduodenectomy; PPPD: pylorus preserving pancreaticoduodenectomy; PJ: pancreaticojejunostomy; CDJ: choledochojejunostomy; HJ: hepaticojejunostomy; CBD: common bile duct; CDD: choledochoduodenostomy; DJ: duodenojejunostomy; TPIAT: total pancreatectomy with islet autotransplantation.

using a single layer of either running or interrupted 3-0 absorbable sutures that include the pancreatic duct and full-thickness bites of the jejunum (*Figure 32.2e*).

OPERATIONS FOR ENLARGED PANCREATIC HEAD

Beger procedure (duodenal preserving pancreatic head resection)

Developed by the German surgeon Hans Beger in 1980, this procedure addresses disease of the pancreatic head by performing a near complete resection of this portion of the gland. The procedure also allows for addressing distal CBD strictures. Of note, the Beger is not a complete ductal drainage procedure as the pancreatic duct is not completely opened and only a simple pancreaticojejunostomy is performed (22,28,29,43).

Brief operative description

The pancreatic head and body are exposed in their entirety by division of the gastrocolic ligament. Caudal mobilization of the hepatic colon flexure is done followed

by a Kocher manoeuvre. The right gastroepiploic vessels are divided to give full exposure of the pancreas as well as the superior mesenteric and portal veins. The pancreas is divided above the portal vein and resection of the pancreatic head is performed focusing on the inflamed fibrotic tissue. It is important to leave a rim of tissue approximately 5 mm wide along the wall of the duodenum to preserve the pancreaticoduodenal arterial arcades. Reconstruction is achieved by means of a Roux-en-Y jejunal loop with an end-to-side anastomosis to the pancreatic body and a side-to-side anastomosis to the excavated pancreatic head. Resection of the fibrotic pancreatic parenchyma is usually sufficient to relieve a CBD stricture. If the obstruction cannot be relieved, a choledochoduodenostomy, choledochojejunostomy, or hepaticojejunostomy can be performed (*Figure 32.2b*).

Frey procedure

The Frey procedure was originally described in 1987 as a novel, hybrid procedure, combining partial resection of the head of the pancreas with the lateral pancreaticojejunostomy. The proposed benefit was an improvement in ductal drainage by decompressing both the duct of Santorini and ducts in the uncinate process while also allowing for removal of ductal calcifications. It is hypothesized that the fibrosis of the pancreatic head drives much of the pain associated with CP and this procedure removes the diseased portion of the gland while also providing adequate drainage. The original indication was for patients with an enlarged fibrotic head of the pancreas and an associated dilated main pancreatic duct. However, it is also now supported in patients who have had prior drainage procedures with no relief of symptoms. Many argue that the Frey procedure is easier to perform than other drainage and resection procedures, as transection of the pancreas neck over the superior mesenteric portal vein confluence is not needed (22,28,29,44,45).

Brief operative description

After opening the lesser sac and fully exposing the anterior pancreas, a Kocher manoeuvre is performed to elevate the duodenum and expose the pancreas. The pancreatic duct is identified with palpation and ductal aspiration, or alternatively with intraoperative ultrasound. The pancreatic duct is opened longitudinally in the same fashion as the Puestow procedure, extending to within 1–2 cm of the distal portion and the incision in the head to within 1 cm of the inner aspect of the duodenum. It is common to divide the anterior pancreaticoduodenal arterial cascade during opening of the duct in the head and these vessels should be suture ligated. The head of the pancreas is cored-out using sharp dissection, with haemostasis obtained using cautery or suture ligation. It is important to preserve a rim of pancreatic tissue along the inner aspect of the duodenum to allow blood supply to the duodenum from superior and inferior pancreaticoduodenal arteries. In patients with a biliary obstructive component, a choledochojejunostomy should be performed. The cored-out head of the pancreas and the open main duct are drained into a Roux-en-Y limb of jejunum of 70–80 cm in length passed through the transverse mesocolon to lie over the pancreas. A single layer pancreaticojejunostomy is performed in a similar fashion to the Puestow procedure described above (*Figure 32.2c*).

In order to avoid unnecessary dissection, or address particular issues, a number of modifications to the above operations have been created. The Berne modification of the Beger procedure was described in Switzerland in 2001 and has shown similar results to the Beger procedure with regards to pain and quality of life, though with shorter operating times and length of hospital stay (46). The modifications include excision of the pancreatic head without transection of the pancreas, along with opening of the CBD and pancreatic ducts. A thin rim of pancreatic tissue is left behind and an end-to-side pancreaticojejunostomy is created with a Roux-en-Y loop. This operation is particularly useful in patients with portal hypertension and dilated collateral veins as it avoids retroperitoneal dissection (*Figure 32.2f*).

The Imaizumi modification of the Beger procedure was described in 2009 and includes removal of the entire pancreatic head, including the intrapancreatic CBD (47). Reconstruction is via end-to-side pancreaticojejunostomy and end-to-side cholecochoduodenostomy or choledochojejunostomy. This operation is useful when CBD stenosis is present and has shown >90% long-term pain relief (*Figure 32.2h*).

Complications of duodenum preserving pancreatic head resections

The most common postoperative complications following pancreatic surgery include: wound infection; haemorrhage; pancreatic fistula and intra-abdominal abscess. Arterial bleeding is the major life-threatening complication and can occur several days postoperatively due to erosion of peripancreatic vessels by pancreatic fluid from an anastomotic leakage, or due to rupture of a pseudoaneurysm. Early postoperative bleeding can also be due to inadequate haemostasis at the time of surgery and retroperitoneal bleeding.

OPERATIONS FOR MINIMAL CHANGE PANCREATITIS

Total pancreatectomy and islet auto-transplantation

The total pancreatectomy with islet autotransplantation (TPIAT) was developed at the University of Minnesota in the 1970s with the goal to remove the pancreas as a nidus for inflammation while preventing, or minimizing, brittle diabetes. The rate of pain relief with this procedure is notable, with 82% reporting pain relief at 10 years and 90% at 15 years at a single, large institution. The procedure also provides frequent success in avoiding the need for insulin support. At 5 years, around one third of patients are insulin independent, one third require insulin supplementation, and one third are insulin dependent. Along with a skilled surgeon, TPIAT requires an islet processing facility and a dedicated multidisciplinary team that would ideally include surgery, gastroenterology, endocrine, pain management, health psychology, genetics, dietician, social work, and specially trained nurse coordinators. At our institution, indications for TPIAT include a diagnosis of chronic, or recurrent, acute pancreatitis, narcotic dependence or pain leading to impaired quality of life, evaluation from a multidisciplinary group, failure of maximal medical/endoscopic management, and adequate islet cell function (22,28,29,38,39).

Brief operative description

The basic operative procedure can be performed laparoscopically or in an open fashion. A Kocher manoeuvre is performed to completely mobilize the duodenum and the pancreatic head. The portal triad is isolated and dissected free. The gastroduodenal artery is dissected and looped but not divided. The short gastric vessels are divided. The spleen is mobilized by dividing the spleno-renal and spleno-colic ligaments. Using the spleen as a handle, the tail and body of the pancreas are mobilized medially to the level of the superior mesenteric and portal veins. The tissue around the splenic artery and splenic vein are dissected, taking care to identify and loop the splenic artery on the superior border of the pancreas. The splenic vein is looped distal to the entry of the inferior mesenteric vein. The duodenum is transected 2–4 cm distal to the pylorus, ensuring the right gastric and gastroepiploic vessels are preserved. The stomach is reflected upwards and laterally to expose the head and body of the pancreas. The proximal jejunum is divided 10–20 cm distal to the ligament of Treitz, then freed proximally until the ligament of Treitz has been taken down (*Figure 32.2d*).

At this point, the pancreas is attached by its vascular supply, the CBD, and the uncinate process. The bile duct is transected at the superior border of the pancreas. Careful examination is done to look for any accessory right hepatic artery arising from the superior mesenteric artery. If one exists, it is carefully preserved. The uncinate process of the pancreas is mobilized off the portal vein by dividing all the small tributaries to the portal vein. The vascular structures are divided in the following order: gastroduodenal artery; splenic artery; splenic vein. The pancreas is then immediately placed in cold sterile preservative solution and transported to the islet isolation laboratory (*Figure 32.3*).

During the processing of the pancreas a Roux-en-Y jejunal loop is created, with each limb of the Roux being 60 cm in length. Both limbs are placed in a retrocolic position and an end-to-side choledocho-jejunostomy is constructed using multiple interrupted absorbable sutures. An end-to-side duodenojejunostomy is constructed in a single layer fashion using multiple interrupted sutures, and a gastrojejunostomy tube is placed in the stomach using a Stamm technique with the tip of the jejunal tube placed in the proximal jejunum.

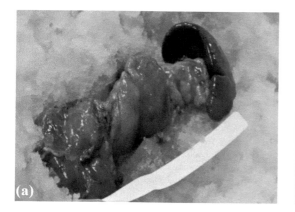
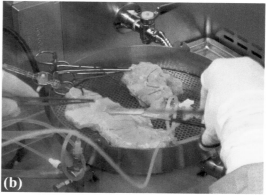
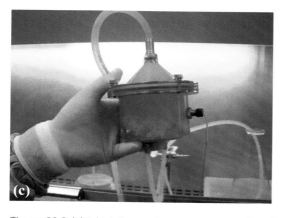
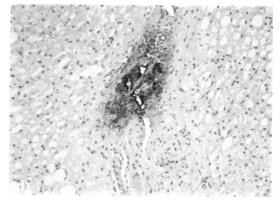

Figure 32.3 Islet isolation and pancreas processing during total pancreatectomy with islet autotransplantation. Surgical specimen: total pancreatectomy, duodenectomy and splenectomy (a). Processing of pancreas in islet laboratory (b). Riccordi chamber enzymatic digestion of pancreas to isolate islets. (c) Islet cells staining with antibody to insulin in liver after islet autotransplant (d).

Once the islet cell preparation is complete, the splenic vein stump or the middle colic vein is cannulated and attached to pressure tubing with an in-line manometer. The islet preparation is infused by gravity into the portal venous system, closely monitoring the portal pressure. The patient receives systemic anticoagulation prior to islet infusion.

The TPIAT operation is a unique surgical procedure that has its own set of postoperative expectations and complications that should be closely monitored. Delayed gastric emptying is common in the early postoperative period, thus the routine placement of a gastrojejunostomy tube intraoperatively. Upon resolution of the ileus, jejunal feeds are initiated. An insulin infusion is started in the operating room immediately following pancreatic resection for tight blood sugar control. Cultures are obtained during the laboratory isolation of the islet cells and pending bacterial growth, patients receive 1 week of intravenous antibiotics.

Many of the postoperative complications are similar to other procedures performed on the pancreas including haemorrhage and fistulae. More specific to TPIAT are hypoinsulinaemia and portal vein thrombosis. The function of the transplanted islet cells often takes months to re-establish with nearly all patients requiring ongoing insulin supplementation at the time of discharge from hospital. Thrombosis of the portal vein is due to the direct infusion of the islet cells and is thought to be due to mechanical obstruction potentially reducing flow as well as a localized inflammatory response providing two of the three factors of Virchow's triad in the portal system. Patients should be routinely screened for portal vein thrombosis (PVT), and if found, placed on anticoagulation for 3–6 months or when the clot is resolved on ultrasound (48).

In 1998, the Hamburg modification of the Frey procedure was introduced as another approach to treat small duct pancreatitis (49). This procedure includes a V-shaped excision longitudinally along the main pancreatic duct that also allows drainage of the secondary and tertiary ductal branches (*Figure 32.2g*). This has shown good pain relief without significant impairment of pancreatic endocrine or exocrine function, however only small studies have been done, and to-date it has not been directly compared to TPIAT.

REFERENCES

1. Beyer G, Habtezion A, Werner J, Lerch MM, Mayerle J. Chronic pancreatitis. *Lancet* 2020;**396(10249)**: 499–512.
2. Wilcox CM, Yadav D, Ye T, Gardner TB, Gelrud A, Sandhu BS, et al. Chronic pancreatitis pain pattern and severity are independent of abdominal imaging findings. *Clin Gastroenterol Hepatol* 2015;**13(3)**:552–29.
3. Guda NM, Muddana V, Whitcomb DC, Levy P, Garg P, Cote G, et al. Recurrent acute pancreatitis: International State of-the-Science conference with recommendations. *Pancreas* 2018;**47(6)**: 653–66.
4. Whitcomb DC, Frulloni L, Garg P, et al. Chronic pancreatitis: An international draft consensus proposal for a new mechanistic definition. *Pancreatology* 2016;**16(2)**:218–24.
5. Strate T, Yekebas E, Knoefel WT, Bloechle C, Izbicki JR. Pathogenesis and the natural course of chronic pancreatitis. *Eur J Gastroenterol Hepatol* 2002;**14(9)**:929–34.
6. Pezzilli R. Etiology of chronic pancreatitis: Has it changed in the last decade? *World J Gastroenterol* 2009;**15(38)**:4737–40.
7. Yadav D, Lowenfels AB. The epidemiology of pancreatitis and pancreatic cancer. *Gastroenterology* 2013;**144(6)**:1252–61.
8. Herreros-Villanueva M, Hijona E, Bañales JM, Cosme A, Bujanda L. Alcohol consumption on pancreatic diseases. *World J Gastroenterol* 2013;**19(5)**: 638–47.
9. Weiss FU, Laemmerhirt F, Lerch MM. Etiology and risk factors of acute and chronic pancreatitis. *Visc Med* 2019;**35(2)**:73–81.
10. Whitcomb DC. Genetic risk factors for pancreatic disorders. *Gastroenterology* 2013;**144(6)**:1292–1302.
11. Fan BG, Andrén-Sandberg A. Autoimmune pancreatitis. *N Am J Med Sci* 2009;**1(4)**:148–51.
12. Asbun HJ, Conlon K, Fernandez-Cruz L, Friess H, Shrikhande SV, Adham M, et al. When to perform a pancreatoduodenectomy in the absence of positive histology? A consensus statement by the International Study Group of Pancreatic Surgery. *Surgery* 2014;**155(5)**:c887–92.
13. Singh VK, Yadav D, Garg PK. Diagnosis and management of chronic pancreatitis: A review. *JAMA* 2019;**322(24)**:2422–34.
14. Drewes AM, Bouwense SAW, Campbell CM, Ceyhan GO, Delhaye M, Demir IE, et al. Guidelines for the understanding and management of pain in chronic pancreatitis. *Pancreatology* 2017;**17(5)**:720–31.
15. Hobbs PM, Johnson WG, Graham DY. Management of pain in chronic pancreatitis with emphasis on exogenous pancreatic enzymes. *World J Gastrointest Pharmacol Ther* 2016;**7(3)**:370–86.
16. Ahmed Ali U, Nieuwenhuijs VB, van Eijck CH, Gooszen HG, van Dam RM, Busch OR, et al. Clinical outcome in relation to timing of surgery in chronic pancreatitis: A nomogram to predict pain relief. *Arch Surg* 2012;**147(10)**:925–32.
17. Ahmed Ali U, Pahlplatz JM, Nealon WH, van Goor H, Gooszen HG, Boermeester MA. Endoscopic or surgical intervention for painful obstructive chronic pancreatitis. *Cochrane Database Syst Rev* 2015;**(3)**:CD007884.
18. Díte P, Ruzicka M, Zboril V, Novotný I. A prospective, randomized trial comparing endoscopic and surgical therapy for chronic pancreatitis. *Endoscopy* 2003;**35(7)**:553–8.
19. Cahen DL, Gouma DJ, Nio Y, Rauws EAJ, Boermeester MA, Busch OR, et al. Endoscopic versus surgical drainage of the pancreatic duct in chronic pancreatitis. *N Engl J Med* 2007;**356(7)**:676–84.
20. Issa Y, Kempeneers MA, Bruno MJ, Fockens P, Poley J-W, Ali UA, et al. Effect of early surgery vs endoscopy-

first approach on pain in patients with chronic pancreatitis: The ESCAPE randomized clinical trial. *JAMA* 2020;**323(3)**:237–47.

21. Kitano M, Gress TM, Garg PK, Itoi T, Irisawa A, Isayama H, et al. International consensus guidelines on interventional endoscopy in chronic pancreatitis. Recommendations from the working group for the international consensus guidelines for chronic pancreatitis in collaboration with the International Association of Pancreatology, the American Pancreatic Association, the Japan Pancreas Society, and European Pancreatic Club. *Pancreatology* 2020;**20(6)**:1045–55.

22. Larsen M, Kozarek R. Management of pancreatic ductal leaks and fistulae. *J Gastroenterol Hepatol* 2014;**29(7)**:1360–70.

23. Ke N, Jia D, Huang W, Nunes QM, Windsor JA, Liu X, et al. Earlier surgery improves outcomes from painful chronic pancreatitis. *Medicine (Baltimore)* 2018;**97(19)**:e0651.

24. Riediger H, Adam U, Fischer E, Keck T, Pfeffer F, Hopt UT, et al. Long-term outcome after resection for chronic pancreatitis in 224 patients. *J Gastrointest Surg* 2007;**11(8)**:949–60.

25. Yang CJ, Bliss LA, Freedman SD, Sheth S, Vollmer CM, Ng SC, et al. Surgery for chronic pancreatitis: The role of early surgery in pain management. *Pancreas* 2015;**44(5)**:819–23.

26. Yang CJ, Bliss LA, Schapira EF, Freedman SD, Ng SC, Windsor JA, et al. Systematic review of early surgery for chronic pancreatitis: Impact on pain, pancreatic function, and re-intervention. *J Gastrointest Surg* 2014;**18(10)**:1863–69.

27. Kempeneers MA, Issa Y, Ali UA, Baron RD, Besselink MG, Büchler M, et al. International consensus guidelines for surgery and the timing of intervention in chronic pancreatitis. *Pancreatology* 2020;**20(2)**:149–57.

28. Strobel O, Büchler MW, Werner J. Surgical therapy of chronic pancreatitis: Indications, techniques and results. *Int J Surg* 2009;**7(4)**:305–12.

29. Neal CP, Dennison AR, Garcea G. Surgical therapy in chronic pancreatitis. *Minerva Gastroenterol Dietol* 2012;**58(4)**:377–400.

30. Büchler MW, Friess H, Müller MW, Wheatley AM, Beger HG. Randomized trial of duodenum-preserving pancreatic head resection versus pylorus-preserving Whipple in chronic pancreatitis. *Am J Surg* 1995;**169(1)**:65–70.

31. Klempa I, Spatny M, Menzel J, et al. Pancreatic function and quality of life after resection of the head of the pancreas in chronic pancreatitis. A prospective, randomized comparative study after duodenum preserving resection of the head of the pancreas versus Whipple's operation. *Chirurg* 1995;**66(4)**:350–9.

32. Farkas G, Leindler L, Daróczi M, Farkas G Jr. Prospective randomised comparison of organ-preserving pancreatic head resection with pylorus-preserving pancreaticoduodenectomy. *Langenbecks Arch Surg* 2006;**391(4)**:338–42.

33. Izbicki JR, Bloechle C, Broering DC, Knoefel WT, Kuechler T, Broelsch CE. Extended drainage versus resection in surgery for chronic pancreatitis: A prospective randomized trial comparing the longitudinal

pancreaticojejunostomy combined with local pancreatic head excision with the pylorus-preserving pancreatoduodenectomy. *Ann Surg* 1998;**228(6)**:771–9.

34. Bachmann K, Tomkoetter L, Kutup A, Erbes J, Vashist Y, Mann O, et al. Is the Whipple procedure harmful for long-term outcome in treatment of chronic pancreatitis? 15-years follow-up comparing the outcome after pylorus-preserving pancreatoduodenectomy and Frey procedure in chronic pancreatitis. *Ann Surg* 2013;**258(5)**:815–21.

35. Izbicki JR, Bloechle C, Knoefel WT, Kuechler T, Binmoeller KF, Broelsch CE. Duodenum-preserving resection of the head of the pancreas in chronic pancreatitis. A prospective, randomized trial. *Ann Surg* 1995;**221(4)**:350–8.

36. Strate T, Taherpour Z, Bloechle C, Mann O, Bruhn JP, Schneider C, et al. Long-term follow-up of a randomized trial comparing the Beger and Frey procedures for patients suffering from chronic pancreatitis. *Ann Surg* 2005;**241(4)**:591–8.

37. Izbicki JR, Bloechle C, Knoefel WT, Kuechler T, Binmoeller KF, Soehendra N, et al. Drainage versus resection in surgical therapy of chronic pancreatitis of the head of the pancreas: A randomized study. *Der Chirurg Zeitschrift fur alle Gebiete der operativen Medizen* 1997;**68(4)**:369–77.

38. Sutherland DE, Radosevich DM, Bellin MD, Hering BJ, Beilman GJ, Dunn TB, et al. Total pancreatectomy and islet autotransplantation for chronic pancreatitis. *J Am Coll Surg* 2012;**214(4)**:409–26.

39. Wilson GC, Sutton JM, Smith MT, Schmulewitz N, Salehi M, Choe KA, et al. Total pancreatectomy with islet cell autotransplantation as the initial treatment for minimal-change chronic pancreatitis. *HPB (Oxford)* 2015;**17(3)**:232–8.

40. Adams DB. The Puestow procedure: How I do it. *J Gastrointest Surg* 2013;**17(6)**:1138–42.

41. Puestow CB, Gillesby WJ. Retrograde surgical drainage of pancreas for chronic relapsing pancreatitis. *AMA Arch Surg* 1958;**76(6)**:898–907.

42. Partington PF, Rochelle RE. Modified Puestow procedure for retrograde drainage of the pancreatic duct. *Ann Surg* 1960;**152(6)**:1037–43.

43. Beger HG, Büchler M, Bittner R. The duodenum preserving resection of the head of the pancreas (DPRHP) in patients with chronic pancreatitis and an inflammatory mass in the head. An alternative surgical technique to the Whipple operation. *Acta Chir Scand* 1990;**156(4)**:309–15.

44. Roch A, Teyssedou J, Mutter D, Marescaux J, Pessaux P. Chronic pancreatitis: A surgical disease? Role of the Frey procedure. *World J Gastrointest Surg* 2014;**6(7)**:129–35.

45. Frey CF, Smith GJ. Description and rationale of a new operation for chronic pancreatitis. **Pancreas** 1987;**2(6)**:701–7.

46. Köninger J, Seiler CM, Sauerland S, Wente MN, Reidel MA, Müller MW, et al. Duodenum-preserving pancreatic head resection--a randomized controlled trial comparing the original Beger procedure with the Berne modification (ISRCTN No. 50638764). *Surgery* 2008;**143(4)**:490–8.

47. Imaizumi T, Hanyu F, Suzuki M, Nakasako T, Harada N, Hatori T. Clinical experience with duodenum-preserving total resection of the head of the pancreas with pancreaticocholedochoduodenostomy. *J Hepatobiliary Pancreat Surg* 1995;**2**:38–44.
48. Robbins AJ, Skube ME, Bellin MD, et al. Portal vein thrombosis after total pancreatectomy and islet autotransplant: Prophylaxis and graft impact. *Pancreas* 2019;**48**(**10**):1329–33.
49. Izbicki JR, Bloechle C, Broering DC, Kuechler T, Broelsch CE. Longitudinal V-shaped excision of the ventral pancreas for small duct disease in severe chronic pancreatitis: Prospective evaluation of a new surgical procedure. *Ann Surg* 1998;**227**(**2**):213–19.

iley & Love's Essential Operations Bailey & Love's Essential Operations
iley & Love's Essential Operations Bailey & Love's Essential Operations
iley & Love's Essential Operations Bailey & Love's Essential Operations

SECTION 6 | PANCREAS

Chapter 33

Pancreatic Adenocarcinoma

Martin Loos and Markus W. Büchler

INTRODUCTION

The prognosis of pancreatic cancer has significantly improved in recent years, although it remains a very aggressive cancer with an utterly devastating prognosis (1). This chapter summarizes the current status of modern pancreatic cancer surgery.

Pancreatic cancer or other terms such as 'pancreatic carcinoma' usually refer to pancreatic ductal adenocarcinoma, which represents 85–90% of all pancreatic neoplasms (2). Surgical resection is the cornerstone of pancreatic cancer treatment providing a chance for prolonged survival or even cure (3–6). However, because of aggressive local tumour invasion of surrounding tissues, including the coeliac axis, the hepatic arteries, the superior mesenteric artery and the superior mesenteric/portal venous axis, and early metastases, predominantly in lymph nodes, liver, peritoneum and lungs, about 30% of patients present with locally advanced disease with a further 50–60% having metastatic disease (1,3,7). Historically these patients were not considered candidates for a surgical approach, explaining why <10% of pancreatic cancer patients were primarily referred for surgical resection (8,9).

Recent advances in both surgical techniques and multimodal treatment concepts have significantly improved the outcome of patients with locally-resectable disease and expanded treatment options with a curative-intent surgical approach even in more advanced disease stages (10–18). Technical refinements that have been implemented in pancreatic cancer surgery include the 'artery-first' and 'uncinate-first' approaches, and radical resection of the so called 'mesopancreas' by complete dissection of the anatomical 'triangle' between the coeliac axis, the superior mesenteric artery, the superior mesenteric/portal vein axis and radical antegrade modular pancreatosplenectomy (RAMPS) (19–25). Resection and reconstruction of the superior mesenteric/portal vein axis has become the surgical standard in patients with venous tumour involvement, with perioperative outcomes comparable to those of standard resections (26–28). The other key components of successful pancreatic cancer treatments are more effective multiagent chemotherapies such as FOLFIRINOX and gemcitabine in combination with nab-paclitaxel (17,29–32). In fact, even in locally unresectable pancreatic cancer, conversion to resectable disease by modern neoadjuvant regimens is possible in up to 60% of patients (33).

EPIDEMIOLOGY

Globally, there were estimated to be nearly 10 million cancer-related deaths in 2020 (34,35). The incidence of pancreatic cancer has increased over the past years approaching 500 000 new cases per year in 2020. Some 466 003 patients were estimated to have died from pancreatic cancer in 2020 representing the seventh most common cause for cancer-related mortality worldwide (36). In the economically developed world, pancreatic cancer is currently the fourth leading cause of cancer mortality (34). There is an estimated incidence of 60 430 new cases in the USA and of 10 300 in the UK with 48 220 and 9 421 deaths, respectively (34,37,38). Within the next decade, pancreatic cancer is predicted to become the second most common cause of cancer-related mortality in the modern Western World (39).

DIAGNOSTIC APPROACH

The clinical signs and symptoms associated with pancreatic cancer are often non-specific which explains why most patients are diagnosed at an advanced disease stage (40–42). Abdominal imaging should be performed in patients where there is a suspicion of pancreatic cancer. The 'gold standard' is a triple-phase contrast-enhanced computed tomography (CECT) of the abdomen (and pelvis) or abdominal magnetic resonance imaging (MRI) (3). Magnetic resonance cholangiopancreatography (MRCP) may be helpful if radiological findings are inconclusive and irregularities of the main pancreatic duct can be accurately detected. Although endoscopic retrograde cholangiopancreatography (ERCP) is a highly sensitive tool for the visualization of the biliary tree and pancreatic ducts, it is less important in the primary diagnosis of pancreatic cancer, principally because of its invasive nature and the risk of post-ERCP pancreatitis. In cases of obstructive jaundice with a significant elevation of serum bilirubin ERCP does offer a therapeutic option to relieve jaundice and is also potentially diagnostic. Although biliary stenting may be required to relieve obstructive jaundice, if neoadjuvant therapy is planned, it should not be routinely performed prior to surgery. Van der Goog et al. have shown that preoperative biliary stenting does not improve perioperative outcomes of pancreatic cancer patients with biliary outflow obstruction and instead this results in an increased perioperative complication rate (43).

DOI: 10.1201/9781003080060-33

Once the diagnosis of pancreatic cancer is radiologically confirmed, resectability should be assessed and metastatic disease must be excluded. Histological confirmation by transcutaneous or endosonographic-guided biopsy is usually not required because radiological criteria are adequate to proceed to surgical exploration (44). Resectability criteria have been defined by several groups (45,46). According to the definitions by the National Comprehensive Cancer Network (NCCN) (47) and the International Study Group (ISGPS) (48), borderline resectable pancreatic cancer (BRPC) is characterized by: 1) Distortion, narrowing, or occlusion of the superior mesenteric vein/portal vein, but with the technical possibility of reconstruction; 2) a semi-circumferential abutment less than 180° of the superior mesenteric artery; or 3) tumour contact with the hepatic artery without extension to the coeliac axis. Locally advanced pancreatic cancer (LAPC) is defined as: 1) More extensive involvement of the aforementioned vessels; 2) any tumour involvement of the aorta or inferior vena cava; or 3) involvement of the mesentericoportal axis without the possibility of venous reconstruction. The International Association of Pancreatology (IAP) additionally identified biological and conditional criteria for borderline resectability which include: 1) Carbohydrate antigen 19-9 (CA 19-9) levels greater than 500 units/mL; 2) presence of regional lymph node metastases confirmed by examination of biopsy samples, or highly suspected on positron emission tomography (PET-CT) scans and 3) when the patient's performance status is significantly reduced (49). Distant metastatic disease is accepted as a strict contraindication for upfront surgery. An advantage of using abdominal CT/MRI as the initial diagnostic modality is that not only local resectability is assessable, but also abdominal metastases can be detected. To rule-out pulmonary metastases, CT imaging of the chest should complete the diagnostic work-up. It is important to note that there remains a risk of under-staging patients with pancreatic cancer if only CT imaging is performed during their work-up. The use of staging laparoscopy can further reduce the post-test probability of unresectable disease following CT from 40% for those patients undergoing CT only, to 18% for patients with CT and laparoscopy (50). The addition of the tumour marker CA 19–9 can further increase the efficacy of staging laparoscopy (51,52), and if there is any suspicion of liver metastases MRI should be considered (53–55). If other metastases are suspected, ^{18}fludeoxyglucose (^{18}FDG)-PET-CT may be helpful because it increases the accuracy compared with CT alone (56). A preoperative biopsy may not be needed in a patient with a potentially resectable pancreatic mass highly suspected of malignancy (44). One major issue following a tissue biopsy is that while a positive biopsy can confirm the suspected diagnosis, a benign sample will not exclude the presence of malignancy.

MODERN PANCREATIC CANCER THERAPY

Surgical strategies in resectable pancreatic cancer

Surgical resection is the only curative-intent treatment option for patients with pancreatic cancer and microscopically complete local resection is one of the most relevant prognostic markers (4). However, complete tumour resection still represents a real challenge in pancreatic cancer surgery and depending on the protocol used for pathological work-up of the resected specimen, high microscopic incomplete resection rates ranging from 28–71%, have been reported (57). Not surprisingly therefore, 20–30% of a patient's tumour will recur at the resection site (58–61) and 50% of pancreatic cancer patients will be found to have systemic tumour recurrence within the first 2 years following resection. The aim of every surgeon should include the prevention of local recurrence which occurs in one or more of three different compartments: 1) The remnant pancreas; 2) regional, mesenteric and retroperitoneal lymph nodes; and 3) perivascular tissue alongside the coeliac trunk, hepatic and superior mesenteric arteries.

To prevent recurrence in the pancreatic remnant, intraoperative frozen section should be performed during pancreatic resection to confirm a microscopically clear resection margin (R0 resection). In case of incomplete tumour resection, re-resection or even total pancreatectomy is necessary (62,63).

To prevent lymph node recurrence, adequate lymph node resection is warranted which usually includes adequate regional lymphadenectomy as defined by the ISGPS (standard lymphadenectomy) (64). According to the Japanese classification, lymph node stations that should be resected during pancreaticoduodenectomy include peripancreatic lymph node (13, 17), supra- and infra-pyloric lymph nodes (5, 6), lymph node in the hepatoduodenal ligament (8, 12), lymph nodes occupying the right aspect of the coeliac axis (9) and the superior mesenteric artery (14,65). A total of 24 lymph nodes should be harvested, a number that can also serve as a quality indicator. The resection of a minimum of 20 regional lymph nodes has been shown to be of prognostic relevance (66,67). In distal pancreatectomy it is recommended that lymph nodes alongside the splenic artery (11), at the splenic hilum (10), lower aspect of the pancreatic tail (18) and coeliac axis (9) should be resected (68). Extended lymphadenectomy is not recommended as there are good data showing that extended lymphadenectomy is not associated with a survival benefit and perioperative morbidity is significantly increased (69).

Most local recurrences are located at the medial, and posterior, aspect of the peripancreatic resection margin towards the coeliac axis, superior mesenteric artery and superior mesenteric/portal vein axis, the so called 'mesopancreas' (70,71). Several surgical strategies have been established to reduce the rate of local recurrences including the 'artery-first' and 'uncinate-first' approaches (19,21). Both manoeuvres intend to facilitate radical resection by: 1) The early assessment of resectability to prevent R2 resections and the reduction of morbidity; 2) by displaying the superior mesenteric artery posteriorly from its aortic origin and medially from the peripheral mesenteric root – which guarantees a very accurate dissection and better control during the resection phase of the pancreatic head; and 3) by enabling better access to the superior mesenteric artery for radical dissection in the periarterial level-III dissection plane (72).

Whether the 'triangle' operation reduces the rate of local recurrences has yet to be assessed within randomized controlled trials (RCT) (24,25). Analogous to the concept of total mesorectal excision (TME) (73) and complete mesocolic excision (CME) (74), the pancreatic resection is not limited to the pancreas but includes the resection of the 'mesopancreas', specifically the tissue between the coeliac axis, the superior mesenteric artery and the superior mesenteric/portal vein axis (24,25). Contrasting however with the TME and CME, the 'mesopancreas' is not embryologically determined and based on the anatomically defined borders, resectable. However, the 'triangle' is the most frequent anatomical site of local recurrence (70,71).

To achieve a complete tumour resection in pancreatic cancer with venous involvement, an *en bloc* pancreatoduodenectomy, distal pancreatectomy or total pancreatectomy with mesentericoportal vein resection may be required. A recent systematic review and meta-analysis of 41 studies demonstrated perioperative morbidity comparable to those of standard resections although 30-day mortality was slightly higher in the venous resection group (3.84% vs. 3.17% p = 0.003) (75). The oncological outcomes after venous resection were significantly worse than those after standard resection. Whether this was attributed to more advanced tumours in the venous resection group remains unclear, although the tumours were larger and the R0 resection rates were lower. A propensity score-matched analysis showed similar survival of patients with venous resection compared to those with standard resection after adjustment for baseline characteristics (76).

Owing to these surgical achievements and advances in adjuvant chemotherapy within the past decade, 5-year survival rates of 38% after resection of tumours located in the pancreatic head and of 56% following resection of tumours situated in the pancreatic body or tail can be achieved in cases where a wide, greater than 1 mm negative resection margin can be achieved and this is combined with adjuvant therapy (77,78). It was the European Study Group of Pancreatic Cancer (ESPAC) that investigated several adjuvant chemotherapy protocols and has provided robust data within the past 3 decades (10,11,14,16,79). In 2017, results of the ESPAC-4 trial demonstrated a significantly longer overall median survival of 28 months after gemcitabine plus capecitabine compared with 25.5 months after gemcitabine monotherapy (p = 0.032) (16). Results from the PRODIGE24/CCTGPA.6 trial showed even better survival after adjuvant modified FOLFIRINOX than after gemcitabine monotherapy (54 vs. 35 months p = 0.003) (29). The role of neoadjuvant therapy in patients with resectable pancreatic cancer has yet to be determined.

Theoretically, neoadjuvant approaches may enable a higher rate of completion of medical therapy. Furthermore, it may also help to identify patients who will have disease progression under medical therapy and are unlikely to benefit from surgical resection. However, thus far, high-level evidence is lacking and most studies comparing upfront surgery with those with neoadjuvant therapy prior to surgical resection display considerable bias and no RCT data is available (80,81). The results of several ongoing RCTs comparing upfront surgery and adjuvant chemotherapy with surgical resection after neoadjuvant therapy are awaited. In summary, the current standard-of-care approach for patients with resectable pancreatic cancer is upfront resection followed by adjuvant multi-agent chemotherapy (gemcitabine plus capecitabine or modified FOLFIRINOX).

Conversion surgery – multimodality approaches in locally advanced and metastatic pancreatic cancer

LAPC is defined by local tumour growth with involvement (partial encasement of greater than 180° or true infiltration) of the coeliac axis or the superior mesenteric artery, according to the NCCN or ISGPS guidelines and has previously been considered an unresectable disease stage (47,48). Data from a meta-analysis showed high postoperative mortality rates of >13% after combined pancreatectomy and arterial resection with disappointing oncological outcomes (82). However, the use of more effective neoadjuvant treatment protocols such as multi-agent FOLFIRINOX or gemcitabine with nab-paclitaxel have changed the view regarding arterial involvement in pancreatic cancer (29). Hackert et al. demonstrated in a 575 patient series that approximately 60% of patients with locally unresectable pancreatic cancer were able to undergo tumour resection after neoadjuvant FOLFIRINOX (33). The median survival was 16 months after resection and 22.5 months after diagnosis. Recently, new surgical dissection techniques have been introduced, including 'arterial divestment' which consists of periadventitial dissection (PAD) of an encased artery (83,84). The idea of this approach is that the remaining tissue encasing arteries does not contain viable tumour cells after neoadjuvant treatment, and that although the artery concerned is still encased on imaging, curative resection can be achieved by sharp dissection along its periadventitial layer of the artery (*Figure 33.1*).

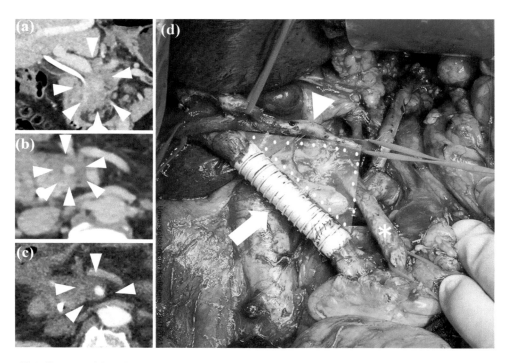

Figure 33.1 Coronary (a) and transverse (b) multidetector CECT images (venous phase) of a patient with locally advanced pancreatic cancer after neoadjuvant FOLFIRINOX therapy. Note the hypodense lesion with occlusion of the portal vein (white arrow heads). Arterial phase (c) of the same patient depicting arterial encasement (270°–360°) of the superior mesenteric artery (white arrow heads). Surgical site after resection (d) with total pancreatectomy, lymphadenectomy, resection of the portal vein confluence and interposition graft reconstruction (white arrow), venous splenorenal shunt, arterial divestment of the coeliac trunk, hepatic arteries (white arrow heads) and superior mesenteric artery (white asterisk). Note the complete dissection of the 'triangle' between the mesentericoportal vein axis, coeliac axis and superior mesenteric artery (white triangle with surrounding dots).

The Heidelberg Group was able to show that a median survival of 21.5% and an overall 5-year survival rate of 15% could be achieved after neoadjuvant treatment and PAD in 190 LAPC patients (85). Even better survival outcomes were reported by Michelakos and co-workers, who found a median overall survival of 31.5 months after neoadjuvant FOLFIRINOX treatment and surgical resection in 110 patients (86). However, the study cohort included not only LAPC (49%), but also Borderline Resectable Pancreas Cancer (BRPC) (51%) patients, and no data on arterial resection or divestment was provided. In another retrospective series, the Boston Group analysed outcomes of 49 LAPC patients treated with total neoadjuvant therapy and aggressive arterial divestment. The authors demonstrated a surgical resection rate of 86%, an R0 resection rate of 69%, a 90-day mortality of 3%, and an overall survival of 31 months from the time of operation (87). Although RCT data is lacking, these convincing results from large cohort studies support the use of neoadjuvant therapy in LAPC patients who should be treated with multi-agent therapy with neoadjuvant intent. If there is no evidence for disease progression during neoadjuvant therapy, patients should undergo surgical exploration. Apart from arterial resection with

vascular reconstruction and the arterial divestment technique, a possible surgical approach in LAPC patients includes distal pancreatectomy with *en-bloc* coeliac axis resection (DP-CAR) (88). In patients with involvement of the coeliac trunk and common hepatic artery, DP-CAR uses the collateral circulation to the liver via the superior mesenteric artery, pancreatoduodenal arcades and gastroduodenal artery to the proper hepatic artery for arterial liver perfusion. This approach is usually possible if the arterial perfusion via the coeliac axis is compromised in terms of tumour-related arterial stenosis. Preoperative interventional arterial embolization of the coeliac trunk can be used to enhance the collateral arterial arc. The coeliac axis is resected and no arterial reconstruction is performed. Results of previous perioperative outcome analyses of different studies are conflicting. Data from a retrospective cohort study within the European-African Hepato-Pancreato-Biliary-Association of 68 patients from 20 hospitals in 12 countries showed a R0 resection rate of 53% and acceptable perioperative morbidity rates (89). The 90-day mortality however, was 16%. In contrast, a recent meta-analysis of seven articles comparing standard DP and PD-CAR reported by Nigri et al. showed that DP-CAR was not associated with an increased postoperative mortality (OR 2.55, 95% CI 0.65–10.08, p = 0.18) whereas overall morbidity was more frequent in the DP-CAR group (OR 1.72, 95% CI 1.115–2.58, p = 0.008) (90). Notwithstanding, oncological outcomes seem favourable and overall survival rates of 25 months have been reported (91).

High-level evidence on the role of neoadjuvant therapy in BRPC patients are likewise limited. To-date, only data from retrospective cohort studies are available with none from RCTs. Murphy et al. reported outcomes of 48 patients with BRPC who underwent total neoadjuvant therapy (92). Thirty-two patients underwent surgical resection and the R0 resection rate was 97%. The median overall survival of all 48 patients was 38 months.

Discussion surrounding conversion surgery for metastatic pancreatic cancer has increased recently and there is a growing body of evidence that patients with metastatic pancreatic cancer may benefit from neoadjuvant therapy and convert to resectable status. The previously mentioned Heidelberg study, included a total of 135 patients undergoing surgical exploration after neoadjuvant therapy for metastatic disease at presentation (33). Fifty-one patients had limited metastatic disease during exploration and underwent pancreatic tumour resection and metastasectomy (liver 69%, peritoneum 17%, or adrenal glands 14%) (33). While metastatic disease was an independent predictor of shorter survival, after both resection and exploration without resection, survival outcome was not separately reported for this subgroup. A bi-institutional study demonstrated a favourable median overall survival in 23 patients with metastatic pancreatic cancer of 18 months after conversion surgery and 34 months after initial diagnosis (93). In a study from Italy, 535 patients with synchronous liver metastases were included and 24 patients underwent surgery after neoadjuvant chemotherapy (94). Selection criteria for surgical exploration were the disappearance of liver metastasis on preoperative imaging and a favourable CA 19-9 response. Intraoperatively, detectable residual metastatic lesions were excluded by intraoperative ultrasound of the liver and tumour resection with metastasectomy was performed. The overall survival was 56 months after diagnosis and 13 months after surgery. Another phase II trial reported conversion surgery results in 33 pancreatic cancer patients with peritoneal carcinomatosis who underwent chemotherapy (95). In 8 patients, conversion surgery resulted in a median survival of 28 months compared with 14 months in non-resected patients. Criteria for conversion surgery were negative cytology, decreasing CA 19-9 levels and the disappearance of macroscopic tumour dissemination assessed by staging laparoscopy. Although these studies mostly report favourable results of conversion surgery in metastatic pancreatic cancer, it has to be acknowledged that only a small sub-cohort who represent a highly selected group of 'super-responders' benefitted from long-term chemotherapy and resection. Further evidence is required to clarify whether favourable survival outcomes were based on individual patient selection and/or surgical resection.

SUMMARY

Pancreatic adenocarcinoma is one of the most aggressive malignancies and it is predicted to become the second most common cause of cancer-related mortality within the next decade. Complete surgical resection with negative margins combined with adjuvant chemotherapy is the treatment of choice for patients with resectable pancreatic cancer. The majority of patients, however, present with locally advanced or even metastatic disease and were previously not considered candidates for surgery.

Owing to enormous advances especially in medical therapy, using more effective multi-agent chemotherapy regimens, and refined surgical techniques, combined in modern multimodality approaches, up to 60% of those patients with locally unresectable tumours and even a selected sub-cohort of patients with metastatic disease can now be converted into resectable pancreatic cancer.

REFERENCES

1. Siegel RL, Miller KD, Jemal A. Cancer statistics, 2018. *CA Cancer J Clin* 2018;**68**:7–30.
2. Hruban RH, Adsay NV, Esposito I, et al. Pancreatic ductal adenocarcinoma. In: *WHO Classification of Tumours: Digestive System Tumours*, 5th ed, WHO Classification of Tumours Editorial Board (Ed), International Agency for Research on Cancer, Lyon; 2019. p.322.
3. Kleeff J, Korc M, Apte M, La Vecchia C, Johnson CD, Biankin AV, et al. Pancreatic cancer. *Nat Rev Dis Primers* 2016;**2**:16022.
4. Wagner M, Redaelli C, Lietz M, Seiler CA, Friess H, Büchler MW, et al. Curative resection is the single most important factor determining outcome in patients with pancreatic adenocarcinoma. *Br J Surg* 2004;**91**:586–94.
5. Schnelldorfer T, Ware AL, Sarr MG, Smyrk TC, Zhang L, Qin R, et al. Long term survival after pancreatoduodenectomy for pancreatic adenocarcinoma: Is cure possible? *Ann Surg* 2008;**247**:456–62.
6. Hartwig W, Werner J, Jäger D, Debus J, Büchler MW. Improvement of surgical results for pancreatic cancer. *Lancet Oncol* 2013;**14**:e476–e485.
7. Strobel O, Lorenz P, Hinz U, Gaida M, König A-K, Hank T, et al. Actual five-year survival after upfront resection for pancreatic ductal adenocarcinoma: Who beats the odds? *Ann Surg* 2022;**275(5)**:962–71.
8. Sener SF, Fremgen A, Menck HR, Winchester DP. Pancreatic cancer: A report of treatment and survival trends for 100,313 patients diagnosed from 1985–1995, using the National Cancer Database. *J Am Coll Surg* 1999;**189**:1–7.
9. Loos M, Kleeff J, Friess H, Büchler MW. Surgical treatment of pancreatic cancer. *Ann N Y Acad Sci* 2008;1**138**:169–80.
10. Neoptolemos JP, Dunn JA, Stocken DD, Friess H, Hickey H, Beger H, et al. Adjuvant chemoradiotherapy and chemotherapy in resectable pancreatic cancer: A randomised controlled trial. *Lancet* 2001;**58**:1576–85.
11. Neoptolemos JP, Stocken DD, Friess H, et al. A randomized trial of chemoradiotherapy and chemotherapy after resection of pancreatic cancer. *NEJM* 2004;**350**:1200–10.

12. Oettle H, Post S, Neuhaus P, Gellert K, Langrehr J, Ridwelski K, et al. Adjuvant chemotherapy with gemcitabine vs observation in patients undergoing curative-intent resection of pancreatic cancer: A randomized controlled trial. *JAMA* 2007;**297**:267–77.

13. Cunningham D, Chau I, Stocken DD, Valle JW, Smith D, Steward W, et al. Phase III randomized comparison of gemcitabine versus gemcitabine plus capecitabine in patients with advanced pancreatic cancer. *J Clin Oncol* 2009;**27**:5513–18.

14. Neoptolemos JP, Stocken DD, Bassi C, Ghaneh P, Cunningham D, Goldstein D, et al. Adjuvant chemotherapy with fluorouracil plus folinic acid versus gemcitabine following pancreatic cancer resection: A randomized controlled trial. *JAMA* 2010;**304**:1073–81.

15. Uesaka K, Boku N, Fukutomi A, Okamura Y, Konishi M, Matsumoto I, et al. Adjuvant chemotherapy of S-1 versus gemcitabine for resected pancreatic cancer: A phase 3, open-label, randomised, non-inferiority trial (JASPAC 01). *Lancet* 2016;**388**:248–57.

16. Neoptolemos JP, Palmer DH, Ghaneh P, Psarelli EE, Valle JW, Halloran CM, et al. Comparison of adjuvant gemcitabine and capecitabine with gemcitabine monotherapy in patients with resected pancreatic cancer (ESPAC-4): A multicentre, open-label, randomised, phase 3 trial. *Lancet* 2017;**389**:1011–24.

17. Suker M, Beumer BR, Sadot E, Marthey L, Faris JE, Mellon EA, et al. FOLFIRINOX for locally advanced pancreatic cancer: A systematic review and patient-level meta-analysis. *Lancet Oncol* 2016;**17**:801–10.

18. Conroy T, Desseigne F, Ychou M, Bouché O, Guimbaud R, Bécouarn Y, et al. FOLFIRINOX versus gemcitabine for metastatic pancreatic cancer. *NEJM* 2011;**364**:1817–25.

19. Weitz J, Rahbari N, Koch M, Büchler MW. The 'artery first' approach for resection of pancreatic head cancer. *J Am Coll Surg* 2010;**210**:e1–4.

20. Sanjay P, Takaori K, Govil S, Shrikhande SV, Windsor JA. 'Artery-first' approaches to pancreatoduodenectomy. *Br J Surg* 2012;**99**:1027–35.

21. Hackert T, Werner J, Weitz J, Schmidt J, Büchler MW. Uncinate process first: A novel approach for pancreatic head resection. *Langenbeck's Arch Surg* 2010;**395**:1161–64.

22. Strasberg SM, Drebin JA, Linehan D. Radical antegrade modular pancreatosplenectomy. *Surgery* 2003;**133**:521–7.

23. Sivasanker M, Desouza A, Bhandare M, Chaudhari V, Goel M, Shrikhande SV. Radical antegrade modular pancreatosplenectomy for all pancreatic body and tail tumors: Rationale and results. *Langenbeck's Arch Surg* 2019;**404**:183–90.

24. Hackert T, Strobel O, Michalski CW, Mihaljevic AL, Mehrabi A, Müller-Stich B, et al. The TRIANGLE operation – radical surgery after neoadjuvant treatment for advanced pancreatic cancer: A single arm observational study. *HPB (Oxford)* 2017;**19**:1001–07.

25. Schneider M, Hackert T, Strobel O, Büchler MW. Technical advances in surgery for pancreatic cancer. Br J Surg 2023;108(7):777–85.

26. Kleive D, Sahakyan MA, Berstad AE, Verbeke CS, Gladhaug IP, Edwin B, et al. Trends in indications, complications and outcomes for venous resection during pancreatoduodenectomy. *Brit J Surg* 2017;**104**:1558–67.

27. Javed AA, Wright MJ, Siddique A, Blair AB, Ding D, Burkhart RA, et al. Outcome of patients with borderline resectable pancreatic cancer in the contemporary era of neoadjuvant chemotherapy. *J Gastrointest Surg* 2019;**23**:112–21.

28. Weitz J, Kienle P, Schmidt J, Friess H, Büchler MW. Portal vein resection for advanced pancreatic head cancer. *J Am Coll Surg* 2007;**204**:712–6.

29. Conroy T, Hammel P, Hebbar M, Abdelghani MB, Wei AC, Raoul J-L, et al. FOLFIRINOX or gemcitabine as adjuvant therapy for pancreatic cancer. *NEJM* 2018;**379**:2395–06.

30. Klaiber U, Schnaidt ES, Hinz U, Gaida MM, Heger U, Hank T, et al. Prognostic factors of survival after neoadjuvant treatment and resection for initially unresectable pancreatic cancer. *Ann Surg* 2021;**273**:154–62.

31. Rangelova E, Wefer A, Persson S, Valente R, Tanaka K, Orsini N, et al. Surgery improves survival after neoadjuvant therapy for borderline and locally advanced pancreatic cancer: A single institution experience. *Ann Surg* 2021;**273**:579–86.

32. Gemenetzis G, Groot VP, Blair AB, Laheru DA, Zheng L, Narang AK, et al. Survival in locally advanced pancreatic cancer after neoadjuvant therapy and surgical resection. *Ann Surg* 2019;**270**:340–7.

33. Hackert T, Sachsenmaier M, Hinz U, Xchneider L, Michalski CW, Springfeld C, et al. Locally advanced pancreatic cancer: Neoadjuvant therapy with folfirinox results in resectability in 60% of the patients. *Ann Surg* 2016;**264**:457–63.

34. Siegel RL, Miller KD, Jemal A. Cancer statistics, 2020. *CA Cancer J Clin* 2020;**70**:7–30.

35. Sung H, Ferlay J, Siegel RL, Laversanne M, Soerjomataram I, Jemal A, et al. Global cancer statistics 2020: GLOBOCAN estimates of incidence and mortality worldwide for 36 cancers in 185 Countries. *CA Cancer J Clin* 2021;**71**: 209–49.

36. Huang J, Lok V, Ngai CH, Zhang L, Yuan J, Lao XQ, et al. Worldwide burden of risk factors for and trends in pancreatic cancer. *Gastroenterology* 2021;**160**:744–54.

37. Pancreatic cancer statistics UK. Available from www.pancreaticcancer.org.uk (Accessed 28 August 2024).

38. Exarchakou A, Papacleovoulou G, Rous B, Magadi W, Rachet B, Neoptolemos JP, et al. Pancreatic cancer incidence and survival and the role of specialist centres in resection rates in England, 2000 to 2014: A population-based study. *Pancreatology* 2020;**20**:454–61.

39. Rahib L, Smith BD, Aizenberg R, Rosenzweig AB, Flexhman JM, Matrisian LM. Projecting cancer incidence and deaths to 2030: The unexpected burden of thyroid, liver, and pancreas cancers in the United States. *Cancer Res* 2014;**74**:2913–21.

40. Gonzalez RS, Kuo E. *Pancreas WHO classification.* Available from: https://www.pathologyoutlines.com/topic/pancreasmcn.html (Accessed 3 September 2024)

41. Luchini C, Grillo F, Fassan M, Vanoli A, Capelli P, Paolini G, et al. Malignant epithelial/exocrine tumors of the pancreas. *Pathologica* 2020;**112**:210–26.

42. Yeo CJ, Cameron JL, Sohn TA, Lillemoe KD, Pitt HA, Talamini MA, et al. Six hundred fifty con-

secutive pancreaticoduodenectomies in the 1990s: Pathology, complications, and outcomes. *Ann Surg* 1997;**226**:248–57.

43. van der Gaag NA, Rauws EAJ, van Eijck CHJ, Bruno MJ, van der Harst E, Kubben FJGM, et al. Preoperative biliary drainage for cancer of the head of the pancreas. *NEJM* 2010;**362**:129–37.

44. Asbun HJ, Conlon K, Fernandez-Cruz L, Friess H, Shrikhande SV, Adham M, et al. When to perform a pancreatoduodenctomy in the absence of positive histology? A consensus statement by the International Study Group of Pancreatic Surgery. *Surgery* 2014;**155**:887–92.

45. Varadhachary GR, Tamm EP, Abbruzzese JL, Xiong HQ, Crane CH, Wang H, et al. Borderline resectable pancreatic cancer: Definitions management, and role of preoperative therapy. *Ann Surg Oncol* 2006;**13**:1035–46.

46. Vauthey JN, Dixon E. AHPBA/SSO/SSAT consensus conference on resectable and borderline resectable pancreatic cancer: Rationale and overview of the conference. *Ann Surg Oncol* 2009;**16**:1725–26.

47. Tempero MA, Malafa MP, Al-Hawary M, Asbun H, Bain A, Behrman SW, et al. Pancreatic adenocarcinoma, version 2.2017, NCCN Clinical Practice Guidelines in Oncology. *J Natl Compr Canc Netw* 2017;**15**:1028–61.

48. Bockhorn M, Uzunoglu FG, Adham M, Imrie C, Milicevic M, Sandberg AA, et al. International Study Group of Pancreatic S. Borderline resectable pancreatic cancer: a consensus statement by the International Study Group of Pancreatic Surgery (ISGPS). *Surgery* 2014;**55**:977–88.

49. Isaji S, Mizuno S, Windsor JA, Bassi C, Fernández-Del Castillo C, et al. International consensus on definition and criteria of borderline resectable pancreatic ductal adenocarcinoma 2017. *Pancreatology* 2018;**18**:2–11.

50. Allen VB., Gurusamy KS, Takwoingi Y, Kalia A, Davidson BR. Diagnostic accuracy of laparoscopy following computed tomography (CT) scanning for assessing the resectability with curative intent in pancreatic and periampullary cancer. *Cochrane Database Syst Rev* 2016;7:CD009323.

51. Halloran CM, Ghaneh P, Connor S, Sutton R, Neoptolemos JP, Raraty MGT. Carbohydrate antigen 19.9 accurately selects patients for laparoscopic assessment to determine resectability of pancreatic malignancy. *Br J Surg* 2008;**95**:453–9.

52. Hartwig W, Strobel O, Hinz U, Fritz S, Hackert T, Roth C, et al. CA19-9 in potentially resectable pancreatic cancer: Perspective to adjust surgical and perioperative therapy. *Ann Surg Oncol* 2013;**20**:2188–96.

53. National Institute for Health and Care Excellence. Pancreatic cancer in adults: Diagnosis and management (NICE, 2018). Available from: https://www.nice.org.uk/guidance/ng85 (Accessed 28 August 2024)

54. Motosugi U, Ichikawa T, Morisaka H, Sou H, Muhi A, Kimura K, et al. Detection of pancreatic carcinoma and liver metastases with gadoxetic acid-enhanced MR imaging: Comparison with contrast-enhanced multi-detector row CT. *Radiology* 2011;**260**:446–53.

55. Tsurusaki M, Sofue K, Murakami T. Current evidence for the diagnostic value of gadoxetic acid-enhanced magnetic resonance imaging for liver metastasis. *Hepatol Res* 2016;**46**:853–61.

56. Ghaneh P, Hanson R, Titman A, Lancaster G, Plumpton C, Lloyd-Williams H, et al. PETPANC: Multicentre prospective diagnostic accuracy and health economic analysis study of the impact of combined modality 18fluorine-2-fluoro-2-deoxy-d-glucose positron emission tomography with computed tomography scanning in the diagnosis and management of pancreatic cancer. *Health Technol Assess* 2018;**22**:1–114.

57. Chandrasegaram MD, Goldstein D, Simes J, Gebski V, Kench JG, Gill AJ, et al. Meta-analysis of radical resection rates and margin assessment in pancreatic cancer. *Br J Surg* 2015;**102**:1459–72.

58. Jones RP, Psarelli EE, Jackson R, Ghaneh P, Halloran CH, Palmer DH, et al. Patterns of recurrence after resection of pancreatic ductal adenocarcinoma: A secondary analysis of the ESPAC-4 randomized adjuvant chemotherapy trial. *JAMA Surg* 2019;**154(11)**:1038–1048019.

59. Kim YI, Song KB, Lee Y-J, Park K-M, Hwang DW, Shin SH, et al. Management of isolated recurrence after surgery for pancreatic adenocarcinoma. *Br J Surg* 2019;**106**:898–909.

60. Tanaka M, Mihaljevic AL, Probst P, Heckler M, Klaiber U, Heger U, et al. Meta-analysis of recurrence pattern after resection for pancreatic cancer. *Br J Surg* 2019;**106**:1590–1601.

61. Groot VP, Rezaee N, Wu W, Cameron JL, Fishman EK, Hruban RH, et al. Patterns, timing, and predictors of recurrence following pancreatectomy for pancreatic ductal adenocarcinoma. *Ann Surg* 2018;**267**:936–45.

62. Kooby DA, Lad NL, Squires MH 3rd, Maithel SK, Sarmiento JM, Staley CA, et al. Value of intraoperative neck margin analysis during Whipple for pancreatic adenocarcinoma: A multicenter analysis of 1399 patients. *Ann Surg* 2014;**260**:494–501.

63. Nitschke P, Volk A, Welsch T, Hackl J Reissfelder C, Rahbari M, et al. Impact of intraoperative re-resection to achieve R0 status on survival in patients with pancreatic cancer: A single center experience with 483 patients. *Ann Surg* 2017;**265**:1219–25.

64. Isaji S, Murata Y, Kishiwada M. New Japanese classification of pancreatic cancer. In: Neoptolemos J, Urrutia R, Abbruzzese J, Büchler M (Eds) *Pancreatic cancer*. New York: Springer; 2018.

65. Strobel O, Hinz U, Gluth A, Hank T, Hackert T, Bergmann F, et al. Pancreatic adenocarcinoma: Number of positive nodes allows to distinguish several N categories. *Ann Surg* 2015; **261**:961–9.

66. Warschkow R, Widmann B, Beutner U, Marti L, Steffen T, Schiesser M, et al. The more the better – lower rate of stage migration and better survival in patients with retrieval of 20 or more regional lymph nodes in pancreatic cancer: A population-based propensity score matched and Trend SEER analysis. *Pancreas* 2017;**46**:648–57.

67. Malleo G, Maggino L, Ferrone CR, Marchegiani G, Mino-Kenudson M, Capelli P, et al. Number of examined lymph nodes and nodal status assessment in distal pancreatectomy for body/tail ductal adenocarcinoma. *Ann Surg* 2019;**270**:1138–46.

68. Dasari BV, Pasquali S, Vohra RS, et al. Extended versus standard lymphadenectomy for pancreatic head cancer: Meta-analysis of randomized controlled trials. *J Gastrointest Surg* 2015;**19**:1725–32.

69. Tol JAMG, Gouma DJ, Bassi C, Dervenis C, Montorsi M, Adham M, et al. Definition of a standard lymphadenectomy in surgery for pancreatic ductal adenocarcinoma: A consensus statement by the International Study Group on Pancreatic Surgery (ISGPS). *Surgery* 2014;**156**:591–600.

70. Esposito I, Kleeff J, Bergmann F, Reiser C, Herpel E, Friess H, et al. Most pancreatic cancer resections are R1 resections. *Ann Surg Oncol* 2008;**15**:1651–60.

71. Verbeke C, Löhr M, Karlsson JS, Del Chiaro M, et al. Pathology reporting of pancreatic cancer following neoadjuvant therapy: Challenges and uncertainties. *Cancer Treat Rev* 2015;**41**:17–26.

72. Inoue Y, Saiura A, Yoshioka R, Ono Y, Takahashi M, Arita J, et al. Pancreatoduodenectomy with systematic mesopancreas dissection using a supracolic anterior artery-first approach. *Ann Surg* 2015;**262**:1092–1101.

73. Heald RJ, Ryall RD. Recurrence and survival after total mesorectal excision for rectal cancer. *Lancet* 1986;**1**:1479–82.

74. Hohenberger W, Weber K, Matzel K, Papadopoulos T, Merkel S. Standardized surgery for colonic cancer: Complete mesocolic excision and central ligation—technical notes and outcome. *Colorectal Dis* 2008;**11**:354–64.

75. Giovinazzo F, Turri G, Katz MH, Heaton, Ahmed I. Meta-analysis of benefits of portal-superior mesenteric vein resection in pancreatic resection for ductal adenocarcinoma. *Br J Surg* 2016;**103**:179–91.

76. Xie ZB, Li J, Gu JC, Jin C, Zou C-F, Fu D-L. Pancreatoduodenectomy with portal vein resection favors the survival time of patients with pancreatic ductal adenocarcinoma: A propensity score matching analysis. *Oncol Lett* 2019;**18**:4563–72.

77. Strobel O, Hank T, Hinz U, Bergmann F, Schneider L, Springfeld C, et al. Pancreatic cancer surgery: The new R- status counts. *Ann Surg* 2017;**265**:565–73.

78. Hank T, Hinz U, Tarantino I, Kaiser J, Niesen W, Bergmann F, et al. Validation of at least 1 mm as cut-of for resection margins for pancreatic adenocarcinoma of the body and tail. *Br J Surg* 2018;**105**:1171–81.

79. Neoptolemos JP, Moore MJ, Cox TF, Valle JW, Palmer DH, McDonald AC, et al. Effect of adjuvant chemotherapy with fluorouracil plus folinic acid or gemcitabine vs observation on survival in patients with resected periampullary adenocarcinoma: The ESPAC-3 periampullary cancer randomized trial. *JAMA* 2012;**308**:147–56.

80. Mokdad AA, Minter RM, Zhu H, Augustine MM, Porembka MR, Wang SC, et al. Neoadjuvant therapy followed by resection versus upfront resection for resectable pancreatic cancer: A propensity score matched analysis. *J Clin Oncol* 2017;**35**:515–22.

81. de Geus SW, Eskander MF, Bliss LA, Kasumova GG, Ng SC, Callery MP, et al. Neoadjuvant therapy versus upfront surgery for resected pancreatic adenocarcinoma: a nationwide propensity score matched analysis. *Surgery* 2017;**161**:592–601.

82. Mollberg N, Rahbari NN, Koch M, Hartwig W, Hoeger Y, Büchler MW, et al. Arterial resection during pancreatectomy for pancreatic cancer: A systematic review and meta-analysis. *Ann Surg* 2011;**254**:882–93.

83. Miao Y, Jiang K, Cai B, Z Lu, Wu J, Gao W, et al. Arterial divestment instead of resection for locally advanced pancreatic cancer (LAPC). *Pancreatology* 2016;**16**:S59.

84. Diener MK, Mihaljevic AL, Strobel O, Loos M, Schmidt T, Schneider M, et al. Periarterial divestment in pancreatic cancer surgery. *Surgery* 2021;**169**:1019–25.

85. Loos M, Kester T, Klaiber U, Mihaljevic Al, Mehrabi A, Müller-Stich BM, et al. Arterial Resection in Pancreatic Cancer Surgery: Effective After a Learning Curve. *Ann Surg* 2022;**275**(**4**):759–68.

86. Michelakos T, Pergolini I, Castillo CF, Honselmann KC, Cai L, Deshpande V, et al. Predictors of resectability and survival in patients with borderline and locally advanced pancreatic cancer who underwent neoadjuvant treatment With FOLFIRINOX. *Ann Surg* 2019;**269**:733–40.

87. Murphy JE, Wo JY, Ryan DP, Clark JW, Jiang W, Yeap BY, et al. Total neoadjuvant therapy with FOLFIRINOX in combination with losartan followed by chemoradiotherapy for locally advanced pancreatic cancer: A phase 2 clinical trial. *JAMA Oncol* 2019;**5**:1020–27.

88. Klompmaker S, Boggi U, Hackert T, Salvia R, Weiss M, Yamaue H, et al. Distal pancreatectomy with celiac axis resection (DP-CAR) for pancreatic cancer. How I do it. *J Gastrointest Surg* 2018;**22**:1804–10.

89. Klompmaker S, van Hilst J, Gerritsen SL, Adham M, Quer MTA, Bassi C, et al. Outcomes after distal pancreatectomy with celiac axis resection for pancreatic cancer: A Pan-European Retrospective Cohort study. *Ann Surg Oncol* 2018;**25**:1440–47.

90. Nigri G, Petrucciani N, Belloni E, Lucarni A, Aurello P, D'Angelo F, et al. Distal pancreatectomy with celiac axis resection: Systematic review and meta-analysis. *Cancers (Basel)* 2021;**13**(**8**):1967.

91. Schmocker RK, Wright MJ, Ding D, Beckman MJ, Javed AA, Cameron JL, et al. An aggressive approach to locally confined pancreatic cancer: Defining surgical and oncologic outcomes unique to pancreatectomy with celiac axis resection (DP-CAR). *Ann Surg Oncol* 2021;**28**:3125–34.

92. Murphy JE, Wo JY, Ryan DP, Jiang W, Yeap BY, Drapek LC, et al. Total neoadjuvant therapy with FOLFIRINOX followed by individualized chemoradiotherapy for borderline resectable pancreatic adenocarcinoma: A phase 2 clinical trial. *JAMA Oncol* 2018;**4**:963–69.

93. Wright GP, Poruk KE, Zenati MS, Steve K. Bahary N, Hogg ME, et al. Primary tumor resection following favorable response to systemic chemotherapy in stage IV pancreatic adenocarcinoma with synchronous metastases: A bi-institutional analysis. *J Gastrointest Surg* 2016;**20**:1830–35.

94. Frigeri I, Regi P, Giardino A, Scopelliti F, Girelli R, Bassi C, et al. Downstaging in stage IV pancreatic cancer: A new population eligible for surgery? *Ann Surg Oncol* 2017;**24**:2397–2403.

95. Satoi S, Fujii Y, Yanagimoto H, Motoi F, Kurata M, Takahara N, et al. Multicenter phase II study of intravenous and intraperitoneal paclitaxel with s-1 for pancreatic ductal adenocarcinoma patients with peritoneal metastasis. *Ann Surg* 2017;**265**:397–401.

SECTION 6 | PANCREAS

Bailey & Love's Essential Operations Bailey & Love's Essential Operations
Bailey & Love's Essential Operations Bailey & Love's Essential Operations
Bailey & Love's Essential Operations Bailey & Love's Essential Operations

Chapter 34

Pancreatic Neuroendocrine Neoplasms

Claudia E. Mack, Leonidas Apostolidis, Thilo Hackert and John P. Neoptolemos

INTRODUCTION

Tumours that show similar histological characteristics to islet cells are known as pancreatic neuroendocrine neoplasms (PNENs) (1–3). These account for 1–2% of all pancreatic tumours with a worldwide incidence which has been increasing over the last three decades reflecting improvements in diagnostic techniques (4–6). A distinction is made between functional and non-functional tumours. The majority of PNENs (60–90%) are non-functioning, since they do not cause clinical, hormone-related symptoms (7,8). The two most common functional tumours are insulinomas (causing hypoglycaemia) and gastrinomas (causing Zollinger–Ellison syndrome). Other rare, functional, tumours include vasoactive intestinal peptide (VIP) tumours, glucagonoma and parathyroid hormone-related peptide (PTHrP) omas and calcitoninoma presenting as watery diarrhoea, facial flushing and neurotensinomas, hypotension, flushing, diarrhoea, unintended weight-loss, and diabetes depending on the predominant hormone secretion. Whereas 95% of PNENs are sporadic, approximately 5% of all patients with PNENs have a family history and/or are inherited (9). These include multiple endocrine neoplasia type 1 (MEN1), von Hippel–Lindau syndrome (VHL) and tuberous sclerosis complex (TSC1 and TSC2) (10).

CLINICAL FEATURES

Non-functioning tumours

Non-functioning tumours are defined by the absence of hormone-related symptoms or syndromes. Even though immunohistochemical staining shows positivity for marker molecules like chromogranin A (CgA), neuron-specific enolase (NSE) or synaptophysin which classifies them as neuroendocrine tumours, the concentration of the secreted hormones is either too low to cause symptoms, or the hormones are clinically inert, since they are in an inactive preliminary stage (11–13). Symptoms occur when the tumour causes a compression, or infiltration, of other organs, or if the disease is already in a metastatic stage. While tumours of the pancreatic head can cause jaundice as a result of obstruction of the intrapancreatic bile duct or backpain

due to intrapancreatic nerve infiltration, tumours of the pancreatic tail remain asymptomatic for a long time or cause only non-specific symptoms. Imbalance of blood sugar levels caused by a destruction of healthy pancreatic tissue may occur and eventually lead to the diagnosis (14). Liver failure can occur in advanced stages if extensive hepatic spread is present.

Functioning tumours

An overview of clinical syndromes of these tumours is provided in *Table 34.1*.

Insulinomas

Accounting for 70% of all functioning PNEN, insulinomas are the most common entity, but with an incidence of 2–4 cases/10^6 population/year they count as rare tumours (15). They most frequently arise in the fifth decade of life and occur mostly sporadically (94%) with a benign behaviour (87%) (16). Only 5–10% are associated with MEN-1 syndrome (7,17). Insulinomas are insulin-secreting tumours and their clinical manifestation is defined by Whipple's triad: (i) hypoglycaemia (plasma glucose <40 mg/dL), (ii) symptoms of hypoglycaemia, and (iii) rapid relief of symptoms following the administration of glucose (17). Symptoms resulting from the neuroglycopenia include confusion, behavioural and personality changes, visual disturbances, seizures and coma, while symptoms of the autonomic nervous system include diaphoresis, nausea, anxiety, tremor, and palpitations (17).

Gastrinomas

Among functioning PNEN, gastrinomas are the second most common entity with an incidence of 1–3 cases/10^6 people/year (18). 80% of gastrinomas occur sporadically, whereas 20% show a hereditary association with MEN-1 syndrome (18). Of all gastrinomas, 60–90% are malignant with predominantly lymph node and/or liver metastases (19). Gastrinomas occur three times more commonly in the duodenum than in the pancreas (20). The Zollinger–Ellison syndrome describes a group of symptoms including severe peptic ulcer disease, gastro–esophageal reflux disease and chronic diarrhoea caused by the gastrin-secreting tumour (21).

DOI: 10.1201/9781003080060-34

Table 34.1 Overview of common and rare, functional pancreatic neuroendocrine tumour syndromes (7)

Name	Biologically active peptide(s) secreted	Incidence: New cases/10^6 population/year	Tumour location	Malignancy (%)	Associated with MEN-1 (%)	Main symptoms/signs
Most common functioning pancreatic neuroendocrine neoplasm syndromes						
Insulinoma	Insulin	1–32	Pancreas (>99%)	<10	4–5	Hypoglycaemic symptoms (100%)
Zollinger–Ellison syndrome (ZES)	Gastrin	0.5–21.5	Duodenum (70%) Pancreas (25%) Other sites (5%)	60–90	20–25	Pain (79–100%) Diarrhoea (30–75%) Oesophageal symptoms (31–56%)
Established, rare, functioning pancreatic neuroendocrine neoplasm syndromes (>100 cases)						
VIP tumour (Verner–Morrison syndrome, pancreatic cholera, WDHA)	Vasoactive intestinal peptide	0.05–0.2	Pancreas (90%, adult) Other (10%, neural, adrenal, periganglionic)	40–70	6	Diarrhoea (90–100%) Hypokalaemia (80–100%) Dehydration (83%)
Glucagonoma	Glucagon	0.01–0.1	Pancreas (100%)	50–80	1–20	Rash (6–90%) Glucose intolerance (38–87%) Weight loss (66–96%)
Somatostatinoma (SSoma)	Somatostatin	Rare	Pancreas (55%) Duodenum/jejunum (44%)	>70	45	Diabetes mellitus (63–90%) Cholelithiasis (65–90%) Diarrhoea (35–90%)
GRHoma	Growth hormone-releasing hormone	Unknown	Pancreas (30%) Lung (54%) Jejunum (7%) Other (13%)	>60	16	Acromegaly (100%)
ACTHoma	ACTH	Rare	Pancreas (4–16% all ectopic Cushing's)	>95	Rare	Cushing's syndrome (100%)
PNEN causing carcinoid syndrome	Serotonin? Tachykinins	Rare (43 cases)	Pancreas (<1% all carcinoids)	60–88	Rare	Same as carcinoid syndrome above
PNEN causing hypercalcemia	PTHrP Others unknown	Rare	Pancreas (rare cause of hypercalcaemia)	84	Rare	Abdominal pain due to hepatic metastases

Very rare, functioning pancreatic neuroendocrine neoplasm syndromes (1–5 cases)

PNEN-secreting renin	Renin	Rare	Pancreas	Unknown	No	Hypertension
PNEN-secreting luteinizing hormone	Luteinizing hormone	Rare	Pancreas	Unknown	No	Anovulation Virilization (female), reduced libido (male)
PNEN-secreting erythropoietin	Erythropoietin	Rare	Pancreas	100	No	Polycythaemia
PNEN-secreting insulin–like growth factor 2	Insulin–like growth factor II	Rare	Pancreas	Unknown	No	Hypoglycaemia
PNEN-secreting CCK (CCKoma)	CCK	Rare	Pancreas	Unknown	No	Diarrhoea Ulcer disease Weight loss Cholecystolithiasis
PNEN-secreting GLP-1	GLP-1	Rare	Pancreas	Unknown	No	Hypoglycaemia

Abbreviations: ACTH: adrenocorticotropic hormone; PTHrP: parathyroid hormone-releasing peptide; VIP: vasoactive intestinal peptide; WDHA: watery diarrhoea, hypokalaemia, achlorhydria.

DIAGNOSIS

Histopathology and tumour markers

Histological diagnosis is mandatory and can be carried out on resection specimens or core biopsies. Gastro-entero-pancreatic (GEP) neuroendocrine tumours (NETs) should be classified based on morphology and proliferation according to the WHO 2019 classification into well-differentiated neuroendocrine tumours (NET, G1–G3) and poorly differentiated neuroendocrine carcinomas (NEC, G3) as shown in *Table 34.2* (2).

Chromogranin A (CgA) is the best characterized, and clinically most useful circulating biomarker that identifies most PNENs (22). The sensitivity of CgA measurement is about 60–90% with a specificity of less than 50% due to elevated CgA levels in many other conditions including impaired renal function, gastro-intestinal (chronic atrophic gastritis), cardiovascular (hypertension), pulmonary, rheumatoid or endocrine diseases. Pregnancy can also influence levels but the most common cause is proton pump inhibitor medi-cation (22,23). Even though CgA is more sensitive than neuron specific enolase (NSE) in differentiated PNEN G1 and G2, highly proliferative PNEN CgA is elevated in only 60% of all cases and therefore not recom-mended as a screening marker (24). If present, CgA may correlate with the tumour mass and can conse-quently serve as a prognostic marker during follow up (25). In poorly differentiated PNENs the level of NSE is higher than in well-differentiated PNENs and is sig-nificantly associated with survival (26).

Functional hormonal biomarkers should be mea-sured selectively in PNEN patients with both sporadic and inherited tumours showing respective symptoms. Insulin, gastrin, glucagon, VIP, somatostatin, and adre-nocorticotropic hormone (ACTH) are the most com-mon elevated hormones in functional PNENs (27).

For more than 80 years the standard diagnosis for insulinoma has been a 72-hour fasting test, when elevated serum insulin levels are measured in the pres-ence of hypoglycaemia after prolonged fasting. Newer assays for insulin and proinsulin achieved the diagnosis after 48 hours (28). Additionally, at the end of the test

β-hydroxybutyrate levels or urine ketone bodies should be determined to ensure adequate fasting (29).

The diagnosis of gastrinoma is made by the demon-stration of elevated serum gastrin levels during fasting combined with elevated gastric acid secretion resulting in a low gastric juice pH (24). In cases of Zollinger–Ellison syndrome, gastrin levels are lower in 60% of the cases and a secretin test is necessary (30).

Imaging

All patients with suspected PNEN should undergo appropriate imaging (13,24). Computed tomography (CT) is the first-line imaging modality allowing anatom-ical examination of the pancreas, as well as the disease extension (2,31). Contrast-enhanced CT (CECT) has a sensitivity and specificity of 82% and 96%, respectively, with a detection rate of liver metastasis of 79%. PNENs are expected to show hypervascular enhancement in the arterial scan phase and benign tumours show a homogenous pattern followed by early wash-out in the venous phase (32). Dynamic contrast-enhanced magnetic resonance imaging (DCE-MRI) is also useful with a sensitivity and specificity of 79% and 100% for PNENs, and a sensitivity and specificity of 70–80% and 98% for liver metastasis (33).

The exact presentation of the primary tumour and potential metastases plays an important role in the plan-ning for curative surgical resection and constitutes the basis for further follow-up (24). Additionally, magnetic resonance cholangiopancreatography (MRCP) can help to identify the positional relationship of the tumour to the main pancreatic and bile duct preoperatively (34).

PNENs are characterized by the expression of somatostatin receptors (SSTRs) which allows functional targeted imaging and specific therapy. Five subtypes of SSTRs have been identified, of which SSTR-2 is predominantly expressed in PNENs. In well-differen-tiated PNENs, expression of SSTR is especially pro-nounced compared to poorly differentiated tumours (31,35). Positron emission tomography (PET)/CT scans with ^{68}Ga-labelled somatostatin analogues DOTATE, DOTATOC and DOTANOC with a high-affinity for SSTR-2 achieve the highest sensitivity for localization

Table 34.2 WHO 2019 classification of GEP neuroendocrine tumours (2)

Type	Differentiation	Grading	Ki-67 Index	Mitotic rate
Neuroendocrine tumours (NET)	Well-differentiated	G1	<3%	≤2/10 HPF
	Well-differentiated	G2	3–20%	2–20/10 HPF
	Well-differentiated	G3	>20%	≥20/10 HPF
Neuroendocrine carcinoma (NEC) Small–cell type (SCNEC) Large-cell type (LCNEC)	Poorly differentiated	G3	>20%	≥20/10 HPF
MiNEN (mixed endocrine/nonendocrine neoplasm) Tumour-like lesions				

Abbreviation: 10 HPF: high-power field = 2 mm², at least 40 fields evaluated in areas at highest mitotic density.

of PNENs (7,36,37). If PET/CT is not available, soma-tostatin receptor scintigraphy (SRS) can be performed (7). In poorly differentiated tumours 18-FDG-PET/CT may be considered (24).

In a small subgroup of insulinomas (5–10%) all conventional imaging studies including endosono-graphic ultrasound are negative. MEN-1 patients with insulinoma often have multiple PNENs, most of them non-functional, and identifying the insu-linoma can be difficult (38). Receptor scintigraphy with radiolabelled glucagon-like peptide 1 (GLP-1) receptor analogues is a sensitive method, since insu-linomas frequently overexpress this receptor (39). Alternatively, functional localization of insulinomas after selective intra-arterial injection of calcium with hepatic venous insulin gradients (IACIG) has proven to be a highly sensitive method to localize insulinomas in 90–100% of all cases (40).

TREATMENT

Surgery for pancreatic neuroendocrine tumours

Surgical resection remains the main therapeutical strategy for every PNEN across all disease stages since it is associated with a significant improvement in survival (2,41). The surgical approach to sporadic pancreatic neuroendocrine tumours (NETs) based on the European Society of Medical Oncology (ESMO) guidelines is shown in the algorithm in *Figure 34.1* (2).

Due to improvements in diagnosis, the incidence of small non-functional PNENs is rising and resec-tion, versus a wait-and-watch policy, is controversial. Certain guidelines recommend a wait-and-watch policy for small (<2 cm) non-functioning PNENs (2,7,24). A systematic review, which included 344 patients with small sporadic non-functioning PNENs, showed that only 22% had tumour growth on fol-low-up, none of them developed metastasis, and only 12% required surgery (42). Other studies challenge the wait-and-watch approach, since patients with small non-functioning PNEN, who underwent sur-gical resection showed a significant improvement in survival and 11% already harboured lymph node metastases (43–45).

Even with spread by G1/G2/G3 PNENs to lym-phatics and/or liver, provided a radical (R0) resection can be achieved, then primary tumour resection with additional metastatectomy (multiple if required) should be undertaken. A 5-year survival benefit of 60–80% was described after liver metastasis resection compared to 30% after nonsurgical therapy (46,47). Recurrence rates still remain high at 46–65% within the first 3–5 years after resection (48,49).

There may also be a benefit for primary tumour surgical resection even with irresectable metastases for G1/G2 PNENs because of the slow metastatic tumour growth. A significant prolonged overall survival of around 74 months can be achieved with resection compared to 14 months when managed non-surgically (50–52).

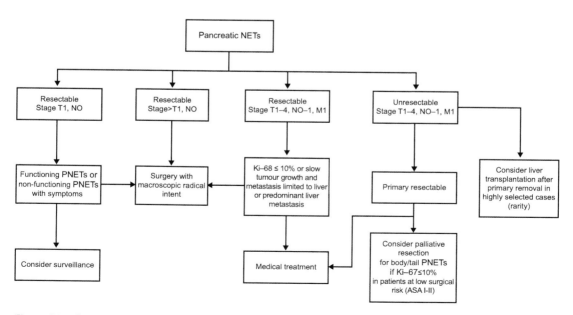

Figure 34.1 Surgical decision-making approach to sporadic pancreatic neuroendocrine tumours (PNETs) based on ESMO guidelines (2).

When liver metastases occur, they are often bilobular and frequently numerous. Reduction of liver metastasis by surgical resection may result in improved symptoms and progression-free survival, in addition to a prolonged overall survival, but requires a cytoreduction of at least 70% (1,53). For patients with diffuse non-resectable liver metastases, not responding to all other treatment options, liver transplantation may be considered. Criteria for transplantation according to the European Neuroendocrine Tumour Society (ENETS) guidelines are; a patient age <50 years, Ki-67 index below 10%, no evidence of extra-hepatic diseases, successfully resected primary tumour, and a stable disease interval of more than 6 months after primary tumour resection (24,54). Five-year survival rates vary between 82–99% (2,55).

The North American Neuroendocrine Tumour Society (NANETS) and ENETS guidelines both recommend the resection of G3 NETs when localized, followed by platinum-based chemotherapy. Cytoreduction of liver metastases may not be indicated because of high recurrence rates and poor survival, in this case chemotherapy remains first-line therapy (1,26). Patients with poorly differentiated pancreatic NEC should not undergo resection, given the aggressive biologic behaviour they exhibit and the extremely poor prognosis, which does not appear to be improved by surgical resection (1,26).

Surgical treatment options for patients with PNENs depend on the anatomic localization of the tumour, size, grading, multifocality, extension of the disease, infiltration of other structures including organs or vessels, and comorbidity of the patient (1). Surgical approaches range from enucleation to atypical (central pancreatectomy) or typical resection with, or without, vessel resection and reconstruction up to multivisceral resection when an R0 situation can be achieved. Accurate assessment of the tumour with the extent of local organ involvement is essential to enable complete resection (*Figures 34.2–34.4*). Since locally advanced tumours may need extended resection, the current guidelines recommend the classification of resectability, according to the criteria for pancreatic adenocarcinomas (56,57).

The extent of lymph node resection is controversial, especially with small non-functioning PNENs. Lymph node involvement is found in 10–27% of small non-functioning PNENs and up to 40% in tumours greater than 1.5 cm (1,45,58). During surgical resection, removal of at least 11–15 lymph nodes is required for accurate nodal staging. If pancreas-sparing surgery is performed, removal of suspicious nodes seen on preoperative imaging, is warranted (1).

Surgical therapy in functioning tumours

Resection of localized, functioning PNENs is indicated to address endocrine symptoms and to prevent

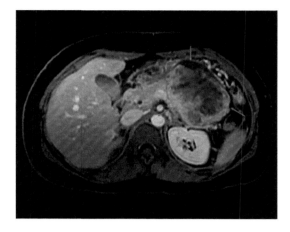

Figure 34.2 Preoperative MRI Imaging showing a neuroendocrine carcinoma located to the pancreatic tail, T2 weighting, transverse plane.

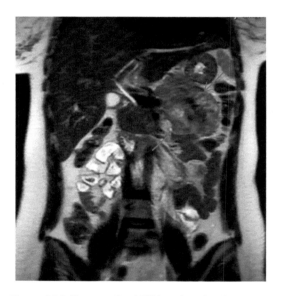

Figure 34.3 Preoperative MRI Imaging showing a neuroendocrine carcinoma located to the pancreatic tail, T1 weighting, frontal plane.

metastatic spread as the majority of PNENs have a strong malignant potential (1). The risk of malignancy varies depending on the type of functioning PNEN, ranging from 5–15% for insulinoma to 60–90% for gastrinoma, glucagonoma and tumours secreting VIP, PTHrP, or ectopic ACTH (1). Cytoreductive surgery may be considered when 70–90% of the visible disease is resectable to facilitate the management of hormone hypersecretion in patients with increasing refractory symptoms (59).

Non-surgical therapy for neuroendocrine tumours

Somatostatin analogues (octreotide or lanreotide) as first-line therapy for tumour-growth control, can be used in patients who have somatostatin receptor positive non-resectable tumours that are well-differentiated and non-functioning with a Ki-67 index <10% and with a low-median hepatic tumour burden (2,54,63,64). Stable disease stage can be achieved in 24–57%, but a partial, or complete, remission can be expected in only 2% of these patients (11,65). For patients with well-differentiated non-functioning non-resectable metastasis, a wait-and-watch strategy with regular follow-up every 3–6 months can be undertaken. However, patients with a high tumour burden and G2 or G3 differentiation are not appropriate for a wait-and-watch strategy (24).

Chemotherapy with (i) streptozotocin and 5-fluorouracil (5FU); (ii) doxorubicin with streptozotocin, or (iii) temozolomide with capecitabine (both given orally) is recommended as first-line therapy for patients with non-functioning PNENs, even G1 and G2 tumours, high hepatic-tumour burden and a significant tumour progression within 6 months, or in G2 tumours with a Ki-67 index higher than 10%. Streptozotocin-based chemotherapy regimens have objective response rates of 45–69% (24). Temozolomide with capecitabine is superior to temozolomide monotherapy with better overall survival as well as a prolonged progression free survival (22.7 vs. 14.4 months, respectively) (66). Targeted therapies with the immunosuppressive mTOR-inhibitor everolimus and the tyrosine-kinase inhibitor sunitinib showed a prolonged, progression free, survival of 11.0 and 11.4 months, respectively, in progressive, non-resectable, non-functioning PNENs (67,68).

Studies of peptide receptor radionuclide therapy using radiolabelled somatostatin analogues have demonstrated a clear anti-tumour efficacy in patients with PNETs. Peptide receptor radionuclide therapy has been considerably effective in controlling hormone-excess states in patients with refractory functioning PNET syndromes (69).

Poorly differentiated G3 and well-differentiated G3 pancreatic neuroendocrine tumours (PNETs) behave paradoxically regarding therapy response and prognosis. In poorly differentiated G3 NECs, cisplatin or carboplatin-based chemotherapy in combination with etoposide is recommended. Despite remission rates of 40–67%, progression free survival is limited to only 4–6 months (70). Second-line treatment options include chemotherapies with folinic acid, 5FU and oxaliplatin (FOLFOX) and folinic acid, 5FU and irinotecan (FOLFIRI). In comparison, well-differentiated G3 PNETs show a better prognosis despite a lower response rate to platinum and etoposide-based chemotherapy. Therefore, alternative chemotherapy regimens like

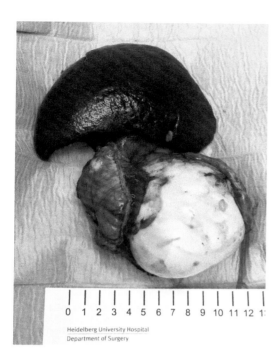

Figure 34.4 Surgical compound after pancreatic tail resection including splenectomy and gastric-wedge resection showing a neuroendocrine carcinoma.

Insulinoma

Due to the low malignancy rate, insulinoma is considered cured after surgical removal (16). Enucleation is indicated for small benign tumours distant at least 2–3 mm from the main pancreatic duct. Formal pancreatic resection is required if the tumour abuts the major pancreatic duct and/or major vessels, or if malignancy is suspected. An aggressive approach is recommended in the presence of metastatic disease with concurrent resection of the primary tumour and synchronous hepatic metastasis. Palliative resection is indicated when more than 90% of the tumour can be removed, and should then be combined with ablative techniques for maximum symptom relief. A perioperative insulin assay is available to determine completeness of tumour excision. If the tumour can't be localized, blind pancreatic resection is not recommended (60).

Gastrinoma

Only 25–35% of patients with Zollinger–Ellison syndrome are cured long-term by surgery, since 25% have MEN-1 with multiple, small gastrinomas, frequently with lymph node metastasis. When resection is performed, regional lymph node removal should also be undertaken, as this increases the chance for biochemical cure and improves overall survival (61,62).

(i) FOLFOX, (ii) streptozotocin + 5FU or, (iii) temozolomide + capecitabine are preferred in well-differentiated G3 PNETs (2,54,71).

In addition to the systemic treatment options mentioned above, most patients with Zollinger–Ellison syndrome require life-long treatment for gastric acid hypersecretion with proton pump inhibitors or histamine H2 receptor antagonists (7). In patients with insulinoma, glucose infusions and diazoxide are used to control hypoglycaemia (59).

For irresectable metastasis of the liver, local ablative procedures as well as trans-arterial embolization (TAE), chemoembolization (TACE), and radioembolization for reduction of the tumour burden may result in improved overall survival (72–74). Liver-directed therapies are especially important for patients with inadequately controlled functional symptoms (59).

FOLLOW-UP

Follow-up for patients who have had resected PNEN is recommended every 3–6 months after curative resection, gradually increasing to every 1–2 years for at least 10 years. Maximum duration of follow-up is not defined and late recurrence can occur in some patients. Therefore, life-long follow-up is mentioned in some guidelines (2). Follow-up for advanced disease is recommended every 3–6 months, lengthening the interval to every 6 months for patients with long duration (>12 months) of stable disease (75) and should include blood tests as well as imaging (75).

SUMMARY

Neuroendocrine neoplasms of the pancreas are rare tumours showing morphologic characteristics which are similar to islet cells. Most pancreatic neuroendocrine neoplasms (PNENs) occur sporadically, few have a family history or are associated with inherited syndromes like multiple endocrine neoplasia type 1 (MEN1) and von Hippel–Lindau syndrome (VHL). A distinction is also made between functional and non-functional tumours. Functional tumours cause symptoms at an early stage related to the hormones they secret. Non-functional tumours are asymptomatic in early stages and only cause symptoms in advanced stages due to their size. Chromogranin A is a circulating biomarker that identifies most PNENs. Functional hormonal biomarkers should be measured selectively in PNEN patients showing respective symptoms. All patients with PNEN should undergo imaging with CT or MRI, which can be complemented by a PET-CT scan. Surgical resection with an R0 resection should be the aim for every resectable PNEN. Alternative therapies are somatostatin analogues, targeted agents, chemotherapy, or peptide receptor radiotherapy. Follow-up for patients who have had resected PNEN is recommended starting every 3–6 months after curative resection, gradually increasing to every 1–2 years for at least 10 years.

REFERENCES

1. Howe JR, Merchant NB, Conrad C, Keutgen XM, Hallet J, Drebin JA, et al. The North American Neuroendocrine Tumor Society Consensus Paper on the surgical management of pancreatic neuroendocrine tumors. *Pancreas* 2020;**9(1)**: 1–33.

2. Pavel M, Öberg K, Falconi M, Krenning EP, Sundin A, Perren A, et al. Gastroenteropancreatic neuroendocrine neoplasms: ESMO Clinical Practice Guidelines for diagnosis, treatment and follow-up. *Ann Oncol* 2020;**31(7)**:844–60.

3. Klöppel G. Neuroendocrine neoplasms: Dichotomy, origin and classifications. *Visc Med* 2017;**33(5)**:324–30.

4. Lawrence B, Gustafsson BI, Chan A, Svejda B, Kidd M, Modlin IM. The epidemiology of gastroenteropancreatic neuroendocrine tumors. *Endocrinol Metab Clin North Am* 2011;**40(1)**:1–18, vii.

5. Modlin IM, Oberg K, Chung DC, Jensen RT, de Herder WW, Thakker RV, et al. Gastroenteropancreatic neuroendocrine tumours. *Lancet Oncol* 2008;**9(1)**:61–72.

6. Dasari A, Shen C, Halperin D, Zhao B, Zhou S, Xu Y, et al. Trends in the incidence, prevalence, and survival outcomes in patients with neuroendocrine tumors in the United States. *JAMA Oncol* 2017;**3(10)**:1335–42.

7. Falconi M, Eriksson B, Kaltsas G, Bartsch DK, Capdevila J, Caplin M, et al. ENETS Consensus Guidelines Update for the management of patients with functional pancreatic neuroendocrine tumors and non-functional pancreatic neuroendocrine tumors. *Neuroendocrinology* 2016;**103(2)**:153–71.

8. Halfdanarson TR, Rabe KG, Rubin J, Petersen GM. Pancreatic neuroendocrine tumors (PNETs): I ncidence, prognosis and recent trend toward improved survival. *Ann Oncol* 2008;**19(10)**:1727–33.

9. Jensen RT, Cadiot G, Brandi ML, de Herder WW, Kaltsas G, Komminoth P, et al. ENETS Consensus Guidelines for the management of patients with digestive neuroendocrine neoplasms: Functional pancreatic endocrine tumor syndromes. *Neuroendocrinology* 2012;**95(2)**:98–119.

10. Schimmack S, Svejda B, Lawrence B, Kidd M, Modlin IM. The diversity and commonalities of gastroenteropancreatic neuroendocrine tumors. *Langenbecks Arch Surg* 2011;**396(3)**:273–98.

11. Falconi M, Plockinger U, Kwekkeboom DJ, Manfredi R, Korner M, Kvols L, et al. Well-differentiate pancreatic nonfunctioning tumors/carcinoma. *Neuroendocrinology* 2006;**84(3)**:196–211.

12. Falconi M, Bartsch DK, Eriksson B, Klöppel G, Lopes JM, O'Connor JM, et al. ENETS Consensus Guidelines for the management of patients with digestive neuroendocrine neoplasms of the digestive system: Well-differentiate pancreatic non-functioning tumors. *Neuroendocrinology* 2012;**95(2)**:120–34.

13. Cloyd JM, Poultsides GA. Non-functional neuro-endocrine tumors of the pancreas: Advances in diagnosis and management. *World J Gastroenterol* 2015;**21(32)**:9512–25.

14. Koshimizu H, Omori H, Funase Y, Tsukada Y, Tauchi K, Furukawa T, et al. Pancreatic nonfunctioning neuroendocrine tumor with the main pancreatic duct obstruction presenting as excessive hyperglycemia: A case report and review of the literature. *Pancreas* 2012;**41(1)**:160–3.

15. Service FJ, McMahon MM, O'Brien PC, Ballard DJ. Functioning insulinoma: Incidence, recurrence, and long–term survival of patients: A 60-year study. *Mayo Clin Proc* 1991;**66(7)**:711–19.

16. Mehrabi A, Fischer L, Hafezi M, Dirlewanger A, Grenacher L, Diener MK, et al. A systematic review of localization, surgical treatment options, and outcome of insulinoma. *Pancreas* 2014;**43(5)**:675–86.

17. de Herder WW, Niederle B, Scoazec JY, Pauwels S, Kloppel G, Falconi M, et al. Well-differentiated pancreatic tumor/carcinoma: Insulinoma. *Neuroendocrinology* 2006;**84(3)**:183–8.

18. Krampitz GW, Norton JA. Current management of the Zollinger-Ellison syndrome. *Adv Surg* 2013;**47**:59–79.

19. Cho MS, Kasi A. *Zollinger-Ellison Syndrome*. Treasure Island (FL): Stat-Pearls Publishing LLC 2021.

20. Cisco RM, Norton JA. Surgery for gastrinoma. *Adv Surg* 2007;**41**:165–76.

21. Zollinger RM, Ellison EH. Primary peptic ulcerations of the jejunum associated with islet cell tumors of the pancreas. *Ann Surg* 1955;**142(4)**:709–23; discussion, 24–8.

22. Modlin IM, Gustafsson BI, Moss SF, Pavel M, Tsolakis AV, Kidd M. Chromogranin A: Biological function and clinical utility in neuro endocrine tumor disease. *Ann Surg Oncol* 2010;**17(9)**:2427–43.

23. Oberg K, Modlin IM, De Herder W, Pavel M, Klimstra D, Frilling A, et al. Consensus on biomarkers for neuroendocrine tumour disease. *Lancet Oncol* 2015;**16(9)**:e435–e46.

24. Practice guideline neuroendocrine tumors – AWMF Reg. 021-27. *Z Gastroenterol* 2018;**56(6)**:583–681.

25. Modlin IM, Kidd M, Malczewska A, Drozdov I, Bodei L, Matar S, et al. The NETest: The clinical utility of multigene blood analysis in the diagnosis and management of neuroendocrine tumors. *Endocrinol Metab Clin North Am* 2018;**47(3)**:485–504.

26. Garcia-Carbonero R, Sorbye H, Baudin E, Raymond E, Wiedenmann B, Niederle B, et al. ENETS Consensus Guidelines for high-grade gastroenteropancreatic neuroendocrine tumors and neuroendocrine carcinomas. *Neuroendocrinology* 2016;**103(2)**:186–94.

27. Halfdanarson TR, Strosberg JR, Tang L, Bellizzi AM, Bergsland EK, O'Dorisio TM, et al. The North American Neuroendocrine Tumor Society Consensus Guidelines for surveillance and medical management of pancreatic neuroendocrine tumors. *Pancreas* 2020;**49(7)**:863–81.

28. Hirshberg B, Livi A, Bartlett DL, Libutti SK, Alexander HR, Doppman JL, et al. Forty-eight-hour fast: The diagnostic test for insulinoma. *J Clin Endocrinol Metab* 2000;**85(9)**:3222–6.

29. Cryer PE, Axelrod L, Grossman AB, Heller SR, Montori VM, Seaquist ER, et al. Evaluation and management of adult hypoglycemic disorders: An Endocrine Society Clinical Practice Guideline. *J Clin Endocrinol Metab* 2009;**94(3)**:709–28.

30. Berna MJ, Hoffmann KM, Serrano J, Gibril F, Jensen RT. Serum gastrin in Zollinger-Ellison syndrome: I. Prospective study of fasting serum gastrin in 309 patients from the National Institutes of Health and comparison with 2229 cases from the literature. *Medicine* 2006;**85(6)**:295–330.

31. Granata V, Fusco R, Setola SV, De Lutio Di Castelguidone E, Camera L, Tafuto S, et al. The multidisciplinary team for gastroenteropancreatic neuroendocrine tumours: The radiologist's challenge. *Radiol Oncol* 2019;**53(4)**:373–87.

32. Cappelli C, Boggi U, Mazzeo S, Cervelli R, Campani D, Funel N, et al. Contrast enhancement pattern on multidetector CT predicts malignancy in pancreatic endocrine tumours. *Euro Radiol* 2015;**25(3)**:751–9.

33. Sundin A, Arnold R, Baudin E, Cwikla JB, Eriksson B, Fanti S, et al. ENETS Consensus Guidelines for the standards of care in neuroendocrine tumors: Radiological, nuclear medicine & hybrid imaging. *Neuroendocrinology* 2017;**105(3)**:212–44.

34. van Essen M, Sundin A, Krenning EP, Kwekkeboom DJ. Neuroendocrine tumours: The role of imaging for diagnosis and therapy. *Nat Rev Endocrinol* 2014;**10(2)**:102–14.

35. Rust E, Hubele F, Marzano E, Goichot B, Pessaux P, Kurtz JE, et al. Nuclear medicine imaging of gastro-entero-pancreatic neuroendocrine tumors. The key role of cellular differentiation and tumor grade: From theory to clinical practice. *Cancer Imaging* 2012;**12(1)**:173–84.

36. Sharma P, Arora S, Dhull VS, Naswa N, Kumar R, Ammini AC, et al. Evaluation of (68)Ga-DOTA NOC PET/CT imaging in a large exclusive population of pancreatic neuroendocrine tumors. *Abdominal Imaging* 2015;**40(2)**:299–309.

37. Schmid–Tannwald C, Schmid-Tannwald CM, Morelli JN, Neumann R, Haug AR, Jansen N, et al. Comparison of abdominal MRI with diffusion-weighted imaging to 68Ga-DOTATATE PET/CT in detection of neuroendocrine tumors of the pancreas. *Eur J Nucl Med Mol Imaging* 2013;**40(6)**:897–907.

38. Thakker RV, Newey PJ, Walls GV, Bilezikian J, Dralle H, Ebeling PR, et al. Clinical practice guidelines for multiple endocrine neoplasia type 1 (MEN1). J Clin Endocrinol Metab 2012;97(9):2990–3011.

39. Christ E, Wild D, Forrer F, Brändle M, Sahli R, Clerici T, et al. Glucagon-like peptide-1 receptor imaging for localization of insulinomas. *J Clin Endocrinol Metab* 2009;**94(11)**:4398–405.

40. Braatvedt G, Jennison E, Holdaway IM. Comparison of two low-dose calcium infusion schedules for localization of insulinomas by selective pancreatic arterial injection with hepatic venous sampling for insulin. *Clin Endocrinol (Oxf)* 2014;**80(1)**:80–4.

41. Hill JS, McPhee JT, McDade TP, Zhou Z, Sullivan ME, Whalen GF, et al. Pancreatic euroendocrine tumors: The impact of surgical resection on survival. *Cancer* 2009;**115(4)**:741–51.

42. Sallinen V, Le Large TY, Galeev S, Kovalenko Z, Tieftrunk E, Araujo R, et al. Surveillance strategy for small asymptomatic non-functional pancreatic neuroendocrine tumors – a systematic review and meta-analysis. *HPB (Oxford)* 2017;**19(4)**:310–20.

43. Chivukula SV, Tierney JF, Hertl M, Poirier J, Keutgen XM. Operative resection in early stage pancreatic neuroendocrine tumors in the United States: Are we over- or undertreating patients? *Surgery* 2020;**167(1)**:180–6.

44. Assi HA, Mukherjee S, Kunz PL, Machiorlatti M, Vesely S, Pareek V, et al. Surgery versus surveillance for well-differentiated, nonfunctional pancreatic neuroendocrine tumors: An 11-year analysis of the National Cancer Database. *Oncologist* 2020;**25(2)**:e276–e83.

45. Tanaka M, Heckler M, Mihaljevic AL, Probst P, Klaiber U, Heger U, et al. Systematic review and metaanalysis of lymph node metastases of resected pancreatic neuroendocrine tumors. *Ann Surg Oncol* 2020;**28(3)**:1614–24.

46. Yuan C-h, Wang J, Xiu D-r, Tao M, Ma Z-l, Jiang B, et al. Meta-analysis of liver resection versus nonsurgical treatments for pancreatic neuroendocrine tumors with liver metastases. *Ann Surg Oncol* 2016;**23(1)**:244–9.

47. Lesurtel M, Nagorney DM, Mazzaferro V, Jensen RT, Poston GJ. When should a liver resection be performed in patients with liver metastases from neuroendocrine tumours? A systematic review with practice recommendations. *HPB (Oxford)* 2015;**17(1)**:17–22.

48. Spolverato G, Bagante F, Aldrighetti L, Poultsides GA, Bauer TW, Fields RC, et al. Management and outcomes of patients with recurrent neuroendocrine liver metastasis after curative surgery: An international multi-institutional analysis. *J Surg Oncol* 2017;**116(3)**:298–306.

49. Zhang XF, Beal EW, Chakedis J, Lv Y, Bagante F, Aldrighetti L, et al. Early recurrence of neuroendocrine liver metastasis after curative hepatectomy: Risk factors, prognosis, and treatment. *J Gastrointest Surg* 2017;**21(11)**:1821–30.

50. Keutgen XM, Nilubol N, Glanville J, Sadowski SM, Liewehr DJ, Venzon DJ, et al. Resection of primary tumor site is associated with prolonged survival in metastatic nonfunctioning pancreatic neuroendocrine tumors. *Surgery* 2016;**159(1)**:311–18.

51. Huttner FJ, Schneider L, Tarantino I, Warschkow R, Schmied BM, Hackert T, et al. Palliative resection of the primary tumor in 442 metastasized neuroendocrine tumors of the pancreas: A population-based, propensity score-matched survival analysis. *Langenbecks Arch Surg* 2015;**400(6)**:715–23.

52. Tierney JF, Chivukula SV, Wang X, Pappas SG, Schadde E, Hertl M, et al. Resection of primary tumor may prolong survival in metastatic gastro-

enteropancreatic neuroendocrine tumors. *Surgery* 2019;**165(3)**:644–51.

53. Mayo SC, de Jong MC, Pulitano C, Clary BM, Reddy SK, Gamblin TC, et al. Surgical management of hepatic neuroendocrine tumor metastasis: Results from an international multi-institutional analysis. *Ann Surg Oncol* 2010;**17(12)**:3129–36.

54. Pavel M, O'Toole D, Costa F, Capdevila J, Gross D, Kianmanesh R, et al. ENETS Consensus Guidelines Update for the management of distant metastatic disease of intestinal, pancreatic, bronchial neuroendocrine neoplasms (NEN) and NEN of unknown primary site. *Neuroendocrinology* 2016;**103(2)**:172–85.

55. Frilling A, Modlin IM, Kidd M, Russell C, Breitenstein S, Salem R, et al. Recommendations for management of patients with neuroendocrine liver metastases. *Lancet Oncol* 2014;**15(1)**:e8–21.

56. Partelli S, Bartsch DK, Capdevila J, Chen J, Knigge U, Niederle B, et al. ENETS consensus guidelines for standard of care in neuroendocrine tumours: Surgery for small intestinal and pancreatic neuroendocrine tumours. *Neuroendocrinology* 2017;**105(3)**:255–65.

57. Bockhorn M, Uzunoglu FG, Adham M, Imrie C, Milicevic M, Sandberg AA, et al. Borderline resectable pancreatic cancer: A consensus statement by the International Study Group of Pancreatic Surgery (ISGPS). *Surgery* 2014;**155(6)**:977–88.

58. Hashim YM, Trinkaus KM, Linehan DC, Strasberg SS, Fields RC, Cao D, et al. Regional lymphadenectomy is indicated in the surgical treatment of pancreatic neuroendocrine tumors (PNETs). *Ann Surg* 2014;**259(2)**:197–203.

59. Öberg K. Management of functional neuroendocrine tumors of the pancreas. *Gland Surg* 2018;**7(1)**:20–7.

60. Tucker ON, Crotty PL, Conlon KC. The management of insulinoma. *Br J Surg* 2006;**93(3)**:264–75.

61. Bartsch DK, Waldmann J, Fendrich V, Boninsegna L, Lopez CL, Partelli S, et al. Impact of lymphadenectomy on survival after surgery for sporadic gastrinoma. *Br J Surg* 2012;**99(9)**:1234–40.

62. Krampitz GW, Norton JA, Poultsides GA, Visser BC, Sun L, Jensen RT. Lymph nodes and survival in pancreatic neuroendocrine tumors. *Arch Surg* 2012;**147(9)**:820–7.

63. Rinke A, Müller HH, Schade-Brittinger C, Klose KJ, Barth P, Wied M, et al. Placebo-controlled, double-blind, prospective, randomized study on the effect of octreotide LAR in the control of tumor growth in patients with metastatic neuroendocrine midgut tumors: A report from the PROMID Study Group. *J Clin Oncol* 2009;**27(28)**:4656–63.

64. Caplin ME, Pavel M, Cwikla JB, Phan AT, Raderer M, Sedláčková E, et al. Lanreotide in metastatic enteropancreatic neuroendocrine tumors. *N Engl J Med* 2014;**371(3)**:224–33.

65. Panzuto F, Di Fonzo M, Iannicelli E, Sciuto R, Maini CL, Capurso G, et al. Long-term clinical outcome of somatostatin analogues for treatment of progresssive, metastatic, well-differentiated entero-pancreatic endocrine carcinoma. *Ann Oncol* 2006;**17(3)**:461–6.

66. Kunz PL, Catalano PJ, Nimeiri H, Fisher GA, Loncinomagacre TA, Suarez CJ, et al. A randomized study of temozolomide or temozolomide and capecitabine in patients with advanced pancreatic neuroendocrine tumors: A trial of the ECOG–ACRIN Cancer Research Group (E2211). *J Clin Oncol* 2018;**36(15_suppl)**:4004.

67. Yao JC, Shah MH, Ito T, Bohas CL, Wolin EM, Van Cutsem E, et al. Everolimus for advanced pancreatic neuroendocrine tumors. *N Engl J Med* 2011;**364(6)**:514–23.

68. Raymond E, Dahan L, Raoul JL, Bang YJ, Borbath I, Lombard-Bohas C, et al. Sunitinib malate for the treatment of pancreatic neuroendocrine tumors. *N Engl J Med* 2011;**364(6)**:501–13.

69. Hicks RJ, Kwekkeboom DJ, Krenning E, Bodei L, Grozinsky-Glasberg S, Arnold R, et al. ENETS consensus guidelines for the standards of care in neuroendocrine neoplasia: Peptide receptor radionuclide therapy with radiolabeled somatostatin analogues. *Neuroendocrinology* 2017;**105(3)**:295–309.

70. Sorbye H, Welin S, Langer SW, Vestermark LW, Holt N, Osterlund P, et al. Predictive and prognostic factors for treatment and survival in 305 patients with advanced gastrointestinal neuroendocrine carcinoma (WHO G3): The NORDIC NEC study. *Ann Oncol* 2013;**24(1)**:152–60.

71. Apostolidis L, Dal Buono A, Merola E, Jann H, Jäger D, Wiedenmann B, et al. Multicenter analysis of treatment outcomes for systemic therapy in well differentiated grade 3 neuroendocrine tumors (NET G3). *Cancers (Basel)* 2021;**13(8)**:1936.

72. Dermine S, Palmieri LJ, Lavolé J, Barré A, Dohan A, Abou Ali E, et al. Non-pharmacological therapeutic options for liver metastases in advanced neuroendocrine tumors. *J Clin Med* 2019;**8(11)**:1907.

73. Mohan H, Nicholson P, Winter DC, O'Shea D, O'Toole D, Geoghegan J, et al. Radiofrequency ablation for neuroendocrine liver metastases: A systematic review. *J Vasc Interv Radiol* 2015;**26(7)**:935–42.e1.

74. Nigri G, Petrucciani N, Debs T, Mangogna LM, Crovetto A, Moschetta G, et al. Treatment options for PNET liver metastases: A systematic review. *World J Surg Oncol* 2018;**16(1)**:142.

75. Kunz PL, Reidy-Lagunes D, Anthony LB, Bertino EM, Brendtro K, Chan JA, et al. Consensus guidelines for the management and treatment of neuroendocrine tumors. *Pancreas* 2013;**42(4)**:557–77.

Bailey & Love's Essential Operations Bailey & Love's Essential Operatio
Bailey & Love's Essential Operations Bailey & Love's Essential Operatio
Bailey & Love's Essential Operations Bailey & Love's Essential Operatio

SECTION 6 | PANCREAS

Chapter 35 Unusual Pancreatic Tumours

Neil Bhardwaj, Deep Malde and Ashley R. Dennison

INTRODUCTION

The most common tumour of the pancreas is ductal adenocarcinoma (PDAC). Pancreatic neuroendocrine tumours (PNETs) occur less frequently but their incidence together with that of cystic lesions, such as intraductal papillary mucinous neoplasm (IPMN), mucinous cystic neoplasms (MCN), and serous cystic neoplasms (SCN) has increased over the past decade due to the wide availability of cross-sectional imaging.

The pancreas is a complex organ containing exocrine and endocrine tissue that may all become neoplastic, and it is also affected by a number of non-neoplastic conditions that mimic tumours including groove pancreatitis (GP) and autoimmune pancreatitis (AIP). Other unusual neoplastic lesions range from relatively well-recognized and described pathologies such as solid pseudopapillary neoplasm and acinar cell carcinoma to very rare tumours including mesenchymal and hepatoid carcinoma. Although non-ductal cancers such as acinar, neuroendocrine, solid-pseudopapillary neoplasms and pancreatoblastoma have distinct clinicopathologic and molecular profiles and presentations, it can be difficult to distinguish them from PDACs. Finally, the pancreas is a potential site for metastatic deposits and can be involved with other conditions such as primary pancreatic lymphoma.

Due to the low incidence of the more unusual pancreatic tumours, there is a paucity of data relating to their diagnosis and treatment. Management is often unclear and confounded by symptoms, principally abdominal discomfort, and jaundice, which are vague or mimic those from PDAC.

Pancreatic adenocarcinoma is discussed in **Chapter 33** and neuroendocrine tumours and cystic lesions in **Chapters 34** and **36**, respectively. In this chapter, we will focus on unusual pancreatic tumours.

HISTORICAL CONTEXT

Giovanni Battista Morgagni (1682–1771) was an Italian anatomist and pathologist whose work helped make pathological anatomy an exact science. He was Professor of Anatomy at the prestigious University of Padua for more than 50 years and in 1761 published his opus *De Sedibus et Causis Morborum per Anatomen Indagatis*, translated as '*The seats and causes of diseases investigated by anatomy*', which marked him as the founder of morbid anatomy. His report identified several cases of '*pancreatic "scirrhus", dry white pancreas of a "scirrhous" nature with pretty hard,*'

Table 35.1 History of pancreatic tumours, not including PDAC

Date	Pathology	Author
1902	First description of an islet cell adenoma	A G Nicholls
1908	Differentiation of alpha and beta cells	M A Lane
1908	Recognition of functioning acinar cell carcinoma and syndrome	P Berner
1922	Isolation and naming of insulin	Banting and Best
1926	Description of 20 cases of islet cell adenoma	Shields Warren
1927	Hyperinsulinism reported with islet cell carcinoma	Wilder, Allen & Power
1938	Whipple's triad associated with insulinoma	A O Whipple
1949	First case of pancreatic squamous cell carcinoma	C C Lowry, H W Whitaker & D J Greiner

(Continued)

DOI: 10.1201/9781003080060-35

Table 35.1 *(Continued)* History of pancreatic tumours, not including PDAC

Date	Pathology	Author
1951	Leiomyosarcoma of the pancreas	C F Ross
1953	First published review of MEN1 syndrome describing 14 cases	L O Underdahl, L B Woolner & B M Black
1954	Phenotype of multiple adenomatosis of endocrine glands	F Wermer
1954	First use of the term inflammatory pseudotumour	Umiker and Iverson
1955	Gastrinoma recognized	R M Zollinger & E H Ellison
1957	Pancreaticoblastoma	W F Becker
1958	Islet cell tumour producing hypokalaemia and diarrhoea	J V Verner & A B Morrison
1959	Solid pseudopapillary neoplasm in a 2-year-old boy	Virginia Kneeland Frantz
1964	Isolation of gastrin from Z-E tumours	R A Gregory & H J Tracy
1966	First report of glucagon-secreting pancreatic tumour	M G McGavran, R H Unger & L Recant
1974	APUD (amine precursor uptake and decarboxylation) concept developed	A G E Pearse & J M Polak
1977	Somatostatinoma defined by radioimmunoassay	O P Ganda, G C Weir & J S Soeldner
1977	Somatostatinoma immunohistochemistry developed	L Larsson, J Holst & J Kuhl
1977	Demonstrated that islet cell tumours secret multiple hormones	S R Bloom, A M West & J M Polak
1987	In 1987, the first classification of mixed neoplasms with neuroendocrine and non-neuroendocrine components was proposed	K Lewin
1996	Solid serous adenoma of the pancreas described	B Perez-Ordonez et al.
1996	Intraductal oncocytic papillary neoplasm of the pancreas	N V Adsay et al.
2010	WHO classification includes mixed serous-neuroendocrine neoplasm	WHO

distinct, lobules', felt to be the earliest recorded accounts of PDAC.

By the late 1800s, the clinical symptoms, signs and histology of pancreatic cancer had been clarified but other pancreatic neoplasms remained unrecognized. The first half of the twentieth century witnessed the development of laboratory techniques which facilitated the identification of neuroendocrine tumours, but unusual and rare pancreatic pathologies and associated syndromes had to wait until the late 1900s (*Table 35.1*).

CLASSIFICATION OF PANCREATIC TUMOURS

Pancreatic tumours are classified by differentiation of the neoplastic cells, as ductal, acinar, or neuroendocrine, and by the macroscopic appearance as solid or cystic lesions. The World Health Organization (WHO) classification is the most widely accepted for primary tumours of the pancreas and in the most recent (5th) edition published in 2019, classification is based on histologic appearance, not molecular characteristics (1). Most of the classification of pancreatic neoplasms remains unchanged from 2010, although there have been important developments in our

understanding of the aetiology and pathogenesis of many tumours. The classification of pancreatic neoplasms by WHO (2019) is shown in *Table 35.2*.

PATHOLOGY, EPIDEMIOLOGY, DIAGNOSIS AND TREATMENT

Benign tumours of the pancreas and premalignant lesions (*Table 35.3*)

Solid serous adenoma (SSCA)

Cystic tumours of the pancreas are defined as serous or mucinous and there are five morphological serous variants. The serous solid adenoma is the rarest with <30 cases reported in the world literature to-date with the first case only described by Perez-Ordonez et al. in 1996 (2).

Microscopically, the serous solid adenoma has the same architectural and cytological characteristics as the serous microcystic cystadenoma, namely, a round or ovoid structure formed of cuboid cells derived from the ductal epithelium. A report from Demesmaker et al. in 2019 described 22 cases from the literature with an average size of 2.7 cm and a capsule in 73% of cases (3). They noted that the absence of a clear benign

Table 35.2 Primary tumours of the pancreas[1]

Benign epithelial tumours and precursors	Malignant epithelial tumours	Pancreatic neuroendocrine neoplasms
Serous cystadenoma: ● Macrocystic (oligocystic) serous cystadenoma ● Solid serous adenoma ● Von Hippel–Lindau syndrome associated serous cystic neoplasm ● Mixed serous-neuroendocrine neoplasm	Ductal adenocarcinoma: ● Colloid carcinoma ● Poorly cohesive carcinoma ● Signet ring carcinoma ● Medullary carcinoma ● Adenosquamous carcinoma ● Epidermoid carcinoma ● Large cell carcinoma with rhabdoid phenotype ● Carcinoma undifferentiated ● Undifferentiated carcinoma with osteoclast-like giant cells	Pancreatic neuroendocrine microadenoma:
Serous cystadenocarcinoma:	Acinar cell carcinoma: ● Acinar cell cystadenocarcinoma ● Mixed acinar-euroendocrine carcinoma ● Mixed acinar-endocrine-ductal carcinoma ● Mixed acinar-ductal carcinoma	Neuroendocrine tumour: ● Neuroendocrine tumour, grade 1 ● Neuroendocrine tumour, grade 2 ● Neuroendocrine tumour, grade 3
Intraepithelial neoplasia: ● Glandular intraepithelial neoplasia, low-grade ● Glandular intraepithelial neoplasia, high-grade	Pancreatoblastoma:	Pancreatic neuroendocrine tumour, non-functioning: ● Oncocytic pancreatic neuroendocrine tumour, non-functioning ● Pleomorphic pancreatic neuroendocrine tumour, non-functioning ● Clear cell pancreatic neuroendocrine tumour, non-functioning ● Cystic pancreatic neuroendocrine tumour, non-functioning
Intraductal papillary mucinous neoplasm: ● Intraductal papillary mucinous neoplasm with low-grade intraepithelial neoplasia ● Intraductal papillary mucinous neoplasm with high-grade intraepithelial neoplasia ● Intraductal papillary mucinous neoplasm with associated invasive carcinoma ● Intraductal oncocytic papillary neoplasm Intraductal oncocytic papillary neoplasm: ● Intraductal oncocytic papillary neoplasm with associated invasive carcinoma ● Intraductal tubulopapillary neoplasm ● Intraductal tubulopapillary neoplasm with associated invasive carcinoma Mucinous cystic neoplasm: ● Mucinous cystic neoplasm with low-grade intraepithelial neoplasia ● Mucinous cystic neoplasm with high-grade intraepithelial neoplasia ● Mucinous cystic neoplasm with associated invasive carcinoma	Solid pseudopapillary neoplasm of the pancreas: ● Solid pseudopapillary neoplasm with high-grade dysplasia	Functioning pancreatic neuroendocrine tumours: ● Insulinoma ● Gastrinoma ● VIPoma ● Glucagonoma ● Somatostatinoma ● ACTH producing tumour ● Enterochromaffin cell carcinoid ● Serotonin-tumour Neuroendocrine carcinoma: ● Large cell neuroendocrine carcinoma ● Small cell neuroendocrine carcinoma Mixed neuroendocrine, non-neuroendocrine neoplasm: ● Mixed acinar-endocrine carcinoma ● Mixed acinar-neuroendocrine carcinoma ● Mixed acinar-neuroendocrine-ductal carcinoma

1 WHO (2019)

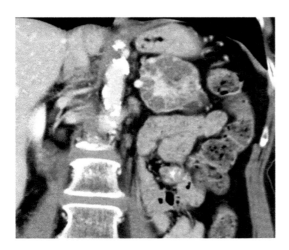

Figure 35.1 CT scan showing a solid serous cystadenoma in a 78-year-old female.

diagnosis frequently led to an aggressive surgical approach (*Figure 35.1*). In the 22 patients reviewed, surgical procedures included a distal pancreatectomy with splenectomy (27.3%) or without (18.2%), pylorus-preserving pancreatoduodenectomy (13.6%), pancreaticoduodenectomy (9.1%), and enucleation (13.6%). A pancreaticoduodenectomy was performed in their case report for 'oncologic reasons' to achieve a lymphadenectomy and because the tumour was obstructing the main pancreatic duct. In the 22 cases reviewed, approximately half were discovered incidentally, and half had abdominal pain.

Mixed serous – neuroendocrine neoplasm (MSNN)

Serous cystic neoplasm (SCN) of the pancreas is a very rare benign lesion, accounting for 1–2% of pancreatic tumours. In 2010, several new types of SCN were added to the WHO criteria for pancreatic tumour classification, including mixed SCNs and pancreatic neuroendocrine tumours. These are termed mixed serous neuroendocrine neoplasms (MSNN) and defined as a tumour containing two components with different pathologies. A number of cases of MSNN have been reported, including distinctly separated and intimately admixed tumours.

In 2016, Li et al. (4) described a case of MSNN and their literature search revealed 14 other studies which included 17 patients. In the case reported by Li et al, the mixed lesion arose in the pancreatic tail and was the first case with a mostly separated mixed SCN and PNET. Among the patients in their literature review, 13 were female and 2 were male. The median age was 52 (range, 28–78) years. The chief complaints were abdominal pain, nausea/vomiting,

weight loss, and jaundice, in 46.7%, 26.7%, 20.0%, and 13.3% of patients, respectively. The symptoms had often been present for several years before diagnosis although there were 5 (33.3%) patients with no symptoms. Due to the co-existence of two types of tumours, as with collision tumours and mixed tumours elsewhere, the prognosis of MSNN depends on the malignant component and MSNNs appear to have a higher malignant potential than SCN alone. Malignant biological behaviour such as perineural, lymphatic, and duodenal invasion appeared in 33.3% (5/15) of all the cases, which is significantly higher than that of SCN or PNET alone. There are three reported cases of MSNN associated with Von Hippel–Lindau disease (VHL) and a high potential for malignant transformation has been reported with VHL-associated PNETs. If a diagnosis of MSNN is established surgical treatment should be considered.

Intraductal oncocytic papillary neoplasm +/– invasive carcinoma

Intraductal oncocytic papillary neoplasms (IOPN-P) are rare, cystic, neoplasms composed of oncocytic cells in a complex papillary arrangement. They were first described in the pancreas by Adsay et al. in 1996 (5). Although intraductal papillary mucinous neoplasm (IPMN) was histologically divided into four subgroups in the WHO classification (4th edition) in 2010, IOPN-P became a separate entity in 2019. They are now classified as 1 of 4 histologic subtypes of intraductal papillary mucinous neoplasm (IPMN). The other three histologic subtypes of IPMN are gastric-type, intestinal-type, and pancreatobiliary-type. Additionally, IOPN-Ps can occur in the intrahepatic and extrahepatic bile duct. Although IOPN is a rare entity with a paucity of data in the literature, significant histologic, immunophenotypic, and potentially biologic differences exist between IOPN-P and other IPMN subtypes. IOPN-P has fewer mutations in *KRAS*, *GNAS*, and *RNF43*. Furthermore, pancreatic and bile duct IOPNs harbour recurrent *ATP1B1-PRKACB*, *DNAJB1-PRKACA*, or *ATP1B1-PRKACA* fusion genes, which do not occur in other tumours of the pancreatobiliary system. IOPN-Ps generates lower quantities of mucin and commonly assemble into intricate configurations with cystic and solid components explaining their misdiagnosis as PDAC (6). Imaging findings suggestive of IOPN-Ps include cystic and solid morphology, absence of peripancreatic invasion, large cyst size, and high FDG uptake. In addition, high-serum CEA and CA19-9 levels may indicate IPMA or IPMC rather than IOPN-P.

Patients with IOPN-P have a more favourable prognosis than those with IPMC and the majority of patients are cured following resection including those with limited invasive disease.

Intraductal tubopapillary neoplasm (ITPN)

IPMN was first described more than 3 decades ago, but more recently, an intraductal neoplasm with a distinctive pattern of growth has been identified. Pancreatic intraductal tubulopapillary neoplasms (ITPN) are rare, premalignant tumours with minimal or no mucin production, first recognized by the WHO in 2010 (7). Histologically, they are characterized by a tubular architecture and only sparse formation of papillary elements. The first case of ITPN in the pancreas (PITPN) was described in 1992 by Shahinian et al. (8), while the first biliary ITPN (BITPN) case was reported by Park et al. in 2010 (9). Typically, ITPN presents with jaundice, abdominal pain, and weight loss, resembling pancreatic adenocarcinoma or cholangiocarcinoma, and is most commonly found in female patients over 50 years of age. ITPN represents <1% of all pancreatic exocrine neoplasms, 3% of pancreatic intraductal neoplasms, and 15% of intraductal neoplasms of the bile duct. Compared with other intraductal neoplasms they have a favourable prognosis.

Due to the malignant potential, ITPNs are frequently treated by radical surgery and pylorus-preserving pancreaticoduodenectomy is the usual procedure as approximately 50% of ITPNs occur in the head of the pancreas.

Malignant lesions of the pancreas (Table 35.4)

Acinar cell carcinoma

Acinar cell carcinoma (ACC) of the pancreas is a rare, malignant neoplasm with distinctive clinical, molecular, and morphological features. Acinar cells are the functional exocrine units of the pancreas, and ACCs arise following malignant transformation of these cells. ACCs represent 1–2% of all exocrine tumours of the pancreas, making it the second most common type of pancreatic cancer. Acinar cell cystadenomas also occur but are considered to be benign.

The tumour most commonly occurs in middle-aged or elderly Caucasian men with an average age of 60 at diagnosis. Patients may present with abdominal pain, or the mass may be found incidentally. Most ACCs produce vague symptoms including weight loss (45%), abdominal pain (60%), back pain (50%), nausea and vomiting (20%), melena (12%), weakness, anorexia, and diarrhoea (8%) (10,11). Biliary obstruction is only seen in 12% of patients and when ACCs cause a mass effect, they displace rather than infiltrate adjacent organs (*Figure 35.2*). Up to 15% of patients will present with widespread subcutaneous fat necrosis, polyarthritis, and eosinophilia (Schmid's triad) due to increased circulating lipase

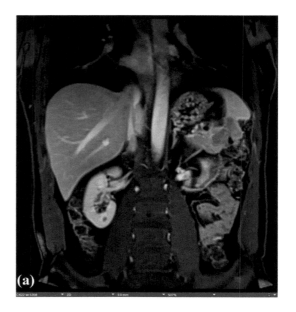

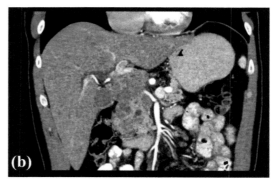

Figure 35.2 CT scans of acinar cell pancreatic tumours. Acinar cell carcinoma (a) invading the spleen. Large acinar cell carcinoma (b) with an enlarged hilar lymph node.

secreted by the tumour and associated with a worse prognosis.

Acinar cell carcinomas can occur in any part of the pancreas. They usually produce a well-circumscribed, partly encapsulated, pink to tan, homogeneous fleshy mass, averaging 11 cm in greatest diameter and occasionally demonstrating extensive haemorrhage and necrosis. Microscopically, most tumours are highly cellular with minimal stroma and lack the desmoplastic response seen with PDACs (12). Four patterns of growth have been described; acinar, solid, trabecular, and glandular. The acinar pattern is the most frequent, often with trabecular and glandular components. On genetic testing, altered genes/proteins are typically found for p53, SMAD4, *APC*, *ARID1A*, and *GNAS*.

Acinar cell carcinomas are aggressive neoplasms, although the long-term survival of ACC patients is superior to that of pancreatic adenocarcinoma with a median survival for patients with localized disease and metastatic disease of 38, and 14 months, respectively, but an overall 5-year survival of <10% (13,14).

Due to the limited data available there is no consensus regarding treatment and management protocols. Early diagnosis is essential to achieve long-term survival and FNA biopsy followed by histological and immunohistochemical analysis usually confirms the diagnosis. Surgical resection is the treatment of choice for patients with the disease restricted to one organ, and when negative margins are achieved appears to improve long-term survival (15). As a result of shared genetic alterations, ACCs are chemosensitive to agents with activity against PDAC and colorectal carcinomas, and although the role of neoadjuvant or adjuvant chemoradiotherapy has not been established, there appears to be some benefit with adjunct treatment.

Pancreatoblastoma

Pancreatoblastoma (PBL) is an extremely rare cancer composed of cells with predominantly acinar differentiation and characteristic squamoid nests. Neuroendocrine, ductal, and less commonly mesenchymal, differentiation can be seen, but is generally less extensive. Neoplastic cells usually demonstrate an organoid arrangement of acinar, solid, trabecular, or ductal formations comparable with acinar cell carcinomas. Due to the rarity of PBL very little is known about its clinical and pathologic features. Although PBL usually occurs in children, more than 70 adult cases have been described. There is a slight male predominance and although PBL may be found throughout the pancreas, it usually occurs in the head or body, and may infiltrate neighbouring structures (*Figure 35.3*). Despite being a very rare tumour, it is the most common pancreatic tumour in children, usually occurring before 10 years-of-age, with the peak incidence at 5 years. The cause is unknown, but some children have a genetic disease called Beckwith–Wiedemann syndrome (a growth disorder variably characterized by macroglossia, hemi-hyperplasia, omphalocele, neonatal hypoglycaemia, macrosomia, embryonal tumours including Wilms tumour, hepatoblastoma, neuroblastoma, and rhabdomyosarcoma, visceromegaly, adrenocortical cytomegaly, and renal kidney abnormalities) and they are rarely associated with familial adenomatous polyposis (FAP).

Genetic investigations and counselling are recommended in children with PBL and genetic syndromes. Children with PBL may present with abdominal pain, vomiting, weight loss, jaundice, and gastrointestinal (GI) bleeding or a palpable mass in the upper abdomen. These symptoms also occur with a number of other childhood conditions and consequently the

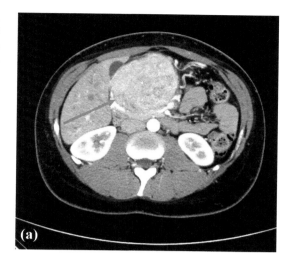

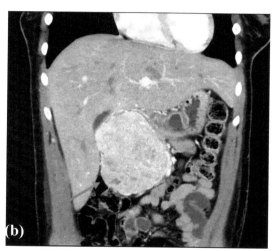

Figure 35.3 Axial (a) and coronal (b) CT scan images demonstrating an adult pancreatoblastoma (red arrow).

initial diagnosis is often delayed. Biological aggressiveness and elevated levels of serum α-fetoprotein (AFP) are comparable with hepatoblastoma. CT and magnetic resonance imaging (MRI) are generally able to differentiate PBL from SPNs of the pancreas (16) but histological confirmation demonstrated the distinctive appearance is important (17). Long-term survival generally follows surgical resection (18,19) but the prognosis is worse where there are metastases or surgical resection is incomplete (20). There is no data to support an agreed standard management, risk stratification or the treatment of relapsed and/or metastatic PBL (21).

Solid pseudopapillary neoplasm

Solid pseudopapillary neoplasm (SPN) of the pancreas is a low-grade malignant tumour with unclear cell of origin and pathogenesis, generally associated with a good prognosis. SPN are also known as solid pseudopapillary tumour, papillary epithelial neoplasm, papillary cystic neoplasm, solid and papillary neoplasm, low-grade papillary neoplasm and Hamoudi or Frantz tumour.

They represent 1–2% of pancreatic neoplasms and may be derived from pluripotent stem cells of the genital ridges which became attached to the pancreas during embryogenesis (22). SPNs show specific morphologic features, but the differential diagnosis with other pancreatic neoplasms, particularly pancreatic neuroendocrine tumours, can be difficult, especially with cytologic or biopsy specimens. Immunohistochemistry is sometimes helpful but is not completely reliable with a relatively low sensitivity.

SPL was first described by V.K. Frantz in 1959 and incorporated into the WHO classification in 1996 (23). They usually present in younger women, in the 3rd or 4th decade of life (mean age 35 years). There is a female: male ratio of 10 : 1 and they account for 30% tumours in women less than 40 years of age. In men, SPN occur at an older age and behave more aggressively. SPL occur throughout the pancreas but usually in the body or tail in adults and the head in children. Macroscopically, they contain varying amounts of solid and cystic components, and microscopically have papillary fronds on a myxoid or hyalinized vascular stalk lined by poorly cohesive, uniform cells.

Most cases are discovered incidentally during cross-sectional imaging when a well circumscribed, encapsulated, heterogeneous pancreatic mass with cystic degeneration is noted in the tail of the pancreas, especially in young women (*Figure 35.4*) (24).

SPN have also been reported from extrapancreatic sites, including the mesocolon, omentum, ovary, and testis. Due to their size, they may be symptomatic with abdominal pain, nausea, vomiting and early satiety and/or a palpable, nontender, upper abdominal mass. Cyst fluid chemistry will demonstrate a low CEA and amylase, and cytology or histology are necessary for confirmation of diagnosis. Poor prognostic factors include size >5 cm, male gender, necrosis, cellular atypia, vascular invasion, perineural invasion and invasion into adjacent structures. Surgical resection is curative in 95% of cases.

Mixed neuroendocrine non-neuroendocrine neoplasms

Mixed neuroendocrine non-neuroendocrine neoplasms (MiNENs) are rare tumours of the gastro-enteropancreatic (GEP) tract. Evidence from the current literature regarding their epidemiology, biology, and management is often conflicting and with the low index of suspicion among clinicians the incidence of MiNENs is probably underestimated. MiNENs are heterogenous neoplasms found in any organ, which by definition must be composed of at least two distinct morphologically recognizable neoplastic components: a neuroendocrine population, either well-differentiated, or more frequently poorly differentiated, and a non-neuroendocrine population. Each component must comprise at least 30% of the whole tumour. Compared with the previous definition of mixed adeno-neuroendocrine carcinomas (MANECs), the term MiNENs better represents the wide spectrum of all the possible combinations, and the variable differentiation and morphology. *Figure 35.5* shows a mixed neuroendocrine and hepatoid tumour.

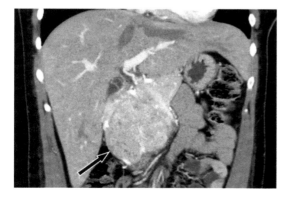

Figure 35.4 Coronal CT scan demonstrating solid pseudopapillary tumour in a 14-year-old female (black arrow).

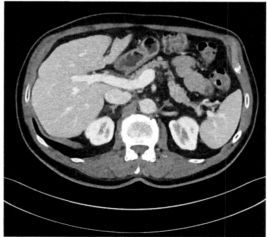

Figure 35.5 Axial CT scan demonstrating mixed neuroendocrine and hepatoid neoplasm in the body of the pancreas (red arrow).

The pathogenesis of MiNENs remains unclear and a number of explanations have been suggested. They may arise from two separate clones, the so-called collision theory, from a common multipotent progenitor stem cell with variable differentiation (common precursor theory), or from a single non-neuroendocrine clone, where neuroendocrine differentiation is the result of the progressive accumulation of genetic alterations and aberrations (25–27). Several studies have recently tried to identify the key genetic and epigenetic changes underlying MiNENs and in a recent systematic review, Frizziero et al. offered a comprehensive overview of the main genetic alterations reported to-date in these tumours (25).

Due to the recent identification of these rare tumours and multiple different descriptions, there is little published data to guide management, and it is impossible to be dogmatic about the pathological features or the most appropriate treatment. Consequently, MiNENs are usually treated according to the standard of care for neuroendocrine carcinomas or adenocarcinomas from the same sites of origin, based on an assumption of biological similarity to their counterparts derived from a single cell line. Treatment generally depends on which of the two components represents the majority of the tumour and/or has the most aggressive histology. When the non-neuroendocrine component is the majority however, especially if the histology is more aggressive, most oncologists will apply the standard of care for epithelial tumours from the same origin. No approach is presently supported by evidence from prospective randomized trials. The outlook is guarded and the prognosis usually poor as MiNENs are aggressive neoplasms driven by their (often high-grade) neuroendocrine component.

Mesenchymal neoplasms

The overwhelming majority of primary tumours of the pancreas are epithelial neoplasms with more than 90% being of ductal origin. Primary mesenchymal tumours, at this site, are exceptionally rare but virtually every sarcoma type has been described and they tend to display different clinicopathological features. The present literature on mesenchymal tumours in the pancreas is essentially limited to individual case reports or analyses of small series, predominantly focusing on their radiologic features. The most common type appears to be GISTs (many of which are secondary involvement from duodenum and stomach, although some may be true primary) and leiomyosarcomas, although different series report conflicting data. In one recent review from the Memorial Sloan Kettering Cancer Center in 2022 (28), Askan and Basturk reported data on 40 cases and found that 25 (63%) tumours were benign/borderline, and the remaining 15 (37%) were malignant. Of the benign/borderline tumours, 9 were

Table 35.3 Different histological types of benign and malignant pancreatic mesenchymal neoplasms

Benign	Malignant
Pancreatic neurofibroma	Pancreatoblastoma *(Figure 35.1)*
Pancreatic ganglioneuroma	Pancreatic lymphoma *(Figure 35.6)*
Pancreatic schwannoma *(Figure 35.4)*	
Pancreatic desmoid tumour	Pancreatic sarcoma
Pancreatic lipoma	Leiomyosarcoma *(Figure 35.5)*
Pancreatic perivascular epithelioid cell tumour (pancreatic PEComa)	Liposarcoma
Pancreatic mature cystic teratoma (pancreatic dermoid)	Rhabdomyosarcoma
Pancreatic lymphangioma	Epithelioid angiosarcoma
Solitary fibrous tumour	Malignant peripheral nerve sheet tumour *(Figure 35.6)*
Gastrointestinal stromal tumour (GIST)	Undifferentiated pleomorphic sarcoma
Inflammatory myofibroblastic tumour	Osteoclastoma *(Figure 35.7)*

solitary fibrous tumours, 6 gastrointestinal stromal tumours (GISTs), 4 schwannomas, 2 desmoid type fibromatosis, 1 lymphangioma, 1 ganglioneuroma, 1 inflammatory myofibroblastic tumour, and 1 low-grade mesenchymal neoplasm. Malignant tumours included 6 cases of leiomyosarcomas, 4 liposarcomas, 2 rhabdomyosarcomas, 1 epithelioid angiosarcoma, 1 malignant peripheral nerve sheet tumour, and 1 undifferentiated pleomorphic sarcoma (see *Table 35.3*). Four cases (multicystic schwannoma, desmoid fibromatosis, lymphangioma and inflammatory myofibroblast tumour) were preoperatively misdiagnosed as a primary epithelial tumour of the pancreas. Primary mesenchymal tumours of the pancreas have an incidence of 0.1% of pancreatic sarcoma diagnosed after autopsy. Benign mesenchymal tumours comprise lymphangiomas, haemangiomas, schwannomas, solitary fibrous tumours (SFTs), adenomatoid tumour, leiomyomas, and hamartomas.

Mesenchymal tumours can mimic epithelial tumours of the pancreas and the patients' demographics, clinical

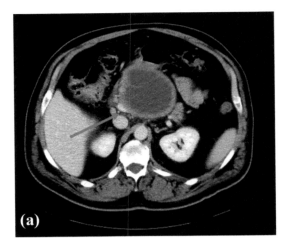

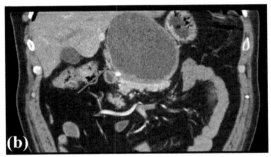

Figure 35.6 Axial (a) and coronal (b) CT scans demonstrating a pancreatic Schwannoma (red arrow).

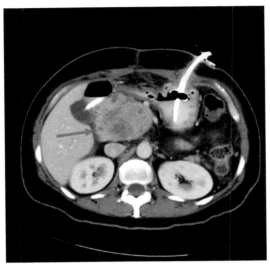

Figure 35.7 Axial CT scan demonstrating a pancreatic leiomyosarcoma (red arrow).

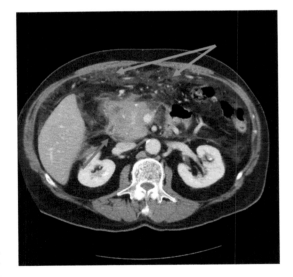

Figure 35.8 Axial CT scan demonstrating a pancreatic lymphoma (red arrow) mimicking autoimmune pancreatitis. The peritoneal disease (green arrows) is lymphomatosis.

symptoms, or tumour location are not helpful in distinguishing between these two pathologies. The mean age at presentation is 55 years, younger than that of PDAC, but the most common presenting symptom is abdominal pain in both groups. Radiologically, mesenchymal tumours may look very similar to pancreatic epithelial tumours, making the preoperative diagnosis difficult. Although a disparate group of tumours with consequently many different imaging appearances, these tumours tend to have clearer margins than the more infiltrative PDACs. A firm diagnosis is often only made after surgical resection and histologic examination.

Cystic mesenchymal tumours may be mistaken for pancreatic epithelial tumours radiologically and histologically. Schwannomas (see *Figure 35.6*) and lymphangiomas are the most common mesenchymal tumours presenting as cystic lesions with appearances similar to IPMNs, MCNs, serous cystadenoma, and cystic NETs. *Figures 35.7–35.10* demonstrate the appearance of a pancreatic leiomyosarcoma, lymphoma mimicking autoimmune pancreatitis an osteoclastic neoplasm and an undifferentiated pleomorphic sarcoma.

Squamous cell carcinoma

This extremely rare, nonendocrine, cancer of the pancreas forms in the pancreatic ducts and is composed of squamous cells which are usually absent from the pancreas. According to recent studies, the incidence of squamous cell carcinoma (SCCP) is low, representing 0.5–5% of exocrine pancreatic tumours (29,30). The histogenesis of pancreatic SCC is unclear and

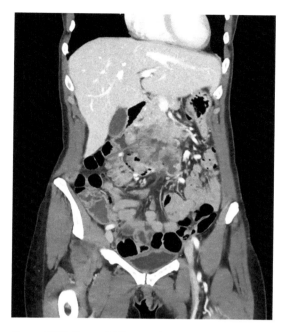

Figure 35.9 Coronal CT scan demonstrating an osteoclastic neoplasm of the pancreas (red arrow).

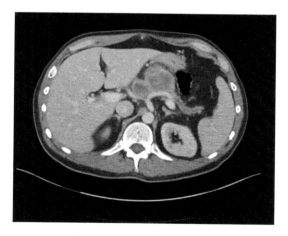

Figure 35.10 CT scan showing an undifferentiated pleomorphic sarcoma of the body of the pancreas.

there are not enough reported cases of this disease for its origins to be fully understood. Nevertheless, there are a number of hypotheses: 1) A bipotential primitive cell capable of differentiating into either squamous or glandular carcinoma undergoes malignant change; 2) Squamous metaplasia of the ductal epithelium undergoes a malignant transformation; 3) Pre-existing adenocarcinoma undergoes squamous

change; 4) An atypical squamous cell undergoes a malignant change (31).

The presenting symptoms with SCCP are similar to PDACs including upper abdominal and back pain, anorexia, weight loss, nausea, fatigue, vomiting, and obstructive jaundice. Local lymph node involvement and liver metastases are common. At present, a tumour blush with angiography or a strongly enhancing tumour on contrast-enhanced computed tomography (CECT) (probably due to the vascularity) are the most useful aids to diagnosis (32–34). Endoscopic ultrasound fine needle aspiration (EUS-FNA) is valuable, and is increasingly accepted for the identification and differentiation of pancreatic malignancies with a high sensitivity and specificity (35). SCCPs behave aggressively and their incidence is gradually increasing. It has a worse survival rate and a lower cure rate than the majority of pancreatic neoplasms with survival from the time of diagnosis similar or worse than that of PDAC. Different treatment protocols including surgical resection, chemotherapeutic regimens, and radiotherapy have not been shown to improve the outcome.

Pancreatic pseudotumours

A number of benign conditions can mimic pancreas cancer and lead to misdiagnosis and unnecessary management. In some series 5–10% of pancreatectomies performed following radiological suspicion of cancer and MDT discussion have revealed non-neoplastic masses referred to as pseudotumours. Pseudotumours are defined as a non-neoplastic space-occupying lesions that may occur almost everywhere in the body and have a varying course and clinical presentation. These tumours present diagnostic problems due to the myriad of radiological and histological patterns, many of which prevent a confident diagnosis of a benign condition. In the pancreas, chronic inflammatory processes are the leading cause of pseudotumours. The most common are paraduodenal, 'groove' pancreatitis and autoimmune pancreatitis both of which are notorious for being mistaken for PDAC. While the aetiology is usually related to these chronic inflammatory conditions, pancreatic pseudotumours may also be the result of trauma, infectious diseases, congenital anomalies, and lymphoproliferative processes (36,37).

Metastatic tumours

Although metastatic lesions of the pancreas only represent about 2% of pancreatic malignancies, at autopsy the pancreas has been found to be a site of metastases in a wide range (3–12%) of patients with disseminated malignant tumours (38).

One of the most challenging aspects of pathologic classification and proper management of pancreatic

Table 35.4 Summary of the pathology, epidemiology and presentation of unusual pancreatic tumours

Tumour type	Pathology	Epidemiology	Presentation
Serous adenoma/ cystadenoma	Numerous small cystic spaces. Microcystic, honeycomb, oligocystic, and solid patterns	Most common in females (M:F, 1:3) and elderly patients	Generally found incidentally but can mimic malignant lesions
Solid serous adenoma (SSA)	Tumour cells are polygonal in shape with small round nuclei and clear or pale cytoplasm, usually without mitosis or necrosis	The serous solid adenoma is the rarest entity of the five subcategories of pancreatic cystadenoma. Only about 30 cases are reported in the world literature. They appear to be slightly more common in females and are distributed throughout the pancreas	The rarity of SSA together with the difficulty of differential diagnosis from pancreatic solid tumours, makes the preoperative diagnosis complex. The absence of malignant behaviour however means that if a diagnosis can be made simple monitoring is appropriate. Presentation is usually with epigastric abdominal pain when symptomatic or as an incidental finding
Mixed serous – neuroendocrine neoplasm	Defined as a tumour containing two components with different pathologies	1–2% of all pancreatic tumours. Several new types added by the WHO in 2010	Usually, non-specific abdominal symptoms or discovered incidentally. Rarely present with palpable abdominal mass
Intraductal oncocytic papillary neoplasm	Pancreatic neoplasm characterized by intraductal growth is forming complex papillae composed of eosinophilic oncocytic cells. Despite its morphologic complexity and often extensive pagetoid spread to adjacent ducts, conventional invasive carcinoma is seen in only 29% and usually as microscopic foci	Rare but distinct type of pancreatic tumour. Mean age: 59-years. Accounts for 4.5% of intraductal neoplasms of the pancreas	Indolent behaviour even if associated with invasive carcinoma and 70% occur in the head, 10% involve whole gland. May also occur in the bile duct and although generally discovered incidentally, may present with jaundice
Acinar cell carcinoma	Most common in the head of the pancreas. Histology demonstrates acinar cell differentiation	1–2% of all pancreatic malignancies and 15% of childhood cancers. M:F, 2:1. Mean age at diagnosis: 59 years (range 22–88)	Non-specific symptoms are abdominal pain, weight loss, vomiting and nausea. 10–15% develop a classic lipase hypersecretion syndrome with fever and subcutaneous fat nodular necrosis
Pancreatoblastoma	Displays at least two pancreatic lines of differentiation, including acinar, ductal, and neuroendocrine elements. Presence of squamoid nests is a pathognomic feature	Rare pancreatic malignancy that is seen most often in children and displays multiple lines of differentiation. Most common pancreatic tumour of children <10 years old. Mean age of presentation in adults: 41 years	About 50% occur in pancreatic head, with the rest in the tail and body. Usually non-specific presentation with abdominal pain. Frequently inoperable at presentation with local extension and metastases to liver, lymph nodes and lungs. Associated with Beckwith–Wiedemann syndrome and familial adenomatous polyposis

Solid pseudopapillary neoplasm	Low-malignant potential tumours with unclear cell of origin and pathogenesis. May be derived from pluripotent stem cells of the genital ridges that become attached to the pancreas during embryogenesis. Variable amount of solid and cystic areas grossly. Papillary fronds on myxoid or hyalinized vascular stalk lined by poorly cohesive, uniform cells with nuclear grooves comprising solid and cystic areas beta catenin nuclear/cytoplasmic positive	Most common in young women (M:F, 1:10) and represents 1–2% of pancreatic tumours. Usually presents in the 3rd–4th decade of life (mean age: 35 years. In men, tends to occur at an older age and has more aggressive behaviour	Presents in younger women, classically as solitary body tail mass. Usually incidental but not infrequently palpable or space-occupying symptoms. When symptomatic generally abdominal pain, nausea, vomiting and early satiety. Located throughout the pancreas but more frequently in the body or tail in adults, while more frequent in the head of the pancreas in children
Mixed neuroendocrine non-neuroendocrine tumours (MiNEN)	Pancreatic, mixed, neuroendocrine, non-neuroendocrine, neoplasms (MiNENs) are heterogeneous malignancies characterized by histologically recognisable neuroendocrine (i.e. carcinoma and rarely, a well-differentiated neuroendocrine tumour) and exocrine (usually ductal carcinoma, acinar carcinoma, or both) components, each composing ≥30% of the volume of the neoplasm	M:F, 1:1. Average age at presentation is 68 years (ranges from 21–84 years). Mixed ductal neuroendocrine carcinomas comprise 0.5–2% of all ductal adenocarcinomas. Mixed acinar neuroendocrine carcinomas comprise 15–20% of all acinar carcinomas	Can occur anywhere in the pancreas. Mixed, ductal neuroendocrine carcinomas are more common in the head of the pancreas. Presentation is non-specific and depends on the tumour size and degree of metastatic disease
Mesenchymal neoplasms	Virtually every sarcoma type can occur in the pancreas. The most common ones appear to be GISTs (many of which are secondary involvement from duodenum and stomach, although some may be true primary), and leiomyosarcomas. Benign mesenchymal tumours comprise lymphangiomas, haemangiomas, schwannomas, solitary fibrous tumours, adenomatoid tumour, leiomyomas, and hamartomas	Primary mesenchymal tumours of the pancreas are rare with a reported incidence of 0.1% of pancreatic sarcoma diagnosed after autopsy. Mean age at presentation is 55 years. M:F is equal	The majority of lesions occur in the tail of the pancreas. The most common presenting symptoms were abdominal pain, loss of appetite, and weight loss although there is considerable variation depending on the histological type. Benign tumours tend to be located in the body/tail of the pancreas, whereas 2/3 of borderline and 1/3 of malignant tumours are located in the body/tail of the pancreas

(Continued)

Table 35.4 (*Continued*) Summary of the pathology, epidemiology, and presentation of unusual pancreatic tumours

Tumour type	Pathology	Epidemiology	Presentation
Squamous cell carcinoma (SCC)	A non-endocrine cancer of the pancreas which forms in the pancreatic ducts. It is composed purely of squamous cells, which are not typically seen in the pancreas. The histogenesis of pancreatic SCC is vague, but there are a number of hypotheses including; a bipotential primitive cell capable of differentiating into either squamous or glandular carcinoma, undergoes malignant change; squamous metaplasia of the ductal epithelium undergoes a malignant transformation; pre-existing adenocarcinoma undergoes squamous change; an atypical squamous cell undergoes a malignant change	Pancreatic SCC is a rare exocrine pancreatic carcinoma. There are different reports for the incidence of SCC, ranging from 0.5–5%	Presentation of pancreatic SCC is similar to ductal adenocarcinoma including upper abdominal and back pain, anorexia, weight loss, nausea, fatigue, vomiting, and obstructive jaundice. Local lymph node involvement and liver metastases are common
Pancreatic pseudotumours	A wide variety of benign conditions can mimic pancreatic tumours including paraduodenal (groove) pancreatitis and autoimmune pancreatitis	In some series 5–10% of pancreatectomies performed following a radiological suspicion of cancer will demonstrate non-neoplastic masses, defined as pseudotumours	Symptoms and presentation depend on the underlying aetiology and are frequently that of an inflammatory process. Treatment generally occurs when confirmation of a benign pathology is not possible
Metastatic tumours	Renal cell cancer is the most frequent primary site (62%) followed by non, small-cell lung cancer and melanoma	Will depend on the primary site and behaviour of the primary tumour	Usually found during investigation of the primary tumour. If origin not recognized may be mistaken for a pancreatic primary

cancers is the problem in distinguishing them from secondary malignancies, both clinically and pathologically. Ampullary/duodenal and CBD cancers often secondarily invade the pancreas and imitate a PDAC. Any unusual histological findings such as signet ring, mucinous or medullary histology should suggest the tumour is an ampullary or duodenal primary unless proven otherwise.

There are a variety of secondary tumours which metastasize to the pancreas which may mimic primary neoplasms. These include metastases from solid primaries such as renal cell (RCC), lung, colon and rectum, breast, liver, ovary, urinary bladder, stomach, prostate, and uterine cancer, Merkel cell carcinoma, lymphoma, and melanoma. Among these, especially lymphomas, renal cell RCCs and gastric cancers are prone to be misdiagnosed as PDACs preoperatively.

Although many patients will usually have widespread disease, isolated metastases can occasionally be identified and surgical management in these patients appears to be associated with improved survival (39,40). Resection is appropriate when patients present following a long disease-free interval after treatment of the primary cancer, suggesting favourable biological behaviour. The interval from diagnosis of an extrapancreatic primary tumour to subsequent detection of a pancreatic metastasis varies but is usually between 1–3 years (41).

A review of resection for metastases to the pancreas found renal cell carcinoma to be the most frequent primary histopathology (62%), followed by non-small-cell lung cancer, and melanoma (42). In series from Hiotis et al., postoperative morbidity was 25%, mortality 6%, and the overall actuarial survival rate for 2–5 years was 62% and 25%, respectively, confirming that resection of metastatic disease to the pancreas is safe, and may offer some survival benefit in selected patients.

Metastases from renal cell carcinoma may present many years after resection of the primary tumour and consequently not be entertained as a possible primary site. McNichols et al. (43) reported that 11% of patients developed metastases 10 or more years after nephrectomy, even with early-stage disease. The longest interval was reported by Muranaka et al. (44), who detected pancreatic metastases 27 years after treatment of an RCC. Rarely, a pancreatic metastasis may be discovered prior to a primary site being identified (41).

MULTIPLE ENDOCRINE NEOPLASIA (MEN) AND MULTIPLE ENDOCRINE ADENOMATOSIS (MEA)

Multiple endocrine neoplasia type 1 (MEN1) is one of the most common familial cancer syndromes. It is an autosomal dominant hereditary syndrome caused by a germline mutation in the *MEN1* tumour suppressor gene with a prevalence of 2–3 per 100 000 (45). MEN1 is characterized primarily by tumours of the parathyroid glands (95%), endocrine GEP tract (30–80%) and anterior pituitary (15–90%) (45).

Although the most common manifestation of MEN1 is the development of primary hyperparathyroidism, approximately 1/3 of patients affected with MEN1 will die early from MEN1-related cancer or associated malignancy. Entero-pancreatic gastrinomas and thymic- and bronchial-carcinoids are the leading cause of morbidity and mortality. Consequently, the average age of death in untreated individuals with MEN1 is significantly lower (55.4 years for men and 46.8 years for women) than that of the general population (46). When a diagnosis of MEN1 has been made based on clinical manifestations and/or genetic testing, an active surveillance program is mandatory for early detection and treatment of MEN1-associated tumours, with malignant potential such as gastrointestinal and pancreatic NETs.

SUMMARY

PDAC, PNET, IPMN, mucinous cystic neoplasm, and serous cystic neoplasm account for the vast majority of solid and cystic lesions of the pancreas. Other unusual neoplasms with very different behaviours may involve the pancreas and a high index of suspicion is required to ensure that benign or low-grade tumours are not mistaken for more aggressive neoplasms.

Due to the increasing availability and use of abdominal cross-sectional imaging, unusual pancreatic lesions are being diagnosed with greater frequency. Patients who present with a cystic, or solid, pancreatic mass with, or without, jaundice and no history of pancreatitis have a 1 in 10 chance of having a potentially curable benign or malignant pancreatic neoplasm. Although a number of these tumours have pathognomonic imaging characteristics, presentations, and demographic features a confident diagnosis remains challenging. In addition, many of these tumours will have features in common with PDACs and it is important to avoid unnecessary major surgical procedures with the inevitable morbidity and potential mortality. CT is the modality with which rare pancreatic tumours are incidentally detected in the majority of cases. MRI is often performed as a subsequent examination for further characterisation and additional modalities including endoscopic retrograde cholangiopancreatography (ERCP), EUS, FNA and tumour markers have increased the likelihood of clinicians being able to accurately identify these unusual tumours. The most important contributor to a correct diagnosis in patients presenting with unusual syndromes (very long symptom history; outside the usual PDAC demographic; atypical imaging features in those detected incidentally) is an informed awareness of the wide range of other pathologies that may affect the pancreas.

REFERENCES

1. Gonzalez RS. Pancreas WHO classification, 2002. Available from: https://www.pathologyoutlines.com/topic/pancreaswho.html PathologyOutlines.com DL (Ed) (Accessed 31 July 2024).

2. Perez-Ordonez B, Naseem A, Lieberman PH, Klimstra DS. Solid serous adenoma of the pancreas. The solid variant of serous cystadenoma? *Am J Surg Pathol* 1996;**20(11)**:1401–5.

3. Demesmaker V, Abou-Messaoud F, Parent M, Vanhoute B, Maassarani F, Kothonidis K. Pancreatic solid serous cystadenoma: A rare entity that can lead to a futile surgery. *J Surg Case Rep* 2019;**2019(12)**:rjz360.

4. Li Y, Dai M, Chang X, Hu W, Chen J, Guo J, et al. Mixed serous neuroendocrine neoplasm of the pancreas: Case report and literature review. *Medicine (Baltimore)* 2016;**95(34)**:e4205.

5. Adsay NV, Adair CF, Heffess CS, Klimstra DS. Intraductal oncocytic papillary neoplasms of the pancreas. *Am J Surg Pathol* 1996;**20**:980–94.

6. Nakaya M, Nakai Y, Takahashi M. , Fukukura Y, Sato K, Kameda A, et al. Intraductal oncocytic papillary neoplasm of the pancreas: Clinical and radiological features compared to those of intraductal papillary mucinous neoplasm. *Abdom Radiol* 2023;**48**:2483–93.

7. Kuan LL, Dennison AR, Garcea G. Intraductal tubulopapillary neoplasm of the pancreas and bile duct: A review. *Pancreas* 2020;**49**:498–502.

8. Shahinian HK, Sciadini MF, Springer DJ, Reynolds VH, Lennington WJ. Tubular adenoma of the main pancreatic duct. Arch Surg 1992;127:1254–55.

9. Park HJ, Jang KT, Heo JS, Choi YL, Han J, Kim SH. A potential case of intraductal tubulopapillary neoplasms of the bile duct. *Pathol Int* 2010;**60**: 630–35.

10. Fontenot J, Spieler B, Hudson C, Boulmay B. Pancreatic acinar cell carcinoma – literature review and case report of a 56-year-old man presenting with abdominal pain. *Radiol Case Rep* 2019;**15(1)**:39–43.

11. Calimano-Ramirez LF, Daoud T, Gopireddy DR, Morani AC, Waters R, Gumus K, et al. Pancreatic acinar cell carcinoma: A comprehensive review. *World J Gastroenterol* 2022;**28(40)**:5827–44.

12. Holen KD, Klimstra DS, Hummer A, Gonen M, Conlon K, Brennan M, et al. Clinical characteristics and outcomes from an institutional series of acinar cell carcinoma of the pancreas and related tumors. *J Clin Oncol* 2002;**20**:4673–78.

13. Sridharan V, Mino-Kenudson M, Cleary JM, Rahma OE, Perez K, Clark JW, et al. Pancreatic acinar cell carcinoma: A multi-center series on clinical characteristics and treatment outcomes. *Pancreatology* 2021;**21(6)**:1119–26.

14. Schmidt CM, Matos JM, Bentrem DJ, Talamonti MS, Lillemoe KD, Bilimoria KY. Acinar cell carcinoma of the pancreas in the United States: Prognostic factors and comparison to ductal adenocarcinoma. *J Gastrointest Surg* 2008;**12**:2078–86.

15. Klimstra DS, Heffess CS, Oertel JE, Rosai J. Acinar cell carcinoma of the pancreas. A clinicopathologic study of 28 cases. *Am J Surg Pathol* 1992;**16**:815–37.

16. Yang Z, Gong Y, Ji M, Yang B, Qiao Z. Differential diagnosis of pancreatoblastoma (PB) and solid pseudopapillary neoplasms (SPNs) in children by CT and MR imaging. *Eur Radiol* 2021;**31(4)**:2209–17.

17. Omiyale AO. Adult pancreatoblastoma: Current concepts in pathology. *World J Gastroenterol* 2021;**27(26)**:4172–81.

18. Xu C, Zhong L, Wang Y, Wang W, Yang Z, Kang X, et al. Clinical analysis of childhood pancreatoblastoma arising from the tail of the pancreas. *J Pediatr Hematol Oncol* 2012;**34(5)**:e177–e181.

19. Défachelles AS, Martin De Lassalle E, Boutard P, Nelken B, Schneider P, Patte C. Pancreatoblastoma in childhood: Clinical course and therapeutic management of seven patients. *Med Pediatr Oncol* 2001;**37(1)**:47–52.

20. Dall'igna P, Cecchetto G, Bisogno G, Conte M, Chiesa PL, D'Angelo P, et al. Pancreatic tumors in children and adolescents: The Italian TREP project experience. *Pediatr Blood Cancer* 2010;**54(5)**:675–80.

21. Huang Y, Yang W, Hu J, Zhu Z, Qin H, Han W, et al. Diagnosis and treatment of pancreatoblastoma in children: A retrospective study in a single pediatric center. *Pediatr Surg Int* 2019;**35(11)**:1231–38.

22. Terris B, Cavard C. Diagnosis and molecular aspects of solid-pseudopapillary neoplasms of the pancreas. *Semin Diagn Pathol* 2014;**31(6)**:484–90.

23. Frantz VK. Section VII, Fascicles 27 and 28. Tumors of the Pancreas. In: *Atlas of Tumor Pathology*. Washington, DC: Armed Forces Institute of Pathology, 1959; pp. 32–33.

24. La Rosa S, Bongiovanni M. Pancreatic solid pseudopapillary neoplasm: Key pathologic and genetic features. *Arch Pathol Lab Med* 2020;**144(7)**:829–37.

25. Frizziero M, Chakrabarty B, Nagy B, Lamarca A, Hubner RA, Valle JW, et al. Mixed neuroendocrine non-neuroendocrine neoplasms: A systematic review of a controversial and underestimated diagnosis. *J Clin Med* 2020;**9(1)**:273.

26. Guerrera LP, Suarato G, Napolitano R, Perrone A, Caputo V, Ventriglia A, et al. Mixed neuroendocrine non-neuroendocrine neoplasms of the gastrointestinal tract: A case series. *Healthcare (Basel)* 2022;**10(4)**:708.

27. La Rosa S, Sessa F, Uccella S. Mixed neuroendocrine-non-neuroendocrine neoplasms (MiNENs): Unifying the concept of a heterogeneous group of neoplasms. *Endocr Pathol* 2016;**27**:284–311.

28. Askan G, Basturk O. Mesenchymal Tumors involving the pancreas: A clinicopathologic analysis and review of the literature. *Turk Patoloji Derg* 2022;**38(1)**:46–53.

29. Baylor SM, Berg JW. Cross-classification and survival characteristics of 5000 cases of cancer of the pancreas. *J Surg Oncol* 1973;**5**:335–58.

30. Beyer KL, Marshall JB, Metzler MH, Poulter JS, Seger RM, Díaz-Arias AA. Squamous cell carcinoma of the pancreas. Report of an unusual case and review of the literature. *Dig Dis Sci* 1992;**37**:312–18.

31. Motojima K, Tomioka T, Kohara N, Tsunoda T, Kanematsu T. Immunohistochemical characteristics of adenosquamous carcinoma of the pancreas. *J Surg Oncol* 1992;**49**:58–62.

32. Sprayregen S, Schoenbaum SW, Messinger NH. Angiographic features of squamous cell carcinoma of the pancreas. *J Can Assoc Radiol* 1975;**2**:122–4.

33. Koduri VG, Ravi TJ. Squamous cell carcinoma of the pancreas: Report of a case and review of ERCP findings. *J Endoscopy* 1994;**26**:333–4.

34. Al-Shehri A, Silverman S. Squamous cell carcinoma of the pancreas. *J Curr Oncol* 2008;**15**:293–7.

35. Lai LH, Romagnuol J, Adams D, Yang J. Primary squamous cell carcinoma of pancreas diagnosed by EUS-FNA: A case report. *World J Gastroenterol* 2009;**15**:4343–45.

36. Adsay NV, Basturk O, Klimstra DS, Klöppel G. Pancreatic pseudotumors: Non-neoplastic solid lesions of the pancreas that clinically mimic pancreas cancer. *Semin Diagn Pathol* 2004;**21**(**4**):260–7.

37. Patnana M, Sevrukov AB, Elsayes KM, Viswanathan C, Lubner M, Menias CO. Inflammatory pseudotumor: The great mimicker. *AJR Am J Roentgenol* 2012;**198**(**3**):W217–27.

38. Rumancik WM, Megibow AJ, Bosniak MA, Hilton S. Metastatic disease to the pancreas: Evaluation by computed tomography. *JCAT* 1984;**8**:829–34.

39. Sperti C, Pasquali C, Liessi G, Pinciroli L, Decet G, Pedrazzoli S. Pancreatic resection for metastatic tumours to the pancreas. *J Surg Oncol* 2003;**83**:161–6.

40. Crippa S, Angelini C, Mussi C, Bonardi C, Romano F, Sartori P, et al. Surgical treatment of metastatic tumours to the pancreas: A single center experience and review of the literature. *World J Surg* 2006;**30**:1536–42.

41. Merkle EM, Boaz T, Kolokythas O, Haaga JR, Lewin JS, Brambs HJ et al. Metastases to the pancreas. *Br J Radiol* 1998;**71**:1208–14.

42. Hiotis SP, Klimstra DS, Conlon KC, Brennan MF. Results after pancreatic resection for metastatic lesions. *Ann Surg Oncol* 2002;**9**:675–9.

43. McNichols DW, Segura JW, Deweerd JH. Renal cell carcinoma. Long term survival and late recurrence. *J Urol* 1981;**126**:17–23.

44. Muranaka T, Teshima K, Honda H, Nanjo T, Hanada K, Oshiumi Y, et al. Computed tomography and histologic appearance of pancreatic metastases from distant sources. *Acta Radiol* 1989;**30**:615–19.

45. Pieterman CR, Schreinemakers JM, Koppeschaar HP, Vriens MR, Borel Rinkes IHM, Zonnenberg BA, et al. Multiple endocrine neoplasia type 1 (MEN1): Its manifestations and effect of genetic screening on clinical outcome. *Clin Endocrinol (Oxf)* 2009;**70**:575–81.

46. Triponez F, Dosseh D, Goudet P, Cougard P, Bauters C, Murat A, et al. Epidemiology data on 108 MEN 1 patients from the GTE with isolated nonfunctioning tumors of the pancreas. *Ann Viswa Surg* 2006;**243**:265–72.

Bailey & Love's Essential Operations Bailey & Love's Essential Operation
Bailey & Love's Essential Operations Bailey & Love's Essential Operation
Bailey & Love's Essential Operations Bailey & Love's Essential Operation

SECTION 6 | PANCREAS

Chapter 36

Pancreatic Cystic Lesions

Giampaolo Perri, Giovanni Marchegiani, Roberto Salvia and Claudio Bassi

INTRODUCTION

The prevalence of pancreatic cystic neoplasms in the general population is high and increases with age. Most pancreatic cystic neoplasms are intraductal papillary mucinous neoplasms (IPMN). Whilst, in most of the cases, pancreatic cystic neoplasms can be safely surveilled over time, some are at risk of malignant progression and surgery is indicated. In this chapter, the main clinical features of the most common pancreatic cystic neoplasms (PCNs), IPMNs, mucinous cystic neoplasms (MCNs), and serous cystic neoplasms (SCNs) will be reviewed and discussed together with their clinical management. Available consensus guidelines for pancreatic cystic neoplasms will be also critically reviewed, highlighting the most recent scientific literature updates, and addressing the existing controversial aspects of their clinical management.

Due to the extensive use of cross-sectional imaging techniques such as computed tomography (CT) scan and magnetic resonance imaging (MRI) among the general population, the prevalence of PCNs is constantly rising (1). Most of the PCNs are diagnosed incidentally in asymptomatic individuals, with IPMNs representing around the 80% of these entities (2). Given

their propensity for malignant progression via the adenoma-to-carcinoma sequence, and consequently the potential development of pancreatic cancer, PCNs represent an ideal population to study to help develop strategies for prevention and early diagnosis (3–5). In the first years after their discovery, PCNs were treated aggressively due to a lack of reliable data on their biology and a high presumed risk of malignancy, which was mainly extrapolated from surgical series. The progressive availability of new evidence from large observational studies has highlighted how most cases can be safely surveilled over time due to a low risk of malignant progression (6–9). Contextually, surgical management has evolved towards a more conservative approach in the attempt to balance effective prevention of pancreatic cancer and unnecessary harmful surgery. Besides IPMNs, PCNs account for different biological entities, as listed in the WHO classification, ranging from completely benign SCNs to potentially pre-malignant MCNs lesions (*Figure 36.1*) (10). Other rare pancreatic tumours may present with a cystic morphology, such as cystic neuroendocrine pancreatic tumours (cystic PNETs) or solid pseudopapillary tumours (SPTs), and other non-epithelial lesions such as pancreatic pseudocysts or retention cysts may mimic a PCN.

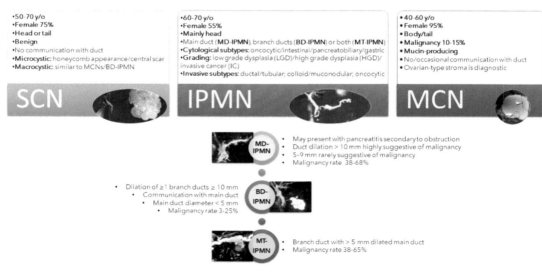

Figure 36.1 Clinical and pathological characteristics of the most frequent PCNs.

DOI: 10.1201/9781003080060-36

CLINICAL CHARACTERISTICS

The first evaluation of a PCN should always take into account epidemiological and clinical aspects, together with cross-sectional imaging and endoscopic ultrasound (EUS) data. Of note, some PCNs are more likely to develop in females, present at a specific age, and be more commonly found in a specific location. The main epidemiological features and likelihood of malignant progression of the most common PCNs are listed in *Figure 36.1*, while their common appearance at gross pathological examination is shown in *Figure 36.2*.

Serous cystic neoplasms

SCNs are more frequently diagnosed in females (75%) between the age of 50–70, with no preferential location between pancreatic head or body/tail (11,12). Most patients are generally asymptomatic, but larger cysts may be associated with abdominal discomfort, or rarely, a palpable mass and causes bile duct or gastric outlet obstruction. Imaging of SCNs reveal a lobulated shape often with a fine honeycomb pattern, which is indicative of a microcystic morphology. In some cases, a pathognomonic central calcified scar is also present. Their macrocystic variants can be indistinguishable from other PCNs and particularly MCNs. SCNs are invariably benign, as clarified in a critical review of their pathological features which highlighted the misinterpretation of a small number of cases reported as malignant (the so-called 'serous cystadenocarcinomas') (13). However, oncological

issues aside, surgical resection still has a place in the management of SCNs if they become sufficiently large to cause symptoms due to a mass effect or in cases of uncertain diagnosis during surveillance (mainly in younger individuals and with pancreatic body or tail lesions) (14).

Mucinous cystic neoplasms

Ninety-five percent of MCNs are found in females between the ages of 40–60 and are located in the pancreatic body or tail (11,12). They are often asymptomatic, but as they increase in size, they may produce pain, present with an abdominal mass, or cause weight loss, which can be insidious and occurring for years before the diagnosis is made (15). MCNs usually appear as round lesions, either uni- or multi-locular and always lack a communication with the main pancreatic duct. The cystic wall and the septa are usually thick and peripheral 'eggshell' calcification may be seen occasionally. The rate of malignant MCNs found in surgical series ranges from 0–34% due to the different histological criteria used historically. The reported rate was considerably higher in older studies, as the series included larger lesions, inadvertently incorporating several cases of IPMNs (usually showing a more aggressive biological behavior) and surgically resected tumours (producing an obvious selection bias). Conversely, recent data have suggested that the risk of malignant transformation of MCNs may be low, especially for smaller tumours (16–18). In a large series of 424 presumed MCNs, less than 50 mm in size

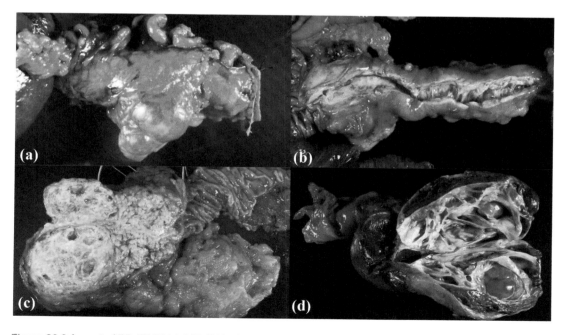

Figure 36.2 Aspect of BD-IPMN (a), MD-IPMN (b), SCN (c) and MCN (d) at gross pathology.

with no mural nodules or enhancing walls, observed at the Verona and San Raffaele University Hospitals, the incidence of malignancy was negligible, favouring surveillance in selected cases given the low risk of the development of cancer and the high rate of misdiagnosis (19).

Intraductal papillary neoplasms

IPMNs represent the most frequent PCN. Their prevalence increases with age, with no significant gender difference or pancreatic location (11,12). The vast majority of IPMNs are incidentally discovered during radiographic cross-sectional imaging but they may present with a plethora of non-specific symptoms such as abdominal pain, bloating, heartburn, and early post-prandial satiety (20,21). While these non-specific symptoms do not help in predicting the risk of malignancy (and are not, probably, even IPMN-related in many of the cases), there are a few signs and symptoms which can be directly related to the presence of IPMNs (particularly in the case of malignant degeneration). These include obstructive jaundice, recurrent acute pancreatitis, new-onset or worsening diabetes mellitus, and steatorrhea due to endocrine or exocrine insufficiency.

From a morphological point of view, IPMNs can be distinguished on the basis of the involvement, or not, of the main pancreatic duct (MPD) (*Figure 36.1*). This allows IPMNs to be categorized as: 1) A main duct type (MD-IPMN) originating directly from the MPD and associated with ductal dilation of greater than 5 mm; 2) The branch duct type (BD-IPMN) originating from a secondary duct of ≥10 mm and not involving the MPD; and 3) The mixed type (MT-IPMN), where the involvement of MPD is associated with a side branch dilation. The risk of malignancy differs significantly between different IPMN subtypes, with BD-IPMNs having the lowest risk (3–25%) and MD- or MT-IPMN being the highest (38–68%) (22,23), although it is important to note that malignancy rates are largely derived from surgical series. The pathological classification of IPMNs also has important implications in predicting the risk of malignant progression. Four subtypes of IPMNs can be distinguished based on immunohistochemical characteristics (24,25): 1) intestinal; 2) pancreato-biliary; 3) gastric; and 4) oncocytic. Intestinal and gastric subtypes are the most common and are principally associated with MD- and BD-IPMNs, respectively, while the pancreato-biliary subtype is associated with higher rates of invasive carcinoma (up to 90% of cases). The oncocytic variant displays different characteristics compared with the other three types and is classed as a separate entity (26,27). Currently, the grading of IPMNs is reported using a two-tier classification system proposed by the WHO in an attempt to improve pathological reporting, including only low-(LGD) and high-grade (HGD) dysplasia (28).

Invasive cancer in IPMNs also represents a heterogenous group of entities with different histological differentiations (29): 1) colloid/muco-nodular (usually arising from intestinal type and with indolent behavior); 2) ductal/tubular (often associated with gastric and pancreato-biliary subtypes, with a prognosis similar to pancreatic ductal adenocarcinoma); and 3) oncocytic (deriving from the homonymous subtype, with a better prognosis when compared with pancreatic cancer).

GUIDELINES

The management of PCNs remains controversial. Three main guidelines exist: the International Guidelines of the International Association of Pancreatology (IAP), published in 2006 and updated in 2012 and 2016, the European Evidence-based Guidelines (EEG) published in 2013 and updated in 2017, and the guidelines of the American Gastroenterological Association (AGA) published in 2015 (30–32). All three guidelines tend to be consistent regarding the main absolute, or relative, indications for surgery (*Figure 36.3*), represented by specific features conferring an implicit high-risk of malignancy (worrisome features [WF] and high-risk stigmata [HRS] for IAP guidelines). With regards to surveillance, the consistency is considerably lower (*Figure 36.4*). The AGA suggests stopping surveillance once the patient is no longer fit for surgery or if there has been no change in the features of the cyst for 5 years. Of note, the indications for ceasing follow-up were based on expert consensus.

Guidelines remain a fundamental tool to guide, and uniform, clinical practice, raising awareness among nonspecialized physicians, and lowering the risk for treatment disparities. However, they are mostly based on low-quality evidence and rely on expert opinion or data extrapolated from surgical series, with only a few observational studies (no randomized controlled trials are currently available for IPMNs). Furthermore, a recent analysis of the application of PCN guidelines in clinical practice demonstrated that three levels of discrepancies exist, between the three existing guidelines themselves, between guidelines and available evidence, and between guidelines and clinical practice (33). A major concern, regarding their actual application, is resource availability, as more than half of physicians responding to the survey do not have access to contrast-enhanced EUS (CE-EUS). The primary low-evidence areas highlighted by the survey were represented by the role of MPD dilatation, mural nodules, cyst size and growth rate, cyst-related symptoms and surveillance discontinuation. Future research lines should aim at increasing the level of available evidence, possibly with large observational studies to capture the true biology of PCNs.

EEG 2018

Absolute indications:
- Positive cytology for malignancy/HGD
- Solid mass
- Jaundice (IPMN related)
- Enhancing mural nodule (≥ 5 mm)
- MPD dilation ≥ 10 mm

Relative indications:
- Growth-rate ≥ 5 mm/year
- Increased levels of serum CA19.9 (> 37 U/m)
- MPD dilation between 5 and 9.9 mm
- Cyst diameter ≥ 40 mm
- New onset of diabetes mellitus
- Acute pancreatitis (caused by IPMN)
- Enhancing mural nodule (> 5 mm)

IAP 2017

Absolute indications: (HIGH RISK STIGMATA)
- Cytology suspicious or positive for malignancy
- Jaundice (IPMN related)
- Enhancing mural nodule (≥ 5 mm)
- MPD dilation ≥ 10 mm

Relative indications: (WORRISOME FEATURES)
- Growth-rate ≥ 5 mm/2 years
- Increased levels of serum CA19.9
- MPD dilation between 5 and 9 mm
- Cyst diameter ≥ 30 mm
- Acute pancreatitis (caused by IPMN)
- Enhancing mural nodule (< 5 mm)
- Lymphadenopathy
- Thickened/enhancing cyst walls

AGA 2015*

Absolute indications:
MPD ≥ 5 mm (on MRI AND EUS) **AND** solid component **OR** cytology positive for malignancy

Relative indications:

* Asymptomatic PCNs

Figure 36.3 Surgical indications for PCNs according to current guidelines.

EEG 2018

Follow-up indications:
- Cyst size < 40 mm
- MPD < 6 mm
- No mural nodules
- Asymptomatic
- Cyst growth rate < 2 mm/year
- Normal serum CA 19-9

Follow-up schedule:
MRI or EUS
- Year 1: every 6 months
- Year 2–5: every 12 months
- Year >5: every 6 months
- In case of increase in size: every 6 months

IAP 2017

Follow-up indications:
- Absence of WF/HRS

Follow-up schedule:
MRI/CT or EUS
- > 30 mm: MRI/CT scan every 3–6 months; consider surgery in young patients
- 20–30 mm: EUS in 3–6 months; then up to 1 year alternating MRI to EUS; consider surgery in young patients
- 10–20 mm: CT/MRI every 6 months for 1 year, then every 12 months for 2 years, then every 2 years
- < 10 mm: CT/MRI in 6 months, then every 2 years

AGA 2015*

Follow-up indications:
- Size < 30 mm
- No solid component
- Absence of concerning features at EUS performed when indicated by guidelines

Follow-up schedule:
MRI
- After 1 year from diagnosis, then every 2 years
- Surveillance should be discontinued after 5 years from diagnosis

* Asymptomatic PCNs

Figure 36.4 Indications for surveillance for PCNs according to current guidelines.

SURGICAL INDICATIONS

MPD dilation ≥10 mm, pancreas-specific symptoms (in particular obstructive jaundice), and enhancing mural nodules are the most recognized and validated predictors of malignant degeneration, and therefore represent indications for surgical resection. In particular, vascularized mural nodules are the strongest predictor of either high-grade dysplasia or invasive carcinoma for all types of suspected IPMNs (34). No evidence for a cut-off related to the size of mural nodules is available, but the risk of malignancy appears to be directly proportional to the size, and according to the guidelines, dimensions ≥5 mm represents an absolute indication for surgery (34). While the presence of a MPD dilation ≥10 mm is associated with a 40% risk of IPMN-related death, supporting the policy of surgical resection, in the absence of other features suggesting malignancy, MPD dilation alone (especially between 5–9 mm) is associated with a considerable risk of misdiagnosis and possible overtreatment (35–37). For this reason, some authors suggested surveillance in asymptomatic patients who have 'worrisome' MPD dilation (5–9 mm) but lacking other absolute or relative indications (36,38). PCNs size has always driven surgical management in the past, as the most simple and obvious feature to observe. However, a cut-off for definitively recommending surgery based on size alone does not exist in the literature and for this reason, growth rate during follow-up has been recently recognized as a more accurate parameter when predicting the risk of progression, rather than cyst size at first observation (39). In general, many of the features of concern listed as 'relative' indications are not strong standalone predictors of malignancy and therefore not indications for surgery *per se* after a single observation. Historically, both observational studies (due to the absence of pathologic diagnosis) and surgical series (due to selection bias) have failed to provide comprehensive information about the malignant transformation of IPMNs. To overcome these limitations, a recent multicentre observational study included a cohort of 292 BD-IPMNs enrolled in a surveillance program for a minimum of 12 months before undergoing surgical resection, and explored dynamic variables associated with the development of high-grade dysplasia and invasive cancer (40). While harboring a stable WF carried the lowest risk of malignant disease, the development of an additional WF or HRS was associated with the presence of high-grade dysplasia, whereas the occurrence of jaundice was associated with invasive cancer. Further similar observational studies focusing on PCNs 'crossing-over' from observation to surgery will hopefully identify further dynamic predictors of malignant change, with the aim of treating high-grade dysplasia before the occurrence of overt pancreatic cancer.

Besides clinical and radiographic indications, surgical decision making should always take into account the patient-related parameters represented by 'fitness' for surgery, such as age and life expectancy, frailty, overall health status and comorbidities, and the will and motivation for surgery. Considering the low overall rate of malignancy of PCNs, this parameter is especially important. This cautious approach aims to select only candidates with a high likelihood of high-grade dysplasia or invasive cancer, sparing the burden of unnecessary surgery to patients who are not showing clinical or radiographic signs of malignancy. Pancreatic surgery is still a procedure with high rates of major morbidity and mortality, ranging from 24–30% and from 1–5%, respectively (41–44). Each case should always be carefully evaluated with input from the patient after adequate counselling. In general, guidelines are valuable tools for identifying patients at high risk for high-grade dysplasia or invasive cancer, but they must be applied with flexibility and in the understanding that they are mostly based on 'expert opinion' with a number of remaining grey areas in respect of scientific evidence. For these reasons, the final decision should be tailored individually to each patient (*Figure 36.5*).

The clinical management of PCNs proposed by the authors is displayed in *Figure 36.6* (20,45). Cyst-related jaundice, vascularized mural nodules or solid components, and malignant cytology are absolute, standalone indications for surgery in all fit patients. Surgery is also recommended for patients showing an MPD dilation greater than 1 cm, but only if the high suspicion of MD- or MT-IPMN is confirmed by EUS (differential diagnoses are MPD-obstruction or chronic pancreatitis). Other features represent relative indications for surgery including a progressively increasing MPD dilation or an MPD between 5–9 mm, recurrent acute pancreatitis, cyst size ≥30 mm or rapid growth rate (>2.5 mm/year), thick vascularized cyst walls, and increased serum levels of CA19.9. Patients with such concerning features but no absolute indications should undergo adequate

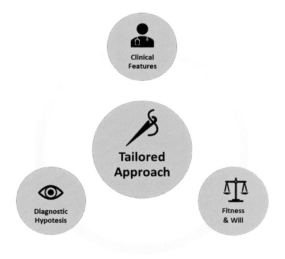

Figure 36.5 A tailored approach for PCN management.

counselling and CE-EUS. If the finding is not confirmed endoscopically, patients should undergo close surveillance with MRI and MRCP, oncological markers and/or CE-EUS when considered appropriate. The worsening of a single parameter or the appearance of a second suspect feature are strong criteria for reconsidering a surgical approach during surveillance (40). In cases of suspected IPMNs, MCNs, and SPTs, surgical resection should always aim to achieve complete tumour removal together with appropriate lymphadenectomy. Intraoperative frozen sections should be evaluated to achieve negative resection margins. If 'free margins' can be achieved from the frozen section, an acceptable risk of recurrence and related death seems preferable to the morbidity and mortality of a total pancreatectomy. Since PCNs that are surgically resected are presumed to be malignant, parenchyma sparing pancreatectomy does not represent a safe procedure and should be avoided.

SURVEILLANCE

As retrospective surgical series represented the historic backbone of scientific literature regarding PCNs, an important selection bias has probably led to an overestimation of IPMNs potential for malignant transformation. In recent years, large observational series of IPMNs undergoing surveillance became available, defining a 'new era' of evidence shedding new light on IPMNs biology and natural history (6–9,46,47). Most of these studies considered long-term surveillance as safe

for BD-IPM without WF or HRS. However, despite a decrease in the presumed overall malignancy risk, discontinuation of surveillance cannot be recommended in general based on current evidence. After 5 years of follow-up, patients with cystic lesions of the pancreas are still at risk for cyst growth, cross-over to operation, and the development of malignancy. This is also true for patients who were stable at the 5-year time point. However, the cost of surveilling thousands of patients is a significant burden for healthcare systems and safe discontinuation of surveillance for presumed BD-IPMN represents an urgent issue that needs to be resolved. It is still not clear yet which cases to select for follow-up cessation without introducing a significative risk of these patients developing a malignancy. The identification of an ideal target for follow-up discontinuation has been introduced with the concept of 'trivial' IPMNs (39). Trivial IPMNs are defined as presumed BD-IPMNs not developing WF or HRS for at least 5 years from the baseline observation. The incidence of pancreatic cancer in trivial BD-IPMNs is as low as 1–6%, in line with the general population and similar to the postoperative mortality following pancreatic surgery in high-volume centers. This study suggested that patients older than 65 with trivial BD-IPMNs may represent a potential target for surveillance discontinuation. To-date, several follow-up schedules have been proposed, but none of them have emerged and been unequivocally accepted as the most cost effective. In the absence of suspicious features (*Figure 36.6*), the authors usually recommend follow-up with MRI/MRCP and oncological markers every 6

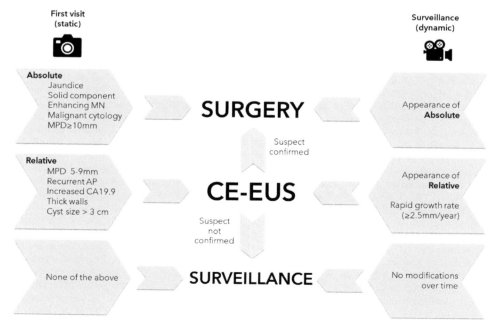

Figure 36.6 The clinical management of PCNs at Verona University Hospital.

months for the first year. In the absence of progression, follow-up with MRI/MRCP and serum markers at 12 or 18 months is maintained until the patient is no longer a surgical candidate.

REFERENCES

1. Moris M, Bridges MD, Pooley RA, Raimondo M, Woodward TA, Stauffer JA, et al. Association between advances in high-resolution cross-section imaging technologies and increase in prevalence of pancreatic cysts from 2005 to 2014. *Clin Gastroenterol Hepatol* 2016;**14**:585–93.e3.
2. Chang YR, Park JK, Jang J-Y, Kwon W, Yoon JH, Kim S-W.. Incidental pancreatic cystic neoplasms in an asymptomatic healthy population of 21,745 individuals. *Medicine (Baltimore)* 2016;**95(51)**:e5535.
3. Sugiyama M, Suzuki Y. Natural History of IPMN: Adenoma–Carcinoma Sequence in IPMN. In: Beger HG, Nakao A, Neoptolemos JP, Peng SY, Sarr MG (eds). *Pancreatic Cancer, Cystic Neoplasms and Endocrine Tumors.* Chichester: John Wiley & Sons, Ltd; 2015, Chapter 30, pp. 225–8.
4. Tanaka M. Intraductal papillary mucinous neoplasm of the pancreas as the main focus for early detection of pancreatic adenocarcinoma. *Pancreas* 2018;**47**:544–50.
5. Konings ICAW, Canto MI, Almario JA, Harinck F, Saxena P, Lucas AL, et al. Surveillance for pancreatic cancer in high-risk individuals. *BJS Open* 2019;**3**:656–65.
6. Pergolini I, Sahora K, Ferrone CR, Morales-Oyarvide V, Wolpin BM, Mucci LA, et al. Long term risk of pancreatic malignancy in patients with branch duct intraductal papillary mucinous neoplasm in a referral center. *Gastroenterology* 2017;**153**:1284–94.e1.
7. Lawrence SA, Attiyeh MA, Seier K, Gönen M, Schattner M, Haviland DL, et al. Should patients with cystic lesions of the pancreas undergo long-term radiographic surveillance? Results of 3024 patients evaluated at a single institution. *Ann Surg* 2017;**266**:536–44.
8. Crippa S, Pezzilli R, Bissolati M, Capurso G, Romano L, Brunori MP, et al. Active surveillance beyond 5 years is required for presumed branch-duct intraductal papillary mucinous neoplasms undergoing non-operative management. *Am J Gastroenterol* 2017;**112**:1153–61.
9. Han Y, Lee H, Kang JS, Kim JR, Kim HS, Lee JM,et al. Progression of pancreatic branch duct intraductal papillary mucinous neoplasm associates with cyst size. *Gastroenterology* 2018;**154**:576–84.
10. Board WC of TE. *Digestive System Tumours*, 5th edition. WHO, Geneva: IARC Publications, 2019.
11. Karoumpalis I, Christodoulou DK. Cystic lesions of the pancreas. *Ann Gastroenterol* 2016;**29**:155–61.
12. Stark A, Donahue TR, Reber HA, Hines OJ. Pancreatic cyst disease: A review. *JAMA* 2016;**315**:1882–93.
13. Reid MD, Choi H-J, Memis B, Krasinskas AM, Jang K-T, Akkas G, et al. Serous neoplasms of the pancreas: A clinicopathologic analysis of 193 cases and literature review with new insights on macrocystic and solid variants and critical reappraisal of so-called "Serous Cystadenocarcinoma." *Am J Surg Pathol* 2015;**39**:1597–610.
14. Marchegiani G, Caravati A, Andrianello S, Pollini T, Bernardi G, Biancotto M, et al. Serous cystic neoplasms of the pancreas management in the real-world: Still operating on a benign entity. *Ann Surg* 2022;**276(6)**:e868–75.
15. Nilsson LN, Keane MG, Shamali A, Bocos JM, van Zanten MM, Antila A, et al. Nature and management of pancreatic mucinous cystic neoplasm (MCN): A systematic review of the literature. *Pancreatology* 2016;**16**:1028–36.
16. Park JW, Jang J-Y, Kang MJ, Kwon W, Chang YR, Kim S-W, et al. Mucinous cystic neoplasm of the pancreas: Is surgical resection recommended for all surgically fit patients? *Pancreatology* 2014;**14**:31–6.
17. Crippa S, Salvia R, Warshaw AL, Domínguez I, Bassi C, Falconi M, et al. Mucinous cystic neoplasm of the pancreas is not an aggressive entity: Lessons from 163 resected patients. *Ann Surg* 2008;**247**:571–79.
18. Keane MG, Shamali A, Nilsson LN, Antila A, Bocos JM, van Zanten MM, et al. Risk of malignancy in resected pancreatic mucinous cystic neoplasms. *Br J Surg* 2018;**105**:439–46.
19. Marchegiani G, Andrianello S, Crippa S, Pollini T, Belfiori G, Gozzini L, et al. Actual malignancy risk of either operated or non-operated presumed mucinous cystic neoplasms of the pancreas under surveillance. *Br J Surg* 2021;**108(9)**:1097–104.
20. Perri G, Marchegiani G, Frigerio I, Dervenis CG, Conlon KC, Bassi C, et al. Management of pancreatic cystic lesions. *Dig Surg* 2020;**37**:1–9.
21. Marchegiani G, Andrianello S, Miatello C, Pollini T, Secchettin E, Tedesco G, et al. The actual prevalence of symptoms in pancreatic cystic neoplasms: A prospective propensity matched cohort analysis. *Dig Surg* 2019;**36**:522–9.
22. Sahora K, Castillo CF, Dong F, Marchegiani G, Thayer SP, Ferrone CR, et al. Not all mixed type intraductal papillary mucinous neoplasms behave like main-duct lesions: Implications of minimal involvement of the main pancreatic duct. *Surgery* 2014;**156**:611–21.
23. Sahora K, Mino-Kenudson M, Brugge W, Thayer SP, Ferrone CR, Sahani D, et al. Branch duct intraductal papillary mucinous neoplasms: Does cyst size change the tip of the scale? A critical analysis of the Revised International Consensus Guidelines in a large single-institutional series. *Ann Surg* 2013;**258**:466–75.
24. Adsay V, Mino-Kenudson M, Furukawa T, Basturk O, Zamboni G, Marchegiani G, et al. Pathologic evaluation and reporting of intraductal papillary mucinous neoplasms of the pancreas and other tumoral intraepithelial neoplasms of pancreatobiliary tract: Recommendations of Verona Consensus Meeting. *Ann Surg* 2016;**263**:162–77.
25. Furukawa T, Hatori T, Fujita I, Yamamoto M, Kobayashi M, Ohike N, et al. Prognostic relevance of morphological types of intraductal papillary mucinous neoplasms of the pancreas. *Gut* 2011; **60**:509–16.
26. Distler M, Kersting S, Niedergethmann M, Aust DE, Franz M, Rückert F, et al. Pathohistological subtype predicts survival in patients with intraductal papillary mucinous neoplasm (IPMN) of the pancreas. *Ann Surg* 2013;**258**:324–30.

27. Basturk O, Tan M, Bhanot U, Allen P, Adsay NV, Scott SN, et al. The oncocytic subtype is genetically distinct from other pancreatic intraductal papillary mucinous neoplasm subtypes. *Mod Pathol* 2016; **29**:1058–69.

28. Basturk O, Hong S-M, Wood LD, Adsay NV, Albores-Saavedra J, Biankin AV, et al. A revised classification system and recommendations from the Baltimore Consensus Meeting for Neoplastic Precursor Lesions in the Pancreas. *Am J Surg Pathol* 2015;**39**:1730–41.

29. Mino-Kenudson M, Castillo CF, Baba Y, Valsangkar NP, Liss AS, Hsu M, et al. Prognosis of invasive intraductal papillary mucinous neoplasm depends on histological and precursor epithelial subtypes. *Gut* 2011;**60**:1712–20.

30. Tanaka M, Fernández-Del Castillo C, Kamisawa T, Jang JY, Levy P, Ohtsuka T, et al. Revisions of international consensus Fukuoka guidelines for the management of IPMN of the pancreas. *Pancreatology* 2017;**17**:738–53.

31. European Study Group on Cystic Tumours of the Pancreas. European evidence-based guidelines on pancreatic cystic neoplasms. *Gut* 2018;**67**:789–804.

32. Vege SS, Ziring B, Jain R, Moayyedi P, Clinical Guidelines Committee, American Gastroenterology Association. American Gastroenterological Association Institute guideline on the diagnosis and management of asymptomatic neoplastic pancreatic cysts. *Gastroenterology* 2015;**148**:819–22;quize12–13.

33. Marchegiani G, Salvia R. Guidelines on pancreatic cystic neoplasms: Major inconsistencies with available evidence and clinical practice: Results From an international survey. *Gastroenterology* 2021;**160(7)**:2234–38.

34. Marchegiani G, Andrianello S, Borin A, Borgo CD, Perri G, Pollini T, et al. Systematic review, meta-analysis, and a high-volume center experience supporting the new role of mural nodules proposed by the updated 2017 international guidelines on IPMN of the pancreas. *Surgery* 2018;**163**:1272–79.

35. Crippa S, Bassi C, Salvia R, Malleo G, Marchegiani G, Rebours V, et al. Low progression of intraductal papillary mucinous neoplasms with worrisome features and high-risk stigmata undergoing non-operative management: A mid-term follow-up analysis. *Gut* 2017;**66**:495–506.

36. Marchegiani G, Andrianello S, Morbin G, Secchettin E, D'Onofrio M, De Robertis R, et al. Importance of main pancreatic duct dilatation in IPMN undergoing surveillance. *Br J Surg* 2018;**105**:1825–34.

37. Dal Borgo C, Perri G, Borin A, Marchegiani G, Salvia R, Bassi C, et al. The clinical management of main duct intraductal papillary mucinous neoplasm of the pancreas. *Dig Surg* 2019;**36**:104–10.

38. Crippa S, Pergolini I, Rubini C, Castelli P, Partelli S, Zardini C, et al. Risk of misdiagnosis and overtreatment in patients with main pancreatic duct dilatation and suspected combined/main-duct intraductal papillary mucinous neoplasms. *Surgery* 2016;**159**:1041–9.

39. Marchegiani G, Andrianello S, Pollini T, Caravati A, Biancotto M, Secchettin E, et al. 'Trivial' cysts redefine the risk of cancer in presumed branch-duct intraductal papillary mucinous neoplasms of the pancreas: A potential target for follow-Up discontinuation? *Am J Gastroenterol* 2019;**114**:1678–84.

40. Marchegiani G, Pollini T, Andrianello S, Tomasoni G, Biancotto M, Javed AA, et al. Progression vs cyst stability of branch-duct intraductal papillary mucinous neoplasms after observation and surgery. *JAMA Surg* 2021;**156(7)**:654–61.

41. van Rijssen LB, Koerkamp BG, Zwart MJ, Bonsing BA, Bosscha K, van Dam RM, et al. Nationwide prospective audit of pancreatic surgery: Design, accuracy, and outcomes of the Dutch Pancreatic Cancer Audit. *HPB (Oxford)* 2017;**19**:919–26.

42. McMillan MT, Allegrini V, Asbun HJ, Ball CG, Bassi C, Beane JD, et al. Incorporation of procedure-specific risk into the ACS NSQIP surgical risk calculator improves the prediction of morbidity and mortality after pancreatoduodenectomy. *Ann Surg* 2017;**265**:978–86.

43. de Wilde RF, Besselink MGH, van der Tweel I, de Hingh IHJT, van Eijack CHJ, Dejong CHC, et al. Impact of nationwide centralization of pancreaticoduodenectomy on hospital mortality. *Br J Surg* 2012;**99**:404–10.

44. Vollmer CM, Sanchez N, Gondek S, McAuliffe J, Kent TS, Christein JD, et al. A root cause analysis of mortality following major pancreatectomy. *J Gastrointest Surg* 2012;**16**:89–102; discussion 102–3.

45. Pollini T, Andrianello S, Caravati A, Perri G, Malleo G, Paiella S, et al. The management of intraductal papillary mucinous neoplasms of the pancreas. *Minerva Chir* 2019;**74**:414–21.

46. Del Chiaro M, Ateeb Z, Hansson MR, Rangelova E, Segersvärd R, Kartalis N, et al. Survival analysis and risk for progression of intraductal papillary mucinous neoplasia of the pancreas (IPMN) under surveillance: A single-institution experience. *Ann Surg Oncol* 2017;**24**:1120–26.

47. Ohno E, Hirooka Y, Kawashima H, Ishikawa T, Kanamori A, Ishikawa H,et al. Natural history of pancreatic cystic lesions: A multicenter prospective observational study for evaluating the risk of pancreatic cancer. *J Gastroenterol Hepatol* 2018;**33**:320–28.

Bailey & Love's Essential Operations Bailey & Love's Essential Operatic
Bailey & Love's Essential Operations Bailey & Love's Essential Operatic
Bailey & Love's Essential Operations Bailey & Love's Essential Operatic
SECTION 6 | PANCREAS

Chapter
37

Pancreatic Ductal Stones

Zaheer Nabi and D. Nageshwar Reddy

INTRODUCTION

Chronic pancreatitis (CP) is an inflammatory process characterized by irreversible morphological changes in the pancreas (1). In patients with CP, pancreatic calcifications develop in almost half of the cases at 5 years and the majority of cases within 14 years of onset of the disease (2). The most common symptom in CP is pain which is experienced by the majority of patients during the course of the disease. Pancreatic ductal stones (PDS) lead to obstruction of the pancreatic duct and intraductal hypertension which is one of the major hypotheses proposed for the generation of pain in these cases. Consequently, ductal decompression via endotherapy or surgery have been the mainstays of treatment in cases with symptomatic PDS although the pathogenesis of pain in chronic pancreatitis is complex and not simply due to raised intraductal pressure. The multifactorial nature of the pain also explains the lack of response, in a proportion of cases, irrespective of the treatment modality used.

PATHOGENESIS

The pathogenesis of PDS is not well understood. One of the proposed theories states that the inciting event is the formation of a 'protein plug' composed of pancreatic stone protein, or other proteins such as GP2 (3). Increased secretion of protein, without a concomitant increase in fluid and bicarbonate along with partial proteolysis, results in its precipitation.

This 'plug', in turn, acts as a nidus for the deposition of calcium carbonate over the 'protein plug' resulting in the formation of PDS. Of note, pancreatic stone protein known as lithostathine prevents the precipitation of calcium under normal conditions (4). Low levels of lithostathine, in cases with chronic pancreatitis, may be the trigger leading to the precipitation of calcium (3).

Although the majority of PDS are radiopaque, a minority may be radiolucent and they are classified according to the type (radiopaque or radiolucent), location (main duct, side branches or parenchyma), size (small <5 mm or large) and number (single or multiple). The characterization of PDS influences the choice of therapy and the management strategy.

DIAGNOSIS

The diagnosis of chronic pancreatitis with PDS is established by clinical symptoms and imaging. Clinical symptoms are not only restricted to pancreatic-type pain but may include those related to exocrine and endocrine insufficiency associated with chronic pancreatitis. Patients may also exhibit signs and symptoms related to deficiencies of fat-soluble vitamins and micronutrients.

Imaging modalities for the evaluation of PDS include plain x-ray of the abdomen, transabdominal ultrasound, endoscopic ultrasound (EUS), computed tomography (CT) and magnetic resonance imaging (MRI) with cholangiopancreatography (MRCP).

Contrast-enhanced CT (CECT) is the preferred, initial modality, in cases with chronic pancreatitis (*Figure 37.1*).

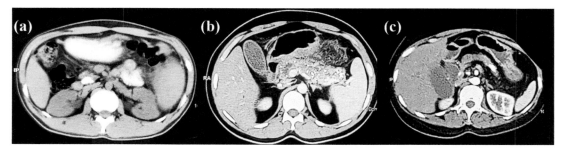

Figure 37.1 CT images in three cases with pancreatic ductal stones. CT image (a) revealing a large intraductal calculus in the head of pancreas (suitable for endoscopic treatment). CT image (b) revealing intraductal and parenchymal calculi in head, body and tail of pancreas (not suitable for endoscopic treatment). CT image (c) revealing large intraductal calculus in the tail of pancreas (not suitable for endoscopic treatment).

DOI: 10.1201/9781003080060-37

MRCP is superior in defining the pancreatic duct (PD) anatomy (5). As the information provided by CT and MRCP is complimentary in delineating pancreatic calcifications and defining pancreatic ductal anatomy, both modalities will usually be required. EUS is usually reserved for cases where the diagnosis of chronic pancreatitis is in question, or a co-existing mass lesion needs to be biopsied for histopathological examination to exclude malignancy. In addition to establishing the diagnosis, information provided by cross-sectional imaging is essential to guide further management. Important observations will include the diameter of the PD, the presence and distribution of PDS and PD strictures, the density of stones, the presence of a mass in the head of the gland and complications associated with chronic pancreatitis such as pseudocysts, biliary strictures and pancreatic ductal leaks.

MANAGEMENT

Overview

The management of chronic pancreatitis with PDS requires a multidisciplinary and multifaceted approach which should not only address the patient's pain, but also exocrine and endocrine insufficiencies, as well as nutritional deficiencies and lifestyle modifications such as alcohol and smoking cessation (*Table 37.1*). The

involvement of gastrointestinal (GI) physicians, radiologists, GI surgeons and nutritionists is essential for the successful management of CP with PDS.

The non-surgical treatment modalities for PDS include endoscopic retrograde pancreatography (ERP), extracorporeal shockwave lithotripsy (ESWL) and per-oral pancreatoscopy (POP)-guided intraductal lithotripsy. It is important to note that intervention (endoscopic or surgical) is indicated only in symptomatic cases with PDS. Although ductal interventions may delay the development of diabetes in cases with PDS, endotherapy and surgery are not recommended exclusively for these indications due to the lack of a strong evidence base (6). Endotherapy will provide short-term relief in the majority of cases and long-term relief in about two thirds of cases with chronic obstructive pancreatitis (7). Endoscopic treatment is therefore initially preferred over surgery as the treatment modality in suitable cases with PDS. Nevertheless, the choice of treatment, endoscopic or surgical, is based on multiple factors: stone burden; the distribution of the stones along the pancreatic duct; associated complications including pseudocysts or biliary strictures; available expertise, and patient preference. Endotherapy may not be suitable in cases with diffuse stone burden, such as those with PDS extending the whole length of the pancreatic duct or where there are multifocal strictures. These cases are best managed surgically.

Table 37.1 Treatment options in chronic pancreatitis with pancreatic ductal stones

Treatment options	Indications	Comment
General		
Enzyme replacement Nutritional therapy Lifestyle interventions	Indicated in all	Endocrine and exocrine insufficiency should be managed; cessation of smoking and alcohol
Endoscopic		
ERP	Small calculi (<5 mm)	Modest success rate, not suitable in large and impacted calculi
ESWL	Large calculi localized to head and body	First-line treatment in suitable candidates with PDS
Intraductal lithotripsy Laser lithotripsy Electrohydraulic lithotripsy	ESWL not available or failed	Performed under per-oral pancreatoscopy guidance, technical expertise required, limited data
Surgery		
Resection Drainage Combined	Unsuitable for endotherapy, failed endotherapy	Early surgery may be preferred in non-responders to endotherapy

Abbreviations: ERP: endoscopic retrograde pancreatography; ESWL: extracorporeal shock wave lithotripsy.

ENDOSCOPIC TREATMENT

Endoscopic retrograde pancreatography

Endoscopic retrograde pancreatography (ERP) is an excellent diagnostic and therapeutic modality in cases with PDS. Non-invasive imaging modalities including CECT and MRI produce high-quality images which guide the choice of therapeutic techniques and management. As a therapeutic tool, ERP alone may be successful in cases with PDS < 5 mm (1) and in these cases, extraction of PDS is accomplished with the help of a balloon or basket during ERP. Prior to extraction of PDS, endoscopic pancreatic sphincterotomy is performed to facilitate their removal and if the duct can be successfully cleared a PD stent is not usually required except in cases with a pre-existing stricture. The main limitation of ERP is that it is relatively ineffective in the removal of large or impacted calculi and those with an upstream PD stricture. Mechanical lithotripsy, useful in large biliary calculi, is avoided in cases where there are large PDS due to the high risk of complications, including a trapped basket, attributed mainly to a tortuous PD configuration (8). These cases are best managed with ESWL which allows fragmentation of the calculi.

Lithotripsy (ESWL and intraductal)

The main modalities available for fragmentation of PDS include ESWL and intraductal lithotripsy systems. ESWL was initially utilized in the early 1980s for the fragmentation of renal calculi. It was adapted in the early 1990s for the management of biliary and pancreatic ductal stones (9–12). Over the last 30 years, the role

for ESWL has been established for the treatment of PDS over 5 mm in size. The subsequent sections discuss the principle, technique, outcomes and adverse events associated with ESWL.

Principles and technique of ESWL

Lithotripters generate shock waves by one of several different methods, including spark discharge, piezoelectric systems, and electromagnetic deflection depending on the type of system being used. Lithotripters equipped with an electromagnetic shock wave generator release electromagnetic energy in an enclosed space such as the PD which results in the generation of shock waves (13). These shock waves generate compressive stresses on the outer surface of PDS resulting in their fragmentation. After initial fragmentation, the shock waves pass through the stones and get reflected from the posterior surface resulting in further fragmentation (14). The localization of the stones is achieved using the fluoroscopy or ultrasound function available with the lithotripters. In a small number of cases with radiolucent PDS, a nasopancreatic tube is placed endoscopically prior to ESWL to facilitate the targeting of stones.

During ESWL, up to 5 000 to 6 000 shocks are delivered per session with an intensity of 15 to 16 kV at a frequency of 90 shocks per minute (14). Larger and multiple PDS may require multiple sessions of ESWL to achieve the required fragmentation. ESWL can be performed under epidural anaesthesia, intravenous sedation or general anaesthesia, depending on the operator's preference (14). The goal of ESWL is to fragment PDS to less than 2–3 mm in size which can be confirmed by a decrease in the radiographical density of the stones or heterogenous appearance on x-ray (*Figure 37.2*) (14).

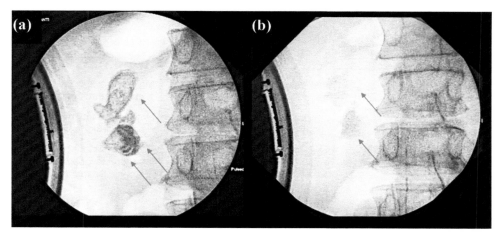

Figure 37.2 Fluoroscopy images before and after ESWL in a case with pancreatic ductal stones. Pre-ESWL image (a) revealing large, dense, and radiopaque calculi towards the right of spine. Post-ESWL image (b) in the same case revealing heterogenous appearance of the stone with reduced radiographical density suggesting adequate fragmentation.

Outcomes

Successful fragmentation can be achieved in 70–100% of patients with PDS (*Table 37.2*). Although effective fragmentation of PDS is attained in the majority of cases, complete ductal clearance is achieved in only 50–75% of cases. It is important to note that complete clearance of the PD may not be required for pain relief (15). Partial and complete pain relief with ESWL has been reported in 70–95% and 50–80%, respectively, at a mean follow-up ranging from 6–77 months (1,16–24). After successful fragmentation of PDS, ERP may be performed to clear residual fragments and place one or more PD stents in those with a co-existent PD stricture. However, the decision to perform ERP subsequent to ESWL should be individualized as the outcomes have not been found to be superior to ESWL alone (23–25).

The predictive factors suggesting good outcomes after ESWL, include short disease duration, limited stone burden, PDS localized to the head or body, the absence of a PD stricture, and cessation of alcohol and smoking (2). Besides these factors, lower stone density (<820.5 or <1000.45 Hounsefield units) on non-contrast CT has also been found to be associated with better outcomes (20,26).

Adverse events

ESWL is a safe procedure and major adverse events are uncommon. In a large series of 634 patients having 1470 ESWL procedures, adverse events were reported in 6.7% of cases including moderate to severe adverse events in only 1.1% of cases (27). Reported adverse events include post-ESWL pancreatitis (4.4%), infection (1.4%), steinstrasse, literally meaning 'stone street' or 'street of stones' coined by the German pioneers of lithotripsy (0.4%), perforation (0.3%), bleeding (0.3%), and pancreatic fistulae (0.1%) (27). The risk factors for complications, after ESWL, include pancreas divisum, and length of the interval between diagnosis of chronic pancreatitis and ESWL (27). Contraindications for ESWL include coagulopathies, pregnancy, the presence of bone, calcified aneurysm and lung tissue in the path of ESWL but ESWL can be safely performed in cases with a co-existing pseudocyst (22).

Table 37.2 Outcomes of ESWL in patients with chronic calcific pancreatitis[1]

Study, year	N	Stone location	ERCP	Complete fragmentation (ductal clearance)	Pain relief: Overall (complete relief)	Follow-up
Inui et al. 2005 (16)	555	NR	42.7%	92.4% (72.6%)	91.1% (NR)	44.3 months (3–141)
Tadenuma et al. 2005 (17)	117	Head (85.5%), body-tail (14.5%)	55.6%	96.6%	68.2% (NR)	77.5±30.9 months
Seven et al. 2012 (18)	120	Head (66.7%), head-body (1.6%), body (2.5%), head-body-tail (29.2%)	100%	NR	85% (50%)	4.3±3.7 years
Suzuki et al. 2013 (19)	479	NR	53.2%	92.1% (74.3%)	90.8% (NR)	31.4 months (1–83)
Ohyama et al. 2015 (20)	128	Head (76.6%), body-tail (23.4%)	100%	NR (51.6%)	89.9% (NR)	42.4± 35.8 months
Hu et al. 2016 (21)	214	Head (75.7%), head-body (6.1%), body (2.3%), head-body-tail (15.9%)	96.7%	100% (72.4%)	95.4% (71.3%)	18.5±3.3 months
Li et al. 2016 (22)	849 (PC 59)	Head (23.7%), head+other location (72.3%), tail (3.4%)	PC group: 98.3%	PC group: 100% (67.2%)	89.1% (63.6%)	21.9 months (12–45.1)
Vaysse et al. 2016 (23)	146	NR	73.5%	NR (56.8%)	NR	23 months (6–90)
Tandan et al. 2019 (24)	5124	Head (55.1%), body (21.4%), tail (7.4%), diffuse (15.9%)	EPS 98% PD stent 69%	72.6%	94.5% (82.6%)	6 months

Abbreviations: EPS: extrapyramidal side effects; NR: not reported; PC: pseudocyst; PD: pancreatic duct.

[1] Reprinted with permission from (1).

Intraductal lithotripsy

ESWL is the mainstay of treatment in suitable candidates with intraductal pancreatic calculi but more recently, per-oral pancreatoscopy (POP)-guided intraductal lithotripsy has emerged as a safe and effective alternative to ESWL for the fragmentation of PDS (28–30). Intraductal lithotripsy involves the fragmentation of PDS with electrohydraulic lithotripsy (EHL) or laser lithotripsy (LL) under the guidance of POP. During intraductal lithotripsy, a POP catheter is introduced, through the working channel of the standard ERP scopes, for cannulation of the pancreatic duct and targeted fragmentation of PDS under direct vision. The current generation POPs (Spyglass Direct Visualization System, Boston Scientific Corp, Natick, MA, USA), provide superior image quality compared with the older fiberoptic cholangioscopy systems, and consequently, the utilisation of intraductal lithotripsy has increased in recent years.

With POP-guided lithotripsy, adequate fragmentation of intraductal calculi and subsequent pain relief can be expected in about three quarters of patients (28–31). In a systematic review, technical and clinical success with intraductal lithotripsy (EHL or LL) was achieved in 76.4% (95% CI: 65.9–84.5) and 76.8% (95% CI: 65.2–85.4) of cases, respectively (32). Both EHL and LL appear comparable with regards to technical success, fragmentation rates and single session duct clearance (33). Major adverse events are uncommon with intraductal lithotripsy, and in one systematic review the pooled rate of adverse events was 14.9% (95% CI: 9.2–23.2), with no significant difference between EHL and LL (11.2% vs. 13.1%) (32).

Post-ERCP pancreatitis is the most commonly reported adverse event (7%), followed by abdominal pain (4.7%), fever (3.7%), perforation (4.3%), and hemorrhage (3.4%) (32).

The advantages of intraductal lithotripsy over ESWL include the fragmentation of PDS under direct vision, potentially reducing the chances of PD injury and the documentation of ductal clearance at the completion of the treatment. Significant issues include the additional cost and technical difficulty if there is a very tortuous PD. Intraductal lithotripsy is not suitable in cases with PDS proximal to a PD stricture, and in those with minimally dilated PD as the insertion of pancreatoscope may not be possible.

Intraductal lithotripsy may be considered in cases where ESWL is not available or adequate fragmentation is not achieved using ESWL. It is important to acknowledge the limitations of the data available regarding the safety and efficacy of intraductal lithotripsy. There is no randomized trial comparing ESWL with intraductal lithotripsy and the choice of modality for the fragmentation of PDS should be based on the available expertise and equipment.

ENDOTHERAPY VERSUS SURGERY

Endotherapy and surgery are the two major modalities utilized for the management of chronic pancreatitis with PDS. Several randomized trials have compared these approaches and demonstrated the superiority of surgery with regards to pain relief (*Table 37.3*) (34–37). In these trials, complete pain relief with endotherapy and surgery was achieved in 14–39% and 37–80%

Table 37.3 Endoscopic treatment versus surgery in chronic pancreatitis[¶]

	Study design	n	Intervention	Mean pain score (Izbicki)	Pain relief (%)	Follow-up
Dite 2003 (35)	RCT	72	E: stenting, stone removal S: resection (80%), drainage (20%)	NR	37% versus 14%	5 years
Cahen 2007 (34)	RCT	39	E: ESWL ± PD stenting, stricture dilatation S: drainage	25 versus 51	75% versus 32%	24 months
Cahen 2011 (36)	RCT	39*	Same as above	22 versus 39	80% versus 38%	79 months
Jiang 2018 (38)	R	86	E: ESWL ± ERCP S: Drainage	NR	82.6% versus 80%	65 ± 13.6 months
Issa 2020 (37)	RCT	88	E: ESWL, PD stenting, stricture dilatation S: resection or drainage procedures	37 versus 49	58% versus 39%	18 months

Abbreviations: RCT: randomized controlled trial; R: retrospective; E: endoscopy; S: surgery; PD: pancreatic duct; ESWL: extracorporeal shock wave lithotripsy; NR: not reported.

* 31 patients were available for long-term follow-up (endoscopy: 16, surgery: 15).

¶ Reprinted with permission from (1).

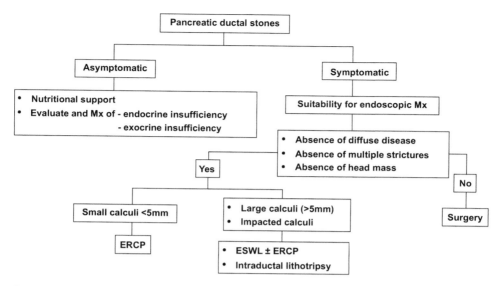

Figure 37.3 Algorithmic, decision-making approach to treatment options for PDS.

of patients, respectively. There has been criticism of these data for improper randomization, suboptimal treatment in the endotherapy arm (without ESWL) and inclusion of opiate dependent patients (35). In the most recent randomized trial, the ESCAPE trial, early surgery within 6 weeks was superior to endoscopy as a first approach and resulted in lower pain scores when integrated over 18 months (37). Of note, the majority of patients had combined stones and PD strictures which may have affected the ductal clearance in these cases and a number of patients in the endotherapy group did not receive optimum endoscopic treatment including no ESWL for large PDS or sequential stenting in those with PD strictures. Pain relief was better and equivalent to surgery in those with complete ductal clearance in this trial.

The management of CP with PDS must be individualized and based on the suitability for endotherapy, the patient's preferences and the available expertise (*Figure 37.3*). In properly selected cases, endotherapy is a relatively minimally invasive treatment option but early surgery is the treatment of choice in non-responders and those unsuitable for endotherapy (38).

SUMMARY

Pancreatic ductal stones (PDS) are a common feature of chronic pancreatitis. Pain is the main presenting feature in the vast majority and results from intraductal hypertension related to obstruction by the intraductal calculi. The management of chronic calcific pancreatitis requires a multidisciplinary approach involving physicians, surgeons and nutrition experts, and endoscopic or surgical treatment is indicated in cases with

painful disease or complications. Endotherapy is the preferred initial modality due to its minimally invasive nature, and satisfactory outcomes are achieved in the majority of cases. The main modalities for PDS are ERP-, ESWL- and POP-assisted lithotripsy. With recent advances in therapeutic endoscopy, a large proportion of cases with PDS can be managed without surgery but endotherapy may not be suitable for all the cases with PDS. It should be emphasized that a proportion of cases will not respond, despite optimal endotherapy and complete ductal clearance supporting the multifactorial pathogenesis of pain in chronic pancreatitis.

Poor candidates for endotherapy include those with diffuse intraductal stones throughout the head, body and tail, or those with isolated calculi in the tail of the pancreas. Endoscopic interventions include the clearance of intraductal stones using balloon or basket, and pancreatic ductal stenting for co-existing main duct strictures. Extracorporeal shock wave lithotripsy is recommended in cases with large or impacted intraductal calculi not amenable to endoscopic extraction. Intraductal lithotripsy (laser or electrohydraulic) is an emerging modality for fragmenting large intraductal calculi with encouraging results. Overall, endotherapy provides long-term pain relief in nearly two-thirds of the patients with PDS. Surgery can be performed either 'upfront' in cases not suitable for endotherapy or as a second-line option in those not responding to endoscopic interventions.

REFERENCES

1. Nabi Z, Lakhtakia S. Endoscopic management of chronic pancreatitis. *Dig Endosc* 2021;**33(7)**:1059–72.

2. Dumonceau JM, Delhaye M, Tringali A, Arvanitakis M, Sanchez-Yague A, Vaysse T, et al. Endoscopic treatment of chronic pancreatitis: European Society of Gastrointestinal Endoscopy (ESGE) Guideline – Updated August 2018. *Endoscopy* 2019;**51**:179–93.

3. Freedman SD. New concepts in understanding the pathophysiology of chronic pancreatitis. *Int J Pancreatol* 1998;**24**:1–8.

4. Multigner L, Sarles H, Lombardo D, De Caro A. Pancreatic stone protein. II. Implication in stone formation during the course of chronic calcifying pancreatitis. *Gastroenterology* 1985;**89**:387–91.

5. Anaizi A, Hart PA, Conwell DL. Diagnosing chronic pancreatitis. *Dig Dis Sci* 2017;**62**:1713–20.

6. Talukdar R, Reddy DN, Tandan M, Gupta R, Lakhtakia S, Ramchandani M, et al. Impact of ductal interventions on diabetes in patients with chronic pancreatitis. *J Gastroenterol Hepatol* 2021;**36**(5):1226–34.

7. Jafri M, Sachdev A, Sadiq J, Lee D, Taur T, Goodman A, et al. Efficacy of endotherapy in the treatment of pain associated with chronic pancreatitis: A systematic review and meta-analysis. *JOP* 2017;**18**:125–32.

8. Thomas M, Howell DA, Carr-Locke D, Wilcox CM, Chak A, Raijman I, et al. Mechanical lithotripsy of pancreatic and biliary stones: Complications and available treatment options collected from expert centers. *Am J Gastroenterol* 2007;**102**:1896–902.

9. Chaussy C, Schmiedt E, Jocham D, Brendel W, Forssmann B, Walther V, et al. First clinical experience with extracorporeally induced destruction of kidney stones by shock waves. *J Urol* 1982;**127**:417–20.

10. Kerzel W, Ell C, Schneider T, Matek W, Heyder N, Hahn EG, et al. Extracorporeal piezoelectric shockwave lithotripsy of multiple pancreatic duct stones under ultrasonographic control. *Endoscopy* 1989;**21**:229–31.

11. Sauerbruch T, Stern M. Fragmentation of bile duct stones by extracorporeal shock waves. A new approach to biliary calculi after failure of routine endoscopic measures. *Gastroenterology* 1989;**96**:146–52.

12. Neuhaus H. Fragmentation of pancreatic stones by extracorporeal shock wave lithotripsy. *Endoscopy* 1991;**23**:161–5.

13. Sharzehi K. Management of pancreatic duct stones. *Curr Gastroenterol Rep* 2019;21:63.

14. Tandan M, Talukdar R, Reddy DN. Management of pancreatic calculi: An update. *Gut Liver* 2016;**10**:873–80.

15. Issa Y, van Santvoort HC, van Goor H, Cahen DL, Bruno MJ, Boermeester MA, et al. Surgical and endoscopic treatment of pain in chronic pancreatitis: A multidisciplinary update. *Dig Surg* 2013;**30**:35–50.

16. Inui K, Tazuma S, Yamaguchi T, Ohara H, Tsuji T, Miyagawa H, et al. Treatment of pancreatic stones with extracorporeal shock wave lithotripsy: Results of a multicenter survey. *Pancreas* 2005;**30**:26–30.

17. Tadenuma H, Ishihara T, Yamaguchi T, Tsuchiya S, Kobayashi A, Nakamura K, et al. Long term results of extracorporeal shockwave lithotripsy and endoscopic therapy for pancreatic stones. *Clin Gastroenterol Hepatol* 2005;**3**:1128–35.

18. Seven G, Schreiner MA, Ross AS, Lin OS, Gluck M, Gan I, et al. Long-term outcomes associated with pancreatic extracorporeal shock wave lithotripsy for chronic calcific pancreatitis. *Gastrointest Endosc* 2012;**75**:997–1004.e1.

19. Suzuki Y, Sugiyama M, Inui K, Igarashi Y, Ohara H, Tazuma S, et al. Management for pancreatolithiasis: A Japanese multicenter study. *Pancreas* 2013;**42**:584–8.

20. Ohyama H, Mikata R, Ishihara T, Tsuyuguchi T, Sakai Y, Sugiyama H, et al. Efficacy of stone density on noncontrast computed tomography in predicting the outcome of extracorporeal shock wave lithotripsy for patients with pancreatic stones. *Pancreas* 2015;**44**:422–8.

21. Hu LH, Ye B, Yang YG, Ji J-T, Zou W-B, Du T-T, et al. Extracorporeal shock wave lithotripsy for Chinese patients with pancreatic stones: A prospective study of 214 Cases. *Pancreas* 2016;**45**:298–305.

22. Li BR, Liao Z, Du TT, Ye B, Chen H, Ji J-T, et al. Extracorporeal shock wave lithotripsy is a safe and effective treatment for pancreatic stones coexisting with pancreatic pseudocysts. *Gastrointest Endosc* 2016;**84**:69–78.

23. Vaysse T, Boytchev I, Antoni G, Sainte Croix D, Choury AD, Laurent V, et al. Efficacy and safety of extracorporeal shock wave lithotripsy for chronic pancreatitis. *Scand J Gastroenterol* 2016;**51**:1380–5.

24. Tandan M, Nageshwar Reddy D, Talukdar R, Vinod K, Kiran SVVS, Santosh D, et al. ESWL for large pancreatic calculi: Report of over 5000 patients. *Pancreatology* 2019;**19**:916–21.

25. Dumonceau JM, Costamagna G, Tringali A, Vahedi K, Delhaye M, Hittelet A, et al. Treatment for painful calcified chronic pancreatitis: Extracorporeal shock wave lithotripsy versus endoscopic treatment: A randomised controlled trial. *Gut* 2007;**56**:545–52.

26. Liu R, Su W, Gong J, Zhang Y, Lu J. Noncontrast computed tomography factors predictive of extracorporeal shock wave lithotripsy outcomes in patients with pancreatic duct stones. *Abdom Radiol (NY)* 2018;**43**:3367–73.

27. Li BR, Liao Z, Du TT, Ye B, Zou W-B, Chen H, et al. Risk factors for complications of pancreatic extracorporeal shock wave lithotripsy. *Endoscopy* 2014;**46**:1092–100.

28. Trikudanathan G, Freeman ML. Electrohydraulic lithotripsy of large pancreatic duct stones by using digital pancreatoscopy. *Gastrointest Endosc* 2016;**83**:1285-6.

29. Bekkali NL, Murray S, Johnson GJ, Bandula S, Amin Z, Chapman MH, et al. Pancreatoscopy-directed electrohydraulic lithotripsy for pancreatic ductal stones in painful chronic pancreatitis using SpyGlass. *Pancreas* 2017;**46**:528–30.

30. Gerges C, Pullmann D, Bahin F, Schneider M, Siersema PD, Neuhaus H, et al. SpyGlass DS-guided lithotripsy for pancreatic duct stones in symptomatic treatment-refractory chronic calcifying pancreatitis. *Endosc Int Open* 2019;**7**:E99–E103.

31. Attwell AR, Patel S, Kahaleh M, Raijman IL, Yen R, Shah RJ. ERCP with per-oral pancreatoscopy-guided laser lithotripsy for calcific chronic pan-

creatitis: A multicenter U.S. experience. *Gastrointest Endosc* 2015;**82**:311–18.

32. Saghir SM, Mashiana HS, Mohan BP, Dhindsa BS, Dhaliwal A, Chandan S, et al. Efficacy of pancreatoscopy for pancreatic duct stones: A systematic review and meta-analysis. *World J Gastroenterol* 2020;**26**:5207–19.

33. McCarty TR, Sobani Z, Rustagi T. Pancreatoscopy with intraductal lithotripsy for difficult pancreatic duct stones: A systematic review and meta-analysis. *Endosc Int Open* 2020;**8**:E1460–E1470.

34. Cahen DL, Gouma DJ, Nio Y, Rauws EAJ, Boermeester MA, Busch OR, et al. Endoscopic versus surgical drainage of the pancreatic duct in chronic pancreatitis. *N Engl J Med* 2007;**356**:676–84.

35. Dite P, Ruzicka M, Zboril V, Novotný I, et al. A prospective, randomized trial comparing endoscopic and surgical therapy for chronic pancreatitis. *Endoscopy* 2003;**35**:553–8.

36. Cahen DL, Gouma DJ, Laramee P, Nio Y, Rauws EAJ, Boermeester MA, et al. Long-term outcomes of endoscopic vs surgical drainage of the pancreatic duct in patients with chronic pancreatitis. *Gastroenterology* 2011;**141**:1690–5.

37. Issa Y, Kempeneers MA, Bruno MJ, Fockens P, Poley J-W, Ali UA, et al. Effect of early surgery vs endoscopy-first approach on pain in patients with chronic pancreatitis: The ESCAPE randomized clinical trial. *JAMA* 2020;**323**:237–47.

38. Jiang L, Ning D, Cheng Q, Chen X-P. Endoscopic versus surgical drainage treatment of calcific chronic pancreatitis. *Int J Surg* 2018;**54**:242–7.

Chapter 38
Intraductal Papillary Mucinous Neoplasms

Giuseppe Kito Fusai, Dimtri Aristotle Raptis and Camila Hidalgo Salinas

INTRODUCTION

Intraductal papillary mucinous neoplasms (IPMNs) of the pancreas are tumours of mucin-producing, columnar epithelial cells, that cause a grossly visible dilatation of the main- or branch-pancreatic ducts (1). As an entity, it received various names from an initial description in the early 1980s until the World Health Organization (WHO) unified the diagnosis as intraductal papillary mucinous tumour in 1996 (2–6) and classified it among neoplastic precursor lesions of the pancreas (7). In view of their prognosis and clinical management, premalignant lesions are currently classified into low-grade or high-grade IPMNs, and malignant lesions are termed IPMN with an associated invasive carcinoma (7), further removing them from the adenoma to carcinoma classification as they were once described (8).

PREVALENCE, CLINICAL PRESENTATION AND RISK FACTORS

Owing to the increased use of cross-sectional imaging, the incidental finding of pancreatic cystic lesions has revealed a high prevalence of IPMN in the general population (9,10). It is estimated that IPMNs make up between 20–50% of all pancreatic cystic lesions (11,12). While the incidence rises with increasing age (13), diagnosis is usually made from the fifth to seventh decades of life (14). Although IPMNs are most often diagnosed incidentally, some patients will present with recurrent pancreatitis, jaundice, weight loss, diarrhoea, new-onset diabetes mellitus, or non-specific symptoms (15,16). Most large series, report an equal distribution between men and women in the US and Europe, however, some have suggested a male preponderance in Asian populations (17–20). IPMNs are usually sporadic, but they can be associated with hereditary syndromes such as Peutz–Jeghers syndrome, McCune–Albright syndrome, and familial adenomatous polyposis (21–23). A family history of pancreatic cancer, previous history of diabetes, and cigarette smoking have all been suggested as predisposing factors (24–26).

MORPHOLOGY

IPMNs are primarily localized to the head of the pancreas, however they have been described as a process that involves the entire pancreatic ductal system (27,28). Not only have different series reported multifocality at the time of diagnosis in as many as 40% of cases (27,29,30), but the risk of synchronous and metachronous progression to the whole pancreas is also well documented (31,32). Morphologically, IPMNs are classified according to the anatomical involvement within the pancreatic ducts into main-duct, branch-duct, or mixed-duct IPMN, if both the main and branch ducts are involved (33,34). It is important for the patient to be fully assessed radiologically at the time of diagnosis, as this classification is an important predictor of outcome and plays a key role in the clinical management of IPMNs (35).

Main-duct IPMN is most commonly found in the head of the pancreas, but may also extend along the pancreatic body and tail (28). On imaging this is seen as a segmental main pancreatic duct dilatation, typically greater than 5 mm, or as a diffuse dilatation if it extends along the length of the pancreas (34) (*Figure 38.1a,b*). Endoscopically, an uncommon but pathognomonic sign of main duct IPMN is a bulging of the ampulla and mucus extrusion, the so-called 'fish mouth ampulla' sign. (12,28,36,37). Branch-duct IPMNs are usually found in the uncinate process and, while in continuity with the main pancreatic duct, they do not involve the main duct (*Figure 38.1c*). Radiologically, they are identified as segmental dilatations of side ducts, often multilocular, resembling a bunch of grapes (*Figure 38.1d*). Mixed-duct IPMNs are characterized by dilatations of both the main- and branch-ducts (*Figure 38.1e*). It is important to note that this is a radiological diagnosis and considerable discrepancy has been reported with subsequent histopathological analyses in patients that proceed to surgical resection (38).

PATHOLOGY

Microscopically, like other premalignant lesions of the pancreas, IPMNs are classified into low-grade and high-grade based on the highest degree of epithelial atypia (7). The previously labelled 'IPMN with intermediate-grade dysplasia' is now grouped together with low-grade IPMN (7,8). The presence of mild- to moderate-atypia, with or without mitosis, and papillary projections is categorized as low-grade IPMN. In

DOI: 10.1201/9781003080060-38

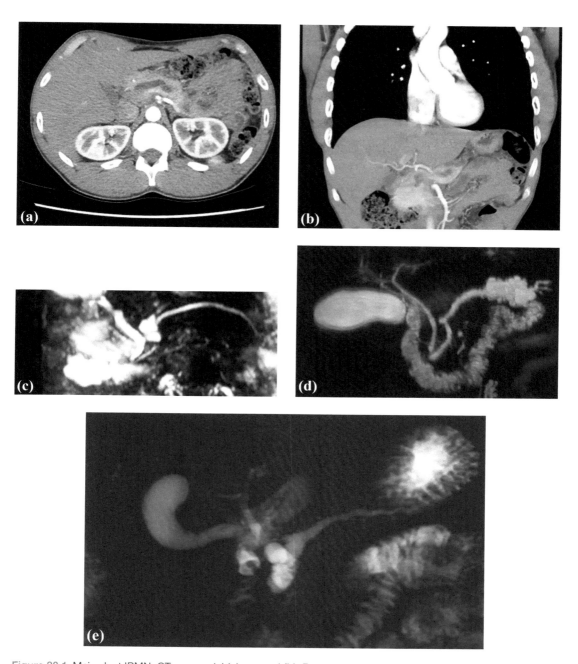

Figure 38.1 Main-duct IPMN. CT scan, axial (a), coronal (b). Branch-duct IPMN in MRCP (c). A mixed-duct IPMN, note multilocular dilatations of side-ducts in the tail of pancreas (d) and in MRCP (e).

contrast, severe atypia, papillae with branching and budding into the lumen, loss of nuclear polarity with prominent nucleoli, and atypical mitoses characterize a high-grade IPMN (1,33) (*Figure 38.2*). While some guidelines discourage the use of the term carcinoma *in situ*, the WHO regards it an acceptable term if used as a parenthetical statement after high-grade IPMN (34). However, caution should be taken when interpreting

older reports using the term malignancy together with this definition. The identification of both IPMN and invasive carcinoma on histopathology falls into two distinct categories. Either carcinoma arising separately from the IPMN or that arising within the IPMN, which is regarded as the direct precursor (7). The former is termed IPMN with concomitant invasive carcinoma and the latter IPMN with an associated invasive carcinoma

(7,39). In terms of staging, high-grade IPMNs are classed as Tis, for *in situ* carcinoma, while the presence of invasive carcinoma follows the staging of pancreatic ductal adenocarcinoma, with the substages pT1a-c for invasive lesions smaller than 2 cm (33,40).

The prevailing cell differentiation pattern also allows the identification of intestinal, gastric, and pancreaticobiliary subtypes (41–43). Each of the three morphological subtypes is associated with a distinct prognosis (44) and it is the second most important predictor of survival after staging (45). Despite being primarily a morphological stratification, immunohistochemistry is advised to differentiate subtypes in undetermined cases, following a set of mucin expression patterns outlined by the WHO classification (1). However, a small cohort of IPMNs are still reported as mixed IPMN because of the overlap in immunohistochemical expression patterns and a lack of single predominant cellular architectural subtype (33,46).

The gastric subtype is characterized by tall columnar cells with pale, mucin-rich cytoplasm and basally oriented nuclei (47). This subtype is most often found in branch ducts and makes up the majority of IPMNs (46). The risk of harboring invasive carcinoma in the gastric-type IPMN is the lowest among all subtypes and estimated at around 10% in review series (41). The intestinal subtype is recognized by the presence of villous, papillae-forming, tall columnar cells with basophilic cytoplasm, apical mucin, and cigar-shaped nuclei (48,49). It is usually found in the main pancreatic duct and it is the second most prevalent subtype with a risk of harbouring malignancy of just over 40% (50). The pancreaticobiliary subtype forms a complex cellular architecture of interconnecting papillae made up of cuboidal cells with enlarged nuclei and prominent nucleoli (19,51). Although this is the least common subtype, it is associated with the highest risk of harboring high-grade lesions and malignancy, close to 70% (51) (*Figure 38.2*). Intraductal oncocytic papillary neoplasm (IOPN), although once grouped as an IPMN subtype, is a distinct tumour entity with a different immunoprofile that develops via a separate mechanism (52). IOPNs are not only morphologically distinct but have a more indolent clinical behavior than IPMNs (53,54).

IPMN with an associated invasive carcinoma, meaning that the invasive lesion arises within the area of the IPMN, may be a colloid or tubular variant. IPMN with a concomitant invasive carcinoma, meaning that the invasive lesion is not in continuity with the IPMN, is ubiquitously tubular adenocarcinoma (45,55). Colloid carcinoma is associated with the intestinal subtype IPMN (56) and has a better prognosis with an estimated 5-year survival of 87% (50), whereas tubular adenocarcinoma is associated with the gastric and pancreatobiliary subtype IPMNs (45,57,58) and has an estimated 5-year survival of 55% (50).

As pancreatic cancer precursors, IPMNs harbor many mutations seen in classic pancreatic adenocarcinoma, including KRAS and TP53 (55,59,60). However, sequencing studies have highlighted differences in their incidence as well identifying new somatic mutations that appear specific to the IPMN precursor pathway (42,61). Guanine nucleotide binding protein, alpha-stimulating (GNAS) oncogene activation is a key genetic alteration (62). GNAS normally functions to maintain body glucose haemostasis, but when mutated it becomes overactive and is involved in the formation of a number of cancers. While present in around 60% of all IPMNs, it

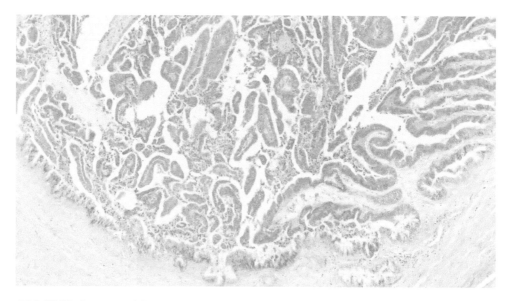

Figure 38.2 IPMN of pancreatobiliary type with high-grade dysplasia – irregular branching papillae, lined by cuboidal cells with loss of nuclear polarity.

is most frequently seen in the intestinal subtype, with a prevalence of 80% (63,64). RNF43-inactivating mutations are detected in about 50% of IPMNs and are also common in mucinous cystic neoplasms (65,66).

Investigation

The evaluation of a suspected pancreatic cyst primarily relies on cross-sectional imaging but may also require endoscopic ultrasound (EUS) and cytology (67,68). Magnetic resonance cholangiopancreatography (MRCP) appears to be of higher diagnostic accuracy than computed tomography (CT) in identifying the specific cyst type (69,70) and is particularly useful in identifying communications between a side branch lesion and the main pancreatic duct (71), which is key to distinguish IPMNs from other cystic lesions of the pancreas. However, both CT and magnetic resonance imaging (MRI) are useful for the evaluation of lymph node involvement and the presence of metastatic disease (72,73). The diameter of the main-duct and cyst dimensions, enhancing mural nodules, and solid components are key radiological features to evaluate in the assessment of IMPNs. These features are essential when predicting the risk of advanced neoplasia, which is important when deciding on the most appropriate management for each patient. In equivocal cases or in the presence of concerning features detected on cross-sectional imaging, EUS can contribute to the characterization of pancreatic cysts and is particularly good at visualizing the cyst wall (74), with contrast-enhanced EUS reported as superior to standard EUS in the characterization of mural nodules (75). Combined with fine needle aspiration (FNA), EUS can also contribute valuable information through the analysis of cystic fluid markers and cytology (76). Although carcinoembryonic antigen (CEA) and mutations such as KRAS/GNAS have been extensively studied to help distinguish the different pancreatic cyst types (77), proteomic analysis of cystic fluid has also been proposed to identify markers that could improve the accuracy of predicting the risk of malignancy, specifically in IPMNs (78–80). Another emerging approach that could provide a greater diagnostic accuracy is through-the-needle biopsy sampling of cyst tissue, however presently this remains an experimental technique with limited supporting evidence (81,82).

Management

Management recommendations are based on the individual risk of malignancy. The goal is to achieve early, curative, treatment in invasive IPMN or cancer prevention in high-grade IPMN, while avoiding major surgery in low-grade IPMN. The Sendai Consensus guidelines, proposed in 2006 by the International Association of Pancreatology (IAP), was the first attempt to devise standardized management recommendations (83). Today, three different working groups have drafted

independent pertinent guidelines: the European Study Group on Cystic Tumours of the Pancreas (84), last updated in 2018; the IAP, most recently updated in 2017 (34); and the American Gastroenterological Association (AGA), published in 2015 (85). While it is known that the vast majority of IPMNs will never progress and develop into carcinoma, and most patients should not be subjected to the burden of pancreatic surgery, these guidelines have demonstrated their usefulness albeit with a higher sensitivity than specificity for the risk of malignancy. The management of IPMNs therefore leans towards overtreatment (86) and the presence of a feature which is highly predictive for advanced neoplasia in a surgically fit patient is deemed an indication for surgery. Patients regarded as unfit for surgery should not undergo follow-up, irrespective of their age. Consensus with regards to diagnostic work-up, indications for surgery, and surveillance remain areas of debate. A recent international survey highlighted substantial discrepancies, not only among the three current management guidelines, but also between these guidelines and the clinical practice, and between the guidelines and the evidence available (87).

Due to the high risk of an occult malignancy, surgical resection is the treatment of choice for main-duct and mixed-duct IPMNs with a main pancreatic duct diameter over 10 mm, in patients who are deemed surgically fit. Main-duct dilatation between 5–9.9 mm, however, remains a relative indication, according to the guidelines, despite increasing evidence of high malignancy rates (88) and there should be careful consideration on a case-by-case basis. The management of branch-duct IPMN should involve MDT discussion and a careful assessment of all the patient and cyst features. Surgery is indicated in patients with evidence of high-grade dysplasia or carcinoma on cytology, malignant jaundice, contrast enhancing mural nodules larger than 5 mm, or a solid component, all of which are regarded as absolute indicators for surgery if at least one is present in any IPMN lesion. Elevated serum CA19-9 >37 U/mL, cyst diameter over 40 mm and growth rate over 5 mm/year, contrast enhancing mural nodule smaller than 5 mm, acute pancreatitis caused by the IPMN, and new-onset diabetes are relative indications for surgery (34,84) (*Table 38.1*). In multifocal branch-duct IPMNs, all the above risk features must be assessed for each individual lesion, and the management indications apply to each lesion as a single entity (89, 90), while considering further characterization with EUS in the presence of concerning features.

If surgery is indicated, then resection with lymphadenectomy is regarded as the 'gold standard' oncological procedure (91,92). Pancreatoduodenectomy is the surgery of choice for lesions in the head and uncinate of the pancreas, and distal pancreatectomy for lesions in the body or tail. Controversy also remains regarding the management of main-duct IMPN with dilatation of the main pancreatic duct along the entire length of

Table 38.1 Comparison of management guideline-indications for surgery, surveillance, and follow-up

Guidelines	Features predictive of cancer progression – indication for surgery	Features associated with high risk of cancer progression – relative indication for surgery	Surveillance of non-resected IPMN
European (2018)	• Jaundice • Enhancing mural nodule >5mm or solid component • Main pancreatic duct measuring >10mm • Cytology positive for cancer	• Symptoms • Serum CA19-9 >37 U/mL • Enhancing mural nodule <5mm and/or cyst diameter >=40mm • Cyst growth-rate >=5mm/year • Main pancreatic duct measuring between 5–9.9mm	In presence of relative indications for surgery: • Every 6 months In absence of any indication for surgery • 6 months from diagnosis and yearly thereafter
IAP (2017)	• Jaundice • Enhancing mural nodule >=5mm • Main pancreatic duct measuring >10mm • Cytology positive or suspicious for cancer	• Acute pancreatitis • Increased serum CA19-9 • Enhancing mural nodule <5mm • Cyst >3cm • Thickened/enhancing cyst walls • Cyst growth-rate >=5mm/2 years • Main pancreatic duct measuring >=5mm and <10mm • Abrupt change in caliber of pancreatic duct with distal pancreatic atrophy • Lymphadenopathy • New onset or recent exacerbation of diabetes mellitus within the past year	According to diameter of largest cyst: • <20 mm in 6 months, then every 18 months if stable • 20–30 mm in 6 months, 1 year, then every 12 months if stable • >30 mm every 12 months if stable • Preferably with MRI, physical examination, tumour markers, and assessment of new onset diabetes
AGA (2015)	• Solid component • Main pancreatic duct measuring >5mm • Cytology positive for cancer		In 1 year, then every 2 years, for up to 5 years, then stop follow-up

the pancreas. The dilemma lies on the fine-line between curative or preventative treatment versus overtreatment with the long-term consequences of exocrine insufficiency and brittle diabetes following extensive resections or a total pancreatectomy. In such cases, supporting endoscopic evidence of diffuse IPMN involvement and detailed assessment of other risk factors for malignancy are mandatory to inform the preoperative planning process. Consensus leans towards pancreatoduodenectomy and full lymph node dissection with frozen section biopsy and possibly extension of resection, while total pancreatectomy is advised by some authors in the presence of mural nodules or a familial history of pancreatic cancer. Pancreas sparing resections are regarded as non-oncological procedures and are deemed inappropriate in lesions at risk of harboring malignancy.

In the presence of a relative feature, different guidelines advise varying different surveillance protocols or surgery (*Table 38.1*) (93). Recommendations for EUS in the follow-up of patients without definite indications for surgery range from every 6 months in the first year after diagnosis, and yearly thereafter to every 3–6 months depending on the cyst size according to the European and the International Guidelines, respectively. Cross-sectional imaging, particularly MRI, serum CA19-9, clinical examination, and new-onset

diabetes play a key role in the surveillance of patients managed conservatively for as long as they remain fit for surgery. This serves to delay the risks of pancreatic surgery without excluding the option of a curative resection in patients with evolving IPMN lesions (80,94). The duration of surveillance in patients with IPMN lesions without features of malignant potential is indefinite and determined by each patient's fitness directing whether they remain surgical candidates.

In the presence of invasive carcinoma, adjuvant chemotherapy is associated with an improved overall survival compared with surgery alone (95). The regimen of choice is most commonly that for pancreatic adenocarcinoma. Neoadjuvant chemotherapy, however, is not generally recommended as there is insufficient evidence. Surveillance, after surgery, is advised in all patients undergoing subtotal pancreatic resections for as long as they remain fit for further surgery, as disease recurrence can occur 5–10 years after surgery (96).

SUMMARY

PMNs are increasingly diagnosed premalignant lesions of the pancreas. The majority will never develop into invasive carcinoma and, therefore, their management relies on a balance between the risks associated with surgery and the objective established benefits of a curative resection. Assessment and advice have to also consider the burden of life-long surveillance if unresected or follow-up of the remnant pancreas following subtotal resections. Consensus is still lacking on how to consistently and safely achieve this balance. Clear evidence and the development of new tools to predict malignancy should both contribute to establishing global management guidelines in the near future.

REFERENCES

1. Basturk O, Esposito I, Klöppel G, Zamboni G, Furukawa T, Fukushima N, et al. Digestive system tumours. *WHO Classification of Tumours*, 5th Edition, Gemeva: IARC Publications;2019.

2. Itai Y, Ohhashi K, Nagai H, Murakami Y, Kokubo T, Makita K, et al. "Ductectatic" mucinous cystadenoma and cystadenocarcinoma of the pancreas. *Radiology* 1986;**161(3)**:697–700.

3. Ohashi K, Murakami Y, Maruyama M, Takekoshi T, Ohta H, Ohashi I. Four cases of "mucin-producing" cancer of the pancreas on specific findings of the papilla of Vater. *Prog Dig Endosc* 1982;**20**:348–51.

4. Klöppel G, Solcia E, Longnecker DS, Capella C, Sobin LH. *Histological Typing of Tumours of the Exocrine Pancreas.* 2nd edition, New York: Springer Nature;1996.

5. Ohashi K, Tajiri H, Gondo M, Yokoyama Y, Maruyama M, Takekoshi T, et al. A case of cystadenocarcinoma of the pancreas forming bilio-pancreatic fistula. *Prog Dig Endosc* 1980;**17**:261–64.

6. Tanaka M. Thirty years of experience with intraductal papillary mucinous neoplasm of the pancreas: From discovery to international consensus. *Digestion* 2014;**90(4)**:265–72.

7. Basturk O, Hong SM, Wood LD, Adsay NV, Al bores-Saavedra J, Biankin AV, et al. A revised classification system and recommendations from the Baltimore Consensus Meeting for Neoplastic Precursor Lesions in the Pancreas. *Am J Surg Pathol* 2015;**39(12)**:1730–41.

8. Hruban RH, Takaori K, Klimstra DS, Adsay NV, Albores-Saavedra J, Biankin AV, et al. An illustrated consensus on the classification of pancreatic intraepithelial neoplasia and intraductal papillary mucinous neoplasms. *Am J Surg Pathol* 2004;**28(8)**:977–87.

9. Zaheer A, Pokharel SS, Wolfgang C, Fishman EK, Horton KM. Incidentally detected cystic lesions of the pancreas on CT: Review of literature and management suggestions. *Abdom Imaging* 2013;**38(2)**:331–41.

10. Moris M, Bridges MD, Pooley RA, Raimondo M, Woodward TA, Stauffer JA, et al. Association between advances in high-resolution cross-section imaging technologies and increase in prevalence of pancreatic cysts From 2005 to 2014. *Clin Gastroenterol Hepatol* 2016;**14(4)**:585–93.e3.

11. Allen PJ, D'Angelica M, Gonen M, Jaques DP, Coit DG, Jarnagin WR, et al. A selective approach to the resection of cystic lesions of the pancreas: Results from 539 consecutive patients. *Ann Surg* 2006;**244(4)**:572–82.

12. Kosmahl M, Pauser U, Peters K, Sipos B, Luttges J, Kremer B, et al. Cystic neoplasms of the pancreas and tumor-like lesions with cystic features: A review of 418 cases and a classification proposal. *Virchows Arch* 2004;**445(2)**:168–78.

13. Kromrey ML, Bulow R, Hubner J, Paperlein C, Lerch MM, Ittermann T, et al. Prospective study on the incidence, prevalence and 5-year pancreatic-related mortality of pancreatic cysts in a population-based study. *Gut* 2018;**67(1)**:138–45.

14. Brugge WR, Lauwers GY, Sahani D, Fernandez-del Castillo C, Warshaw AL. Cystic neoplasms of the pancreas. *N Engl J Med* 2004;**351(12)**:1218–26.

15. de Wilde RF, Hruban RH, Maitra A, Offerhau GJA. Reporting precursors to invasive pancreatic cancer: Pancreatic intraepithelial neoplasia, intraductal neoplasms and mucinous cystic neoplasm. *Diagn Histopathol* 2012;**18(1)**:17–30.

16. Lennon AM, Wolfgang CL, Canto MI, Klein AP, Herman JM, Goggins M, et al. The early detection of pancreatic cancer: What will it take to diagnose and treat curable pancreatic neoplasia? *Cancer Res* 2014;**74(13)**:3381–9.

17. Ingkakul T, Warshaw AL, Fernandez-del Castillo C. Epidemiology of intraductal papillary mucinous neoplasms of the pancreas: Sex differences between 3 geographic regions. *Pancreas* 2011;**40(5)**:779–80.

18. Hwang DW, Jang JY, Lee SE, Lim CS, Lee KU, Kim SW. Clinicopathologic analysis of surgically proven intraductal papillary mucinous neoplasms of the pancreas in SNUH: A 15-year experience at a single academic institution. *Langenbecks Arch Surg* 2012;**397(1)**:93–102.

19. Fernandez-del Castillo C, Adsay NV. Intraductal papillary mucinous neoplasms of the pancreas. *Gastroenterology* 2010;**139(3)**:708–13, 13.e2.

20. Schnelldorfer T, Sarr MG, Nagorney DM, Zhang L, Smyrk TC, Qin R, et al. Experience with 208 resections for intraductal papillary mucinous neoplasm of the pancreas. *Arch Surg* 2008;**143(7)**:639–46; discussion 46.

21. Sato N, Rosty C, Jansen M, Fukushima N, Ueki T, Yeo CJ, et al. STK11/LKB1 Peutz-Jeghers gene inactivation in intraductal papillary-mucinous neoplasms of the pancreas. *Am J Pathol* 2001;**159(6)**:2017–22.

22. Wood LD, Noe M, Hackeng W, Brosens LA, Bhaijee F, Debeljak M, et al. Patients with McCune-Albright syndrome have a broad spectrum of abnormalities in the gastrointestinal tract and pancreas. *Virchows Arch* 2017;**470(4)**:391–400.

23. Maire F, Hammel P, Terris B, Olschwang S, O'Toole D, Sauvanet A, et al. Intraductal papillary and mucinous pancreatic tumour: A new extracolonic tumour in familial adenomatous polyposis. *Gut* 2002;**51(3)**:446–9.

24. Canto MI, Hruban RH, Fishman EK, Kamel IR, Schulick R, Zhang Z, et al. Frequent detection of pancreatic lesions in asymptomatic high-risk individuals. *Gastroenterology* 2012;**142(4)**:796–804; quiz e14–15.

25. Capurso G, Boccia S, Salvia R, Del Chiaro M, Frulloni L, Arcidiacono PG, et al. Risk factors for intraductal papillary mucinous neoplasm (IPMN) of the pancreas: A multicentre case-control study. *Am J Gastroenterol* 2013;**108**(**6**):1003–9.

26. Fukushima N, Mukai K. Pancreatic neoplasms with abundant mucus production: Emphasis on intraductal papillary-mucinous tumors and mucinous cystic tumors. *Adv Anat Pathol* 1999;**6**(**2**):65–77.

27. Basturk O, Coban I, Adsay NV. Pancreatic cysts: Pathologic classification, differential diagnosis, and clinical implications. *Arch Pathol Lab Med* 2009;**133**(**3**): 423–38.

28. Kloppel G, Basturk O, Schlitter AM, Konukiewitz B, Esposito I. Intraductal neoplasms of the pancreas. *Semin Diagn Pathol* 2014;**31**(**6**):452–66.

29. Jang JY, Kim SW, Ahn YJ, Yoon YS, Choi MG, Lee KU, et al. Multicenter analysis of clinicopathologic features of intraductal papillary mucinous tumor of the pancreas: Is it possible to predict the malignancy before surgery? *Ann Surg Oncol* 2005;**12**(**2**):124–32.

30. Pelaez-Luna M, Chari ST, Smyrk TC, Takahashi N, Clain JE, Levy MJ, et al. Do consensus indications for resection in branch duct intraductal papillary mucinous neoplasm predict malignancy? A study of 147 patients. *Am J Gastroenterol* 2007;**102**(**8**):1759–64.

31. Pea A, Yu J, Rezaee N, Luchini C, He J, Dal Molin M, et al. Targeted DNA sequencing reveals patterns of local progression in the pancreatic remnant following resection of intraductal papillary mucinous neoplasm (IPMN) of the pancreas. *Ann Surg* 2017;**266**(**1**):133–41.

32. Luchini C, Pea A, Yu J, He J, Salvia R, Riva G, et al. Pancreatic cancer arising in the remnant pancreas is not always a relapse of the preceding primary. *Mod Pathol* 2019;**32**(**5**):659–65.

33. Adsay V, Mino-Kenudson M, Furukawa T, Basturk O, Zamboni G, Marchegiani G, et al. Pathologic evaluation and reporting of intraductal papillary mucinousneoplasms of the pancreas and other tumoral intraepithelial neoplasms of pancreatobiliary tract: Recommendations of Verona Consensus Meeting. *Ann Surg* 2016;**263**(**1**):162–77.

34. Tanaka M, Fernandez-del Castillo C, Kamisawa T, Jang JY, Levy P, Ohtsuka T, et al. Revisions of international consensus Fukuoka guidelines for the management of IPMN of the pancreas. *Pancreatology* 2017;**17**(**5**):738–53.

35. Attiyeh MA, Fernandez-del Castillo C, Al Efisha M, Eaton AA, Gonen M, Batts R, et al. Development and validation of a multi-institutional preoperative nomogram for predicting grade of dysplasia in intraductal papillary mucinous neoplasms (IPMNs) of the pancreas: A report from the Pancreatic Surgery Consortium. *Ann Surg* 2018;**267**(**1**):157–63.

36. Azar C, Van de Stadt J, Rickaert F, Deviere M, Baize M, Kloppel G, et al. Intraductal papillary mucinous tumours of the pancreas. Clinical and therapeutic issues in 32 patients. *Gut* 1996;**39**(**3**):457–64.

37. Zhang TT, Sadler TJ, Whitley S, Brais R, Godfrey E. The CT fish mouth ampulla sign: A high-

ly specific finding in main duct and mixed intraductal papillary mucinous neoplasms. *Br J Radiol* 2019;**92**(**1103**):20190461.

38. Baiocchi GL, Portolani N, Missale G, Baronchelli C, Gheza F, Cantu M, et al. Intraductal papillary mucinous neoplasm of the pancreas (IPMN): Clinico-pathological correlations and surgical indications. *World J Surg Oncol* 2010;**8**:25.

39. Yamaguchi K, Kanemitsu S, Hatori T, Maguchi H, Shimizu Y, Tada M, et al. Pancreatic ductal adenocarcinoma derived from IPMN and pancreatic ductal adenocarcinoma concomitant with IPMN. *Pancreas* 2011;**40**(**4**):571–80.

40. Allen PJ, Kuk D, Castillo CF, Basturk O, Wolfgang CL, Cameron JL, et al. Multi-institutional Validation Study of the American Joint Commission on Cancer (8th Edition) Changes for T and N Staging in Patients With Pancreatic Adenocarcinoma. *Ann Surg* 2017;**265**(**1**):185–91.

41. Koh YX, Zheng HL, Chok AY, Tan CS, Wyone W, Lim TK, et al. Systematic review and meta-analysis of the spectrum and outcomes of different histologic subtypes of noninvasive and invasive intraductal papillary mucinous neoplasms. *Surgery* 2015;**157**(**3**):496–509.

42. Patra KC, Bardeesy N, Mizukami Y. Diversity of precursor lesions For pancreatic cancer: The genetics and biology of intraductal papillary mucinous neoplasm. *Clin Transl Gastroenterol* 2017;**8**(**4**):e86.

43. Reid MD, Lewis MM, Willingham FF, Adsay NV. The evolving role of pathology in new developments, cassification, terminology, and diagnosis of pancreatobiliary neoplasms. *Arch Pathol Lab Med* 2017;**141**(**3**):366–80.

44. Distler M, Kersting S, Niedergethmann M, Aust DE, Franz M, Ruckert F, et al. Pathohistological subtype predicts survival in patients with intraductal papillary mucinous neoplasm (IPMN) of the pancreas. *Ann Surg* 2013;**258**(**2**):324–30.

45. Furukawa T, Hatori T, Fujita I, Yamamoto M, Kobayashi M, Ohike N, et al. Prognostic relevance of morphological types of intraductal papillary mucinous neoplasms of the pancreas. *Gut* 2011;**60**(**4**):509–16.

46. Schaberg KB, DiMaio MA, Longacre TA. Intraductal papillary mucinousneoplasms often contain epithelium from multiple subtypes and/or are unclassifiable. *Am J Surg Pathol* 2016;**40**(**1**):44–50.

47. Ban S, Naitoh Y, Mino-Kenudson M, Sakurai T, Kuroda M, Koyama I, et al. Intraductal papillary mucinous neoplasm (IPMN) of the pancreas: Its histopathologic difference between 2 major types. *Am J Surg Pathol* 2006;**30**(**12**):1561–9.

48. Adsay NV, Merati K, Basturk O, Iacobuzio-Donahue C, Levi E, Cheng JD, et al. Pathologically and biologically distinct types of epithelium in intraductal papillary mucinous neoplasms: Delineation of an "intestinal" pathway of carcinogenesis in the pancreas. *Am J Surg Pathol* 2004;**28**(**7**):839–48.

49. Nakamura A, Horinouchi M, Goto M, Nagata K, Sakoda K, Takao S, et al. New classification of pan-

creatic intraductal papillary-mucinous tumour by mucin expression: Its relationship with potential for malignancy. *J Pathol* 2002;**197(2)**:201–10.

50. Yopp AC, Katabi N, Janakos M, Klimstra DS, D'Angelica MI, DeMatteo RP, et al. Invasive carcinoma arising in intraductal papillary mucinous neoplasms of the pancreas: A matched control study with conventional pancreatic ductal adenocarcinoma. *Ann Surg* 2011;**253(5)**:968–74.

51. Adsay NV, Merati K, Andea A, Sarkar F, Hruban RH, Wilentz RE, et al. The dichotomy in the preinvasive neoplasia to invasive carcinoma sequence in the pancreas: Differential expression of MUC1 and MUC2 supports the existence of two separate pathways of carcinogenesis. *Mod Pathol* 2002;**15(10)**:1087–95.

52. Basturk O, Tan M, Bhanot U, Allen P, Adsay V, Scott SN, et al. The oncocytic subtype is genetically distinct from other pancreatic intraductal papillary mucinous neoplasm subtypes. *Mod Pathol* 2016;**29(9)**:1058–69.

53. Basturk O, Chung SM, Hruban RH, Adsay NV, Askan G, Iacobuzio-Donahue C, et al. Distinct pathways of pathogenesis of intraductal oncocytic papillary neoplasms and intraductal papillary mucinous neoplasms of the pancreas. *Virchows Arch* 2016;**469(5)**:523–32.

54. Marchegiani G, Mino-Kenudson M, Ferrone CR, Warshaw AL, Lillemoe KD, Fernandez-del Castillo C. Oncocytic-type intraductal papillary mucinous neoplasms: A unique malignant pancreatic tumor with good long-term prognosis. *J Am Coll Surg* 2015;220(5):839–44.

55. Tan MC, Basturk O, Brannon AR, Bhanot U, Scott SN, Bouvier N, et al. GNAS and KRAS mutations define separate progression pathways in intraductal papillary mucinous neoplasm-asociated carcinoma. *J Am Coll Surg* 2015;**220(5)**:845–54.e1.

56. Ideno N, Ohtsuka T, Kono H, Fujiwara K, Oda Y, Aishima S, et al. Intraductal papillary mucinous neoplasms of the pancreas with distinct pancreatic ductal adenocarcinomas are frequently of gastric subtype. *Ann Surg* 2013;**258(1)**:141–51.

57. Poultsides GA, Reddy S, Cameron JL, Hruban RH, Pawlik TM, Ahuja N, et al. Histopathologic basis for the favorable survival after resection of intraductal papillary mucinous neoplasm-associated invasive adenocarcinoma of the pancreas. *Ann Surg* 2010;**251(3)**:470–6.

58. Mino-Kenudson M, Fernandez-del Castillo C, Baba Y, Valsangkar NP, Liss AS, Hsu M, et al. Prognosis of invasive intraductal papillary mucinous neoplasm depends on histological and precursor epithelial subtypes. *Gut* 2011;**60(12)**:1712–20.

59. Jones S, Zhang X, Parsons DW, Lin JC, Leary RJ, Angenendt P, et al. Core signaling pathways in human pancreatic cancers revealed by global genomic analyses. *Science* 2008;**321(5897)**:1801–6.

60. Kuboki Y, Shimizu K, Hatori T, Yamamoto M, Shibata N, Shiratori K, et al. Molecular biomarkers for progression of intraductal papillary mucinous neoplasm of the pancreas. *Pancreas* 2015;**44(2)**:227–35.

61. Panarelli NC, Sela R, Schreiner AM, Crapanzano JP, Klimstra DS, Schnoll-Sussman F, et al. Commercial molecular panels are of limited utility in the classification of pancreatic cystic lesions. *Am J Surg Pathol* 2012;**36(10)**:1434–43.

62. Furukawa T, Kuboki Y, Tanji E, Yoshida S, Hatori T, Yamamoto M, et al. Whole-exome sequencing uncovers frequent GNAS mutations in intraductal papillary mucinous neoplasms of the pancreas. *Sci Rep* 2011;**1**:161.

63. Springer S, Wang Y, Dal Molin M, Masica DL, Jiao Y, Kinde I, et al. A combination of molecular markers and clinical features improve the classification of pancreatic cysts. *Gastroenterology* 2015;**149(6)**:1501–10.

64. Mas L, Lupinacci RM, Cros J, Bachet JB, Coulet F, Svrcek M. Intraductal papillary mucinous carcinoma versus conventional pancreatic ductal adenocarcinoma: A comprehensive review of clinical-pathological features, outcomes, and molecular insights. *Int J Mol Sci* 2021;**22(13)**:6756.

65. Wu J, Matthaei H, Maitra A, Dal Molin M, Wood LD, Eshleman JR, et al. Recurrent GNAS mutations define an unexpected pathway for pancreatic cyst development. Sci Transl Med 2011;3(92):92ra66.

66. Sakamoto H, Kuboki Y, Hatori T, Yamamoto M, Sugiyama M, Shibata N, et al. Clinicopathological significance of somatic RNF43 mutation and aberrant expression of ring finger protein 43 in intraductal papillary mucinous neoplasms of the pancreas. *Mod Pathol* 2015;**28(2)**:261–7.

67. Jang DK, Song BJ, Ryu JK, Chung KH, Lee BS, Park JK, et al. Preoperative diagnosis of pancreatic cystic lesions: The accuracy of endoscopic ultrasound and cross-sectional imaging. *Pancreas* 2015;**44(8)**:1329–33.

68. Hecht EM, Khatri G, Morgan D, Kang S, Bhosale PR, Francis IR, et al. Intraductal papillary mucinous neoplasm (IPMN) of the pancreas: Recommendations for standardized Imaging and reporting from the Society of Abdominal Radiology IPMN disease focused panel. *Abdom Radiol* (NY) 2021;**46(4)**:1586–606.

69. Lee HJ, Kim MJ, Choi JY, Hong HS, Kim KA. Relative accuracy of CT and MRI in the differentiation of benign from malignant pancreatic cystic lesions. *Clin Radiol* 2011;**66(4)**:315–21.

70. Song SJ, Lee JM, Kim YJ, Kim SH, Lee JY, Han JK, et al. Differentiation of intraductal papillary mucinous neoplasms from other pancreatic cystic masses: Comparison of multirow–detector CT and MR imaging using ROC analysis. *J Magn Reson Imaging* 2007;**26(1)**:86–93.

71. Waters JA, Schmidt CM, Pinchot JW, White PB, Cummings OW, Pitt HA, et al. CT vs MRCP: Optimal classification of IPMN type and extent. *J Gastrointest Surg* 2008;**12(1)**:101–9.

72. Sahani DV, Kadavigere R, Blake M, Fernandez-del Castillo C, Lauwers GY, Hahn PF. Intraductal papillary mucinous neoplasm of pancreas: Multi-detector row CT with 2D curved reformations – correlation with MRCP. *Radiology* 2006;**238(2)**:560–9.

73. Kim JH, Eun HW, Kim KW, Lee JY, Lee JM, Han JK, et al. Intraductal papillary mucinous neoplasms with associated invasive carcinoma of the pancreas: Imaging findings and diagnostic performance of MDCT for prediction of prognostic factors. *AJR Am J Roentgenol* 2013;**201(3)**:565–72.

74. Lisotti A, Napoleon B, Facciorusso A, Cominardi A, Crino SF, Brighi N, et al. Contrast–enhanced EUS for the characterization of mural nodules within pancreatic cystic neoplasms: Systematic review and meta-analysis. *Gastrointest Endosc* 2021;**94(5)**:881–9.

75. Harima H, Kaino S, Shinoda S, Kawano M, Suenaga S, Sakaida I. Differential diagnosis of benign and malignant branch duct intraductal papillary mucinous neoplasm using contrast-enhanced endoscopic ultrasonography. *World J Gastroenterol* 2015;**21(20)**:6252–60.

76. Gilani SM, Adeniran AJ, Cai G. Endoscopic ultrasound-guided fine needleaspiration cytologic evaluation of intraductal papillary mucinous neoplasm and mucinous cystic neoplasms of pancreas. *Am J Clin Pathol* 2020;**154(4)**:559–70.

77. Gillis A, Cipollone I, Cousins G, Conlon K. Does EUS-FNA molecular analysis carry additional value when compared to cytology in the diagnosis of pancreatic cystic neoplasm? A systematic review. *HPB (Oxford)* 2015;**17(5)**:377–86.

78. Do M, Han D, Wang JI, Kim H, Kwon W, Han Y, et al. Quantitative proteomic analysis of pancreatic cyst fluid proteins associated with malignancy in intraductal papillary mucinous neoplasms. *Clin Proteomics* 2018;**15**:17.

79. Do M, Kim H, Shin D, Park J, Kim H, Han Y, et al. Marker identification of the grade of dysplasia of intraductal papillary mucinous neoplasm in pancreatic cyst fluid by quantitative proteomic profiling. *Cancers (Basel)* 2020;**12(9)**:2383.

80. Salvia R, Marchegiani G. Evolving management of pancreatic cystic neoplasms. *Br J Surg* 2020;**107(11)**:1393–5.

81. Basar O, Yuksel O, Yang DJ, Samarasena J, Forcione D, DiMaio CJ, et al. Feasibility and safety of microforceps biopsy in the diagnosis of pancreatic cysts. *Gastrointest Endosc* 2018;**88(1)**:79–86.

82. McCarty T, Rustagi T. Endoscopic ultrasound-guided through-the-needle microforceps biopsy improves diagnostic yield for pancreatic cystic lesions: A systematic review and meta-analysis. *Endosc Int Open* 2020;**8(10)**:e1280–e90.

83. Tanaka M, Chari S, Adsay V, Fernandez-del Castillo C, Falconi M, Shimizu M, et al. International consensus guidelines for management of intraductal papillary mucinous neoplasms and mucinous cystic neoplasms of the pancreas. *Pancreatology* 2006;**6(1–2)**:17–32.

84. European Study Group on Cystic Tumours of the Pancreas. European evidence-based guidelines on pancreatic cystic neoplasms. *Gut* 2018;**67(5)**:789–804.

85. Vege SS, Ziring B, Jain R, Moayyedi P, Clinical Guidelines Committee, American Gastroenterology Association American gastroenterological association institute guideline on the diagnosis and management of asymptomatic neoplastic pancreatic cysts. *Gastroenterology* 2015;**148(4)**:819–22; quize12–13.

86. Grippa S, Fogliati A, Valente R, Sadr-Azodi O, Arnelo U, Capurso G, et al. A tug-of-war in intraductal papillary mucinous neoplasms management: Comparison between 2017 International and 2018 European guidelines. *Dig Liver Dis* 2021;**53(8)**:998–1003.

87. Marchegiani G, Salvia R, Verona EBMoI. Guidelines on pancreatic cystic neoplasms: Major inconsistencies with available evidence and clinical practice – Results from an international survey. *Gastroenterology* 2021;**160(7)**:2234–8.

88. Del Chiaro M, Beckman R, Ateeb Z, Orsini N, Rezaee N, Manos L, et al. Main duct dilatation is the best predictor of high–grade dysplasia or invasion in intraductal papillary mucinous neoplasms of the pancreas. *Ann Surg* 2020;**272(6)**:1118–24.

89. Matthaei H, Norris AL, Tsiatis AC, Olino K, Hong SM, dal Molin M, et al. Clinicopathological characteristics and molecular analyses of multifocal intraductal papillary mucinous neoplasms of the pancreas. *Ann Surg* 2012;**255(2)**:326–33.

90. Fritz S, Schirren M, Klauss M, Bergmann F, Hackert T, Hartwig W, et al. Clinicopathologic characteristics of patients with resected multifocal intraductal papillary mucinous neoplasm of the pancreas. *Surgery* 2012;**52(3 Suppl 1)**:S74–80.

91. Tol JA, Gouma DJ, Bassi C, Dervenis C, Montorsi M, Adham M, et al. Definition of a standard lymphadenectomy in surgery for pancreatic ductal adenocarcinoma: A consensus statement by the International Study Group on Pancreatic Surgery (ISGPS). *Surgery* 2014;**156(3)**:591–600.

92. Partelli S, Fernandez-del Castillo C, Bassi C, Mantovani W, Thayer SP, Crippa S, et al. Invasive intraductal papillary mucinous carcinomas of the pancreas: Predictors of survival and the role of lymph node ratio. *Ann Surg* 2010;**251(3)**:477–82.

93. Ohtsuka T, Fernandez-del Castillo C, Furukawa T, Hijioka S, Jang J-Y, Lennon AM, et al. International evidence-based Kyoto guidelines for the management of intraductal papillary mucinous neoplasm of the pancreas. *Pancreatology* 2024;**24(2)**:255–70.

94. Marchegiani G, Andrianello S, Pollini T, Caravati A, Biancotto M, Secchettin E, et al. 'Trivial' cysts redefine the risk of cancer in presumed branch-duct intraductal papillary mucinous neoplasms of the pancreas: A potential target for follow-up discontinuation? *Am J Gastroenterol* 2019;**114(10)**:1678–84.

95. Chong E, Ratnayake B, Dasari BVM, Loveday BPT, Siriwardena AK, Pandanaboyana S. Adjuvant chemotherapy in the treatment of intraductal papillary mucinous neoplasms of the pancreas: Systematic review and meta-analysis. *World J Surg* 2021;**46(1)**:223–34.

96. Moriya T, Traverso W. Fate of the pancreatic remnant after resection for an intraductal papillary mucinous neoplasm: A longitudinal level II cohort study. *Arch Surg* 2012;**147(6)**:528–34.

Chapter
39

Technical Aspects of Pancreatoduodenectomy

John Keith Roberts and Stefan Burgdorf

INTRODUCTION

Pancreatic ductal adenocarcinoma (PDAC) is the twelfth most common cancer worldwide, the seventh cause of cancer-related deaths, and responsible for 4% of all cancer-related mortality (1). In 1898, the first pancreaticoduodenectomy (PD) was performed by an Italian surgeon, Alessandro Codivilla (21 March 1861–28 February 1912), from Bologna who was head of the surgical department of the hospital of Castiglion Fiorentino (2). In his report, he describes removal of part of the pancreas, duodenum, distal stomach and distal bile duct with reconstruction using a Roux-en-Y gastrojejunostomy following a cholecystojejunostomy. He did not anastomose or occlude the pancreatic duct or stump and the patient died at 18 days from cachexia due to steatorrhea. Codivilla's technique was modified by Walhter Kausch in 1912, who was the first to attempt the resection of the duodenum *en bloc* with a segment of the pancreas, re-establishing continuity with a pancreaticoduodenostomy (3). Pancreatic resection was subsequently performed as a two-stage procedure by the American surgeon Allen Oldfather Whipple (September 2, 1881–April 6, 1963). He began work on the procedure for resection of the pancreas (pancreaticoduodenectomy) and in 1935 Whipple, Parsons and Mullins published the first report of three patients from Columbia Presbyterian Hospital in New York. The first patient died after 2 days due to an anastomotic breakdown but the second and third patients lived for 9 and 24 months, respectively, ultimately dying from cholangitis and liver metastases. In 1940, Whipple modified the procedure to facilitate a one-stage operation and during his lifetime performed 37 pancreaticoduodenectomies (4). To-date, surgical resection remains the only potentially curative approach to PDAC, due to the almost ubiquitous late presentation. Only 10–20% of patients are candidates for resection initially, with 5-year reported survival rates of 11–27% (5). With the advent of effective chemotherapy protocols, the concept of neoadjuvant treatment emerged and developed in parallel with technical advances that facilitated radical vessel resection and dissection of the mesopancreas to reduce the risk of local recurrence. The aim was to obtain a complete surgical resection (R0), in borderline resectable and locally advanced disease, in the hope that it would result in prolonged survival or potential cure. There is also early data suggesting that patients with PDAC, who have residual margin positive

(R1) disease, have an improved survival compared with those treated non-surgically, especially when associated with neoadjuvant treatment (5).

In 1951, Moore et al. described the first cases of PD with superior mesenteric vein (SMV) and portal vein (PV) resection (6), only just over a decade after Whipple described his one-stage PD. Subsequently, in 1963 Asada et al. also reported venous reconstruction during PD (7), but vascular resection as a routine component of PD did not gain acceptance until the work of Joseph G. Fortner from Memorial Sloan Kettering Cancer Center, described a series of patients who underwent total pancreatectomy with venous, or venous and arterial, resection and reconstruction (8,9). In 1984, Fortner described the results following regional pancreatectomy for PDAC or ampullary and periampullary cancers in 61 patients. The mortality was 32% from 1972–1978, and 8% between 1979 and 1982 (10). As a consequence of the high morbidity and mortality rates, and the lack of data demonstrating improved survival until the 1990s, very few surgeons were performing vascular resections as part of a PD. During the 1990s, however, with improved anaesthetic and surgical techniques, the morbidity and mortality related to vascular resections improved and a number of authors suggested that localized PV involvement, when there was no evidence of additional local invasion, should not contraindicate pancreatic resection in patients with PDAC (11–13). Subsequently, venous resection has become routine, although arterial resection and surgery where there is combined vascular involvement remains controversial.

Pancreatic adenocarcinoma is discussed in **Chapter 33**, and in this chapter, we will focus on the technical aspects of pancreatoduodenectomy. This will include surgical approaches to the open procedure and recent advances in the surgical treatment of PDAC, relating to the management of peripancreatic vessels, with illustrations of various anastomotic techniques and the methods employed in cases where there is vascular involvement.

INCISION

The two main incisions used when performing pancreatic surgery are midline or bilateral subcostal. The advantage of a midline incision is that it provides sufficient access to mobilize the small and large bowel, to perform a Cattell-Braasch manoeuvre (medial visceral rotation *with mobilization of the colon and duodenum through*

DOI: 10.1201/9781003080060-39

the embryological plane of Toldt's coalescence fascia), to resect porto-mesenteric structures, and to dissect the superior mesenteric artery (SMA). With a bilateral subcostal incision, access to lower abdominal structures and the root of the small bowel mesentery is more challenging, but the surgeon has good direct sight of the duodenum, inferior vena cava and hilum. There appears little difference in clinical outcomes (incision hernia, respiratory complications, analgesic requirements) between the two when evaluated in clinical trials, although a recent study suggests that wound complications are less common with a subcostal incision (14). A hybrid reverse L incision technique which is claimed to give many of the benefits of both approaches is used by some surgeons.

LYMPHADENECTOMY

The prognosis, following pancreatoduodenectomy, for patients with pancreatic cancer depends on a number of factors including: tumour biology; resection margins; socio-economic status; the availability, and provision of, adjuvant chemo and radiotherapy; lymph node status. Of the prognostic factors, the single most important is lymph node status. Lymphadenectomy is important for correct staging and to achieve optimal outcomes. The most recent International Study Group on Pancreatic Cancer (ISGPS) guidelines recommend that resected lymph node stations should include 5, 6, 8A, 12, 13, 14 and 17 (15). If a complete harvesting of these lymph node stations is performed, the number of harvested lymph nodes identified will depend on the thoroughness and experience of the pathologist and the length of the resected jejunal limb. Some studies have suggested survival benefits following extended lymphadenectomy, especially in those patients with borderline resectable tumours (16), and this is likely to evolve with developments in modern multimodal therapy, where more patients are offered neoadjuvant and downsizing chemotherapy.

PYLORUS PRESERVING VERSUS PYLORUS RESECTING PANCREATODUODENECTOMY

Pylorus resecting pancreatoduodenectomy (PRPD) has in some studies been associated with post-gastrectomy syndrome. Symptoms of which include post-prandial dumping, diarrhoea, dyspepsia, nausea and vomiting, which are reduced after pylorus preserving pancreatoduodenectomy (PPPD). Other studies however, have found the two methods are similar in terms of postoperative complications and have suggested that delayed gastric emptying (DGE) is dependent on other factors including: age; the occurrence of postoperative pancreatic fistulae; intra-abdominal abscess formation; pancreatitis. Debate continues with no clear consensus. Data continue to emerge supporting each approach and there is even a recent publication from Cai et al. suggesting that DGE is reduced following PRPD (17–20).

REDUCING DELAYED GASTRIC EMPTYING

Delayed gastric emptying (DGE) is associated with various factors unrelated to technical aspects of surgical practice, such as a history of pancreatitis and postoperative complications, particularly postoperative pancreatic fistulae (POPF) (21,22). It is also associated with prolonged operation times and increased blood loss, which suggests a possible link with the conduct of surgery. Pylorus resections are associated with reduced rates of DGE (20) in meta-analysis, but when only randomized control trials (RCTs) are considered, the effect is not significant. Antecolic or retrocolic gastrojejunostomy, pancreatogastrostomy, or pancreatojejunostomy and a Billroth II or Roux-en-Y reconstructions do not appear to affect rates of DGE (23–26). Early oral feeding appears to reduce DGE in non-randomized trials, a result not reproduced in randomized studies.

A focus on the physiology of gastric emptying, contractions and control is helpful. The duodenal pacemaker lies 0.5–1 cm distal to the pylorus and in a large cohort study, a reduced length of duodenum (with presumably resection of the pacemaker) with pylorus preservation was associated with DGE. The pylorus requires both a blood supply and neural control to work effectively and it is highly likely that DGE, following pylorus preservation, relates to failure to appreciate this. The autonomic nerve supply to the pylorus is supplied via the right-gastric and the right-gastroepiploic arteries, which are divided at surgery, and thus the majority of neural control is lost (*Figure 39.1*). Arterial supply is from the same vessels and

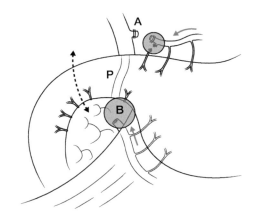

Figure 39.1 Pylorus preservation – autonomic nerves and arterial supply to the pylorus via the right gastric artery **(A)** and the right gastroepiploic artery **(B)**. Reverse arterial flow through the arterial arcades on the greater and lesser curves (red arrows) will continue to supply the pylorus; however, if tissue is ligated around the pylorus (P) (red circles) then it is left without a neural or arterial supply and risks delayed gastric emptying.

so is also lost, but the arcades on the lesser, and greater, curve will ensure continued flow as long as tissue around the pylorus is preserved. If this is resected, then the pylorus will lose both arterial and neural supply (27).

The route of the small bowel and orientation of the anastomosis are also important as kinking of the anastomosis can lead to severe symptoms of gastric outlet obstruction which mimic DGE.

REDUCING POSTOPERATIVE PANCREATIC FISTULA

The primary determinant of morbidity and mortality following PD is the development of a postoperative pancreatic fistula (POPF). Given the nature and complexity of the surgical reconstruction, it is not possible to neglect the role and contribution of surgical technique in either causing, or reducing, the risk of POPF. However, many RCTs have been conducted that focus on common variations of anastomotic technique (28) which include: pancreatogastrostomy versus pancreatojejunostomy; one versus two-layer; invagination versus duct to mucosa; Blumgart versus Cattell Warren pancreatojejunostomy (29). Adjuncts to the anastomosis have also been evaluated and include: somatostatin analogues; internal and external pancreatic ductal stents; autologous barriers such as the falciform ligament; pharmaceutical barriers, such as haemostatic patches or fibrin glue. Several RCTs show positive associations, but often others examining the same intervention show conflicting results. At meta-analysis, only external pancreatic duct drainage reduces rates of all- and clinically relevant POPF (28). Avoidance of abdominal drainage reduces rates of all-POPF, but it is likely that this is an effect of failing to detect biochemical POPFs, as rates of clinically relevant POPFs are not reduced and recent RCTs suggest a

higher rate of mortality in patients without abdominal drainage (28). One major problem with the conduct of these trials is that they overestimate the impact of the intervention, leading to underpowered trials and unsurprisingly the majority yield a negative result. For those trials with positive results, frequently the observed effect is not confirmed by further studies.

Despite the lack of clarity over which technique is optimal, it is clear that there is inter-surgeon variation supporting the premise that technique is important (29–31). Risk adjustment with a cumulative sum chart (CUSUM) analysis can be useful to determine if outcomes are expected (*Figure 39.2*).

The impact of these tools is not yet clear, but critical evaluation of surgical technique by individual surgeons could help them critically appraise their outcomes and changes of technique. These tools also allow pooled data and platforms for the conduct of large, real-world trials. In colorectal surgery, for example, standardization of techniques is being evaluated in a similar way.

SURGICAL APPROACH

In pancreatic cancer surgery, radicality is of uttermost importance. As a consequence, early focus on the vascular structures surrounding the pancreas is necessary. If resection is being considered for tumours involving the portomesenteric veins, the venous system must be able to be reconstructed in a way that ensures sufficient venous flow to, and through, the PV.

Regarding the arteries, it is important to be familiar not only with the traditional anatomical configuration, but also to be aware of potential variations. If arteries are involved by the tumour, this must be realised as early as possible during surgery, and in all circumstances prior to 'burning any bridges' where division or sacrificing structures commits the surgeon to completing

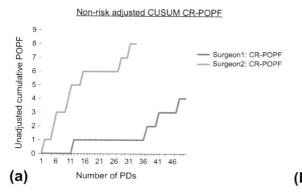
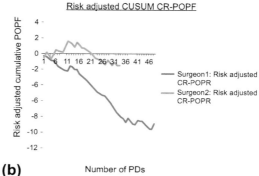

(a)

(b)

Figure 39.2 The importance of risk adjustment using real examples of two surgeons in the same department. The newly-appointed consultant, surgeon 1 (orange line), has a higher rate of clinically-relevant postoperative pancreatic fistula (CR-POPF) than the experienced surgeon 2 (blue line) (a). However, using risk adjustment (see https://paranoiastudy.wixsite.com/website for the method) (b), the outcome of surgeon 1 is acceptable with one fewer occurrence of CR-POPF after operating on 33 patients than expected. Surgeon 2 is the outlier, with 9 fewer cases of CR-POPF than expected, after operating on 49 patients.

the PD. The most reliable way to achieve this is the 'artery-first-approach'. By initially identifying and dissecting the SMA from its origin on the aorta, tumour involvement can be excluded, and this approach also ensures that any SMA bleeding is easy controlled by clamping at its root. In addition, the 'artery-first-approach' ensures complete resection of the station 16 lymph nodes and prepares the surgical field for 'arterial divestment' and extended pancreatoduodenectomy (Heidelberg triangle operation). Arterial divestment refers to the technique of dissecting all the soft tissue, and neuro-lymphatic tissue, off the tunica adventitia of the involved artery using a combination of blunt and sharp dissection (some surgeons also describe the use of energy devices such as bipolar diathermy and the harmonic scalpel). There is also a sub-adventitial technique described by Cai et al. (32), where the plane between the tunica adventitia and the external elastic lamina is identified at the arterial segment, proximal or distal, to the area of tumour involvement, and the dissection performed along the plane superficial to the external elastic lamina. The Heidelberg triangle operation ensures radical tumour removal by sharp dissection along the coeliac axis and SMA, with complete removal of all soft tissue between both arteries and the superior mesenteric and PVs (the right border of the triangle).

ARTERIAL RESECTION

In borderline, and locally-advanced, pancreatic cancers, it is recommended that patients are treated with neoadjuvant chemotherapy (33). If there is no progression during chemotherapy, patients should undergo exploration and if residual tissue surrounding the arteries remains, and is suspicious, frozen samples should be performed prior to deciding on a surgical strategy. In many cases R1/R0 resections can be achieved with arterial divestment, and in a small number of selected cases arterial resection can be performed (34) but this should be in the setting of a previously agreed protocol or a clinical trial.

TECHNICAL ASPECTS OF PANCREATIC AND UPPER ABDOMINAL ARTERIAL SUPPLY

The pancreas is intimately related to major arteries, but technical advances have facilitated the safe performance of increasingly complex surgery and vascular resections. These advances have been largely enabled by neoadjuvant therapies but due to an ageing and increasingly comorbid population (especially cardiovascular issues) a detailed understanding of arterial anatomy and potential limiting pathology is essential for the pancreatic surgeon.

COELIAC STENOSIS

Prior to the ubiquitous availability of computed tomography (CT) scanning, intraoperative assessment of the flow

in the hepatic artery was assessed by initially clamping the gastroduodenal artery, to ensure continued flow to the liver, in case there was a coeliac artery occlusion when the liver would be supplied by flow from the inferior to superior pancreatoduodenal arteries, and then to the hepatic via the gastroduodenal artery. More rarely, coeliac artery compression by the crura of the diaphragm (also known as median arcuate ligament syndrome) is a cause of impaired arterial flow (35). In either situation, ligation of the gastroduodenal artery impairs or completely interrupts hepatic arterial flow, with the subsequent risk of liver failure. Since the advent of CT scans, these features can, and should, be identified preoperatively. It is to be noted that at radiology meetings, the focus is often the vascular network in the immediate vicinity of the pancreas and not at the coeliac axis. The surgeon must be vigilant and ensure that attention is also paid to this area. Coeliac occlusion by atheromatous disease can be explored and treated employing interventional angiographic techniques (36). Surgical treatment is now rarely required and can be associated with high rates of mortality.

ACCIDENTAL DIVISION OF ARTERIES DURING PANCREATODUODENECTOMY

The right- and left-hepatic arteries have an anastomotic network around the central hilar ducts. Thus, accidental or planned, division of one of the hepatic arteries is usually inconsequential if the hilum is preserved (*Figure 39.3*). This explains however, why associated

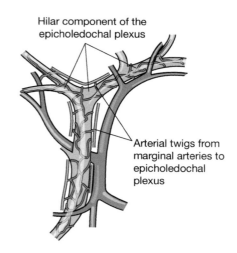

Figure 39.3 Arterial anastomosis around the bile duct and hilum. Note that flow from left- to right-arteries can occur via this network. A planned, or accidental, division of a right- or left-hepatic artery is thus possible without harm in the majority of cases, as long as the remaining hepatic artery is unharmed.

right-hepatic artery injury at cholecystectomy is associated with much worse outcomes when the hilum is also damaged or resected.

Efforts to reconstruct the damaged, or sacrificed, artery are not recommended due to risks of subsequent pseudoaneurysm formation and the increased duration and complexity of the operation. Back bleeding of arterialized blood is invariably seen from the liver side of the cut artery, confirming successful cross-flow of arterial blood (*Figure 39.4*). Division of the common hepatic, coeliac or SMA will almost certainly require reconstruction, with the exception of a divided common hepatic or coeliac axis, if the gastroduodenal artery has not been ligated.

Gastroduodenal artery

During pancreatoduodectomy most surgeons leave the gastroduodenal artery (GDA) stump long. In the event of post-pancreatectomy haemorrhage, bleeding is usually from a pseudoaneurysm of this artery. If there is a sufficient length of preserved stump then it is sometimes possible for the interventional radiologists to embolize the bleeding vessel with coils. An alternative strategy is to occlude the origin of the GDA with a stent, but this approach potentially compromises the patency of the hepatic artery, and a long GDA stump facilitates safer and potentially less invasive options. The falciform ligament, if left long, can be wrapped around the hepatic artery and GDA stump to create a barrier between the stump and the pancreatic anastomosis. An RCT with 445 patients suggests that there may be a reduction in bleeding risk with this strategy (37).

Venous resection

When venous resection may be required to achieve a potentially curative resection, three factors must be considered: 1) Is the disease resectable and constructible? 2) Is a graft required to reconstruct the defect due to the length of vein requiring resection and if so, what is available locally? 3) Finally, what strategies are available to minimize postoperative complications? The definition of unresectable venous disease remains unclear. Long segment involvement and/or occlusion with no reconstruction possible is usually considered an indicator of inoperability, but although the basic principles of vascular surgery must apply, assessment will vary from centre to centre and be influenced by

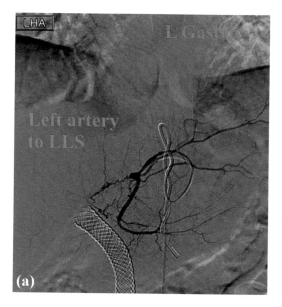
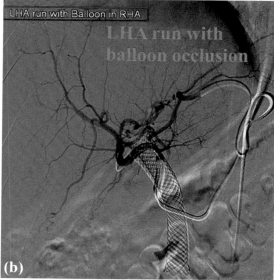

Figure 39.4 This patient had a locally advanced cancer and received neoadjuvant therapy. The main hepatic artery arose from the SMA and was encased in tumour for 4 cm. There was a left-hepatic artery arising from the left-gastric artery. The initial angiogram (a) via the left-gastric artery, only segments 2 and 3 were perfused. The same angiogram (b), but this time with a balloon occlusion of the hepatic artery arising from the SMA. Here, filling of the entire intrahepatic arterial tree was briskly observed and demonstrated excellent cross-flow. At surgery, the major hepatic artery arising from the SMA was ligated at its origin and sacrificed. Intraoperative Doppler demonstrated flow in the intrahepatic right arteries, there was good back bleeding from the distal end of the cut artery and finally, at the end of the operation there was a palpable pulse in the right artery at the hilum.

experience. A defect in the resected vein of 2–3 cm is the maximum that can be brought together with primary anastomosis without a graft. The right liver should be mobilized to the vena cava and that will allow the hilum to come down. If further mobilization is required, a Cattell-Braasch manoeuvre will provide additional mobility and allow tension-free approximation. However, it is important to note that tension on the vein risks sutures cutting through and narrows the vein due to traction along its length. A further consideration is the proximal (SMV) extent of the venous resection, which is more important than the distal, PV component. The distal vein is wide and quite robust, while the SMV is narrower, thinner, and more fragile. The ileal and jejunal branches which form the SMV are even smaller and equally fragile, and any tension on those structures leads to sutures tearing through.

If the splenic and/or inferior mesenteric veins are involved, it is recommended that they are reimplanted into the main portomesenteric vein. This is to enable venous outflow from the bowel and inflow to the liver, which may be useful if the primary anastomosis is in any way compromised (*Figures 39.5* and *39.6*).

It is generally believed that a resection, which would necessarily include the superior mesenteric main branches, is not possible but this is not always true. The reconstruction of one but not both, of the ileal or jejunal branches is feasible with careful technique and the avoidance of any tension and the non-reconstructed branch is sutured/ligated. Venous drainage is enabled via the small bowel arcades and the inferior mesenteric vein. Important considerations when performing venous resections are summarized in *Table 39.1*.

Pancreatic tumours where there is complete PV occlusion with associated varices in the mesentery are considered unresectable. However, if the SMV can be dissected in the mesentery, then a temporary mesentericocaval shunt will allow venous drainage from the small bowel and greatly reduce flow in the varices. A standard resection is then performed, followed by the final-step in the resection which is to ligate the shunt at its insertion to the cava, then upturn the graft and anastomose it to the PV to reinstate hepatic venous flow (*Figure 39.7*).

PV clamping and subsequent resection is associated with an increased risk of PV thrombosis. The risk of venous thrombosis after a PV/SMV resection is estimated to be as high as 21–26% in some series (38–40). There are no published guidelines regarding anticoagulation following venous resection during pancreatic surgery, and no current systematic review. The need for long-term anticoagulation is presently the focus of ongoing international registry work.

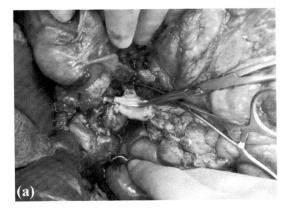

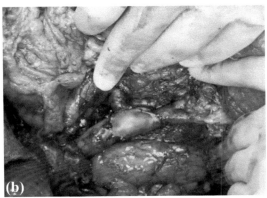

Figure 39.5 Reimplantation of the splenic vein to a vein graft (a – partial reimplantation of the splenic vein complete; b – completed anastomosis). This will optimize venous drainage of the spleen, avoid left upper-quadrant venous hypertension and also provide venous flow to the liver, in the event of a reduction of venous flow from the SMV.

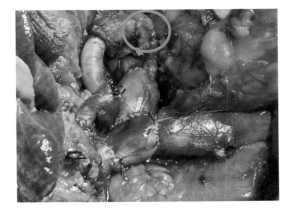

Figure 39.6 Two vein grafts, one to bridge the gap between SMV and PV and one to bridge the gap between the splenic vein and the PV graft. Note the inferior mesenteric vein included in the anastomosis (green circle).

Table 39.1 Important considerations when performing venous resections during pancreaticoduodenectomy

Manoeuvre	Potential complications
Mobilize the liver and if needed small bowel and colon	Avoids tension during reconstruction
Cattell–Braasch manoeuvre	Avoid a complete rotation of the bowel as this will lead to occlusion of the vein graft after the bowel is returned to its normal position
The PV is forgiving, it is wide, and the thickness of its wall makes it robust	The SMV less so and the ileal/jejunal branches of the SMV are very fragile. Avoidance of tension is essential and vein grafts must be immediately available to reduce the clamp time and ensure a successful anastomosis
There is a temptation to perform a wedge resection, rather than full circumferential resection	The former reduces the rate of thrombosis but risks creating an acute angle in the vein, or narrowing, whilst the latter will create a straighter vein
If the splenic and/or inferior mesenteric veins are ligated, it is recommended that they are reimplanted to the main portomesenteric system	This provides alternative routes for venous outflow from the bowel and inflow to the liver

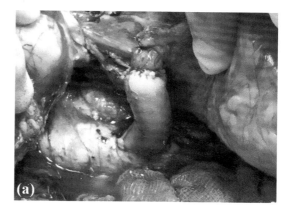

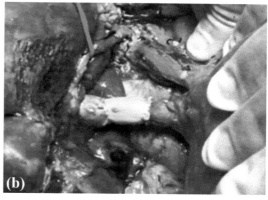

Figure 39.7 Temporary mesenteric-caval shunt for complete occlusion of the PV with associated varices. A vein graft (a) between the SMV in the small bowel mesentery is crated to the vena cava (middle of image). The resection (b) then proceeds, as normal, followed by ligation of the shunt on the cava with the graft upturned and anastomosed to the PV.

CENTRALIZATION OF PANCREATIC SURGICAL SERVICES

Pancreatic surgery is technically challenging, but excellent surgical technique alone does not guarantee good results. Pancreatic units must have a sufficient volume of complex cases and the necessary infrastructure and support to correctly select patients and be able to rapidly recognize and deal with intraoperative and postoperative complications. The value of centralization of pancreatic surgery in high-volume centres is clear with data confirming higher resection rates, a lower incidence of morbidity and mortality and improved long-term survival (41–43).

SUMMARY

The majority of patients with pancreatic cancer have locally-advanced or metastatic disease at presentation. For the 15–20% of patients who are potentially operable with curative intent, a PD is the standard of care and results in an improved 5-year survival of 15–25%. Nevertheless, PD is a complex abdominal procedure and although results have improved, especially in high-volume centres with mortality rates of less than 5%, morbidity remains high at approximately 30–45%.

The number of vascular resections and reconstructions involving the SMV and PV, coeliac axis, SMA, and hepatic artery have significantly increased in the last decade, with the consequence of improved resection rates for pancreatic cancer. Initially, vascular resections raised concerns about increased morbidity and mortality, but despite the increased complication rates, if an R0 resection could be achieved then survival was improved.

More recent results, however, have demonstrated that venous and some arterial resections can be performed with morbidity rates which are equivalent to PD alone. Venous resection is now widely accepted for local involvement of the PV and SMV, but the value of arterial resections in borderline resectable, and locally advanced PDAC, remains controversial. Short- and long-term vessel patency varies with the type of reconstruction, the conduit used, and the surgeon's and unit's experience. Higher resectability rates and satisfactory long-term results have been reported following neoadjuvant therapy for borderline resectable and locally advanced pancreatic cancers which require vascular resection.

REFERENCES

1. Schnelldorfer T, Ware AL, Sarr MG, Smyrk TC, Zhang L, Qin R, et al. Long-term survival after pancreatoduodenectomy for pancreatic adenocarcinoma: Is cure possible? *Ann Surg* 2008;**247**:456–62.
2. Søreide K, Olsen F, Nymo LS, Kleive D, Lassen K. A nationwide cohort study of resection rates and short-term outcomes in open and laparoscopic distal pancreatectomy. *HPB (Oxford)* 2019;**21**:669–78.
3. Asbun HJ, Moekotte AL, Vissers FL, Kunzler F, Cipriani F, Alseidi AD, et al. The Miami International Evidence-based Guidelines on Minimally Invasive Pancreas Resection. *Ann Surg* 2020;**271**:1–14.
4. Vollmer CM, Asbun HJ, Barkun J, Besselink MG, Boggi U, Conlon KCP, et al. Proceedings of the First International State-of-the-Art Conference on Minimally-Invasive Pancreatic Resection (MIPR). *HPB (Oxford)* 2017;**19**:171–7.
5. Abu Hilal M, van Ramshorst TME, Boggi U, Dokmak S, Edwin B, Keck T, et al. The Brescia Internationally Validated European Guidelines on Minimally Invasive Pancreatic Surgery (EGUMIPS). *Ann Surg* 2023;**279(1)**:45–57.
6. Cuschieri A, Jakimowicz JJ, Van Spreeuwel J. Laparoscopic distal 700 pancreatectomy and splenectomy for chronic pancreatitis. *Ann Surg* 1996;**223(3)**: 280–5.
7. Melvin WS, Needleman BJ, Krause KR, Ellison EC. Robotic resection of pancreatic neuroendocrine tumor. *J Laparoendosc Adv Surg Tech A.* 2003;**13**:33–6.
8. NICE. *Guidelines on laparoscopic distal pancreatectomy.* Available from: https://www.nice.org.uk/guidance/ipg204 (Accessed 7 August 2024).
9. Lof S, Moekotte AL, Al-Sarireh B, Ammori B, Aroori S, Durkin D, et al. Multicentre observational cohort study of implementation and outcomes of laparoscopic distal pancreatectomy. *Br J Surg* 2019;**106**:1657–65.
10. Esposito A, Ramera M, Casetti L, De Pastena M, Fontana M, Frigerio I, et al. 401 consecutive minimally invasive distal pancreatectomies: Lessons learned from 20 years of experience. *Surg Endosc* 2022;**36(9)**: 7025–37.
11. Ota M, Asakuma M, Taniguchi K, Ito Y, Komura K, Tanaka T, et al. Short-term outcomes of laparoscopic and open distal pancreatectomy using propensity-score analysis: A real-world retrospective cohort study. *Ann Surg* 2023; **278(4)**: e805-e811.
12. Rehman S, John SKP, Lochan R, Jaques BC, Manas DM, Charnley RM, et al. Oncological feasibility of laparoscopic distal pancreatectomy for adenocarcinoma: A single-institution comparative study. *World J Surg* 2014;**38**:476–83.
13. Björnsson B, Larsson AL, Hjalmarsson C, Gasslander T, Sandström P. Comparison of the duration of hospital stay after laparoscopic or open distal pancreatectomy: Randomized controlled trial. *Br J Surg* 2020;**107**:1281–88.
14. de Rooij T, van Hilst J, van Santvoort H, Boerma D, van den Boezem P, Daams F, et al. Minimally invasive versus open distal pancreatectomy (LEOPARD). *Ann Surg* 2019;**269**:2–9.
15. Korrel M, Jones LR, van Hilst J, Balzano G, Björnsson B, Boggi U, et al. Minimally invasive versus open distal pancreatectomy for resectable pancreatic cancer (DIPLOMA): An international randomised non-inferiority trial. *Lancet Reg Heal – Eur* 2023;**31**: 100673.
16. Kamarajah SK, Sutandi N, Robinson SR, French JJ, White SA. Robotic versus conventional laparoscopic distal pancreatic resection: A systematic review and meta-analysis. *HPB (Oxford)* 2019;**21**:1107–18.
17. Chen JW, van Ramshorst TME, Lof S, Al-Sarireh B, Bjornsson B, Boggi U, et al. Robot-assisted versus laparoscopic distal pancreatectomy in patients with resectable pancreatic cancer: An international, retrospective, cohort study. *Ann Surg Oncol* 2023;**30**:3023–32.
18. Kamarajah SK, Sutandi N, Sen G, Hammond J, Manas DM, French JJ, et al. Comparative analysis of open, laparoscopic and robotic distal pancreatic resection: The United Kingdom's first single-centre experience. *J Minim Access Surg* 2022;**18**:77–83.
19. Shoup M, Brennan MF, McWhite K, Leung DHY, Klimstra D, Conlon KC. The value of splenic preservation with distal pancreatectomy. *Arch Surg* 2002; **137**:164.
20. Sahara K, Tsilimigras DI, Moro A, Mehta R, Dillhoff M, Heidsma CM, et al. Long-term outcomes after spleen-preserving distal pancreatectomy for pancreatic neuroendocrine tumors: Results from the US Neuroendocrine Study Group. *Neuroendocrinology* 2021;**111**:129–38.
21. Kimura W, Fuse A, Hirai I, Suto K, Suzuki A, Moriya T, et al. Spleen-preserving distal pancreatectomy with preservation of the splenic artery and vein for intraductal papillary-mucinous tumor (IPMT): Three interesting cases. *Hepatogastroenterology* 2003;**50**:2242–5.
22. Warshaw AL. Conservation of the spleen with distal pancreatectomy. *Arch Surg* 1988;**123(5)**:550–3.
23. Jain G, Chakravartty S, Patel AG. Spleen-preserving distal pancreatectomy with and without splenic vessel ligation: A systematic review. *HPB (Oxford)* 2013;**15**:403–10.
24. Korrel M, Lof S, Al Sarireh B, Björnsson B, Boggi U, Butturini G, et al. Short-term outcomes after spleen-preserving minimally invasive distal pancreatectomy with or without preservation of splenic vessels. *Ann Surg* 2023;**277**:e119–e125.

25. Gagner M, Pomp A. Laparoscopic pylorus-preserving pancreatoduodenectomy. *Surg Endosc* 1994; **8**:408–10.

26. Giulianotti PC, Coratti A, Angelini M, Sbrana F, Cecconi S, Balestracci T, et al. Robotics in general surgery. *Arch Surg* 2003;**138**:777.

27. van Hilst J, de Rooij T, Bosscha K, Brinkman DJ, van Dieren S, Dijkgraaf MG, et al. Laparoscopic versus open pancreatoduodenectomy for pancreatic or periampullary tumours (LEOPARD-2): A multicentre, patient-blinded, randomised controlled phase 2/3 trial. *Lancet Gastroenterol Hepatol* 2019;**4**: 199–207.

28. Palanivelu C, Senthilnathan P, Sabnis SC, Babu NS, Srivatsan Gurumurthy S, Anand Vijai N, et al. Randomized clinical trial of laparoscopic versus open pancreatoduodenectomy for periampullary tumours. *Br J Surg* 2017;**104**:1443–50. bjs.10662.

29. Poves I, Burdío F, Morató O, Iglesias M, Radosevic A, Ilzarbe L, et al. Comparison of perioperative outcomes between laparoscopic and open approach for pancreatoduodenectomy: The PADULAP randomized controlled trial. *Ann Surg* 2018;**268**:731–9,

30. Wang M, Li D, Chen R, Huang X, Li J, Liu Y, et al. Laparoscopic versus open pancreatoduodenectomy for pancreatic or periampullary tumours: A multicentre, open-label, randomised controlled trial. *Lancet Gastroenterol Hepatol* 2021;**6**:438–47.

31. Kamarajah SK, Bundred J, Marc O, Saint Jiao LR, Manas D, Abu Hilal M, et al. Robotic versus conventional laparoscopic pancreaticoduodenectomy a systematic review and meta-analysis. *Eur J Surg Oncol* 2020;**46**:6–14.

32. Salehi O, Vega EA, Kutlu OC, Alarcon Velasco SV, Krishnan S, Ricklan D, et al. Combining Appleby with RAMPS – laparoscopic radical antegrade modular pancreatosplenectomy with celiac trunk resection. *J Gastrointest Surg* 2020;**24**:2700–01.

33. Napoli N, Kauffmann EF, Menonna F, Iacopi S, Cacace C, Boggi U. Robot-assisted radical antegrade modular pancreatosplenectomy including resection and reconstruction of the spleno-mesenteric junction. *J Vis Exp* 2020;**155**:e60370.

34. Thomaschewski M, Zimmermann M, Honselmann K, Müller-Debus CF, Jacob F, Wellner UF, et al. Robot-assisted distal pancreatectomy with enbloc celiac axis resection (modified Appleby Procedure) after neoadjuvant therapy. *Zentralbl Chir* 2021;**146**:552–9.

35. Giulianotti PC, Addeo P, Buchs NC, Ayloo SM, Bianco FM. Robotic extended pancreatectomy with vascular resection for locally advanced pancreatic tumors. *Pancreas* 2011;**40**:1264–70.

36. Low T-Y, Goh BKP. Initial experience with minimally invasive extended pancreatectomies for locally advanced pancreatic malignancies: Report of six cases. *J Minim Access Surg* 2019;**15**:204–9.

37. Marino MV Latteri MA Ahmad A. Tangential venous resections during robotic-assisted pancreaticoduodenectomy: The results of a case series (with Video). *J Gastrointest Surg* 2020;**24**:1920–21.

38. Kauffmann EF, Napoli N, Menonna F, Vistoli F, Amorese G, Campani D, et al. Robotic pancreatoduodenectomy with vascular resection. *Langenbeck's Arch Surg* 2016;**401**:1111–22.

39. Allan BJ, Novak SM, Hogg ME, Zeh HJ. Robotic vascular resections during Whipple procedure. *J Vis Surg* 2018;**4**:13.

40. Marino MV, Giovinazzo F, Podda M, Gomez Ruiz M, Gomez Fleitas M, Pisanu A, et al. Robotic-assisted pancreaticoduodenectomy with vascular resection. Description of the surgical technique and analysis of early outcomes. *Surg Oncol* 2020;**35**:344–50.

41. Robertson FP, Parks RW. A review of the current evidence for the role of minimally invasive pancreatic surgery following neo-adjuvant chemotherapy. *Laparosc Endosc Robot Surg* 2022;**5**:47–51.

42. Kowalewski K-F, Schmidt MW, Proctor T, Pohl M, Wennberg E, Karadza E, et al. Skills in minimally invasive and open surgery show limited transferability to robotic surgery: Results from a prospective study. *Surg Endosc* 2018;**32**:1656–67.

43. Hogg ME, Besselink MGH, Clavien P-A, Fingerhut A, Jeyarajah DR, Kooby DA, et al. Training in minimally invasive pancreatic resections: A paradigm shift away from "See one, Do one, Teach one". *HPB (Oxford)* 2017;**19**:234–45.

44. Lof S, Claassen L, Hannink G, Al-Sarireh B, Björnsson B, Boggi U, et al. Learning curves of minimally invasive distal pancreatectomy in experienced pancreatic centers. *JAMA Surg* 2023;**158(9)**:927–33.

45. McMillan MT, Malleo G, Bassi C, Sprys MH, Vollmer CM. Defining the practice of pancreatoduodenectomy around the world. *HPB (Oxford)* 2015;**17**:1145–54.

46. Zwart MJW, van den Broek B, de Graaf N, Suurmeijer JA, Augustinus S, te Riele WW, et al. The feasibility, proficiency, and mastery learning curves in 635 robotic pancreatoduodenectomies following a multicenter training program. *Ann Surg* 2023;**278(6)**:e1232–e1241.

47. de Rooij T, van Hilst J, Topal B, Bosscha K, Brinkman DJ, Gerhards MF, et al. Outcomes of a multicenter training program in laparoscopic pancreatoduodenectomy (LAELAPS-2). *Ann Surg* 2019;**269**:344–50.

48. Zwart MJW, Nota CLM, de Rooij T, van Hilst J, Te Riele WW, van Santvoort HC, et al. Outcomes of a multicenter training program in robotic pancreatoduodenectomy (LAELAPS-3). *Ann Surg* 2022;**276**:e886–e895.

49. Joechle K, Conrad C. Cost-effectiveness of minimally invasive pancreatic resection. *J Hepatobiliary Pancreat Sci* 2018;**25**:291–8.

Chapter 40

Minimally Invasive Pancreatic Surgery

Francis P. Robertson and Cheng-Hong Peng

INTRODUCTION

Pancreatic resection remains a key component in the treatment pathways of various benign and malignant diseases (1). As with the majority of many surgical specialties, minimally invasive surgery, in the form of both laparoscopic and more recently robotic assisted, has been introduced to pancreatic surgery. Again, similar to other surgical specialties, minimally invasive pancreatic resection was introduced in a phased fashion with initial attempts preserved for patients with benign disease (mucous cystic neoplasms or neuro-endocrine tumours) and predominantly in patients requiring a distal pancreatectomy without the need for an anastomosis. The incidence of minimally invasive pancreatic surgery (MIPS) varies per unit, but there has been a clear documentation from studies investigating national registry studies of an increase in its use (2). The International Study Group on Minimally Invasive Pancreatic Surgery (I-MIPS) met in Miami in March 2019 (3) and updated the guidelines on the safe implementation of MIPS from Sao Paulo in 2017 (4), highlighting current areas of controversy and areas for future clinical research. This was further updated in Brescia, and the Brescia Internationally Validated European Guidelines on MIPS have been recently published (5). In this chapter we describe the current evidence, trends, outcomes, and controversies in minimally invasive pancreatic resection. Management of necrotic complications from acute pancreatitis has largely shifted towards an endoscopic approach and therefore this chapter focuses on minimally invasive pancreatic resection.

DISTAL PANCREATECTOMY

The first description of a laparoscopic distal pancreatectomy in the medical literature was by Cuschieri et al. in Dundee in 1996, in which he published their experience of laparoscopic distal pancreatectomy for intractable pain in 5 patients with chronic pancreatitis (6) and demonstrated safety combined with a shorter postoperative stay. The first robotic distal pancreatectomy was described in a case report in 2003 (7), with the patient discharged on the 2nd postoperative day. Minimally invasive distal pancreatectomy (MIDP) has become more common. In the UK, the National

Institute of Clinical Excellence (NICE) published guidelines that laparoscopic distal pancreatectomy was a safe and acceptable technique to be used in specialized pancreatic centres (8). A review of the practice in UK centres carried out in 2019 found that post-2009, 46% of distal pancreatectomies were performed laparoscopically, compared to 24% pre-2009 (9). Similarly, a review of the Norwegian national database identified 554 patients and has shown that since 2012, 59% of distal pancreatectomies are now performed laparoscopically, with a significant increase year-on-year (2). This is reflected in a case series carried out in two Italian centres, demonstrating a clear annual increase in the number of minimally invasive procedures performed since 2012 (10).

MIDP has been shown to be a safe technique. A retrospective nationwide review on laparoscopic distal pancreatectomy in Japan demonstrated that the laparoscopic approach was associated with superior short-term outcomes, and the open approach with significantly lower rates of postoperative morbidity, re-operation rates, and length of hospital stay (11). Similar oncological outcomes were seen in a retrospective UK study including lymph node yield, R0 resection rates and 3-year survival rates (12). Results from two prospective, randomized clinical trials (RCTs) (*Table 40.1*) comparing laparoscopic and open distal pancreatectomy have shown that laparoscopic distal pancreatectomy carries similar morbidity rates as open distal pancreatectomy (13,14). The LEOPARD trial included both benign and malignant lesions and demonstrated a lower length of stay (6 [4–7] days vs. 8 [6–9] days, p < 0.001) with better overall quality of life, up to 30 days postoperatively in patients undergoing laparoscopic distal pancreatectomy (14). More recently, the DIPLOMA trial which was recently published included 258 patients from 35 centres across Europe. Patients were randomly assigned to either open, distal pancreatectomy or minimally invasive (laparoscopic or robotic). This study has demonstrated that MIDP was comparable in terms of R0 resections (73% vs. 69%) with similar lymph node yield (22.0 [16.0–30.0] nodes vs. 23.0 [14.0–32.0] nodes, p = 0.86) and risk of intraperitoneal recurrence (41% vs. 38%, p = 0.45) (15). There is now a growing body of evidence (level 1) to support the use of MIDP, as it is associated with improved short-term outcomes and similar oncological outcomes.

DOI: 10.1201/9781003080060-40

A meta-analysis comparing laparoscopic and robotic distal pancreatectomy demonstrated a reduced risk of conversion in robotic surgery (8% vs. 21%, p < 0.0001) and a reduced hospital stay by 1-day (16). However, this was offset by a lengthier procedure. An international retrospective cohort study carried out by the European Consortium on Minimally Invasive Pancreatic Surgery (E-MIPS), compared 542 patients undergoing MIDP across 33 European centres and found that the robotic approach was associated with a longer operating time (290 min vs. 240 min, p < 0.001] and hospital stay (10 days vs. 8 days, p < 0.001), and more major complications (22.6% vs. 16.3%, p = 0.019]. There was a higher rate of vascular resection performed robotically (7.6% vs. 2.7%, p = 0.03) and a lower conversion rate (4.9% vs. 17.3%, p = 0.001). The R0, 90-day mortality and overall survival rates were similar between the groups (17). A single-centre study from the UK compared their experience of open, laparoscopic and robotic distal pancreatectomies in 125 patients. They demonstrated that robotic surgery was associated with a higher rate of splenic preservation (30% vs. 2%, p < 0.001) and a shorter operating time than laparoscopic surgery

(284 min vs. 300 min, p < 0.001). Patients undergoing robotic surgery had a shorter length of hospital stay (8 days vs. 9 days vs. 10 days, p = 0.001) (18). There is currently insufficient published evidence to support the use of robotic surgery over a laparoscopic approach. In the author's institution a robotic approach is preferred, and it is likely that it provides a greater possibility of splenic-preserving surgery and the ability to progress to more complicated resections, including major vascular resections.

Spleen preserving distal pancreatectomy

In patients undergoing distal pancreatectomy (DP) for reasons other than pancreatic malignancy, splenic preservation is associated with a reduction in postoperative morbidity, particularly infective complications (19) and equivalent long-term oncological outcomes in patients with neuroendocrine tumours (20). Splenic preservation during distal pancreatectomy can be performed using either the Kimura technique, where the splenic vessels are preserved (21), or the Warshaw technique, where the splenic vessels are resected as part of the specimen,

Table 40.1 Published RCTs in minimally invasive distal pancreatectomy

Study	Year of publication	Country	Patients	Procedures			Main outcomes
				Open	Laparoscopic	Robotic	
Bjornsson et al. (13)	2020	Sweden	58	29	29	n/a	• Hospital stay ⇓ 1 day • Functional recovery ⇓ 3 days • Blood loss ⇓ 50 mL • Length of surgery ⇔ • Complications ⇔
De Rooij et al. (14)	2019	Netherlands	102	42	5	55	• Functional recovery ⇓ 2 days • Quality of life (3–30 days) ⇓ • Conversion rate 8% • Blood loss ⇓ 250 mL • Operative time ⇑ 38 min • Complications ⇓ 13% • Postoperative pancreatic fistula (B/C) ⇑ 16% • Delayed gastric emptying ⇓ 14%
Korrel et al. (15)	2023	Europe	227	110	86	31	• Functional recovery ⇔ • Conversion rate 12% • Overall survival ⇔ • R0 resection ⇔ • Lymph node yield ⇔ • Serious adverse events ⇓ 4%

⇓ Improved outcomes in minimally invasive group.
⇑ Poorer outcomes in minimally invasive group.
⇔ No difference.

and the short gastric vessels are preserved to supply the spleen (22). To-date, no RCT exists comparing the short- and long-term outcomes of either technique. The Warshaw technique is easier to perform, however. A systematic review published in 2013 found a higher incidence of splenic infarction (22% vs. 2%, p < 0.001) and resulting splenectomy (2% vs. 0%, p = 0.001) (23). A more recent multicentre study by E-MIPS across 29 European centres demonstrated equivalent short-term outcomes between the techniques with similar rates of clinically relevant splenic ischaemia (0.6% vs. 1.6%, p = 0.127) (24).

Spleen preserving distal pancreatectomy should therefore be considered in all suitable patients, including those undergoing surgery for chronic pancreatitis, mucinous cystic neoplasms, and neuroendocrine tumours. There is no strong evidence to support either technique for splenic preservation over others, and this therefore comes down to individual preference and experience.

PANCREATODUODENECTOMY

The first laparoscopic pancreaticoduodenectomy was described in a case report of a single patient with chronic pancreatitis by Gagner and Pomp in 1994 (25) and demonstrated feasibility, but no difference in outcomes. The first robotic pancreaticoduodenectomy was described in 2001 (26). In this study they described eight procedures, but the first six were performed as a combination of laparoscopic resection and robotic reconstruction. The final two cases in the series were performed fully robotically, so meaningful conclusions cannot be taken. This, however, does represent an example of the learning curve required in the more complex resections. The introduction of minimally invasive pancreatoduodenectomy has not been without controversy. The LEOPARD-2 study was a RCT investigating laparoscopic pancreaticoduodenectomy versus open, but had to be stopped prematurely due to excess 90-day mortality (10%) in the laparoscopic group (27). Further studies, however, have demonstrated conflicting results with a shorter hospital stay (7 days vs. 13 days, p = 0.001) and similar complication rates between the groups (28). Equal, oncological outcomes, were seen between the groups including lymph node yield and R0 resection rates. Results from the PADULAP trial were similar and demonstrated a shorter hospital stay (13.5 days vs. 17 days, p = 0.024) and equivalent complication rates, lymph node yield, and resection margin status between the groups (29). The largest trial from China included 656 patients (328 laparoscopic and 328 open), and has again confirmed equivalent morbidity and mortality between the procedures, with a significantly shorter postoperative stay (15 days vs. 16 days, p = 0.02) (30).

Despite initial reservations following the LEOPARD-2 trial, there is growing evidence to support the use of a minimally invasive approach in suitable patients undergoing pancreatoduodenectomy, as long

as the surgeons' experience is sufficient (level 2) (*Table 40.2*). No randomized trial has yet been carried out that compares laparoscopic and robot pancreatoduodenectomy. A meta-analysis of non-randomized studies has shown a lower rate of conversion in the robotic group (odds ratio [OR] 0.41 [0.30–0.57]) and a reduced hospital stay by 1 day (31). There is, therefore, insufficient evidence to support the use of one approach over the other. This depends on the individual surgeon's preference and the equipment available.

Vascular resections and neoadjuvant chemotherapy

A perceived benefit of the introduction of robotic pancreatic surgery is the ability to progress to more complex resections, including vascular resection for advanced tumours. The published data on vascular resections in MIDP is limited to case reports (32–34) and small case series (35,36), as is the case with pancreatoduodenectomy (36–40). As such, there is currently insufficient evidence to comment on safety and the role of minimally invasive vascular resections in patients undergoing pancreatic resection.

There has been a paradigm shift, in the management of patients with pancreatic ductal adenocarcinoma, to the delivery of upfront chemotherapy which is associated with a more difficult pancreatoduodenectomy. A systematic review has analysed the current evidence for minimally invasive pancreatic resection following neoadjuvant chemotherapy (41). This included eight studies and concluded that the current evidence base was poor, but that there was evidence that it could be performed safely in high-volume centres with good patient selection.

LEARNING CURVE

Much consideration has been given to training in MIPS and whether skills are transferable between different approaches (42). It is accepted that, between 50–80 pancreaticoduodenectomies are required to surpass the training curve (43).

Distal pancreatectomy

A retrospective review of outcomes in MIDP in European centres demonstrated a learning curve of 85 procedures to achieve textbook outcomes or mastery (44). With earlier time points required for operative time (laparoscopic 16, robotic 15) and complications (laparoscopic 25, robotic 40) (5). A review of training numbers in US residency programmes has shown that many fellows will not achieve this number in open resections (45), let alone minimally invasive pancreatic resection (43). In 2014, a 1-year nationwide training programme in MIDP was initiated in the Netherlands. This demonstrated a seven–fold increase in the use of a minimally invasive route and a significant increase in

Table 40.2 Published RCTs in minimally invasive pancreatoduodenectomy

Study	Year of publication	Country	Patients	Procedures			Main outcomes
				Open	Laparoscopic	Robotic	
Van Hilst et al. (27)	2019	Netherlands	99	50	49	n/a	• 90-day mortality ⇑ 8% • Trial stopped early due to safety concerns • Functional recovery ⇑ 2 days • Complications ⇑ 11% • Postoperative pancreatic fistula (B/C) ⇔
Palanivelu et al. (28)	2017	India	64	32	32	n/a	• Hospital stay ⇓ 6 days • Conversion rate 3% • Blood loss ⇓ 150 mL • Operative time ⇑ 39 min • Complications ⇔ • Postoperative pancreatic fistula (B/C) ⇔ • Delayed gastric emptying ⇔
Poves et al. (29)	2018	Spain	66	32	34	n/a	• Hospital stay ⇓ 3.5 days • Conversion rate 24% • Operative time ⇑ 119 min • Complications ⇓ 19% • R0 resection ⇔ • Lymph node yield ⇔ • Serious adverse events ⇓ 4%
Wang et al. (30)	2021	China	656	328	328	n/a	• Hospital stay ⇓ 1 day • Conversion rate 4% • Operative time ⇑ 25 min • Complications ⇔ • 90-day mortality ⇔ • Blood loss ⇓ 100 mL • Postoperative pancreatic fistula (B/C) ⇔ • Delayed gastric emptying ⇔

⇓ Improved outcomes in minimally invasive group.

⇑ Poorer outcomes in minimally invasive group.

⇔ No difference.

its use for patients with adenocarcinoma (20% vs. 10%, p = 0.03). Conversion rates, blood loss, and length of hospital stay were significantly reduced over this time period.

Pancreatoduodenectomy

The training curve for pancreatoduodenectomy has been described as 84 procedures to achieve mastery or textbook outcomes (46). With earlier time points required for operative time (laparoscopic 25; robotic 21) and complications (laparoscopic 25–80; robotic 25–40) (5).

A minimally invasive training programme was initiated in laparoscopic (47) and robotic (48) pancreatoduodenectomy in the Netherlands, and demonstrated that with sufficient training this can be carried out with acceptable morbidity and mortality rates. These training programmes include a mixture of video tutorial, simulation and proctorship. The introduction of the robot with dual-platform operating and the robotic simulator bring a fantastic opportunity for early training and the optimizing of surgical outcomes in these procedures that may be associated with a higher risk of major morbidity.

COST EFFECTIVENESS OF MINIMALLY INVASIVE PANCREATIC SURGERY

A perceived, increased perioperative cost, has been associated with minimally invasive surgery. A systematic review included 14 studies analysing the cost effectiveness of laparoscopic, open distal pancreatectomy, and pancreatoduodenectomy. The review demonstrated that higher operative costs were outweighed by reduced postoperative costs, and the laparoscopic route represented a cost saving of on average $2,008 for distal pancreatectomies and $1,268 for pancreatoduodenectomies (49).

SUMMARY

There is strong evidence (level 2) to support non-inferiority of minimally invasive pancreatic resection, for both distal pancreatectomy and pancreatoduodenectomy, in terms of postoperative complications and long-term oncological outcomes. Results from well-designed RCTs have confirmed that minimally invasive pancreatic resection is associated with favourable short-term outcomes, including reduced length of stay and faster return to functional status.

The training curve for minimally invasive pancreatic resection is long, but is feasible in high-volume centres. The introduction of nationwide training programmes, such as those introduced in the Netherlands, has allowed the safe introduction of robotic pancreatic surgery, ensuring optimal outcomes for patients during the incorporation of this novel, and exciting, surgical approach.

REFERENCES

1. Schnelldorfer T, Ware AL, Sarr MG, Smyrk TC, Zhang L, Qin R, et al. Long-term survival after pancreatoduodenectomy for pancreatic adenocarcinoma: Is cure possible? *Ann Surg* 2008;**247**:456–62.
2. Søreide K, Olsen F, Nymo LS, Kleive D, Lassen K. A nationwide cohort study of resection rates and short-term outcomes in open and laparoscopic distal pancreatectomy. *HPB (Oxford)* 2019;**21**:669–78.
3. Asbun H J, Moekotte AL, Vissers FL, Kunzler F, Cipriani F, Alseidi AD, et al. The Miami International Evidence-based Guidelines on minimally invasive pancreas resection. *Ann Surg* 2020;**271**:1–14.
4. Vollmer C M, Asbun HJ, Barkun J, Besselink MG, Boggi U, Conlon KCP, et al. Proceedings of the first international state-of-the-art conference on minimally-invasive pancreatic resection (MIPR). *HPB (Oxford)* 2017;**19**:171–77.
5. Abu Hilal M, van Ramshorst TME, Boggi U, Dokmak S, Edwin B, Keck T, et al. The Brescia Internationally Validated European Guidelines on minimally invasive pancreatic surgery (EGUMIPS). *Ann Surg* 2023;**279(1)**:45–57.
6. Cuschieri A, Jakimowicz JJ, Van Spreeuwel J. Laparoscopic distal 700 pancreatectomy and splenectomy for chronic pancreatitis. *Ann Surg* 1996;**223(3)**:280–5.
7. Melvin WS, Needleman BJ, Krause KR, Ellison EC. Robotic resection of pancreatic neuroendocrine tumor. *J Laparoendosc Adv Surg Tech A* 2003;**13**:33–6.
8. Laparoscopic distal pancreatectomy | Guidance |NICE, 2007. Available from: https://www.nice.org.uk/guidance/ipg204 (Accessed 2 September 2024).
9. Lof S, Moekotte AL, Al-Sarireh B, Ammori B, Aroori S, Durkin D, et al. Multicentre observational cohort study of implementation and outcomes of laparoscopic distal pancreatectomy. *Br J Surg* 2019;**106**:1657–65.
10. Esposito A, Ramera M, Casetti L, De Pastena M, Fontana M, Frigerio I, et al. 401 consecutive minimally invasive distal pancreatectomies: Lessons learned from 20 years of experience. *Surg Endosc* 2022;**36**:7025–37.
11. Ota M, Asakuma M, Taniguchi K, Ito Y, Komura K, Tanaka T, Y. et al. Short-term outcomes of laparoscopic and open distal pancreatectomy using propensity-score analysis: A real-world retrospective cohort study. *Ann Surg* 2023;**278(4)**:e805–e811.
12. Rehman S, John SKP, Lochan R, Jaques BC, Manas DM, Charnley RM, et al. Oncological feasibility of laparoscopic distal pancreatectomy for adenocarcinoma: A single-institution comparative study. *World J Surg* 2014;**38**:476–83.
13. Björnsson B, Larsson AL, Hjalmarsson C, Gasslander T, Sandström P. Comparison of the duration of hospital stay after laparoscopic or open distal pancreatectomy: randomized controlled trial. *Br J Surg* 2020;**107**:1281–88.
14. de Rooij T, van Hilst J, van Santvoort H, Boerma D, van den Boezem P, Daams F, et al. Minimally invasive versus open distal pancreatectomy (LEOPARD). *Ann Surg* 2019;**269**:2–9.
15. Korrel M, Jones LR, van Hilst J, Balzano G, Björnsson B, Boggi U, et al. Minimally invasive versus open distal pancreatectomy for resectable pancreatic cancer (DIPLOMA): an international randomised non-inferiority trial. *Lancet Reg Heal Eur* 2023;**31**:100673.
16. Kamarajah SK, Sutandi N, Robinson SR, French JJ, White SA. Robotic versus conventional laparoscopic distal pancreatic resection: A systematic review and meta-analysis. *HPB (Oxford)* 2019;**21**:1107–18.
17. Chen JW, van Ramshorst TME, Lof S, Al-Sarireh B, Bjornsson B, Boggi U, et al. Robot-assisted versus laparoscopic distal pancreatectomy in patients with resectable pancreatic cancer: An international, retrospective, cohort study. *Ann Surg Oncol* 2023;**30**:3023–32.
18. Kamarajah SK, Sutandi N, Sen G, Hammond J, Manas DM, French JJ, et al. Comparative analysis of open, laparoscopic and robotic distal pancreatic resection: The United Kingdom's first single-centre experience. *J Minim Access Surg* 2022;**18**:77–83.

19. Shoup M, Brennan MF, McWhite K, Leung DHY, Klimstra D, Conlon KC. The value of splenic preservation with distal pancreatectomy. *Arch Surg* 2002;**137**:164.

20. Sahara K, Tsilimigras DI, Moro A, Mehta R, Dilhoff M, Heidsma CM, et al. Long-term outcomes after spleen-preserving distal pancreatectomy for pancreatic neuroendocrine tumors: Results from the US Neuroendocrine Study Group. *Neuroendocrinology* 2021;**111**:129–38.

21. Kimura W, Fuse A, Hirai I, Suto K, Suzuki A, Moriya T, et al. Spleen-preserving distal pancreatectomy with preservation of the splenic artery and vein for intraductal papillary-mucinous tumor (IPMT): Three interesting cases. *Hepatogastroenterology* 2003;**50**:2242–5.

22. Warshaw AL. Conservation of the spleen with distal pancreatectomy. Arch Surg 1988;123:550–3.

23. Jain G, Chakravartty S, Patel AG. Spleen-preserving distal pancreatectomy with and without splenic vessel ligation: A systematic review. *HPB (Oxford)* 2013;**15**:403–10.

24. Korrel M, Lof S, Al Sarireh B, Björnsson B, Boggi U, Butturini G, et al. Short-term outcomes after spleen-preserving minimally invasive distal pancreatectomy with or without preservation of splenic vessels. *Ann Surg* 2023;**277**:e119–e25.

25. Gagner M, Pomp A. Laparoscopic pylorus-preserving pancreatoduodenectomy. *Surg Endosc* 1994;**8**:408–10.

26. Giulianotti PC, Coratti A, Angelini M, Sbrana F, Cecconi S, Balestracci T, et al. Robotics in general surgery. *Arch Surg* 2003;**138**:777.

27. van Hilst J, de Rooij T, Bosscha K, Brinkman DJ, van Dieren S, Dijkgraaf MG, et al. Laparoscopic versus open pancreatoduodenectomy for pancreatic or periampullary tumours (LEOPARD-2): A multicentre, patient-blinded, randomised controlled phase 2/3 trial. *Lancet Gastroenterol Hepatol* 2019;**4**: 199–207.

28. Palanivelu C, Senthilnathan P, Sabnis SC, Babu NS, Srivatsan Gurumurthy S, Anand Vijai N, et al. Randomized clinical trial of laparoscopic versus open pancreatoduodenectomy for periampullary tumours. *Br J Surg* 2017;**104**:1443–50.

29. Poves I, Burdío F, Morató O, Iglesias M, Radosevic A, Ilzarbe L, et al. Comparison of perioperative outcomes between laparoscopic and open approach for pancreatoduodenectomy: The PADULAP randomized controlled trial. *Ann Surg* 2018;**268**:731–9.

30. Wang M, Li D, Chen R, Huang X, Li J ,Liu Y, et al. Laparoscopic versus open pancreatoduodenectomy for pancreatic or periampullary tumours: A multicentre, open-label, randomised controlled trial. *Lancet Gastroenterol Hepatol* 2021;**6**:438–47.

31. Kamarajah SK, Bundred J, Marc O, Saint Jiao LR, Manas D, Abu Hilal M, et al. Robotic versus conventional laparoscopic pancreaticoduodenectomy: A systematic review and meta-analysis. *Eur J Surg Oncol* 2020;**46**:6–14.

32. Salehi O, Vega EA, Kutlu OC, Alarcon Velasco SV, Krishnan S, Ricklan D, et al. Combining Appleby with RAMPS – laparoscopic radical antegrade modular pancreatosplenectomy with celiac trunk resection. *J Gastrointest Surg* 2020;**24**:2700–1.

33. Napoli N, Kauffmann EF, Menonna F, Iacopi S, Cacace C, Boggi U. Robot-assisted radical antegrade modular pancreatosplenectomy including resection and reconstruction of the spleno-mesenteric junction. *J Vis Exp* 2020;e60370.

34. Thomaschewski M, Zimmermann M, Honselmann K, Müller-Debus CF, Jacob F, Wellner UF, et al. Robot-assisted distal pancreatectomy with enbloc celiac axis resection (modified Appleby Procedure) after neoadjuvant therapy. *Zentralbl Chir* 2021;**146**:552–9.

35. Giulianotti PC, Addeo P, Buchs NC, Ayloo SM, Bianco FM. Robotic extended pancreatectomy with vascular resection for locally advanced pancreatic tumors. *Pancreas* 2011;**40**:1264–70.

36. Low T-Y, Goh BKP. Initial experience with minimally invasive extended pancreatectomies for locally advanced pancreatic malignancies: Report of six cases. *J Minim Access Surg* 2019;**15**:204–9.

37. Marino MV Latteri MA Ahmad A. Tangential venous resections during robotic-assisted pancreaticoduodenectomy: The results of a case series (with Video). *J Gastrointest Surg* 2020;**24**:1920–21.

38. Kauffmann EF, Napoli N, Menonna F, Vistoli F, Amorese G, Campani D, et al. Robotic pancreatoduodenectomy with vascular resection. *Langenbeck's Arch Surg* 2016;**401**:1111–22.

39. Allan BJ, Novak SM, Hogg ME, Zeh HJ. Robotic vascular resections during Whipple procedure. *J Vis Surg* 2018;**4**:13.

40. Marino MV, Giovinazzo F, Podda M, Gomez Ruiz M, Gomez Fleitas M, Pisanu A, et al. Robotic-assisted pancreaticoduodenectomy with vascular resection. Description of the surgical technique and analysis of early outcomes. *Surg Oncol* 2020;**35**:344–50.

41. Robertson FP, Parks RW. A review of the current evidence for the role of minimally invasive pancreatic surgery following neo-adjuvant chemotherapy. *Laparosc Endosc Robot Surg* 2022;**5**:47–51.

42. Kowalewski K-F, Schmidt MW, Proctor T, Pohl M, Wennberg E, Karadza E, et al. Skills in minimally invasive and open surgery show limited transferability to robotic surgery: Results from a prospective study. *Surg Endosc* 2018;**32**:1656–67.

43. Hogg ME, Besselink MGH, Clavien P-A, Fingerhut A, Jeyarajah DR, Kooby DA, Moser AJ, et al. Training in minimally invasive pancreatic resections: A paradigm shift away from "See one, Do one, Teach one". *HPB (Oxford)* 2017;**19**:234–245.

44. Lof S, Claassen L, Hannink G, Al-Sarireh B, Björnsson B, Boggi U, et al. Learning curves of minimally invasive distal pancreatectomy in experienced pancreatic centers. *JAMA Surg* 2023;**158(9)**:927–33.

45. McMillan MT, Malleo G, Bassi C, Sprys MH, Vollmer CM. Defining the practice of pancreatoduodenectomy around the world. *HPB (Oxford)* 2015;**17**:1145–54.

46. Zwart MJW, van den Broek B, de Graaf N, Suurmeijer JA, Augustinus S, Te Riele WW, et al. The feasibility, proficiency, and mastery learning curves

in 635 robotic pancreatoduodenectomies following a multicenter training program. *Ann Surg* 2023;**278**(6):e1232–e1241.

47. de Rooij T, van Hilst J, Topal B, Bosscha K, Brinkman DJ, Gerhards MF, et al. Outcomes of a multicenter training program in laparoscopic pancreatoduodenectomy (LAELAPS-2). *Ann Surg* 2019:**269**:344–50.

48. Zwart MJW, Nota CLM, de Rooij T, van Hilst J, Te Riele WW, van Santvoort HC, et al. Outcomes of a multicenter training program in robotic pancreatoduodenectomy (LAELAPS-3). *Ann Surg* 2022;**276**:e886–e95.

49. Joechle K, Conrad C. Cost-effectiveness of minimally invasive pancreatic resection. *J Hepatobiliary Pancreat Sci* 2018;**25**:291–8.

Chapter
41

Management of Surgical Complications Following Pancreatectomy

Donna Marie L. Alvino and Tara S. Kent

INTRODUCTION

With the rise of pancreatectomy: pancreaticoduo-denectomy (PD); distal pancreatectomy (DP); and total pancreatectomy (TP) as a mainstay of treatment for numerous pancreatic pathologies, including benign and malignant lesions, as well as pancreatitis, it has become increasingly important for surgeons to accurately anticipate, identify, and effectively manage the most commonly encountered surgical complications in this setting. This is especially true as pancreatic surgery still has a significant, associated morbidity, despite an overall decline in operative mortality in recent decades. When faced with the most frequent and most dreaded complications of pancreatectomy, including delayed gastric emptying (DGE), postoperative pancreatic fistula, and post-pancreatectomy hemorrhage, fundamental knowledge of the aetiologies, risk factors, preventive measures and management strategies associated with each, is required. In reviewing several well-known complications of pancreatectomy in detail, this chapter seeks to provide surgeons with contemporary evidence to guide decision-making for post-pancreatectomy patients.

Prior to the late 19th century, surgical intervention for pancreatic pathology remained largely theoretical, in part, because related anatomical knowledge was limited at the time. Early segmental pancreatic resections performed by Billroth and Senn in the 1880s paved the way for surgical intervention as a mainstay of treatment for pancreatic neoplasms, cysts, trauma, and pancreatitis (1). Despite this longstanding history of exploration into pancreatic surgical resection, pancreatectomy remains one of the most complex, and technically challenging, procedures for surgeons.

Mortality, following pancreatic resection, has drastically fallen over the years to approximately 1%. This follows centralization of complex pancreatic surgery to high-volume centers equipped to provide the necessary multidisciplinary and critical care (2–4). But postoperative morbidity remains quite high, with complications occurring in up to 50% of cases (5–6). In the face of such statistics, surgeons must have a clear understanding of their approach to the identification, and management,

of the most frequent complications encountered following pancreatic resection.

The term 'pancreatectomy' is broad, and denotes a wide range of procedures related to pancreatic resection, which vary depending on the site and nature of the pathology. Within the context of this chapter, pancreatectomy refers to several major types of pancreatic resection: PD; DP with, or without, splenectomy; and TP. Central pancreatectomy (CP) is **not** separately addressed. Indications for these procedures are numerous, ranging from pancreatic malignancies and cystic pancreatic lesions to chronic pancreatitis. The choice of procedure is primarily dictated by diagnosis and disease location within the organ. Similarly, complications following pancreatectomy are often procedurally related, and a better understanding of this topic can help surgeons improve postoperative management strategies. This chapter will outline the most frequently encountered surgical complications following pancreatectomy, and discuss relevant diagnostic and management approaches.

DELAYED GASTRIC EMPTYING

DGE ranks as one of the most common complications following pancreatectomy, with reported incidence rates of 15–61% (7–9). The occurrence of DGE following PD was first described in the 1980s, as a state of gastroparesis requiring prolonged gastric decompression and delay in oral food tolerance potentially necessitating nutritional support (10). More recently, the International Study Group in Pancreatic Surgery (ISGPS) developed a standardized definition of DGE to allow a common language in research efforts investigating complication rates and outcomes of new operative approaches and techniques (7).

In the confirmed absence of mechanical obstruction, via imaging or endoscopic studies, DGE is diagnosed and classified based upon its clinical course and postoperative management with respect to symptoms: nausea and vomiting; by mouth (PO) intolerance; time to solid food intake; duration of nasogastric tube (NGT) decompression; NGT reinsertion in the immediate postoperative period (*Table 41.1*) (7). While DGE grade A (mild) does not typically influence hospital

DOI: 10.1201/9781003080060-41

Table 41.1 Consensus definition of DGE after pancreatic surgery*

DGE grade	NGT required	Unable to tolerate solid oral intake by POD	Vomiting/ gastric distention	Use of prokinetics
A	4–7 days or reinsertion >POD 3	7	±	±
B	8–14 days or reinsertion >POD 7	14	+	+
C	>14 days or reinsertion >POD 14	21	+	+

Abbreviations : DGE: delayed gastric emptying; POD: postoperative day; NGT: nasogastric tube.

Note: To exclude mechanical causes of abnormal gastric emptying, the patency of either the gastrojejunostomy of the deodenojejunostomy should be confirmed by endoscopy or upper gastrointestinal gastrograffin series.

* Table adapted from (7).

discharge, grade B (moderate) requires adjustment of patient's clinical pathway, and grade C (severe) often necessitates major changes in clinical management, potentially including parenteral nutrition, and leads to a significant prolongation of hospital stay and delays in adjuvant chemotherapy (7,11). When considering the negative impact on hospital costs and patient outcomes, in relation to increased length of stay (12) and postponement of adjuvant treatments (13), the need to efficiently identify and treat patients with postoperative DGE becomes apparent.

Despite the fact that DGE is among the most commonly encountered postoperative complications following pancreatectomy, the mechanisms leading to DGE are not entirely understood. Intra-abdominal complications, such as anastomotic leak at the pancreaticojejunostomy (PJ) or abscess formation, have been described as causes for DGE in relevant patient subsets (14,15). Decreased plasma motilin levels following duodenal resection, extended lymph node dissection with disruption of antropyloric innervation, and relative devascularization of the pylorus during pylorus-preserving PD (PPPD) have also been described (7,16,17). In considering an operative approach, studies have demonstrated variable rates of DGE when comparing PPPD versus classic PD (16–21), antecolic versus retrocolic gastric drainage reconstruction (8,22), or Billroth II versus Roux-en-Y reconstruction (9,23). Preoperative risk factors for DGE following pancreatectomy include: patient age; male sex; ASA class; BMI; increased operative time; intraoperative blood loss, among others (13,24).

By understanding the perioperative factors influencing DGE, surgeons can appropriately anticipate and address this clinical challenge. In pancreatectomy involving duodenal resection (PD or TP), prophylactic initiation of a prokinetic agent, such as erythromycin, has been shown to reduce postoperative rates of DGE by up to 75% (25), and metoclopramide may also be used. Balzano et al. discovered that patients enrolled in a fast-track recovery program following PD, including earlier postoperative feeding and mobilization, had

significantly lower rates of DGE compared with their unenrolled counterparts (13.9% vs. 24.6%) (26), while other studies have demonstrated an increased association of DGE with early, enteral feeding (27,28). The authors have a strong preference for early feeding and self-regulation by patients, as long as clinically appropriate.

The mainstay of treatment for DGE following pancreatectomy involves NGT decompression combined with use of promotility agents as needed (25,29), assuming that mechanical obstruction has been excluded. At our institution, NGT removal typically occurs on postoperative day 2 (POD2), unless the patient's clinical status precludes this step, and prokinetic agents are routinely initiated. In cases of DGE grade B or C, supplemental nutrition should be considered either enterally via nasojejunal tube, or an intraoperatively placed jejunostomy tube, parenterally with the use of TPN, or a combination of both (29). Enteral access should be the preferred route of nutrition administration, whenever possible, and intraoperative placement of a feeding jejunostomy tube should be considered in patients at high risk of malnutrition and postoperative DGE (30). Earlier recognition and intervention for DGE, via initiation of supplemental nutrition, has been associated with earlier return to regular diet, decreased hospital readmissions, and decreased hospital costs (29).

POSTOPERATIVE PANCREATIC FISTULA

Clinically relevant postoperative pancreatic fistula (POPF) remains a highly morbid and costly complication of pancreatectomy, with estimated incidence rates between 3–45% at high-volume centers (12,31), and an associated mortality rate of ~1% in recent decades (32). Moreover, POPF development after pancreatectomy for pancreatic ductal adenocarcinoma (PDAC) is one of the strongest predictors of failing to receive adjuvant chemotherapy, with significant implications for patient survival (33). In the updated guidelines published by the ISGPS in 2016, clinically relevant POPF is defined as 'an abnormal communication between the pancreatic ductal system and another epithelial surface containing pancreas-derived, enzyme-rich fluid' (7). Current POPF classification parameters are outlined in *Table 41.2* (31). Grade A POPF has been re-classified as 'biochemical leak' given its overall lack of clinical impact on the patient's course, while grade B necessitates changes in postoperative management (duration of drain placement, drain repositioning), and grade C requires reoperation or directly leads to organ failure and/or mortality.

Numerous predisposing factors, attributed to POPF formation, have been utilized in formulating highly predictive fistula risk scores to help surgeons anticipate, manage and even determine financial outcomes for POPF (34–37). Patient factors, such as male sex, advanced age, increased BMI, coronary artery disease, and poor nutritional status, are predictive of POPF, while a history of diabetes mellitus and neoadjuvant therapy seem to confer some protective benefit (3,38–40). Disease-related risk factors include small pancreatic duct diameter, soft gland texture, and high-risk disease pathology (34–35). Additionally, operative time, intraoperative blood loss and surgeon experience all variably impact the risk of POPF (35–38). Procedure-specific factors, such as pancreatico-enteric reconstruction (pancreaticogastrostomy vs. PJ), anastomotic technique (duct-to-mucosa vs.

invagination PJ) and PJ stent placement for PD (38–42), as well as pancreatic stump closure (handsewn vs. stapled closure), staple line reinforcement (fibrin sealants vs. autologous tissue patches), and intraperitoneal drain placement for DP, have all been rigorously studied as potential mitigating strategies for POPF (43–47). TP has been suggested as an operative approach to obviate the risk of POPF, though obligatory development of insulin-dependent diabetes mellitus and complete loss of pancreatic exocrine function have prevented this approach from being more broadly adopted (25,38).

Timely diagnosis, and treatment initiation, are crucial to minimizing the potentially devastating impact of POPF. A high clinical suspicion for POPF should be maintained for patients who develop unexpected abdominal pain or distention, DGE, fever, leukocytosis, elevated C-reactive protein, increasing tachycardia, high volume or change in quality of drain output, or other deviation from 'normal' postoperative recovery (37–38). Early postoperative testing of drain-amylase levels is crucial in predicting the occurrence of POPF (25) and any measurable volume of drain fluid on, or after, POD3 with amylase levels >3 times the upper-limit of normal serum amylase concentration and affecting patient's clinical course is diagnostic (31). Indeed, McMillan et al. demonstrated the significant clinical impact of immediate postoperative (POD1) drain-amylase testing for patients deemed moderate/

Table 41.2 The revised 2016 ISGPS classification and grading of POPF, a checklist for clinical use[¶]

Event	Biochemical leak (no POPF)	Grade B POPF*	Grade C POPF*
Increased amylase activity >3 times upper limit institutional normal serum value	Yes	Yes	Yes
Persisting peripancreatic drainage >3 weeks	No	Yes	Yes
Clinically relevant change in management of POPF	No	Yes	Yes
POPF percutaneous- or endoscopic-specific interventions for collections	No	Yes	Yes
Angiographic procedures for POPF-related bleeding	No	Yes	Yes
Reoperation for POPF	No	No	Yes
Signs of infection related to POPF	No	Yes, without organ failure	Yes, with organ failure
POPF-related organ failure^	No	No	Yes
POPF-related death	No	No	Yes

Abbreviations: ISGPS: International Study Group of Pancreatic Surgery; POPF: postoperative pancreatic fistula.

* A clinically relevant POPF is defined as a drain output of any measurable volume of fluid with amylase level greater than three times the upper institutional normal serum amylase level, associated with a clinically relevant development/condition related directly to the POPF.

\# Suggests prolongation of hospital or ICU stay, includes use of therapeutic agents specifically employed for fistula management or its consequences (of these: somatostatin analogues; TPN/TEN; blood product transfusion or other medications).

^ Postoperative organ failure is defined as the need for re-intubation, haemodialysis, and/or inotropic agents >24 hours for respiratory, renal, or cardiac insufficiency, respectively.

¶ Table adapted from (31).

high risk for POPF by fistula risk score calculation in a recent randomized controlled trial. For patients with POD1 drain-amylase <5000 U/L and benign-appearing output, rates of POPF were found to be lower by POD3. Early postoperative drain removal is recommended for these patients, highlighting the degree to which drain-surveillance can impact POPF diagnosis and management (48). While the use of routine CT imaging for POPF surveillance has been suggested (25), it is difficult to distinguish normal postoperative fluid accumulations from POPF, and systematic imaging of post-pancreatectomy patients is not generally recommended (38,49).

Generally, POPF management is dictated by the volume of output and the patient's clinical status. Non-operative management of high-output POPF resembles treatment of postoperative ileus and intra-abdominal collections. Patients are kept nothing-by-mouth (NPO) with hydration, and initiation of supplemental enteral or parenteral nutrition is considered for patients unable to tolerate sufficient oral intake by POD10 (25,38). Enteral nutrition initiation is preferred, when possible, given higher rates of fistula closure (50). For low output POPF (<200 cc/day), patients should continue oral nutrition, as tolerated, and be advised to reduce their fat intake as far as possible. Empiric antibiotics are started if there is a clinical suspicion of infection (fever, leukocytosis, purulent discharge or drain output, wound erythema, warmth or tenderness) and are subsequently adjusted based on a Gram stain, culture, and sensitivity data. High rates of microbial growth are observed in POPF (up to 82%) and subsequent development of infected POPF (~67%), which is defined as microbial growth and clinical evidence of infection, highlighting the importance of maintaining a high index of suspicion for infection (51,52). Surgical drains can be removed as early as POD3, as previously discussed (48), but are typically removed at the surgeon's discretion (the authors recommend removal when volumes diminish to <25 cc/day). Patients can be safely discharged home as long as their drain output is stable or decreasing, and has consistent output character, with cautious drain management advised for high-output (>200 cc/day) drainage. Somatostatin analogue use, a prior mainstay of conservative therapy for POPF, is no longer considered standard treatment given the lack of demonstrable advantage for fistula closure rates (37,53). Altogether, utilizing this conservative management strategy, in the appropriate setting, has a published success rate of ~85% within 1 month (25).

Interventional approaches to POPF management include computed tomography (CT)- or ultrasound (US)-guided repositioning of surgical drains and insertion of percutaneous drains for large fluid collections, unresponsive to conservative therapy. This is more frequently employed for POPF after DP, which typically follow a more protracted course. While uncommon, surgical re-intervention is necessary when percutaneous access to abdominal collections is not possible, when anastomotic dehiscence is suspected, or for patients with rapid clinical deterioration in the setting of sepsis or multiple organ dysfunction (25,54). Operative approaches to POPF include wide external peripancreatic drainage of fluid collections, bridge-stent in combination with external drainage (55), or completion (total) pancreatectomy. As previously mentioned, TP is definitive in treating POPF, but in the setting of high morbidity and exceedingly high mortality rates (75–100%), it is mainly employed as a radical salvage procedure (25,38,54).

POST-PANCREATECTOMY HAEMORRHAGE

As a relatively rare, but potentially fatal, complication of pancreatectomy, post-pancreatectomy haemorrhage (PPH) occurs in approximately 1–8% of all pancreatic resections (4–16% after PD, 2–3% after DP) and accounts for 11–38% of overall mortality (25,38,54). The ISGPS defines PPH by postoperative onset (early vs. late), location (intraluminal vs. extraluminal) and severity (mild vs. severe), with grading of PPH (A, B and C) assigned according to these parameters (*Table 41.3*) (56). While early PPH is associated with technical failure in achieving appropriate intraoperative haemostasis, or an underlying perioperative coagulopathy, late PPH typically arises from operative complications days to weeks following surgery. Anastomotic leak or POPF, bile leak, intra-abdominal abscess, and generalized sepsis have all been described in relation to PPH occurrence and the pathogenesis appears to be multifactorial. PPH is believed to arise from enzymatic digestion or infection of iatrogenic injury to vessel walls leading to pseudoaneurysm formation and subsequent rupture, direct erosion into vessel walls by intra-abdominal drains or POPF, or marginal ulceration at the anastomosis (25,43,56–59). Vascular structures serving as common sources of PPH include the gastroduodenal artery (GDA) stump for PD, splenic artery after DP, superior mesenteric artery branches and, rarely, an intrapancreatic artery (43,56).

Because of the significant morbidity and mortality associated with PPH, surgeons must maintain a high index of suspicion in order to facilitate rapid management. A meta-analysis by Limongelli et al. (58), identified that 62% of post-pancreatectomy patients were found to present with intra-abdominal, extraluminal bleeding rather than gastrointestinal bleeding (~28%), highlighting the importance of stringent postoperative drain observation, while acknowledging that evidence of bleeding in drains is not always present. Careful assessment of patients' clinical status remains imperative and any patients with haematemesis or melaena, unexplained hypotension or tachycardia, or decreasing hemoglobin concentration on laboratory studies should undergo immediate evaluation and treatment for PPH

(56). Appearance of a 'sentinel bleed', or small volume of blood loss via intra-abdominal drains or NGT, in a haemodynamically stable patient should merit significant concern for impending PPH. Contrast-enhanced CT (CECT)-imaging or upper endoscopy should be obtained immediately in these patients as prompt intervention is key in preventing severe, potentially fatal outcomes (25,56,57).

While the management of early PPH involves resuscitative efforts and surgical re-intervention, as needed, to address causative technical errors, the management of late PPH is somewhat more controversial (25). Repeat laparotomy had been the traditional management strategy for PPH prior to the rise of newer interventional approaches, and still remains the procedure of choice in most haemodynamically unstable patients

(58). Currently, interventional angioembolization of bleeding vessels or ruptured pseudoaneurysms using Gelfoam® (Pfizer Inc, New York, US), arterial stents, or coils is the initial preferred treatment modality in the appropriate clinical setting (patients' clinical stability, availability of interventional radiology) and is highly effective in stopping PPH in up to 80% of cases, with operative re-intervention necessary only in instances of conservative failure (43,56,60). Within our institution, angioembolization is often initially attempted even in the setting of relative haemodynamic instability, given the technical prowess of our interventional radiology department and surgeons and operating room (OR) staff remain on standby in these instances. Nonetheless, given the lack of evidence in the literature demonstrating the clear superiority of endovascular modalities over surgical intervention (58), careful consideration must be given to the individual clinical scenario in management decision-making.

OTHER COMPLICATIONS

Intra-abdominal abscess (IAA) is observed in approximately 3–8% of pancreatectomy patients and is most frequently associated with POPF formation or bile leak. Associations with preoperative biliary drainage and intraoperative PJ stenting have also been reported (25,61). After obtaining CT imaging to confirm the presence of IAA, management options include: conservative observation and antibiotics for smaller IAA (<4 cm) in clinically non-toxic patients; percutaneous drainage with antibiotics for larger IAA (≥4 cm) or systemically ill patients; surgical debridement and/or operative drain placement for IAA not amenable to percutaneous drainage, or for patients in whom conservative measures have failed (61). Management of any abscess after pancreatectomy, other than TP, should also include assessment of amylase levels (if aspiration or drainage occurs). Incidence rates of bile leak or fistula are cited around 1–5%, and management typically involves either observation, percutaneous drainage and/or, for DP, endoscopic stenting (25). The incidence of surgical site infections (SSI) is approximately 12% following pancreatectomy. SSIs are usually managed in the standard conservative fashion of observation with, or without, antibiotics and/or wound exploration/opening (62). Regarding IAA and SSI, proper management should ameliorate any long-term effects on morbidity and mortality.

SUMMARY

Despite continued regionalization and technical advances in the field of pancreatic surgery, pancreatectomy still has a significant associated morbidity, even as mortality has declined to 1% at high-volume centers (2–4). While research efforts continue to strengthen

Table 41.3 Proposed definition of PPH*

Time of onset

- Early haemorrhage (≤24 h after the end of the index operation)
- Late haemorrhage (>24 h after the end of the index operation)

Location

- Intraluminal (intraenteric, e.g. anastomotic suture line at stomach or duodenum or pancreatic surface at anastomosis, stress ulcer, pseudoneurysm)
- Extraluminal (extraenteric, bleeding into the abdominal cavity, e.g. from arterial or venous vessels, diffuse bleeding from resection area, anastomosis suture lines, pseudoaneurysm

Severity of haemorrhage

Mild

- Small- or medium-volume blood loss (from drains, nasogastric tube, or on ultrasonography, decrease in haemoglobin concentration <3 g/dL)
- Mild clinical impairment of the patient, no therapeutic consequence, or at most, the need for non-invasive treatment with volume resuscitation or blood transfusions (2–3 units packed red cells within 24 h of end of operation or 1–3 units if later than 24 h after operation)
- No need for reoperation or interventional angiographic embolization; endoscopic treatment of anastomotic bleeding may occur provided the other conditions apply

Severe

- Large volume blood loss (drop of haemoglobin level by ≥3 g/dL)
- Clinically significant impairment (e.g. tachycardia, hypotension, oliguria, hypovolemic shock), need for blood transfusion (>3 units packed cells)
- Need for invasive treatment (interventional angiographic embolization or relaparotomy

* Adapted table reproduced from (7).

understanding of pathogenesis and prevention in the arena of postoperative complications following pancreatectomy, a sound knowledge of the contemporary evidence for diagnosis and management of these complications remains integral in guiding decision-making for the care of post-pancreatectomy patients.

REFERENCES

1. McClusky DA, Skandalakis LJ, Colborn GL, Skandalakis JE. Harbinger or hermit? Pancreatic anatomy and surgery through the ages – Part 1. *World J Surg* 2002;**26**:1175–85.
2. Birkmeyer JD, Siewers AE, Finlayson EV, Stukel TA, Lucas FL, Batista I, et al. Hospital volume and surgical mortality in the United States. *N Engl J Med* 2002;**346(15)**:1128–37.
3. Ecker BL, McMillan MT, Allegrini V, Bassi C, Beane JD, Beckman RM, et al. Risk factors and mitigation strategies for pancreatic fistula after distal pancreatectomy: Analysis of 2026 resections from the International, Multi-institutional Distal Pancreatectomy Study Group. *Ann Surg* 2019;**269(1)**:143–9.
4. Stoop TF, Ateeb Z, Ghorbani P, Scholten L, Arnelo U, Besselink MG, et al. Surgical outcomes after total pancreatectomy: A high-volume center experience. *Ann Surg Oncol* 2021;**28(3)**:1543–51.
5. Kent TS, Sachs TE, Callery MP, Vollmer CM Jr. Readmission after major pancreatic resection: A necessary evil? *J Am Coll Surg* 2011;**213(4)**:515–23.
6. Winter JM, Cameron JL, Campbell KA, Arnold MA, Change DC, Coleman J, et al. 1423 Pancreaticoduodenectomies for pancreatic cancer: A single-institution experience. *J Gastrointest Surg* 2006;**10(9)**:1199–211.
7. Wente MN, Bassi C, Dervenis C, Fingerhut A, Guma DJ, Izbicki JR, et al. Delayed gastric emptying (DGE) after pancreatic surgery: A suggested definition by the International Study Group of Pancreatic Surgery (ISGPS). *Surgery* 2007;**142(5)**:761–8.
8. Eshuis WJ, van Eijck CHJ, Gerhards MF, Coene PP, de Hingh IJJT, Karsten TM, et al. Antecolic versus retrocolic route of the gastroenteric anastomosis after pancreatoduodenectomy: A randomized controlled trial. *Ann Surg* 2014;**259**:45–51.
9. Glowka TR, Webler M, Matthaei H, Matthaei H, Schäfer N, Schmitz V, et al. Delayed gastric emptying following pancreatoduodenectomy with alimentary reconstruction according to Roux-en-Y or Billroth-II. *BMC Surg* 2017;**17(1)**:24.
10. Warshaw AL, Torchiana DL. Delayed gastric emptying after pylorus-preserving pancreaticoduodenectomy. *Surg Gynecol Obstet* 1985;**160(1)**:1–4.
11. Klaiber U, Probst P, Strobel O, Michalski CW, Dörr-Harim C, Kiener MK, et al. Meta-analysis of delayed gastric emptying after pylorus-preserving versus pylorus-resecting pancreatoduodenectomy. *Br J Surg* 2018;**105(4)**:339–49.
12. Wang J, Ma R, Churilov L, Eleftheriou P, Nikfarjam M, Christophi C, et al. The cost of perioperative complications following pancreaticoduodenectomy: A systematic review. *Pancreatology* 2018;**18(2)**:208–20.
13. Futagawa Y, Kanehira M, Furukawa K, Kitamura H, Yoshida S, Usuba T, et al. Impact of delayed gastric emptying after pancreaticoduodenectomy on survival. *J Hepatobiliary Pancreat Sci* 2017;**24(8)**:446–74.
14. Welsch T, Bonn M, Degrate L, Welsch T, Borm M, Degrate L, et al. Evaluation of the International Study Group of Pancreatic Surgery definition of delayed gastric emptying after pancreatoduodenectomy in a high-volume centre. *Br J Surg* 2010;**97(7)**:1043–50.
15. Park JS, Hwang HK, Kim JK, Cho SI, Yoon D-S, Lee WJ, et al. Clinical validation and risk factors for delayed gastric emptying based on the International Study Group of Pancreatic Surgery (ISGPS) Classification. *Surgery* 2009;**146(5)**:882–7.
16. van Berge Henegouwen MI, van Gulik TM, DeWit LT, Allema JG, Rauws, EA, Obertop H, et al. Delayed gastric emptying after standard pancreaticoduodenectomy versus pylorus-preserving pancreaticoduodenectomy: An analysis of 200 consecutive patients. *J Am Coll Surg* 1997;**185(4)**:373–9.
17. Sadowski C, Uhl W, Baer HU, Reber P, Seiler C, Büchler MW. Delayed gastric emptying after classic and pylorus-preserving Whipple procedure: A prospective study. *Dig Surg* 1997;**14**:159–64.
18. Seiler CA, Wagner M, Sadowski C, Kulli C, Büchler MW. Randomized prospective trial of pylorus-preserving vs. classic duodenopancreatectomy (Whipple Procedure): Initial clinical results. *J Gastrointest Surg* 2000;**4**:443–52.
19. Tran KTC, Smeenk HG, van Eijck CHJ, Kazemier G, Hop WC, Greve JWG, et al. Pylorus preserving pancreaticoduodenectomy versus standard Whipple procedure: A prospective, randomized, multicenter analysis of 170 patients with pancreatic and periampullary tumors. *Ann Surg* 2004;**240(5)**:738–45.
20. Horstmann O, Markus PM, Ghadimi MB, Becker H. Pylorus preservation has no impact on delayed gastric emptying after pancreatic head resection. *Pancreas* 2004;**1**:69–74.
21. Jimenez RE, Fernandez-Del Castillo C, Rattner DW, Chang Y, Warshaw AL. Outcome of pancreaticoduodenectomy with pylorus preservation or with antrectomy in the treatment of chronic pancreatitis. *Ann Surg* 2000;**231**:293–300.
22. Bell R, Pandanaboyana S, Shah N, Bartlett A, Windsor JA, Smith AM. Meta-analysis of antecolic versus retrocolic gastric reconstruction after a pylorus-preserving pancreatoduodenectomy. *HPB (Oxford)* 2015;**17(3)**:202–8.
23. Kamarajah SK, Bundred JR, Alessandri G, Robinson SM, Wilson CH, French JJ, et al. A systematic review and network-meta-analysis of gastro-enteric reconstruction techniques following pancreatoduodenectomy to reduce delayed gastric emptying. *World J Surg* 2020;**44(7)**:2314–22.
24. Snyder RA, Ewing JA, Parikh AA. Delayed gastric emptying after pancreaticoduodenectomy: A study

of the national surgical quality improvement program. *Pancreatology* 2020;**20(2)**:205–10.

25. Lermite E, Sommacale D, Piardi T, Arnaud J-P, Sauvanet A, Dejong CHC, et al. Complications after pancreatic resection: Diagnosis, prevention and management. *Clin Res Hepatol Gastroenterol* 2013;**37(3)**:230–9.

26. Balzano G, Zerbi A, Braga M, Rocchetti S, Beneduce AA, Di Carlo V. Fast-track recovery programme after pancreaticoduodenectomy reduces delayed gastric emptying. *Br J Surg* 2008;**95(11)**:1387–93.

27. Martignoni ME, Friess H, Sell F, Ricken L, Shrikhande S, Kulli C, et al. Enteral nutrition prolongs delayed gastric emptying in patients after whipple resection. *Am J Surg* 2000;**180(1)**:18–23.

28. Watters JM, Kirkpatrick SM, Norris SB, Shamji FM, Wells GA. Immediate postoperative enteral feeding results in impaired respiratory mechanics and decreased mobility. *Ann Surg* 1997;**226(3)**:369–77.

29. Beane JD, House MG, Miller A, Nakeeb A, Schmidt CM, Zyromski NJ, et al. Optimal management of delayed gastric emptying after pancreatectomy: An analysis of 1089 patients. *Surgery* 2014;**156(4)**:939–46.

30. Gianotti L, Besselink MG, Sandini M, Hackert T, Conlon K, Gerritsen A, et al. Nutritional support and therapy in pancreatic surgery: A position paper of the International Study Group on Pancreatic Surgery (ISGPS). *Surgery* 2018;**164(5)**:1035–48.

31. Bassi C, Marchegiani G, Dervenis C, Sarr M, Abu Hilal M, Adham M, et al. The 2016 update of the International Study Group (ISGPS) definition and grading of postoperative pancreatic fistula: 11 years after. *Surgery* 2017;**161(3)**:584–91.

32. Pedrazzoli S. Pancreatoduodenectomy (PD) and postoperative pancreatic fistula (POPF): A systematic review and analysis of the POPF-related mortality rate in 60,739 patients retrieved from the English literature published between 1990 and 2015. *Medicine (Baltimore)* 2017;**96(19)**:e6858.

33. Mackay TM, Smits FJ, Roos D, Bonsing BA, Bosscha K, Busch OR, et al. The risk of not receiving adjuvant chemotherapy after resection of pancreatic ductal adenocarcinoma: A nationwide analysis. *HPB (Oxford)* 2020;**22(2)**:233–40.

34. Callery MP, Pratt WB, Kent TS, Chaikof EL, Vollmer CM Jr. A prospectively validated clinical risk score accurately predicts pancreatic fistula after pancreatoduodenectomy. **J Am Coll Surg** 2013;**216(1)**:1–14.

35. Mungroop TH, van Rijssen LB, van Klaveren D, Smits FJ, van Woerden V, Linnemann RJ, et al. Alternative fistula risk score for pancreatoduodenectomy (a-FRS): Design and international external validation. *Ann Surg* 2019;**269(5)**:937–43.

36. Abbott DE, Tzeng CWD, McMillan MT, Callery MP, Kent TS, Christein JD, et al. Pancreas fistula risk prediction: Implications for hospital costs and payments. *HPB (Oxford)* 2017;**19**:(2):140–6.

37. Malleo G, Vollmer CM Jr. Postpancreatectomy complications and management. *Surg Clin North Am* 2016;**96(6)**:1313–36.

38. Machado N. Pancreatic fistula after pancreatectomy: Definitions, risk factors, preventive measures, and management: Review. *Int J Surg Oncol* 2012;**2012**:602478.

39. Williamsson C, Stenvall K, Wennerblom J, Andersson R, Andersson B, Tingstedt B. Predictive factors for postoperative pancreatic fistula: A Swedish nationwide register-based study. *World J Surg* 2020;**44(12)**:4207–13.

40. Lin JW, Cameron JL, Yeo CJ, Riall TS, Lillemoe KD. Risk factors and outcomes in postpancreaticoduodenectomy pancreaticocutaneous fistula *J Gastrointest Surg* 2004;**8(8)**:951–9.

41. Kawaida H, Kono H, Hosomura N, Amemiya H, Itakura J, Fujii H, et al. Surgical techniques and postoperative management to prevent postoperative pancreatic fistula after pancreatic surgery. *World J Gastroenterol* 2019;**25(28)**:3722–37.

42. Berger AC, Howard TJ, Kennedy EP, Sauter PK, Bower-Cherry M, Dutkevitch S, et al. Does type of pancreaticojejunostomy after pancreaticoduodenectomy decrease rate of pancreatic fistula? A randomized, prospective, dual-institution trial. *J Am Coll Surg* 2009;**208(5)**:738–49.

43. Parikh PY, Lillemoe KD. Surgical management of pancreatic cancer: Distal pancreatectomy. *Semin Oncol* 2015;**42(1)**:110–22.

44. Diener MK, Seiler CM, Rossion I, Kleeff J, Glanemann M, Butturini G, et al. Efficacy of stapler versus hand-sewn closure after distal pancreatectomy (DISPACT): A randomised, controlled multicentre trial. *Lancet* 2011;**377**:1514–22.

45. Hassenpflug M, Hinz U, Strobel O, Volpert J, Knebel P, Diener MK, et al. Teres ligament patch reduces relevant morbidity after distal pancreatectomy (the DISCOVER randomized controlled trial). *Ann Surg* 2016;**264(5)**:723–30.

46. Sarr MGL, Pancreatic Surgery Group. The potent somatostatin analogue vapreotide does not decrease pancreas-specific complications after elective pancreatectomy: A prospective, multicenter, double-blind ed, randomized, placebo-controlled trial. *J Am Coll Surg* 2003;**196(4)**:556–64.

47. van Buren II G, Bloomston M, Schmidt CR, Behrman SW, Zyromski NJ, Ball CG, et al. A prospective randomized multicenter trial of distal pancreatectomy with and without routine intraperitoneal drainage. *Ann Surg* 2017;**266(3)**:421–31.

48. McMillan MT, Malleo G, Bassi C, Butturini H, Salvia R, Roses RE, et al. Drain management after pancreatoduodenectomy: Reappraisal of a prospective randomized trial using risk stratification. *J Am Coll Surg* 2015;**221(4)**:798–809.

49. Bruno O, Brancatelli G, Sauvanet A, et al. Utility of CT in the diagnosis of pancreatic fistula after pancreaticoduodenectomy in patients with soft pancreas. *AJR Am J Roentgenol* 2009;**193(3)**:W175–180.

50. Klek S, Sierzega M, Turczynowski L, Szybinski P, Szczepanek K, Kulig J. Enteral and parenteral nutrition in the conservative treatment of pancreatic fistula: A randomized clinical trial. *Gastroenterology* 2011;**141(1)**:157–63.

51. Loos M, Strobel O, Legominski M, Dietrich M, Hinz U, Brenner T, et al. Postoperative pancreatic fistula: Microbial growth determines outcome. *Surgery* 2018;**164**(**6**):1185–90.

52. Kent TS, Sachs TE, Callery MP, Vollmer CM Jr. The burden of infection for elective pancreatic resections. *Surgery* 2013;**153**(**1**):86–94.

53. Adiamah A, Arif Z, Berti F, Singh S, Laskar N, Gomez D. The use of prophylactic somatostatin therapy following pancreaticoduodenectomy: A meta-analysis of randomised controlled trials. *World J Surg* 2019;**43**(**7**):1788–801.

54. Callery MP, Pratt WB, Vollmer CM Jr. Prevention and management of pancreatic fistula. *J Gastrointest Surg* 2009;**13**(**1**):163–73.

55. Kent TS, Callery MP, Vollmer CM Jr. The bridge stent technique for salvage of pancreaticojejunal anastomotic dehiscence. *HPB (Oxford)* 2010;**12**(**8**):577–82.

56. Wente MN, Veit JA, Bassi C, Dervenis C, Fingerhut, A, Gouma DJ, et al. Postpancreatectomy hemorrhage (PPH): An International Study Group of Pancreatic Surgery (ISGPS) definition. *Surgery* 2007;**142**(**1**):20–5.

57. Sledzianowski JF, Duffas JP, Muscari F, Suc B, Fourtanier F. Risk factors for mortality and intra-abdominal morbidity after distal pancreatectomy. *Surgery* 2005;**137**(**2**):180–5.

58. Limongelli P, Khorsandi SE, Pai M, Jackson JE, Tait P, Tierris J, et al. Management of delayed postoperative hemorrhage after pancreaticoduodenectomy: A meta-analysis. *Arch Surg* 2008;**143**(**10**): 1001–7.

59. Chipaila J, Kato H, Iizawa Y, Motonori N, Noguchi D, Gyoten K, et al. Prolonged operating time is a significant perioperative risk factor for arterial pseudoaneurysm formation and patient death following hemorrhage after pancreaticoduodenectomy. *Pancreatology* 2020;**20**(**7**):1540–9.

60. Yekebas EF, Wolfram L, Cataldegirmen G, Habermann CR, Bogoevski D, Koenig AM, et al. Postpancreatectomy hemorrhage: diagnosis and treatment: An analysis in 1669 consecutive pancreatic resections. *Ann Surg* 2007;**246**(**2**):269–80.

61. Schulick RD. Complications after pancreaticoduodenectomy: Intraabdominal abscess. *J Hepatobiliary Pancreat Surg* 2008;**15**(**3**):252–6.

62. Sanford DE, Strasberg SM, Hawkins WG, Fields RC. The impact of recent hospitalization on surgical site infection after a pancreatectomy. *HPB (Oxford)* 2015;**17**(**9**):819–23.

Chapter

42

Ampullary Tumours: Endoscopic Treatment, Dysplasia, Benign Tumours and Submucosal Lesions

Raja R. Narayan and Brendan C. Visser

INTRODUCTION

With the expanded use of endoscopy, the incidence of tumours of the ampulla of Vater has increased in the last decade (1). Although most lesions are incidentally diagnosed and benign, early detection of malignant tumours can enable prompt intervention and long-term survival. Due to the regional anatomy (*Figure 42.1*), many ampullary masses will present early with features of biliary or pancreatic duct obstruction such as jaundice, cholangitis, or pancreatitis (2). Although ampullary lesions have historically been managed by surgical intervention, the increased use of advanced

endoscopic techniques presents less invasive opportunities for management of benign ampullary tumours. With respect to malignant tumours, as a result of early diagnosis, these masses are more commonly amenable to surgical resection compared with similarly malignant lesions arising in the duodenum, bile duct, or pancreatic head (3,4). Additionally, sporadic lesions bear different implications for management compared to those associated with familial syndromes. In this chapter, the variety of masses that may present at the ampulla of Vater and their management options are described.

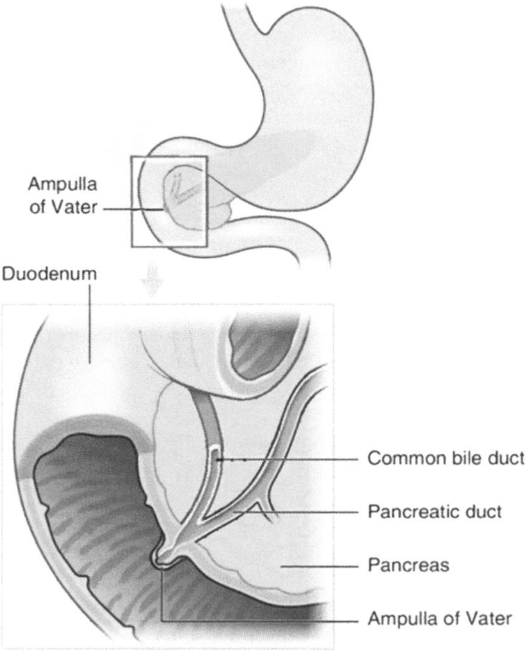

BENIGN AMPULLARY MASSES

Ampullary adenoma

Ampullary adenomas are the most common benign lesion occurring at the ampulla of Vater. These tumours are detected in the 6th–8th decades of life and noted in 0.04–0.12% on autopsy studies (5). Although benign, ampullary adenomas have been noted to undergo malignant degeneration in 30% of patients (6). Most patients will be asymptomatic at incidental diagnosis (1) and unfortunately, there is a paucity of data informing the risk of malignant degeneration with respect to size, degree of dysplasia, and time. For those presenting with symptoms, the majority have jaundice followed by pancreatitis, abdominal pain, weight loss, and dyspepsia (1).

Diagnostic work-up, especially in the case of jaundice, begins with abdominal ultrasound which has a poor sensitivity for the detection of ampullary masses. In one report, <8% had their ampullary mass detected on ultrasound (US) (7). Abdominal computed tomography (CT) is a more sensitive imaging modality but may be inadequate to identify small lesions. Magnetic resonance cholangiopancreatography (MRCP) may better define the ampullary adenoma by demonstrating a stricture, or filling defect, in or near the distal common bile duct (CBD). Ultimately, endoscopic ultrasound (EUS) and endoscopic retrograde cholangiopancreatography

Figure 42.1 Anatomy of the ampulla of Vater.

DOI: 10.1201/9781003080060-42

(ERCP) with fine needle aspiration (FNA) is the optimal diagnostic study to confirm the presence of an ampullary mass, obtain a pathological diagnosis, and stage the depth of invasion as well as identify adjacent lymph node involvement in case of malignancy. Clinicians need to be aware that superficial biopsies of ampullary lesions may miss invasive cancers. Patients who have low grade dysplasia with malignant clinical features such as obstructive jaundice or concerning imaging features such as a double-duct sign are best managed assuming they harbor malignancy.

MALIGNANT AMPULLARY MASSES

Ampullary adenocarcinoma

Malignant lesions arising at the ampulla of Vater make up 0.5% of all gastrointestinal cancers (8). Cattell and Pyrtek first theorized that mucosa along the Vaterian system was prone to develop adenocarcinoma because this represents 'an area of epithelium transition which is constantly being irritated chemically and mechanically' (9). Kimura described two subtypes of adenocarcinoma defined as the pancreatobiliary and intestinal subtypes (10). Pancreatobiliary ampullary adenocarcinoma is identified on microscopy as aberrant glands nested within desmoplastic stroma (11). This subtype tends to have a worse prognosis associated with lymph node involvement, perineural invasion, and poor differentiation. As a result, patients with pancreatobiliary ampullary adenocarcinoma have three-fold worse survival compared with patients with the intestinal subtype. Conversely, intestinal ampullary adenocarcinoma is the more common invasive subtype (11). The intestinal subtype is distinguished by the presence of tubular or cribriform glands, although some versions can have a mix of these features. Variants of the adenocarcinoma histopathology also include adenosquamous carcinoma, colloid carcinoma, signet-ring cell carcinoma, undifferentiated carcinoma, papillary adenocarcinoma, and neuroendocrine tumours (11).

In addition to this pathologic classification, anatomic subtypes of ampullary adenocarcinoma have been described based on the extension of local disease (12–14). Intra-ampullary neoplasms represent malignancies with prominent intraluminal growth that extend into the duodenal lumen from a patulous orifice of the Vaterian system. Peri-ampullary neoplasms are more prominently exophytic, with ulcerated and vegetating components involving the duodenal surface of the ampulla. The vegetating aspect of the tumour signifies pre-invasive disease, whereas the ulcerating component represents the invasive portion. As a result, the presence of ulceration is associated with a worse survival (15). Lastly, mixed features of the aforementioned types can exist.

Patients with ampullary adenocarcinoma will most commonly present with obstructive jaundice or CBD dilation which is noted in up to 85% (16–18). Similarly,

the pancreatic duct is dilated in about half of presenting patients (14). Over half will present with weight loss, fatigue, and abdominal pain (19) while a third may have an occult gastrointestinal (GI) bleed (20). The most commonly associated tumour markers for ampullary adenocarcinoma include carcinoembryonic antigen (CEA) and carbohydrate antigen 19-9 (CA 19-9), both of which have been shown to be markers of survival in this patient population (21,22). In fact, CA 19-9 has been reported to be elevated in 86% of ampullary adenocarcinoma patients (23).

Imaging is next pursued to make the diagnosis of ampullary adenocarcinoma, often beginning with abdominal ultrasound which is reported to have a sensitivity for detecting ampullary tumours in 5–15% (7,24–26). Indirect features of an ampullary mass can also be detected in 70% at the time of US, such as pancreatic or CBD dilation (24). If the suspicion of a solid mass remains, CT is the next appropriate investigation which has a reported sensitivity of 19–69% and specificity of 20–76% for an ampullary tumour (24–29). Some centres give 'negative contrast' or water to distend the duodenum at the time of imaging to better define the ampulla (14). Alternatively, if a cystic mass is seen, MRCP is recommended as the next imaging study to better identify concerning features that may be harbored in the cyst. Compared to EUS, only 75% undergoing MRCP will have their tumour identified on that scan (30). If present, a mildly hyperenhancing lobulated mass can be seen on T2-weighted half-Fourier single-shot turbo spin-echo MRI (HASTE-MRI) (*Figure 42.2a*) (31). If no mass is seen on abdominal US and there remains a high index of clinical suspicion, EUS-ERCP is recommended. While cross-sectional imaging is the most accurate modality for staging nodal and metastatic disease, EUS-ERCP is superior for tumour, or T, staging and pathologic diagnosis (*Table 42.1*). Unfortunately, EUS-ERCP carries a false negative rate of 50% on biopsy (32,33). Several endoscopic features can also suggest a lesion is malignant, such as firmness, ulceration, areas of depression, and failure to lift the lesion with submucosal injection (34,35). Ultimately, there may be circumstances where there is inadequate radiographic detail to make a preoperative diagnosis, and a constellation of clinical features may indicate proceeding to surgical exploration if there is a high index of suspicion.

For diagnosed ampullary malignancies, the 'gold standard' of management remains the Whipple pancreaticoduodenectomy (PD). Reports on the natural history of disease has found that the 5-year overall survival for ampullary adenocarcinoma patients is approximately 45% following resection, which exceeds that of pancreatic adenocarcinoma or bile duct cancer (36). The PD provides an opportunity to sample local lymph nodes and prior reports have found that sampling over 12 lymph nodes is associated with improved survival for patients with N0 or N1 disease (37). One retrospective review led by Moekotte et al. incorporating

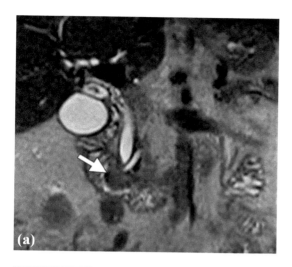

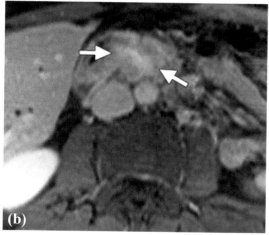

Figure 42.2 Features of ampullary adenoma on T2-weighted HASTE-MRI (a). A hypo-enhancing lobulated lesion is labelled (white arrows) arising from the ampulla with associated mild dilation of the common bile duct and pancreatic duct (b). (Reproduced from Nikolaidis P et al. [31].)

887 ampullary adenocarcinoma patients, that underwent resection at nine European tertiary centres, found that lymph node status was the single greatest predictor of overall, and disease-free, survival independent of histologic subtype or tumour stage (38). For those with node-negative disease, a nomogram designed by Huang et al. using the Surveillance, Epidemiology, and End Results (SEER) database notes that tumour grade, T stage, and number of examined lymph nodes are principal predictors of overall survival (39).

Although no level 1 data exists to support the use of systemic chemotherapy in the neoadjuvant period, several reports are available to inform oncologists on the use of adjuvant chemotherapy for ampullary

adenocarcinoma. The European Study Group for Pancreatic Cancer (ESPAC)-3 trial incorporated 428 patients that underwent surgery for periampullary cancer from 100 centres around the world, including 297 with ampullary adenocarcinoma (40). This trial compared groups undergoing postoperative observation versus either fluorouracil or gemcitabine-based chemotherapy. Although, ampullary cancer patients had the best overall survival (median survival: 53 months, 95% CI=42–73) compared with patients with pancreatic (median survival: 33 months, 95% CI = 17–∞) or bile duct cancer (median survival: 21 months, 95% CI = 17–28). No difference in overall survival was noted between those observed versus those receiving adjuvant chemotherapy. As a follow-up, Neoptolemos and colleagues performed a sub-analysis of this data, showing that resected ampullary adenocarcinoma patients with negative microscopic margins treated with adjuvant chemotherapy had a nearly significant improvement in survival over those not treated with adjuvant chemotherapy (median survival: 58 vs 45 months, p = 0.057) (41). Additionally, an international multicentre trial is underway to compare the effect of adjuvant gemcitabine with capecitabine as compared to gemcitabine alone for periampullary cancer patients (ESPAC-4). The relative rarity of this malignancy, compared to others with better randomized data guiding adjuvant therapy, leads many to extrapolating data from other well-known malignant GI entities. As a result, practice patterns have shifted to the bulk of patients receiving adjuvant therapy unless they have very early disease. For now, the role of adjuvant therapy for ampullary adenocarcinoma patients remains unclear.

Ampullary neuroendocrine tumours

In addition to adenocarcinoma, the ampulla is the site of less than 1% of gastroenteropancreatic neuroendocrine tumours (NET) (42,43). Given the rarity of these lesions, the American Joint Committee on Cancer (AJCC) groups the staging of ampullary NETs with duodenal NET (44). Despite this, existing reports on ampullary NETs suggests these entities may be more aggressive than their duodenal or pancreatic counterparts. A retrospective cohort study of the SEER database, by Randle and colleagues, compared 120 patients with ampullary NETs with 1360 patients with duodenal NET and found the former to have a larger burden of, and higher-grade, disease at presentation that portends a worse overall survival (98 vs. 143 months, p = 0.037) (45). As a follow-up to this study, Ruff et al. reported on the largest number of ampullary NETs patients to-date in their review of the National Cancer Database (NCD) for all patients with a NET arising in the ampulla (n = 872), duodenum (n = 9692), and pancreatic head (n = 6561) (43). Therein, ampullary NET patients were again found to have larger tumours and higher-grade disease at presentation. Additionally, a larger proportion of ampullary NET

Table 42.1 Comparing 7th and 8th editions of the AJCC TNM staging for ampullary adenocarcinoma

7th Edition		8th Edition	
T			
T1	Limited to ampulla or sphincter of Oddi	T1a	Limited to sphincter of Oddi
		T1b	Invasion into duodenal submucosa
T2	Invasion into duodenal wall	T2	Invasion into duodenal muscularis propria
		T3a	Invasion into pancreas ≤0.5 cm
		T3b	Invasion into pancreas >0.5 cm or duodenal subserosa
T4	Invasion into peripancreatic soft tissue or other adjacent organs	T4	Involvement of coeliac or superior mesenteric artery
N			
N0	No lymph node involvement	N0	No lymph node involvement
N1	Lymph node involvement	N1	Metastasis in 1–3 lymph nodes
		N2	Metastasis in ≥4 lymph nodes
AJCC stage			
IA	T1, N0, M0	IA	T1a, N0, M0
IB	T2, N0, M0	IB	T1b–2, N0, M0
IIA	T3, N0, M0	IIA	T3a, N0, M0
IIB	T1–3, N2, M0	IIB	T3b, N0, M0
III	T4, any N, M0	IIIA	T1a–T3, N1, M0
		IIIB	Any T, N2, M0

patients had positive lymph nodes despite presenting with early T-stage disease (T1 associated with 21% bearing at least N1 disease). Among those undergoing resection, patients with ampullary NET had the worst median and 5-year overall survival (121 months and 62%) compared to NET patients with primary disease in the pancreatic head (132 months and 76%) and duodenum (145 months and 78%), respectively. With the growing understanding of this entity, in the future it may be prudent to separately stage and define the management strategy for ampullary NETs relative to duodenal and pancreatic head NETs. Consequently, as a result of the natural history of this disease, ampullary NETs likely demand a more aggressive operative approach than similarly sized ampullary adenocarcinomas.

GENETIC PREDISPOSITION TO AMPULLARY MASSES

Familial adenomatous polyposis

Although the majority of ampullary adenomas are sporadic, a large proportion occur in patients with genetic disorders such as familial adenomatous polyposis (FAP) (46). Similar to the adenoma-to-carcinoma sequence known to drive malignant transformation in polyps found on screening colonoscopy (47),

ampullary adenomas warrant excision in patients with these familial syndromes. These lesions tend to occur around, or just distal to, the ampulla of Vater in the duodenal mucosa and are present in nearly all FAP patients (48). Although presenting sporadically in elderly patients, FAP patients tend to develop ampullary adenomas earlier by their 20s or 30s (49). Among FAP patients, the prevalence of ampullary cancer is reported to be 3–12%. After colorectal cancer, periampullary or ampullary adenocarcinoma is the most common cause of death in patients with FAP warranting close surveillance (50–53). Noting this, the European Society of Gastrointestinal Endoscopists (ESGE) have recommended surveillance upper endoscopy for FAP patients to begin at the age of 25, at intervals determined by the number of lesions detected (54). Based on prior reports suggesting that FAP patients have a 100–330-fold increased risk for malignant transformation, this more aggressive surveillance strategy is advised as opposed to those with sporadic lesions (48,53,55–58). These FAP-related ampullary adenomas have a more indolent pattern of growth, thus warranting close surveillance rather than resection. As a result, there is a limited role for endoscopic resection of polyps in patients with this familial disorder, as the genetic predisposition results in both diffuse disease along the duodenal mucosa and near-certain recurrence after endoscopic resection.

On cross-sectional imaging, ampullary adenomas appear as lobulated, and hypoenhancing, masses often associated with CBD or pancreatic duct dilation (*Figure 42.2b*) (31). Ultimately, EUS-ERCP is needed to make the diagnosis.

MANAGEMENT OF AMPULLARY MASSES

Surgical management

As noted earlier, PD remains the 'gold standard' for management of ampullary adenocarcinoma. Given the opportunity for lymph node sampling and the survival advantage from obtaining 12 or more lymph nodes, most centres will offer PD for patients with T1 or greater disease (37). Additionally, for FAP patients that have a blanket of duodenal polyps with the potential for malignancy, PD reduces the risk for cancer by clearing the patient of these predisposing lesions. For Tis lesions or benign disease, some centres will offer transduodenal ampullectomy (TDA) to avoid the postoperative morbidity and impaired quality of life that can follow PD (59–61). William Halsted first reported the technical feasibility for ampullectomy in 1899 (62). Since then, wide acceptance of this technique has been limited by reports of high recurrence rates (20–100% in some studies) when performed for malignant lesions (63–66). Other than single-centre reports, no guidelines or level 1 evidence exist to indicate which lesions are best managed by PD or TDA. Winter and colleagues, at the Johns Hopkins Hospital, reported the largest series on techniques for operatively managing ampullary lesions in 450 patients between 1970–2007 reporting on PD (97%) and TDA (3%) (67). In this report, no difference in postoperative morbidity or mortality was noted between the two operative approaches, although patients were discharged significantly earlier following TDA at 7 days as opposed to 11 days after PD. Of note, among patients with ampullary adenocarcinoma, lymph node metastases were present in 28%, even with T1 disease. Citing the absence of an association between symptoms or lesion size with benign or malignant disease, the authors concluded that all ampullary lesions should be considered malignant and thus, PD should be the standard of care in all circumstances. Interpretation of their data is difficult, due to their clear institutional bias in favor of PD, but other studies to-date have not included a larger, or more modern, cohort.

Endoscopic management

Other than TDA or PD, some centres have been moving to perform endoscopic mucosal resection (EMR) when deemed feasible. In addition to EMR, some reports have described a 'piecemeal' approach to removing ampullary lesions as either treatment

for malignant lesions staged node-negative with T1 disease (68), or as a 'macrobiopsy' and bridge to an eventual operation (69,70). If either of these endoscopic strategies are pursued in the case of a malignant lesion, concerns regarding procedural complications, disease recurrence, and worse survival need to be weighed against the morbidity of pursuing an operation. To address this, a systematic review and meta-analysis was carried out by a European group that pooled 59 studies to compare outcomes following EMR, TDA, and PD for patients with ampullary lesions (71). The authors reported that microscopic resection (R0) was significantly more common on pooled proportion-meta-analysis and transformation analysis by the surgical approaches (TDA = 94.6%, PD = 99.2%) as compared with EMR (77.3%). Moreover, the pooled proportion-meta-analysis transformation rate for complications was significantly lower for EMR (24.5%) compared to PD (44.7%), but not TDA (28.7%). A similar analysis was lastly performed for the risk of recurrence finding no significant difference between the three different resection modalities (EMR = 13.2%, TDA = 11.0%, PD = 14.4%). Despite the limitations of this study, these findings raise concerns about the use of EMR for the resection of malignant lesions. For well-selected patients, EMR may be an option to remove small benign ampullary lesions, however, further research and consensus is necessary.

Guidelines released by the American Society of Gastrointestinal Endoscopy (ASGE) in 2015 supports the endoscopic removal of benign ampullary lesions less than 5 cm and/or Tis lesions (*Figure 42.3*) (72). Additionally, cannulation of the pancreatic duct is advised to reduce the risk of pancreatitis following endoscopic ampullary mass resection. Once the anatomy and trajectory of the pancreatic duct is identified from cannulation, the wire is removed to perform endoscopic resection. After the mass is removed, the pancreatic duct is re-cannulated to confirm no injury using fluoroscopic images obtained at the time of initial canulation. Up to a fifth of patients experience complications after endoscopic ampullary mass resection including bleeding, cholangitis, pancreatitis, ductal stenosis, and perforation (69,73). After a successful endoscopic resection, a 4-week follow-up EUS-ERCP is performed to remove a pancreatic duct stent placed at the time of resection. Thereafter, most centres will repeat EUS-ERCP every 3 months, up to a year, to monitor for ampullary stenosis and recurrent disease (1).

SUMMARY

Due to the complexity of its regional anatomy, multiple tumours (benign or malignant) can develop at the ampulla of Vater, due to either a sporadic or familial predisposition. Although the size and, if malignant, stage of the lesion will guide the optimal approach for

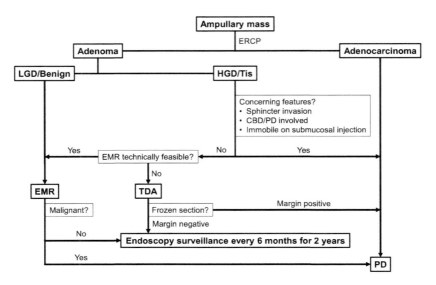

Figure 42.3 Management, decision-making, algorithm for ampullary masses. *Abbreviations:* CBD/PD: common bile duct/pancreatic duct; EMR: endoscopic mucosal resection; ERCP: endoscopic retrograde cholangiopancreatography; HGD: high-grade dysplasia; LGD: low-grade dysplasia; TDA: transduodenal ampullectomy; Tis: Tumour *in situ*; PD: pancreaticoduodenectomy.

management, the ultimate strategy must be tailored to the patient, the biology of their tumour, and the implications for morbidity following an anatomic or endoscopic resection. The understanding of how to best manage ampullary tumours is still in its infancy, but with greater experience, and collaboration, better patient selection for interventions and therapies can be achieved.

REFERENCES

1. Campbell DR Jr, Lee JH. A comprehensive approach to the management of benign and malignant ampullary lesions: Management in hereditary and sporadic settings. *Curr Gastroenterol Rep* 2020;**22(9)**:46.
2. Westgaard A, Tafjord S, Farstad IN, Cvancarova M, Eide TJ, Mathisen O, et al. Pancreatobiliary versus intestinal histologic type of differentiatiois an independent prognostic factor in resected periampullary adenocarcinoma. *BMC Cancer* 2008;**8**:170.
3. Michelassi F, Erroi F, Dawson PJ, Peitrabissa A, Noda S, Handcock M, et al. Experience with 647 consecutive tumors of the duodenum, ampulla, head of the pancreas, and distal common bile duct. *Ann Surg* 1989;**210(4)**:544–54;discussion 554–46.
4. Howe JR, Klimstra DS, Moccia RD, Conlon KC, Brennan MF. Factors predictive of survival in ampullary carcinoma. *Ann Surg* 1998;**228(1)**:87–94.
5. Sato T, Konishi K, Kimura H, Maeda K, Yabushita M, Tsuji M, et al. Adenoma and tiny carcinoma in adenoma of the papilla of Vater–p53 and PCNA. *Hepatogastroenterology* 1999;**46(27)**:1959–62.
6. Seifert E, Schulte F, Stolte M. Adenoma and carcinoma of the duodenum and papilla of Vater: A clinicopathologic study. *Am J Gastroenterol* 1992;**87(1)**:37–42.
7. Qiao QL, Zhao YG, Ye ML, Yang Y-M, Zhao J-X, Huang Y-T, et al. Carcinoma of the ampulla of Vater:

Factors influencing long-term survival of 127 patients with resection. *World J Surg* 2007;**31(1)**:137–43;discussion 144–36.
8. Kimura W, Ohtsubo K. Incidence, sites of origin, and immunohistochemical and histochemical characteristics of atypical epithelium and minute carcinoma of the papilla of Vater. *Cancer* 1988;**61(7)**:1394–402.
9. Cattell RB, Pyrtek LJ. Premalignant lesions of the ampulla of Vater. *Surg Gynecol Obstet* 1950;**90(1)**:21–30.
10. Kimura W, Futakawa N, Yamagata S, Wada Y, Kuroda A, Muto T, et al. Different clinicopathologic findings in two histologic types of carcinoma of papilla of Vater. *Jpn J Cancer Res* 1994;**85(2)**:161–6.
11. Panzeri F, Crippa S, Castelli P, Aleotti F, Pucci A, Partelli S, et al. Management of ampullary neoplasms: A tailored approach between endoscopy and surgery. *World J Gastroenterol* 2015;**21(26)**:7970–87.
12. Tasaka K. Carcinoma in the region of the duodenal papilla. A histopathologic study (author's transl). *Fukuoka Igaku Zasshi* 1977;**68(1)**:20–44.
13. Cubilla AL, Fitzgerald PJ. Surgical pathology aspects of cancer of the ampulla-head-of-pancreas region. *Monogr Pathol* 1980;**21**:67–81.
14. Albores–Saavedra J. Tumors of the gallbladder, extrahepatic bile ducts, and ampulla of Vater. *Atlas Tumor Pathol* 2000;**27**:259–316.
15. Kayahara M, Nagakawa T, Ohta T, Kitagawa H, Miyazaki I. Surgical strategy for carcinoma of the papilla of Vater on the basis of lymphatic spread and mode of recurrence. *Surgery* 1997;**121(6)**:611–17.
16. Walsh DB, Eckhauser FE, Cronenwett JL, Turcotte JG, Lindenauer SM. Adenocarcinoma of the ampulla of Vater. Diagnosis and treatment. *Ann Surg* 1982;**195(2)**:152–7.
17. Neoptolemos JP, Talbot IC, Carr-Locke DL, Shaw DE, Cockleburgh R, Hall AW, et al. Treatment and

outcome in 52 consecutive cases of ampullary carcinoma. *Br J Surg* 1987;**74(10)**:957–61.

18. Bakkevold KE, Arnesjo B, Kambestad B. Carcinoma of the pancreas and papilla of Vater-assessment of resectability and factors influencing resectability in stage I carcinomas. A prospective multicentre trial in 472 patients. *Eur J Surg Oncol* 1992;**18(5)**:494–507.

19. Ponchon T, Berger F, Chavaillon A, Bory R, Lambert R. Contribution of endoscopy to diagnosis and treatment of tumors of the ampulla of Vater. *Cancer* 1989;**64(1)**:161–7.

20. Tsukada K, Takada T, Miyazaki M, Miyakawa S, Nagino M, Kondo S, et al. Diagnosis of biliary tract and ampullary carcinomas. *J Hepatobiliary Pancreat Surg* 2008;**15(1)**:31–40.

21. Todoroki T, Koike N, Morishita Y, Kawamoto T, Ohkohchi N, Shoda J, et al. Patterns and predictors of failure after curative resections of carcinoma of the ampulla of Vater. *Ann Surg Oncol* 2003;**10(10)**:1176–83.

22. Smith RA, Ghaneh P, Sutton R, Raraty M, Campbell F, Neoptolemos JP. Prognosis of resected ampullary adenocarcinoma by preoperative serum CA19–9 levels and platelet–lymphocyte ratio. *J Gastrointest Surg* 2008;**12(8)**:1422–8.

23. Chen YF, Mai CR, Tie ZJ, Feng ZT, Zhang J, Lu XH, et al. The diagnostic significance of carbohydrate antigen CA 19-9 in serum and pancreatic juice in pancreatic carcinoma. *Chin Med J (Engl)* 1989;**102(5)**:333–7.

24. Skordilis P, Mouzas IA, Dimoulios PD, Alexandrakis G, Moschandrea J, Kouroumalis E. Is endosonography an effective method for detection and local staging of the ampullary carcinoma? A prospective study. *BMC Surg* 2002;**2**:1.

25. Chen CH, Tseng LJ, Yang CC, Yeh YH. Preoperative evaluation of periampullary tumors by endoscopic sonography, transabdominal sonography, and computed tomography. *J Clin Ultrasound* 2001;**29(6)**:313–21.

26. Chen WX, Xie QG, Zhang WF, Zhang X, Hu T-T, Xu P, et al. Multiple imaging techniques in the diagnosis of ampullary carcinoma. *Hepatobiliary Pancreat Dis Int* 2008;**7(6)**:649–53.

27. Komorowski RA, Beggs BK, Geenan JE, Venu RP. Assessment of ampulla of Vater pathology. An endoscopic approach. *Am J Surg Pathol* 1991;**15(12)**:1188–96.

28. Rosch T, Braig C, Gain T, et al. Staging of pancreatic and ampullary carcinoma by endoscopic ultrasonography. Comparison with conventional sonography, computed tomography, and angiography. *Gastroenterology* 1992;**102(1)**:188–99.

29. Midwinter MJ, Beveridge CJ, Wilsdon JB, Bennett MK, Baudouin CJ, Charnley RM. Correlation between spiral computed tomography, endoscopic ultrasonography and findings at operation in pancreatic and ampullary tumours. *Br J Surg* 1999;**86(2)**:189–93.

30. Manta R, Conigliaro R, Castellani D, Messerotti A, Bertani H, Sabatino G, et al. Linear endoscopic ultrasonography vs magnetic resonance imaging in ampullary tumors. *World J Gastroenterol* 2010;**16(44)**:5592–7.

31. Nikolaidis P, Hammond NA, Day K, Yaghmai V, Wood CG 3rd, Mosback DS, et al. Imaging features of benign and malignant ampullary and periampullary lesions. *Radiographics* 2014;**34(3)**:624–41.

32. Yamaguchi K, Enjoji M, Kitamura K. Endoscopic biopsy has limited accuracy in diagnosis of ampullary tumors. *Gastrointest Endosc* 1990;**36(6)**:588–92.

33. Sauvanet A, Chapuis O, Hammel P, Fléjou JF, Ponsot P, Bernades P, et al. Are endoscopic procedures able to predict the benignity of ampullary tumors? *Am J Surg* 1997;**174(3)**:355–8.

34. Kahaleh M, Shami VM, Brock A, Conaway MR, Yoshida C, Moskaluk CA, et al. Factors predictive of malignancy and endoscopic resectability in ampullary neoplasia. *Am J Gastroenterol* 2004;**99(12)**:2335–39.

35. Cheng CL, Sherman S, Fogel EL, McHenry L, Watkins JL, Fukushima T, et al. Endoscopic snare papillectomy for tumors of the duodenal papillae. *Gastrointest Endosc* 2004;**60(5)**:757–64.

36. Albores-Saavedra J, Schwartz AM, Batich K, Henson DE. Cancers of the ampulla of Vater: Demographics, morphology, and survival based on 5,625 cases from the SEER program. *J Surg Oncol* 2009;**100(7)**:598–605.

37. Partelli S, Crippa S, Capelli P, Neri A, Bassi C, Zamboni G, et al. Adequacy of lymph node retrieval for ampullary cancer and its association with improved staging and survival. *World J Surg* 2013;**37(6)**:1397–404.

38. Moekotte AL, Malleo G, van Roessel S, Bonds M, Halimi A, Zarantonello L, et al. Gemcitabine-based adjuvant chemotherapy in subtypes of ampullary adenocarcinoma: International propensity score-matched cohort study. *Br J Surg* 2020;**107(9)**:1171–82.

39. Huang XT, Huang CS, Chen W, Cai J-P, Gan T-T, Zhao Y, et al. Development and validation of a nomogram for predicting overall survival of node-negative ampullary carcinoma. *J Surg Oncol* 2020;**121(3)**:518–23.

40. Neoptolemos JP, Moore MJ, Cox TF, Valle JW, Palmer DH, McDonald AC, et al. Effect of adjuvant chemotherapy with fluorouracil plus folinic acid or gemcitabine vs observation on survival in patients with resected periampullary adenocarcinoma: The ESPAC-3 periampullary cancer randomized trial. *JAMA* 2012;**308(2)**:147–56.

41. Neoptolemos JP, Moore MJ, Cox TF, Valle JW, Palmer DH, McDonald AC, et al. Ampullary cancer ESPAC-3 (v2) trial: A multicentre, international, open-label, randomized controlled phase III trial of adjuvant chemotherapy versus observation in patients with adenocarcinoma of the ampulla of Vater. J Clin Oncol 2011;**29(18_suppl)**:LBA4006–LBA4006.

42. Kleinschmidt TK, Christein J. Neuroendocrine carcinoma of the ampulla of Vater: A case report, review and recommendations. *J Surg Case Rep* 2020;**2020(6)**:rjaa119.

43. Ruff SM, Standring O, Wu G, Levy A, Anantha S, Newman E, et al. Ampullary neuroendocrine tumors: Insight into a rare histology. *Ann Surg Oncol* 2021;**28(13)**:8318–28.

44. Herman JM, Pawlik TM, Merchant NB. Ampulla of Vater. In: Amin MB (ed). *AJCC Cancer Staging Manual*, 8th edition, Springer International Publishing, American Joint Commission on Cancer, 2017, pp. 327.

45. Randle RW, Ahmed S, Newman NA, Clark CJ. Clinical outcomes for neuroendocrine tumors of the duodenum and ampulla of Vater: A population-based study. *J Gastrointest Surg* 2014;**18(2)**:354–62.

46. van Stolk R, Sivak MV Jr, Petrini JL, Petras R, Ferguson DR, Jagelman D. Endoscopic management of upper gastrointestinal polyps and periampullary lesions in familial adenomatous polyposis and Gardner's syndrome. *Endoscopy* 1987;**19 (Suppl 1)**:19–22.

47. Stolte M, Pscherer C. Adenoma-carcinoma sequence in the papilla of Vater. *Scand J Gastroenterol* 1996;**31(4)**:376–82.

48. Groves CJ, Saunders BP, Spigelman AD, Phillips RK. Duodenal cancer in patients with familial adenomatous polyposis (FAP): Results of a 10 year prospective study. *Gut* 2002;**50(5)**:636–41.

49. Matsumoto T, Iida M, Nakamura S, Hizawa K, Yao T, Tsuneyoshi M, et al. Natural history of ampullary adenoma in familial adenomatous polyposis: Reconfirmation of benign nature during extended surveillance. *Am J Gastroenterol* 2000;**95(6)**:1557–62.

50. Jagelman DG, DeCosse JJ, Bussey HJ. Upper gastrointestinal cancer in familial adenomatous polyposis. *Lancet* 1988;**1(8595)**:1149–51.

51. Brosens LA, Keller JJ, Offerhaus GJ, Goggins M, Giardiello FM. Prevention and management of duodenal polyps in familial adenomatous polyposis. *Gut* 2005;**54(7)**:1034–43.

52. de Campos FG, Perez RO, Imperiale AR, Seid VE, Nahas SC, Cecconello I. Evaluating causes of death in familial adenomatous polyposis. *J Gastrointest Surg* 2010;**14(12)**:1943–9.

53. Jaganmohan S, Lynch PM, Raju RP, Ross WA, Lee JE, Raju GS, et al. Endoscopic management of duodenal adenomas in familial adenomatous polyposis: A single-centre experience. *Dig Dis Sci* 2012;**57(3)**:732–7.

54. van Leerdam ME, Roos VH, van Hooft JE, Dekker E, Jover R, Kaminski MF, et al. Endoscopic management of polyposis syndromes: European Society of Gastrointestinal Endoscopy (ESGE) Guideline. *Endoscopy* 2019;**51(9)**:877–95.

55. Offerhaus GJ, Giardiello FM, Krush AJ, Booker SV, Tersmette AC, Kelley NC, et al. The risk of upper gastrointestinal cancer in familial adenomatous polyposis. *Gastroenterology* 1992;**102(6)**:1980–82.

56. Debinski HS, Spigelman AD, Hatfield A, Williams CB, Phillips RK. Upper intestinal surveillance in familial adenomatous polyposis. *Eur J Cancer* 1995;**31A(7–8)**:1149–53.

57. Bjork J, Akerbrant H, Iselius L, Bergman A, Engwall Y, Wahlström J, et al. Periampullary adenomas and adenocarcinomas in familial adenomatous polyposis: Cumulative risks and APC gene mutations. *Gastroenterology* 2001;**121(5)**:1127–35.

58. Latchford AR, Neale KF, Spigelman AD, Phillips RK, Clark SK. Features of duodenal cancer in patients with familial adenomatous polyposis. *Clin Gastroenterol Hepatol* 2009;**7(6)**:659–63.

59. Rattner DW, Fernandez-del Castillo C, Brugge WR, Warshaw AL. Defining the criteria for local resection of ampullary neoplasms. *Arch Surg* 1996;**131(4)**:366–71.

60. Yoon SM, Kim MH, Kim MJ, Jang SJ, Lee TY, Kwon S, et al. Focal early stage cancer in ampullary adenoma: Surgery or endoscopic papillectomy? *Gastrointest Endosc* 2007;**66(4)**:701–7.

61. Grobmyer SR, Stasik CN, Draganov P, Hemming AW, Dixon LR, Vogel SB, et al. Contemporary results with ampullectomy for 29 "benign" neoplasms of the ampulla. *J Am Coll Surg* 2008;**206(3)**:466–71.

62. Halsted WS. Contributions to the surgery of the bile passages, especially of the common bile-duct. *Bost Med Surg* 1899;**141(26)**:645–54.

63. Knox RA, Kingston RD. Carcinoma of the ampulla of Vater. *Br J Surg* 1986;**73(1)**:72–3.

64. Asbun HJ, Rossi RL, Munson JL. Local resection for ampullary tumors. Is there a place for it? *Arch Surg* 1993;**128(5)**:515–20.

65. Alstrup N, Burcharth F, Hauge C, Horn T. Transduodenal excision of tumours of the ampulla of Vater. *Eur J Surg* 1996;**162(12)**:961–7.

66. Patel R, Varadarajulu S, Wilcox CM. Endoscopic ampullectomy: Techniques and outcomes. *J Clin Gastroenterol* 2012;**46(1)**:8–15.

67. Winter JM, Cameron JL, Olino K, Herman JM, de Jong MC, Hruban RH, et al. Clinicopathologic analysis of ampullary neoplasms in 450 patients: Implications for surgical strategy and long-term prognosis. *J Gastrointest Surg* 2010;**14(2)**:379–87.

68. Ito K, Fujita N, Noda Y, Kobayashi G, Obana T, Horaguchi J, et al. Impact of technical modification of endoscopic papillectomy for ampullary neoplasm on the occurrence of complications. *Dig Endosc* 2012;**24(1)**:30–35.

69. Bohnacker S, Seitz U, Nguyen D, Thonke F, Seewald S, deWeerth A, et al. Endoscopic resection of benign tumors of the duodenal papilla without and with intraductal growth. *Gastrointest Endosc* 2005;**62(4)**:551–60.

70. Perez-Cuadrado-Robles E, Piessevaux H, Moreels TG, Yeung R, Aouattah T, Komuta M, et al. Combined excision and ablation of ampullary tumors with biliary or pancreatic intraductal extension is effective even in malignant neoplasms. *United European Gastroenterol J* 2019;**7(3)**:369–76.

71. Heise C, Abou Ali E, Hasenclever D, Auriemma F, Gulla A, Regner S, et al. Systematic review with meta–analysis: Endoscopic and surgical resection for ampullary lesions. *J Clin Med* 2020;**9(11)**:3622.

72. Committee ASoP, Chathadi KV, Khashab MA, Acosta RD, Chandrasekhara V, Eloubeidi MA, et al. The role of endoscopy in ampullary and duodenal adenomas. *Gastrointest Endosc* 2015;**82(5)**:773–81.

73. Yamao T, Isomoto H, Kohno S, Mizuta Y, Yamakawa M, Nakao K, et al. Endoscopic snare papillectomy with biliary and pancreatic stent placement for tumors of the major duodenal papilla. *Surg Endosc* 2010;**24(1)**:119–24.

Chapter 43

Resection Principles of Hepatectomy

Wei-Ren Liu, Wei-Feng Qu, Jun Gao, Xiao-Ling Wu and Ying-Hong Shi

INTRODUCTION

Compared to other surgical specialties, liver surgery and especially hepatectomy were late to appear, due to their complexity. The first recorded hepatectomy was performed by Berta in 1716. In 1886, Lius removed a tumour from the left lobe of the liver of a patient who unfortunately died of haemorrhage 6 hours later. Langenbuch is credited with the first successful hepatectomy (1). In 1887, he performed a hepatectomy on a 30-year-old woman with abdominal pain and removed a benign tumour. In 1899, Keen carried out the first anatomic hepatectomy (2) and in 1910, Wendel performed a right hepatic lobectomy following formal ligation of the right hepatic artery and the right hepatic duct in the porta hepatis.

After the outbreak of World War II, the use of anti-biotics and anaesthetic advances facilitated the development of formal and more extensive hepatectomy procedures. In 1952, Lortat-Jocob and Robert performed the first 'classical' right hepatectomy with initial ligation of the vessels in the porta hepatis to control intraoperative bleeding. In 1955, Claude Couinaud, in Paris, proposed the concept of defining the anatomical regions of liver based on the distribution of the portal vein and carried out detailed studies on the anatomical structure of the liver. His research enabled the development of hepatectomy from the original lobectomies and local resections, to surgical procedures based on an understanding of the intrahepatic segmental anatomy. These changes heralded the modern era of liver surgery with improved safety and better outcomes, due to the more precise nature of the operative procedure. Couinaud's anatomical segmentation of liver remains the framework upon which surgical approaches to liver resection are based (3–6).

In 1991, Reich pioneered the use of laparoscopy for hepatectomy (7). In the first 10 years, the adoption and development of laparoscopic hepatectomy was cautious, mainly due to a lack of surgical familiarity with minimally invasive procedures, other than chole-cystectomy, and the technical difficulty particularly with access to the porta hepatis and posteriorly placed lesions (8). However, with increased familiarity and training, more surgeons have started to perform laparoscopic hepatectomy and it has become a routine procedure in tertiary centres. In addition, preoperative imaging

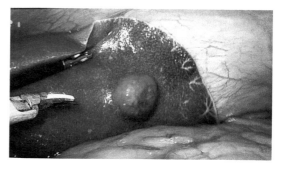

Figure 43.1 Surgical image showing the use of indocyanine green (ICG) fluorescence imaging to guide a hepatectomy of a posteriorly based lesion.

evaluation, intraoperative fluorescence imaging and the application of 3D-laparoscopic technology have aided the development of laparoscopic liver surgery and the location of liver tumours is no longer an absolute contraindication (9,10). Developments in the field continue, and indocyanine green (ICG) fluorescence imaging is now available to guide surgeons performing resections for malignant tumours and is especially valuable to facilitate the segmental resection (*Figure 43.1*) of posteriorly based lesions (segments 4a, 7 and 8).

PREOPERATIVE EVALUATION FOR HEPATECTOMY

Preoperative patient evaluation

As with all surgical procedures, the preoperative evaluation of the patient's overall condition is essential. This is particularly true for those patients with liver pathology and concomitant parenchymal disease, either constitutional, such as cirrhosis, or as a consequence of treatment, including chemotherapy. The preoperative work-up must include an assessment of the cardiovascular, respiratory, renal and endocrine systems and nutritional status. For older patients and those with significant comorbidity, the Eastern Cooperative Oncology Group (ECOG) performance status (11) and American Society of Anesthesiologists (ASA) grades are recommended (12).

DOI: 10.1201/9781003080060-43

The evaluation of liver function and tumour characteristics are essential. For patients who have hepatitis B infection with a high viral-load and elevated serum alanine transaminase (ALT), preoperative active anti-viral therapy should be initiated (13). Major hepatic resection in patients with portal hypertension and advanced cirrhosis will need to be carefully considered and planned. For patients with obstructive jaundice for more than 2 weeks, or serum total bilirubin over 200 μmol/L, percutaneous transhepatic drainage (PTCD) should be performed in order to improve the chance of an uneventful postoperative course (14).

For the evaluation of liver lesions, imaging should include: 1) Colour Doppler ultrasound (US); 2) contrast-enhanced computed tomography (CECT); 3) magnetic resonance imaging (MRI); 4) positron emission tomography CT (PET-CT); 5) digital image reconstruction in cases where tumours are located in difficult positions and 6) liver biopsy when doubt concerning the nature of the lesion remains. Lesions should always be initially evaluated non-invasively and assessment should include: 1) The need to perform multiple resections; 2) the potential involvement of adjacent organs; 3) the possibility of a synchronous approach; 4) which important vessels are involved; 5) whether the vascular structures, which can be preserved, will be adequate to ensure recovery following the surgery and/or 6) the need to consider vascular reconstruction.

Evaluation of hepatic functional reserve

Preoperative evaluation of liver functional reserve is performed to predict whether a tumour can be completely resected safely. A comprehensive assessment of liver function reserve should be based on serological tests, Child-Pugh grade and ICG excretion test. Important serological tests include: 1) ALT; 2) aspartate aminotransferase (AST); 3) alkaline phosphatase (ALP) and 4) γ-glutamyltransferase (r-GGT). Bilirubin and albumin are useful in patients undergoing general surgical procedures but are inadequate for the assessment of patients prior to liver resection, especially if the patient has cirrhosis. An ICG excretion test, combined with the Child-Pugh grade, is the most accurate method to predict the response of patients after a liver resection and ensure an uneventful postoperative recovery (15).

Evaluation of liver lesions

The planning of a safe and potentially curative liver resection requires information about the nature of the lesion and anatomical details. For asymptomatic benign liver lesions, such as hepatic haemangioma and focal nodular hyperplasia, considerable care must be exercised when deciding whether surgery is indicated. For malignant tumours, the performance of a complete R0 resection should always be the aim to avoid a non-curative hepatectomy and careful preoperative planning is required. The quantitative hepatectomy decision-making system (QHD-MS) is the key to determining whether a hepatectomy can be carried out safely in the context of patients with different liver diseases. A number of 3D-interactive quantitative surgical planning approaches (IQSP) now exist to guide abdominal surgery decision-making. The QHD-MS combines the ICG R15 level, Child-Pugh

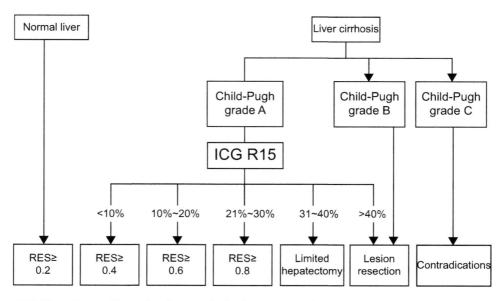

Figure 43.2 Flow diagram illustrating the quantitative hepatectomy decision-making system. *Abbreviation:* RES: essential functional standardized liver volume ratio.

grade, imaging examination and evaluation of liver parenchyma and vascular anatomies with the calculation of liver volume and uses R_{ES} to set the safety limit of liver resection (SLLR) (*Figure 43.2*) (16).

Evaluation of surgical approaches

For benign lesions, the maturity of laparoscopic liver surgery means it should be the preferred approach. Non-anatomical resections are safe and will allow the maximum amount of liver parenchyma to be preserved. For malignant lesions, where vascular invasion is evident, to achieve an adequate clearance and to ensure an R0 resection, a vascular reconstruction will be needed and open surgery is recommended. A formal anatomical hepatectomy is recommended for most advanced malignant liver lesions and large benign lesions involving a number of liver segments. However, a non-anatomical hepatectomy may need to be performed even for malignant lesions when the liver functional reserve is borderline (17). Finally, extracorporeal hepatectomy is technically feasible and can be considered when liver tumours invade multiple vessels, especially when the tumour is so large that *in vivo* hepatectomy and reconstruction would not be technically feasible or if massive bleeding control would not be possible due to the size or location of the tumour.

HEPATECTOMY

Basic principles of hepatectomy

Tumour-free principle

The 'tumour-free principle' is an important concept, the aim of which is to reduce the chance of local recurrence. It includes non-contact surgery, the early isolation of any intraluminal tumour thrombus and macroscopically clear margins to achieve an R0 resection and avoid iatrogenic dissemination (18). In patients with vascular invasion, combined vascular resection and reconstruction can significantly improve the chance of a potentially curative resection. Radiofrequency ablation (RFA) and other *in situ* ablative techniques can be employed as an adjunct to address possible residual disease after the resection of the main lesions.

Maximizing residual functional liver volume

If during preoperative imaging, vascular reconstruction is anticipated, it is essential that the perfusion, and drainage, of the residual liver at the end of the procedure are adequate to ensure postoperative recovery is uneventful (19). Intermittent inflow occlusion is acceptable, but should be performed for as short a time as possible to minimize the effect of liver ischaemia-reperfusion on the future liver remnant (FLR).

Injury control during surgery

Control of bleeding is important during liver surgery. Careful selection of the parenchymal transection plane, recognition of the location of major inflow and outflow vessels (aided by the use of intraoperative US) and the use of the Pringle manoeuvre will minimize blood loss. Vascular structures must also be dealt with securely using a combination of suture ligation, locking clips and stapling devices. The surgical incision should be chosen to ensure adequate access for the proposed procedure and to reduce the risk of inadvertent injury to the FLR. Surgical technique should emphasize gentle tissue handling, the avoidance of unnecessary retraction and the use of large ligatures or suture material.

Selection of surgical incision and approach

Selection of surgical incision

The choice of surgical incision, both the extent and the position, should be based on the tumour characteristics including size and texture, and for multiple lesions, the need to access different parts of the liver. It is important to remember that for tumours which are likely to be soft and potentially rupture, an appropriate incision will need to be larger to facilitate gentle handling and control (20).

When lesions are unequivocally benign, the need to avoid handling wherever possible is not as important and incisions can consequently be relatively limited to reduce the associated morbidity. A right reverse 'L' incision is the most common incision for the majority of resections. When the left side of the liver needs to be fully exposed, a left 'L' or 'Mercedes-Benz' incision can be used. When the target lesion is located in the hilar region, in patients with an acute V-shaped costal margin, for lesions involving the diaphragm or hepatic veins and when patients have a very deep chest, resection of xiphoid process and full retraction of both costal margins will improve the exposure. For very large lesions high in the right upper quadrant applied to and potentially involving the diaphragm, especially when the right hepatic vein and inferior vena cava are compressed or involved, a combined thoracoabdominal incision can be used to obtain the maximum exposure and control and consequently the safest operating field.

Anatomical or non-anatomical hepatectomy

When performing an anatomic hepatectomy, the Glissonean sheath (Glisson's capsule was discovered by Johannis Walaeus in 1640 and described by Francis Glisson in 1654) investing the inflow vessels to the target lesion should be controlled and disconnected prior to transection of the liver parenchyma (21). Non-anatomic hepatectomy is based on a resection line determined by preoperative imaging and intraoperative assessment, both manually and with intraoperative US. The resection line is marked to ensure a clear macroscopic margin and an R0 resection, avoiding major vessels where possible, and preserving the inflow and drainage of all the segments of the FLR.

Determining the hepatic parenchyma transection plane

Surgical resection of liver for malignant tumours should include a margin of non-tumour containing liver tissue. Identifying the extent of the tumour with intraoperative US is very valuable and facilitates a clear understanding to its relationship to intrahepatic vessels and bile ducts, while ensuring an adequate resection margin. A number of methods are available to identify the correct transection plane.

Anatomical landmarks such as the ligamentum teres or falciform ligament identify the plane between segments 2 and 3 and segment 4. Cantlie's line (first described by the Scottish surgeon James Cantlie in 1887) describes the boundary between the left- and right-liver lobes and extends from the middle hepatic vein (or the inferior vena cava) to the middle of the gallbladder fossa (22). The root of the main hepatic vein can predict its intrahepatic direction and mark the boundary between liver segments. Pathological changes can be used if the liver parenchyma has been affected by involvement of vascular structures, resulting in perfusion abnormalities. This may be due to invasion of vessels, intrahepatic stones, and previous surgery, including portal vein ligation for staged procedures. These changes may produce a natural boundary or landmark due to atrophy or hypertrophy, or clear demarcation indicated by the colour of the different parts of the liver.

The extent of the ischaemia resulting from inflow occlusion when performing anatomical resections will determine the resection plane. Portal vein puncture staining techniques are performed under intraoperative US guidance, and the portal vein branch supplying the target lesion is identified and injected with a biological dye (positive staining), or the adjacent liver segment(s) which are to be preserved can be injected (reverse staining).

Digital off-plane image determination technology can be employed to accurately delineate the transection plane. Intraoperative US scans, CT, and MRI images can be combined using fusion navigation technology and 3D image-augmented reality technology to identify the real-time position of lesions and intrahepatic vessels. Finally, virtual fluoroscopy which uses image-guided computer technology to enhance a standard C-arm fluoroscope, allowing pre-acquired fluoroscopic images to be used for real-time surgical localization and instrument tracking, can greatly improve the accuracy of determining parenchymal transection planes.

Liver parenchyma transection

Principles

Surgery must be performed delicately, and the loss of liver parenchyma minimized, by carefully preserving the hepatic vascular structure supplying the proposed FLR. Clear objectives of the operation should be decided at the outset. Liver surgery commences on the surface of the organ and proceeds centrally, identifying the sectoral and segmental vessels and bile ducts. It is important to avoid opening a deep plane with narrow access as this limits the ability to dissect gently and makes the control of bleeding difficult.

Techniques of liver parenchyma transection

Parenchymal transection techniques can be divided into three groups:

1 Initially transect the liver parenchyma using a waterjet and Peng's dissector and then clamp the vessels, the classical 'clamp method'. In 1990, SY Peng and JT Li of Sir Run Run Shaw Hospital, Zhejiang University in China, developed a versatile electrosurgical instrument called Peng's multifunction operative dissector (PMOD) (Hangzhou Shuyou Medical Instrument Co, Hangzhou, Zhejiang, PR China) (23)

2 Simultaneous transection of liver parenchyma and vascular closure using devices which cut and coagulate, or cut and seal vessels, including the Harmonic™ scalpel, TissueLink™ and LigaSure™ (*Figure 43.3*)

3 First seal the vessel and then transect the liver parenchyma using the Habib® radiofrequency ablation (RFA)-assisted hepatectomy device. The Habib 4X is a bipolar, hand-held, disposable RF device consisting of two pairs of opposing electrodes with an active end of 6 or 10 cm in length. The device is connected to a 500 kHz generator (Model 1500X), (AngioDynamics, New York, USA)

Control of bleeding

Application of hepatic vascular occlusion

Vascular occlusion is the most effective means of controlling bleeding during liver parenchyma transection (24). The impact of repeated vascular inflow occlusion is significantly less than that of massive bleeding and infusion of allogeneic blood or blood products. Vascular occlusion can be selective or non-selective, and the surgeon should choose a technique depending on the operative approach and developments during the operation. The Pringle method, which is simple and effective, is the most

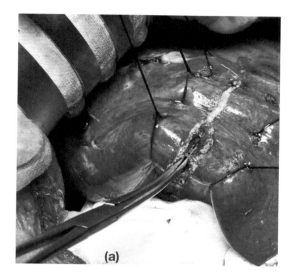

(a)

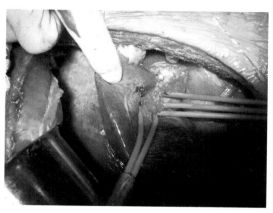

Figure 43.4 In-surgery image showing an extrahepatic Glissonean pedicle transection technique for a selective inflow occlusion.

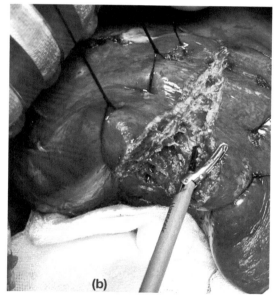

(b)

Figure 43.3 In-surgery images demonstrating two liver parenchyma transection techniques; the classical clamp-crush (a) and using a Harmonic scalpel dissection (b).

Low central venous pressure

The central venous pressure should be controlled at ≤5 cm H_2O. As long as the patient is cardiovascularly stable, a lower central venous pressure will significantly reduce blood loss from backflow in hepatic veins. It can be achieved by a reverse Trendelenberg position, reducing the tidal volume, controlling the rate and volume of any intravenous fluids, and the use of diuretics and/or vasodilators as appropriate (25).

Vascular reconstruction

Vascular reconstructions are occasionally required to comply with the requirements for a well-vascularized FLR following a major resection, or where tumours are awkwardly (often centrally) placed. With the aid of operating loupes, surgeons who are experienced in vascular surgical techniques can complete the reconstruction of arteries, thin veins, and even subsegmental components of the of liver (19).

Technique of vessel reconstruction

Non-absorbable PROLENE™ sutures are generally used for vascular anastomosis, and the appropriate size selected according to the diameter and thickness of the vessel wall. Presently the classic fixed-point method is used, where two or three equidistant sutures are placed along the vascular circumference and tension is applied while the remaining sutures are inserted. A continuous or intermittent suture technique can be used depending on the diameter of the vessel. Surgeons should avoid the distortion or twisting of the vessel which should be under moderate tension when the anastomosis has been completed. During the reconstruction of the hepatic artery, the intima of both sides must be kept intact to avoid the formation of aneurysm and delayed bleeding. For portal vein anastomoses, excessive tightening of the suture must be avoided to prevent narrowing

commonly used occlusion technique. It is performed by clamping the hepatic pedicle containing the hepatic artery and portal vein for intermittent periods of 10–15 minutes, with unclamping for 5 minutes between each period. The extrahepatic Glissonean pedicle transection method is another popular method to achieve selective inflow occlusion during hepatic resection (*Figure 43.4*).

and iatrogenic portal hypertension. The angle of the anastomotic plane should be carefully constructed to ensure that the venous outflow tract has no angulation, tension or folding, and lies in a natural position.

Biliary reconstruction

Ideally biliary reconstructions replicate the original anatomy and physiology as far as possible. When an end-to-end reconstruction is not technically possible, or there is a risk of leak or stricture due to concerns about the blood supply, a Roux-en-Y hepaticojejunostomy should be performed using full thickness mucosa apposing sutures (26).

POSTOPERATIVE MANAGEMENT FOLLOWING A LIVER RESECTION

Prevention and management of postoperative complications

Post-hepatectomy liver failure

In 2011, the International Study Group of Liver Surgery (ISGLS) proposed a standardized definition and severity classification of post-hepatectomy liver failure (PHLF) (27). The definition states that 'if after excluding biliary obstruction and other non-hepatocellular abnormalities if the international normalized ratio (INR) and serum bilirubin continued to increase on or after 5-postoperative days PHLF is present'. If the preoperative values of INR and serum bilirubin are above the normal range, the values on or after 5-postoperative days should be higher to comply with the definition.

Grade A PHLF is a transient, temporary decline in liver function. Generally, there are no obvious clinical symptoms and patients do not need targeted treatment. Grade B refers to patients with abnormal clinical manifestations, such as a minor degree of ascites, mild respiratory insufficiency, and hepatic encephalopathy. Patients should be given a fresh frozen plasma infusion, albumin supplementation, diuretics, and other medical treatments to maintain normal coagulation and electrolyte levels. Invasive treatments are not required at this stage. Grade C is characterized by massive ascites, cardiovascular instability, renal failure, respiratory compromise, and confusion. These patients will require mechanical ventilation, haemodialysis, artificial liver support, and possibly liver transplantation depending on the indication for the liver resection (benign or malignant pathology).

The incidence of PHLF depends on: 1) The degree of any liver cirrhosis; 2) the presence of active hepatitis; 3) the FLR volume; 4) the severity of intraoperative bleeding; 5) the method and duration of portal vein occlusion; 6) the type of anaesthesia, and 7) the use of perioperative medication (28). Diabetic patients have an increased risk of PHLF after surgery and malnutrition, especially when their BMI is <18.5 kg/m^2;

an independent risk factor leading to poor prognosis following liver resections.

Bile leakage

The incidence of postoperative bile leakage is in the order of 4.0–17% (29). Common causes are incomplete ligation of the distal truncated bile duct at the margin of the remaining liver, leakage from the common bile duct anastomosis, incomplete sutures around a biliary T-tube, and bile duct injury due to poor surgical technique. Following parenchymal transection, the surgeon should use clean gauze to cover the cut surface of the remnant liver to check for any overlooked bile leaks.

Postoperative bile leaks may present as abdominal pain, tenderness, and rebound pain or be identified in drains. Most minor bile leaks will settle if there is no distal biliary obstruction. However, if patients have symptoms of peritonitis, open surgery should be performed as soon as possible to clean the abdominal cavity thoroughly and repair any damaged bile ducts. Antibiotics should be administered if there is any suggestion of infection (16).

Postoperative haemorrhage

The incidence of intraperitoneal haemorrhage usually occurs within 48 hours is 4.2–10% (30). The most common cause is bleeding from the resection margin following incomplete haemostasis during the operation. The resection margin of liver should be covered with gelatin sponge or haemostatic gauze to aid long-term stable haemostasis, and surgeons should examine the whole operative field at the end of operation to confirm that there is no bleeding.

Persistent postoperative haemorrhage can usually be seen in abdominal drains, but blood clots may block the drainage tube leading to persistent abdominal distention and abnormal vital signs, a falling haemaglobin, and abnormal coagulation profile. Patients with uncontrolled bleeding should be operated on urgently (31).

Postoperative infection

The most common sites of infection following liver resections are the abdominal cavity and lungs (32). The causes of abdominal infection include effusions accumulating in the surgical area, bile leakage, and intestinal flora displacement due to acute intraoperative haemorrhage. Pulmonary infections are mainly caused by prolonged bed rest and a reduced willingness to cough and breathe deeply due to postoperative pain.

Tracheal intubation should be removed as soon as possible, pain relief must be adequate and carefully monitored, and patients should be mobilized early and regularly.

Application of Enhanced Recovery After Surgery

Enhanced Recovery After Surgery (ERAS®) protocols have been introduced to optimize perioperative management, reduce traumatic stress, promote functional recovery, reduce postoperative complications, and shorten the recovery time and hospital stay (33,34).

ERAS protocols propose a number of postoperative measures following liver resection including early removal of drainage tubes, removal of urinary catheters within 24–48 hours of surgery, and the use of non-steroidal anti-inflammatory drugs for postoperative pain relief. ERAS also suggests oral feeding should be restarted as soon as possible following recovery of gastrointestinal function. Research has shown that ERAS protocols accelerate the return of gastrointestinal function, do not increase the incidence of complications, morbidity or mortality, reduce the length of hospital stays, and reduce hospital costs.

Postoperative nutritional support

Early enteral nutritional support is recommended following liver resections. Nutritional supplements containing short-chain-length peptide formulations with a lower energy density should be prescribed initially, followed by those containing whole protein formulation with higher energy density. Intravenous nutritional support is occasionally required in patients who are unable to tolerate oral or supplementary nasogastric tube (NG) feeding for prolonged periods (35).

REFERENCES

1. Hardy KJ. Liver surgery: The past 2000 years. *Aust N Z J Surg* 1990;**60(10)**:811–17.
2. Keen WW. IV. Report of a case of resection of the liver for the removal of a neoplasm, with a table of seventy-six cases of resection of the liver for hepatic tumors. *Ann Surg* 1899;**30(3)**:267–83.
3. Bismuth H. A new look on liver anatomy: Needs and means to go beyond the Couinaud scheme. *J Hepatol* 2014;**60(3)**:480–1.
4. Ichida H, Imamura H, Yoshioka R, Mizuno T, Mise Y, Kuwatsuru R, et al. Re-evaluation of the Couinaud classification for segmental anatomy of the right liver, with particular attention to the relevance of cranio-caudal boundaries. *Surgery* 2021;**169(2)**:333–40.
5. Lyu F, Ma AJ, Yip TC-F, Wong GL-H, Yuen PC. Weakly supervised liver tumor segmentation using Couinaud segment annotation. *IEEE Trans Med Imaging* 2022;**41(5)**:1138–49.
6. Han H-S, Yoon Y-S, Cho JY, Hwang DW. Laparoscopic liver resection for hepatocellular carcinoma: Korean experiences. *Liver Cancer* 2013;**2(1)**:25–30.
7. Reich H, McGlynn F, DeCaprio J, Budin R. Laparoscopic excision of benign liver lesions. *Obstet Gynecol* 1991;**78(5 Pt 2)**:956–8.
8. Descottes B, Lachachi F, Sodji M, Valleix D, Durand-Fontanier S, de Laclause BP, et al. Early experience with laparoscopic approach for solid liver tumors: Initial 16 cases. *Ann Surg* 2000;**232(5)**:641–5.
9. Costi R, Capelluto E, Sperduto N, Bruyns J, Himpens J, Cadière GB. Laparoscopic right posterior hepatic bisegmentectomy (Segments VII-VIII). *Surg Endosc* 2003;**17(1)**:162.
10. Han H-S, Cho JY, Yoon Y-S. Techniques for performing laparoscopic liver resection in various hepatic locations. *J Hepatobiliary Pancreat Surg* 2009;**16(4)**:427–32.
11. Young J, Badgery-Parker T, Dobbins T, Jorgensen M, Gibbs P, Faragher I, et al. Comparison of ECOG/WHO performance status and ASA score as a measure of functional status. *J Pain Symptom Manage* 2015;**49(2)**:258–64.
12. Doyle DJ, Hendrix JM, Garmon EH. 2023. American Society of Anesthesiologists Classification. Available from: www.ncbi.nlm.nih.gov/books/NBK441940. (Accessed March 2024).
13. Huang G, Lau WY, Shen F, Pan Z-Y, Fu S-Y, Yang Y, et al. Preoperative hepatitis B virus DNA level is a risk factor for postoperative liver failure in patients who underwent partial hepatectomy for hepatitis B-related hepatocellular carcinoma. *World J Surg* 2014;**38(9)**:2370–6.
14. Umeda J, Itoi T. Current status of preoperative biliary drainage. *J Gastroenterol* 2015;**50(9)**:940–54.
15. Tralhao JG, Hoti E, Oliveiros B, Botelho MF, Castro Sousa F. Study of perioperative liver function by dynamic monitoring of ICG-clearance. *Hepatogastroenterology* 2012;**59(116)**:1179–83.
16. Lau L, Christophi C, Nikfarjam M, Starkey G, Goodwin M, Weinberg L, et al. Assessment of liver remnant using ICG clearance intraoperatively during vascular exclusion: Early experience with the ALIIVE Technique. *HPB Surg* 2015;**2015**:757052.
17. Dai X-M, Xiang Z-Q, Wang Q, Li H-J, Zhu Z. Oncological outcomes of anatomic versus non-anatomic resections for small hepatocellular carcinoma: Systematic review and meta-analysis of propensity-score matched studies. *World J Surg Oncol* 2022;**20(1)**:299.
18. Orcutt ST, Anaya DA. Liver resection and surgical strategies for management of primary liver cancer. *Cancer Control* 2018;**25(1)**:1073274817744621.
19. Radulova-Mauersberger O, Weitz J, Riediger C. Vascular surgery in liver resection. *Langenbecks Arch Surg* 2021;**406(7)**:2217–48.
20. Gaujoux S, Goéré D. Surgical approach for hepatectomy. *J Visc Surg* 2011;**148(6)**:e422–e6.
21. Launois B, Maddern G, Tay KH. The Glissonian approach of the hilum. *Swiss Surg* 1999;**5(3)**:143–6.
22. van Gulik TM, van den Esschert JW. James Cantlie's early messages for hepatic surgeons: How the concept of pre-operative portal vein occlusion was defined. *HPB (Oxford)* 2010;**12(2)**:81–3.
23. Peng SY, LI JT. "Currettage and aspiration dissection technique" using PMOD for liver resection. *HPB (Oxford)* 2008;**10(4)**:285–8.
24. van Gulik TM, de Graaf W, Dinant S, Busch ORC, Gouma DJ. Vascular occlusion techniques during liver resection. *Dig Surg* 2007;**24(4)**:274–81.
25. Hughes MJ, Ventham NT, Harrison EM, Wigmore SJ. Central venous pressure and liver resection: A systematic review and meta-analysis. *HPB (Oxford)* 2015;**17(10)**:863–71.

26. Carmody IC, Romano J, Bohorquez H, Bugeaud E, Bruce DS, Cohen AJ, et al. Novel biliary reconstruction techniques during liver transplantation. *Ochsner J* 2017;**17(1)**:42–5.

27. Rahbari NN, Garden OJ, Padbury R, Brooke-Smith M, Crawford M, Adam R, et al. Posthepatectomy liver failure: A definition and grading by the International Study Group of Liver Surgery (ISGLS). *Surgery* 2011;**149(5)**:713–24.

28. Xing Y, Liu Z-R, Yu W, Zhang H-Y, Song M-M. Risk factors for post-hepatectomy liver failure in 80 patients. *World J Clin Cases* 2021;**9(8)**:1793–802.

29. Yamashita Y, Hamatsu T, Rikimaru T, Tanaka S, Shirabe K, Shimada M, et al. Bile leakage after hepatic resection. *Ann Surg* 2001;**233(1)**:45–50.

30. López-Guerra D, Santos-Naharro J, Rojas-Holguín A, Jaen-Torrejimeno I, Prada-Villaverde A, Blanco-Fernández G. Postoperative bleeding and biliary leak after liver resection: A cohort study between two different fibrin sealant patches. *Sci Rep* 2019;**9(1)**:12001.

31. Rahbari NN, Garden OJ, Padbury R, Maddern G, Koch M, Hugh TJ, et al. Post-hepatectomy haemorrhage: A definition and grading by the International Study Group of Liver Surgery (ISGLS). *HPB (Oxford)* 2011;**13(8)**:528–35.

32. Jin S, Fu Q, Wuyun G, Wuyun T. Management of post-hepatectomy complications. *World J Gastroenterol* 2013;**19(44)**:7983–91.

33. Joliat G-R, Kobayashi K, Hasegawa K, Thomson J-E, Padbury R, Scott M, et al. Guidelines for perioperative care for liver surgery: Enhanced recovery after surgery (ERAS®) society recommendations 2022. *World J Surg* 2023;**47(1)**:11–34.

34. Wang C, Zheng G, Zhang W, Zhang F, Lv S, Wang A, et al. Enhanced recovery after surgery programs for liver resection: A Meta-analysis. *J Gastrointest Surg* 2017;**21(3)**:472–86.

35. Chen L, Chen X, Li G. Nutritional management after hepatopancreatobiliary surgery. *Hepatobiliary Surg Nutr* 2021;**10(2)**:273–5.

Chapter
44

Hepatic Parenchymal Transection

Li Lian Kuan and Guy J. Maddern

INTRODUCTION

In the last few decades, technological advances have led to rapid developments in a number of techniques employed during liver resection. Hepatic parenchymal transection is the most crucial phase of the operation, and morbidity and mortality seem to be related to complications associated with the liver remnant (1). Intraoperative haemorrhage remains one of the major risks during hepatic resections, and operative blood loss and perioperative blood transfusion are two of the most important factors influencing postoperative morbidity and mortality (2–4).

This chapter aims to provide an overview of the surgical techniques currently utilized in hepatic surgery and will discuss the most widely used methods and techniques presently used for hepatic parenchymal transection. The existing randomized data comparing the different approaches will be presented while acknowledging that there isn't 'one size fits all'.

Early hepatic resections were associated with significant mortality due to haemorrhage. The first partial hepatectomy attempted in 1886 by Lius for a hepatic adenoma died 6 hours after surgery due to postoperative haemorrhage (5). The first successful hepatic resection was performed by a German surgeon Carl Johann August Langenbuch in 1888 (6). Technological innovation has allowed for enormous improvements in the safety of hepatic parenchymal resections, and novel techniques have since emerged with the primary aim of reducing blood loss. The various energy devices facilitate the different aspects of liver surgery and play a role in vascular control, haemostasis, and parenchymal transection. Minimally invasive techniques are increasingly utilized for hepatic resection, and while currently only applied in selected patients, the indications are increasing.

Various modalities for hepatic resection have been tested and compared, but the complexity of liver resections and the location of tumours often requires approaches tailored to the individual patient. Although there are a number of different approaches available during hepatic parenchymal transection, the preferred approach remains controversial among liver surgeons and a constant source of debate. There are a range of devices available for hepatic parenchymal transection and in recent years, novel instruments using different types of energy for coagulation or sealing of vessels

have been developed. Methods presently employed range from basic finger fracture or clamp-crushing, to devices based on more complex technology, such as ultrasonic or radiofrequency energy, water-jet technology developed from industrial applications, tissue-sealing devices and surgical staplers (7). These strategies all aim to reduce blood loss and transfusion requirements, and facilitate safe dissection in difficult areas (the hilum and hepatic veins), especially when dealing with malignant pathologies.

With advances in surgical techniques and the perioperative management in liver surgery over the last 30 years, outcomes after hepatic resection have improved substantially and the mortality of large hepatic resections has decreased to 3–5% (8). The evolution of operative techniques is one of the major contributors to the reduction of haemorrhage during the hepatic transection phase of the procedure. Specific examples include the use of intraoperative ultrasound (US), to better delineate transection planes, finer hepatic venous control, both of the inflow and outflow, and stringent central venous pressure monitoring to ensure where possible a CVP of 2–5 mmHg.

It is also important to consider other crucial factors when deciding on a particular technique including: 1) Operative time; 2) a team with the requisite experience; 3) the availability of essential equipment and knowledge of its use, and 4) cost. During the surgery, the type of hepatic resection, extent of thermal injury, and state of the liver parenchyma due to underlying issues such as cirrhosis or non-alcoholic steatohepatitis (NASH), or following chemotherapy (CASH), will also be factors that will guide the surgeon when selecting the most appropriate approach and equipment.

PARENCHYMAL TRANSECTION

Finger fracture and Kelly-clamp crushing

These are the original and oldest techniques for hepatic parenchymal transection and to-date are still widely used by experienced surgeons. Lin et al. first introduced the finger fracture technique in 1958, and described the crushing of the liver parenchyma between the surgeon's fingers under inflow occlusion to isolate vessels and bile radicles for ligation (9). The introduction of the clamp-crushing technique (CCT) in the 1970s served

DOI: 10.1201/9781003080060-44

as a refinement of the finger fracture technique by employing basic surgical clamps to crush the tissue and provides the inexperienced surgeon with a technique of hepatic resection which can be performed rapidly and safely in an almost bloodless field (10,11). Once the hepatic parenchyma is crushed, the exposed vessels and bile ducts can be divided using suture ligation, bipolar electrocautery, vessel sealing devices, or vascular clips (7). This technique is simple, quick, efficient, easy to learn and perform, and cost-effective. It is most often used in combination with the Pringle manoeuvre (total inflow occlusion).

A series of randomized controlled trials (RCTs) and subsequent meta-analyses have examined and compared the finger fracture technique with newer modalities. A meta-analysis by Rahbari et al. included seven RCTs with 554 patients and demonstrated no clinically important benefit of an alternative transection technique in terms of blood loss, parenchymal injury, transection time, and hospital stay (12). A Cochrane review of randomized data advocated for the CCT as the method of choice in hepatic parenchymal transection because it avoids the need for any special equipment and expertise by surgeons and theatre staff. The newer methods which have been examined confer no obvious benefit in respect of decreasing the morbidity or transfusion requirements (13). The review also concluded that the CCT was faster and less expensive (13). Lesurtel et al. performed an RCT which included 100 patients, and compared CCT with the cavitron ultrasonic surgical aspirator (CUSA®), hydro-jet, and a dissecting sealer (14). The CCT was most efficient in respect of resection time, blood loss, and blood transfusion frequency as well as being the most cost-effective (14). The oldest described method, therefore, remains the reference technique for parenchymal transection (15).

Ultrasonic dissection

The CUSA (Integra LifeSciences, New Jersey, USA) is a widely used technology as an alternative to CCT. The CUSA is an ultrasonic surgical dissection and aspiration system that allows tissue to be removed efficiently and selectively. It works by performing three functions which are described as: 1) Fragmentation; 2) irrigation, and 3) aspiration. The hepatic parenchyma is initially fragmented by ultrasonic energy generated through vibration at its tip at 23 kHz which exposes tougher fibrous tissues (Glisson's triads, hepatic veins) (16). The device simultaneously irrigates with saline, and as vascular structures have different water content, they are spared due to their intrinsic properties and fragmentation at different supersonic frequencies. The exposed blood vessels and bile ducts are then carefully isolated atraumatically and subsequently ligated or clipped depending on their size (very small vessels can also be diathermied) (17). The presently available CUSA machines are sophisticated and the power, irrigation, and suction modes can all be adjusted to ensure

selective tissue fragmentation. In patients with cirrhosis, a significant increase in the power setting is frequently required for the transection to be effective.

One of the main advantages of using the CUSA is the precision achievable. This enables a very clear transection plane to be developed with the identification of major structures when they are in close proximity to large, or awkwardly placed, tumours. This ability to delicately dissect adjacent to vital structures or tumours is equally applicable in minimally invasive procedures and ensures that the maximum clearance margin can be achieved safely. CUSA use is associated with low blood loss, has a well-established and documented safety record, and postoperative bile leak rates are low (18). Negative aspects of CUSA use are that it is more time consuming, has a learning curve (albeit relatively short), the expense of the equipment, and it does not produce coagulation.

Water-jet dissector

Papachristou first reported the use of a water-jet (Hydro-Jet) surgical dissector in 1972 (19). The water-jet dissector works by using high pressure (up to 30 atmospheres) to produce a very fine jet of water (a diameter of 0.15 mm). travelling at 62.5 m/s. The technology is based on industrial use, where water-jets are used to cut large pipes using a coherent jet. The design of medical water-jets uses a modified nozzle which allows slight divergence of the jet as the distance from the nozzle increases. In this way the cutting effect is maximal near to the nozzle and dissipates within 10–1 cm, reducing the cutting action and allowing the surgeon to control the effect by movement of the handpiece towards, and away from, the tissue. The fine jet of water disrupts the liver parenchyma and exposes the vascular and ductal structures. (*Figure 44.1*). The jet power is simply adjusted by fine movements according to the consistency of the hepatic parenchyma and requires no adjustment of the machine. Water-jet dissection is also a no-touch technique and the thin laminar liquid-jet effect provides precise, controllable, tissue-selective dissection with excellent visualization, minimal trauma to the surrounding fibrous structures, and limited blood loss (20). However, there is a potential, albeit theoretical, infection risk as a water-jet device produces a considerable aerosol which could contain viral or bacterial particles.

A prospective RCT comparing the water-jet and CUSA devices demonstrated that there were significantly fewer blood transfusions with the water-jet dissector, that it was a rapid and safe surgical technique for hepatic resection, and concluded that it offered an attractive alternative approach (21). Nevertheless, the technique has not gained widespread support and is presently used in far fewer units than CUSA, possibly because newer technologies have emerged, hindering the adoption due to their ability to dissect and coagulate. A meta-analysis of RCTs on techniques

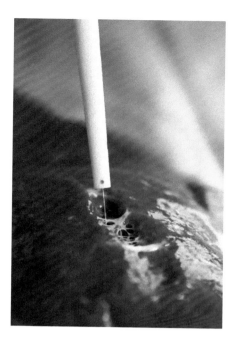

Figure 44.1 Demonstration of a water-jet dissector. (Reprinted with permission from Erbe Elektromedizin GmbH, Georgia, USA.)

of hepatic resection again showed similar results and concluded that 'CCT is more rapid and is associated with lower rates of blood loss and otherwise similar outcomes when compared with other methods of parenchymal transection. It represents the reference standard against which new methods may be compared' (16).

VESSEL SEALING ENERGY DEVICES

The Harmonic™ scalpel

The Harmonic scalpel (J&J Med Tech, New Jersey, USA) uses the principle of ultrasound energy applied to vibrating ultrasonic shears to seal and divide blood vessels up to 3 mm in diameter. The vibration of the blades at 55 500 cycles/second simultaneously cuts and coagulates tissues by causing denaturation of proteins, rather than heat (although some heat is produced). This allows for a more precise transection plane and reduces lateral thermal damage. The Harmonic scalpel and similar devices are ideally suited to use during laparoscopic hepatic resections. In a non-randomized study by Kim et al. the use of the Harmonic scalpel was associated with decreased operative times and a trend toward decreased blood loss and transfusion requirement, although with a significant increase in biliary fistula rates (22). A more recent RCT in living donors did not demonstrate any benefit of the Harmonic scalpel in comparison to CCT (23).

LigaSure™ vessel sealing system

This bipolar device uses a combination pressure and energy to seal vessels, and is claimed to safely occlude arteries, veins, and lymphatics up to 7 mm in diameter. This is achieved using the body's own collagen and elastin to create a permanent fusion zone. When used in hepatic transection, LigaSure (Medtronic, Minnesota, USA) can seal and cut vessels more rapidly, usually within 1–4 seconds, than manual ligation and is more consistent and reliable than conventional electric cautery while delivering less energy to the tissues. This device is useful during hepatic resection in patients with a normal liver parenchyma, where it achieves good haemostasis and seals bile ducts, but its use should be avoided in cirrhosis (24,25).

An RCT conducted in Japan on 120 patients comparing the LigaSure with conventional clamping methods, demonstrated that it was safe but failed to show any significant decrease in operation time or blood loss (26). However, another RCT found that the LigaSure system was an effective and safe tool for decreasing liver resection times compared with conventional clamping methods, and morbidity rates were similar (27).

Thunderbeat™

The Thunderbeat (Olympus Medical Systems Corp., Tokyo, Japan), is the first device to simultaneously integrate electrically generated bipolar energy and ultrasonically generated frictional heat energy. The ultrasonic technology is used for rapid cutting and precise dissection, while the bipolar technology performs reliable vessel sealing (28) (*Figure 44.2*). The Thunderbeat technology is based on its claimed ability to produce a rapid surge in temperature with minimal thermal spreading (29). Aryal et al. demonstrated that the hepatic resection time in the Thunderbeat group in minor hepatectomy was significantly reduced compared with hepatic resection using basic techniques (CCT and CUSA). However, there was no observed difference between the groups in terms of blood transfusion ratio, postoperative complications, and hepatic dysfunction (28).

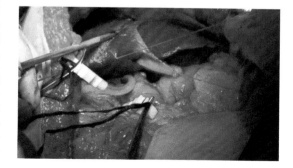

Figure 44.2 Demonstration of technique of parenchymal transection with Thunderbeat. Liver parenchyma being divided using Thunderbeat in a patient with left hepatectomy. (Reprinted with permission from [28].)

RADIOFREQUENCY ABLATION DEVICES

Radiofrequency ablation (RFA) probes work by coagulative necrosis of the hepatic parenchyma and thrombosis and coagulation of small blood vessels. A radiofrequency (RF)-assisted device works by creating a thermal coagulative necrosis along the transection plane to create a bloodless plane. The transection of the hepatic parenchyma is then performed using a scalpel.

Habib™-4X

The RF-based device Habib-4X (AngioDynamics, New York, USA) is used to produce coagulative necrosis along the line of intended hepatic parenchymal transection without vascular clamping of either portal triads or major vessels (30). Firstly, a line is made on the liver surface with diathermy to mark the periphery of the tumour, assisted with bimanual palpation and intraoperative US (*Figure 44.3*). This has to be performed

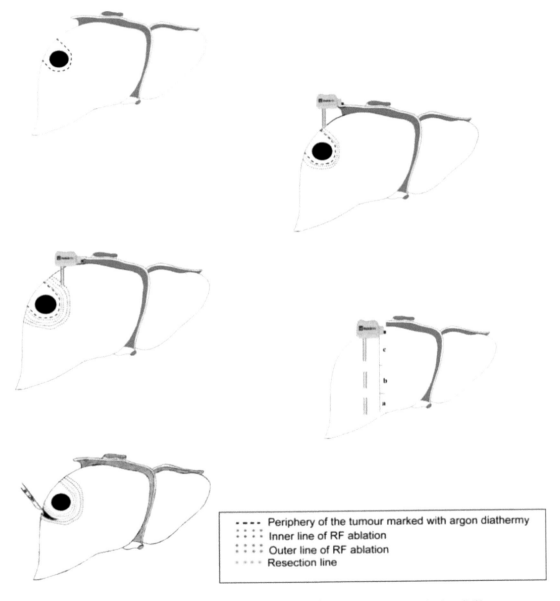

- - - -	Periphery of the tumour marked with argon diathermy
::::	Inner line of RF ablation
::::	Outer line of RF ablation
· · · ·	Resection line

Figure 44.3 The steps to achieve liver resection using Habib 4X. (Reprinted with permission from [31].)

prior to use of the device, as the parenchyma hardens during treatment, making it impossible to visualize the tumour edge with intraoperative US or identify the margins by palpation.

Some compelling evidence has shown that the device has the ability to induce systemic and local immunomodulatory changes that further expand the boundaries of survival outcomes following hepatic resection (32,33). Unfortunately, RF-assisted resection is associated with a significantly higher rate of postoperative complications, particularly bile leak and abdominal abscess formation, compared with CCT (34).

The thermal technique of RF-assisted resection may prevent blood loss by inducing necrotic coagulation along the resection plane, and is a unique, simple, and safe and feasible surgical resection technique for patients with cirrhosis and concomitant HCC (35). A systematic review conducted on laparoscopic RF-assisted hepatic resection for benign and malignant disease showed that RF is a safe and feasible technique associated with a reduction in blood loss, low morbidity, and lower hospital mortality rates (36).

TissueLink™

The TissueLink is a saline-linked RF-dissecting sealer which employs proprietary technology to coagulate and seal tissues to provide haemostasis before and after transection. It delivers RF energy through a conductive fluid (saline) to coagulate and seal tissue. This device may also be used in laparoscopic hepatic resection. A meta-analysis on four clinical trials with 276 patients was unable to demonstrate that the TissueLink device was superior to CCT during hepatic transection (37).

VASCULAR STAPLER

Stapling devices have primarily been used in liver surgery for the control of inflow and outflow vessels. Their use has however expanded and they are now employed for the transection of the parenchyma when performing a liver resection (38). Their increasing acceptance and popularity are based on the ease of manipulation and it enables rapid and efficient transection of the hepatic parenchyma (39–41) (*Figure 44.4*). It is particularly useful in dividing major hepatic duct pedicles in hemi-hepatectomies or large hepatic veins deep within the transection plane (*Figure 44.5*). Stapling devices have become an acceptable alternative, and are essentially indispensable in laparoscopic liver operations due to the convenience, time saved, and security of closure following deployment, especially for minimally invasive major hepatectomy procedures (43,44).

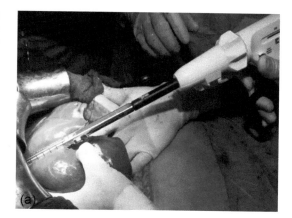

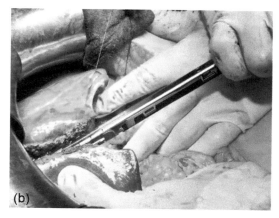

Figure 44.4 Demonstration of vascular staple use, initial (a) and continued (b) during a hepatic parenchymal transection. (Reprinted with permission from [42].)

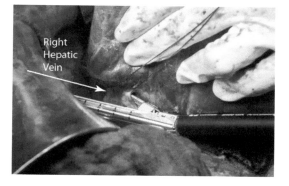

Figure 44.5 Dissection of the right hepatic vein with a 45 mm vascular stapler. (Reprinted with permission from [42].)

One frequent approach is to combine CCT and a stapling device. The parenchyma is crushed with a straight clamp and subsequently transection with a stapler, which again utilizes the easy manipulation and rapid application of the stapling devices. There are limitations, however, and these advantages must be weighed against the known increase in the rate of bile leakage, since the stapler is not very effective in sealing small bile ducts (45). Stapling devices should only be used in select cases and appropriate areas, as large bundles of tissue or abnormally fibrotic parenchyma often result in the device failing to fire properly, resulting in an incomplete or insecure closure potentially with significant bleeding. The appropriate use of a stapler for transection of the hepatic parenchyma is in minor wedge resection or left lateral segmentectomy where the liver tissue is not too bulky (19). A retrospective study of 1174 patients found that the use of a stapling device for hepatic resections was safe and effective, but it is important to note that the uncommon instances (1.1%) of a misfiring stapling device have resulted in adverse outcomes (45).

The CRUNSH trial is an RCT, which compared CCT versus stapled hepatectomy for transection of the parenchyma in elective hepatic resection (46). The trial concluded that stapler transection is a safe technique, but does not reduce intraoperative blood loss in elective hepatic resection compared with the CCT (47).

Another RCT performed by Fritzmann et al. showed that stapled hepatectomy was associated with reduced blood loss and a shorter operating time compared with the LigaSure device when used for parenchymal transection in elective partial hepatectomy (48). There is also an RCT comparing the use of CUSA and a stapling device, which concluded that the stapler offers an attractive alternative for division of the hepatic parenchyma during routine hepatic surgery without adding extra cost (49). The overall conclusion from presently available studies is that the use of endoscopic vascular staplers in hepatic surgery is feasible and safe.

Advances in the techniques used during hepatic surgery have produced dramatic improvements in the safety of hepatic parenchymal resections. There are a number of modalities currently available but CCT and CUSA are currently the two most widely used techniques. Surgeons desire to improve the outcomes for their patients, and their interest in new and emerging technologies often means that novel and expensive devices are introduced in surgical procedures without sufficient evidence for their efficacy, safety or superiority over simpler, traditional techniques. The economic burden associated with medical devices and their impact on healthcare costs means that they should be closely scrutinized when considering their introduction and during the early stage of their adoption.

There remains a paucity of good quality data comparing the various hepatic transection techniques, and the method used is almost inevitably based on the individual surgeon's preference. Nevertheless, certain general recommendations can be made based on existing data. The CCT or CUSA-based techniques in hepatic resection are conventional, validated, safe, and widely utilized. The CCT is a low-cost technique but it requires substantial experience to be used effectively for hepatic transections. Novel instruments lend themselves to quicker transection, and enhance the capability of haemostasis, but lack the precision of CUSA in the dissection around major hepatic veins and may be associated with an increased risk of bile leak. When used alone, they are more suited to wedge or segmental resection where dissection of the major hepatic veins is not required, and they are particularly useful for laparoscopic liver resections (50). All the described approaches and devices can of course be used in combination but this increases the cost substantially. RFA-assisted transection is probably the most rapid method for hepatic transection, but the risk of thermal injury to major bile ducts is a significant adverse effect.

The preferred approach remains, and will remain, controversial among liver surgeons. There is still insufficient evidence for one energy device to be considered superior, and each device has relative advantages and disadvantages. A fundamental understanding of the utility of any of the devices is crucial in deciding which energy source is best suited for a specific procedure. Hepatic parenchymal transection will continue to be a technical challenge in hepatic resections. Liver surgeons should select techniques based on their familiarity with a technique and an understanding of the instruments, and tailor their approach to the individual patient (51). Liver resection remains a formidable operation, and novel developments in the field require multidisciplinary efforts to provide the safest and most efficient treatment to patients (52).

SUMMARY

In the last few decades, technological advancements have led to remarkable developments in the surgical techniques employed for hepatic resection, enabled largely by developments which have expanded the armamentarium available to surgeons. The various surgical energy devices now available, facilitate different aspects of hepatic operations and play a role in vascular control, haemostasis, and parenchymal transection. Several modalities have been tested and compared, but the complexity of hepatic resections, coupled with the location of tumours, often requires various approaches tailored to the individual patient and surgeons must be familiar with a number of approaches. Technological advances have led to the development of diverse and novel instruments for hepatic transection, such as the ultrasonic dissector, water-jet dissector, vessel sealing devices (Thunderbeat, Harmonic scalpel, LigaSure), radiofrequency ablation-based devices, TissueLink dissecting sealer, and staplers. The preferred approach remains controversial among liver surgeons and is likely to remain so for the foreseeable future. Despite the technological advances, hepatic parenchymal transection continues to be a technical challenge. The appropriate use, and a better understanding, of each device will contribute to a safer resection and liver surgeons should select techniques based on their (and the theatre teams) familiarity with, and understanding of, instruments available.

REFERENCES

1. Takayama T, Makuuchi M, Kubota K, Harihara Y, Hui AM, Sano K, et al. Randomized comparison of ultrasonic vs clamp transection of the liver. *Arch Surg* 2001;**136(8)**:922–8.
2. Jarnagin WR, Gonen M, Fong Y, DeMatteo RP, Ben-Porat L, Little S, et al. Improvement in perioperative outcome after hepatic resection: Analysis of 1,803 consecutive cases over the past decade. *Ann Surg* 2002;**236(4)**:397–406.
3. Yang T, Zhang J, Lu J-H, Yang G-S, Wu M-C, Yu W-F. Risk factors influencing postoperative outcomes of major hepatic resection of hepatocellular carcinoma for patients with underlying liver diseases. *World J Surg* 2011;**35(9)**:2073–82.
4. McNally SJ, Revie EJ, Massie LJ, McKeown DW, Parks RW, Garden OJ, et al. Factors in perioperative care that determine blood loss in liver surgery. *HPB (Oxford)* 2012;**14(4)**:236–41.
5. Keen WW. IV. Report of a case of resection of the liver for the removal of a neoplasm, with a table of seventy-six cases of resection on the liver for hepatic tumors. *Ann Surg* 1899;**30(3)**:267–83.
6. Langenbuch C. Ein Fall von Resection eines links seitigen Schnürlappens der Leber. Heilung. In: Schmiedebach H, Winau R, Häring R (ed) Erste Operationen Berliner Chirurgen 1817–1931. De Gruyter, 2015, pp. 59–61.
7. Aragon RJ, Solomon NL. Techniques of hepatic resection. *J Gastrointest Oncol* 2012;**3(1)**:28–40.
8. Li L, Wang H-Q, Wang Q, Yang J, Yang J-Y. Anterior vs conventional approach hepatectomy for large liver cancer: A meta-analysis. *World J Gastroenterol* 2014;**20(45)**:17235–43.
9. Lin TY, Chen KM, Lin TK. Study on lobectomy of the liver: A new technical suggestion on hemihepatectomy and report of three cases of primary hepatoma treated with total left lobectomy of the liver. *J Formos Med Assoc* 1958;**57**:742–61.
10. Lin TY. A simplified technique for hepatic resection: The crush method. *Ann Surg* 1974;**180(3)**:285–90.
11. Lin TY. Results in 107 hepatic lobectomies with a preliminary report on the use of a clamp to reduce blood loss. *Ann Surg* 1973;**177(4)**:413–21.
12. Rahbari NN, Koch M, Schmidt T, Motscall E, Bruckner T, Weidmann K, et al. Meta-analysis of the clamp-crushing technique for transection of the parenchyma in elective hepatic resection: Back to where we started? *Ann Surg Oncol* 2009;**16(3)**:630–9.
13. Gurusamy KS, Pamecha V, Sharma D, Davidson BR. Techniques for liver parenchymal transection in liver resection. *Cochrane Database Syst Rev* 2009;**(1)**:CD006880.
14. Lesurtel M, Selzner M, Petrowsky H, McCormack L, Clavien P-A. How should transection of the liver be performed?: A prospective randomized study in 100 consecutive patients: Comparing four different transection strategies. *Ann Surg* 2005;**242(6)**:814–22, discussion 822–3.
15. Sun H-C, Qin L-X, Lu L, Wang L, Ye Q-H, Ren N, et al. Randomized clinical trial of the effects of abdominal drainage after elective hepatectomy using the crushing clamp method. *Br J Surg* 2006;**93(4)**:422–6.
16. Pamecha V, Gurusamy KS, Sharma D, Didson BR. Techniques for liver parenchymal transection: A meta-analysis of randomized controlled trials. *HPB (Oxford)* 2009;**11(4)**:275–81.
17. Honda G, Ome Y, Yoshida N, Kawamoto Y. How to dissect the liver parenchyma: Excavation with cavitron ultrasonic surgical aspirator. *J Hepatobiliary Pancreat Sci* 2020;**27(11)**:907–12.
18. Poon RTP. Current techniques of liver transection. *HPB (Oxford)* 2007;**9(3)**:166–73.
19. Papachristou DN, Barters R. Resection of the liver with a water jet. *Br J Surg* 1982;**69(2)**:93–4.
20. Vollmer CM, Dixon E, Sahajpal A, Cattral MS, Grant DR, Gallinger S, et al. Water-jet dissection for parenchymal division during hepatectomy. *HPB (Oxford)* 2006;**8(5)**:377–85.
21. Rau HG, Duessel AP, Wurzbacher S. The use of water-jet dissection in open and laparoscopic liver resection. *HPB (Oxford)* 2008;**10(4)**:275–80.
22. Kim J, Ahmad SA, Lowy AM, Buell JF, Pennington LJ, Soldano DA, et al. Increased biliary fistulas after liver resection with the harmonic scalpel. *Am Surg* 2003;**69(9)**:815–19.
23. Sultan AM, Shehta A, Salah T, Elshoubary M, Elghawalby AN, Said R, et al. Clamp-Crush technique versus harmonic scalpel for hepatic parenchymal transection in living donor hepatectomy: A randomized controlled trial. *J Gastrointest Surg* 2019;**23(8)**:1568–77.
24. Romano F, Franciosi C, Caprotti R, Uggeri F, Uggeri F. Hepatic surgery using the ligasure vessel sealing system. *World J Surg* 2005;**29(1)**:110–12.
25. Romano F, Garancini M, Caprotti R, Bovo G, Conti M, Perego E, et al. Hepatic resection using a bipolar vessel sealing device: Technical and histological analysis. *HPB (Oxford)* 2007;**9(5)**:339–44.
26. Ikeda M, Hasegawa K, Sano K, Imamura H, Beck Y, Sugawara Y, et al. The vessel sealing system (LigaSure) in hepatic resection: A randomized controlled trial. *Ann Surg* 2009;**250(2)**:199–203.
27. Saiura A, Arita J, Takahashi Y, Yamaguchi T. Faster liver transection using ligasure combined with clamp crush technique. *HPB (Oxford)* 2014;**16**:719.
28. Aryal B, Komokata T, Yasumura H, Kamiimabeppu D, Inoue M, Yoshikawa K, et al. Evaluation of THUNDERBEAT® in open liver resection – A single-center experience. *BMC Surg* 2018;**18(1)**:86.
29. Obonna GC, Mishra RK. Differences between Thunderbeat, Ligasure and Harmonic Scalpel Energy System in minimally invasive surgery. *World J Lap Surg* 2014;**7(1)**:41–4.
30. Pai M, Navarra G, Ayav A, Sommerville C, Khorsandi SK, Damrah O, et al. Laparoscopic HabibTM 4X: A bipolar radiofrequency device for bloodless laparoscopic liver resection. *HPB (Oxford)* 2008;**10(4)**:261–4.

31. Pai M, Jiao LR, Khorsandi S, Canelo R, Spalding DR, Habib NA. Liver resection with bipolar radiofrequency device: Habib® 4X. *HPB (Oxford)* 2008;**10(4)**:256–60.

32. Mazmishvili K, Jayant K, Janikashvili N, Kikodze N, Mizandari M, Pantsulaia I, et al. Study to evaluate the immunomodulatory effects of radiofrequency ablation compared to surgical resection for liver cancer. *J Cancer* 2018;**9(17)**:3187–95.

33. Jayant K, Sodergren MH, Reccia I, Kusano T, Zacharoulis D, Spalding D, et al. A systematic review and meta-analysis comparing liver resection with the Rf-Based Device Habib™-4X with the Clamp-Crush technique. *Cancers (Basel)* 2018;**10(11)**:428.

34. Lupo L, Gallerani A, Panzera P, Tandoi F, Di Palma G, Memeo V. Randomized clinical trial of radiofrequency-assisted versus clamp-crushing liver resection. *Br J Surg* 2007;**94(3)**:287–91.

35. Li M, Zhang W, Li Y, Li P, Li J, Gong J, et al. Radiofrequency-assisted versus clamp-crushing parenchyma transection in cirrhotic patients with hepatocellular carcinoma: A randomized clinical trial. *Dig Dis Sci* 2013;**58(3)**:835–40.

36. Reccia I, Kumar J, Kusano T, Zanellato A, Draz A, Spalding D, et al. A systematic review on radiofrequency assisted laparoscopic liver resection: Challenges and window to excel. *Surg Oncol* 2017;**26(3)**:296–304.

37. Zhang S, Zheng Y, Wu B, Ji S, Yu Z, Zhang Q. Is the TissueLink dissecting sealer a better liver resection device than clamp-crushing? A meta-analysis and system review. *Hepatogastroenterology* 2012;**59(120)**:2602–8.

38. Fong Y, Blumgart LH. Useful stapling techniques in liver surgery. *J Am Coll Surg* 1997;**185(1)**:93–100.

39. Delis SG, Bakoyiannis A, Karakaxas D, Athanassiou K, Tassopoulos N, Manesis E, et al. Hepatic parenchyma resection using stapling devices: Peri-operative and long-term outcome. *HPB (Oxford)* 2009;*11(1)*:38–44.

40. Schemmer P, Friess H, Dervenis C, Schmidt J, Weitz J, Uhl W, et al. The use of Endo-GIA Vascular staplers in liver surgery and their potential benefit: A review. *Dig Surg* 2007;**24(4)**:300–5.

41. Yoh T, Cauchy F, Soubrane O. Techniques for laparoscopic liver parenchymal transection. *Hepatobiliary Surg Nutr* 2019;**8(6)**:572–81.

42. Mehrabi A, Hoffmann K, Nagel AJ, Ghamarnejad O, Khajeh E, Golriz M, Büchler MW. Technical aspects of stapled hepatectomy in liver surgery: How we do it. *J Gastrointest Surg* 2019;**23(6)**:1232–9.

43. Scuderi V, Troisi RI. Tissue management with tri-staple technology in major and minor laparoscopic liver resections. *Int Surg* 2014;**99(5)**:606–11.

44. Buell JF, Gayet B, Han H-S, Wakabayashi G, Kim K-H, Belli G, et al. Evaluation of stapler hepatectomy during a laparoscopic liver resection. *HPB (Oxford)* 2013;**15(11)**:845–50.

45. Schemmer P, Friess H, Hinz U, Mehrabi A, Kraus TW, Z'graggen K, et al. Stapler hepatectomy is a safe dissection technique: Analysis of 300 patients. *World J Surg* 2006;**30(3)**:419–30.

46. Raoof M, Aloia TA, Vauthey J-N, Curley SA. Morbidity and mortality in 1174 patients undergoing hepatic parenchymal transection using a stapler device. *Ann Surg Oncol* 2014;**21(3)**:995–1001.

47. Rahbari NN, Elbers H, Koch M, Vogler P, Striebel F, Bruckner T, et al. Randomized clinical trial of stapler versus clamp-crushing transection in elective liver resection. *Br J Surg* 2014;**101(3)**:200–7.

48. Fritzmann J, Kirchberg J, Sturm D, Ulrich AB, Knebel P, Mehrabi A, et al. Randomized clinical trial of stapler hepatectomy versus Liga-SureTM transection in elective hepatic resection. *Br J Surg* 2018;**105(9)**:1119–27.

49. Savlid M, Strand AH, Jansson A, Agustsson T, Söderdahl G, Lundell L, et al. Transection of the liver parenchyma with an ultrasound dissector or a stapler device: Results of a randomized clinical study. *World J Surg* 2013;**37(4)**:799–805.

50. Romano F, Garancini M, Uggeri F, Gianotti L, Nespoli L, Nespoli A, et al. The aim of technology during liver resection — A strategy to minimize blood loss during liver surgery. In: Abdeldayem H (ed) *Hepatic Surgery*. IntechOpen, 2013, pp. 147–54.

51. Otsuka Y, Kaneko H, Cleary SP, Buell JF, Cai X, Wakabayashi G. What is the best technique in parenchymal transection in laparoscopic liver resection? Comprehensive review for the clinical question on the 2nd International Consensus Conference on Laparoscopic Liver Resection. *J Hepatobiliary Pancreat Sci* 2015;**22(5)**:363–70.

52. Bismuth H, Eshkenazy R, Arish A. Milestones in the evolution of hepatic surgery. *Rambam Maimonides Med J* 2011;**2(1)**:e0021.

Chapter

45

Formal Liver Resections

Derek A. O'Reilly and Zhai Meng Yao

INTRODUCTION

Records describing operations on the liver date back to 1870, but the procedures performed were either removal of a protruding portion following trauma, or attempts to control bleeding. Formal attempts to resect liver began in 1886 when Antonio Luis resected a large adenoma, but Carl Langenbuck is credited with the first successful procedure 2 years later. It was another 64-years before Lortat-Jacob and Robert, in Paris, were able to complete a formal right hepatectomy (*Table 45.1*).

The modern era of liver surgery required considerable developments in anaesthesia and intensive care, imaging, surgical technique, and the understanding of liver anatomy and physiology, but formed the basis for remarkable progress (*Figure 45.1*).

Current liver surgery has evolved from traditional surgical resections performed as open operations, when the indications were relatively conservative, and formal resections based on anatomical watersheds. Today liver surgery focuses on what will remain behind, rather than the burden of disease within the liver, namely a functional future liver remnant (FLR). Currently, hepatic colorectal metastases or primary liver tumours should be defined as resectable when it is anticipated that disease can be completely removed, two adjacent liver segments can be spared, adequate vascular inflow

Table 45.1 Milestones in the development of modern liver surgery

Date	Surgeon	Procedure
1886	Antonio Luis	First hepatectomy in a 67-year-old female patient with a giant adenoma (15.5 x 11 cm). The patient died 6 hours later due to bleeding
1888	Carl Johann August Langenbuch, Lazarus Hospital Berlin	Hepatectomy. Resected a 370 g mass in the left lobe of the liver and controlled bleeding with mass sutures. The patient required a further laparotomy for bleeding
1890	McLane-Tiffany, Baltimore, Maryland	Liver tumour resected at Johns Hopkins Hospital
1891	T Lucke	First removal of malignant tumour
1896	Michel Kousnetzoff and Jules Pensky	Described the 'suture fracture technique' using a continuous suture sufficiently far from the wound edge to avoid it cutting out
1899	William Williams Keen, Philadelphia	First anatomical left lateral segmentectomy. Reported 76 liver resections (3 of his own and 73 from the literature), 37 for benign or malignant tumours
1911	Walter Wendel	First anatomical resection in a patient with an HCC. Following a right lobectomy, the patient survived 9 years
1943	Cattell, Boston Massachusetts	First colorectal metastasectomy at the Lahey Clinic
1952	Lortat-Jacob and Robert, Paris	First formal right hepatectomy performed for colorectal liver metastases in a 58-year-old woman
1953	Julian K Quattlebaum, Savannah Georgia	Pioneer of American liver surgery. Reported 3 hepatectomies using the scalpel handle
1957	Claud Couinaud, Paris	The Couinaud classification of liver anatomy divides the liver into eight functionally independent segments. Each segment has its own vascular inflow, outflow and biliary drainage. Paris: Masson, 1957. *Le foie. Etudes anatomiques et chirurgicales*
1958	Tien-Yu Lin, Taipei Taiwan	Described the finger fracture technique for major hepatectomy

Abbreviation: HCC: hepatocellular carcinoma.

DOI: 10.1201/9781003080060-45

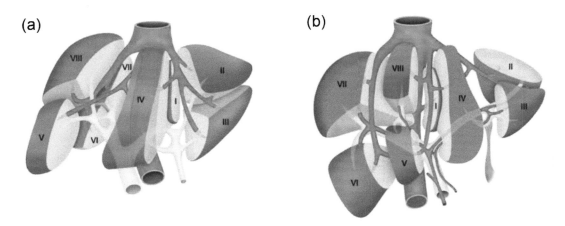

Figure 45.1 The functional division of the liver and of the liver segments according to Couinaud's nomenclature, as seen in the patient (a) and in the *ex vivo* position (b).

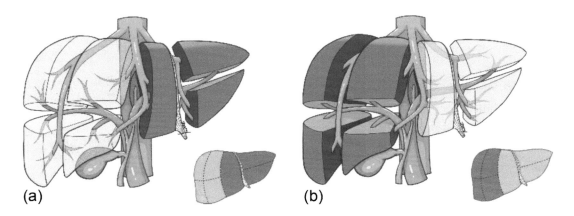

Figure 45.2 First-order division of the liver is through the midplane of the liver. Right hemi-hepatectomy (a) consists of the formal resection of liver segments 5, 6, 7 and 8 (coloured lilac), preserving the FLR, segments 1, 2, 3 and 4, (coloured brown). Left hemi-hepatectomy (b) consists of the formal resection of liver segments 2, 3 and 4 (coloured lilac), preserving the FLR, segments 5, 6, 7 and 8, (coloured brown). If segment 1 is ever resected, this should be stipulated in addition.

and outflow and biliary drainage can be preserved, and the volume of the liver remaining after resection will be adequate (at least 20% of the total estimated liver volume) (1).

More recently, especially with the appreciation of the adverse effects of preoperative chemotherapy on the liver, an 'organ-preserving' approach has been increasingly adopted. Parenchymal-preserving resections can achieve adequate oncological clearance margins, reduce the risk of postoperative liver failure, and facilitate re-do surgery. However, formal liver resections, particularly right and left hemi-hepatectomies and extended operations (tri-sectionectomies), are still common when the tumour burden demands it, to achieve oncological clearance margins, for resection of liver metastases, hepatocellular carcinoma, and cholangiocarcinoma. This chapter will discuss formal liver resections (segmental

resections are covered in **Chapter 46**) and include: 1) The anatomical basis; 2) preoperative assessment; 3) technical aspects, and 4) future developments.

ANATOMY AND TERMINOLOGY OF FORMAL LIVER RESECTIONS

The Brisbane 2000 terminology of liver anatomy and resections, forms the basis of the modern nomenclature for formal liver resections (2). The border or watershed of the first-order division, which separates the two hemi-livers, is a plane that intersects the gallbladder fossa and the fossa for the inferior vena cava (IVC) and is referred to as the midplane of the liver (also known as Cantlie's line). The terms used for surgical resections based on this division is either a right or left hepatectomy (or hemi-hepatectomy) (*Figure 45.2*).

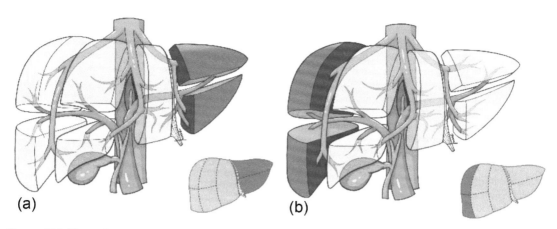

Figure 45.3 The preferred term for resection of the right hemi-liver, segments 5, 6, 7, 8, plus the left medial section, segment 4, is a right tri-sectionectomy (a) (coloured lilac), preserving the FLR, segments 2 and 3 (coloured brown). If segment 1 is ever resected, this should be stipulated in addition. Left tri-sectionectomy (b) applies to resection of the left hemi-liver, segments 2, 3, 4 plus the right anterior section, segments 5 and 8 (coloured lilac), preserving the FLR, segments 6 and 7 (coloured brown). If segment 1 is ever resected, this should be stipulated in addition.

Second-order divisions of the hemi-liver divides the right side into anterior and posterior sections, and the left side into medial and lateral sections. The term for surgical resection is to add sectionectomy to the anatomical term. The preferred term for resection of the right hemi-liver plus the left medial section is a right tri-sectionectomy, while the term left tri-sectionectomy applies to resection of the left hemi-liver plus the right anterior section. If segment 1 is ever resected, this should be stipulated in addition (*Figure 45.3*).

Third-order division of the liver into Couinaud segments results in surgical resections called segmentectomies, or if contiguous but not part of the same section, a bi-segmentectomy (for example, resection of segments 5 and 6).

Unlike the right hemi-liver, where the watersheds of the hepatic artery, bile duct, and portal vein are identical, the arterial and biliary watersheds divide the left side of the liver through the umbilical fissure, while the portal vein watershed divides the left side of the liver through the plane between Couinaud segments 2 and 3. Hence, acceptable alternative nomenclature for resection, based on second-order division of the left portal vein, are left medial-sectorectomy for segments 3 and 4 and left lateral-sectorectomy for resection of segment 2.

PREOPERATIVE CONSIDERATIONS

Careful global- and liver-specific preoperative assessment is required in order to reduce complications and postoperative death. These risks are especially pertinent when undertaking major liver surgery, such as the formal liver resections.

Preoperative assessment of liver function

Post-hepatectomy liver failure (PHLF) remains one of the most frequent causes of major morbidity, with a reported incidence of 9–30% after extended resections, and is a major determinant of postoperative mortality. Hence, preoperative liver function assessment is essential to identify patients at increased risk of PHLF (3).

Preoperative liver function assessment should be considered in patients: 1) Scheduled for major, extended major, or complex hepatectomy; 2) with suspected or known underlying liver disease; 3) suspected or known drug-induced or chemotherapy-associated liver injury, such as sinusoidal obstructive syndrome or chemotherapy-associated steatohepatitis (CASH). In patients at risk, liver volumetry, for accurate estimation of the FLR volume, using computed tomography (CT) or magnetic resonance imaging (MRI) should be performed. Functional liver MRI with hepatocyte-specific, hepatobiliary contrast media provides an estimation of the function of the FLR and can be used to further improve prediction of PHLF. Measurement of hepatic venous pressure gradient (HVPG) can be considered in patients in whom liver cirrhosis with portal hypertension is suspected. Indocyanine green (ICG) clearance and the LiMAx test, the latter based on the liver-specific metabolism of the ^{13}C-labelled substrate methacetin, can both be used to estimate overall liver function, and may improve risk stratification and outcomes.

Prehabilitation

The process of enhancing physical fitness before an operation to enable the patient to withstand the stress of surgery has been termed 'prehabilitation'. It aims to reduce the complications and side effects associated with treatment, aid recovery, and improve quality of life, with the greatest benefits potentially being seen in high-risk groups, such as people who are older and frail. The main elements are preoperative exercise, nutritional optimization, and psychological support. Increasing evidence indicates that prehabilitation improves perioperative physical function in major abdominal surgery. In a randomized clinical trial (RCT) of prehabilitation before planned liver resection, a 4-week programme of high-intensity interval training delivered improvements in cardiopulmonary exercise testing scores and quality of life before liver resection (4). Although individual studies of prehabilitation have shown inconsistent results, a recent systematic review and meta-analysis demonstrated that prehabilitation improves overall complications, postoperative pulmonary complications, and pneumonia in patients undergoing major abdominal surgery (5).

BASIC TECHNIQUES FOR FORMAL LIVER RESECTIONS

Access

For open surgery, an incision 2–3 cm below the right costal margin is made. Alternatively, a roof-top incision may be performed with a vertical extension (Mercedes-Benz). Many modifications of the Makuuchi incision are also used. This incision begins cephalad to the xiphoid, extends to a variable degree above the umbilicus, and then extends laterally to the right or left. Fixed retraction under the ribs improves access. Intraoperative ultrasound (IUS) is the standard of care for hepatobiliary surgery, and is used with bimanual palpation to assess the extent of the tumour(s).

A Pringle manoeuvre involves occlusion of the hepatoduodenal ligament to interrupt blood flow into the liver. A tape is placed around the portal vein, common

bile duct and hepatic artery, and a clamping system used to enable a Pringle manoeuvre if required (*Figure 45.4*).

Although many protocols for clamping and releasing exist, and not all resections require inflow occlusion, 10–15 minutes clamping with 5-minutes release is the most common. For formal right-sided resections, the gallbladder is usually removed.

Liver mobilization

The falciform ligament is divided, using diathermy close to the liver capsule followed along the anterosuperior surface of the liver towards the supra-hepatic IVC, until it begins to bifurcate. At this point, careful dissection is used to identify the IVC and anterior surfaces of the right and left hepatic veins. If a left hepatectomy is planned, the left triangular ligament is divided, freeing the left lobe from the diaphragm. The left phrenic vein is found on the inferior surface of the diaphragm and used to identify the left hepatic vein, into which it drains, at the upper surface of the liver.

The right triangular ligament is divided by retracting the liver inferiorly and to the left, away from the diaphragm, exposing the bare area of the liver. The IVC may also be slung, supra-hepatically above the main hepatic veins, and infra-hepatically above the renal veins. Approach to the small inferior hepatic veins, connecting the liver to the IVC, is facilitated by lifting the liver anteriorly and rotating it to the left. They can then be ligated and divided to clear the anterior surface of the IVC from the level of the renal veins, superiorly to the main hepatic veins. Care must be taken to identify the right adrenal gland and ensure that this is separated and falls away. As the dissection proceeds towards the right hepatic vein, the right-sided part of a small band of fibrous tissue, posteriorly surrounding the retro-hepatic IVC (Makuuchi ligament), needs to be carefully divided. Once this is achieved it is possible to isolate and loop the right hepatic vein.

The liver 'hanging manoeuvre' is a technique passing a tape along the retro hepatic avascular space and suspending the liver during parenchymal transection. It is done classically by creating a space between the caudate lobe and the IVC, starting on the edge of the caudate lobe and extending cranially, in a para-caval fashion, towards the space between the right and middle hepatic veins. It facilitates the anterior approach during major hepatectomy. Proponents argue that it facilitates liver transection, guides anatomical resections, decreases blood loss, and also has oncological advantages.

The liver is now ready for hepatic resection with inflow control, if required, and with the right and left hepatic veins identified and controlled.

Hilar dissection

After cholecystectomy, the common bile duct is identified in the free edge of the lesser omentum. The tissue in the right free border of the hepatoduodenal ligament is dissected and removed by ligation and division, to avoid

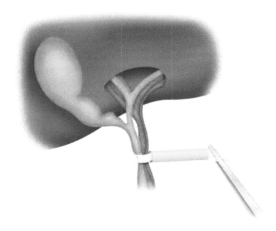

Figure 45.4 Illustration of the Pringle manoeuvre.

lymphatic leaks, and the portal vein is identified and slung. Developing the plane anterior to the vein allows the bile duct and artery to be mobilized forwards and the bifurcation of the vein to be identified (the branch to the side to be retained must be clearly identified). At this point, anterior tissue (the hilar plate) should be freed from the base of the liver, lowering the structures which bifurcate.

Hilar arterial and biliary anatomy is highly variable; thus confirmation of the vascular anatomy is essential. The commonest anomalies include a replaced right hepatic artery, arising from the superior mesenteric artery and lying posterior to the bile duct (occurs in 25% of people) and an accessory left hepatic artery from the left gastric artery running through the lesser omentum, which also occurs in 25% of people.

Attention is then turned to division of the bile duct and, depending on the planned resection, the ducts and arteries to that side are identified and slung. Lifting the hepatic artery and bile duct forward, allows the portal vein bifurcation to be fully exposed and the side to be ligated slung. Soft clamps are applied to the artery and vein(s), producing a clear line of demarcation. The division of the structures should always occur as far away from the hilum as possible. After division of the major structures of the liver, the operative field should be further cleared of any small accessory vessels or ducts.

Alternatively, a posterior intrahepatic (Glissonean) approach may be used, as it offers a more rapid method of gaining control of the inflow to the right side of the liver. The portal vein, hepatic artery, and bile ducts are contained within an extrusion of the Glissonean sheath (a continuation of the liver capsule which forms a tough fibrous outer layer holding the contents in tight apposition). The hilar plate is mobilized, bringing down the confluence of the left and right sheaths. Small 1–2 cm incisions are made in front and behind this sheath as it enters the liver. It is

then possible to use two fingers to separate the sheath from the liver parenchyma and, with gentle dissection, two fingertips can be made to meet intra-hepatically. By staying as close as possible to the sheath, significant bleeding is avoided and a large, curved clamp can be passed around the right hepatic inflow sheath. The liver parenchyma can be detached from the sheath, appearing to render it extra hepatic. Occlusion with a vascular clamp and clear demarcation will confirm that the right main pedicle has been identified and it is then divided.

Liver parenchymal transection

An array of techniques and technologies have been developed to aid parenchymal dissection, by facilitating identification of vascular and biliary structures, to enable accurate diathermy, ligation or clipping (*see* Chapter 44). Safe transection with minimal blood loss and an adequate tumour clearance can be achieved using a crushing clamp, cavitating ultrasonic suction and aspiration (CUSA®), and energy devices, such as the Harmonic™ scalpel or radio frequency ablation/transection devices. These techniques allow a safe resection, with adequate clearance, to be performed, including for centrally placed tumours near the confluence of the hepatic veins and the IVC or the inflow sheaths.

As the parenchyma is divided, vessels and bile ducts are diathermized, clipped, or ligated depending on their size. Hepatic veins and the Glissonean sheath are now commonly stapled with a vascular stapler.

Close co-operation with the anaesthetist is essential in order to achieve a central venous pressure between 0–4 mmHg, which represents the ideal compromise, minimizing the risk of air embolus and venous bleeding.

Further details of individual formal liver resections can be found in *Table 45.2*, as well as potential specific problems that may be encountered and how to avoid them.

Table 45.2 Traditional formal liver resections

Formal resection	Approach	Potential problems and how to avoid them
Right hepatectomy	The liver is mobilized, and right sided structures divided. The clamp should be placed as laterally as possible and either an endoscopic vascular stapler or ligation and transfixion used, to divide the inflow structures. Once the inflow has been divided, the right hepatic vein can also be divided, reducing the blood loss during the dissection significantly and providing greater control	The transection line should be placed as laterally as possible, to avoid damage to bile ducts that may be passing along the right lateral aspect, prior to giving off the main right hepatic duct and becoming the left hepatic duct
Left hepatectomy	For a left lobectomy (segments II, III and IV) mobilization and division of the hilar structures are as described in the text. The posterior approach can be used to isolate the left hepatic sheath, which can be encircled with a vascular tape. The procedure is easier than on the right side, as the sheath is more extrahepatic at the confluence	Following occlusion and division of the inflow, dissection is down through the main fissure avoiding the middle hepatic vein to enable it to continue to drain the right side of the liver. The caudate lobe can be included or spared depending on the clinical situation

(Continued)

Table 45.2 *(Continued)* Traditional formal liver resections

Formal resection	Approach	Potential problems and how to avoid them
Right tri-sectionectomy or extended right hepatectomy	After mobilization, if a caudate lobe resection is required, it is freed from its caval attachments left to right. After the right inflow structures are divided, the sheath to segment 4 is identified and ligated. The right hepatic vein is divided, and the demarcation is along the line of segment 4 and the right hepatic vein ligation	Avoid significant bleeding by ensuring a full mobilization of the liver from the IVC. Avulsion of small inferior right hepatic veins is also avoided
Left tri-sectionectomy or extended left hepatectomy	A formal extended left hepatectomy including segments II, III, IV, V, VIII and I is not frequently performed and because the dissection is performed deep within the posterior aspect of the liver, it is the most difficult of the major resections. The liver is fully mobilized, and the caudate lobe freed from the IVC, left to right. The left inflow structures are divided as well as those to segments VIII and V. The left and middle hepatic veins are divided after the right hepatic vein has been isolated and slung	Once the right lateral fissure has been demonstrated, dissection should take place as medially as possible to avoid damage to the right hepatic veins

MINIMALLY INVASIVE SURGERY

Laparoscopic liver resection

International consensus conferences (Louisville, Morioka and most recently, Southampton) have emphasized the benefits of laparoscopic liver resection. In trained teams and when clinically appropriate, laparoscopic liver resection can be recommended, since it reduces postoperative length of stay and complication rates (6).

In experienced hands, laparoscopic right hemi-hepatectomies are associated with reduced hospital stay and blood loss. Mortality and completeness of resection are comparable with an open approach. For left hemi-hepatectomy, compared with an open approach, a laparoscopic approach is associated with reduced blood loss, morbidity, and hospital stay with comparable operative times, completeness of resection, and mortality.

As in open surgery, intra-operative ultrasound (IUS) is a necessary tool to investigate liver anatomy and tumour location, and to plan transection lines and margins. Inflow control can be achieved with either a hilar or a Glissonean approach. There is no universal agreement regarding the optimal transection technique during laparoscopic liver transection.

During laparoscopic right hemi-hepatectomy, although the anterior approach to liver transection, without prior liver mobilization, has been recommended by many, a conventional approach with liver mobilization before transection is also possible and recommended by others. The choice between the two techniques depend on surgeon's preference, tumour size, and liver fragility. The 'hanging manoeuvre' has also been successfully used in many centres.

The use of a Pringle manoeuvre has been reported to have no detrimental effects on postoperative liver function. Several technical papers highlight the importance of a sufficient cuff of tissue when applying clips and endovascular staplers. Lower intraoperative blood loss is reported in patients with a central venous pressure (CVP) lower than 5 cm H_2O.

Risk factors for conversion include an increased body mass index (BMI), tumour size, extent of resection, and in cirrhosis. In case of conversion for a significant vascular injury, temporary control of the bleeding source before conversion is highly recommended.

Guidelines suggest that the learning curve for minor resections is 60 cases, which shortens the learning curve for major resections such that, for major resections it is 55 cases.

It is important to note that the majority of the evidence underpinning guidelines report data from high-volume, specialist liver centres, which may represent a publication bias. Laparoscopic liver surgery is complex and requires advanced laparoscopic skills, comprehensive experience of open liver surgery, and the support of an experienced team before embarking on the introduction of a laparoscopic liver programme.

Robotic surgery

To-date, robotic liver surgery has mainly been associated with non-inferior outcomes compared to laparoscopy, although it has been suggested that the robotic approach has a shorter learning curve, lower conversion rates, and less intraoperative blood loss (7). Robotic surgical systems offer a more realistic image with integrated 3D systems. In addition, the improved dexterity offered by robotic surgical systems can lead to improved intra and postoperative outcomes. In the future, integrated and improved haptic feedback mechanisms, artificial intelligence, and the introduction of more liver-specific dissectors will likely be implemented, further enhancing the robots' abilities and subsequent uptake.

POSTOPERATIVE CARE

Enhanced Recovery After Surgery (ERAS®) is a multi-modal and perioperative management pathway that has been widely adopted for major abdominal surgery. For liver surgery, strong recommendations include carbohydrate loading the evening before liver surgery and 2–4 hours before induction of anaesthesia. Low molecular weight heparin or unfragmented heparin reduces the risk of thromboembolic events and should be started routinely postoperatively. Although thoracic epidural analgesia can provide excellent analgesia for open liver surgery, it has significant disadvantages, such as hypotension and decreased mobility. Multimodal analgesia (including continuous local anaesthetic wound infiltration and potential use of intrathecal opiates) is preferred. The routine use of nasogastric tubes and abdominal drain placement is not recommended. Early oral intake with normal diet should be implemented after hepatectomy. Early mobilization after liver surgery should be established from the operative day until hospital discharge (8).

FUTURE DEVELOPMENTS

Artificial intelligence (AI) in medicine consists of several subfields. Computer vision is a specific area of AI that enables computers to effectively perceive and understand visual things, like x-rays, CT or MRI scans, pathology slides, and operative video. Enhanced computer vision with augmented reality, virtual reality, and mixed reality are fields of AI that are considered to have the greatest potential to positively improve surgical outcomes and reduce complications. One clear use of AI in liver surgery involves the use of 3D visualization, to delineate complex liver anatomy and its relationship to the tumour. Opportunities exist to improve outcomes, such as operative time, duration of liver inflow occlusion and complications, especially if the opportunity is taken to perform virtual surgery before the real event. Intraoperative use of AI in liver surgery involves associating the 3D-reconstructed images or physical models to the actual surgery. Augmented reality (AR) can be used to display virtual information based on real images of the patient to improve oncological surgery, delineating the ideal dissection plane and anatomical landmarks in real time, to help achieve safe margins with maximum functional preservation. Ultimately, the promise of AI is to solve the urgent problems inherent to our specialty and make our lives, and patients' lives, 'easier and better' (9).

SUMMARY

Formal liver resections, particularly right and left hemi-hepatectomies and extended operations (trisectionectomies), are still common when the tumour burden demands it, to achieve oncological clearance margins, for liver metastases, hepatocellular carcinoma,

and cholangiocarcinoma. The Brisbane 2000 terminology of liver anatomy and resections, forms the basis of the modern nomenclature for formal liver resections. Careful global- and specific-preoperative assessment of liver function is required in order to reduce complications and postoperative death. Basic techniques for formal liver resections include adequate access, liver mobilisation, hilar dissection or a Glissonean approach for inflow division, and liver parenchymal transection. In trained teams, laparoscopic liver resection can be recommended since it reduces postoperative length of stay and complication rates. Robotic liver surgery has mainly been associated with non-inferior outcomes compared to laparoscopy, although it is suggested that the robotic approach has a shorter learning curve, lower conversion rates, and less intraoperative blood loss. Enhanced recovery after surgery is a multimodal and perioperative management pathway that has been widely adopted after major abdominal surgery and is strongly recommended for liver surgery. In the future, AI, in particular computer vision, has the potential to positively improve surgical outcomes and reduce complications.

REFERENCES

1. Charnsangavej C, Clary B, Fong Y, Grothey A, Pawlik TM, Choti MA. Selection of patients for resection of hepatic colorectal metastases: Expert consensus statement. *Ann Surg Oncol* 2006;**13(10)**:1261–8.
2. The Brisbane 2000 Terminology of Liver Anatomy and Resections. Terminology Committee of the International Hepato-Pancreato-Biliary Association. *HPB* 2000;2(3):333–9.
3. Primavesi F, Maglione M, Cipriani F, Denecke T, et al. E-AHPBA-ESSO-ESSR Innsbruck consensus guidelines for preoperative liver function assessment before hepatectomy. *Br J Surg* 2023;**110(10)**:1331–47.
4. Dunne DF, Jack S, Jones RP, Jones L, Lythgoe DR, Malik HZ, et al. Randomized clinical trial of prehabilitation before planned liver resection. *Br J Surg* 2016;**103**:504–12.
5. Kamarajah SK, Bundred J, Weblin J, Tan BHL. Critical appraisal on the impact of preoperative rehabilitation and outcomes after major abdominal and cardiothoracic surgery: A systematic review and meta-analysis. *Surgery* 2020;**167**:540–9.
6. Abu Hilal M, Aldrighetti L, Dagher I, Edwin B, Troisi RI, Alikhanov R, et al. The Southampton Consensus Guidelines for laparoscopic liver surgery: From indication to implementation. *Ann Surg* 2018;**268(1)**:11–18.
7. Bozkurt E, Sijberden JP, Hilal MA. What is the current role and what are the prospects of the robotic approach in liver surgery? *Cancers (Basel)* 2022;**14(17)**:4268.
8. Joliat GR, Kobayashi K, Hasegawa K, Thomson J-E, et al. Guidelines for perioperative care for liver surgery: Enhanced recovery after surgery (ERAS®) society recommendations 2022. *World J Surg* 2023;**47(1)**:11–34.
9. O'Reilly DA, Pitt HA. Artificial intelligence HPB surgery – current problems, future solutions? *AIS* 2022;**2(3)**:173–6.

Bailey & Love's Essential Operations Bailey & Love's Essential Operatic
Bailey & Love's Essential Operations Bailey & Love's Essential Operatic
Bailey & Love's Essential Operations Bailey & Love's Essential Operatic

SECTION 8 | LIVER

Chapter 46 — Segmental Liver Resection

Mohammed Ghallab, Daniel Cherqui and Henri Bismuth

INTRODUCTION

Liver resection strategies have evolved over the past two decades, with a marked shift from major hepatectomies to parenchyma-sparing resections (*Figure 46.1*). Historically, major resections were the norm, with the practice driven by the belief that they were necessary for the treatment of large tumours or extensive disease. Although still often required, they carry a higher risk of post-hepatectomy liver failure (PHLF) and recent studies demonstrate that in western hepato-pancreato-biliary (HPB) centres, the proportion of major hepatectomies has declined to 25–30% of all liver resections. Segmental and local resections are invaluable when managing benign pathologies, dealing with metastases with potential for repeat hepatectomy, and preserving non-tumoral parenchyma in cirrhotic patients.

This chapter describes the basic principles of segmental liver resections, defined by H. Bismuth in 1982 as procedures involving fewer than three anatomical segments (1). Aspects of major liver resections such as postoperative liver failure and remnant liver volume are covered in **Chapters 43** and **44**.

Laparoscopic liver resections began in the early 2000s and the indications have expanded, especially following the 2014 consensus meeting in Morioka. The laparoscopic approach offers potential benefits such as: 1) Enhanced visualization; 2) reduced blood loss; 3) smaller incisions; 4) diminished postoperative pain; 5) faster recovery, and 6) shorter hospital stays. Laparoscopic surgery with an extraction incision remains the most common technique. Hand-assisted and laparoscopic-assisted procedures, which were common initially, have largely been abandoned. Recently, robotic surgery has emerged as a serious competitor to the purely laparoscopic approach. Robotic enthusiasts emphasise the potential advantages such as better image quality, the 360° range of movement, and a reportedly shorter learning curve, which may facilitate the transition from open to minimally invasive surgery (MIS) (2).

PREOPERATIVE CONSIDERATIONS

Indications

Segmental liver resection should always be considered when there is a localized lesion confined to a specific liver segment, enabling the removal of the affected portion while preserving as much healthy liver tissue as possible. Indications for such interventions encompass a spectrum of benign and malignant conditions, including hepatocellular carcinoma, metastatic colorectal cancer, intrahepatic cholangiocarcinoma, benign tumours, localized infections or stones and trauma involving a particular liver segment.

Preoperative investigations and patient selection

Preoperative and intraoperative planning to assess the patient's anatomy are essential for successful segmental liver resection. Cross-sectional modalities, including computed tomography (CT) and magnetic resonance imaging (MRI), must be reviewed during multidisciplinary team meetings. 3D reconstructions are helpful to accurately localize lesions within one or several liver segments, determine their proximity to major vessels, and identify any important anatomical variations. Tumour extension assessed by chest CT, and in selected cases positron emission tomography (PET) scans, are also important to exclude the presence of extrahepatic disease. We employ 3D-image reconstruction software to assist preoperative planning and research is underway to develop augmented reality solutions to allow these 3D models to be used as real-time navigation tools during surgery. Other advanced intraoperative techniques, such as ultrasound (US) scanning and indocyanine green (ICG) fluorescence imaging, facilitate real-time visualization and offer improved precision in demarcating segmental boundaries and conserving vital structures.

Preoperative assessment must also include blood tests for liver function (serum bilirubin, clotting factors/prothrombin time and international normalized ratio [PT INR], albumin), and Child-Pugh and MELD scores to evaluate hepatic function, particularly in the presence of liver disease. The presence of portal hypertension should also be assessed using the hepatic vein pressure gradient or surrogate markers, such as varices, spleen size, low platelet count, and liver stiffness. Patient-specific considerations, such as overall health status, existing medical conditions, and functional capabilities, are additional crucial parameters when determining surgical suitability and in anticipating postoperative recovery.

DOI: 10.1201/9781003080060-46

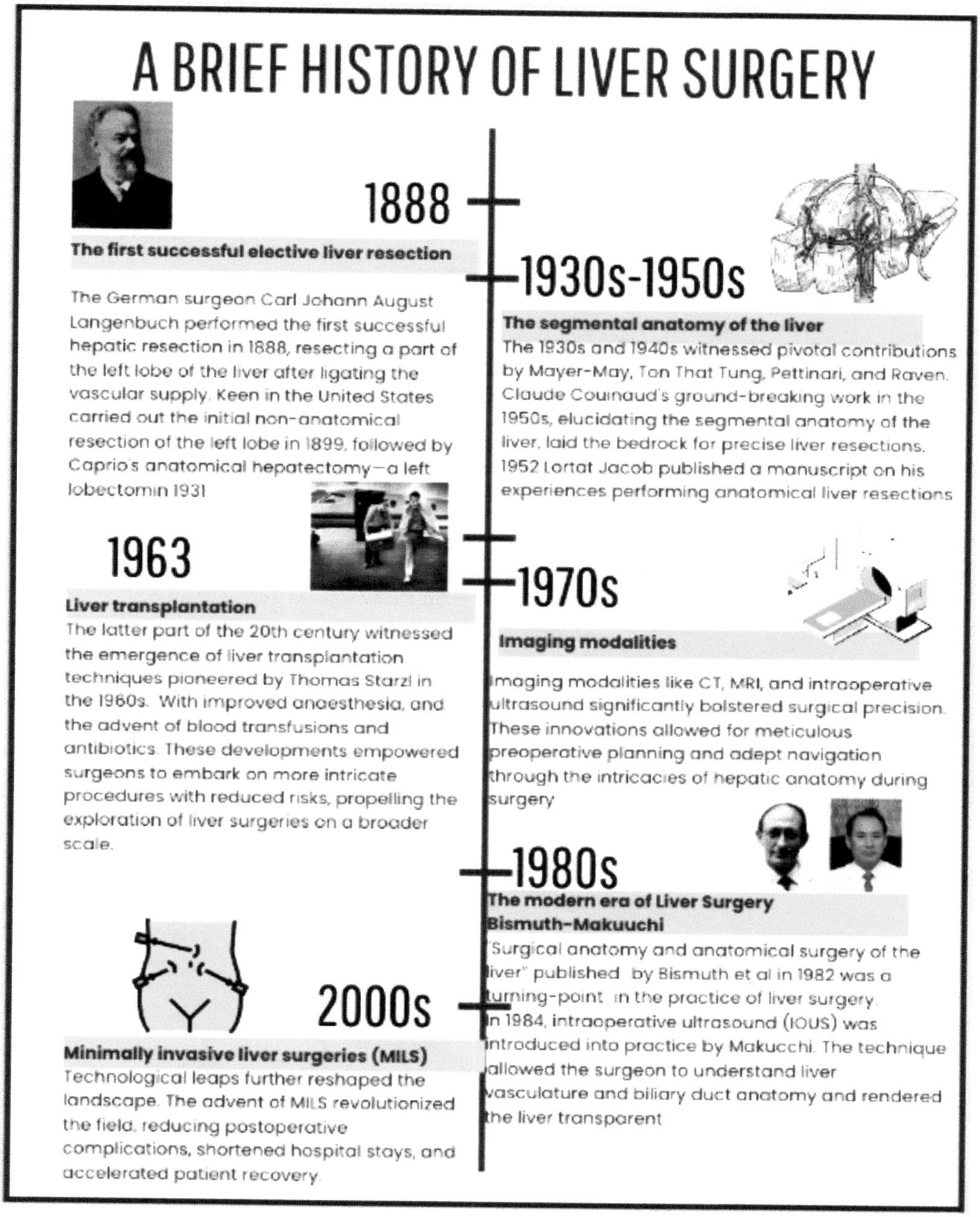

A BRIEF HISTORY OF LIVER SURGERY

1888

The first successful elective liver resection

The German surgeon Carl Johann August Langenbuch performed the first successful hepatic resection in 1888, resecting a part of the left lobe of the liver after ligating the vascular supply. Keen in the United States carried out the initial non-anatomical resection of the left lobe in 1899, followed by Caprio's anatomical hepatectomy—a left lobectom in 1931

1930s-1950s

The segmental anatomy of the liver

The 1930s and 1940s witnessed pivotal contributions by Mayer-May, Ton That Tung, Pettinari, and Raven. Claude Couinaud's ground-breaking work in the 1950s, elucidating the segmental anatomy of the liver, laid the bedrock for precise liver resections. 1952 Lortat Jacob published a manuscript on his experiences performing anatomical liver resections

1963

Liver transplantation

The latter part of the 20th century witnessed the emergence of liver transplantation techniques pioneered by Thomas Starzl in the 1960s. With improved anaesthesia, and the advent of blood transfusions and antibiotics. These developments empowered surgeons to embark on more intricate procedures with reduced risks, propelling the exploration of liver surgeries on a broader scale.

1970s

Imaging modalities

Imaging modalities like CT, MRI, and intraoperative ultrasound significantly bolstered surgical precision. These innovations allowed for meticulous preoperative planning and adept navigation through the intricacies of hepatic anatomy during surgery

1980s

The modern era of Liver Surgery Bismuth-Makuuchi

"Surgical anatomy and anatomical surgery of the liver" published by Bismuth et al in 1982 was a turning-point in the practice of liver surgery. In 1984, intraoperative ultrasound (IOUS) was introduced into practice by Makucchi. The technique allowed the surgeon to understand liver vasculature and biliary duct anatomy and rendered the liver transparent

2000s

Minimally invasive liver surgeries (MILS)

Technological leaps further reshaped the landscape. The advent of MILS revolutionized the field, reducing postoperative complications, shortened hospital stays, and accelerated patient recovery.

Figure 46.1 Infographic highlighting the milestones in the evolution of hepatic surgery.

Anaesthetic considerations

Refinements in perioperative care have markedly improved the outcome following liver resections. The critical role of anaesthetists in managing intraoperative fluids during liver surgeries has been a significant advance in the field of HPB surgery (*see* **Chapter 15**). This management requires an accurate orchestration of intraoperative fluid and transfusion criteria, and pharmacological interventions. A key strategy in mitigating blood loss is avoiding fluid overload and maintaining a low central venous pressure (CVP) (*Figure 46.2*). This technique has been extensively investigated and a direct correlation between blood loss and CVP levels demonstrated, diverging from historical pre-resection fluid loading methods. Initial concerns regarding potential risks, including air embolisation or renal complications, have been shown to be unfounded.

A collaborative approach between surgeon and anaesthetist prevents fluid and allows the maintenance of a low CVP (0–4 mmHg). With strict adherence to meticulous transfusion guidelines, red blood cells are administered to maintain a minimum haematocrit of 25% in patients under 60 years of age and 30% in older patients or those at heightened risk of coronary disease.

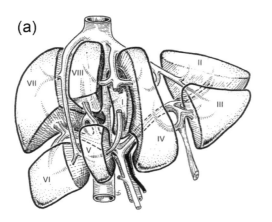

Figure 46.2 In-surgery image showing low CVP surgery. Note the collapsed IVC during segmental liver resection.

Anatomical considerations and terminology

A thorough understanding of the Couinaud liver segmentation system, as described by Claude Couinaud in his seminal descriptions in 1952 (*Figure 46.3a*), underpins all liver resections. Couinaud's original description outlining eight distinct functional segments characterized by unique vascular and biliary arrangements (3) was subsequently modified by Henri Bismuth (*Figure 46.3b,c*).

An alternative anatomical surgical principle, the 'Glissonean pedicle transection,' was introduced by Takasaki in the 1990s and was responsible for a change of hepatectomy techniques (4). Within the hepatoduodenal ligament, a collective structure, encased in connective tissue and sheathed by peritoneum envelops the portal vein, artery, and bile duct forming the Glissonean pedicle (*Figure 46.4*). It maintains a uniform structure inside and outside the liver. At the liver hilum, the structures in the hepatoduodenal ligament divide into right- and left-primary branches and then secondary branches. A single Couinaud segment receives blood supply from one or more tertiary branches, emphasising that a segment isn't a solitary unit. In 2017, Sugioka et al. expanded this concept and identified the six 'gates' indicated by the four anatomical landmarks: 1) The Arantius plate; 2) the umbilical plate; 3) the cystic plate and 4) the Glissonean pedicle of the caudate process. A gap exists between Laennec's capsule and Glissonean pedicle which allows us to isolate them extrahepatically (5).

The traditional hepatic nomenclature is still based on Couinaud's segments. The Brisbane terminology, introduced by Pang in 2002, aimed to alleviate confusion inherent in American, European, and Japanese descriptions, eschewing intricate lobes and sectors.

(a)

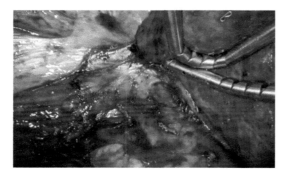

(b)

(c)

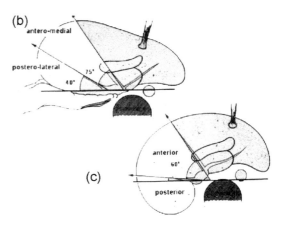

Figure 46.3 Illustration of Claude Couinaud's segmental liver anatomy showing eight distinct functional segments (a) which was later revised by Henri Bismuth. The direction of the main and middle scissurae: *ex vivo* in the flat liver according to the initial description of Couinaud (b), and *in situ* in the body (c). (1).

(a)

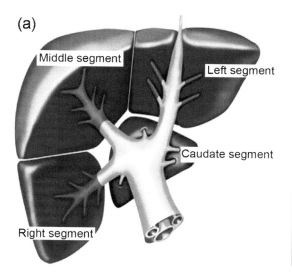

Middle segment

Left segment

Caudate segment

Right segment

(b)

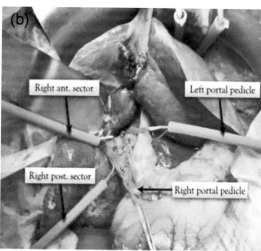

Right ant. sector

Left portal pedicle

Right post. sector

Right portal pedicle

Figure 46.4 Labelled illustration (a) and in-surgery image (b) showing Glissonean pedicle anatomy as introduced by Takasaki (4).

The categorisations of 'hemi-liver' (primary division), 'sector' (secondary division), and 'segment' (tertiary division) offered consistent terminology, facilitated communication among liver surgeons and consistent descriptions in the published literature. Nevertheless, there are issues with the Brisbane terminology, including multiple descriptions for formal resections, for example: 1) Right tri-sectoriectomy; 2) extended right hepatectomy; 3) extended right hemi-hepatectomy, and 4) non-anatomical resections. In addition, multiple resections and combined bilio-vascular resections were not described.

More recently, a new descriptive system called 'New World terminology', based on Couinaud's anatomy, has been suggested following an international consensus meeting (6). In the new nomenclature described by Nagino et al. the letter 'H' indicates hepatectomy. Non-anatomical resections are named according to the segment number and apostrophe ('). For *en bloc* resection of multiple segments, the number of resected segments is mentioned in ascending order, while separate resections of multiple segments are separated by a slash (/). Finally, the number of non-anatomically resected segments is mentioned. The add-ons express the combined resection of: 1) '-B,' (extrahepatic bile duct); 2) '-PV,' (portal vein); 3) '-HA,' (hepatic artery); '-RHV,' (right hepatic vein); '-MHV' (middle hepatic vein); or '-IVC' (inferior vena cava). The authors did not include subsegment resections and lymphadenectomy to the nomenclature to keep it simple (6). Examples of the 'New World' terminology for hepatectomy are shown in *Figure 46.5*.

OPERATIVE TECHNIQUE

There is a lack of consensus in the literature regarding the various technical aspects of segmental liver resection. Rather than an exhaustive description of all existing methods, our intention is to recognize the diversity in techniques practiced by different surgical teams, emphasising this chapter's purpose to elucidate a preferred methodology, rather than impose a singular definitive approach (*Figure 46.6*).

Surgical approach and patient positioning

Laparotomy

For segmental liver resections, the patient is positioned supine with the right arm by the side. The right subcostal incision, commonly favoured for access, has historically been placed a short distance (3–4 cm) from the costal margin. However, this approach has gradually transitioned to a lower position accompanied by an upper midline extension, creating a 'J-shaped' or 'hockey stick' incision. Extensions to the left are seldom required for segmental resections, but an upper midline incision may be employed, particularly for interventions on the left side of the liver (*see* **Chapter 45**).

Minimally invasive approach

There is no universally accepted standardization for port placement techniques corresponding to the varied types of resections in MIS. Port placement is determined by surgeon preference and is discussed further

Minor hepatectomy

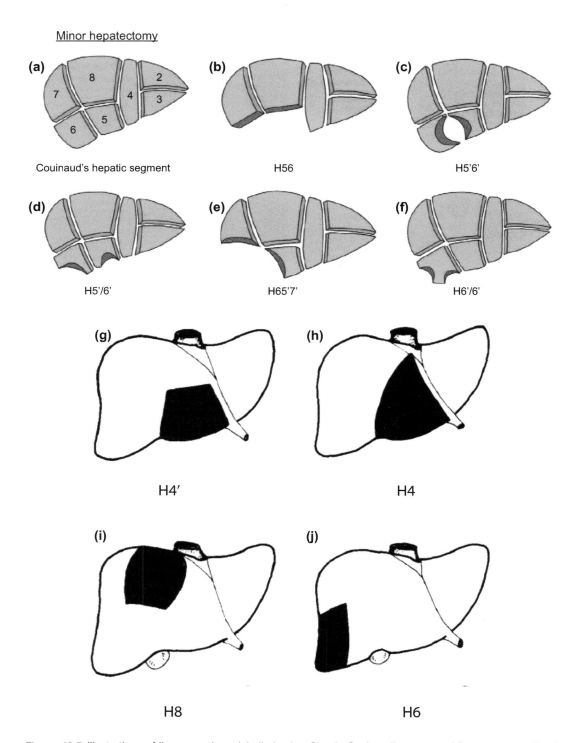

Figure 46.5 Illustrations of liver resections, labelled using Claude Couinaud's segmental liver anatomy, showing eight distinct functional segments (a) and according to 'New World' terminology after Nagino et al. Non-anatomical resections are named according to the segment number and apostrophe ('). Shown are H56 (b), H5'6' (c), H5'/6' (d), H65'7' (e), H6'/6' (f), H4' (g), H4 (h), H8 (i) and H6 (j).

Concepts

Technical Concept for segmental liver resection

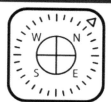

Preoperative planning

- Type of segmental resection
- Choice of open or MIS approach

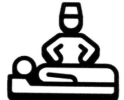

Intraoperatively

- Exploration including IOUS
- Defining segments for resection
- Inflow control for ischemic and/or ICG delineation
- Outflow control if needed

Surgical oncological principles

- Precise parenchymal transection including a margin for malignant tumours (R0)
- HCC prefer anatomic resection or wide margin (ideally 2 cm or more)
- Colorectal metastases: anatomic resection can be applied but non anatomic resection is sufficient margin > 1 mm 1 cm preferable
- R1 vascular resection is considered acceptable for CRLM

Parynchymal transection

- Avoidance of bleeding using low CVP and liberal use of inflow occlusion
- Intrahepatic control of venous/glissonian structures with cautery, clips, ties or sutures according to size
- Avoidance of leaving devascularized liver tissue

Figure 46.6 An example of an infographic compiled by the authors which covers basic technical principles for segmental liver resection.

in Chapter 48. However, irrespective of the sites chosen for the ports, the basic principles of MIS should apply allowing for triangulation, access to target region and flexibility to change the camera ports and working ports depending on the particular step in the operation. Laparoscopic liver surgery is now widely practiced, and more recently there has been increasing use of robotic assisted surgery. This was recently addressed in Paris at the first international consensus conference on robotic HPB surgery (7).

Scoring systems, such as the Iwate and Southampton scores (8,9), have been adopted to guide patient selection for minimally-invasive (MI) liver surgery. These systems evaluate factors including tumour location, size, and proximity to major vessels in addition to anticipated technical challenges. Typically, lesions smaller than 5 cm in the anterolateral segments (namely segments 2–6) are ideal candidates for an MI approach. Conversely, lesions in the posterosuperior segments (1, 4A, 7, and 8) present a significant challenge requiring greater surgeon and unit expertise. Despite the technical issues, there is a growing trend to manage these lesions with MI segmental liver resection, facilitated by advances in surgical techniques and instrumentation. It is vital to initially ascertain the type of resection required, which will determine the possible surgical approaches and avoid a major a hepatectomy, where possible.

Exploration of abdominal cavity and mobilisation of the liver

The liver resection commences with a thorough exploration of the abdominal cavity, inspecting key areas such as the lesser omentum and relevant lymph nodes. Overcoming difficulties in examining the lower abdomen, particularly in those with previous pelvic surgery, relies on careful palpation complemented by preoperative imaging. The initial steps involve dividing the ligamentum teres and incising the falciform ligament. This provides access to the liver's under surface and critical fissure areas. Bimanual palpation is vital for identifying deep parenchymal lesions, and the lesser omentum may be incised for improved palpation of the caudate lobe. Mobilization of the right liver involves careful division of the coronary and triangular ligaments, identification of the right hepatic vein, and sequential division of retro hepatic veins. Division of the vena caval ligament is done with clips or an endoscopic vascular stapler. On the left side, the left lateral sector is mobilized by division of the apex of the left triangular ligament, ensuring protection of the stomach and spleen during the process.

Use of intraoperative adjuncts

Intraoperative ultrasound

Intraoperative ultrasound (IUS) of the liver is essential, transcending surface landmarks with real-time intrahepatic visualisation, establishing anatomical relationships, and guiding precise resections. Recent technological advances, such as real-time virtual sonography (RVS) may improve intraoperative navigation, but is still not yet widely available. RVS integrates preoperative CT or MRI scans with IUS, merging the preoperative imaging data with real-time ultrasound images (see Chapter 14). This innovative technology enhances surgical guidance by providing a direct visualization of the preoperative plan during surgery.

Indocyanine green fluorescence imaging

Although used during open surgery, ICG fluorescence-guided surgery has found its main application in laparoscopic surgery, due to availability of near-infrared imaging systems. ICG fluorescence imaging in segmental liver surgery, facilitates a number of important functions including hepatic segmentation mapping, tumour identification (primary, secondary, and metastatic), and real-time cholangiography. There are two techniques which involve systemic venous injection after portal vein clamping (negative staining) or direct portal puncture and injection (positive staining). Negative staining provides uniform, reproducible results, while positive staining results in wider, less discriminating ICG perfusion. ICG is effective in detecting tumours, including those not seen preoperatively, but has depth and reliability limitations, especially in chronic liver disease. Administration typically occurs within 14 days of the planned surgery, with many studies administering it within 3 days prior to the resection (10).

Vascular control during segmental liver resection

Pringle manoeuvre

Despite the ongoing controversy regarding the advantages and disadvantages of hepatic inflow control during hepatectomy, the Pringle manoeuvre (PM) remains the most commonly used, the simplest and the most evidence-based method of hepatic inflow control. In the literature, there is no clear evidence that PM decreases the blood transfusion requirements, however evidence suggests it significantly decreases intraoperative blood loss, the amount of blood products transfused, and operation time, especially when performed in combination with a low central venous pressure (Figure 46.7).

While using the PM, it's essential to search for, and clamp, a potential left hepatic artery within the lesser omentum, which could be responsible for the apparent inefficacy of pedicle clamping. The clamping of the hepatic pedicle can be applied continuously or intermittently. In the former case, the clamp is applied from the beginning to the end of the parenchymal transection. In non-cirrhotic livers, there have been reports of continuous pedicular clamping for up to 1 hour. We

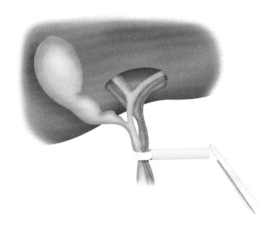

Figure 46.7 Illustration of the Pringle manoeuvre.

tend to avoid continuous clamping when we anticipate that the parenchymal transection will take longer than 30 minutes. In the intermittent method, clamping periods of 15 minutes are interspersed with 5-minutes of de-clamping. Although the vast majority of segmental resections can be performed in four clamping sessions or less, studies have indicated that the total duration of intermittent pedicular clamping can extend to over 300 minutes in a healthy liver and around 200 minutes in a cirrhotic liver.

During de-clamping, the hepatectomy generally pauses, and the sectioned area is compressed to ensure haemostasis, and assess any major vascular bleeding that was not visible during the PM.

We use the Rummel tourniquet technique, temporarily occluding the hilar structures using tape (cotton, nylon, or umbilical), which is then passed through a rigid tube and clamped when required. In cases of laparoscopic resections, we use the extracorporeal technique, passing the tape through a small skin incision but not through a port.

Glissonean pedicle approach selective clamping

We will now describe the technique that we use for the isolation, and selective clamping, of the three secondary Glissonean pedicles. Selective clamping can be performed in isolation, or in combination, with inflow and/or outflow clamping during parenchymal transection. When performed in isolation, it has the advantage of not interrupting splanchnic venous return and thus allows continuous clamping, whilst avoiding intestinal congestion with improved postoperative recovery.

The procedure commences with the performance of a cholecystectomy and subsequent exposure of the hilum by lowering the gallbladder (cystic) plate. The control of the right- and left-Glissonean pedicles is achieved through the creation of small parenchymal incisions above the cystic plate and at the junction of the

caudate process with liver substance. A curved, smooth-tip clamp is delicately introduced above the hilar plate through these incisions, ensuring a gentle manoeuvre to prevent potential harm to the Glissonean sheath or associated structures.

Two tapes are then passed through the tunnel formed by these incisions, one directed to the right side and the other to the left, securing control over the left and right portal pedicles. Identification of the anterior and posterior Glissonean pedicles follows, noting their varying division locations. IUS and manipulation of the right portal pedicle tape aid in pinpointing the division.

A further parenchymal incision is made above the identified division, allowing the passage of a smooth-tip clamp between the anterior and posterior pedicles without force. Introduction of two additional tapes completes the control of the right anterior and posterior pedicles. This sequence of actions, termed 'the taping game', facilitates nuanced control of the portal sheaths.

Selective clamping of one of the three secondary Glissonean pedicles will induce ischaemic demarcation within the right anterior or posterior sector (segments 5 and 8 or 6 and 7) or the left branch (segments 2, 3, 4), as per the planned surgical strategy. The future transection line is marked along the ischaemic demarcation line with monopolar cautery.

Outflow control

Classic hepatic vascular exclusion (HVE) involves clamping the portal triad and the IVC, leading to significant haemodynamic disturbances that require careful intraoperative management. Some patients do not tolerate this approach well and an alternative method, HVE with preservation of caval flow hepatic vascular exclusion with preservation of the caval flow (HVEPC), obviates the hemodynamic challenges of complete HVE by clamping major hepatic veins while preserving flow in the IVC. This technique allows for intermittent, or partial, application based on the required extent of occlusion. Total HVEPC is achieved by clamping the porta hepatis, the left hepatic artery if present, the three principal hepatic veins, and a significant right inferior hepatic vein (*Figure 46.8*). Left partial HVEPC excludes the left liver (segments II to IV) and part of the right anterior sector (segments V and VIII), necessitating clamping of the porta hepatis, the left hepatic artery if present, and the left and MHV. Right posterior partial HVEPC omits the right posterior sector (segments VI and VII), and entails clamping the porta hepatis or the right portal pedicle along with the right hepatic vein, together with clamping or division of the right inferior hepatic vein if present. Exclusion of the right lobe (segments V to VIII) through right partial HVEPC is feasible only when distinct caval insertions exist for the left- and middle-hepatic veins, involving clamping of the porta hepatis and the right- and middle-hepatic veins.

Controlling the hepatic veins commences with the complete division of the falciform ligament to reveal

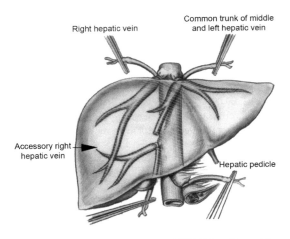

Figure 46.8 Illustration of a total HVEPC achieved by clamping the porta hepatis, the left hepatic artery if present, the three principal hepatic veins, and a significant right inferior hepatic, preserving the caval flow.

the suprahepatic IVC and the confluence of the principal hepatic veins. Identifying the right hepatic vein requires complete separation from the liver's anterior aspect, achieved by division of minor hepatic veins and the hepatocaval ligament, progressing cranially until it is possible to encircle the right hepatic vein at its entry into the IVC. Similarly, mobilization of the left- and middle-hepatic veins began with the left hepatic lobe's mobilization and division of the lesser omentum. The IVC's upper left aspect is revealed following division of the peritoneal reflection above the caudate lobe, followed by ligation and division of the ligamentum venosum, exposing the left hepatic vein's junction with the IVC. Vascular structures are encircled using umbilical tapes and clamping by use of a tourniquet.

When dealing with segments VI and VII resections, applying right posterior partial HVEPC entails clamping of the porta hepatis, or the right portal pedicle, and clamping of the right hepatic vein(s). Central resections involving two transection lines, one on the left and the other on the right liver, allowed for alternate sequential partial HVEPC. Complete removal of segment I mandates its complete detachment from the IVC, by dividing all minor hepatic veins until the liver is entirely pedicled on the three principal hepatic veins. Achieving complete hepatic vascular exclusion necessitates systematic mobilization of segment I from the IVC, effectively disconnecting the liver from the systemic circulation.

Though potentially elongating operative duration, this approach did not occur in practice, as demonstrated in our experience, and in contrast to conventional HVE, avoided retrocaval dissection and adrenal vein ligation (11).

Parenchymal transection

Efficient parenchymal transection aims at excising defined liver segments, achieving oncological margins, and preserving adjacent segmental blood supply to avoid remnant liver ischemia. The avoidance of hepatic vein injury is crucial to prevent significant bleeding and potential gas embolism. Gentle handling of liver tumours is important to prevent tumour rupture or venous dissemination.

The histological anatomy of the liver demonstrates soft epithelial hepatocyte plates and the firmer stromal tissue enveloping them. This stromal layer is in continuity with the Glissonean Laennec's capsule, housing arterial, venous, and biliary structures and facilitating parenchymal division, while preserving crucial vascular elements. Historical methods such as blunt dissection using the finger-fracture technique or Kelly clamp-crushing, have been largely replaced by the use of ultrasonic dissection, the most frequent of which is the cavitron ultrasonic surgical aspirator (CUSA®). This selectively disrupts liver parenchyma, while sparing denser fibrotic tissue, housing the hepatic veins and Glissonean structures. Other techniques such as in-line radiofrequency ablation (Habib® 4X), linear cutting staplers, or energy devices (Harmonic™ or Liga-Sure™) have been described. These methods, however, indiscriminately divide liver tissue, disregarding its distinctive histologic architecture, potentially leading to postoperative bile leaks, liver necrosis, or uncontrollable bleeding from inadequately dissected venous branches.

Transection strategies involve two components. One focuses on reducing blood loss through vascular occlusion and performing the transection carefully, but as quickly as possible, while the other aims to prevent vascular injury by dissecting structures from the surrounding parenchyma. Our preferred approach combines both philosophies. Beginning with inflow/outflow vascular control, liver transection involves cautery incision of the liver capsule, followed by division using CUSA. This controlled transection in a bloodless field allows for intricate dissection of intrahepatic vascular structures and prompt management of any bleeding. Energy devices such as LigaSure, Thunderbeat, or the Harmonic scalpel may be used to assist in dividing superficial liver parenchyma (up to 2 cm) before deeper transection with CUSA.

Minor bleeding from small vessels along the remnant edge is controlled by bipolar or monopolar diathermy. Medium, or larger, venous branches are controlled by suture ligation. A final inspection, following the transection, is performed to check for any visible bile leaks, which are also controlled by suture ligation. The use of an argon beam coagulator, various types of fibrin sealant or haemostatic patches have been described, but we rarely use them in our practice.

This methodology is appropriate for both open, and minimally invasive, approaches. Mastery of these techniques in open surgery paves the way for executing advanced, minimally invasive, liver surgery under precise vascular control, establishing a bloodless field, and upholding the integrity of hepatic vascular landmarks.

Specific technical features of monosegment and bisegment resections

Segment I resection

An isolated resection of segment 1 poses significant surgical challenges, due to its location adjacent to the retro hepatic IVC and the presence of numerous accessory hepatic veins. Segment 1 is also known as the caudate lobe, lobus caudatus and Spigelian lobe. The caudate process represents the portion that continues from the Spiegel lobe to the parenchyma of the right posterior sector, behind the main portal trunk and the right portal vein. There is no consensus on the extent of the caudate lobe. It lies behind the left lobe of the liver and its blood supply originates from multiple small pedicles branching from its posterior aspect of portal bifurcation, but predominately from the left side. Tumours arising in the caudate lobe are closely related to the posterior aspect of the left- and middle-hepatic veins, and the oncological margin is what determines the choice of a left hepatectomy or an isolated resection of segment I (H1).

Complete mobilization of the liver from both the right and left sides is essential. To access the caudate lobe along the left edge of the IVC division of the lesser omentum's pars flaccida is necessary. Additionally, the right triangular ligament is incised until it reaches the right margin of the IVC, and the left triangular ligament is also dissected. Sequential ligation of small caudate veins that drain into the anterior aspect of the vena cava, progressing from right to left, allows complete separation of the anterior vena cava from the caudate lobe. The demarcation between segment 1 and segment 4 presents a surgical challenge due to the absence of a distinct anatomical fissure or structure. An approach encircling the vena cava from the right to the left, around the insertion of the ligament of Arantius (also known as the ligamentum venosum, which is the obliterated ductus venosus, which joins the left portal vein to left hepatic vein), is recommended for this separation.

Resection of segments II and/or III

The combined resection of segments II and III, also known as left lobectomy in Couinaud-Bismuth terminology, and left lateral resection in other terminologies, is one of the most straightforward liver resections. It is mostly performed laparoscopically nowadays and is a recommended early procedure for training surgeons (12). Segments II-III are facing the laparoscope, there are few anatomical variations and the transection surface is usually thin in the normal liver. If present, an accessory left hepatic artery, originating from the left gastric, can be either clamped or divided.

The left lobe is mobilized by division of the left triangular ligament. If present, the parenchymal bridge between segments III and V should be divided early to gain access to the inferior part or the Rex recessus, giving vision to the Glissonean pedicles to segments III and II (ventral to caudal). The line of transection is marked with cautery on the liver surface on the right border of the right and falciform ligaments up to the level of the left hepatic vein. At this stage, liver parenchymal division is started. It is safe to prepare for a Pringle manoeuvre. The latter can often be omitted when the liver is normal, but is usually required in the presence of diseased liver (e.g. steatosis, cirrhosis). Parenchymal transection is performed as described earlier in the chapter. Inflow to segment III is the first encountered and it is divided using a linear stapler. Parenchymal transection is continued cephalad, giving access to inflow to segment II which is also divided with a linear stapler. A rim of parenchyma anterior to the caudate lobe is divided in the fissure for ligamentum venosum preserving segment I blood supply. The specimen is now only attached by the left hepatic vein and a rim of parenchyma. It is controlled, taking care to avoid venous injury and divided with a linear stapler completing the resection.

Isolated segment III resection is a parenchymal-sparing resection particularly indicated for HCC in a cirrhotic liver. The operation begins as decribed above. Glisonnean pedicle for segment III is individually dissected and clamped marking the anatomical ischaemic margin of segment III. ICG can be injected at this stage to create negative staining. Parenchymal transection is carried out along the ischaemic/stained margin.

Isolated segment II resection is rarely performed.

Segment IV resection

Segment 4 is delineated by the ligamentum teres and the falciform ligament on the left, the gallbladder and MHV on the right and posteriorly by the hilar plate and IVC. Venous outflow is to the MHV, but occasionally to a separate scissural vein, which either drains directly into the IVC, or the posterior aspect of the common trunk of MHV and LHV.

Once the ligamentum teres and falciform ligament are incised, the parenchymal transection on their right anterior side, and the segment IVa and IVb pedicles can be isolated, encircled, and divided individually or together depending on the resection planned (H4, H4a or H4b).

Transection continues superiorly to the level of the suprahepatic IVC at the junction of the LHV and MHV, or lower when the LHV and MHV join within the liver. Venous tributaries from segment 4 to the LHV are identified and ligated. On the right, detachment of the left half of the gallbladder's insertion or performing a cholecystectomy often facilitates access to the right part of the hilum. The transection line is along Cantile's line a vertical plane that divides the liver into left and right lobes creating the principal plane used for hepatectomy. It extends from the IVC posteriorly to the middle of the gallbladder fossa anteriorly and the transection is performed to the left of the MHV. This can be facilitated by selective clamping to detect the demarcation of liver parenchyma. Once both transection lines are opened, segment 4 is only connected to the liver by its posterior part. Lifting it reveals a transverse plane connecting the hilum to the rest of the hepatic parenchyma. Numerous secondary vessels, portal branches, and hepatic veins may need to be ligated at this point. The hilar plate is lowered, and the separation of segment 4 is completed. Sometimes, aberrant right-anterior and posterior sectional ducts cross in this position, and these should be preserved during resection.

Resection of segment 4a (H4a) is not common and it was initially described by Champeau in 1964, to access the hilar convergence on its superior aspect during biliary repairs.

Segment V and VIII resection

Right anterior sectoriectomy (RAS) consists of removing segments 5 and 8, which is the liver territory lying between the RHV and the MHV. The pedicular control is performed, employing the hilar Glissonean approach, together with the precise delineation facilitated by the 'taping game' technique, ensuring a distinct boundary between the anterior and posterior sectors. Transection demarcations are guided by capsular incision using monopolar cautery. The procedure meticulously encompasses two transection lines. Initially, the first delineation is executed between the right anterior sector and segment 4, positioned to the right of the MHV along the main portal fissure, Cantlie's line. This initial transection is conducted under super-selective clamping of the right anterior pedicle or employing the full PM, depending on the particular intraoperative conditions. While the MHV is supplied by both the right and left pedicles on either side of the main portal fissure, selective or super-selective clamping of the right anterior pedicle is often sufficient for a successful transection. In the event of significant bleeding, the full PM is employed. Preservation of the MHV requires division of its right tributaries, V5 and V8, encountered during the process. Subsequently, the division of the right anterior pedicle is accomplished using a stapler or suture ligation, with care being taken to avoid injury to the posterior bile duct. The ensuing stage involves the right transection plane, between the anterior and posterior sections, while ensuring preservation of the right hepatic vein. This involves selective clamping of the right portal pedicle, eliminating the necessity for a full PM, provided the right anterior pedicle has been divided. Clamping of the right hepatic vein can be considered, particularly in the concluding stages of transection when dissecting in close proximity to the vein. Upon the removal of the anterior segments, a comprehensive exposure of both the middle- and right-hepatic veins is achievable. Cholangiography should be undertaken to ensure the integrity of the right posterior bile duct.

Segment VI and VII resection

Right posterior sectoriectomy involves the resection of segments 6 and 7 situated behind the RHV. Ideally, preservation of the RHV is preferred to ensure adequate outflow for the anterior sector. However, in cases of oncological necessity, its removal should be considered.

The meticulous control of vascular structures follows the initial steps outlined above, including the intra-hepatic control known as the 'taping game' and the identification and encircling of the right hepatic vein. Full mobilization of the right lobe is performed, and branches that drain into the IVC are carefully divided, including the inferior right hepatic vein, if present.

After managing the portal pedicles, the clamping of the right posterior pedicle (RPP) is performed to establish a demarcation zone for the posterior sector. This ischaemic line corresponds to the right fissure, marking the initiation point for transection. Employing super-selective clamping of the right posterior pedicle or intermittent selective clamping of the entire right portal pedicle, effectively mitigates blood loss. In RPS, the use of the PM is generally unnecessary. However, clamping of the right hepatic vein can be useful particularly in the final stages of transection involving contact with the RHV. Division of the RPP may occur before transection and is often exposed and divided during transection for better exposure and precision.

Drainage of abdominal cavity

Franco and colleagues initially recommended hepatic resection without routine drainage, a notion supported by the prospective trial of Fong et al. (13). Drain insertion may prolong hospital stays and heighten infection risks. While simultaneous liver and colorectal resections may warrant a drain near the liver bed, cautious consideration for cirrhotic patients is crucial due to potential prolonged fluid loss. In cases of biliary reconstruction, drainage is advocated, with careful management to avoid underestimating negative pressure from closed-suction drains. Typically, drain removal in such cases occurs after 4–5 days if no bile leakage is detected.

POSTOPERATIVE CARE (ERAS®)

Enhanced Recovery After Surgery (ERAS) represents a comprehensive approach aimed at mitigating the adverse impacts of perioperative stress following surgery, and specific guidelines have been established for liver surgery (14). These guidelines advocate for the consideration of minimally invasive techniques, provided suitable expertise is available. Moreover, they recommend the cessation of routine practices involving nasogastric tubes and prophylactic abdominal drains, while promoting early initiation of oral intake and mobilization. Although thoracic epidural catheters are still widely used following open liver surgery, there is an increasing trend for the utilization of wound infusion catheters.

POSSIBLE COMPLICATIONS AND POSTOPEARTIVE OUTCOME MEASURES

The principal risks associated with hepatic resection primarily involve biliary leakage and bleeding. Biliary leakage poses a specific challenge, particularly in those patients requiring a biliary reconstruction such as following a resection of a hilar cholangiocarcinoma. However, this risk persists even following segmental liver resection when dissection occurs near the Glissonean pedicles. Additionally, significant problems can arise from bleeding occurring from the hepatic veins and the IVC during parenchymal transection.

The common complications used when assessing postoperative outcomes are bile leak, delayed gastric emptying, postoperative haemorrhage, portal vein thrombosis, relaparotomy rates, and hospital readmission. For cancer patients, disease recurrence and overall survival are important outcomes measures that depend on surgical technique as well as disease biology. Post-hepatectomy liver failure is still a potential complication although it is rare following segmental resections.

CONCLUSION

The success of a hepatectomy mirrors the precision and coordination observed in an orchestral performance. Achieving optimal patient outcomes and upholding oncological integrity require the meticulous mastery of each technical aspect, akin to individual musicians, perfecting their roles in achieving harmonious music.

From careful ergonomic positioning to comprehensive preoperative planning and understanding of the individual anatomical configuration, from precise anaesthetic preparation to adept vascular control and judicious parenchymal transection, each factor plays a vital part in the surgical ensemble. These components all contribute significantly and cohesively rather than independently.

The seasoned HPB surgeon assumes the role of a conductor, orchestrating this surgical symphony. Their expertise lies in adroitly manoeuvring and adapting each instrument or technique, akin to musical instruments, to achieve harmony, ultimately leading to the best patient-centred outcomes.

REFERENCES

1. Bismuth H. Surgical anatomy and anatomical surgery of the liver. *World J Surg* 1982;**6(1)**:3–9.
2. Hobeika C, Pfister M, Gellar D, Tsung A, Chan A, Troisi RI, et al. Recommendations on robotic hepato-pancreato-biliary surgery. The Paris jury-based consensus conference. *Ann Surg* 2024;doi: 10.1097/SLA.0000000000006365. Online ahead of print.
3. Couinaud C. Lobes et segments hépatiques: Notes sur l'architecture anatomiques et chirurgicale du foie (Liver lobes and segments: notes on the anatomical architecture and surgery of the liver). *Presse Med (1893)* 1954;**62(33)**:709–12.
4. Takasaki K. Glissonean pedicle transection method for hepatic resection: A new concept of liver segmentation. *J Hepatobiliary Pancreat Surg* 1998;**5(3)**:286–91.
5. Sugioka A, Kato Y, Tanahashi Y. Systematic extra-hepatic Glissonean pedicle isolation for anatomical liver resection based on Laennec's capsule: Proposal of a novel comprehensive surgical anatomy of the liver. *J Hepatobiliary Pancreat Sci* 2017;**24(1)**:17–23.
6. Nagino M, DeMatteo R, Lang H, Cherqui D, Malago M, Kawakatsu S, et al. Proposal of a new comprehensive notation for hepatectomy: The 'New World' terminology. *Ann Surg* 2021;**274(1)**:1–5.
7. Liu R, Wakabayashi G, Kim HJ, Choi GH, Yiengpruksawan A, Fong Y, et al. International consensus statement on robotic hepatectomy surgery in 2018. *World J Gastroenterol* 2019;**25(12)**:1432–44.
8. Labadie KP, Droullard DJ, Lois AW, Daniel SK, McNevin KE, Gonzalez JV, et al. IWATE criteria are associated with perioperative outcomes in robotic hepatectomy: A retrospective review of 225 resections. *Surg Endosc* 2022;**36(2)**:889–5.
9. Sucandy I, Kang RD, Adorno J, Goodwin S, Crespo K, Syblis C, et al. Analysis of clinical outcomes after robotic hepatectomy applying the Western Model Southampton Laparoscopic Difficulty Scoring System. An experience from a tertiary US hepatobiliary center. *Am Surg* 2023;**89(9)**:3788–93.
10. Wakabayashi T, Cacciaguerra AB, Yuta A, Bona ED, Nicolini D, Mocchegiani F, et al. Indocyanine green fluorescence navigation in liver surgery: A systematic review on dose and timing of administration. *Ann Surg* 2022;**275(6)**:1025–34.
11. Cherqui D, Malassagne B, Colau PI, Brunetti F, Rotman N, Fagniez PL. Hepatic vascular exclusion with preservation of the caval flow for liver resections. *Ann Surg* 1999;**230(1)**:24–30.
12. Chang S, Laurent A, Tayar C, Karoui M, Cherqui D. Laparoscopy as a routine approach for left lateral sectionectomy. *Br J Surg* 2007;**94(1)**:58–63.
13. Fong Y, Brennan MF, Brown K, Heffernan N, Blumgart LH. Drainage is unnecessary after elective liver resection. *Am J Surg* 1996;**171(1)**:158–62.
14. Agarwal V, Divatia JV. Enhanced recovery after surgery in liver resection: Current concepts and controversies. *Korean J Anesthesiol* 2019;**72(2)**:119–29.

FURTHER READING

Bismuth H. Revisiting liver anatomy and terminology of hepatectomies. *Ann Surg* 2013;**257(3)**:383–6.
Bismuth H. Geopolitics of liver anatomy: It's Cantlie's Fault! *Ann Surg* 2021;**274(1)**:4–5.
Figueroa R, Laurenzi A, Laurent A, Cherqui D. Perihilar Glissonian approach for anatomical parenchymal sparing liver resections: Technical aspects: The taping game. *Ann Surg* 2018;**267(3)**:537–43.

Bailey & Love's Essential Operations Bailey & Love's Essential Operatic
Bailey & Love's Essential Operations Bailey & Love's Essential Operatic
Bailey & Love's Essential Operations Bailey & Love's Essential Operatic

SECTION 8 | LIVER

Chapter
47

Local Liver Resection
Rachel V. Guest and Rowan W. Parks

INTRODUCTION

The principle of parenchymal-sparing liver surgery, whereby the future liver remnant (FLR) is maximized by removing the minimum amount of liver tissue to achieve a safe oncological margin, has led to the increasing adoption of non-anatomical liver resection (NAR) for a range of liver pathologies (1,2). NAR, also referred to as local, wedge or atypical liver resection is promulgated as an alternative operative approach to the traditional observance of the segmental anatomy as described by Couinaud (3), particularly in patients with colorectal liver metastases (CRLM) (4). NAR enables the removal of multiple tumours, whilst preserving the maximum possible amount of functional hepatic parenchyma, to reduce the risk of postoperative liver failure and/or allow opportunity for two-stage hepatectomy or re-resection, should intrahepatic recurrence occur. This is pertinent in a patient population where many individuals facing surgery receive perioperative chemotherapy, may have a degree of chemotherapy associated liver injury (CALI) or in the case of patients with hepatocellular carcinoma (HCC), who have underlying liver disease. NAR, in combination with 3D-volumetry software to plan resection lines and quantify volumes of tumours, cysts and ablation zones to accurately calculate the FLR, has enabled an individualized surgical approach to patients with CRLM (*Figure 47.1*).

COLORECTAL LIVER METASTASES

Initial studies comparing outcomes between NAR and anatomical resection (AR) including segmental resection, hemi-hepatectomy and tri-sectionectomy, raised concerns regarding the potential for inferior survival

with NAR, thought likely to be secondary to the higher rates of margin positivity (5–7). However, subsequent large retrospective series have demonstrated non-inferiority of survival after NAR compared with AR (8–10). A meta-analysis of 21 such studies has examined short- and long-term pooled outcomes in patients with CRLM undergoing NAR versus AR (11) (*Figure 47.2*). In 12 of the 21 studies reporting short-term outcomes, no difference in blood loss was observed, however NAR was associated with a significantly reduced requirement for transfusion (OR 2.94, CI 1.87–4.62), shorter operating time (weighted mean difference 43.62 minutes, CI 5.25–81.99), lower 30-day morbidity (OR 1.68, CI 1.13–2.50) and lower 30-day mortality (OR 3.74, CI 1.60–8.75). In studies describing long-term outcomes in 1803 patients, no significant difference was observed in either overall survival (HR 1.06, CI 0.95 – 1.18) or disease-free survival (HR 1.11, CI 0.99–1.24).

As regards margin status, the above meta-analysis by Tang et al. found a small, pooled effect in favour of AR in terms of R0 rate (OR 0.79, CI 0.49–1.29), however the 95% confidence interval intercepted the no-effects line. The largest of the 10 series in this systematic review included 582 patients undergoing AR and 409 undergoing NAR, and reported that the rate of intrahepatic recurrence was similar between the groups (AR 17.5% NAR 22%, P = 0.08), although the need for re-do liver surgery was higher in the NAR group (AR 8.7% NAR 15.4%, P < 0.001) (12). A large multicentre retrospective series from Pawlik and colleagues examined survival and recurrence in patients undergoing both AR and NAR. Overall, they observed no difference in survival, but concluded that across all groups margin involvement negatively impacted disease-free

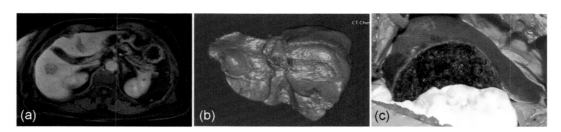

Figure 47.1 Panel demonstrating CT (a), volumetric reconstruction (b) and intraoperative image (c) of patient undergoing non-anatomical liver resections (NAR) for colorectal liver metastases (CRLM).

DOI: 10.1201/9781003080060-47

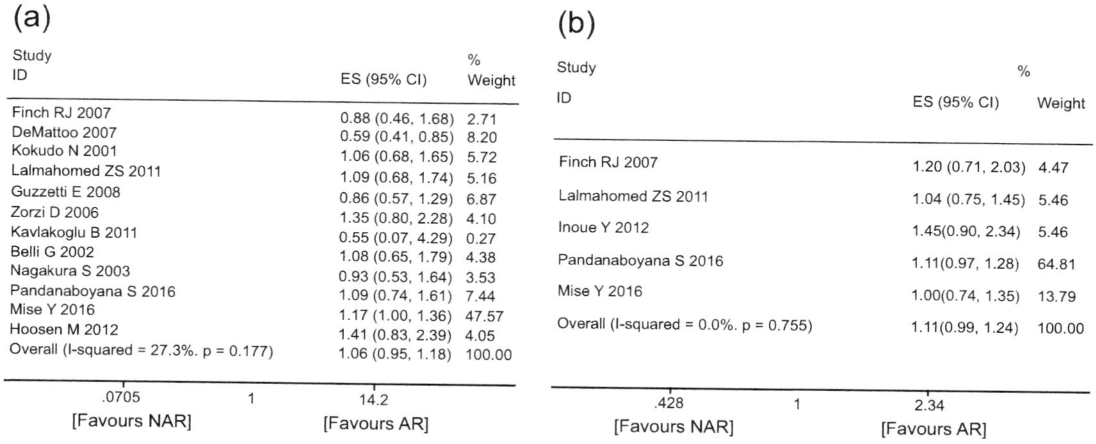

(a)

Study ID	ES (95% CI)	% Weight
Finch RJ 2007	0.88 (0.46, 1.68)	2.71
DeMattoo 2007	0.59 (0.41, 0.85)	8.20
Kokudo N 2001	1.06 (0.68, 1.65)	5.72
Lalmahomed ZS 2011	1.09 (0.68, 1.74)	5.16
Guzzetti E 2008	0.86 (0.57, 1.29)	6.87
Zorzi D 2006	1.35 (0.80, 2.28)	4.10
Kavlakoglu B 2011	0.55 (0.07, 4.29)	0.27
Belli G 2002	1.08 (0.65, 1.79)	4.38
Nagakura S 2003	0.93 (0.53, 1.64)	3.53
Pandanaboyana S 2016	1.09 (0.74, 1.61)	7.44
Mise Y 2016	1.17 (1.00, 1.36)	47.57
Hoosen M 2012	1.41 (0.83, 2.39)	4.05
Overall (I-squared = 27.3%. p = 0.177)	1.06 (0.95, 1.18)	100.00

.0705   1   14.2

[Favours NAR]   [Favours AR]

(b)

Study ID	ES (95% CI)	% Weight
Finch RJ 2007	1.20 (0.71, 2.03)	4.47
Lalmahomed ZS 2011	1.04 (0.75, 1.45)	5.46
Inoue Y 2012	1.45 (0.90, 2.34)	5.46
Pandanaboyana S 2016	1.11 (0.97, 1.28)	64.81
Mise Y 2016	1.00 (0.74, 1.35)	13.79
Overall (I-squared = 0.0%. p = 0.755)	1.11 (0.99, 1.24)	100.00

.428   1   2.34

[Favours NAR]   [Favours AR]

Figure 47.2 Forest plots illustrating non-inferiority of NAR vs AR on overall survival (a) and disease-free survival (b) in patients undergoing surgery for CRLM from a meta-analysis of 21 studies. (Reproduced with permission from [11].)

survival. On stratification, according to resection margin width (≥1 cm, 5–9 mm, 1–4 mm), recurrence rates were similar (8). This and other studies led the Expert Group on OncoSurgery Management of Liver Metastases (EGOSLIM) to advocate a minimum resection margin of 1 mm (13). Consequently, many institutions use this 1 mm margin as the initial surgical approach of choice for patients with CRLM, particularly when tumours are small and peripherally sited.

Surgical margins in CRLM continue to be hotly debated, with some recent studies suggesting that in patients with good biological characteristics such as *RAS* wild-type and chemoresponsive tumours, sub-millimetre R1 margins do not necessarily result in inferior survival (14,15). It has been observed that patients with *RAS* mutant tumours have higher rates of liver micrometastases (16) and that fewer micrometastases are observed histologically following treatment with perioperative chemotherapy with, or without, the monoclonal antibodies bevacizumab or cetuximab (17). This interface between tumour biology and surgical outcomes has been further explored in a retrospective analysis of 389 patients undergoing liver resection at Johns Hopkins, where patients with *KRAS* mutant and wild-type tumours were compared (18). AR was associated with significantly improved disease-free survival and tumour recurrence in patients with *KRAS* mutant tumours, whereas in patients with *KRAS* wild-type tumours, survival and recurrence were similar between AR and NAR after correction for tumour number, bilobar disease and the use of ablation. A recent dual-centre European study by Andreou and colleagues proposes identification of the site of recurrence as an important distinction in patients undergoing surgery. In their cohort, local recurrence at the resection margin was no more common in R1 compared to R0 resections compared with intrahepatic recurrence arising elsewhere in the liver, and that margin recurrence did not confer

inferior survival (15). The corollary of this for patients with borderline resectable disease is evident and further large, multi-institutional or randomized studies are required to determine the latent importance of resection margin status in the modern era of chemotherapeutics and biological agents.

Few major studies have compared the resectability of intrahepatic CRLM recurrences following initial AR or NAR. Kokudo and colleagues analysed patterns of first recurrence following hepatectomy in 174 patients with CRLM (19). They found no statistical difference between the rate of intrahepatic recurrence between patients who had undergone NAR compared to AR, however when recurrence occurred within the ipsilateral lobe to that on which surgery had been performed, 90% patients in the NAR cohort proceeded to repeat hepatectomy. This contrasted with just 20% overall (ipsilateral and contralateral) in the AR group. Survival was significantly greater in patients undergoing repeat surgery for ipsilateral recurrence compared with contralateral disease (log rank 0.047), with a 5-year survival of 58.3% in patients undergoing ipsilateral re-resection. This option for re-resection following NAR is a strong determinant of strategy when multidisciplinary teams plan treatment pathways for patients, especially in those with bilobar disease, and indeed NAR has become a cornerstone of the two-stage hepatectomy approach described in **Chapter 43**.

THE DISAPPEARING LIVER METASTASIS

A complete radiological response with lesion disappearance on cross-sectional imaging is observed in 5–25% of patients undergoing systemic chemotherapy for CRLM, a phenomenon known as the disappearing liver metastasis (DLM) (20). This issue has been brought to the fore by the increased adoption of NAR/

parenchymal-preserving liver resection as well as advances in systemic chemotherapy, biological agents, and manoeuvres to boost the FLR (21). DLMs occur more frequently in patients with lesions less than 2 cm in size, when there are three or more tumours, with synchronous disease, and in those patients who have undergone multiple cycles of chemotherapy, especially oxaliplatin-based regimens. The reported rate of corresponding complete pathological response or the absence of recurrence in patients with DLM is highly variable (4–80.5%), which in part might reflect the variable use of magnetic resonance imaging (MRI) for staging between institutions (22–24). The optimal strategy for the management of DLMs remains controversial, although there is consensus that this must be determined via a multidisciplinary team approach (20,25,26). Currently no randomized data exist comparing resection of DLM sites versus observation or further systemic therapy, however observational studies show that an active surgical approach lengthens the time to recurrence and enhances recurrence-free survival (RFS), although to-date no effect on overall survival has been demonstrated (27,28).

OTHER SECONDARY MALIGNANCIES

The evidence for the optimal type of liver resection for non-colorectal secondary tumours is less concrete. In patients with hepatic metastases from neuroendocrine tumours (NETs), non-randomized data support the use of resection to control symptoms and prolong survival regardless of the site of the primary, although only a minority of patients are suitable for surgery at diagnosis due to tumour volume and/or the distribution of disease (29). Although NET metastases tend to follow a more indolent course than CRLM, particularly 'low grade' or well differentiated tumours, recurrence after resection occurs in the vast majority of patients (30). One large multicentre retrospective study has directly compared AR with NAR in 250 patients undergoing surgery with curative intent (31). They found NAR was associated with a higher rate of microscopic margin positivity (R1), and a two-fold risk of recurrence although after controlling for relevant patient and tumour related co-variates, OS and RFS were not significantly different between the groups (*Table 47.1*). Stronger determinants

Table 47.1 Hazard regression analysis of factors associated with overall survival after resection of hepatic metastases from NETs

Variables	Median survival (months)	P value	Hazard ratio	95% CI	P value
		Multivariable survival analysis			
Age			0.50		
• <65 years	Not reached				
• ≥65 years	Not reached		1.28	0.75–2.18	0.36
Race		0.28			
• White	Not reached				
• Black	88.1				
• Other	86.2				
Gender		0.93			
• Male	Not reached				
• Female	Not reached				
Location of primary tumour		0.06			
• Pancreas	151.0			–	
• Small intestine	Not reached				
• Large intestine	Not reached				
Symptomatic disease	Not reached	0.24	0.76	0.42–1.39	0.38
Primary tumour grade		0.11			
• Low	Not reached			–	
• Intermediate	151.02		1.92	1.04–3.56	0.04
• High	Not reached		1.55	0.73–3.29	0.25

(Continued)

Table 47.1 (*Continued*) Hazard regression analysis of factors associated with overall survival after resection of hepatic metastases from NETs

Variables	Median survival (months)	Multivariable survival analysis			
		P value	Hazard ratio	95% CI	P value
Lymph node status		0.001			
• No lymph node metastasis	Not reached			–	
• Lymph node metastasis	138.3		1.95	1.01–3.76	0.05
Liver disease presentation		0.11			
• No synchronous disease	Not reached			–	
• Synchronous disease	Not reached		1.27	0.68–2.83	0.35
Liver metastasis location		0.79			
• Unilateral metastases	138.3				
• Bilateral metastases	124.4				
Estimated liver involvement		0.003			
• <50%	151.0			–	
• ≥50%	Not reached		1.40	0.69–2.83	0.94
Type of liver resection		0.005			
• Non-anatomic	138.3			–	
• Anatomic	Not reached		0.94	0.12–7.44	0.96
Resection margin		0.04			
• R0	Not reached				
• R1	151.02		2.92	1.65–5.17	<0.001

Source: Reproduced with permission from (31).

of prognosis in patients with hepatic metastases from NETs appear to be the histological grade of the tumour, the presence of extrahepatic disease and the response to systemic therapies (32).

For non-colorectal non-neuroendocrine (NCNN) metastases, liver resection also offers long-term survival benefit in highly selected patients with favourable biology. The best outcomes are observed in patients with primaries of the reproductive tract, breast and genitourinary tract (*see* Chapter 51) (33–35). To-date, no studies in patients with NCNN have directly compared NAR with AR, however the evidence suggests that macroscopic negative margins are associated with the most favourable outcomes (36).

HEPATOCELLULAR CARCINOMA

The use of NAR in the context of HCC is much more controversial. Orthodox opinion posits that HCC propagates along portal tributaries and intersegmental branches and therefore AR is necessary to ensure systematic removal of the tumour-bearing portal territories, with exposure of the landmark veins framing the segmental territories (*Figure 47.3*) (37).

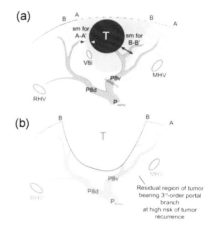

Figure 47.3 Anatomic resection (a) (A-A') removes entirely the tumour-bearing portal branches bordered by the landmark veins, while non-anatomic resection (B-B') is any other type of resection in which the tumour-bearing third-order portal region is not fully removed. After non-anatomic resection of HCC (b) some part of the tumour-bearing region is left, which is thought to be at high risk of recurrence. *Abbreviations*: MHV: middle hepatic vein; P8v: ventral branch of P8; PRPM: right paramedial pedicle; RHV: right hepatic vein; V8i: intermediate vein from segment VIII. (Reproduced with permission from [37] and [38].)

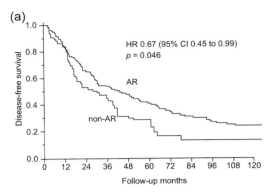
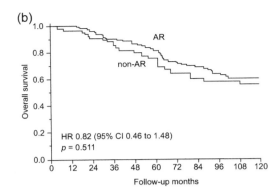

Figure 47.4 Long-term survival outcomes after anatomic resection and non-anatomic resection of HCC in a propensity score adjusted population. Disease-free survival rate (a). Overall survival rate (b). (Reproduced with permission from [38].)

Traditionally, AR has therefore been the most commonly adopted surgical approach for patients with HCC meeting criteria for resection (39). Although no randomized data exists, several observational studies have examined this question, often with conflicting results. A retrospective observational study from the University of Tokyo used multivariate analysis to compare AR and NAR in 210 patients undergoing potentially curative resection for solitary HCC (40). The group reported superior 5-year overall and disease-free survival in the AR group (66% vs. 35%, P=0.01), however they acknowledged that the rate of ascites and cirrhosis was worse in the NAR group, and this group also had worse liver function. A further prospective cohort of 209 patients with Child-Pugh A cirrhosis and solitary HCC ≤5 cm maximal diameter undergoing AR or NAR were compared in a later study from Japan (*Figure 47.4*) (38). Superior DFS was again observed in the AR group (HR 0.67, 95% CI 0.45–0.99, p=0.046), but there was no difference in OS (HR 0.82, 95% CI 0.46–1.48, p=0.511). Regression analysis revealed AR to be associated with significantly reduced recurrence (HR 0.12, 0.05–0.30, p<0.001). It should be noted that a significant number of patients scheduled to undergo AR preoperatively were re-classified into the NAR group due to the presence of cirrhosis, ascites, or unexpectedly widespread indigo carmine staining, used for intraoperative detection of tumour-bearing portal branches. A recent study used propensity score matching (PSM) in 51 patients undergoing laparoscopic resection for large HCC and concluded that DFS was significantly better in patients undergoing AR compared with NAR (52.3% vs. 27.0%, p=0.042), as was 3-year OS (59.4% vs. 38.7%, p=0.045) (41).

Others have highlighted the issues with selection bias and heterogeneity in these observational data (42), and have argued that the oncological advantages of an extensive AR might not necessarily confer benefit, particularly in situations where parenchymal preservation to boost the FLR is desirable. For example, in a cohort of 546 patients with HCC exceeding Milan criteria, AR and

NAR achieved comparable survival outcomes following propensity score matching for variables including tumour burden and liver function reserve (43). In the largest propensity score matching study to date, 1102 patients undergoing resection at Osaka Medical Centre were compared (577 AR; 525 NAR) (44). After PSM, 329 patients were included in each group and matched for age, tumour size, indocyanine green (ICG) retention rate at 15 minutes and prothrombin time. No significant difference was observed in recurrence-free and overall survival between the two matched groups, or in the recurrence rate at 2 years. As the rate of microvascular invasion (MVI) was higher in the AR group, the authors performed a subset analysis of patients with and without MVI and found no difference in recurrence-free survival (*Figure 47.5*).

A meta-analysis conducted in 2012 included 18 observational studies involving 9036 patients and concluded that AR offered superior 5-year OS (RR 1.14, p=0.001) and DFS (RR 1.38, p=0.010), but found that this was accounted for by a higher rate of cirrhosis and hepatic dysfunction in the AR group (45). The 2018 European Association for the Study of the Liver (EASL) clinical practice guidelines recommend that either AR or NAR is advocated and selection should be made according to the relevant patient and tumour related factors in each individual's case (37).

OPERATIVE CONSIDERATIONS

NAR is most frequently utilized in the setting of small and/or peripherally sited tumours. Early concerns regarding the safety of parenchymal-preserving techniques pertained to haemorrhage due to a relative lack of vascular control of the portal segmental pedicle and/or venous outflow, particularly in tumours sited more deeply, in steatotic livers and for segment VII/VIII/IVa lesions in close proximity to the caval confluence. Novel systems for parenchymal transection, including vessel-sealing energy devices (LigaSure™, Harmonic™ scalpel, Thunderbeat™)

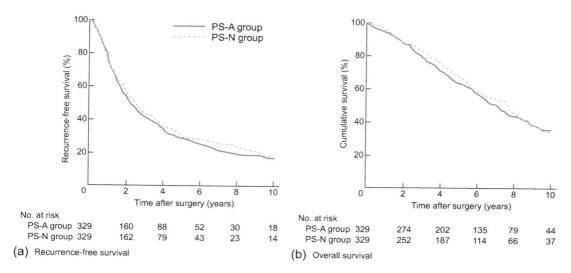

Figure 47.5 Recurrence-free (a) and overall (b) survival after hepatectomy with curative intent for hepatocellular carcinoma. (Reproduced with permission from [44].) Hazard ratio (HR) for part (a) 0.95, 95% (CI=0.74–1.22), stratified Cox proportional hazard regression analysis; P=0.704 (stratified log rank test). HR for part (b) 1.14, (0.85–1.51; P=0.381). Propensity score matched for age, tumour size, ICG clearance and prothrombin time. *Abbreviations:* PS-A: propensity-matched anatomical resection; PS-N: propensity-matched non-anatomical resection.

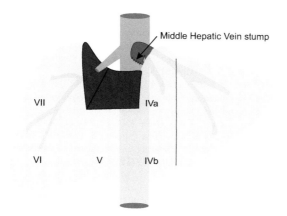

Figure 47.6 Schematic of mini-mesohepatectomy; initially described by Torzilli et al. (46) involves US-guided partial resection of segment VIII and IVa at the hepatocaval confluence, preserving the remaining right anterior and left median sections and excising the involved segment of middle hepatic vein.

and CUSA®, can aid in minimising blood loss and the intraoperative use of ultrasound (US) and Doppler to delineate tumour-threatened tributaries assists the determination of safe resectability. The development of novel techniques such as the 'mini-mesohepatectomy', a US-guided partial resection of segments IV, V and VIII for tumours involving the middle hepatic vein within 4 cm of the caval confluence, has broadened the armament of potential approaches for tumours that traverse segmental boundaries or which would otherwise have not been previously considered suitable for parenchymal-sparing approaches (46) (*Figure 47.6*).

SUMMARY

NAR enables parenchymal preservation in patients with CRLM whose tumours traverse the segmental boundaries of the liver, where tumours are multiple and/or bilobar and when maximising the FLR is desirable, without compromising oncological outcomes. The use of NAR in HCC is more controversial and further data are required. Novel technologies and operative techniques and various adjuncts have accelerated the widespread popularity of NAR throughout the (HPB) community.

REFERENCES

1. Moris D, Ronnekleiv-Kelly S, Rahnemai-Azar AA, Felekouras E, Dillhoff M, Schmidt C, et al. Parenchymal-sparing versus anatomic liver resection for colorectal liver metastases: A systematic review. *J Gastrointest Surg* 2017;**21(6)**:1076–85.
2. Gold JS, Are C, Kornprat P, Jarnagin WR, Gönen M, Fong Y, et al. Increased use of parenchymal-sparing surgery for bilateral liver metastases from colorectal cancer is associated with improved mortality without change in oncologic outcome: Trends in treatment over time in 440 patients. *Ann Surg* 2008;**247(1)**:109–17.

3. Couinaud C. Lobes et segments h.patiques: Notes sur l'architecture anatomiques et chirurgicale du foie (Liver lobes and segments: Notes on the anatomical architecture and surgery of the liver). *Presse Med (1893)* 1954;**62(33)**:709–12.

4. Pawlik TM, Schulick RD, Choti MA. Expanding criteria for resectability of colorectal liver metastases. *Oncologist* 2008;**13(1)**:51–64.

5. DeMatteo RP, Palese C, Jarnagin WR, Sun RL, Blumgart LH, Fong Y. Anatomic segmental hepatic resection is superior to wedge resection as an oncologic operation for colorectal liver metastases. *J Gastrointest Surg* 2000;**4(2)**:178–84.

6. Wanebo HJ, Chu QD, Vezeridis MP, Soderberg C. Patient selection for hepatic resection of colorectal metastases. *Arch Surg* 1996;**131(3)**:322–9.

7. Ekberg H, Tranberg KG, Andersson R, Lundstedt C, Hägerstrand I, Ranstam J, et al. Determinants of survival in liver resection for colorectal secondaries. *Br J Surg* 1986;**73(9)**:727–31.

8. Pawlik TM, Scoggins CR, Zorzi D, Abdalla EK, Andres A, Eng C, et al. Effect of surgical margin status on survival and site of recurrence after hepatic resection for colorectal metastases. *Ann Surg* 2005;**241(5)**:715–22, discussion 22–4.

9. Yamamoto J, Shimada K, Kosuge T, Yamasaki S, Sakamoto M, Fukuda H. Factors influencing survival of patients undergoing hepatectomy for colorectal metastases. *Br J Surg* 1999;**86(3)**:332–7.

10. Fong Y, Cohen AM, Fortner JG, Enker WE, Turnbull AD, Coit DG, et al. Liver resection for colorectal metastases. *J Clin Oncol* 1997;**15(3)**:938–46.

11. Tang H, Li B, Zhang H, Dong J, Lu W. Comparison of anatomical and nonanatomical hepatectomy for colorectal liver metastasis: A meta-analysis of 5207 patients. *Sci Rep* 2016;**6**:32304.

12. Pandanaboyana S, Bell R, White A, Pathak S, Hidalgo E, Lodge P, et al. Impact of parenchymal preserving surgery on survival and recurrence after liver resection for colorectal liver metastasis. *ANZ J Surg* 2018;**88**(1–2):66–70.

13. Adam R, de Gramont A, Figueras J, Kokudo N, Kunstlinger F, Loyer E, et al. Managing synchronous liver metastases from colorectal cancer: A multidisciplinary international consensus. *Cancer Treat Rev* 2015;**41(9)**:729–41.

14. Xu D, Wang H-W, Yan X-L, Li J, Wang K, Xing B-C. Sub-millimeter surgical margin is acceptable in patients with good tumor biology after liver resection for colorectal liver metastases. *Eur J Surg Oncol* 2019;**45(9)**:1551–8.

15. Andreou A, Knitter S, Schmelzle M, Kradolfer D, Maurer MH, Auer TA, et al. Recurrence at surgical margin following hepatectomy for colorectal liver metastases is not associated with R1 resection and does not impact survival. *Surgery* 2021;**169(5)**:1061–8.

16. Zhang Q, Peng J, Ye M, Weng W, Tan C, Ni S, et al. KRAS mutation predicted more mirometastases and closer resection margins in patients with colorectal cancer liver metastases. *Ann Surg Oncol* 2020;**27(4)**:1164–73.

17. Nishioka Y, Shindoh J, Yoshioka R, Gonoi W, Abe H, Okura N, et al. Clinical impact of preoperative chemotherapy on microscopic cancer spread surrounding colorectal liver metastases. *Ann Surg Oncol* 2017;**24(8)**:2326–33.

18. Margonis GA, Buettner S, Andreatos N, Sasaki K, Ijzermans JNM, van Vugt JLA, et al. Anatomical resections improve disease-free survival in patients with KRAS-mutated colorectal liver metastases. *Ann Surg* 2017;**266(4)**:641–9.

19. Kokudo N, Tada K, Seki M, Ohta H, Azekura K, Ueno M, et al. Anatomical major resection versus nonanatomical limited resection for liver metastases from colorectal carcinoma. *Am J Surg* 2001;**181(2)**: 153–9.

20. Tsilimigras DI, Ntanasis-Stathopoulos I, Paredes AZ, Moris D, Gavriatopoulou M, Cloyd JM, et al. Disappearing liver metastases: A systematic review of the current evidence. *Surg Oncol* 2019;**29**:7–13.

21. Elias D, Goere D, Boige V, Kohneh-Sharhi N, Malka D, Tomasic G, et al. Outcome of posthepatectomy-missing colorectal liver metastases after complete response to chemotherapy: impact of adjuvant intra-arterial hepatic oxaliplatin. *Ann Surg Oncol* 2007;**14(11)**:3188–94.

22. Adam R, Wicherts DA, de Haas RJ, Aloia T, Lévi F, Paule B, et al. Complete pathologic response after preoperative chemotherapy for colorectal liver metastases: myth or reality? *J Clin Oncol* 2008;**26(10)**: 1635–41.

23. Ono T, Ishida H, Kumamoto K, Okada N, Ishibashi K. Outcome in disappearing colorectal cancer liver metastases during oxaliplatin-based chemotherapy. *Oncol Lett* 2012;**4(5)**:905–9.

24. Benoist S, Brouquet A, Penna C, Julié C, El Hajjam M, Chagnon S, et al. Complete response of colorectal liver metastases after chemotherapy: Does it mean cure? *J Clin Oncol* 2006;**24(24)**:3939–45.

25. Kuhlmann K, van Hilst J, Fisher S, Poston G. Management of disappearing colorectal liver metastases. *Eur J Surg Oncol* 2016;**42(12)**:1798–805.

26. Bischof DA, Clary BM, Maithel SK, Pawlik TM. Surgical management of disappearing colorectal liver metastases. *Br J Surg* 2013;**100(11)**:1414–20.

27. Goèré D, Gaujoux S, Deschamp F, Dumont F, Souadka A, Dromain C, et al. Patients operated on for initially unresectable colorectal liver metastases with missing metastases experience a favorable longterm outcome. *Ann Surg* 2011;**254(1)**:114–18.

28. van Vledder MG, de Jong MC, Pawlik TM, Schulick RD, Diaz LA, Choti MA. Disappearing colorectal liver metastases after chemotherapy: Should we be concerned? *J Gastrointest Surg* 2010;**14(11)**:1691–700.

29. Pavel M, O'Toole D, Costa F, Capdevila J, Gross D, Kianmanesh R, et al. ENETS Consensus Guidelines Update for the Management of Distant Metastatic Disease of Intestinal, Pancreatic, Bronchial Neuroendocrine Neoplasms (NEN) and NEN of Unknown Primary Site. *Neuroendocrinology* 2016;**103(2)**:172–85.

30. Sarmiento JM, Heywood G, Rubin J, Ilstrup DM, Nagorney DM, Que FG. Surgical treatment of

neuroendocrine metastases to the liver: A plea for resection to increase survival. *J Am Coll Surg* 2003;**197(1)**:29–37.

31. Sham JG, Ejaz A, Gage MM, Bagante F, Reames BN, Maithel S, et al. The impact of extent of liver resection among patients with neuroendocrine liver metastasis: An international multi-institutional study. *J Gastrointest Surg* 2019;**23(3)**:484–91.

32. Saxena A, Chua TC, Perera M, Chu F, Morris DL. Surgical resection of hepatic metastases from neuroendocrine neoplasms: A systematic review. *Surg Oncol* 2012;**21(3)**:e131–41.

33. Adam R, Chiche L, Aloia T, Elias D, Salmon R, Rivoire M, et al. Hepatic resection for noncolorectal nonendocrine liver metastases: Analysis of 1,452 patients and development of a prognostic model. *Ann Surg* 2006;**244(4)**:524–35.

34. Hoffmann K, Bulut S, Tekbas A, Hinz U, Büchler MW, Schemmer P. Is hepatic resection for non-colorectal, non-neuroendocrine liver metastases justified? *Ann Surg Oncol* 2015;**22(Suppl 3)**:S1083–92.

35. Fitzgerald TL, Brinkley J, Banks S, Vohra N, Englert ZP, Zervos EE. The benefits of liver resection for non-colorectal, non-neuroendocrine liver metastases: A systematic review. *Langenbecks Arch Surg* 2014;**399(8)**:989–1000.

36. Weitz J, Blumgart LH, Fong Y, Jarnagin WR, D'Angelica M, Harrison LE, et al. Partial hepatectomy for metastases from noncolorectal, nonneuroendocrine carcinoma. *Ann Surg* 2005;**241(2)**:269–76.

37. European Association for the Study of the Liver. EASL Clinical Practice Guidelines: Management of hepatocellular carcinoma. *J Hepatol* 2018;**69(1)**:182–236.

38. Shindoh J, Makuuchi M, Matsuyama Y, Mise Y, Arita J, Sakamoto Y, et al. Complete removal of the tumor-bearing portal territory decreases local tumor recurrence and improves disease-specific survival of patients with hepatocellular carcinoma. *J Hepatol* 2016;**64(3)**:594–600.

39. Llovet JM, Brú C, Bruix J. Prognosis of hepatocellular carcinoma: The BCLC staging classification. *Semin Liver Dis* 1999;**19(3)**:329–38.

40. Hasegawa K, Kokudo N, Imamura H, Matsuyama Y, Aoki T, Minagawa M, et al. Prognostic impact of anatomic resection for hepatocellular carcinoma. *Ann Surg* 2005;**242(2)**:252–9.

41. Xu H, Liu F, Hao X, Wei Y, Li B, Wen T, et al. Laparoscopically anatomical versus non–anatomical liver resection for large hepatocellular carcinoma. *HPB (Oxford)* 2020;**22(1)**:136–43.

42. Huang X, Lu S. A Meta–analysis comparing the effect of anatomical resection vs. non–anatomical resection on the long–term outcomes for patients undergoing hepatic resection for hepatocellular carcinoma. *HPB (Oxford)* 2017;**19(10)**:843–9.

43. Li S-Q, Huang T, Shen S-L, Hua Y-P, Hu W-J, Kuang M, et al. Anatomical versus non–anatomical liver resection for hepatocellular carcinoma exceeding Milan criteria. *Br J Surg* 2017;**104(1)**:118–27.

44. Marubashi S, Gotoh K, Akita H, Takahashi H, Ito Y, Yano M, et al. Anatomical versus non–anatomical resection for hepatocellular carcinoma. *Br J Surg* 2015;**102(7)**:776–84.

45. Cucchetti A, Cescon M, Ercolani G, Bigonzi E, Torzilli G, Pinna AD. A comprehensive meta-regression analysis on outcome of anatomic resection versus nonanatomic resection for hepatocellular carcinoma. *Ann Surg Oncol* 2012;**19(12)**:3697–705.

46. Torzilli G, Palmisano A, Procopio F, Cimino M, Botea F, Donadon M, et al. A new systematic small for size resection for liver tumors invading the middle hepatic vein at its caval confluence: Mini-mesohepatectomy. *Ann Surg* 2010;**251(1)**:33–9.

Bailey & Love's Essential Operations Bailey & Love's Essential Operatio
Bailey & Love's Essential Operations Bailey & Love's Essential Operatio
Bailey & Love's Essential Operations Bailey & Love's Essential Operatio

SECTION 8 | LIVER

Chapter
48

Minimally Invasive Liver Surgery

Lulu Tanno and Rong Liu

INTRODUCTION

This chapter reviews current practices in laparoscopic liver surgery, beginning with details of the three international consensus meetings on minimally invasive liver surgery, followed by a discussion of the indications and technical aspects including patient positioning and port placement.

The first minimally invasive liver surgery (MILS) was reported in 1991 by H Reich and colleagues from Wyoming Valley, Kingston, Pennsylvania. Over the last three decades, the field has evolved at an astonishing rate due to advances in techniques and instruments and most recently the introduction of robotic-assisted procedures (1). Several published studies have demonstrated the safety of MILS compared to open surgery in selected patients and demonstrated reductions in blood loss, hospital stays and a quicker return to full functional recovery (2,3).

To reflect the development of this technique, the first international conference on minimally invasive

liver surgery was held in Louisville in 2008 (4). This meeting helped to standardize terminologies and techniques used in MILS and lead to the global acceptance of MILS by the international hepato-pancreato-biliary (HPB) community. The International Consensus Conference on Laparoscopic Liver Resection (ICCLLR) at Morioka in 2014 achieved a consensus on techniques including parenchymal transection, the use of energy devices and haemorrhage control. It concluded that a minimally invasive approach should be considered for minor liver resections involving less than two segments. However, it proposed the use of a difficulty scoring system (*Figure 48.1*) because at that time the minimally invasive approach was still considered to be an innovative and unproven technique for major resections involving more than three segments (5). The latest consensus guidelines from Southampton in 2017 focus on the safe progression

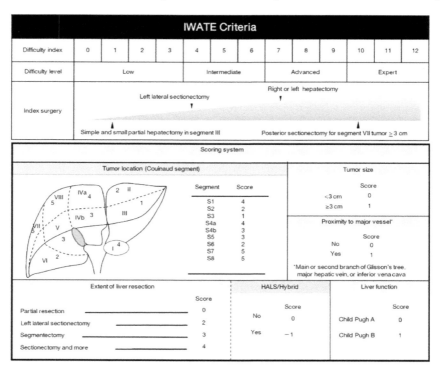

Figure 48.1 IWATE criteria proposed at the 2nd ICCLLR in Morioka as an up-versioned difficulty scoring system (20).

DOI: 10.1201/9781003080060-48

and dissemination of MILS and recognized the need for training in advanced MILS (6).

TERMINOLOGY

The Louisville consensus defined minor liver resections as either a simple wedge resection, left lateral sectionectomy (segments 2 and 3) or anterior segments (segments 4b, 5, and 6). Major liver resections were defined as hemi-hepatectomies, posterio-superior segments (segments 1, 4a, 7, and 8), and tri-sectionectomies (4). The terminology for major resection in MILS deviates from that used for conventional open surgery where the resection of three or more contiguous lesions is considered major. Currently, it is considered standard practice to approach minor resections by minimally invasive methods, although an increasing numbers of major liver resections are being performed by MILS. Nevertheless, major resections remain technically more demanding and should only be performed by those with advanced skills and expertise in a unit with the necessary infrastructure and support.

INDICATIONS

Internationally, primary liver cancer still remains the single most common indication for liver surgery, although in North America and Europe the number of cases is higher for metastatic colorectal cancer. Indications for MILS also include benign liver lesions and donor hepatectomy. The location of the lesion, technical difficulty in exposing the involved segment laparoscopically, and plans for potential haemorrhage control need to be considered when planning MILS, irrespective of the pathology. The Louisville consensus stated that ideal lesions for a minimally invasive approach (4) should be: 1) Solitary; 2) less than 5 cm in size and 3) in a peripheral location (segments 2 to 6).

However, with the increasing experience and expertise in MILS, numerous centres have now published their outcomes involving resections of major and more difficult segments including the caudate lobe, posterior segments (segment 7, 8 and 4a), and major hepatectomies (7,8). It is clear, however, that the surgical approach must be carefully planned based on the tumour location and its relationships to hepatic vessels whether it is to be performed open or by MILS. In high-volume centres with expertise in MILS, indication for a laparoscopic or open approach frequently do not differ, but has not yet become the norm in all centres.

The size of the lesion still needs to be considered when planning MILS, but certainly over the last decade large tumours have become less of an absolute contra-indication. What is important is to remain mindful of potential damage resulting from retraction with the risk of tumour exposure and consequent dissemination.

Due to the shortage of donors for liver transplantation, resection remain the first-choice treatment for patients with solitary HCCs, even in those with a background of liver cirrhosis. The cirrhotic liver involves additional challenges for the MILS approach due to distorted anatomy, the rigidity of the diseased organ limiting mobility and mobilization and the altered liver parenchyma with an increased echogenicity leading to difficulty in identifying lesions using intraoperative ultrasound (IUS) (*Figure 48.2*). Other challenges to

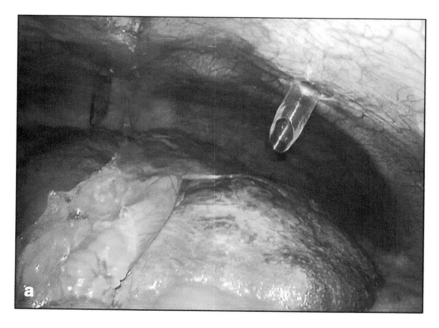

Figure 48.2 Intraoperative image of liver demonstrating congestive hepatomegaly and cirrhosis.

consider include the unpredictable response to energy devices during parenchymal dissection (both cauterizing devices and dissecting instruments), the increased risk of bleeding and potential difficulty of haemorrhage control. Patients with advanced cirrhosis also pose significant management challenges postoperatively with the morbidity and mortality from fulminant decompensated liver failure, hepatic insufficiency and ascites, and Child-Pugh C cirrhosis is a contraindication to resection. There have been a number of publications from high-volume centres demonstrating longer operative time with MILS in carefully selected Child-Pugh A liver cirrhosis, but with equivalent intraoperative blood loss, morbidity and disease-free survival compared with the open surgery groups. The presently available data demonstrate that MILS is an acceptable treatment option for patients with Child-Pugh A and low-B liver cirrhosis (9,10).

Laparoscopic living liver donation

In the context of living-donor liver transplantation (both adult-to-paediatric or adult-to-adult), MILS has been enthusiastically adopted due to the significant postoperative benefits, with improved cosmetic and functional outcomes and the often significantly shorter lengths of hospital stay for the donors (11). Laparoscopic living-donor left lateral sectionectomy has been shown to be safe and repeatable and has become a standard of care in experienced centres. However, right donor hepatectomy is still considered to be an immature MILS technique and currently there is insufficient evidence to support its adoption as the standard of care (12).

PATIENT POSITION AND PORT PLACEMENTS

A diligent approach to patient positioning and port placements for MILS are two essential components required to achieve the optimal ergonomics for a surgeon which leads to improved visualization, safer dissection, shorter procedures and improved results. However, there are no ubiquitously accepted standard patient positions or port placements and these practices are still very much based on the individual centres and surgeon's preferences. In addition, the patient's position and port placements vary significantly between laparoscopic and robotic resections.

The most common patient position for laparoscopic resections is supine with a straight split-leg position, commonly referred to as the 'French position' (13). This positioning allows the main operating surgeon to stand between the patient's legs with the assistant and the scrub nurse on either side. If a surgical table does not allow the legs to be split then a modified Lloyd-Davies position where the patient's legs are held in stirrups is an acceptable alternative. This position may also be an advantage in cases of combined colorectal and liver resections where access to the pelvis is required.

In the straight split-leg position, the first port which is also the optical (camera) port is most commonly placed in the supra-umbilical position. To perform a wedge resection, additional ports are placed in a concentric circle radiating from the target lesion, using the 12 mm ports as the working ports for the use of a parenchymal dissection or stapling device. Based on the xiphisternum to umbilical distance, the position of the supra-umbilical port can vary, and you may need to insert the port higher in some patients where this distance is unusually long. Particularly for those with a high BMI, port placements are best assessed from fixed bony landmarks. In a cirrhotic patient, an option for an infra-umbilical port may be considered to avoid potential haemorrhage from the re-cannulated umbilical vein. For the insertion of the first port, an open cut-down technique is recommended, particularly in those patients who have had previous surgery, and it should be placed away from the previous incision. It may be necessary to insert additional ports for adhesiolysis prior to proceeding with the planned liver resection if patients had previous surgery.

The resected specimen is normally extracted using a retrieval bag device either through an extension of the para-umbilical port incision, or a separate incision such as Pfannenstiel for larger specimens (14). Below are some examples of laparoscopic approaches.

Anterolateral segments

For the resections of the anterior-lateral segments, such as left lateral sectionectomy (LLS), the supine with straight leg split position is most commonly employed. There are no standardized port placements for LLS but typically between 4–6 ports are used, with or without the 5 mm epigastric port and at least two 12 mm working ports (*Figure 48.3a*) (13).

For posterior and superior lesions, and major resections

There is no standardized patient position for posterior-superior or right hepatectomy procedures. Several options exist including a left lateral decubitus position which may be ideal for posterior lesions (segment 6, 7 and dorsal aspect of segment 8). This position may lead to reduced venous bleeding during transection due to the position of the right hepatic vein being higher than the IVC. A semi-prone position has also been described, but this position may make mobilization and manipulation of the right hemi-liver challenging, particularly in those with a large tumour. One must also be prepared for open conversion in an emergency, and for this reason this position may not be ideal for all cases especially those where technical difficulty is anticipated. A further option is supine with a straight leg split position and using an inflatable balloon or a cushion to raise the right posterior costal margin (14,15).

Typical port positions are along the 'reverse L' incision (*Figure 48.3b*), which allows for adequate right-sided liver mobilization, and 12 mm working ports for medial and inferior dissection (15).

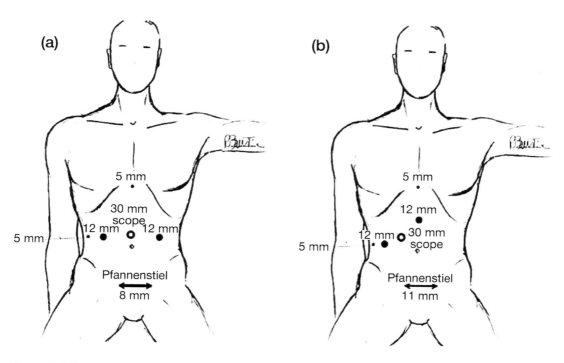

Figure 48.3 Illustrations showing laparoscopic port placements in left lateral sectionectomies (a) and right hepatectomy in an 'reverse L' pattern (b) (13).

PRINGLE MANOEUVRE

Various methods of applying the Pringle manoeuvre for MILS have been described, either intra- or extracorporeally and this is again based very much on the surgeon's preference (16). A 5 mm nylon tape around the hilum is commonly passed through a rubber snugger, trocar or appropriately sized NG tube. The tape can then be passed extracorporeally through the abdominal wall which allows for rapid application and release of the inflow control without interfering with the resection (15).

INTRAOPERATIVE ULTRASONOGRAPHY AND FLUORESCENCE IMAGING SYSTEM

Intraoperative ultrasound (IUS) has been increasingly used in both open and MILS to aid real-time decision-making, to assess the extent of the tumour and its relationship to major vessels, and to mark the proposed transection plane. Due to the limitation in tactile feedback during MILS, the importance of the use of IUS has been supported by international consensus (6).

More recently, indocyanine green (ICG) has been used by some centres to mark the boundaries of individual segments. ICG can be either injected directly into the portal branch of the target resection segment (positive staining technique) or the target segment can be identified by an area of ischaemia (negative staining technique) by injection of ICG after clamping or ligation and division of the portal pedicle (17). The negative staining technique is thought to be technically more straightforward during the MILS approach, where injection of ICG directly into the portal vein can be technically challenging.

ENHANCED RECOVERY AFTER SURGERY (ERAS®) PROGRAMME

The Enhanced Recovery After Surgery (ERAS) programme in colorectal surgery has been shown to reduce postoperative morbidity and hospital stay and has been expanded and modified for use in other specialities, including open liver surgery. With the increasing application of MILS, and the additional potential benefits of the laparoscopic approach compared with open liver surgery, many centres are starting to use ERAS programs for MILS. The ORANGE II and the ORANGE segments trials aimed to assess oncological outcomes in laparoscopic liver surgery versus open liver resections within ERAS protocols. Unfortunately, the ORANGE II trial was closed prematurely due to poor recruitment but there was a suggestion of a slightly shorter functional recovery following MILS in an ERAS protocol in the laparoscopic group (18,19).

It is most likely that with wider acceptance and increasing practices in minimally invasive liver surgery, more and more centres will adopt the ERAS program to standardize pre, intra, and postoperative care for patients to improve outcomes.

SUMMARY

In 1991, the first minimally invasive liver surgical procedure was reported and supported by technological advances and the evolution of surgical techniques. Since then, indications have expanded and outcomes have all improved. With the recent introduction of robotic-assisted surgery (RAS), previously inaccessible tumours in superior and posterior positions have been successfully and safely resected (20). A number of published studies have demonstrated the safety of MILS compared with open surgery, highlighted the reduced blood loss, shorter hospital stays and return to full functional recovery. These data have encouraged more units to integrate MILS into traditional HPB practice (21). This trend shows no sign of slowing down and in the foreseeable future it is likely that data will be available to identify those patients where MILS and RAS are the preferred option and the number of tumours and intrahepatic locations, currently considered 'unsuitable' will diminish further.

REFERENCES

1. Reich H, McGlynn F, DeCaprio J, Budin R. Laparoscopic excision of benign liver lesions. *Obstet Gynecol* 1991;**78(5 Pt 2)**:956–8.
2. Nguyen KT, Laurent A, Dagher I, Geller DA, Steel J, Thomas MT, et al. Minimally invasive liver resection for metastatic colorectal cancer: A multi-institutional, international report of safety, feasibility, and early outcomes. *Ann Surg* 2009;**250(5)**:842–8.
3. Lo WM, Tohme ST, Geller DA. Recent advances in minimally invasive liver resection for colorectal cancer liver metastases—a review. *Cancers (Basel)* 2022;**15(1)**:142.
4. Buell JF, Cherqui D, Geller DA, O'Rourke N, Iannitti D, Dagher I, et al. The international position on laparoscopic liver surgery: The Louisville statement, 2008. *Ann Surg* 2009;**250(5)**:825–30.
5. Wakabayashi G, Cherqui D, Geller DA, Buell JF, Kaneko H, Han HS, et al. Recommendations for laparoscopic liver resection: A report from the second international consensus conference held in Morioka. *Ann Surg* 2015;**261(4)**:619–29.
6. Hilal MA, Aldrighetti L, Dagher I, Edwin B, Troisi RI, Alikhanov R, et al. The Southampton consensus guidelines for laparoscopic liver surgery: From indication to implementation. *Ann Surg* 2018;**68(1)**:11–8.
7. Kasai M, Cipriani F, Gayet B, Aldrighetti L, Ratti F, Sarmiento JM, et al. Laparoscopic versus open major hepatectomy: A systematic review and meta-analysis of individual patient data. *Surgery* 2018;**163(5)**:985–95.
8. Ciria R, Cherqui D, Geller DA, Briceno J, Wakabayashi G. Comparative short-term benefits of laparoscopic liver resection: 9000 cases and climbing. *Ann Surg* 2016;**263(4)**:761–77.
9. Witowski J, Rubinkiewicz M, Mizera M, Wysocki M, Gajewska N, Sitkowski M, et al. Meta-analysis of short- and long-term outcomes after pure laparoscopic versus open liver surgery in hepatocellular carcinoma patients. *Surg Endosc* 2019;**33(5)**:1491–1507.
10. Seehofer D, Sucher R, Schmelzle M, Öllinger R, Lederer A, Denecke T, et al. Evolution of laparoscopic liver surgery as standard procedure for HCC in cirrhosis? *Z Gastroenterol* 2017;**55(5)**:453–60.
11. Gao Y, Wu W, Liu C, Liu T, Xiao H. Comparison of laparoscopic and open living donor hepatectomy: A meta-analysis. *Medicine (Baltimore)* 2021;**100(32)**:e26708.
12. Cherqui D, Ciria R, Kwon CHD, Kim KH, Broering D, Wakabayashi G, et al. Expert consensus guidelines on minimally invasive donor hepatectomy for living donor liver transplantation from innovation to implementation: A joint initiative from the international laparoscopic liver society (ILLS) and the Asian-Pacific hepato-pancreato-biliary association (A-PHPBA). *Ann Surg* 2021;**273(1)**:96–108.
13. Goumard C, Farges O, Laurent A, Cherqui D, Soubrane O, Gayet B, et al. An update on laparoscopic liver resection: French hepato-bilio-pancreatic surgery association statement. *Journal de Chirurgie Viscerale* 2015;**152(2)**:107–12.
14. Thiruchelvam N, Lee SY, Chiow AKH. Patient and port positioning in laparoscopic liver resections. *Hepatoma Res* 2021;**7**:22.
15. Abu Hilal M, Tschuor C, Kuemmerli C, López-Ben S, Lesurtel M, Rotellar F. Laparoscopic posterior segmental resections: How I do it: Tips and pitfalls. *Int J Surg* 2020;**82S**:178–186.
16. Piardi T, Lhuaire M, Memeo R, Pessaux P, Kianmanesh R, Sommacale D. Laparoscopic Pringle maneuver: How we do it? Hepatobiliary Surg Nutr 2016;5(4):345.
17. Ishizawa T, Saiura A, Kokudo N. Clinical application of indocyanine green-fluorescence imaging during hepatectomy. *Hepatobiliary Surg Nutr* 2016;**5(4)**:322–8.
18. Wong-Lun-Hing EM, Van Dam RM, Van Breukelen GJP, Tanis PJ, Ratti F, Van Hillegersberg R, et al. Randomized clinical trial of open versus laparoscopic left lateral hepatic sectionectomy within an enhanced recovery after surgery programme (ORANGE II study) behalf of the ORANGE II. *Br J Surg* 2017;**104(5)**:525–35.
19. Fung AKY, Chong CCN, Lai PBS. ERAS in minimally invasive hepatectomy. *Ann Hepatobiliary Pancreat Surg* 2020;**24(2)**:119–26.
20. Zhao ZM, Yin ZZ, Pan LC, Liu R. Robotic isolated partial and complete hepatic caudate lobectomy: A single institution experience. *Hepatobiliary Pancreat Dis Int* 2020;**19(5)**:435-9.
21. Wakabayashi G. What has changed after the Morioka consensus conference 2014 on laparoscopic liver resection? *Hepatobiliary Surg Nutr* 2016;**5(4)**:281–9.

Chapter 49

Ablation Techniques

Ali Arshad and Clare Bent

INTRODUCTION

Hepatocellular carcinoma (HCC) and liver metastases, particularly secondary to colorectal carcinoma (CLM), represent the two most common malignant tumours of the liver. Only a small proportion of patients, 20% for HCC and 10–25% for CLM, are suitable for radical surgical treatment at the time of diagnosis (1,2) and when left untreated, the prognosis for patients with such disease is dismal, approaching 100% mortality at 5 years (3). Conventional systemic therapies including chemotherapy and radiotherapy have also shown limited survival benefit.

The large proportion of patients with unresectable but treatable liver disease has driven the development and innovation of alternative therapies including chemoembolization and ablation. This chapter aims to provide an overview of both chemical and thermal ablative techniques and irreversible electroporation, in addition to combination treatments.

BACKGROUND

In 1891, d'Arsonval demonstrated that radiofrequency waves could pass through living tissue, causing an elevation in tissue temperature in the absence of neuromuscular excitation (4). In 1928, radiofrequency ablation was introduced into medical practice in the form of the surgical Bovie® knife (Symmetry Surgical Inc. Tennessee, USA) (5).

Interest in targeted liver treatment gained momentum in the mid-1980s, when image-guided chemical ablation with ethanol or acetic acid was described and accepted as a treatment option for patients with malignant liver disease. From 1990, percutaneous and laparoscopic thermal ablative techniques were also introduced into this arena, including the application of radiofrequency ablation, and subsequently many of these options have been adopted into consensus practice guidelines worldwide.

When compared to surgical resection, local ablation (both chemical and thermal) is frequently of lower cost, has minimal morbidity and can be performed on a day case basis, making it an attractive option to many patients. However, clinicians must be cognisant that all techniques within the treatment armamentarium are not mutually exclusive, and there is increasing evidence to support the role of ablation in conjunction with surgery and chemoembolization and/or immunotherapy

as combination treatments to improve survival outcomes further.

Local ablative techniques serve as a potentially curative option with an ability to induce complete cell death due to cytotoxicity and coagulative necrosis in the targeted tumour.

MECHANISMS OF ACTION

Chemical ablation most commonly involves ethanol instillation via percutaneous injection (PEI) into the tumour site. This results in cellular dehydration, protein denaturation and occlusion of small vessels with resultant coagulative necrosis. The amount of ethanol required can be calculated by using the formula of a sphere: $V = \frac{4}{3} \pi r^3$ (3).

Thermal ablation involves either freezing (cryoablation) or heating (radiofrequency [RFA], microwave [MWA] and high-intensity focused ultrasound [HIFU] techniques).

Cryoablation

Cryoablation (CA) circulates liquid nitrogen or argon to a percutaneously or laparoscopically placed probe. The probe tip is active and uses a freeze-thaw process (based on the Joule-Thomson effect) to induce rapid cooling of tissue and intracellular ice crystal formation. Damage to the surrounding microvasculature disrupts tissue perfusion, leading to ischaemia. Cell death is achieved by freezing at temperatures below -40°C or lower secondary to osmotic shock, with resultant cell membrane rupture (6).

Radiofrequency ablation

RFA involves the application of energy to a tissue target via an RFA probe with a frequency of <900 kHz. An alternating current is used to cause rapid oscillation of adjacent dipole molecules. Frictional energy losses between neighbouring molecules result in local energy deposition and tissue hyperthermia, with growth of the ablation zone being attributed primarily to thermal diffusion. The objective is to reach temperatures of greater than 60°C to ensure protein denaturation and instantaneous cell death. Temperatures of between 42–60°C result in irreversible cell damage due to microvascular thrombosis, ischaemia and hypoxia.

DOI: 10.1201/9781003080060-49

Microwave ablation

Microwave ablation (MWA) uses propagating electromagnetic waves in the region of 900 MHz and 2.4 GHz to induce targeted tissue hyperthermia via dielectric hysteresis, most commonly via a percutaneously placed probe. Polar molecules continuously realign with the oscillating microwave field, increasing kinetic energy and tissue temperature. In contrast to electric currents, microwaves radiate through all biological tissues, including those with high impedance such as bone, lung and charred or desiccated tissues. Consequently, MWA can produce faster, hotter and larger ablation zones than when compared to RFA. The process of cell death in MWA is almost identical to that observed in RFA.

High-intensity focused ultrasound

High-intensity focused ultrasound (HIFU) uses multiple ultrasound beams, produced by piezoelectric or piezoceramic transducers, to target a 3D focal point typically 1–5 mm in diameter and 10–50 mm in length (7). A degassed water bath couples the ultrasound source to the patient to achieve minimal reflection or absorption of sound waves prior to reaching their target. The ultrasound beams' focal point is thermally ablative and causes cavitation within the targeted treatment site.

Irreversible electroporation

Irreversible electroporation (IRE) technology, e.g. NanoKnife® system (AngioDynamics, New York, USA), is a non-thermal modality where electrode placement is used to create a pulsed direct current, thereby inducing cytotoxicity within tumour cells by altering trans membrane potential, creating permanent cell membrane pores, irreversibly disrupting cell membrane integrity with resultant lysis and cell death.

TECHNICAL FACTORS
Anaesthesia

The majority of percutaneous ablation techniques can be completed on an outpatient basis requiring a short period of post-procedural recovery. Consequently, percutaneous ablation is associated with significantly less morbidity and shorter length hospital stay when compared with surgical alternatives, including intraoperative ablation or laparoscopic techniques.

Percutaneous ablation is performed either under conscious ablation or general anaesthesia. The decision regarding the type of anaesthesia is dependent upon patient preference, patient comorbidity, complexity of ablation (including the need for additional protective manoeuvres such as hydrodissection) and physician preference or local practice.

Image guidance and technical aspects

The operator's ability to visualize the target tumour using imaging is key to a technically and clinically successful procedure. Geographical variation in clinical practice exists with ultrasound being the preferred method in Asia, versus computed tomography (CT) in the USA. Many centres use a combination of both, largely as ultrasound allows for real-time visualization of probe placement followed by CT to confirm exact probe positioning and ensure sufficient ablation margins to achieve complete tumour targeting. More recently, positron emission tomography CT (PET/CT) has been developed to guide ablation due to its ability to highlight biologically active tumour sites, further improving the accuracy of targeting.

A safe ablation zone is vital to eliminate the risk of collateral organ damage during thermal ablation, particularly if adjacent to the gallbladder, stomach, diaphragm or bowel. Technical steps to increase safety include the introduction of air causing either an artificial pneumothorax or localized air dissection, or instillation of fluid (sterile water or 5% dextrose depending on the thermal ablation modality in use) to create additional space and distance between the target site and non-target organs, protecting the latter from thermal injury.

Other considerations include 'heat sink' effect, whereby ablation temperatures may be compromised by perfusion-mediated cooling of vessels adjacent to the tumour target, and non-visible tumours on imaging, whereby anatomical planning may be required, rather than focused tumour targeting, to achieve the required outcome.

CLINICAL OUTCOMES
Chemical ablation

Percutaneous ethanol injection (PEI) and percutaneous acetic acid injection (PAI) are well-tolerated, low-cost and low-risk procedures. Two trials have compared PEI to PAI in early liver cancer revealing no significant difference in overall survival (OS) or recurrence-free survival (RFS) (8,9). PEI did demonstrate a significantly shorter hospital stay, and perhaps consequently, the majority of evidence focuses solely on PEI of malignant liver disease in clinical practice.

For HCC less than 3 cm, 5-year survival post-PEI ranges from 38–60% (10), and a large Japanese study of 685 patients published 5-, 10- and 20-year survival rates of 49%, 18% and 7.2%, respectively (10). Survival rates are therefore comparable to patients with cirrhosis but with no demonstrable evidence of HCC. Local tumour progression ranges between 6–31% and is directly proportional to tumour size. PEI is proven to be a safe procedure with morbidity and mortality rates of 0–3.2% and 0–0.4%, respectively (11).

For CLM, the effectiveness of PEI is unclear. One study reported that greater than 50% of patients with liver metastases larger than 4 cm treated with PEI achieved complete tumour necrosis (12). However, another study reported PEI to be ineffective in metastatic disease due to the inherent scirrhous nature of liver metastases and consequent preferential diffusion of ethanol into 'softer' adjacent normal liver parenchyma (13).

In summary, clinical outcomes of PEI are limited by the unpredictable distribution of ethanol within heterogeneous tumoral tissue, therefore during injection, ethanol dispersion requires real-time ultrasound monitoring and frequent repositioning of the needle to ensure complete treatment. Consequently, PEI is used primarily for treatment of HCCs less than 2 cm and when thermal ablative techniques are not feasible due to high-risk locations or enterobiliary reflux.

Thermal ablation

Cryoablation

Cryoablation (CA) allows real-time monitoring of ice-ball formation improving both accuracy of ablation and procedural safety profile, which are critical when treating lesions in close proximity to high-risk structures.

Early concerns regarding 'cryoshock', a life-threatening syndrome of multi-organ failure and coagulopathy with a 40% mortality, led to reduced utilization of CA within the liver, however, advances in technology including thinner probes and argon-helium systems have re-ignited clinical interest in its use (14).

For HCC, one large series of 866 patients with 1197 HCCs undergoing 1401 CA sessions, demonstrated no procedure-related mortality. Major complications were reported in 2.8% patients and local recurrence was 24.2%, at a median of 30.9 months, indicating a performance and safety profile similar to both RFA and MWA. Specifically, advantages of CA include less pain during and post-procedure and increased immunological effects (15).

Clinical outcome comparisons of CA with alternative thermal ablation techniques are conflicting. One meta-analysis concluded that RFA was superior to CA when examining complications and local recurrence, although no difference in mortality was demonstrated (16). Subsequently, Wang et al. published a randomized controlled trial (RCT) comparing CA with RFA in patients with cirrhosis, Child-Pugh A or B liver function and one or two HCC nodules measuring ≤4 cm. Treatment groups were similar and according to the study, local tumour progression at 3-years was found to be significantly lower in the CA group (p = 0.043) for tumours measuring between 3.1–4 cm in diameter. However, complication rates and survival, overall and tumour-free, were comparable (17). No study has as yet compared procedural cost differences, an important factor in today's economy.

For CLM, CA evidence is limited. A 2013 Cochrane review identified only one trial examining outcomes in this setting. The trial included 123 patients with solitary or multiple unilobar or bilobar liver metastases who underwent either cryotherapy (via cryoextirpation, cryoresection or cryodestruction) or conventional surgery. In the cryotherapy group, survival rates were 60%, 44%, and 19% at 3, 5, and 10 years, respectively, compared to 51%, 36% and 8% in the conventional surgery group (Hazard ratio [HR] = 0.71). No statistically significant difference was found regarding tumour recurrence between groups. The review stated that in this setting cryotherapy should not be recommended outside RCTs (18).

In conclusion, there has been a redirection of focus into the use of CA for malignant liver disease, however more evidence is required to justify its use and determine its role in this setting.

Radiofrequency ablation

RFA is the most established and evidence-based thermal ablative technique for use within the liver, however MWA and CA are increasingly utilized.

For HCC, a Cochrane database review published evidence from 11 RCTs involving 1819 participants. Four comparison groups were compared with RFA: 1) Hepatic resection; 2) PEI; 3) MWA, and 4) laser ablation. Conclusions were that there was: 1) moderate-quality evidence that hepatic resection is superior to RFA regarding survival, however RFA is associated with fewer complications and a shorter hospital stay; 2) moderate-quality evidence showing RFA is superior to PEI regarding survival (19). This latter finding is supported by Lencioni et al. who published the treatment outcomes of HCCs greater than 2 cm, showing RFA was associated with higher rates of complete necrosis and improved long-term outcomes than when compared to PEI (20). Major complication rates of RFA are reported as approximately 4.1%.

For CLM, similar conclusions can be drawn for the clinical utility of RFA with surgical resection being preferable when feasible. However, RFA is frequently used in patients ineligible for resection or for post-surgical tumour recurrence with good outcomes. Evidence suggests that RFA of small tumours that can be ablated with clear margins can provide outcomes similar to surgery (21). One study reported a local tumour progression rate of 3% within 12-months, and a local tumour progression-free survival of over 95% at 30-months post-ablation within margins over 5 mm and biopsy-proven complete tumour necrosis (22). A further study demonstrating the benefit of RFA, compared a combination treatment using RFA plus systemic treatment, versus systemic treatment alone. The actuarial patient survival at 8 years was significantly prolonged (p = 0.01) for the ablation group (39%) when compared with the chemotherapy-only group (9%). This is the only level 1 evidence illustrating the impact of RFA on oncologic outcomes (23).

Microwave ablation

In recent years, MWA has become the favoured thermal ablation technique for use within the liver due to shorter ablation times and increased efficacy, despite a lack of prospective evidence (*Figures 49.1* and *49.2*).

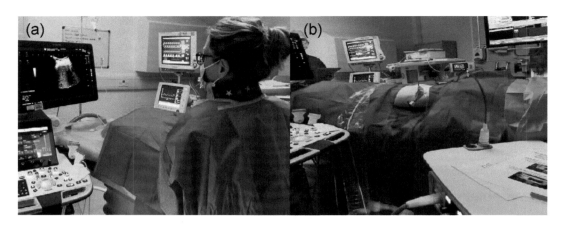

Figure 49.1 US and CT imaging in use to guide a liver microwave ablation procedure, using the Emprint™ ablation system with Thermosphere™ technology (Medtronic, Minnesota, USA).

Two RCTs have compared MWA with RFA (24,25). The reported therapeutic outcomes of MWA for HCC included technical success rates of 99.6%, local tumour progression rates of 1.1%, 4.3% and 11.4%, and overall survival rates of 96.4%, 81.9% and 67.3% at 1, 3 and 5 years, although no significant difference was noted when compared to RFA. Microwave ablation-associated mortality is reported to occur in 0.002% with major complication rates of approximately 4.6%, significantly higher than seen with RFA, although more recent data suggest no difference in complications between the modalities (26). For CLM, the clinical utility of MWA replicates that of RFA.

High-intensity focused ultrasound

Early reports of use in primary and secondary liver malignancy indicate HIFU to be an excellent local ablative treatment. However, logistical requirements remain a significant barrier to implementation within the cancer setting.

For HCC, in a series of 49 patients unfit for surgical treatment with a median tumour size 2.2 cm and a range 0.9–8 cm, Ng et al. reported 1- and 3-year overall survival rates of 87.7% and 62.4%, respectively (27).

Limited data are available for HIFU in the context of CLM. One recent clinical trial examined HIFU in 13 patients with 1–3 CLMs, unsuitable for treatment by surgical resection or thermal ablation (28). The authors reported a median progression-free survival of 9 months and a 2-year overall survival of 77.8%. More data is required to support the use of HIFU in this setting.

Irreversible electroporation

The use of irreversible electroporation (IRE) in humans was first reported as safe in 2011 by Thomson et al. (29). This was supported by Kingham and colleagues who studied its use in patients with small hepatic tumours,

all of which were adjacent to and within 1 cm of a major vascular structure. The 65 tumours treated had a median diameter of 1 cm (range = 0.5–5 cm) and only one demonstrated persistent disease (1.9%) and three tumours (5.7%) recurred locally with no life-threatening events being reported (30). This technique is promising for future treatment at anatomical sites previously considered prohibitively dangerous for thermal ablation. Most recently, the COLDFIRE-2 trial examined the safety and feasibility of this technique for unresectable colorectal liver metastases. Fifty-one participants with tumours smaller than 5.0 cm were enrolled and local control was achieved in 74% of patients. There was a median overall survival of 2.7 years and an acceptable safety profile (31).

Combination treatment

The efficacy of thermal ablation may vary depending on the anatomical location of the tumour within the liver. The synergistic use of local ablative techniques in combination with other treatment options has already been proven in the literature with improved overall survival following combination RFA and chemoembolization when compared to RFA alone (32). Improved outcomes are in part hypothesized to be due to reduced blood flow from primary chemoembolization, reducing heat loss during ablative therapy and potentiating the heat destruction effect of RFA. Chemoembolization can also potentially help control any adjacent non-visible satellite lesions.

In patients with unresectable disease, a hybrid approach of surgical resection and ablation is also reasonable. Liu et al. compared 67 patients undergoing a hybrid approach versus 268 undergoing standard resectional surgery. Overall survival, progression-free survival, and local recurrence-free survival were not statistically different despite a higher tumour burden in the hybrid group (33,34).

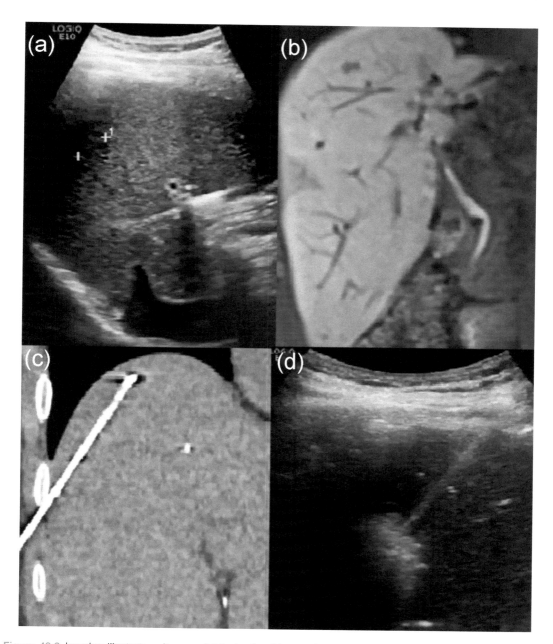

Figure 49.2 Imaging illustrates ultrasound (a) of a focal hypoechoic colorectal liver metastasis identified during surveillance post a left hemicolectomy and liver metastectomy. Coronal T1 fat-saturated volumetric interpolated breath-hold examination (VIBE) MRI sequence (b) 20 minutes post-Primovist® injection (Bayer AG, Leverkusen, Germany), confirming a solitary segment 8 liver metastasis. Coronal CT (c) confirming MWA needle position pre-ablation of liver metastasis. Ultrasound (d) demonstrating MWA needle in position during ablation treatment (100 Watts for 10 minutes) with hyperechoic change at the site of the lesional ablation.

More recently, interest has focused on localized radiation in combination with ablation. Hyperthermia is proven to heighten the cytotoxic effect of radiation, and several animal trials have indicated that RFA and radiation of liver lesions resulted in improved tumour control than when compared with RFA alone. One hypothesis suggests free radical formation after radiation results in inhibition of tumour cell recovery, which enhances the thermal ablative effects. Such combination treatment is an exciting new avenue of treatment for future research and investigation.

SUMMARY

Local ablative therapies are well established and have been incorporated in consensus guidelines including the European Association for the Study of Liver. Treatment is aimed at patients who present with nonsurgical primary and metastatic liver tumours with low disease burden and the treatment objective is with curative intent.

RFA has the greatest volume of evidence supporting its use to improve overall survival for both primary and secondary liver malignancy. MWA and CA are gaining popularity due to technical advantages and possible improved local tumour-free progression. Further evidence should help clinically validate both their roles and place within the treatment algorithm. HIFU and IRE remain exciting innovations, although they remain reliant on being able to overcome implementation challenges, both regarding technique, technical aspects, and cost. Combination treatments to exploit inherent immunological responses and promote a synergistic effect resulting in cytotoxicity also offer a focus for future research and advances in treatment to further improve survival benefit within the ablative setting.

REFERENCES

1. Borie F, Bouvier A-M, Herrero A, Faivre J, Launoy G, Delafosse P, et al. Treatment and prognosis of hepatocellular carcinoma: A population based study in France. *J Surg Oncol* 2008;**98(7)**:505–9.
2. Hill CR, Chagpar RB, Callender GG, Brown RE, Gilbert JE, Martin RCG 2nd, et al. Recurrence following hepatectomy for metastatic colorectal cancer: Development of a model that predicts patterns of recurrence and survival. *Ann Surg Oncol* 2012;**19(1)**:139–44.
3. McGhana JP, Dodd GD. Radiofrequency ablation of the liver current status. *AJR* 2001;**176(1)**:3–16.
4. d'Arsonval MA. Action physiologique des courants alternatifs. *CR Soc Biol* 1891;**43**:283–6.
5. Cushing H, Bovie WT. Electro-surgery as an aid to the removal of intracranial tumours. *Surg Gynaecol Obstet* 1928;**47**:751–84.
6. Rubinsky B. Cryosurgery. *Annu Rev Biomed Eng* 2000;**2**:157–87.
7. Mearini L. High intensity focused ultrasound, liver disease and bridging therapy. *World J Gastroenterol* 2013;**19(43)**:7494–9.
8. Ohnishi K, Yoshioka H, Ito S, Fujiwara K. Prospective randomised controlled trial comparing percutaneous acetic acid and percutaneous ethanol injection for small hepatocellular carcinoma. *Hepatology* 1998;**27(1)**:67–72.
9. Lin S-M, Lin C-J, Lin C-C, Hsu C-W, Chen Y-C. Randomised controlled trial comparing percutaneous radiofrequency thermal ablation, percutaneous ethanol injection and percutaneous acetic acid injection to treat hepatocellular carcinoma of 3 cm or less. *Gut* 2005;**54(8)**:1151–6.
10. Shiina A, Tateishi R, Imamura M, Teratani T, Koike Y, Sato S, et al. Percutaneous ethanol injection for hepatocellular carcinoma: 20-year outcome and prognostic factors. *Liver Int* 2012;**32(9)**:1434–42.
11. Shiina A, Sato K, Tateishi R, Shimizu M, Ohama H, Hatanaka T, et al. Percutaneous ablation for hepatocellular carcinoma: Comparison of various ablation techniques and surgery. *Can J Gastroenterol Hepatol* 2018;**2018**:4756147.
12. Giovannini M. Percutaneous alcohol ablation for liver metastasis. *Semin Oncol* 2002;**29(2)**:192–5.
13. Livraghi T, Vettori C, Lazzaroni S. Liver metastases: Results of percutaneous ethanol injection in 14 patients. *Radiology* 1991;**179(3)**:709–12.
14. Eochagáin AN. Cryoshock following cryoablation for hepatocellular carcinoma. *J Clin Anaesth* 2022;**77**:110641.
15. Littrup PJ, Aoun HD, Adam B, Krycia M, Prus M, Shields A. Percutaneous cryoablation of hepatic tumours: Long-term experience of a large US series. *Abdom Radiol (NY)* 2016;**41(4)**:767–80.
16. Huang Y-Z, Zhou S-C, Zhou H, Tong M. Radiofrequency ablation versus cryosurgery ablation for hepatocellular carcinoma: A meta-analysis. *Hepatogastroenterology* 2013;**60(125)**:1131–35.
17. Wang C, Wang H, Yang W, Hu K, Xie H, Hu K-Q, et al. Multicentre randomized controlled trial of percutaneous cryoablation versus radiofrequency ablation in hepatocellular carcinoma. *Hepatology* 2015;**61(5)**:1579–90.
18. Bala MM, Riemsma RP, Wolff R, Pedziwiatr M, Mitus JW, Storman Dawid, et al. Cryotherapy for liver metastases. *Cochrane Database Syst Rev* 2019;**7(7)**:CD009058.
19. Weis S, Franke A, Mössner J, Jakobsen JC, Schoppmeyer K. Radiofrequency (thermal) ablation versus no intervention or other interventions for hepatocellular carcinoma. *Cochrane Database Syst Rev* 2013:**(12)**:CD003046.
20. Lencioni RA, Allgaier H-P, Cioni D, Olschewski M, Deibert P, Crocetti L, et al. Small hepatocellular carcinoma in cirrhosis: Randomised comparison of radiofrequency thermal ablation versus percutaneous ethanol injection. *Radiology* 2003;**228(1)**:235–40.
21. Hur H, Ko YT, Min BS, Kim KS, Choi JS, Sohn SK, et al. Comparative study of resection and radiofrequency ablation in the treatment of solitary colorectal liver metastases. *Am J Surg* 2009;**197(6)**:728–36.
22. Sotirchos VS, Petrovic LM, Gönen M, Klimstra D, Do RKG, Petre EN, et al. Colorectal cancer liver metastases: Biopsy of the ablation zone and margins can be used to predict oncologic outcome. *Radiology* 2016;**280(3)**:949–59.
23. Ruers T, Punt C, Van Coevorden F, Pierie JPEN, Borel-Rinkes I, Ledermann JA, et al. Radiofrequency ablation combined with systemic treatment versus systemic treatment alone in patients with non–resectable colorectal liver metastases: A randomized EORTC Intergroup phase II study (EORTC 40004). *Ann Oncol* 2012;**23(10)**:2619–26.
24. Shibata T, Iimuro Y, Yamamoto Y, Maetani Y, Ametani F, Itoh K, et al. Small hepatocellular carcinoma: Comparison of radio-frequency ablation and percutaneous microwave coagulation therapy. *Radiology* 2002;**223(2)**:331–7.

25. Yu J, Yu X-L, Han Z-Y, Cheng Z-G, Liu F-Y, Zhai H-Y, et al. Percutaneous cooled-probe microwave versus radiofrequency ablation in early-stage hepatocellular carcinoma: A phase III randomised controlled trial. *Gut* 2017;**66**(**6**):1172–3.

26. Radosevic A, Quesada R, Serlavos C, Sánchez J, Zugazaga A, Sierra A, et al. Microwave versus radiofrequency ablation for the treatment of liver malignancies: A randomized controlled phase 2 trial. *Sci Rep* 2022;**12**(**1**):316.

27. Ng KK, Poon RT, Chan SC, Chok KSH, Cheung TT, Tung H, et al. High-intensity focused ultrasound for HCC: A single centre experience. *Ann Surg* 2011;**253**(**5**):981–7.

28. Yang T, Ng DM, Du N, He N, Dai X, Chen P, et al. HIFU for the treatment of difficult colorectal liver metastases with unsuitable indications for resection and radiofrequency ablation: A phase 1 clinical trial. *Surg Endosc* 2021;**35**(**5**):2306–15.

29. Thomson KR, Cheung W, Ellis SJ , Federman D, Kavnoudias H, Loader-Oliver D, et al. Investigation of the safety of irreversible electroporation in humans. *J Vasc Interv Radiol* 2011;**22**(**5**):611–21.

30. Kingham TP, Karkar AM, D'Angelica MI, Allen PJ, Dematteo RP, Getrajdman GI, et al. Ablation of perivascular hepatic malignant tumours with irreversible electroporation. *J Am Coll Surg* 2012;**215**(**3**):379–87.

31. Meijerink MR, Ruarus AH, Vroomen LGPH, Puijk RS, Geboers B, Nieuwenhuizen S, et al. Irreversible Electroporation to treat unresectable colorectal liver metastases (COLDFIRE-2): A Phase II, two centre, single arm clinical trial. *Radiology* 2021;**299**(**2**):470–80.

32. Chen Q-W, Ying H-F, Gao S, Shen Y-H, Meng Z-Q, Chen H, et al. Radiofrequency ablation plus chemoembolization versus radiofrequency ablation alone for hepatocellular carcinoma: A systematic review and meta-analysis. *Clin Res Hepatol Gastroenterol* 2016;**40**(**3**):309–14.

33. Liu M, Wang K, Wang Y, Bao Q, Wang H, Jin K, et al. Short- and longterm outcomes of hepatectomy combined with intraoperative radiofrequency ablation for patients with multiple primarily unresectable colorectal liver metastases: a propensity matching analysis. *HPB (Oxford)* 2021;**23**(**10**):1586–94.

34. Dai Y, Zhang Y, He W, Peng C, Qiu J, Zheng N, et al. Long-term outcome for colorectal liver metastases: combining hepatectomy with intraoperative ultrasound guided open microwave ablation versus hepatectomy alone. *Int J Hyperthermia* 2021;**38**(**1**):372–81.

Bailey & Love's Essential Operations Bailey & Love's Essential Operatio
Bailey & Love's Essential Operations Bailey & Love's Essential Operatio
Bailey & Love's Essential Operations Bailey & Love's Essential Operatio

SECTION 8 | LIVER

Chapter 50

Hepatocellular Cancer

Yazan S. Khaled and Ahmed Kotb

INTRODUCTION

Hepatocellular carcinoma (HCC) is a malignant transformation of the primary functional cells within the liver known as hepatocytes. It accounts for 90% of all primary liver cancers and worldwide its incidence continues to rise. HCC is a true major health burden since it is the 5th most common cause of cancer death in men and the 7th in women, accounting for a third of all cancer-related deaths. Five-year overall survival for patients with HCC is approximately 20% with only pancreatic cancer being worse. Geographical variations in the incidence of HCC are significant, with more than 80% of cases occurring in Asia and sub-Saharan Africa. The incidence in these regions is much higher compared with Europe, reflecting the prevalence of specific aetiological factors including chronic hepatitis B virus (HBV) and hepatitis C virus (HCV) infections, which are the primary risk factors for HCC in these high-risk areas (1,2).

RISK FACTORS FOR HCC

Liver cirrhosis is the main aetiological factor for HCC, as 90% of the cases develop in patients with a background of liver disease. Chronic liver inflammation associated with necrosis and fibrosis, followed by cellular regeneration (either solitary as one dominant mass or with daughter nodules), is the underlying pathophysiology. HBV is a major risk factor for HCC, accounting for over 50% of cases worldwide. Chronic HBV/HCV infections can cause chronic liver inflammation, leading to fibrosis, cirrhosis, and ultimately HCC. Other risk factors that can lead to chronic liver inflammation, cirrhosis and subsequent HCC include excessive alcohol consumption, haemochromatosis, Wilson's disease, aflatoxin, diabetes mellitus type 2 and hepatocellular adenoma. Non-alcoholic fatty liver disease (NAFLD) can also progress to cause fibrosis and liver cirrhosis with a significantly increased risk of developing HCC. The underlying mechanisms involve chronic inflammation, oxidative stress, insulin resistance, and dysregulated lipid metabolism (3–5).

DIAGNOSIS OF HCC

HCC may be diagnosed in several clinical scenarios. As an incidental finding on imaging, during the investigation of deranged liver function tests (LFTs) or as a consequence of management of liver-related symptoms. HCC can cause abdominal pain, weight loss, fatigue and malaise, and as the tumour enlarges mass effects occur which can lead to jaundice, portal vein thrombosis, portal hypertension, ascites and in 5–15% of patients there is spontaneous rupture and haemobilia.

Several serum biomarkers are useful in the diagnosis of HCC. Alpha-fetoprotein (AFP) is the most commonly used biomarker, although the sensitivity of approximately 62% and specificity of 86% limits its diagnostic usefulness particularly in early-stage HCC. Other biomarkers, such as des-gamma-carboxy prothrombin (DCP) and glypican-3 (GPC3) have been investigated and shown to have diagnostic value for HCC and can be used alone or in combination with AFP to improve the accuracy.

Imaging in the context of HCC is aimed at differentiating HCC from other pathologies and for screening high-risk patients. Ultrasound (US) scan is considered the first-line imaging tool for identifying focal liver nodules and plays a significant role in screening. However, dynamic phase-contrast imaging computed tomography (CT) and magnetic resonance imaging (MRI) are the standard imaging modality for the diagnosis of HCC. Since arterial neoangiogenesis is a pathognomonic feature of HCC, radiological investigations are characterized by hyperarterialization of the nodule in the arterial phase and washout during the portal or venous phases. Other diagnostic features on imaging include the presence of capsule enhancement, fat content, and hyperintensity on T2-weighted images on MRI. Positron emission tomography CT (PET-CT) has a very low sensitivity of about 60% for the detection of small or well-differentiated nodules but PET-CT is useful for the detection of metastases and poorly differentiated HCC.

Liver biopsy may be performed when imaging and biomarkers are inconclusive, or when a histological confirmation is required before commencing aggressive treatment. The current guidelines suggest that for nodules greater than 1 cm, and in the absence of liver cirrhosis or atypical vascular features on imaging, a pathological confirmation is recommended. A significant false-negative rate has been reported with fine needle biopsy and therefore a negative biopsy cannot exclude malignancy. In addition, concerns remain about the potential for seeding. Immune staining for GPC3, HSP70, and GS in the hands of experienced

DOI: 10.1201/9781003080060-50

pathologists are highly recommended to confirm the diagnosis particularly for small lesions.

STAGING OF HCC

Accurate staging of HCC is critical to predict outcome and hence determine treatment selection. Various staging systems have evolved including the Liver Cancer Study Group of Japan (LCSGJ) and the American Joint Committee on Cancer (AJCC), but the Barcelona Clinic Liver Cancer (BCLC) staging system remains the most widely used. Unlike other staging systems, the BCLC incorporates tumour stage, liver function, performance status, and cancer-related symptoms (2,6–10). The BCLC staging system classifies HCC into five stages (*Figure 50.1*):

1   *Very early stage (0)*: Solitary tumour <2 cm or up to three nodules, each <3 cm. No vascular invasion or extrahepatic spread. Good liver function (Child-Pugh A) and performance status
2   *Early stage (A)*: Solitary tumour <5 cm or up to three nodules, each <3 cm. No vascular invasion or

extrahepatic spread. Good liver function and performance status
3   *Intermediate stage (B)*: Large or multifocal tumours, or presence of vascular invasion. Good liver function and performance status
4   *Advanced stage (C)*: Presence of vascular invasion, extrahepatic spread, or both. Any tumour size. Performance status may be preserved or impaired
5   *Terminal stage (D)*: Presence of advanced stage symptoms, such as cancer-related symptoms and/or impaired liver function (Child-Pugh C). The tumour burden and vascular invasion may vary.

TREATMENT OPTIONS

Treatment options for HCC range from curative therapies, such as ablation, resection and transplantation, for early-stage HCC to palliative treatments, such as chemoembolization, systemic therapies including sorafenib or best supportive care, for advanced-stage disease. The management of HCC should be considered in a multidisciplinary team (MDT) setting involving expert

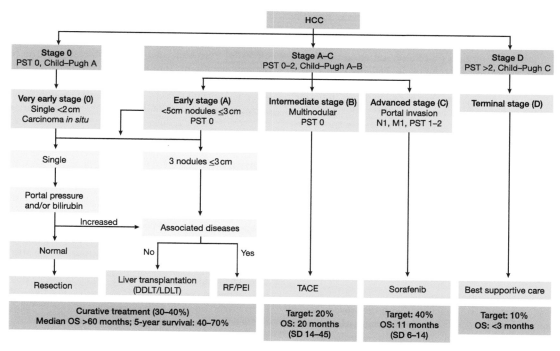

Figure 50.1 The Barcelona Clinic Liver Group staging system for the management of HCC. Patients with asymptomatic early tumours (stage 0-A) are candidates for curative therapies (resection, transplantation or local ablation). Asymptomatic patients with multinodular HCC (stage B) are suitable for chemoembolization (TACE), whereas patients with advanced symptomatic tumours and/or an invasive tumoral pattern (stage C) are candidates for sorafenib. End-stage (stage D) includes patients with grim prognosis who should be treated by best supportive care. *Abbreviations:* DDLT: deceased donor liver transplantation; LDLT: living donor liver transplantation; OS: overall survival; PEI: percutaneous ethanol injection; ECOG PST: Eastern Cooperative Oncology Group performance status; RF: radiofrequency ablation; SD: standard deviation; TACE: transarterial chemoembolization.

liver surgeons, radiologists, oncologists, hepatologists, pathologists and cancer nurses and should adhere to validated guidelines.

SURGICAL RESECTION

HCC in normal liver accounts for only a small percentage of patients and surgical resection is the treatment of choice. The estimated operative mortality and morbidity is <1% and 15%, respectively, with a 5-year survival rate of >50%. Lymphadenectomy is advocated as 15% of cases are associated with positive lymph node disease. Ablative therapy is often not feasible due to tumour size while transplantation is reserved for cases where resection is impeded by the anatomical location of the tumour, or as a salvage treatment for recurrent nodule not amenable to repeat resection.

Surgical resection of HCC in patients with liver cirrhosis is challenging with an estimated mortality rate of 6% and careful patient selection is essential taking into account a number of recognized criteria:

1 *Tumour characteristics*: a single tumour or up to three tumours, each less than 5 cm in size. The presence of major vascular invasion or extrahepatic metastasis are absolute contraindications for resection

2 *Liver function*: adequate liver function, typically evaluated using the Child-Pugh classification, is necessary to predict that patients will be able to tolerate the surgical procedure and ensure sufficient postoperative liver function. Patients with Child-Pugh class A are considered for resection. The presence of portal hypertension is an important consideration in the preoperative evaluation. Measurement of portal pressure gradients and assessment of oesophageal varices will help determine the risk of postoperative complications and guide perioperative management

3 *Resection margins (R0)*: the goal of surgical resection is to achieve an R0 resection with wide margins whilst preserving an adequate amount of healthy liver tissue to maintain sufficient liver function postoperatively. The risk of recurrence remains high due to persistent cirrhosis.

Surgical techniques

Evolving evidence has clearly indicated that anatomical resection is associated with improved overall survival (OS) and disease-free survival (DFS) when compared with a non-anatomical resection. Anatomical resection entails the removal of the tumour and adjacent segments with the same portal tributaries (*Figure 50.2*). This approach aims to achieve a wide resection margin of at least 2 cm which reduces risk of recurrence from satellite nodules. Several steps have been taken recently to optimize the management of the future liver remnant (FLR) including the measurement of the total liver volume and proposed liver remnant with CT scans, selective portal vein embolization and minimizing the mobilization of the liver during surgery. When considering a major hepatectomy, preoperative portal vein embolization is essential to evaluate the regenerative capacity of the FLR. Emerging evidence suggests that the functional evaluation of a proposed FLR is as important as volumetry assessment to determine the extent of resection that can be safely performed. Due to advances in surgical technologies, laparoscopic resection of HCCs has gained wide acceptance amongst surgeons. In addition to the advantages of reduced blood loss and postoperative pain, laparoscopic surgery may also reduce the risk of ascites and adhesions, should transplantation be required in the future.

Prognosis after resection

The prognosis after surgical resection depends on a number of factors including resection margins, tumour size, the presence of microvascular invasion, and underlying liver function. The 5- and 10-year survival rates are estimated at 43.9% and 28.7%, respectively, in patients who have their tumours resected and as high as 70% at 5 years, in patients with tumours ≤2 cm in diameter. Regular surveillance and close follow-up with 6-monthly CT scans are essential to detect recurrence at an early stage. Unfortunately, even following successful resection, the risk of disease recurrence remains significant. Intrahepatic recurrence occurs in approximately 80% of patients within 5 years of their surgery. Adjuvant therapy options, such as transarterial chemoembolization (TACE) or systemic therapies, may be considered to reduce the risk of recurrence and improve long-term outcomes.

Management of recurrence

The management of recurrent HCC is dependent on the location and extent of the disease and the patient's liver function and performance status. Early recurrent HCC, which is confined to the liver, can be treated with repeat curative resection highlighting the importance of regular surveillance. Other treatment options may include ablative techniques, TACE, targeted therapies, or supportive care. The incidence of recurrence is 40% in the 1st year, 60% in the 2nd year and ~80% at 5 years. The high risk of recurrence in cirrhotic patients is not unexpected since the aetiology is not removed. To date, there remains a paucity of evidence supporting the role of neoadjuvant or adjuvant therapy to reduce the risk of recurrence including chemotherapy. While liver transplantation remains the most effective approach for the prevention of recurrence in carefully selected patients, management of the underlying cause of chronic liver disease, such as the treatment of hepatitis, will improve survival and reduce the incidence of recurrence (8,9,11,12).

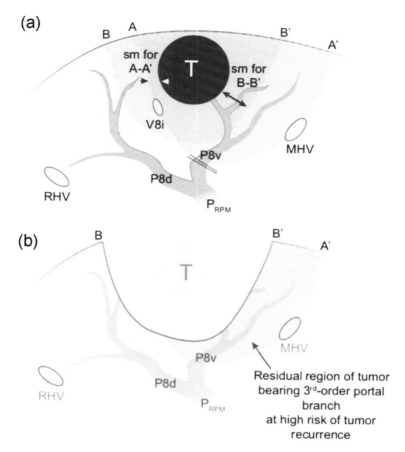

Figure 50.2 Principles of anatomic versus non-anatomic liver resection for HCC. Anatomic resection (a) (A-A') removes entirely the tumour-bearing portal branches bordered by the landmark veins, while non-anatomic resection (B-B') is any other type of resection in which the tumour-bearing third-order portal region is not fully removed. After non-anatomic resection of HCC (b) some part of the tumour-bearing portal region is left, which is at high-risk of tumour recurrence (12). *Abbreviations:* HCC: hepatocellular carcinoma; MHV: middle hepatic vein; P8v: ventral branch of P8; P8d: dorsal branch of P8; PRPM: right para-median pedicle; RHV: right hepatic vein; V8i: intermediate vein for segment VIII.

Transplantation

Liver transplantation is considered for patients with unresectable HCC, or those who meet specific transplant criteria, such as the Milan criteria or extended Milan University of California San Francisco (UCSF) Criteria (*Table 50.1*). Transplantation confers the advantage of removing all the detectable and non-detectable nodules and treating the underlying liver disease, thus being potentially curative and the 5-year survival following liver transplantation for HCC ranges from 60–75%. While the patient is on the waiting list, downstaging treatment such as resection, ablation, or TACE can be offered to prevent tumour progression and drop-out from the waiting list.

Table 50.1 Characteristics of liver transplant criteria for HCC

Milan criteria	UCSF criteria
Single tumour ≤5 cm, or	Single tumour ≤6.5 cm, or
2–3 tumours, none exceeding 3 cm, and	2–3 tumours, none exceeding 4.5 cm, with a total tumour diameter ≤8 cm, and
No vascular invasion and/ or extrahepatic spread	No vascular invasion and/or extrahepatic spread

Transarterial chemoembolization

Unlike the liver parenchyma, HCCs receive all their blood supply from the hepatic artery. Exploiting this unique feature, TACE combines the delivery of cytotoxic molecules directly into the feeding artery, consequently embolising those vessels, and tumour cells become ischaemic and necrose producing local control. TACE is recommended as first-line palliative treatment for BCLC stage B. Conventional TACE involves the injection of a chemotherapeutic agent, such as doxorubicin or cisplatin, mixed with a lipiodol-based contrast agent into the hepatic artery. This is followed by embolization of the tumour-feeding vessels with particles or gelatin sponge. Transarterial radioembolization (TARE), also known as selective internal radiation therapy (SIRT), involves the delivery of radioactive microspheres such as Yttrium-90 into the tumour's arterial blood supply. These microspheres deliver localized radiation to the tumour, causing cell death comparable with TACE (13).

Ablative therapies

Ablative therapies involve control and destruction of tumour cells using heat, cold, or chemical agents such ethanol or acetic acid (*see* **Chapter 49**). Radiofrequency ablation (RFA) is the most commonly used ablative technique for HCC. A needle electrode is inserted into the tumour, which converts electromagnetic energy to heat to achieve tumour cell death from coagulative necrosis. Microwave ablation (MWA) uses microwave energy to create heat leading to tumour destruction and has demonstrated comparable efficacy to RFA in terms of tumour control. Percutaneous ethanol injection (PEI) involves injecting ethanol directly into the tumour, causing tumour cell destruction by dehydration and protein denaturation. While ablative therapies were initially used to treat HCCs in non-surgical candidates, their application has been expanded recently and they are used as neoadjuvant therapy for primary tumours <2 cm and recurrent tumours (8).

FIBROLAMELLAR CARCINOMA

Fibrolamellar carcinoma (FLC) is a rare variant of HCC and accounts for 1% of all primary liver cancers. Microscopically, FLC is a well-differentiated polygonal hepatic tumour with cells that display eosinophilic cytoplasm surrounded by lamellated fibrous stroma. FLCs tends to occur in patients who are 20–35 years of age, with higher incidence in western countries. The underlying aetiology of FLC is not fully understood as these patients will not have a history of chronic liver disease or cirrhosis.

CT imaging often shows a large hypervascular, heterogeneous liver mass with central necrosis or fibrosis, while MRI shows low attenuation on T2 images due to a central scar. The margins are well defined, and calcification can be seen in up to 68% of cases. Metastasis to locoregional lymph nodes is common (60%) and serum biomarkers lack sensitivity and specificity for FLC. Surgical resection is the treatment of choice and in the presence of lymph nodes disease, simultaneous lymphadenectomy is strongly recommended. Despite surgery with curative intent, recurrent disease occurs in over 60% of patients. Repeat surgical resection can be offered to treat recurrent FLC in young patients and occasionally liver transplantation. However, the prognosis of FLC is superior to that of HCC with 5-year survival rates of 50–75% following resection. Considering the high risk of recurrence, intensive surveillance is necessary for early detection of this aggressive tumour. Accurate differentiation between FLC and FLC-HCC (HCC with nodules characteristic of FLC) is essential to plan personalized treatment (14).

SUMMARY

Liver cancer is a global challenge both clinically and to healthcare systems, with predictions of more than one million cases worldwide by 2025. The incidence of HCC in the USA is anticipated to increase by 122% between 2016 and 2030 as a consequence of increased rates of obesity and diabetes. Hepatocellular carcinoma is the most common form of liver cancer and accounts for at least 90% of cases. Infection with hepatitis B and C are the principle risk factors, and universal hepatitis B vaccination should decrease the worldwide incidence. NAFLD is now another important aetiological factor especially in western countries. The 5-year overall survival rates for patients with HCC is approximately 20%, with only pancreatic cancer being worse. The treatment of HCC requires the input from a number of specialities, in the context of an MDT, if optimal outcomes are to be achieved. There are a number of new trials investigating the use of combination therapies and it is hoped that they will improve the outcome for this devastating and costly disease.

REFERENCES

1. World Health Organization. (2018). Cancer Fact Sheets: Liver. Available from: https://www.who.int/news-room/fact-sheets/detail/cancer (Accessed 13 March 2023).
2. Villanueva A, Hernandez-Gea V, Llovet JM. Medical therapies for hepatocellular carcinoma: A critical view of the evidence. *Nat Rev Gastroenterol Hepatol* 2013;**10(1)**:34–42.
3. El-Serag HB, Kanwal F. Epidemiology of hepatocellular carcinoma in the United States: Where are we? Where do we go? *Hepatology* 2014;**60(5)**:1767–75.
4. Liu Z, Jiang Y. Hepatitis B virus infection: Epidemiology and vaccination. *Epidemiol Infect* 2018;**146(13)**: 1636–44.
5. Llovet JM, Zucman-Rossi J, Pikarsky E, Sangro B, Schwartz M, Sherman M, et al. Hepatocellular carcinoma. *Nat Rev Dis Primers* 2016;**2**:16018.

6. Fang Y-S, Wu Q, Zhao H-C, Zhou Y, Ye L, Liu S-S, et al. Do combined assays of serum AFP, AFP-L3, DCP, GP73, and DKK-1 efficiently improve the clinical values of biomarkers in decision-making for hepatocellular carcinoma? A meta-analysis *Expert Rev Gastroenterol Hepatol* 2021;**15(9)**:1065–76.

7. Forner A, Reig M, Bruix J. Hepatocellular carcinoma. *Lancet* 2018;**391(10127)**:1301–14.

8. European Association for the Study of the Liver. EASL Clinical Practice Guidelines: Management of hepatocellular carcinoma. *J Hepatol* 2018;**69(1)**: 182–236.

9. Bruix J, Sherman M. Management of hepatocellular carcinoma: An update. *Hepatology* 2011;**53(3)**:1020–2.

10. Reig M, Forner A, Rimola J, Ferrer-Fábrega J, Burrel M, Garcia-Criado A, et al. BCLC strategy for prognosis prediction and treatment recommendation: The 2022 update. *J Hepatol* 2022;**76(3)**:681–93.

11. Pang TC, Lam VW, Yeh MM. Surgical treatment of hepatocellular carcinoma. *HPB* 2015;**17(5)**:422–30.

12. Shindoh J, Makuuchi M, Matsuyama Y, Mise Y, Arita J, Sakamoto Y, et al. Complete removal of the tumor-bearing portal territory decreases local tumor recurrence and improves disease- specific survival of patients with hepatocellular carcinoma. *J Hepatol* 2016;**64(3)**:594–600.

13. Abdalla EK. Portal vein embolization (prior to major hepatectomy) effects on regeneration, resectability, and outcome. *J Surg Oncol* 2010;**102(8)**:960–7.

14. Simon SM. Fighting rare cancers: Lesson from fibrolamellar hepatocellular carcinoma. *Nat Rev Cancer* 2023;**23(5)**:335–46.

Bailey & Love's Essential Operations Bailey & Love's Essential Operatio
Bailey & Love's Essential Operations Bailey & Love's Essential Operatio
Bailey & Love's Essential Operations Bailey & Love's Essential Operatio

SECTION 8 | LIVER

Chapter
51

Liver Metastases

Ajith K. Siriwardena

INTRODUCTION

This chapter discusses the management of patients with liver metastases. The principal focus is on the care of those with liver metastases from colorectal cancer. Here, the importance of a thorough assessment of disease distribution and patient fitness is emphasized together with the involvement of a multidisciplinary team. The importance of multimodal therapy including systemic chemotherapy is also discussed. The selection of patients for surgery, approach to liver resection and current nomenclature are reviewed. The chapter also provides an overview of the management of patients with non-colorectal liver metastases.

INCIDENCE AND MORTALITY RATES

Liver metastases are common. The European commission estimated that colorectal cancer accounted for 12.7% of all new cancer diagnoses in 2020, and 12.4% of all deaths due to cancer, making this the second most frequently occurring cancer (1). Incidence rates were highest in Australia/New Zealand and European regions (40.6 per 100 000 males) and lowest in several African regions and Southern Asia (4.4 per 100 000 females). Similar patterns were observed for mortality rates, with the highest observed in Eastern Europe (20.2 per 100 000 males) and the lowest in Southern Asia (2.5 per 100 000 females) (2). About one-fifth of patients with colorectal cancer have metastases, either exclusively or predominantly, within the liver at the time of presentation and liver metastases may also become apparent later in the course of the disease (3).

In relation to non-colorectal liver metastases, true incidence figures are less clear and depend on the nature of the primary tumour.

CURRENT TERMINOLOGY

Accurate terminology is important for the description of disease, selection of optimal treatment and reporting of outcomes. There is significant variation in the terminology used for liver metastases from colorectal cancer. Although it is likely that variation will persist, a recent consensus report produced by a collaboration of the European-African Hepato-Pancreato-Biliary Association (E-AHPBA), the European Society of Surgical Oncology (ESSO), the European Society of Coloproctology (ESCP), the European Society of

Gastrointestinal and Abdominal Radiology (ESGAR), and the Cardiovascular and Interventional Radiological Society of Europe (CIRSE) promises to standardize the terminology used for synchronous and metachronous liver metastases (*Table 51.1*) (4). In addition, variation in the description of liver metastases from colorectal cancer which respond to chemotherapy is heterogeneous and the consensus report also addressed the reporting of the so called 'disappearing' liver metastases (*Table 51.2*).

MODES OF PRESENTATION

Liver metastases are typically asymptomatic until they reach an advanced stage when jaundice can occur, either as a result of hepatic parenchymal replacement by tumour resulting in liver insufficiency or by nodal obstruction of the common bile duct at the hilum of the liver.

More usually, liver metastases are detected on cross-sectional imaging undertaken as part of cancer surveillance or because of elevation of the cancer biomarker carcinoembryonic antigen (CEA) (5).

ASSESSMENT OF THE PATIENT WITH LIVER METASTASES

History and clinical examination

A detailed history is an important cornerstone of management. Information on current symptoms, previous symptoms, prior cancer history, co-morbidity, activity levels, medication and allergies are all important. Physical examination should focus on general signs of anaemia, jaundice or muscle wasting and abdominal signs including scars of previous surgery, distension and ascites.

Routine blood tests

These include blood count and assessment of liver function including clotting and renal function.

Biomarkers

CEA is routinely measured in colorectal cancer post-resection surveillance. Although it is not sufficiently sensitive to be used as a stand-alone diagnostic test, evidence of elevation, after previously normal values, can be used to trigger further investigations (5).

DOI: 10.1201/9781003080060-51

Table 51.1 Consensus terminology for synchronous and metachronous liver metastases (4)

i	Liver metastases detected at the time of diagnosis of the primary are termed 'synchronous'
ii	The definition of synchronous liver metastases also includes patients with incidental liver metastases detected intraoperatively
iii	To be termed 'metachronous' disease, liver metastases should have been excluded on cross-sectional imaging at the time of diagnosis of the primary tumour
iv	Liver metastases detected up to 12 months after diagnosis of the primary tumour – but absent at presentation – are termed 'Early metachronous' metastases
v	Liver metastases detected more than 12 months after diagnosis of the primary are termed 'Late metachronous' metastases

Table 51.2 Consensus definitions of 'disappearing' liver metastases (4)

i	The term 'disappearing' in reference to metastases is defined in this study as lesions present on baseline contrast MRI which are **no longer visible** on hepatobiliary contrast MRI after systemic chemotherapy
ii	The presence of a 'scar' on cross-sectional imaging is termed 'evidence of treatment response' but, if visible on hepatobiliary contrast MRI, the lesion is not regarded as 'disappearing'

Transabdominal ultrasonography

The presence of liver metastases can be detected on ultrasonography (6). Lesions typically show as hypodense areas. The addition of intravenous contrast agents can increase the accuracy of transabdominal ultrasonography (7). Although contrast-enhanced ultrasound (CEUS) is cheaper than computed tomography (CT) or magnetic resonance imaging (MRI), it is operator dependent. Undertaken prior to surgery, it is not useful in treatment planning. There may be a role for intraoperative CEUS in the detection of small lesions in patients treated by systemic chemotherapy (8). CEUS is insufficiently accurate for the planning of interventions such as liver resection and for this more detailed cross-sectional imaging is required.

Computed tomography

Intravenous contrast-enhanced triple phase (referring to non-contrast, arterial and portal phases) CT (CECT) is the mainstay of diagnosis and management of patients with liver metastases (9). CECT of the thorax, abdomen and pelvis is the standard of care to be undertaken as part of the initial work-up of patients with suspected liver metastases and is also the most commonly used mode of surveillance after resection (9). Assessment of treatment response can be undertaken using the response evaluation criteria in solid tumours (RECIST version 1.1) although more often disease stability, progression or response are simply reported using descriptive terminology (10).

Magnetic resonance imaging

MRI offers greater accuracy in the diagnosis of liver metastases and in many centres is the standard

procedure undertaken for treatment planning (9). T1 and T2 phases help to distinguish solid from cystic lesions, and liver metastases restrict the diffusion of contrast agents. Diffusion weighted imaging (DWI) is useful in assessing the location and size of lesions (9). The limitations of MRI include patients with metallic implants, and those who suffer from claustrophobia and who may not be able to tolerate the time required in the machine.

^{18}Fluro-deoxyglucose positron emission tomography

Preferential uptake of labelled glucose is seen in cancer cells and in areas of inflammation which can be used to detect tumours. An important randomized clinical trial (RCT) assessed the management of patients with colorectal liver metastases comparing the use of ^{18}fluro-deoxyglucose positron emission tomography (^{18}FDG-PET) to management without this test. The trial results showed that although there was no difference in overall survival, the ^{18}FDG-PET changed management by reducing unnecessary surgery and helped to better plan resection in other patients (11).

Biopsy of liver lesions

Liver biopsy is not recommended for the diagnosis of liver metastases from colorectal cancer. The two reasons for this are: 1) It is unnecessary, lesions can be diagnosed with sufficient certainty to plan management by cross-sectional imaging, especially MRI, and 2) percutaneous passage of a needle into a liver metastasis can result in seeding of the tumour in up to 10% of cases (12).

Amalgamating diagnostic tests into a clinical management algorithm

From a practical perspective it is important to assemble a management algorithm from the available list of tests. For the patient newly diagnosed with colorectal cancer and liver metastases, necessary tests should include (in addition to clinical assessment): 1) Biopsy confirmation of malignancy from the primary tumour; 2) CT scan of thorax, abdomen and pelvis; 3) baseline liver MRI prior to chemotherapy in those patients who are potential candidates for surgery and 4) baseline measurement of CEA to facilitate future surveillance.

MULTIDISCIPLINARY TEAM ASSESSMENT

A mainstay of modern surgical oncological care is the involvement of a multidisciplinary team assessment (MDT) in providing guidance on management. It is important that the MDT has expertise in the management of patients with liver metastases and should include hepatobiliary surgery, interventional radiology and oncology specialists. Management of these patients must involve a specialist liver surgeon to ensure appropriate management (13).

Selection of patients with colorectal liver metastases for surgical intervention

Liver resection to remove the hepatic burden of metastases has been shown to have a positive effect on survival (14). It has been argued, even relatively recently, that there is no RCT evidence to support liver resection (15). However, evidence from clinical cohorts and large registries, such as the LiverMetSurvey data, show a convincing survival benefit in favour of patients who can undergo liver resection (16,17).

Hepatic criteria for selection for surgery

The principle of liver resection for colorectal hepatic metastases is to ensure complete resection of the tumour with a cuff of non-cancer liver parenchyma of 1 cm, although there are data suggesting that a smaller resection margin may be acceptable (18). Modern resectional liver surgery for colorectal hepatic metastases uses a 'parenchyma-preserving' approach (19). The extent of safe liver resection is not precisely delineated, but older patients, those with underlying liver parenchymal disease, and patients who have been pre-treated by chemotherapy are less able to tolerate extensive liver resections. Conventional guides to the extent of safe liver resection typically advise that resection of up to 70% of parenchyma is feasible in a patient with normal parenchyma, whilst 50% is said to be the safe threshold for those with underlying parenchymal liver disease (20,21). However,

these guidelines are not practical in current practice for two reasons. Firstly, in the era of parenchyma-preserving surgery, blind, major resection is often not indicated and second, a far more important consideration is to ensure that after resection, the future remnant liver has adequate arterial and portal inflow, together with biliary drainage and hepatic venous outflow.

Assessment of risk of recurrence after hepatic resection

Synchronous disease

Systemic chemotherapy should be considered prior to liver or colorectal resection in patients with extra-hepatic metastases in addition to liver metastases, those with a locally advanced colonic tumour, patients with a rectal tumour which requires radiotherapy or chemoradiotherapy and those with an extensive liver metastatic burden (4).

Metachronous disease

There are a range of prognostic scores which predict the risk of recurrence after hepatectomy. Of these, probably the most widely utilized is the Fong score based on 1001 patients treated in New York (22). In this score, patients were allocated a point if they had: 1) Liver metastases within 12 months of diagnosis of the primary; 2) a liver metastasis >5 cm in size; 3) number of liver lesions >1; 4) positive lymph nodes in the primary tumour, and 5) an elevated CEA level >200 ng/mL. The total score was highly predictive of outcome and no patient with a score of 5 was a long-term survivor.

Nomenclature for hepatic resection

The current liver resection nomenclature was standardized at a conference held in Brisbane in 2000, and is based on an understanding of the segmental anatomy of the liver (23). The eight segments of the liver are arranged in sections. The left hemi-liver has a lateral (segment II and III) and a medial section (segment IV a and b), whereas the right hemi-liver has an anterior (segments V and VIII) and a posterior section (segments VI and VII) (*Figure 51.1*). Thus, an anatomical resection of the left lobe of the liver, previously termed left lobectomy, involves resection of segments II and III and as these two constitute the left lateral section of the liver, the procedure is known as left lateral sectionectomy (*Figure 51.2*). Formal right hepatectomy is termed a right bi-sectionectomy, as it involves resection of the right anterior and posterior sections (*Figure 51.2*). Resection of the right lobe of the liver involves removal of the right anterior and posterior sections, together with the left medial section (segment IV a and b), and is thus termed a right tri-sectionectomy. In practice, some of these terms, such as left lateral sectionectomy and right (and left) tri-sectionectomy have become accepted in standard terminology whilst others such as right

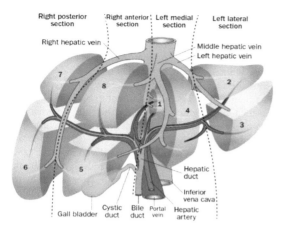

Figure 51.1 Segments of the human liver and current surgical nomenclature of liver sections. The human liver is divided by the falciform ligament into an anatomical right lobe and left lobe. However, the liver also has a functional right and left side divided by Cantlie's line (a hypothetical line from the gallbladder fossa to the middle hepatic vein). Each functional hemi-liver is composed of two sections. On the right, an anterior section (segments V and VIII) and a posterior section (segments VI and VII). On the left, a lateral section (segments II and III) and a medial section (segment IV). The black dashed lines show the demarcation between sectors. (Reproduced with permission from *Nature* publications.)

bi-sectionectomy are not adopted. Right hepatectomy remains the preferred term and central hepatectomy is more widely used than left medial sectionectomy.

In an effort to improve the accuracy of this terminology, the 'New World' classification system was proposed. This uses nomenclature such as V', VI to denote partial resection of V and complete resection of VI (24). Although this terminology undoubtedly represents an advance in precision of description, it is not universally accepted and the reader is referred to the original source reference for further information on this nomenclature (24).

Practical work-up for hepatectomy

After MDT discussion, it is vitally important to involve the patient (and depending on the individual, any relatives) in the outcome of the deliberations. Once a decision is taken to proceed with surgery, further planning can include both oncologic and physiologic assessment. Oncologic assessment may use more scans such as [18]FDG-PET. Physiologic assessment involves additional tests of cardiorespiratory reserve and can be valuable in selection of patients for surgery. Tests such as echocardiography and respiratory spirometry are static tests of cardiac and respiratory function and thus may be limited in value. Predictive scoring systems such as that of the American Society of Anaesthesiology are of value (25). Functional testing of cardiorespiratory

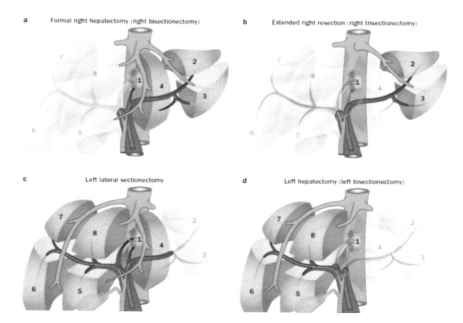

Figure 51.2 'New World' terminology for major liver resections illustrating sections and segments removed at each procedure. (a) In a formal right hepatectomy, the right anterior and posterior sections, comprising segments V to VIII are resected; the procedure could also be termed right bi-sectionectomy. (b) Liver sections removed in an extended right resection. In addition to the right anterior and posterior section, the left medial section is removed with a transection line to the right of the falciform ligament. This is termed a right tri-sectionectomy. (c) Left lateral sectionectomy. (d) Anatomical left hepatectomy. (Reproduced with permission from *Nature* publications.)

reserve can be undertaken by cardiopulmonary exercise testing (CPET) which detects the point of transition from aerobic to anaerobic metabolism, together with respiratory effort. CPET has been demonstrated to be of value in helping to select patients for liver resection (26).

PRINCIPLES AND PRACTICE OF HEPATECTOMY FOR LIVER METASTASES

Open or minimally invasive liver surgery

Current evidence indicates that oncologically appropriate liver resection can be undertaken by open or minimally invasive approaches, and selection is dependent on the expertise of the operating team (27,28). Worldwide, open liver resection remains the most widely practiced technique and the principles of this will be described here.

Perioperative preparation and anaesthesia

Avoidance of overnight fasting by the use of carbohydrate drinks prevents liver resection being undertaken in a glycogen-depleted liver and may help to reduce postoperative liver dysfunction. The evening before, and 2 hours before the operation, intake of a carbohydrate-rich drink is recommended (excluding patients with obstruction, diabetes, and neuropathy) (29). General anaesthesia with monitoring by arterial and central venous pressure (CVP) lines is standard preoperative preparation. A discussion of the choice of anaesthetic agents for liver surgery is out of the scope of this chapter but is discussed in **Chapter 15**.

Although epidural analgesia was widely used in liver surgery, there is RCT evidence that wound catheters can provide effective analgesia for patients undergoing open liver resection (30). A cornerstone of modern liver surgical practice is the maintenance of a low CVP. This can be achieved by avoidance of overfilling with intravenous fluids during induction/maintenance.

Choice of incision

Typically, an epigastric midline incision with a right transverse extension is used for liver surgery. This is combined with fixed costal margin retraction.

Liver mobilization

Adequate mobilization of the liver is the key to safe liver surgery. For right-sided resection, the falciform and right triangular ligaments are divided and depending on location and extent of resection, the liver may need to be mobilized from the inferior vena cava, dividing a variable number of short inferior hepatic veins. The

hepatoduodenal ligament is slung to permit intermittent inflow occlusion (Pringle manoeuvre). The hepatocaval ligament usually contains short hepatic veins and may need to be divided to complete mobilization of the right lobe. Before division, the ligament must be separated from the cava typically by passing a sling around the ligament. This allows the ligament to be divided with a vascular stapling device. Finally, the right hepatic vein can also be slung. The vein wall is thin and can easily be damaged and thus it can often be safer to divide the right hepatic vein intrahepatically. Even in those cases where it is slung outside the liver, the transection should be undertaken during division of the liver parenchyma and not before to avoid venous congestion of the liver being resected.

Mobilization of the left lobe of the liver requires division of the left triangular ligament, taking care not to injure the oesophagus and proximal lesser curve of the stomach which lie immediately below. If necessary, the left hepatic vein can be encircled outside the liver but note that in about two-thirds of cases, the left and middle hepatic veins have a joint ostium. Thus, care must be taken to avoid inadvertent damage to the middle hepatic vein. The pars flaccida can be divided and, if required, selective inflow control of the left hepatic artery and left portal vein can be achieved.

Intraoperative ultrasonography

Intraoperative ultrasonography (IUS) is a standard component of modern liver surgery (31). IUS is utilized to confirm the location of lesions, assess the nature of liver parenchyma, to visualize vascular structures in the proposed hepatic transection plane, and to demonstrate that there are no lesions in the proposed future remnant liver.

Hepatic transection

The liver parenchyma can be divided in several ways (32). The author uses the cavitron ultrasonic suction aspirator (CUSA®, Integra LifeSciences, New Jersey, USA) which uses high-frequency ultrasonic energy to break down liver parenchyma and aspiration to remove tissue and expose vessels. Small vessels can be divided between titanium Ligaclips™ (J&J Med Tech, New Jersey, USA), and larger vessels by use of the vascular stapler. It is important to keep the operative field as dry as possible during transection and thus intermittent inflow occlusion (10 minutes of occlusion followed by 5 minutes reperfusion up to a total of 60 minutes) can be used.

Other techniques of liver transection range from early methods, such as the use of a Kelly clamp to crush the parenchyma and expose vessels, to the use of electrocautery and thermal-based transection devices. It is important that a surgeon embarking on liver transection be familiar with a range of techniques of hepatectomy.

Post-transection

Once resection is complete, the anaesthetist will gradually raise the CVP to normal levels allowing any bleeding points to be identified and controlled. Bile leaks must be sought and also controlled. Although liver cut surface haemostats are widely used, there is no substantive evidence that these are of any benefit in preventing postoperative complications (33).

After right hepatectomy, provided that the left lobe has not been mobilized, it is not necessary to re-attach the falciform ligament (although some surgeons do) as the liver will not rotate excessively in the postoperative period. The decision to use a surgical drain is at the discretion of the surgeon with RCTs indicating that there is no difference in outcome with, or without, drainage (34).

Enhanced Recovery After Hepatectomy (ERAS®)

Active postoperative recovery programmes, such as ERAS® have become standard of care after liver surgery (29). Enhanced recovery involves appropriate pre and intraoperative steps but also includes active measures undertaken after surgery. Essentially, these involve early mobilization and institution of diet, incentive spirometry to ameliorate the risks of postoperative atelectasis and early discharge from hospital. Evidence of the increased risk of postoperative deep venous thromboembolic (DVT) phenomena in the first 4–6 weeks after liver resection has resulted in DVT thromboprophylaxis, with a combination of mechanical and pharmacological options being used in this period (35).

SYSTEMIC CHEMOTHERAPY FOR COLORECTAL LIVER METASTASES

Systemic chemotherapy is the mainstay of treatment for the majority of patients with stage IV colorectal cancer (36). The current guidelines of the European Society of Medical Oncology recommend that surgical resection can be considered as the first treatment in patients with a 'favourable' cancer biology and a disease burden that is completely removable by surgery. For the majority of patients, systemic chemotherapy using either a combination of the oral 5-fluorouracil analogue capecitabine combined with oxaliplatin (CAPOX) or 5-FU, leucovorin, oxaliplatin (FOLFOX) should be considered (36). Chemotherapy can also be used to downsize initially unresectable disease to make resection feasible (16). Specific biologic pathway inhibitor therapy has also become established as part of the oncological care of patients with liver metastases. In those who do not carry mutations of the *KRAS* gene, an important component of the epidermal growth factor pathway (EGFR), therapy with anti-EGFR agents such as cetuximab can be incorporated into chemotherapy regimens (37) and inhibitors of the vascular endothelial growth

factor (VEGF) can also be used (36). Recent evidence indicates that patients with mismatch repair-deficient (MMR-deficient) tumours have high microsatellite instability which makes these cancers immunogenic, and specific targeting with immune checkpoint inhibitors such as pembrolizumab has a beneficial effect on survival (38).

Non-colorectal liver metastases

In addition to liver surgery for colorectal hepatic metastases, hepatectomy can be considered in selected patients with non-colorectal liver metastases. These can logically be categorized as those from non-colorectal gastrointestinal sources and non-colorectal, non-gastrointestinal sources.

Non-colorectal, gastrointestinal liver metastases

Foregut tumours

Tumours of the oesophagus, stomach, duodenum, and pancreas can metastasize to the liver. In the majority of patients, liver metastases from these tumours are indicative of advanced, multi-site systemic disease and thus resection of liver metastases is not recommended. There are small case cohort series of patients with solitary liver metastases from gastric cancer, gastro-oesophageal cancer, or pancreatic where benefit from resection is claimed (39–41), but these case series do not reflect the majority view that resection of liver metastases from these foregut tumours is not beneficial.

Midgut tumours

Hepatic resection for carcinoid liver metastases is an accepted indication (42). Although a detailed discussion is outside the scope of this chapter, two important biologic characteristics are of relevance. First, the majority of tumours are slow growing and second, debulking surgery can be considered in patients, especially those with functioning carcinoid tumours which secrete vasoactive compounds and produce carcinoid syndrome (and other syndromes). Effective palliation can be achieved even if complete hepatic metastatic burden clearance cannot.

Non-colorectal, non-gastrointestinal metastases

Liver resection for these tumours which, by definition, have systemic involvement by the time of hepatic involvement must be considered very carefully. As with liver metastases from foregut tumours, the majority of patients have extensive multi-site disease in addition to liver lesions.

Liver resection for breast cancer metastases

This can be considered. It is important to ensure that the primary tumour is adequately treated and that extrahepatic metastases have been excluded. Hormone receptor status likely impacts survival with poorer survival outcomes among those with triple-negative cancer undergoing surgery (43).

LIVER TRANSPLANTATION FOR LIVER METASTASES

A detailed discussion is beyond the scope of this chapter, but there is emerging evidence, together with consensus guidance, that in highly selected patients with liver-dominant, surgically unresectable colorectal hepatic metastases pre-treated with systemic chemotherapy there may be a role for liver transplantation (44).

LOCOREGIONAL TREATMENT FOR COLORECTAL HEPATIC METASTASES

These can be broadly considered in three categories. First, direct ablation of liver metastases either intra-operatively or by image-guided percutaneous access. Second, intra-arterially delivered therapies such as intra-arterial chemotherapy and third, externally delivered therapy such as SABR (stereotactic ablative body radiotherapy).

Ablation of liver metastases

Radiofrequency ablation in combination with systemic chemotherapy was evaluated in the European Organisation for Research and Treatment of Cancer (EORTC) 40004 RCT. It demonstrated a median overall survival of 60 months (45), and more recently, microwave ablation has become widely used [46]. In highly selected patients, a pooled analysis reported 5-year recurrence-free rates of 33% and microwave ablation has the advantage that it can also be combined with hepatic resection. A newer, non-thermal, ablative technique is irreversible electroporation, which involves the passage of a current between probes located in the liver metastasis inducing a strong electrical field to create permanent, and hence lethal, nanopores in the cell membrane to disrupt cellular homeostasis. This new technique has been demonstrated to be effective in causing cell death although further evaluation is required (47).

Intra-arterial therapy

Selective internal radiotherapy (SIRT) using intra-arterially delivered yttrium-90 resin microspheres was evaluated in a combined series of large multi-centre RCTs (48). The pooled analysis in over 1000 patients concluded that addition of SIRT to first-line FOLFOX chemotherapy for patients with liver-only and liver-dominant metastatic colorectal cancer did not improve overall survival compared with that for FOLFOX alone (48). Intra-arterial chemotherapy delivered by infusion

pump has been reported to show beneficial results in patients with surgically unresectable liver metastases and as adjuvant therapy after liver resection (49,50). Hepatic arterial infusion chemotherapy remains a treatment which has not been widely adopted, although recent work on starting an infusion pump programme has quantified the requirements for developing this technique (51).

External radiotherapy

Stereotactic ablative radiotherapy (SABR) is a highly focused form of radiotherapy which targets a tumour with external radiation beams from different angles at the same time. The treatment is delivered in a fewer number of treatments (hypofractionation) than conventional radiotherapy using one, three, five or eight fractions (52).

SUMMARY

This chapter provides an overview of the diagnosis and management of patients with liver metastases. The principal focus is on the care of those with liver metastases from colorectal cancer. Here, the importance of a thorough assessment of disease distribution and patient fitness is emphasized. Modern medical care is multidisciplinary and it is vital that patients with liver metastases from colorectal cancer have their care reviewed at an MDT with expertise in the management of this condition. The importance of multimodal therapy including systemic chemotherapy is emphasized. The aim of surgery is to remove the liver metastatic burden and the safe steps for hepatectomy are described.

REFERENCES

1. European Commission. 2021. *Colorectal cancer burden in EU-27. A factsheet from ECIS – European Cancer Information System.* Available from: https://ecis.jrc.ec.europa.eu/factsheets.php (Accessed August 2024).
2. Morgan E, Arnold M, Gini A, Lorenzoni V, Cabasag CJ, Laversanne M, et al. Global burden of colorectal cancer in 2020 and 2040: Incidence and mortality estimates from GLOBOCAN. *Gut* 2023;72(2):338–44.
3. Siriwardena AK, Mason JM, Mullamitha S, Hancock HC, Jegatheeswaran S. Management of colorectal cancer presenting with synchronous liver metastases. *Nat Rev Clin Oncol* 2014;**11(8)**:446–59.
4. Siriwardena AK, Serrablo A, Fretland AÅ, Wigmore SJ, Ramia-Angel JM, Malik HZ, et al. Multi-societal European consensus on the terminology, diagnosis, and management of patients with synchronous colorectal cancer and liver metastases: An E-AHPBA consensus in partnership with ESSO, ESCP, ESGAR, and CIRSE. *Br J Surg* 2023;**110(9)**:1161–70.
5. Nicholson BD, Shinkins B, Pathiraja I, Roberts NW, James TJ, Mallett S, et al. Blood CEA levels for detecting recurrent colorectal cancer. *Cochrane Database Syst Rev* 2015;**2015(12)**:CD011134.

6. Floriani I, Torri V, Rulli E, Garavaglia D, Compagnoni A, Salvolini L, et al. Performance of imaging modalities in diagnosis of liver metastases from colorectal cancer: A systematic review and meta-analysis. *J Magn Reson Imaging* 2010;**31(1)**:19–31.

7. Westwood M, Joore M, Grutters J, Redekop K, Armstrong N, Lee K, et al. Contrast-enhanced ultrasound using SonoVue® (sulphur hexafluoride microbubbles) compared with contrast- enhanced computed tomography and contrast-enhanced magnetic resonance imaging for the characterisation of focal liver lesions and detection of liver metastases: A systematic review and cost-effectiveness analysis. *Health Technol Assess* 2013;**17(6)**:1–243.

8. Leen E, Ceccotti P, Moug SJ, Glen P, MacQuarrie J, Angerson WJ, et al. Potential value of contrast-enhanced intraoperative ultrasonography during partial hepatectomy for metastases: An essential investigation before resection? *Ann Surg* 2006;**243(2)**:236–40.

9. Benson AB, Vernook AP, Al-Hawary MM, Arain MA, Chen Y-J, Ciombor KK, et al. Colon Cancer, Version 2.2021, NCCN Clinical Practice Guidelines in Oncology. *J Natl Compr Canc Netw* 2021;**19(3)**:329–59.

10. Eisenhauer EA, Therasse P, Bogaerts J, Schwartz LH, Sargent D, Ford R, et al. New response evaluation criteria in solid tumours: Revised RECIST guideline (version 1.1). *Eur J Cancer* 2009;**45(2)**:228–47.

11. Moulton C-A, Gu C-S, Law CH, Tandan VR, Hart R, Quan D, et al. Effect of PET before liver resection on surgical management for colorectal adenocarcinoma metastases: A randomized clinical trial. *JAMA* 2014;**311(18)**:1863–69.

12. Chen I, Lorentzen T, Linnemann D, Nolsøe CP, Skjoldbye B, Jensen BV, et al. Seeding after ultrasound-guided percutaneous biopsy of liver metastases in patients with colorectal or breast cancer. *Acta Oncol* 2016;**55(5)**:638–43.

13. Jones RP, Vauthey J-N, Adam R, Rees M, Berry D, Jackson R, et al. Effect of specialist decision-making on treatment strategies for colorectal liver metastases. *Br J Surg* 2012;**99(9)**:1263–69.

14. Stangl R, Altendorf-Hofmann A, Charnley RM, Scheele J. Factors influencing the natural history of colorectal liver metastases. *Lancet* 1994;**343(8910)**:1405–10.

15. Treasure T. Metastasectomy for colorectal cancer: Are there clothes on the emperor? *J R Soc Med* 2017;**110(6)**:227–30.

16. Innominato PF, Cailliez V, Allard M-A, Lopez-Ben S, Ferrero A, Marques H, et al. Impact of preoperative chemotherapy features on patient outcomes after hepatectomy for initially unresectable colorectal cancer liver metastases: A livermetsurvey analysis. *Cancers (Basel)* 2022;**14(17)**:4340.

17. Giuliante F, Viganò L, De Rose AM, Mirza DF, Lapoihte R, Kaiser G, et al. Liver-first approach for synchronous colorectal metastases: Analysis of 7360 patients from the livermetsurvey registry. *Ann Surg Oncol* 2021;**28(13)**:8198–208.

18. Hamady ZZR, Lodge JPA, Welsh FK, Toogood GJ, White A, John T, et al. One-millimeter cancer-free margin is curative for colorectal liver metastases: A propensity score case-match approach. *Ann Surg* 2014;**259(3)**:543–48.

19. Torzilli G, McCormack L, Pawlik T. Parenchyma-sparing liver resections. *Int J Surg* 2020;**82(Suppl)**:192–7.

20. Stewart GD, O'Súilleabháin CB, Madhavan KK, Wigmore SJ, Parks RW, Garden OJ. The extent of resection influences outcome following hepatectomy for colorectal liver metastases. *Eur J Surg Oncol* 2004;**30(4)**:370–6.

21. Ethun CG, Maithel SK. Hepatic resection for benign disease and for liver and biliary tumors. In: Jarnagin W (ed). Blumgart's Surgery of the Liver, Biliary Tract and Pancreas, 6th edition, Elsevier, 2017, Chapter 103B, pp.1522–71.

22. Fong Y, Fortner J, Sun RL, Brennan MF, Blumgart LH. Clinical score for predicting recurrence after hepatic resection for metastatic colorectal cancer: Analysis of 1001 consecutive cases. *Ann Surg* 1999;**230(3)**:309–18; discussion 318–21.

23. Strasberg SM, Belghiti J, Clavien P-A, Gadžijev E, Garden J-O, Lau W-Y, et al. The Brisbane 2000 Terminology of Liver Anatomy and Resections. *HPB (Oxford)* 2000;**2**:333–9.

24. Nagino M, DeMatteo R, Lang H, Cherqui D, Malago M, Kawakatsu S, et al. Proposal of a new comprehensive notation for hepatectomy: The "New World" Terminology. *Ann Surg* 2021;**274(1)**:1–3.

25. Dripps RD. New classification of physical status. *Anesthesiol* 1963;**24**:111.

26. Junejo MA, Mason JM, Sheen AJ, Moore J, Foster P, Atkinson D, et al. Cardiopulmonary exercise testing for preoperative risk assessment before hepatic resection. *Br J Surg* 2012;**99(8)**:1097–104.

27. Beppu T, Wakabayashi G, Hasegawa K, Gotohda N, Mizuguchi T, Takahashi Y, et al. Long-term and perioperative outcomes of laparoscopic versus open liver resection for colorectal liver metastases with propensity score matching: A multi-institutional Japanese study. *J Hepatobiliary Pancreat Sci* 2015;**22(10)**:711–20.

28. Morise Z. Current status of minimally invasive liver surgery for cancers. *World J Gastroenterol* 2022;**28(43)**:6090–8.

29. Melloul E, Hübner M, Scott M, Snowden C, Prentis J, Dejong CHC, et al. Guidelines for Perioperative Care for Liver Surgery: Enhanced Recovery After Surgery (ERAS) Society Recommendations. *World J Surg* 2016;**40(10)**:2425–40.

30. Revie EJ, McKeown DW, Wilson JA, Garden OJ, Wigmore SJ. Randomized clinical trial of local infiltration plus patient-controlled opiate analgesia vs. epidural analgesia following liver resection surgery. *HPB (Oxford)* 2012;**14(9)**:611–18.

31. Gluskin JS. Ultrasound of the liver, biliary tract, and pancreas. In: Jarnagin W (ed). *Blumgart's Surgery of the Liver, Biliary Tract and Pancreas*, 6th edition, Elsevier, 2017, Chapter 15, pp. 245–75.

32. Yoh T, Cauchy F, Soubrane O. Techniques for laparoscopic liver parenchymal transection. *Hepatobiliary Surg Nutr* 2019;8(6):572–81.

33. Kobayashi S, Takeda Y, Nakahira S, Tsuije M, Shimizu J, Miyamoto A, et al. Fibrin sealant with polyglycolic acid felt vs fibrinogen-based collagen fleece at the liver cut surface for prevention of postoperative bile leakage and hemorrhage: A prospective, randomized, controlled study. *J Am Coll Surg* 2016;**222(1)**:59–64.

34. Dezfouli SA, Ünal UK, Ghamarnejad O, Khajeh E, Ali-Hasan-Al-Saegh S, Ramouz A, et al. Systematic review and meta-analysis of the efficacy of prophylactic abdominal drainage in major liver resections. *Sci Rep* 2021;**11(1)**:3095.

35. Lancellotti F, Coletta D, de'Liguori Carino N, Satyadas T, Jegatheeswaran S, Maruccio M, et al. Venous thromboembolism (VTE) after open hepatectomy compared to minimally invasive liver resection: A systematic review and meta-analysis. *HPB (Oxford)* 2023;**25(8)**:872–80.

36. Van Cutsem E, Cervantes A, Adam R, Sobrero A, Van Krieken JH, Aderka D, et al. ESMO consensus guidelines for the management of patients with metastatic colorectal cancer. *Ann Oncol* 2016;**27(8)**:1386–422.

37. Bridgewater JA, Pugh SA, Maishman T, Eminton Z, Mellor J, Whitehead A, et al. Systemic chemotherapy with or without cetuximab in patients with resectable colorectal liver metastasis (New EPOC): Long-term results of a multicentre, randomised, controlled, phase 3 trial. *Lancet Oncol* 2020;**21(3)**:398–411.

38. Saberzadeh-Ardestani B, Jones JC, Hubbard JM, McWilliams RR, Halfdanarson TR, Shi Q, et al. Association between survival and metastatic site in mismatch repair-deficient metastatic colorectal cancer treated with first–line pembrolizumab. *JAMA Netw Open* 2023;**6(2)**:e230400.

39. Sato S, Tanabe K, Ota H, Saeki Y, Ohdan H. Successful management of multiple liver metastasis from gastric cancer with second conversion surgery: A case report. *Int J Surg Case Rep* 2023;**107**:108340.

40. Weiss ARR, Donlon NE, Schlitt HJ, Hackl C. Resection of oesophageal and oesophagogastric junction cancer liver metastases – A summary of current evidence. *Langenbecks Arch Surg* 2022;**407(3)**:947–55.

41. Pausch TM, Liu X, Cui J, Wei J, Miao Y, Heger U, et al. Survival benefit of resection surgery for pancreatic ductal adenocarcinoma with liver metastases: A propensity score-matched SEER database analysis. *Cancers (Basel)* 2021;**14(1)**:57.

42. Cloyd JM, Ejaz A, Konda B, Makary MS, Pawlik TM. Neuroendocrine liver metastases: A contemporary review of treatment strategies. *Hepatobiliary Surg Nutr* 2020;**9(4)**:440–51.

43. Calpin GG, Davey MG, Calpin P, Browne F, Lowery AJ, Kerin MJ. The impact of liver resection on survival for patients with metastatic breast cancer – A systematic review and meta- analysis. *Surgeon* 2022;**21(4)**:242–9.

44. Bonney GK, Chew CA, Lodge P, Hubbard J, Halazun KJ, Trunecka P, et al. Liver transplantation for non-resectable colorectal liver metastases: The International Hepato-Pancreato-Biliary Association consensus guidelines. *Lancet Gastroenterol Hepatol* 2021;**6(11)**:933–46.

45. Ruers T, Punt C, Van Coevorden F, Pierie JPEN, Borel-Rinkes I, Ledermann JA, et al. Radiofrequency ablation combined with systemic treatment versus systemic treatment alone in patients with non-resectable colorectal liver metastases: A randomized EORTC Intergroup phase II study (EORTC 40004). *Ann Oncol* 2012;**23(10)**:2619–26.

46. Mimmo A, Pegoraro F, Rhaiem R, Montalti R, Donadieu A, Tashkandi A, et al. Microwave ablation for colorectal liver metastases: A systematic review and pooled oncological analyses. *Cancers (Basel)* 2022;**14(5)**:1305.

47. Spiers HVM, Lancellotti F, de Liguori Carino N, Pandanaboyana S, Frampton AE, Jegatheeswaran S, et al. Irreversible electroporation for liver metastases from colorectal cancer: A systematic review. *Cancers (Basel)* 2023;**15(9)**:2428.

48. Wasan HS, Gibbs P, Sharma NK, Taieb J, Heinemann V, Ricke J, et al. First-line selective internal radiotherapy plus chemotherapy versus chemotherapy alone in patients with liver metastases from colorectal cancer (FOXFIRE, SIRFLOX and FOXFIRE-Global): A combined analysis of three multicentre, randomised, phase 3 trials. *Lancet Oncol* 2017;**18(9)**:1159–71.

49. Connell LC, Kemeny NE. Intraarterial chemotherapy for liver metastases. *Surg Oncol Clin N Am* 2021;**30(1)**:143–58.

50. Kemeny NE, Chou JF, Capanu M, Chatila WK, Shi H, Sanchez-Vega F, et al. A randomized phase II trial of adjuvant hepatic arterial infusion and systemic therapy with or without panitumumab after hepatic resection of KRAS wild-type colorectal cancer. *Ann Surg* 2021;**274(2)**:248–54.

51. McDonald HG, Patel RA, Ellis CS, Gholami S, Barry-Hundeyin M, Pandalai PK, et al. Starting a successful hepatic artery infusion pump program: A practical guide. *Surgery* 2023;**174(1)**:101–5.

52. Chalkidou A, Macmillan T, Grzeda MT, Peacock J, Summers J, Eddy S, et al. Stereotactic ablative body radiotherapy in patients with oligometastatic cancers: A prospective, registry-based, single-arm, observational, evaluation study. *Lancet Oncol* 2021;**22(1)**:98–106.

Chapter 52

Benign Liver Tumours

Samrat Ray, Eyad Issa and Trevor W. Reichman

INTRODUCTION

Benign liver tumours (BLTs) comprise a group of lesions frequently diagnosed incidentally during routine abdominal imaging. They comprise a heterogeneous group of lesions with varied and distinct cellular origins, characterized by an indolent, non-metastasizing and non-invasive behaviour. Most commonly, they are defined by a benign proliferation of hepatocytes presenting as mass-forming lesions, namely the hepatocellular adenoma (HCA) and focal nodular hyperplasia (FNH). In addition, hepatic haemangiomas, arising from the proliferation of the endothelial cells constitute another group of common benign liver tumours.

BLTs have a prevalence of about 15% in the general population, with up to 30% of affected patients being >40 years of age (1,2) with the majority being encountered in the adult population (30–40 years of age) (3). They are very rare in the paediatric population, comprising 4–5% of all intra-abdominal tumours and <2% of all pediatric malignancies (4). Clinical symptoms range from an inconspicuous incidental mass lesion to life-threatening situations due to rupture and haemorrhage. Differentiation of these lesions on standard imaging such as ultrasonography (US), computed tomography (CT) and magnetic resonance imaging (MRI) is essential for diagnosis but can be challenging. In the subsequent sections of this chapter, we will elaborate upon the classification, pathogenesis and risk factors and describe a detailed approach based on available guidelines for the diagnosis and management of the three most commonly encountered BLTs, namely HCA, FNH and cavernous haemangioma. In the latter part of the chapter will give a brief overview of the miscellaneous or less commonly encountered benign liver tumours.

CLASSIFICATION OF BLTs

The nomenclature and classification of benign liver tumours were defined in 1994 by the international consensus meeting at the World Congress of Gastroenterology (Los Angeles, CA) (5). *Table 52.1* outlines the classification of these tumours based on the histological cells of origin.

Detailed discussion of the bile duct adenomas and cystic lesions is beyond the scope of this chapter (*see* **Chapters 60, 64** and **66**). From a practical standpoint, the most common benign hepatic tumours are hepatocytic adenoma, focal nodular hyperplasia and cavernous haemangioma. The salient demographic and radiologic features facilitating differentiation between these three entities are summarized in *Table 52.2*.

Table 52.1 Histological classification of benign liver tumours

Epithelial

Origin: Hepatocytes	• Hepatocellular adenoma (HCA) • Focal nodular hyperplasia (FNH) • Nodular regenerative hyperplasia (NRH) • Focal fatty change
Origin: Biliary cells	• Bile duct adenoma • Biliary hamartomas (Von Meyenburg complexes)

Non-epithelial

Origin: Various	• Haemangiomas (cavernous haemangiomas) • Angiomyolipomas • Lipoma • Heterotopia: Adrenal, spleen and pancreatic tissue • Peliosis hepatis • Inflammatory pseudotumours

DOI: 10.1201/9781003080060-52

Table 52.2 Overview of salient demographic and radiological distinguishing features comparing HCA, FNH and hepatic haemangiomas

	HCA	FNH	Hepatic haemangioma
Demographics			
	• Extremely rare (0.1 per year per 100 000) in general population • Higher incidence in OC users (3–4 per year per 100 000) • M:F ratio 1:9 • 20–30 years age group • Associated with higher rate of complications (bleeding, malignant transformation)	• Second most frequent BLT (Clinical prevalence of 0.03%) • Mostly affecting females 35–50 years age group • Not influenced by OC usage • Mostly solitary, <5cm in size; could be multiple in 20–30% cases • No malignant potential	• Most common BLT (Prevalence of 1–20% in general population) • More common in females (M:F ratio 1:5) • Mostly incidentally detected • Age group of 30–50 years (mean age of 50-years) • Rarely can reach up to 20cm in size (Giant haemangiomas) and could be a part of Kasabach-Merritt syndrome (KMS) • No malignant potential
Imaging (salient features)			
US and contrast-enhanced US (CEUS)	• *Arterial phase:* homogeneous contrast- enhancement (CEUS), rapid complete centripetal filling • *Early portal venous phase:* isoechoic	• *US:* hypo/isoechoic, very rarely could be hyperechoic • *Arterial phase:* strong and homogeneous enhancement • *Colour Doppler US:* central arteries have a 'spoke wheel' pattern	• *US:* homogenous, hyperechoic, sharp rim • *Atypical:* peripheral and globular enhancement followed by central enhancement in delayed phases (CEUS). Absence of halo sign
CT scan	• *Classic type:* clear margins with peripheral enhancement, homogenous >heterogenous • *Steatotic type:* hypodense • *Haemorrhagic type:* hyperdense	• Central vascular supply • *Arterial phase:* homogenous, hyperdense • *Portal phase:* isodense with adjacent liver • Central hypodense scar visible in ⅓ of patients	• Inhomogeneous peripheral nodular enhancement iso-attenuating to the aorta, progressive centripetal contrast filling
MRI scan	Based on molecular subtypes: 1. *HNF1a-inactivated HCA:* diffuse and homogeneous signal dropout on chemical shift T1-weighted sequences 2. *Inflammatory HCAs*; telangiectatic features: strong hyperintense signal on T2-weighted images Persistent enhancement on delayed phase (extracellular contrast agent) 3. *β-catenin mutations in exon:* No specific features 4. *β-catenin mutations in exons 7/8:* No specific features 5. *Unclassified:* No specific features	*T1:* hypointense *T2:* • *Arterial phase:* strongly hyperintense, homogenous • *Portal venous phase:* isointense to the liver. The central scar is hyperintense on T2 and enhances on delayed-phase imaging • *T2 contrast (Primovist):* retention of Primovist in delayed (20min) phase. The central scar does not enhance on the hepatobiliary phase on T2 Primovist scan	*T1:* hypointense *T2:* hyperintense
HIDA scan	Normal flow No uptake	Increased flow; immediate uptake and delayed clearance	Decreased uptake
Tc-99m sulphur colloid scan	Decreased uptake	Normal or increased uptake (may be decreased in up to ⅓ cases)	Decreased uptake

Abbreviations: BLT: benign liver tumours; CEUS: contrast-enhanced ultrasound; CT: computed tomography; HIDA: hepatobiliary iminodiacetic acid; HNF: hepatocyte nuclear factor; MRI: magnetic resonance imaging; OC: oral contraceptives; Tc-99m: Technetium 99m; US: ultrasonography

HEPATOCELLULAR ADENOMA

Hepatocellular adenoma (HCA) is a benign tumour occurring predominantly in women between 30–50 years of age, often with a history of long-term oral contraceptive (OC) use or other steroid medications. In 1973, Baum et al. described the association between OCs and HCA occurrence (6). Between 1918 and 1954, only two HCA cases were found in 48 900 autopsies performed in the Los Angeles General Hospital, making this clinical entity very rare before 1960 when the OC pill was introduced (7). The positive correlation between OCs and HCA incidence is dose dependent, with spontaneous regression of these lesions being observed after oestrogen withdrawal in most clinical scenarios (6). Furthermore, the influence of obesity on the development of HCA is suggested, as supported by a higher incidence of HCAs in patients with non-alcoholic steatohepatitis (NASH) (8). In men, anabolic steroid use, underlying metabolic diseases including type 1 glycogen storage disease (9), iron overload related to β-thalassemia and haemochromatosis (10) have been linked to the pathogenesis of HCAs. Portacaval shunt or portal deprivation is linked to the pathogenesis of HCA and some familial cases have been reported in patients with diabetes mellitus type 3 (11). It is extremely rare in the paediatric population, with a weak association with Fanconi anaemia (a rare disorder in the category of inherited bone marrow failure syndromes), Hurler's syndrome (caused by a deficiency of alpha-L-iduronidase, encoded by the *IDUA* gene, which aids in the breakdown of dermatan and heparin sulphate. This results in the accumulation of large amounts of group-specific antigen in the body, eventually causing the cells to become severely dysfunctional leading to death), Turcot syndrome (a condition characterized by multiple adenomatous colon polyps and an increased risk of colorectal and brain cancer), and as a part of familial adenomatous polyposis (12).

Subtypes of HCA

Histologically, HCAs are identified by the monoclonal proliferation of well-differentiated hepatocytes associated with the absence of a portal triad and interlobular bile ducts (*Figure 52.1a*). They arise in non-cirrhotic livers, appearing as well circumscribed, non-encapsulated yellow-brown lesions with, or without, cystic or haemorrhagic changes (*Figure 52.1b*). In 1985, Flejou et al. defined a specific clinical entity, liver adenomatosis, as the occurrence of more than 10 HCAs, which was interestingly not associated with OC intake (13). Until the early 2000s, HCA was considered a well-defined homogeneous entity. Recent developments in molecular medicine have facilitated the sub-classification of HCA and revealed the heterogeneity of the disease, further refining our understanding of the oncogenic mechanisms activated in benign liver tumorigenesis that are specific to the different molecular subtypes (14–16). HCAs are classified into the following four major molecular subgroups according to their genetic and phenotypical characteristics. *Table 52.3* summarizes the salient points of difference between the four molecular subtypes of HCAs:

1 HNF1α (coding for hepatocyte nuclear factor) mutated adenomas
2 β-catenin-activated adenomas
3 Inflammatory or telangiectatic adenomas
4 Unclassified adenomas

Diagnosis and management of HCAs

Most patients with HCAs are asymptomatic and lesions are diagnosed incidentally during routine abdominal imaging. The most common symptom is abdominal pain (occurring in <10% cases) and the main complication is haemorrhage in 25% of cases (19–21). The risk of haemorrhage is higher in pregnant

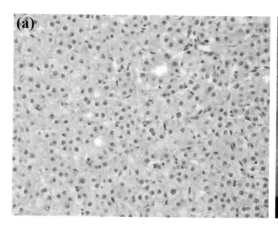
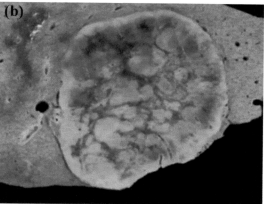

Figure 52.1 Histological appearance of Hepatocellular adenoma (HCA), showing sheets and cords of normal looking well-differentiated hepatocytes with absence of portal triads and bile ducts (a); Cut section of the tumour in right lobe showing well encapsulated yellow tan appearance of the mass (b). (Figure 52.1b Courtesy of Jarnagin WR (ed). *Blumgart's Surgery of the Liver, Biliary Tract and Pancreas*, Elsevier, 2022, with permission.)

Table 52.3 Subtypes of HCA and their salient features of differentiation (molecular classification).

HCA subtype (2017)	Molecular aberration	% Cases	Demographics	Salient clinical features	Salient pathologic features	IHC**
HNF1a inactivated	Biallelic inactivating mutation of HNF1a. Somatic 90% and constitutional 10%	40–50%	Female sex, Oral contraceptives. Associated with liver adenomatosis. Might be related with MODY 3 DM	Majority asymptomatic	Steatosis is a hallmark feature	Absence of staining LFABP
β-catenin activated						
β-catenin exon 7/8	CTNNB1-activating mutations or deletions with differing levels of β-catenin pathway activation	3%	Young age, solitary tumour. Associated with OC use, high alcohol consumption and obesity. Association with GSD type 1a	Majority asymptomatic	Widespread atypia (inconstant). Multiple vessels. Non-specific features	Non-specific
β-catenin exon 3		7%	Young age, Male sex, solitary tumour. Associated with androgens and liver vascular disease	Risk of malignant transformation		GS diffuse/strong staining
IHCA	IL6/JAK/STAT activation (80%) IL6ST (65%) GNAS somatic mutation	30–35%	Older age. OC use. Inflammatory syndromes associated. Association with McCune-Albright syndrome, GSD type 1a	Elevated GGT and ALP on blood chemistry	Sinusoidal dilatation. Inflammation, thick arteries, pseudo-portal tracts	CRP/SAA overexpression
Unclassified hepatocellular adenoma						
Sonic hedgehog variant	No identified mutations	4%	OC use and obesity associated GSD type 1a association	Risk of bleeding	Non-specific	Non-specific
Unclassified variant	Non-specific	7%	Non-specific	Non-specific		

Source: Nault et al. (2017) (17).

** IHC: Bordeaux IHC classification (18).

Abbreviations: ALP: alkaline phosphatase; CRP: C-reactive protein; CTNNB: catenin β; GGT: gamma glutamyl transpeptidase; GS: glutamine synthetase; GSD: glycogen storage disease; HNF: hepatocyte nuclear factor; IHC: immunohistochemistry; IHCA: inflammatory hepatocellular adenoma; LFABP: liver fatty acid binding protein; MODY: maturity onset diabetes of the young; OC: oral contraceptives; SAA: serum amyloid A; UHCA: unclassified hepatocellular adenoma.

women and those taking an OC principally because this demographic usually has large HCAs. In large HCAs defined as >5 cm in diameter, radiographic visualization of arteries within the HCA, location of the lesion in left lateral lobe and an exophytic morphology are risk factors for haemorrhage (21). About 10% of patients will present with acute peritonitis from intraperitoneal rupture and hemoperitoneum, leading in most cases to hypovolemic shock. The overall risk of malignant transformation in HCA is reported to be 5–6% or less (22–24). Distinguishing HCA from well-differentiated hepatocellular carcinoma (HCC) on imaging and on histology remains a challenge and serum analysis reveals a normal α-fetoprotein (AFP) level in most cases. The risk of malignancy is very high in men, occurring in about 50%, irrespective of the size of the tumour. The natural history detailing the progression of an HCA with malignant transformation and the development of a well differentiated HCC is not well understood or described. The risk factors for malignant transformation include sex, androgen use, β-catenin HCA subtype and large size (>5 cm) (25). About one-third of patients diagnosed with HCA will have multiple lesions (defined as more than 3) of various sizes and this is termed liver adenomatosis. Patients with adenomatosis do not carry a higher risk of complications than solitary HCA and the management is identical (26).

It is currently well established that the different molecular subtypes of HCAs correspond to distinct phenotypic features on imaging (summarized in *Table 52.2*). The presence of marked steatosis (clear cells) on pathology constitutes the hallmark findings in HNF1a inactivated HCAs (*Figure 52.2*) (27). They appear homogeneous on MRI and have a variable signal on T2-sequences which is usually slightly hyperintense on non-fat suppressed sequence and iso-or hypointense on fat suppressed T2-weighted sequence (*Figure 52.3*). The striking finding is a diffuse and homogeneous signal dropout on chemical shift T1-weighted sequences (specificity 90–95%) (*Figure 52.3*) (28). They are usually moderately hypervascular and often show washout on portal and/or delayed phases using extracellular MRI contrast agents. Diffusion-weighted (DW) MRI reveals an iso- or moderately hyperintense appearance. Inflammatory type HCAs have certain distinct features on imaging (29) with Doppler signals commonly seen on US and unlike other subtypes, central arteries that mimic FNH may be seen on contrast-enhanced ultrasound (CEUS). They are characterized on MRI by their telangiectatic features, showing a strong hyperintense signal on T2-weighted images (isointense with the spleen), either diffuse or as a rim-like band in the periphery of the lesion – the 'atoll sign'. T1-weighted sequences reveal variable iso- to hyperintensity, which persists on fat suppressed and opposed-phase sequences. These lesions are markedly hypervascular as evidenced by persistent enhancement on delayed phase using extracellular

MR contrast agents. The two striking imaging findings (strong hypersignal on T2-weighted MR images and the persistent enhancement on delayed phase) are associated with a high sensitivity (85–88%) and specificity (88–100%) of MRI for diagnosing inflammatory HCA using extracellular contrast agents (30). Recent studies by Ba-Ssalamah et al. have demonstrated that nearly half of the inflammatory HCAs are iso- or hyperintense on hepatobiliary MR phase using Gd-BOPTA or gadoxetic acid, mimicking that of FNH (sensitivity of 81% and specificity of 77%) (31). A β-catenin HCA is characterized by hyperintensity on T2- and hypointensity on T1-weighted sequences, with a central scar but no signal loss on chemical shift sequences. Contrast-enhanced images reveal strong arterial enhancement with either persistent or decreased signal intensity on a portal venous phase. The unclassified HCAs display strong arterial enhancement but no delayed enhancement after gadolinium injection (CEMR), with no characteristic imaging features described to date.

Treatment of patients with HCA is tailored depending on the patient's gender and the size of the tumour, together with any associated risk factors noted during evaluation. Irrespective of the size, HCAs in men mandate resection, given the high risk of malignancy. In women, however, lesions which are less than 5 cm in diameter irrespective of the number carry a low risk of complications and could be safely observed after cessation of an OC. The influence of discontinuing OC use on the regression of HCA is debated and reports contradictory justifying serial imaging in patients managed conservatively. The algorithm for the management of HCAs is also determined by its molecular phenotype and is summarized in *Figure 52.4*. The essential recommendations in the management of these tumours have been detailed as clinical practice guidelines in August 2016 by the European Association of the Study of Liver (EASL) described below (32,33). Some of the key points of approach to management of HCAs follow.

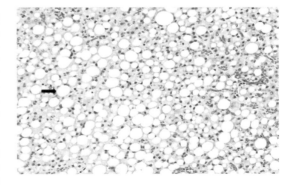

Figure 52.2 Hepatocellular adenoma (HNF1 alpha mutated variant): Note the marked steatosis (arrow) evident on H&E staining by clear cells. (With permission from ref 82.)

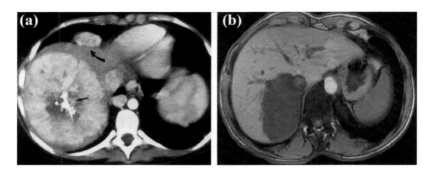

Figure 52.3 Appearance of Hepatocellular adenoma on MRI: (a) hyperintensity on T2 weighted phase; (b) loss of signal on out of phase T1 weighted image. (With permission from ref 83.)

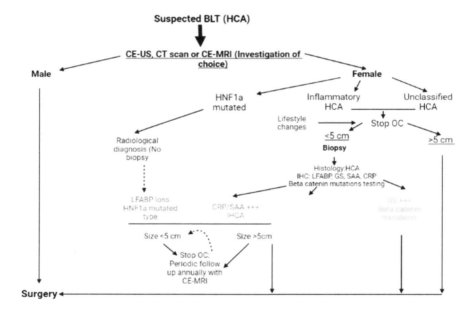

Figure 52.4 Algorithmic approach for the management of suspected hepatocellular adenoma. *Abbreviations:* CEUS: contrast enhanced ultrasound; CEMRI: contrast enhanced MRI; HNF: hepatocyte nuclear factor; HCA: hepatocellular adenoma; OC: oral contraceptives; IHC: immunohistochemistry; LFABP: liver fatty acid binding protein; GS: glutamine synthetase; SAA: serum amyloid A; CRP: C-reactive protein; IHCA: inflammatory HCA.

Liver multidisciplinary team

A dedicated benign liver multidisciplinary team (MDT) forms a key component for the initial approach to all BLTs. The team should be one with expertise in the management of benign liver lesions and should include a hepatologist, a hepatobiliary surgeon, diagnostic and interventional radiologists and a pathologist.

Imaging recommendations

MRI is superior to other imaging modalities. Its intrinsic properties facilitating the detection of fat and vascular spaces, including sinusoids and caverns, allows subtyping of HCAs in up to 80% of patients. The identification

of HNF-1α HCA or inflammatory HCA with MRI is possible with >90% specificity contrasting with the identification and classification of β-catenin activated HCAs and unclassified HCAs, which is not possible by any imaging technique alone.

Treatment recommendations

Treatment decisions are directed by gender, size and the pattern of progression. Lifestyle changes such as stopping OC use and weight loss should be advised. Male gender and proven β-catenin mutations are absolute indications for resection, irrespective of the size. Lesions less than 5 cm in women should be reassessed at 1 year, and subsequently by annual imaging. Non-surgical modalities, such as embolization (transarterial embolization [TAE]) for larger lesions or ablation for smaller lesions are alternatives to resection but should only be performed in poor surgical candidates (34). Ablation without confirmation of the diagnosis is not recommended in small indeterminate lesions.

Emergency management of HCA

If clinically evident haemorrhage occurs, admission for close observation, resuscitation and contrast-enhanced CT (CECT) is recommended. For major haemorrhage, resuscitation with fluids and blood products and referral to a centre where embolization can be performed to control active bleeding is advised. A bleeding HCA with hypovolemic shock should be embolized as the initial treatment and any residual viable lesion on follow-up imaging should be considered for resection.

HCA in pregnancy

HCA in a pregnant woman should be monitored for progression of size by close follow-up using frequent US (every 6–12 weeks). If there is evidence of an increase in the size of the lesion, with associated increased risk of rupture, the obstetric team should be involved in planning the appropriate emergency management. For adenomas <5 cm which are not exophytic, and are stable in size, vaginal delivery is acceptable. Embolization can be considered for lesions which are increasing in size but prior to 24 weeks, surgery is preferred over other modalities to avoid exposure to ionising radiations and intravenous contrast agents.

Multiple HCAs

The term liver adenomatosis, defined as >10 HCAs has been replaced by multiple HCAs owing to the frequent inability to accurately count the number of lesions on cross-sectional imaging. The management of patients with multiple HCA is based on the size of the largest tumour. Hepatic resection might be considered when the disease is confined to one lobe, and in those cases with more widespread or multifocal HCAs, resection of the largest adenomas may be an option. Liver transplantation is not recommended as a treatment for multiple HCA, but might be considered in individuals with background liver disease such as cirrhosis due to another pathology.

Paediatric HCAs

Because of relevant associated risks (intra-tumoral or intra-abdominal haemorrhage and malignant transformation) complete resection is recommended by most authors, especially for tumours larger than 5 cm (35,36). Alternatives to surgical resections include percutaneous procedures such as radiofrequency ablation and are determined on an individual case basis. Optimization of dietary therapy for glycogen storage disease will lead to spontaneous regression in most cases, which are subsequently managed by a close follow-up.

Targeted therapy in HCAs – Future directions

The ability to categorize HCAs into different molecular phenotypes based on the underlying genetic mechanism is a potential area for targeted therapy in these patients. The three important signalling pathways that have emerged from these molecular analyses include inactivation of *HNF-1a* and activation of the *Wnt/ β-catenin* and *IL-6/JAK/STAT3* pathways. Targeted inhibition of these pathways could have a significant, sustainable effect on the molecular pathogenesis of HCAs. Evidence from genetically engineered murine models replicating benign tumorigenesis in the liver is still lacking. Several drugs are known to affect the *IL-6/ JAK/STAT3* pathway and in patients with unresectable IHCA or adenomatosis may prove valuable and are under investigation. One example is Src inhibitors of kinases such as Dasatinib (an ATP-competitive protein tyrosine kinase inhibitor) which have been shown to shut down the JAK/STAT activation induced by *STAT3* mutations. This could lead to a detailed understanding of the tumorigenesis mechanism and could potentially allow targeting of the benign to malignant tumour progression in future experimental models (37,38).

FOCAL NODULAR HYPERPLASIA

Focal nodular hyperplasia (FNH) is the second most common BLT and can be described as an indolent tumour-like condition commonly affecting women between the ages of 35–50 (39). It is extremely rare in the paediatric population, with only around 200 cases being described to date in the world literature, with an age distribution of 7–14 years (40–42). Unlike HCAs, FNH is not influenced by OC use. They are multiple in 20–30% of cases and are associated with vascular disorders of the liver such as haemangiomas in around 20% of cases (43). Some authors report the finding of FNH nodules in 13.7% of patients with hereditary haemorrhagic telangiectasia (HHT), and there are even reports of them in case series of explanted livers with Budd–Chiari syndrome (44,45). In addition, congenital absence of portal flow (PV agenesis and Abernathy syndrome or Abernethy malformation, which is a congenital extrahepatic portosystemic shunt) and portal vein (PV) thrombosis with resultant hepatic arterialization has also been linked with the development of FNH. Involution of FNH lesions after the menopause has also been observed, further supporting the significance of oestrogen receptor expression in FNH tissue samples (46,47).

The pathogenesis of FNH involves a polyclonal hepatocellular proliferation, regarded by some authors as a hyperplastic reaction consequent upon an arterial malformation. This hypothesis is supported by the absence of somatic mutations described in liver tumorigenesis in FNH and the dysregulation of genes, such as angiopoietins (ANGPT) involved in vascular remodelling (48). The regenerative process induced in a specific area or sector supplied by the affected artery could explain the absence of size changes in the majority of cases.

Clinical and biological features

Most cases are asymptomatic and usually discovered incidentally during routine liver US examination (49,50). A small number of patients may present with abdominal pain or discomfort especially with large lesions located in the left lobe of the liver which can cause pressure effects leading to early satiety. In rare cases of pedunculated lesions, presentation may be with acute abdomen pain following torsion of the pedicle. Complications, such as rupture or haemorrhage, are very rare and probably related to atypical forms of FNH with specific imaging and biologic features (telangiectatic FNH), which should actually be classified as an adenoma (45). Malignant transformation of FNH has not been reported and liver function tests are normal in almost 80% of cases (44), although large FNH causing bile duct compression may present with mild elevations of GGT and ALP. Morphologically, an FNH appears as a solitary well-circumscribed, unencapsulated mass, with a central fibrous scar containing dystrophic arterial vessels (*Figure 52.5a*). Histologically, a 'typical' FNH is composed of benign-appearing hepatocytes arranged in nodules, partially delineated by fibrous septa originating from the central scar, and containing varying degrees of ductular proliferation along the septae (*Figure 52.5b*). Several atypical forms of FNH have been recognized, including FNH without a central scar (the most common atypical form) or FNH with significant steatosis, but they are rare (51). Molecular analysis will identify activation of the transforming growth factor beta (TGF-β) signalling pathway (extracellular matrix) and overexpression of *Wnt/β-catenin* target genes. These include *GLUL* which codes for glutamine synthase and results in a typical map-like pattern of glutamine synthase (GS) overexpression in the periphery of the nodules close to the vessels which is specific for FNH (52). GS staining (IHC) should be used to achieve a firm pathological diagnosis in difficult cases.

Imaging features

On US, FNH lesions appears slightly hypoechoic or isoechoic with lobulated contours frequently with a hypoechoic halo (53). The central scar is slightly hyperechoic, but is often difficult to visualize on US and is clearly seen in only 20% of cases. Doppler US will demonstrate the presence of a central feeding artery with a stellate or 'spoke wheel' pattern (a classic feature) corresponding to the artery running from the central scar to fibrous septae (*Figure 52.6a*). A plain CT of the abdomen will demonstrate a focal hypodense or isodense mass in the non-contrast phase. A central hypodense scar is identified in only one-third of patients on a plain scan (54). In most cases, the lesion enhances rapidly during the arterial phase of a CECT (the degree of enhancement is higher than HCA), and decreases during the portal venous phase, where the lesion may become isodense or slightly hyperdense relative to normal background liver. MRI helps in differentiating the classic or typical FNH subtype from the non-classic or atypical FNH (*Table 52.4*). Compared with US and CT, MRI has a much higher sensitivity (95–99%) and specificity (99–100%) for the diagnosis of FNH. The combination of CEUS and MRI yields the highest diagnostic accuracy. CEUS is more accurate than MRI in lesions less than 3 cm whereas the opposite is true for larger lesions. The addition of hepatobiliary MR contrast agents such as Gadolinium, Eovist®, and

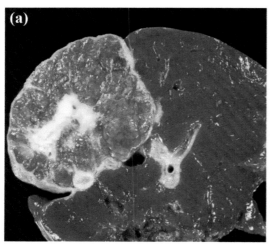
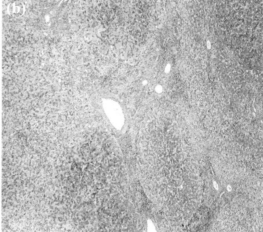

Figure 52.5 Focal nodular hyperplasia, appearance (a) gross and (b) microscopic (5X).

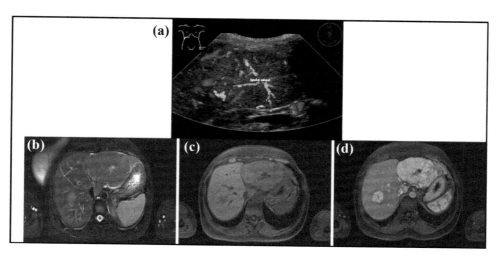

Figure 52.6 Appearance of the FNH lesion on US Doppler (a): Characteristic spoke wheel appearance of the central arterial arcade. Appearance of the typical FNH lesion on MRI: Hypointense on T2 and isointense on T1 on precontrast phase, with bright enhancement on contrast MR. Central stellate scar characteristic.

Table 52.4 MRI findings of FNH subtypes (classic and non-classic) compared

MRI phases	Classic (typical) FNH	Non classic (atypical) FNH
T1W	Iso-/mildly hypointense	Heterogenous (hypo/iso/hyper-intense)
T2W	Iso-/mildly hyperintense	Heterogenous (iso/hyper-intense)
Arterial phase	Intense enhancement	Intense heterogenous enhancement
Portal/delayed venous phase	Persistent enhancement	Heterogenous persistent enhancement; Pseudocapsule present
In and out phase	No signal drop	Rarely, focal signal drop
Central scar	T2 hyperintense scar showing delayed enhancement	Absent/atypical scar

Abbreviations: FNH: focal nodular hyperplasia; MRI: magnetic resonance imaging; T1W: T1-weighted; T2W: T2-weighted.

Primovist® which demonstrate retention of contrast in the late (20 minute) phase increases the sensitivity to 90%. In atypical cases (*see Table 52.4*) on imaging, liver biopsy is indicated (54,55).

Management of FNH

FNH almost always behaves in an indolent fashion, with very few complications and little change over time, although enlargement of these lesions with OC use and during pregnancy have been reported (33). The most common approach to these lesions is watchful waiting (*Figure 52.7*) and follow-up imaging at 6–12 months is usually sufficient to establish the stability of the lesion and its benign nature. A long-term follow-up protocol is not indicated unless there is doubt regarding the diagnosis, and surgery should only be considered for patients with symptomatic or suspicious lesions (malignancy not ruled out on repeated biopsies or imaging). In high-risk symptomatic patients, TAE is an attractive alternative

and has demonstrated the ability to reduce the size of lesions and provide symptom relief. Similarly, RFA has been reported as an effective treatment for symptomatic FNH, but the vast majority of cases are managed conservatively. Definitive treatment is considered only in exceptional cases (pedunculated, expanding, exophytic causing space-occupying issues), where resection is the treatment of choice (*Figure 52.7*).

The essential recommendations for evaluation and management of FNH can be summarized (EASL clinical practice guidelines 2016) (33).

Imaging

CEUS, CT, or MRI in combination have almost 100% specificity for diagnosing FNH, with MRI alone having the highest diagnostic performance when compared with the CEUS and CT. The highest diagnostic accuracy with CEUS is achieved in FNH less than 3 cm.

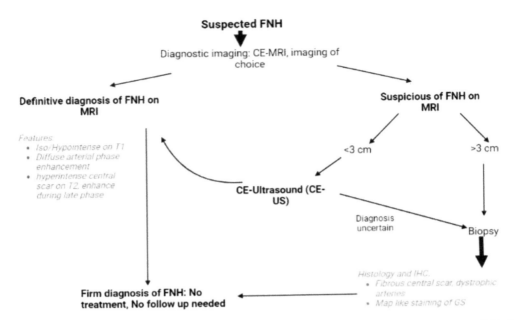

Suspected FNH

Diagnostic imaging: CE-MRI, imaging of choice

Definitive diagnosis of FNH on MRI

Features
- *Iso/Hypointense on T1*
- *Diffuse arterial phase enhancement*
- *hyperintense central scar on T2, enhance during late phase*

Suspicious of FNH on MRI

<3 cm   >3 cm

CE-Ultrasound (CE-US)

Diagnosis uncertain   Biopsy

Histology and IHC:
- *Fibrous central scar, dystrophic arteries*
- *Map like staining of GS*

Firm diagnosis of FNH: No treatment, No follow up needed

Figure 52.7 Algorithmic approach to the management of focal nodular hyperplasia. *Abbreviations:* FNH: focal nodular hyperplasia; ceMRI: contrast-enhanced MRI; IHC: immunohistochemistry; GS: glutamine synthetase.

Treatment

For a typical FNH (defined on imaging or biopsy, in doubtful cases) follow-up is not necessary, unless there is underlying vascular liver disease and no treatment is recommended. For atypical imaging features or symptomatic patients, referral to a benign liver tumour MDT to rule out other causes is advised.

In pediatric populations, observation is indicated in asymptomatic patients (56). In symptomatic cases or those where there is still diagnostic doubt, complete surgical excision is considered. Post-surgical recurrences have been reported but are extremely uncommon. In the presence of mild and continuous abdominal symptoms, follow-up every 6–12 months with repeat imaging and alpha fetoprotein measurement is recommended, since the biological behaviour of FNH can range from involution to growth.

HEPATIC HAEMANGIOMA

Hepatic haemangiomas (HHs) are the most common primary liver tumours, present in 0.4–20% of the general population and usually discovered incidentally during evaluation of non-specific abdominal symptoms (57,58). They occur much more commonly in women with a female/male ratio of 5 : 1 and they affect patients who are 30–50 years of age (57). In the paediatric population it is the most common benign liver tumour of infancy and childhood, with a diagnosis being made within the first 6 months of life in over 80% of cases. However, due to differences in histologic structure between the adult and the infantile forms of haemangioma, they are regarded as separate entities (59). The infantile form shows an increased association with hemi-hypertrophy and Beckwith–Wiedemann syndrome, a growth disorder variably characterized by macroglossia, hemihyperplasia, omphalocele, neonatal hypoglycemia, macrosomia, embryonal tumours including Wilms' tumour, hepatoblastoma, neuroblastoma and rhabdomyosarcoma, visceromegaly, adrenocortical cytomegaly and renal abnormalities (59).

Clinical presentation and pathogenesis

Haemangioma is possibly a congenital disorder, although the pathogenesis is presently not well understood. There is a possible hormonal association as evidenced by the presence of oestrogen receptors in some of these tumours and an accelerated growth observed with high-oestrogen states, such as puberty, pregnancy and OC use (58). Recent reports suggested an increase in vascular endothelial growth factor (VEGF) is involved in the development of haemangiomas. This is supported by a number of case reports demonstrating reduction in size of haemangiomas following anti-VEGF treatment, although this is not demonstrated in other case series (60). In adults, haemangiomas are mostly solitary lesions between 1–30 cm in diameter, with the majority being <5 cm (*Figure 52.8*). An HH with a diameter of greater than 10 cm is referred to as a giant haemangioma (57). Unlike the usual asymptomatic presentation, these may be symptomatic with pain and features of

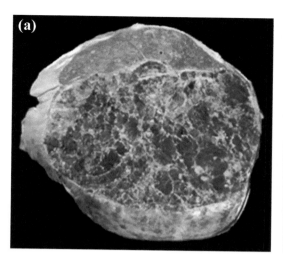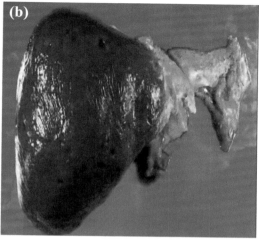

Figure 52.8 Gross morphology of cavernous hepatic hemangioma (a) transverse view, (b) surface view.

an inflammatory reaction syndrome (low-grade fever, weight loss, abdominal pain, accelerated erythrocyte sedimentation rate, normal white blood cell count, anemia, thrombocytosis and increased fibrinogen level) with a coagulopathy referred to as Kasabach-Merritt syndrome (KMS). KMS syndrome is characterized by the combination of a rapidly enlarging vascular tumour, thrombocytopenia, microangiopathic haemolytic anaemia, a consumptive coagulopathy and purpura (61,62). Although KMS may complicate any haemangioma, it is more likely to be associated with haemangiomas over 5 cm. The pathogenesis of KMS involves the interaction of platelets and endothelial cells of the HH leading to platelet trapping, activation and consumption within the abnormal vascular structure (62).

Most haemangiomas, however, are usually asymptomatic and pain accompanying an uncomplicated haemangioma might be associated with the concurrent presence of gallbladder disease, liver cysts, a gastroduodenal ulcer or hiatus hernia, but left lobe lesions can cause pain due to pressure effects on adjacent organs. Liver function tests are usually normal, and when associated with a large hepatic lesion on imaging and mild symptoms, frequently suggests the diagnosis of a haemangioma (58). Complications are extremely rare and mostly observed in large haemangiomas and could be due to inflammation of the internal architecture of the lesion (usually due to acute thrombosis of a part or all the haemangioma), coagulation abnormalities leading to haemorrhage and resultant hemoperitoneum, compression of adjacent structures causing pressure symptoms or high output cardiac failure.

Imaging

The classic appearance of a haemangioma on routine US is that of a homogenous hyperechoic mass usually

less than 3 cm with acoustic enhancement and sharp margins (63). In cases where the US findings are not typical, contrast-enhanced, and cross-sectional imaging modalities are recommended. CEUS shows an early peripheral and globular enhancement of the lesion followed by infilling and central enhancement on delayed phases. The CT criteria for the diagnosis of HH are:

1 *Non-contrast phase*: low attenuation
2 *Contrast phase (early)*: peripheral and globular enhancement of the lesion
3 *Contrast phase (delayed)*: central enhancement of the lesion (*Figure 52.9a*)

The presence of peripheral puddles on the arterial phase has a sensitivity of 67%, a specificity of 99%, and a positive predictive value of 86% for HH (64). On MRI, the classic appearance of a liver haemangioma is that of a hypointense lesion on T1-weighted sequences and a strongly hyperintense lesion on heavily T2-weighted sequences, the so called 'lightbulb pattern' (*Figure 52.9b*) (65). On diffusion-weighted MR sequences, the signal of a haemangioma drops with increasing b-values and consequently, the apparent diffusion co-efficient (ADC) value is high. High-flow haemangiomas may show atypical features using hepatobiliary MR contrast agents (gadoxetic acid) with relatively low signal intensity relative to the surrounding normal liver parenchyma during the equilibrium (3 min delayed) phase, mimicking hypervascular hepatic tumours, a pseudo 'washout pattern' (66). This will allow differentiation due to the observation of a very strong signal intensity on T2-weighted imaging and enhancement on arterial phase-dominant imaging, in the former compared with the latter. Giant haemangiomas are often heterogeneous with marked central areas that correspond

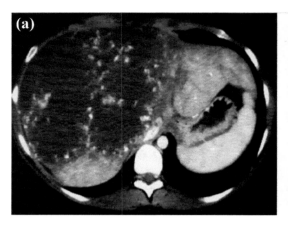
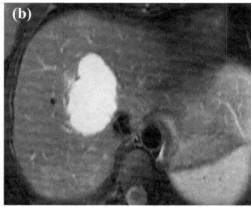

Figure 52.9 Appearance of typical hepatic hemangioma on cross-sectional imaging (a) and (b).

to thrombosis, extensive hyalinization and fibrosis. However, the typical early and progressive peripheral nodular enhancement is usually observed along with strong hyperintensity on T2-weighted MR images, which generally does not lead to complete central filling. When the diagnosis cannot be confirmed with imaging alone, percutaneous biopsy may be required to differentiate HHs from other space-occupying lesions of the liver. Needle biopsy is not contraindicated (a cuff of normal hepatic parenchyma is interposed between the capsule and the margin of a haemangioma) and allows a diagnosis with an overall accuracy of 96% (65).

Treatment

All asymptomatic hepatic haemangiomas are followed up by observation alone, irrespective of the size. Reassurance about the rare occurrence of growth and the extremely low risk of complication (rupture/bleeding/inflammatory syndromes and high output failure) should be given. The need for resection must be weighed against the risk of postoperative complications (albeit low) such as bleeding or biliary fistulae, given the benign nature of the nature. The essential recommendations in management of hepatic haemangiomas are outlined as follows (based on the clinical practice guidelines by the EASL, 2016) (33).

Imaging

A hyperechoic lesion against the background of a healthy liver in an asymptomatic individual is very likely to be a liver haemangioma. With typical imaging findings: homogeneous hyperechoic; sharp margin; posterior enhancement; and absence of halo sign, in a lesion less than 3 cm US is sufficient to establish the diagnosis. In patients with underlying liver disease or with a doubtful diagnosis (malignancy), contrast enhanced imaging

(CEUS, CT, or MRI) is required. Follow-up imaging is not required for a typical haemangioma.

Treatment and follow-up

Conservative management is the rule for all typical asymptomatic cases. Pregnancy and oral contraceptives are not contraindicated. Presence of KMS, enlarging lesions or those which cause symptoms due to pressure effects should be referred to a benign liver tumour MDT.

Surgical and non-surgical options for hepatic haemangioma

Surgical resection is the most common treatment for symptomatic haemangiomas (67). The surgical options range from liver resection (non-anatomical or anatomical) to parenchyma preserving approaches, including preoperative portal vein embolization (PVE), enucleation, hepatic artery ligation, and liver transplantation in very rare cases. Most studies suggest that enucleation is associated with lower morbidity, shorter operation time, reduced blood loss and fewer complications, and it will preserve the maximum amount of hepatic parenchyma compared with resection (67). However, this is contradicted by another single-centre study in 86 patients with giant haemangiomas, which demonstrated no difference between enucleation and resection regarding operation time, blood loss, complications, and hospital stay (68). For centrally located haemangiomas, enucleation is more challenging and will require significantly longer vascular inflow occlusion and operating time with a greater chance of the need for significant blood transfusions. Laparoscopic liver resection has gained widespread acceptance and is considered to be a safe approach for the management of benign liver lesions. A recently conducted systematic review comparing laparoscopic and open surgery for BLTs demonstrated that the laparoscopic approach was associated with less blood loss, shorter postoperative hospital stays and lower complication rates compared to the open approach with no difference in the short-term 'quality of life' outcomes (69). Liver transplantation has rarely been reported for hepatic haemangiomas. The United Network for Organ Sharing (UNOS) database identifies 394 liver transplants performed for BLTs between 1989 and 2008, accounting for only 0.9% of the total number of procedures (70). Most studies are limited to small case reports and series and the most recent report and review of series by Zhao et al. only identified 26 cases of liver transplantation being performed for hepatic haemangiomas 1989–2022 (71). KMS was identified as the most frequent indication accounting for 50% of the cases. Most patients identified from this review had a dominant tumour measuring greater than 4 cm in diameter and presented with abdominal pain and distension (88%), followed by respiratory distress and intra-abdominal bleeding. Liver transplantation should continue to be reserved for unresectable giant haemangiomas causing severe symptoms, failure of previous interventions or complications such as the KMS.

Owing to the associated perioperative complications such as massive intraoperative blood loss, bile leakage, long operating and hospitalization times, nonsurgical treatment options should always be considered where feasible. There are, however, no established guidelines and no consensus for recommending surgery over intervention radiology (IR)-guided therapy. Transcatheter arterial embolization (TAE) has traditionally been indicated to control acute haemorrhage or to reduce the size and vascularity of lesions prior to surgery (72). With improvements in interventional devices and procedures, and the application of super-selective techniques, TAE has become the treatment of choice for HH. It works on the principle of combining a chemotherapy drug and lipiodol. Proliferation of the vascular endothelial cells is inhibited by the chemotherapy drug and lipiodol selectively embolizes the blood vessels leading to concentrated aggregates of the chemotherapy drug with slow release in the haemangioma cavity facilitating its inhibitory effect and achieving the destruction of hepatic sinusoidal lumen by fibrosis and gradual tumour shrinkage (72). A recent study demonstrated a 50% reduction in the haemangioma volume in 17 of 23 patients treated with bleomycin-TAE (73). Radiofrequency ablation (RFA) is another alternative to TAE. RFA is usually performed under ultrasound (US) guidance, but CT guidance for percutaneous RFA is more suitable for haemangiomas located deeply in liver parenchyma (74), and laparoscopic RFA with US guidance is preferred for subcapsular HHs. Percutaneous sclerotherapy is another less commonly used option and involves puncture of the lesion and injection of drugs under IR fluoroscopic guidance (75). Pingyangmycin, anhydrous alcohol and sodium morrhuate are commonly used agents for this purpose. Percutaneous sclerotherapy combined with TAE has been found to benefit ischaemic haemangiomas. Percutaneous argon-helium cryotherapy is a novel option that works on the principle of formation of ice crystals in cells causing necrosis leading to degeneration of proteins and cell membranes, blood stasis, and local ischaemia. It is rarely used in clinical practice because of its questionable long-term effects (76).

A different approach is taken to the management of paediatric haemangiomas depending mainly on the type (unifocal/multifocal/diffuse) and the association of systemic complications, such as high output cardiac failure and compartment syndrome, especially in neonates. Discussion of this is beyond the scope of this chapter and will be dealt with, elsewhere (77,78).

MISCELLANEOUS BLTs

Besides these common forms of BLTs, there are other important uncommon benign liver tumours (of non-epithelial origin) that must be considered in the differential diagnosis of a suspected liver nodule on imaging. The key demographic and imaging points of some of these miscellaneous tumours are summarized in *Table 52.5*.

Table 52.5 Summary and comparison of the features of miscellaneous benign liver tumours which facilitate a differential diagnosis

Lesion	General characteristics	Imaging	Other remarks
Angiomyolipoma (79)	• Composed of smooth muscles, fat, blood vessels • More common in kidney (part of tuberous sclerosis) than liver • Females > Males • 30–50 years age group • Asymptomatic mostly • Malignant transformation reported	• Hyperdense and hypo-attenuated on non-contrast CT • Marked arterial enhancement with central vascular opacification • Large central vessels (*macroaneurysms*) are characteristic	• Needle biopsy with tissue staining by anti-HMB-45 identifies the myoid component • Lesions <5 cm: Close follow-up with serial imaging • Large tumours (>5 cm): Resection recommended (degenerated components within the tumour)

(Continued)

Table 52.5 (*Continued*) Summary and comparison of the features of miscellaneous benign liver tumours which facilitate a differential diagnosis

Lesion	General characteristics	Imaging	Other remarks
Inflammatory pseudotumour of liver (IPL) (80)	• Can mimic cholangiocarcinoma • More common in lung than liver • Males > Females • Age groups: 50s • Presentation with vague constitutional symptoms (fever, abdominal pain, weight loss), normal haematological tests. Inflammatory syndrome in ⅓ of cases • Possible infective aetiology suggested (via portal circulation), some also suggest autoimmune aetiology (IgG4 associated)	• Diffuse and infiltrative pattern on imaging, mostly confined around the GB fossa, mimicking malignant biliary stricture 3 forms: • *Encapsulated form*: mimicking solitary necrotic liver nodule • *Inflammatory form*: Presentation with inflammatory syndrome, ill-defined on imaging • *Infiltrating periportal form*: Presentation with jaundice Progressive enhancement on contrast (Gd) MRI	• Treatment choices not well defined • Most patients end up with surgery (in presumably resectable cases) due to the inability to clearly differentiate from other malignant causes • They have no malignant potential otherwise • In cases with definitive diagnosis of IPL, antibiotics and steroids are recommended
Nodular regenerative hyperplasia (NRH) (81)	• Rare benign diffuse micronodular transformation of liver • Nodules are composed of hyperplastic hepatocytes • *Important DD*: Regenerative nodules of cirrhosis and FNH • Prevalence around 2% • Associated with myeloproliferative and lymphoid disorders, collagen vascular disorders, drugs (oxaliplatin, steroids, azathioprine) • Mostly asymptomatic and detected incidentally • Abnormal liver function tests in two-thirds of cases • Portal hypertension in 30% cases	• Imaging non-specific • Can range from normal imaging to multiple liver nodules with or without portal hypertension • Variable enhancement on MRI • Contrary to FNH, no central scar	• In asymptomatic patients no treatment required • In patients with clinically significant portal hypertension, appropriate medical management is indicated • Liver transplantation in very rare cases of decompensated liver failure with portal hypertension • Oxaliplatin-based chemotherapy in CRLM might be associated with NRH • Presence of NRH nodules in such patients calls for avoiding major liver resection

Abbreviations: CRLM: colorectal liver metastases; DD: differential diagnosis; FNH: focal nodular hyperplasia; GB: gall bladder; Gd: gadolinium; HMB: human melanoma black; IgG: immunoglobulin G.

SUMMARY

Benign liver tumours (BLTs) are mostly an incidental diagnosis on routine abdominal imaging. Haemangiomas are the most frequent type of BLTs in adult and paediatric age groups. The majority of BLTs do not require any treatment, with follow-up by imaging being necessary only in selected patients and pathologies. In asymptomatic HH and FNH regardless of their size, no intervention is required. HCAs are treated based on the gender, size and the genetic phenotype due to the risk of bleeding and malignant transformation. The essential guidelines on diagnostic work up and management of hepatic haemangioma, FNH and HCA advocate the use of a dedicated BLT multidisciplinary team for management decisions, defining the indications for imaging and biopsy, timing and duration of follow-up, and the role of surgery versus conservative management. Future developments will focus on exploring novel and experimental therapeutic targets in these tumours and developing an international consensus on clinical management to achieve a streamlined, safe, evidence-based approach.

REFERENCES

1. Marrero JA, Ahn J, Rajender Reddy K. ACG clinical guideline: The diagnosis and management of focal liver lesions. *Am J Gastroenterol* 2014;**109(9)**: 1328–47.
2. Reddy KR, Schiff ER. Approach to a liver mass. *Semin Liver Dis* 1993;**13(4)**:423–35.

3. Mergo PJ, Ros PR. Benign lesions of the liver. *Radiol Clin North Am* 1998;**36(2)**:319–31.

4. Weinberg AG, Finegold MJ. Primary hepatic tumors of childhood. *Hum Pathol* 1983;**14(6)**:512–37.

5. International Working P. Terminology of nodular hepatocellular lesions. *Hepatology* 1995;**22(3)**:983–93.

6. Baum JK, Bookstein JJ, Holtz F, Klein EW. Possible association between benign hepatomas and oral contraceptives. *Lancet* 1973;**2(7835)**:926–9.

7. Edmondson HA, Steiner PE. Primary carcinoma of the liver: A study of 100 cases among 48,900 necropsies. *Cancer* 1954;**7(3)**:462–503.

8. Bunchorntavakul C, Bahirwani R, Drazek D, Soulen MC, Siegelman ES, Furth EE, et al. Clinical features and natural history of hepatocellular adenomas: The impact of obesity. *Aliment Pharmacol Ther* 2011;**34(6)**:664–74.

9. Labrune P, Trioche P, Duvaltier I, Chevalier P, Odièvre M. Hepatocellular adenomas in glycogen storage disease type I and III: A series of 43 patients and review of the literature. *J Pediatr Gastroenterol Nutr* 1997;**24(3)**:276–9.

10. Brenard R, Chapaux X, Deltenre P, Henrion J, De Maeght S, Horsmans Y, et al. Large spectrum of liver vascular lesions including high prevalence of focal nodular hyperplasia in patients with hereditary haemorrhagic telangiectasia: The Belgian Registry based on 30 patients. *Eur J Gastroenterol Hepatol* 2010;**22(10)**:1253–9.

11. Chiche L, Dao T, Salamé E, Galais MP, Bouvard N, Schmutz G, et al. Liver adenomatosis: Reappraisal, diagnosis, and surgical management: Eight new cases and review of the literature. *Ann Surg* 2000;**231(1)**:74–81.

12. Franchi-Abella S, Branchereau S. Benign hepatocellular tumors in children: Focal nodular hyperplasia and hepatocellular adenoma. *Int J Hepatol* 2013;**2013**:215064.

13. Flejou JF, Barge J, Menu Y, Degott C, Bismuth H, Potet F, et al. Liver adenomatosis. An entity distinct from liver adenoma? *Gastroenterology* 1985;**89(5)**:1132–8.

14. Sasaki M, Yoneda N, Kitamura S, Sato Y, Nakanuma Y. Characterization of hepatocellular adenoma based on the phenotypic classification: The Kanazawa experience. *Hepatol Res* 2011;**41(10)**:982–8.

15. Bellamy CO, Maxwell RS, Prost S, Azodo IA, Powell JJ, Manning JR. The value of immunophenotyping hepatocellular adenomas: Consecutive resections at one UK centre. *Histopathology* 2013;**62(3)**:431–45.

16. van Aalten SM, Verheij J, Terkivatan T, Dwarkasing RS, de Man RA, Izermans JNM. Validation of a liver adenoma classification system in a tertiary referral centre: Implications for clinical practice. *J Hepatol* 2011;**55(1)**:120–5.

17. Nault J-C, Paradis V, Cherqui D, Vilgrain V, Zucman-Rossi J. Molecular classification of hepatocellular adenoma in clinical practice. *J Hepatol* 2017;**67(5)**:1074–83.

18. Bioulac-Sage P, Sempoux C, Frulio N, Le Bail B, Blanc JF, Castain C, et al. Snapshot summary of diagnosis and management of hepatocellular adenoma subtypes. *Clin Res Hepatol Gastroenterol* 2019;**43(1)**:12–19.

19. Bonder A, Afdhal N. Evaluation of liver lesions. *Clin Liver Dis* 2012;**16(2)**:271–83.

20. Karhunen PJ. Benign hepatic tumours and tumour like conditions in men. *J Clin Pathol* 1986;**39(2)**:183–8.

21. Dokmak S, Paradis V, Vilgrain V, Sauvanet A, Farges O, Valla D, et al. A single-center surgical experience of 122 patients with single and multiple hepatocellular adenomas. *Gastroenterology* 2009;**137(5)**:1698–705.

22. van Aalten SM, de Man RA, IJzermans JNM, Terkivatan T. Systematic review of haemorrhage and rupture of hepatocellular adenomas. *Br J Surg* 2012;**99(7)**:911–16.

23. Nault JC, Mallet M, Pilati C, Calderaro J, Bioulac-Sage P, Laurent C, et al. High frequency of telomerase reverse-transcriptase promoter somatic mutations in hepatocellular carcinoma and preneoplastic lesions. *Nat Commun* 2013;**4**:2218.

24. Oldhafer KJ, Habbel V, Horling K, Makridis G, Wagner KC. Benign liver tumors. *Visc Med* 2020;**36(4)**:292–303.

25. Zheng J, Sadot E, Vigidal JA, Klimstra DS, Balachandran VP, Kingham TP, et al. Characterization of hepatocellular adenoma and carcinoma using microRNA profiling and targeted gene sequencing. *PLoS One* 2018;**13(17)**:e0200776.

26. Ribeiro A, Burgart LJ, Nagorney DM, Gores GJ. Management of liver adenomatosis: Results with a conservative surgical approach. *Liver Transpl Surg* 1998;**4(5)**:388–98.

27. Zucman-Rossi J, Jeannot E, Nhieu JT, Scoazec J-Y, Guettier C, Rebouissou S, et al. Genotype- phenotype correlation in hepatocellular adenoma: New classification and relationship with HCC. *Hepatology* 2006;**43(3)**:515–24.

28. Ronot M, Bahrami S, Calderaro J, Valla D-C, Bedossa P, Belghiti J, et al. Hepatocellular adenomas: Accuracy of magnetic resonance imaging and liver biopsy in subtype classification. *Hepatology* 2011;**53(4)**:1182–91.

29. Agarwal S, Fuentes-Orrego JM, Arnason T, Misdraji J, Jhaveri KS, Harisinghani M, et al. Inflammatory hepatocellular adenomas can mimic focal nodular hyperplasia on gadoxetic acid-enhanced MRI. *AJR Am J Roentgenol* 2014;**203(4)**:W408–14.

30. Bieze M, van den Esschert JW, Nio CY, Verheij J, Reitsma JB, Terpstra V, et al. Diagnostic accuracy of MRI in differentiating hepatocellular adenoma from focal nodular hyperplasia: Prospective study of the additional value of gadoxetate disodium. *AJR Am J Roentgenol* 2012;**199(1)**:26–34.

31. Ba-Ssalamah A, Antunes C, Feier D, Bastati N, Hodge JC, Stift J, et al. Morphologic and molecular features of hepatocellular adenoma with gadoxetic acid-enhanced MR imaging. *Radiology* 2015;**277(1)**:104–13.

32. European Association for the Study of the Liver (EASL). EASL Clinical Practice Guidelines on the management of benign liver tumours. *J Hepatol* 2016;**65(2)**:386–98.

33. Haring MPD, Cuperus FJC, Duiker EW, de Haas RJ, de Meijer VE. Scoping review of clinical practice guidelines on the management of benign liver tumours. *BMJ Open Gastroenterol* 2021;**8(1)**:e000592.

34. van Rosmalen BV, Klompenhouwer AJ, de Graeff JJ, Haring MPD, de Meijer VE, Rifai L, et al. Safety and efficacy of transarterial embolization of hepatocellular adenomas. *Br J Surg* 2019;**106(10)**:1362–71.

35. Fuchs J, Warmann SW, Urla C, Schäfer JF, Schmidt A. Management of benign liver tumors. *Semin Pediatr Surg* 2020;**29(4)**:150941.

36. Qureshi SS, Bhagat M, Kembhavi S, Vora T, Ramadwar M, Chinnaswamy G, et al. Benign liver tumors in children: Outcomes after resection. *Pediatr Surg Int* 2015;**31(12)**:1145–9.

37. Rebouissou S, Amessou M, Couchy G, Poussin K, Imbeaud S, Pilati C, et al. Frequent in-frame somatic deletions activate gp130 in inflammatory hepatocellular tumours. *Nature* 2009;**457(7226)**:200–4.

38. Pilati C, Amessou M, Bihl MP, Balabaud C, Van Nhieu JT, Paradis V, et al. Somatic mutations activating STAT3 in human inflammatory hepatocellular adenomas. *J Exp Med* 2011;**208(7)**:1359–66.

39. Nguyen BN, Fléjou JF, Terris B, Belghiti J, Degott C. Focal nodular hyperplasia of the liver: A comprehensive pathologic study of 305 lesions and recognition of new histologic forms. *Am J Surg Pathol* 1999;**23(12)**:1441–54.

40. Towbin AJ, Luo GG, Yin H, Mo JQ. Focal nodular hyperplasia in children, adolescents, and young adults. *Pediatr Radiol* 2011;**41(3)**:341–9.

41. Freidl T, Lackner H, Huber J, Sovinz P, Moser A, Schroettner B, et al. Focal nodular hyperplasia in children following treatment of hemato-oncologic diseases. *Klin Padiatr* 2008;**220(6)**:384–7.

42. Laurent C, Trillaud H, Lepreux S, Balabaud C, Bioulac-Sage P. Association of adenoma and focal nodular hyperplasia: Experience of a single French academic center. *Comp Hepatol* 2003;**2(1)**:6.

43. Buscarini E, Danesino C, Plauchu H, de Fazio C, Olivieri C, Brambilla G, et al. High prevalence of hepatic focal nodular hyperplasia in subjects with hereditary hemorrhagic telangiectasia. *Ultrasound Med Biol* 2004;**30(9)**:1089–97.

44. Rifai K, Mix H, Krusche S, Potthoff A, Manns MP, Gebel MJ. No evidence of substantial growth progression or complications of large focal nodular hyperplasia during pregnancy. *Scand J Gastroenterol* 2013;**48(1)**:88–92.

45. D'Halluin V, Vilgrain V, Pelletier G, Rocher L, Belghiti J, Erlinger S, et al. Natural history of focal nodular hyperplasia. A retrospective study of 44 cases. *Gastroenterol Clin Biol* 2001;**25(11)**:1008–10.

46. Bouyn CI-D, Leclere J, Raimondo G, Le Pointe HD, Couanet D, Valteau-Couanet D, et al. Hepatic focal nodular hyperplasia in children previously treated for a solid tumor. Incidence, risk factors, and outcome. *Cancer* 2003;**97(12)**:3107–13.

47. Cherqui D, Rahmouni A, Charlotte F, Boulahdour H, Métreau JM, Meignan M, et al. Management of focal nodular hyperplasia and hepatocellular adenoma in young women: A series of 41 patients with clinical, radiological, and pathological correlations. *Hepatology* 1995;**22(6)**:1674–81.

48. Paradis V, Benzekri A, Dargère D, Bièche I, Laurendeau I, Vilgrain V, et al. Telangiectatic focal nodular

hyperplasia: A variant of hepatocellular adenoma. *Gastroenterology* 2004;**126(5)**:1323–9.

49. Cazals-Hatem D, Vilgrain V, Genin P, Denninger M-H, Durand F, Belghiti J, et al. Arterial and portal circulation and parenchymal changes in Budd-Chiari syndrome: A study in 17 explanted livers. *Hepatology* 2003;**37(3)**:510–19.

50. Weimann A, Ringe B, Klempnauer J, Lamesch P, Gratz KF, Prokop M, et al. Benign liver tumors: Differential diagnosis and indications for surgery. *World J Surg* 1997;**21(9)**:983–90.

51. Luciani A, Kobeiter H, Maison P, Cherqui D, Zafrani E-S, Dhumeaux D, et al. Focal nodular hyperplasia of the liver in men: Is presentation the same in men and women? *Gut* 2002;**50(6)**:877–80.

52. Bioulac-Sage P, Laumonier H, Rullier A, Cubel G, Laurent C, Zucman-Rossi J, et al. Over-expression of glutamine synthetase in focal nodular hyperplasia: A novel easy diagnostic tool in surgical pathology. *Liver Int* 2009;**29(3)**:459–65.

53. Kehagias D, Moulopoulos L, Antoniou A, Hatziioannou A, Smyrniotis V, Trakadas S, et al. Focal nodular hyperplasia: Imaging findings. *Eur Radiol* 2001;**11(2)**:202–12.

54. Bertin C, Egels S, Wagner M, Huynh-Charlier I, Vilgrain V, Lucidarme O. Contrast-enhanced ultrasound of focal nodular hyperplasia: A matter of size. *Eur Radiol* 2014;**24(10)**:2561–71.

55. Grazioli L, Morana G, Kirchin MA, Schneider G. Accurate differentiation of focal nodular hyperplasia from hepatic adenoma at gadobenate dimeglumine-enhanced MR imaging: Prospective study. *Radiology* 2005;**236(1)**:166–77.

56. Lautz T, Tantemsapya N, Dzakovic A, Superina R. Focal nodular hyperplasia in children: Clinical features and current management practice. *J Pediatr Surg* 2010;**45(9)**:1797–803.

57. Gandolfi L, Leo P, Solmi L, Vitelli E, Verros G, Colecchia A. Natural history of hepatic haemangiomas: Clinical and ultrasound study. *Gut* 1991;**32(6)**:677–80.

58. Glinkova V, Shevah O, Boaz M, Levine A, Shirin H. Hepatic haemangiomas: Possible association with female sex hormones. *Gut* 2004;**53(9)**:1352–5.

59. Iacobas I, Phung TL, Adams DM, Trenor CC 3rd, Blei F, Fishman DS, et al. Guidance document for hepatic hemangioma (infantile and congenital) evaluation and monitoring. *J Pediatr* 2018;**203**:294–300.

60. Lee M, Choi J-Y, Lim JS, Park M-S, Kim M-J, Kim H. Lack of anti-tumor activity by anti-VEGF treatments in hepatic hemangiomas. *Angiogenesis* 2016;**19(2)**:147–53.

61. Hall GW. Kasabach-Merritt syndrome: Pathogenesis and management. *Br J Haematol* 2001;**112(4)**:851–62.

62. O'Rafferty C, O'Regan GM, Irvine AD, Smith OP. Recent advances in the pathobiology and management of Kasabach-Merritt phenomenon. *Br J Haematol* 2015;**171(1)**:38–51.

63. Quaia E, Bertolotto M, Dalla Palma L. Characterization of liver hemangiomas with pulse inversion harmonic imaging. *Eur Radiol* 2002;**12(3)**:537–44.

64. Hanafusa K, Ohashi I, Himeno Y, Suzuki S, Shibuya H. Hepatic hemangioma: Findings with two-phase CT. *Radiology* 1995;**196**(2):465–9.

65. Coumbaras M, Wendum D, Monnier-Cholley L, Dahan H, Tubiana JM, Arrivé L. CT and MR imaging features of pathologically proven atypical giant hemangiomas of the liver. *AJR Am J Roentgenol* 2002;**179**(6):1457–63.

66. Doo KW, Lee CH, Choi JW, Lee J, Kim KA, Park CM. "Pseudo washout" sign in high-flow hepatic hemangioma on gadoxetic acid contrast-enhanced MRI mimicking hypervascular tumor. *AJR Am J Roentgenol* 2009;**193**(6): W490–6.

67. Miura JT, Amini A, Schmocker R, Nichols S, Sukato D, Winslow ER, et al. Surgical management of hepatic hemangiomas: A multi-institutional experience. *HPB (Oxford)* 2014;**16**(10):924–8.

68. Zhang W, Huang Z-Y, Ke C-S, Wu C, Zhang Z-W, Zhang B-X, et al. Surgical treatment of giant liver hemangioma larger than 10 cm: A single center's experience with 86 patients. *Medicine (Baltimore)* 2015;**94**(34):e1420.

69. van Rosmalen BV, de Graeff JJ, van der Poel MJ, de Man IE, Besselink M, Hilal MA, et al. Impact of open and minimally invasive resection of symptomatic solid benign liver tumours on symptoms and quality of life: A systematic review. *HPB (Oxford)* 2019;**21**(9):1119–30.

70. Ercolani G, Grazi GL, Pinna AD. Liver transplantation for benign hepatic tumors: A systematic review. *Dig Surg* 2010;**27**(1):68–75.

71. Zhao Y, Legan CE. Liver Transplantation for giant hemangioma complicated by kKasabach-Merritt syndrome: A case report and literature review. *Am J Case Rep* 2022;**23**:e936042.

72. Liu X, Yang Z, Tan H, Huang J, Xu L, Liu L, et al. Long-term result of transcatheter arterial embolization for liver hemangioma. *Medicine (Baltimore)* 2017;**96**(49):e9029.

73. Akhlaghpoor S, Torkian P, Golzarian J. Transarterial bleomycin-lipiodol embolization (B/LE) for symptomatic giant hepatic hemangioma. *Cardiovasc Intervent Radiol* 2018;**41**(11):1674–82.

74. Gao J, Fan R-F, Yang J-Y, Cui Y, Ji J-S, Ma K-S, et al. Radiofrequency ablation for hepatic hemangiomas: A consensus from a Chinese panel of experts. *World J Gastroenterol* 2017;**23**(39):7077–86.

75. Song YS, Tian YF, Lai WG, et al. Percutaneous injection of cinnamyl foam sclerosing agent in hemangioma of blood supply liver. *J Prac Med* 2016;**32**:4094–7.

76. Silverman SG, Tuncali K, Adams DF, vanSonnenberg E, Zou KH, Kacher DF, et al. MR imaging–guided percutaneous cryotherapy of liver tumors: Initial experience. *Radiology* 2000;**217**(3):657–64.

77. Christison-Lagay ER, Burrows PE, Alomari A, Dubois J, Kozakewich HP, Lane TS, et al. Hepatic hemangiomas: Sub-type classification and development of a clinical practice algorithm and registry. *J Pediatr Surg* 2007;**42**(1):62–7.

78. Rialon KL, Murillo R, Fevurly RD, Kulungowski AM, Christison-Lagay ER, Zurakowski D, et al. Risk factors for mortality in patients with multifocal and diffuse hepatic hemangiomas. *J Pediatr Surg* 2015;**50**(5):837–41.

79. Damaskos C, Garmpis N, Garmpi A, Nonni A, Sakellariou S, Margonis G-A, et al. Angiomyolipoma of the Liver: A rare benign tumor treated with a laparoscopic approach for the first time. *In Vivo* 2017;**31**(6):1169–73.

80. Balabaud C, Bioulac-Sage P, Goodman ZD, Makhlouf HR. Inflammatory pseudotumor of the liver: A rare but distinct tumor-like lesion. *Gastroenterol Hepatol (NY)* 2012;**8**(9):633–4.

81. Hartleb M, Gutkowski K, Milkiewicz P. Nodular regenerative hyperplasia: Evolving concepts on underdiagnosed cause of portal hypertension. *World J Gastroenterol* 2011;**17**(11):1400–9.

82. Abdelmalak M, Pendse A. Liver and intrahepatic bile ducts: Hepatocellular adenoma. Available from: https://www.pathologyoutlines.com/topic/livertumorhepatocellularadenoma.html (Accessed September 2024).

83. Grazioli L, Federle MP, Brancatelli G, Ichikawa T, et al. Hepatic adenomas: Imaging and pathologic findings. *Radiographics* 2001;**21**(4):877–92.

Bailey & Love's Essential Operations Bailey & Love's Essential Operatio
Bailey & Love's Essential Operations Bailey & Love's Essential Operatio
Bailey & Love's Essential Operations Bailey & Love's Essential Operatio

SECTION 8 | LIVER

Chapter

53

Liver Cysts and Polycystic Liver Disease

Rohan Kumar and A. M. James Shapiro

INTRODUCTION

Polycystic liver diseases (PLD) are an inherited cilio-cholangiopathy characterized by multiple and, at least twenty, liver cysts occupying at least half the volume of liver parenchyma (1). The cilio-cholangiopathy results in a malformation within a biliary-type epithelium and a failure to communicate with the biliary tree. This entity is common to all liver cysts irrespective of whether they are isolated and simple, or multiple cysts in PLD. Liver cysts are differentiated histopathologically from the cystic walls of hydatid, biliary cystadenoma, cystic hepatobiliary neoplasia and cystic dilatation of intrahepatic biliary ducts (2,3).

Microscopically, liver cysts are bordered by cuboidal or columnar, uniform cells and resemble biliary epithelium and are benign. Small simple cysts lack stroma, whilst larger ones stretch their stroma to the extent of reducing it to a thin film.

The formation of liver cysts occurs due to an accelerated differentiation of hepatoblasts into cholangiocyte precursors. Hyperproliferation in cholangiocytes leads to enhanced fluid secretion and is combined with a malformation of the biliary ductal plates (4–6).

An aberrant biliary duct loses communication with the biliary tree and progressively dilates with time. Both cellular differentiation and secretory function are maintained and fluid production from the latter leads to positive intraluminal pressures, occasionally in excess of 30 cm H_2O and accounts for symptoms. The secretory fluid contains water, minerals and electrolytes and is similar in composition to bile, although, bile acid salts and bilirubin are absent and it is therefore non-toxic to the peritoneum. The non-toxic nature of secretory fluid is the basis of the rationale for cyst fenestration as one operative solution to the problem of symptomatic, pressurized, large and dominant liver cysts (1–3).

Large cysts produce atrophy of the adjacent liver tissue which leads to compensatory hypertrophy in the contralateral lobe. The areas of atrophy that lie in contact with cysts contain an abundance of bile ducts and blood vessels. These may persist after atrophy and protrude to form folds over the inner surface of the liver cyst. Liver cysts are unilocular and do not contain septations (3).

LIVER CYSTS

Prevalence

Gender, age and the incidence of liver cysts are related. Liver cysts are not common under 40 years of age but the incidence increases sharply thereafter. They are more common in women, with a female to male ratio of 1.5 : 1 at necropsy. This ratio rises to 9 : 1 in symptomatic or complicated liver cysts, and huge cysts almost exclusively affect women in their fifties.

Diagnosis

The majority of liver cysts can be identified with ultrasonography (US) and this is useful for diagnosis in those without symptoms. US identifies sharp, oval or circular shaped anechoic lesions, with a smooth border. Lesions also have a clear posterior acoustic shadow because cysts have a well-defined interface between their fluid and the liver parenchyma. Septations may be falsely over-interpreted, especially when two or more cysts lie immediately next to each other. Computed tomography (CT) scanning contributes little to US for the diagnosis of liver cysts but will give a clearer understanding of the topographical orientation of cysts in relation to each other and to bile ducts and vessels. Usually, with magnetic resonance imaging (MRI), liver cysts are homogeneous, hypointense on T1 and very hyperintense on T2 sequences (*Figures 53.1–53.4*).

The causal relationship between abdominal discomfort or pain with a simple liver cyst is a diagnosis of exclusion. Occasionally, the fluid within a simple cyst is so tense that it may be mistaken for a solid tumour, and although the liver parenchyma and biochemistry *per se* are usually preserved, a cyst may cause extrinsic compression of a bile duct(s). Fluid biochemistry has a high concentration of cancer antigen (CA) 19-9 and carcinoembryonic antigen (CEA) but low levels of glycoprotein-72, and serum CA 19-9 levels may also be raised.

Natural history of liver cysts

Most cases are asymptomatic and the use of serial US for surveillance difficult to justify. This is because most people with simple cysts are stable, often over long periods and, ultrasonography will not demonstrate

DOI: 10.1201/9781003080060-53

any appreciable change, although particularly women in their fifties, may rapidly develop severe pain due to growth and capsular stretching. Complications seldom arise, the most frequent being intra-cyst bleeding, probably secondary to arterial erosion within the liver parenchyma immediately adjacent to a cyst. This results in sudden severe pain from the increased size of the cyst due to the accumulated blood. The severe pain tends to last a few days and is associated with moderate elevations of g-glutamyl-transferase with otherwise normal liver biochemistry. Ultrasonography may reveal clots and other mobile, dependent echoic material within cysts. Bacterial infections however are to be considered the exception and they may occasionally result from cystic erosion into bile ducts, allowing direct inoculation with biliary commensals. Tense cysts, if appropriately located, may compress the inferior vena cava and lead to acute Budd–Chiari syndrome and cystic compression of hepatic veins or biliary radicals are alternative causes for perioperative morbidity (*Figure 53.1*). Pulmonary symptoms are due to cysts that are located in the hepatic dome, particularly on the right side, which elevate the diaphragm occasionally up to the level of the pulmonary hilum. Meanwhile cysts near to the hepatic hilum may compress the portal vein, and while this is relatively common, the development of portal hypertension with secondary porto-systemic collateralization and ascites is fortunately rare (*Figure 53.1*).

Clinical management of liver cysts

Asymptomatic liver cysts require neither treatment nor surveillance. Asymptomatic cysts tend to be less than 8 cm and do not protrude beyond the liver surface or compress neighbouring organs. If this is not the case, or the symptoms are vague, then an empirical trial of US-guided needle aspiration may be undertaken. When aspiration successfully alleviates symptoms, and improvements are transient because of inevitable fluid re-accumulation, then a longer-term solution is sought. Conversely, in asymptomatic patients but with radiological evidence of compression of key structures such as bile ducts, the inferior vena cava, portal and/ or hepatic veins, the correct management is less clear and it is difficult to decide when, and if, to intervene. Intervention may be considered if these abnormalities are unilateral, and the contralateral hemi-liver has its normal biliary drainage preserved and there is no compromise to vascular perfusion or outflow. There are two treatment options for symptomatic hepatic cysts, sclerotherapy *and* fenestration.

Cyst sclerotherapy

The cyst epithelium lining is destroyed with US-guided sclerotherapy, preventing further intra-cyst fluid secretion. Cysts are punctured with small drainage catheters using the Seldinger technique and water-soluble contrast is injected to confirm that there is no

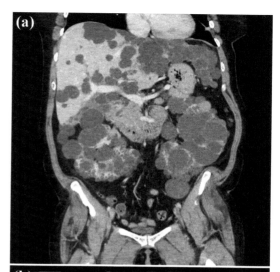
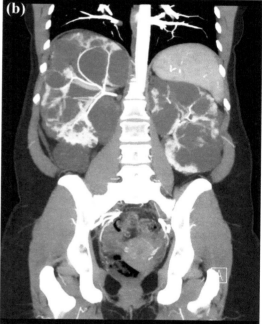

Figure 53.1 Coronal MR images showing (a) compression and stretching of the main portal vein due to cysts around the hilum and (b) stretching and distortion of the segmental arteries as they circumnavigate around two adjacent cysts.

communication with the peritoneal cavity or biliary tract. Both are absolute contraindications to sclerotherapy. The sclerosant of choice is 95% ethanol, with minocycline hydrochloride (pleurodesis), ethanolamine oleate, hypertonic saline and bleomycin being less frequently used alternatives. The volume of 95% ethanol injection is limited to around 100 mL because alcohol sclerotherapy is associated with an increase in blood alcohol levels, although ethanol induced intoxication or coma, are rarely reported. The patient is rolled so that the alcohol may come into contact with the entirety of the epithelial surface and the alcohol is then aspirated and catheter removed. The procedure may be painful and tends to be better tolerated if performed under general anaesthesia. Alcohol sclerotherapy may be repeated, but should be delayed for at least 3 months when cystic communication with biliary ducts has occurred. Inadvertently punctured vessels during the procedure may later bleed and so patients are often observed overnight rather than discharged as a day case (1,2,7).

Cyst fenestration

Alternatively, the cyst is drained by creating a direct communication between the cyst and peritoneum, usually by laparoscopic fenestration. Fenestration prevents fluid re-accumulation and is the treatment of choice for single, large, dominant, symptomatic cysts that protrude beyond the confines of the normal liver parenchyma. Following fenestration, cyst fluid secretion continues and, together with peritoneal reabsorption, the cyst cavity eventually collapses. Postoperative bleeding and biliary peritonitis are less likely because liver parenchymal dissection is avoided. The most severe intraoperative complication is bleeding when the liver parenchyma rather than the cyst wall is opened. The open conversion rate is around 5% with the most frequently quoted reason being intraoperative bleeding. Patients may stay in hospital between 1–3 days as late bleeds or bile leaks may result from the re-expansion of portal pedicles that were previously compressed by a cyst and which were poorly secured intraoperatively. Consideration should be given to either endovascular stapling or intra-corporeal suturing techniques for haemostasis in cyst walls that are particularly thick. Ascites is a very rare complication after fenestration of simple liver cysts (conferatur PLD).

Sclerotherapy versus fenestration

Both sclerotherapy and fenestration techniques have been performed for several decades but they have not been compared with one another in randomized control trials or prospective comparative studies (8,9). Furthermore, the severity of symptoms that lead to intervention has not been standardized and symptom recurrence poorly defined. They would appear to be as effective as each other, and consequently some centres favour offering a 'step-up' approach, with fenestration being reserved as a salvage procedure for recurrence following two previous sclerotherapy sessions (6,8–12).

POLYCYSTIC LIVER DISEASES

Polycystic liver diseases (note: plural, diseases) are genetic disorders that lead to the development of multiple liver cysts. There are two forms of PLD, those that occur with adult polycystic kidney disease (ADPKD) and those without. ADPKD occurs with a preponderance of 1 in 800 live births and it is characterized by progressive development and enlargement of kidney cysts which leads ultimately to renal failure in half those affected. PLD is the most frequent extra-renal manifestation with the liver cysts developing following the kidney cysts. The overall prevalence is similar in men and women, however, as with simple cysts, women tend to follow a more severe course particularly if multiparous, or taking exogenous oestrogen (13).

Isolated PLD is rare with an incidence of less than 0.01%. In clinical series that deal with symptomatic patients only, isolated PLD cases are 2–5 times less frequent than those associated with ADPKD and isolated PLD generally follows a milder clinical course. Two forms of ADPKD are linked to mutations in either the *PKD1* or *PKD2* gene. *PKD1* encodes polycystin-1 and is found on the short arm of chromosome 16, accounting for 85% of PLD cases. *PKD2* is found on chromosome 4 and encodes polycystin-2. *PKD1* mutation is associated with larger renal cysts, a greater prevalence of hypertension and more frequent progression to end stage renal disease than *PKD2* mutations.

Isolated PLD is associated with heterogenous gene mutations. The protein kinase C substrate 80K-H (*PRKCSH*), *SEC63*, or *LRP5* genes affect the secretory function of the endoplasmic reticulum (14). *PRKCSH* encodes hepatocystin which functions as the beta subunit for alpha-glucosidase 2, and is required for protein folding and quality control of newly synthesized glycoproteins. SEC63 protein is involved in transport across the endoplasmic reticulum and polycystin-1 and polycystin-2 cause dysfunctional cilia. In those with isolated PLD, polycystin may be the target of aberrant maturation of glycoproteins PRKCSH or *SEC63* mutations (5). Gene mutations account for a variable 25–40% of cases. PLD has an autosomal dominant inheritance pattern, but at the molecular level they are recessive diseases because they require a second, 'two hit' theory, for cell proliferation and cyst formation. Individuals need a germline mutation and a second, loss of function, somatic mutation in the gene copy. This explains the sporadic nature of affected liver cells, and may in part also explain the clinical heterogeneity (4,14).

Angiogenic factors may promote vascularization in PLD cysts, and direct cholangiocyte stimulation and PLD cysts are both insulin growth factor-1 (IGF-1) and oestrogen receptor positive. These observations explain the rationale for various medical therapies with vasopressin antagonists, somatostatin analogues, inhibition of mammalian target of rapamycin (mTOR) signalling, or inhibition of vascular endothelial growth factor (VEGF) (7,13,15).

Diagnosis

The majority of liver cysts remain small and asymptomatic, but even with massive liver enlargement, because of the number or size of the cysts, significant hepatic complications remain uncommon. Symptoms include abdominal pain or discomfort, early satiety, shortness of breath and lower limb oedema. This is due to a mass effect with compression of the stomach, diaphragm and inferior vena cava occasionally by single or multiple large cysts, but usually because of gross enlargement of the whole liver (*Figure 53.2*). Due to the chronicity of progression, it is not uncommon for patients to become accustomed to significant discomfort and be consciously unaware. They may eat small and light meals more frequently and only offer this symptom upon direct questioning. Clinical examination may reveal cysts that are so tense they are misinterpreted as solid tumours. It is not uncommon for the inferior edge of the liver to be palpable down to the iliac fossae. Periods of self-limiting abdominal pain are not unusual because of spontaneous cyst bleeds or infection, and as the disease progresses abdominal ascites and/or pleural effusions may develop. This is in addition to sarcopoenia from a progressive deterioration of nutritional intake and body weight is initially inaccurate and can be misleading as a marker of sarcopoenia because as skeletal muscle mass declines, the mass of the liver increases, sometimes eventually weighing up to 10 kilograms. It is better to use the abdominal wall and psoas muscle thickness and density on cross-sectional imaging as a surrogate of sarcopoenia (*Figure 53.2*). Typically, the patient is female, referred between the ages of 35 and 50, having been diagnosed with PLD a decade previously with incapacitating symptoms for a few years prior to surgical review. The clinical management is the same irrespective of whether PLD is isolated or as part of ADPKD entities.

Clinical management of PLD

Symptomatic dominant cysts with mass effect based on history and physical examination, corroborated radiologically are managed in a similar fashion to simple liver cysts. Schnelldorfer's and Gigot's classifications aim to identify those patients that may benefit from resection or transplantation (10,11,16). Schnelldorfer's classification takes into account a number of factors: 1) symptoms (absent, moderate, or severe); 2) the number and size of cysts; 3) the presence of normal liver parenchyma (at least two sectors, more than one sector, or less than one sector), and 4) the presence of iso-sectoral portal or hepatic vein occlusion of the preserved sector (*Table 53.1*) (10,11,16).

Medical treatment

Avoidance of oestrogen hormonal replacement appears logical but there is a paucity of evidence and patients should be counselled accordingly (17,18). Somatostatin analogues are considered more useful because somatostatin receptors are expressed on cholangiocytes and when stimulated they activate proliferation via cyclic AMP (cAMP) signals (19). Blocking the secretin induced cAMP cascade with octreotide blunts hepatic cyst expansion (13,15,20,21). Sirolimus inhibits secretion and proliferation of biliary and cystic epithelium via mTOR and it has been shown to be effective in ADPKD kidney transplant recipients. When anti-rejection regimes contain sirolimus, reductions in both the native kidney and liver cystic volumes, have been noted in comparison to similar patients maintained on calcineurin inhibitors alone (20,22). Noteworthy is that the additional benefits of everolimus with octreotide is not supported by any conclusive data (23).

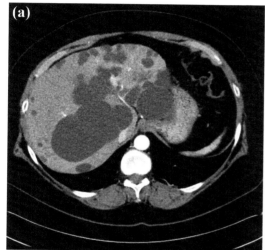

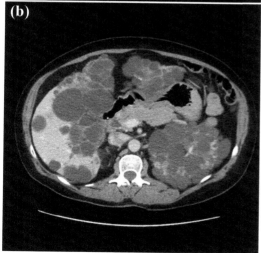

Figure 53.2 Axial MR images showing (a) mass effect caused by extensive polycystic liver disease causing extrinsic compression of the outflow to the stomach. This leads (b) to gradual denutrition (small stomach/poor psoas muscle bulk) and secondary sarcopenia.

Table 53.1 Schnelldorfer and Gigot classification of polycystic liver disease

Schnelldorfer	Type A	Type B	Type C	Type D
Gigot	I	II	III	III
Symptoms	Absent	Moderate or severe	Severe	Severe
Size & number of cysts	Moderate few	Few that are large in size	Few that are large in size and some small multiple cysts	Innumerable
Number of spared liver segments	>3 segments	>= 2 segments	>=1 segment	<1 segment
Prescence of collateral venous circulation in the spared segment	Moderate	Absent	Absent	Present
Recommended treatment	Rx abstention or medical rx	Fenestration	Partial hepatectomy with fenestration of contralateral cysts	Hepatic transplantation

Clinical and other experimental therapeutic approaches to control PLD

Surgical treatment

As a general rule, sclerotherapy and laparoscopic fenestrations are ineffective in highly symptomatic patients with PLD, especially if there is diffuse and massive involvement of the liver. Some patients may, however, have a few (up to five) dominant liver cysts with many smaller clinically less significant cysts (*Figure 53.3*). Even in these patients, sclerotherapy may not control symptoms because they are related to the multiplicity of liver cysts which cannot all be targeted. Fenestrations in the setting of PLD, as compared to simple cyst treatment, are more likely to be complicated by biliary peritonitis and postoperative bleeding. A Glissonean radical containing peripheral branches of the hepatic artery, portal vein and bile ducts typically traverses the cyst walls, and it is easy to inadvertently overlook these radicles in substantial and deep fenestration attempts. Meticulous identification and suture transfixion of these structures may be required to avoid such complications and intra-operative cholangiography to confirm that both hemi-livers have adequate biliary drainage at the end of the procedure is therefore advised. Ascites with, or without, infection may develop postoperatively and, in turn, compromise wound healing. The mechanism for postoperative ascites is multifactorial with persistent cyst fluid secretion from the unablated epithelium compounded by outflow obstruction from non-fenestrated cysts, compressing the terminal hepatic veins especially in patients with impaired renal function (1,24).

Hepatectomy

Partial liver resections may be considered in combination with fenestration of the remnant liver. Resections reduce disease burden and stimulated liver regeneration

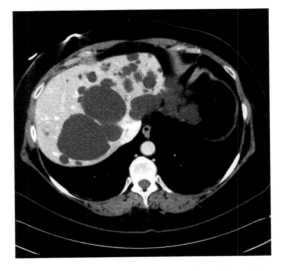

Figure 53.3 Axial MR image of a female patient with a right hemi-hepatectomy resection with some fenestrations to the left lobe. The variable nature of liver cysts in PLD may mean that one hemi-liver is amenable to a resection in the hope that the remaining parenchyma regenerates without cysts.

and it is hoped the new parenchyma will not contain cysts. Resection is possible where there is an asymmetric distribution of cysts and relatively spared segments. Regeneration is associated with the expansion of spared areas while the volume of the remaining small cysts remains unchanged or progress slowly. Hepatectomy is invaluable for certain patients, but it is technically challenging with a high associated morbidity, and indications must be highly selective and restrictive. It is only effective if the quantity of liver to be resected is at least three segments and the future functional liver remnant of sufficient volume to meet the immediate postoperative metabolic and synthetic function requirements. Hepatectomy aims to resect as much cystic liver as possible, caveated with the maintenance of sufficient outflow from the remaining liver. Some patients may have developed venous outflow collaterals between the hepatic veins which may facilitate and dictate the intra-operative resection margin. Often the resection is either a left lateral sectionectomy, left bi-sectionectomy or a right bi-sectionectomy and with left sided resections, caudate resection may be a necessary adjunct.

The technical challenges centre around distortion of the usual landmarks within the parenchyma and important structures may be unrecognized, compounded by intra-operative US imaging which is generally not helpful as peripheral portal structures are often small and compressed. Additionally, anechoic regions and posterior shadows simply confuse the greyscale image and surgeon alike (*Figure 53.4*). The operative solution commences with surface cyst fenestration to facilitate liver mobilization. Transection proceeds in the non-cystic parenchyma or from cyst cavity to cyst cavity in stepwise fashion, and care must be taken when approaching the biliary confluence as Glissonean pedicles are often compressed. A cyst wall should not be divided unless absolute certainty exists about the nature of its contents, if necessary, using intraoperative cholangiography to facilitate the identification of bile ducts. Following hepatectomy, the remnant side is widely fenestrated and consequently bile leaks are relatively common. Particularly following right sided resections, the remnant liver should be secured with the falciform reconstructed to maintain venous outflow and prevent torsion. The most frequent postoperative morbidity arises from the accumulation of ascites and/or the development of pleural effusions with early perioperative mortality often quoted at around 4% and morbidity around 40%. Of note, ascites often resolve

over the course of 3–4 weeks but occasionally it may be refractory and only resolve following stenting of the inferior vena cava or hepatic veins (24,25). Following a resection-fenestration procedure, the average reduction in hepatic volume is between 50–75% which results in considerable subjective and objective improvement in more than three quarters of patients (1,26). Symptoms may unfortunately recur, and in these patients, sclerotherapy may be particularly useful because further surgical fenestration may be technically difficult due to postoperative adhesions. It is estimated that the liver volume increases by 11% on volumetric analyses 4 years after resection surgery (10,16) although over half of these patients have stable volumes which is further testament to the highly variable natural history of PLD (1,25,26).

Liver transplantation

PLD are a set of genetic disorders, therefore it stands to reason that liver transplantation following a complete explant, is the only cure. Liver function is often preserved in PLD and because of its benign nature, there may be some reluctance to undertake transplantation. Truly incapacitated individuals, however, with life-threatening issues such as severe sarcopoenia, where previous treatments have failed or the cyst distribution precludes a surgical approach, should be considered for transplantation. Prospective quality of life and the potential improvement following transplantation, which is reportedly excellent despite the need for lifelong anti-rejection medications, must be considered in the context of the risks associated with transplantation. Especially in countries where the model for end-stage liver disease (MELD) criteria is used to prioritize allografts, exception points are often considered and awarded to wait-listed PLD transplant candidates. This is because these patients, despite a debilitating quality of life, often have preserved liver parenchymal function, reflected in low MELD criteria, and can theoretically (and often do) wait months to several years to access transplantation. Liver transplantation is performed within centre-specific guidelines, and the operation is performed for a variety of indications including decompensated end-stage liver disease and transplantation of PLD patients. When there is a donor organ shortage, this can be difficult to justify. The techniques and common variations described for liver transplantation are described in **Chapter 77**. Consideration of living liver donation for PLD patients can pose a special challenge as the vena cava is often compressed and encased with cystic change, making hepatectomy with caval preservation tedious, time-consuming and fraught with an increased risk of bleeding compared to caval replacement employed for a standard whole liver transplant.

Technically, PLD introduces some particular challenges during liver transplantation. Extensive fenestration may be required to gain access to mobilize the liver and preserve the inferior vena cava in live donor

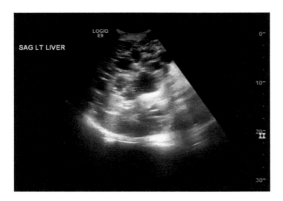

Figure 53.4 US of the liver in the context of PLD. Note the anechoic cysts and their posterior shadows. This image is taken at the level of the hilum, but due to the nature of greyscale artefact, the portal structures were unreportable with any degree of confidence.

allografts using a 'piggy back' technique. However, transient caval clamping may be required to facilitate the preservation of the inferior vena cava or a temporary portocaval shunt may be required, because these recipients often lack portosystemic venous collaterals and are less likely to tolerate the anhepatic phase. PLD transplant recipient hepatectomies are technically some of the most difficult, as the porta hepatis is often stretched and the entire abdomen may be full of adhesions, hindering safe access to the inferior vena cava. Total vascular exclusion may be required to remove the caudate and preserve the cava.

PLD combined with kidney failure due to ADPKD may rarely require a simultaneous kidney with liver transplant. Those with diminished glomerular filtration rates, but above the threshold for routine kidney transplantation, may do well with a liver alone transplant and a renal sparing anti-rejection regime. Secondary renal transplantation will subsequently be required in about half these patients and a kidney after liver transplant has important immunological sequelae associated with receipt of two solid organs from separate donor human leucocyte antigen profiles.

Virtually all PLD transplant patients undergo a blood transfusion intraoperatively and mortality from sepsis can be significant in comparison with other indications, especially if they are catabolic with sarcopoenia. Previous fenestrations, sclerotherapy and resections all increase the technical difficulty of the explant procedure. Where it is anticipated that ultimately a transplant will be inevitable, fenestrations and resections prior to transplant must be judiciously considered because they will increase the complexity and risk (1,27–30).

SUMMARY

Progressive expansion of liver volume in PLD patients produces a variety of symptoms which affect quality of life. These include body image issues, protrusion of the abdominal wall associated with discomfort or pain, gastric compression, recurrent cyst infection and psychological problems which all contribute to the significant associated morbidity. Surgical approaches range from fenestration for decompression and hemi-hepatectomy for focal disease, and where indicated liver transplantation may prove to be the only effective option. Advances in our understanding of the aetiology and novel targets for therapeutic control may in future offer opportunities to stabilize or reverse this disease without surgery, but for the present these largely remain experimental or confined to small case reports.

REFERENCES

1. Aussilhou B, Dokmak S, Dondero F, Joly D, Durand F, Soubrane O, et al. Treatment of polycystic liver disease. Update on the management. *J Visc Surg* 2018;**155(6)**:471–81.

2. Gevers TJ, Drenth JP. Diagnosis and management of polycystic liver disease. *Nat Rev Gastroenterol Hepatol* 2013;**10(2)**:101–8.

3. Blumgart LH. *Surgery of the liver, biliary tract and pancreas.* Elsevier Saunders;2006.

4. Cordi S, Godard C, Saandi T, Jacquemin P, Monga SP, Colnot S, et al. Role of β-catenin in development of bile ducts. *Differentiation* 2016;**91(1–3)**:42–9.

5. Raynaud P, Carpentier R, Antoniou A, Lemaigre FP. Biliary differentiation and bile duct morphogenesis in development and disease. *Int J Biochem Cell Biol* 2011;**43(2)**:245–56.

6. Furumaya A, van Rosmalen BV, de Graeff JJ, Haring MPD, de Meijer VE, van Gulik TM, et al. Systematic review on percutaneous aspiration and sclerotherapy versus surgery in symptomatic simple hepatic cysts. *HPB (Oxford)* 2021;**23(1)**:11–24.

7. Khan S, Dennison A, Garcea G. Medical therapy for polycystic liver disease. *Ann R Coll Surg Engl* 2016;**98(1)**:18–23.

8. Moorthy K, Mihssin N, Houghton PW. The management of simple hepatic cysts: Sclerotherapy or laparoscopic fenestration. *Ann R Coll Surg Engl* 2001;**83(6)**:409–14.

9. Erdogan D, van Delden OM, Rauws EA, Busch OR, Lameris JS, Gouma DJ, et al. Results of percutaneous sclerotherapy and surgical treatment in patients with symptomatic simple liver cysts and polycystic liver disease. *World J Gastroenterol* 2007;**13(22)**:3095–100.

10. Zhang Z-Y, Wang Z-M, Huang Y. Polycystic liver disease: Classification, diagnosis, treatment process, and clinical management. *World J Hepatol* 2020;**12(3)**: 72–83.

11. Gigot JF, Jadoul P, Que F, Van Beers BE, Etienne J, Horsmans Y, et al. Adult polycystic liver disease: Is fenestration the most adequate operation for long-term management? *Ann Surg* 1997;**225(3)**:286–94.

12. Wong MY, McCaughan GW, Strasser SI. An update on the pathophysiology and management of polycystic liver disease. *Expert Rev Gastroenterol Hepatol* 2017;**11(6)**:569–81.

13. van Keimpema L, Nevens F, Vanslembrouck R, van Oijen MGH, Hoffman AL, Dekker HM, et al. Lanreotide reduces the volume of polycystic liver: A randomized, double-blind, placebo-controlled trial. *Gastroenterology* 2009;**137(5)**:1661–8.

14. Lee-Law PY, van de Laarschot LFM, Banales JM, Drenth JPH. Genetics of polycystic liver diseases. *Curr Opin Gastroenterol* 2019;**35(2)**:65–72.

15. van Aerts RMM, Kievit W, D'Agnolo HMA, Blijdorp CJ, Casteleijn NF, Dekker SEI, et al. Lanreotide reduces liver growth in patients with autosomal dominant polycystic liver and kidney disease. *Gastroenterology* 2019;**157(2)**:481–91.

16. Schnelldorfer T, Torres VE, Zakaria S, Rosen CB, Nagorney DM. Polycystic liver disease: A critical appraisal of hepatic resection, cyst fenestration, and liver transplantation. *Ann Surg* 2009;**250(1)**:112–18.

17. Gimpel C, Bergmann C, Bockenhauer D, Breysem L, Cadnapaphornchai MA, Cetiner M, et al. International consensus statement on the diagnosis and

management of autosomal dominant polycystic kidney disease in children and young people. *Nat Rev Nephrol* 2019;**15(11)**:713–26.

18. Aapkes SE, Bernts LHP, van den Berg M, Gansevoort RT, Drenth JPH. Tamoxifen for the treatment of polycystic liver disease: A case report. *Medicine (Baltimore)* 2021;**100(32)**:e26797.

19. Caroli A, Antiga L, Cafaro M, Fasolini G, Remuzzi A, Remuzzi G, et al. Reducing polycystic liver volume in ADPKD: Effects of somatostatin analogue octreotide. *Clin J Am Soc Nephrol* 2010;**5(5)**:783–9.

20. Shillingford JM, Murcia NS, Larson CH, Low SH, Hedgepeth R, Brown N, et al. The mTOR pathway is regulated by polycystin-1, and its inhibition reverses renal cystogenesis in polycystic kidney disease. *Proc Natl Acad Sci (USA)* 2006;**103(14)**:5466–71.

21. Hogan MC, Masyuk TV, Page LJ, Kubly VJ, Bergstralh EJ, Li X, et al. Randomized clinical trial of long-acting somatostatin for autosomal dominant polycystic kidney and liver disease. *J Am Soc Nephrol* 2010;**21(6)**:1052–61.

22. Weimbs T, Shillingford JM, Torres J, Kruger SL, Bourgeois BC. Emerging targeted strategies for the treatment of autosomal dominant polycystic kidney disease. *Clin Kidney J* 2018;**11(Suppl 1)**:i27–i38.

23. Chrispijn M, Gevers TJ, Hol JC, Monshouwer R, Dekker HM, Drenth JP. Everolimus does not further reduce polycystic liver volume when added to long acting octreotide: Results from a randomized controlled trial. *J Hepatol* 2013;**59(1)**:153–9.

24. Barbier L, Ronot M, Aussilhou B, Cauchy F, Francoz C, Vilgrain V, et al. Polycystic liver disease: Hepatic venous outflow obstruction lesions of the noncystic parenchyma have major consequences. *Hepatology* 2018;**68(2)**:652–62.

25. Boillot O, Cayot B, Guillaud O, Crozet-Chaussin J, Hervieu V, Valette P-J, et al. Partial major hepatectomy with cyst fenestration for polycystic liver disease: Indications, short and long-term outcomes. *Clin Res Hepatol Gastroenterol* 2021;**45(3)**:101670.

26. Aussilhou B, Douflé G, Hubert C, Francoz C, Paugam C, Paradis V, et al. Extended liver resection for polycystic liver disease can challenge liver transplantation. *Ann Surg* 2010;**252(5)**:735–43.

27. Ueno T, Barri YM, Netto GJ, Martin A, Onaca N, Sanchez EQ, et al. Liver and kidney transplantation for polycystic liver and kidney-renal function and outcome. *Transplantation* 2006;**82(4)**:501–7.

28. Dan AA, Younossi ZM. Quality of life and liver transplantation in patients with polycystic liver disease. *Liver Transpl* 2006;**12(8)**:1184–5.

29. Gedaly R, Guidry P, Davenport D, Daily M, Ronsenau J, Shah M, et al. Peri-operative challenges and long-term outcomes in liver transplantation for polycystic liver disease. *HPB (Oxford)* 2013;**15(4)**:302–6.

30. van Keimpema L, Nevens F, Adam R, Porte RJ, Fikatas P, Becker T, et al. Excellent survival after liver transplantation for isolated polycystic liver disease: An European Liver Transplant Registry study. *Transpl Int* 2011;**24(12)**:1239–45.

Bailey & Love's Essential Operations Bailey & Love's Essential Operatio
Bailey & Love's Essential Operatic tions Bailey & Love's Essential Operatio
Bailey & Love's Essential Operations Bailey & Love's Essential Operatio

SECTION 8 | LIVER

Chapter

54

Synchronous Colorectal and Liver Metastases

Sanjay Pandanaboyana and Derek M. Manas

INTRODUCTION

At the time of their primary colorectal cancer diagnosis, 15–25% of patients present with synchronous liver metastasis (SCRLM) (1). Surgical resection of the primary tumour and the liver metastasis remains the only potential treatment for cure, with 5-year survival rates between 25–40% (2,3).

The traditional treatment algorithm for SCRLM is a staged approach that includes primary colonic tumour resection, followed by systemic chemotherapy then resection of liver metastases for patients without progression of disease. The benefits of this approach are thought to reduce the risk of new metastatic disease and avoid the development of complications such as obstruction, perforation, or bleeding. In addition, it is suggested that pre-hepatectomy chemotherapy improves selection of patients with optimal tumour biology. Many proponents of this traditional approach argue that the morbidity of simultaneous colorectal and liver resection is prohibitive (4).

In recent years, the safety of hepatic surgery has markedly improved, and as a result the surgical management of SCRLM has begun to experience a paradigm shift. Many specialist centres are now reporting that simultaneous procedures can be safely performed in selected patients, with perioperative results comparable to staged resections. With this approach patients can avoid a second surgical procedure and mitigate the risk of interval progression of liver disease, thus permitting an earlier initiation of adjuvant chemotherapy (5–7). At present, most authors still consider that simultaneous colorectal resections and minor hepatectomy are usually safe and should be preferred in selected patients with limited liver disease (7–9), while patients requiring simultaneous colorectal and major liver resection should undergo staged resections due to the increased morbidity and mortality rates being reported (10). A consensus statement published in 2015 endorsed this view that simultaneous resection be discouraged when the hepatectomy involved three or more adjacent liver segments or when complex rectal surgery was to be performed, due to significantly higher postoperative mortality and morbidity (11).

However, more recently, authors suggest that simultaneous colorectal and major liver resection (LR) have similar perioperative risks compared to major LR alone, so that even simultaneous resection of rectal tumours and major hepatectomies are considered reasonable in appropriate patients (12–14).

SYNCHRONOUS COLON AND LIVER RESECTION

In a study by Martin et al. 134 patients who underwent SCRLM combined resections were compared to 106 patients who underwent staged resections. Patients with right-sided colon tumours, and smaller and fewer liver metastases undergoing less extensive LR, were more likely to undergo a simultaneous approach. The simultaneous resection group had fewer complications (49% vs. 67%, P < 0.003) and had a shorter median hospital length of stay (10 vs. 18 days, P = 0.001), with lower mortality rates (14). A large multicentre study by Reddy et al. (10) included 327 patients requiring major LR for SCRLM. Patients who underwent simultaneous colorectal resection and major hepatectomy (n = 36) had higher rates of severe morbidity (36% vs. 15% P < 0.05) and mortality (8% vs. 1%, P < 0.05) compared to the staged approach (n = 291) (10). Therefore, the authors recommend that caution be exercised when considering a combined approach to SCRLM for cases requiring a major LR.

Bodjema et al. (15) undertook the first randomized controlled trial (RCT) of synchronous versus delayed resection of initially resectable colorectal cancer and liver metastasis. Of the 105 patients included, around 60% received preoperative chemotherapy (across both groups). The distribution of the colonic tumours (right colon, left colon and rectum) was comparable between both groups. Major postoperative complications were similar between both groups (49% vs 46%) with complications rates of 28% and 13% at the colorectal site and 15% and 17% at the liver site, respectively. The simultaneous resection group tended to have improved overall survival (OS) and disease-free survival (DFS) at 2 years, a tendency which persisted for OS after a median follow-up of 47 months. The trial, however, was not powered to explore the feasibility of major hepatectomies in conjunction with rectal resection. Nevertheless, this is the first RCT comparing resection strategies, suggesting it is acceptable for patients presenting with synchronous CRLM to undergo simultaneous resection of the primary tumour and liver metastasis. Having said that, the overall recruitment time was a decade and did not reach the calculated sample size (estimated at 222 patients),

DOI: 10.1201/9781003080060-54

in spite of the broad inclusion criteria, (major hepatectomy, bilobar liver metastases and patients with rectal cancer). The authors also argued that colorectal cancer, with initially resectable synchronous liver metastases, is a rare event and patients being referred were in poor health and the majority of patients were referred after the primary tumour had been resected (16).

It is also understandable that many surgeons have concerns regarding the perceived risks of combining pelvic surgery with hepatectomy. Few studies, however, have reported the actual clinical outcome of such combined rectal and liver resections. Silberhumer et al. (17) reported on 198 patients who underwent surgical treatment for stage IV rectal cancer. In 145 (73%) patients, a simultaneous procedure was performed. A subpopulation of 69 (35%) patients underwent major LR (3 segments or more) and 30 (44%) patients with simultaneous surgery. Complication rates were comparable for simultaneous or staged resections, even in the group subjected to major LR.

Yin et al. (18) conducted a systematic review of all observational studies to define the safety and efficacy of simultaneous versus delayed resection of the colon and liver. Long-term oncological pooled estimates of overall survival (hazard ratio [HR]: 0.96) and recurrence-free survival (HR = 1.04) showed similar outcomes for both simultaneous and delayed resections. A lower incidence of postoperative complications was attributed to the simultaneous group when compared with the delayed group (modified relative ratio [RR] 5 0.77), whereas in terms of mortality within the first 60 days after surgery showed no statistical difference (RR 5 1.12) between the two groups. They concluded that in SCRLM patients, simultaneous resection is an acceptable and safe option with carefully selected criteria.

The published evidence suggests a synchronous colon and liver resection is associated with comparable short- and long-term outcomes to staged resection. The evidence to support a synchronous resection for rectal tumours and liver metastases, particularly those liver metastases warranting a major hepatectomy, is lacking. A staged approach or a 'liver first' approach may still be the preferred approach in this group of patients. Driedger et al. (19) recently published their 17-year experience of combining a major liver with major colorectal resection. This was associated with a significant increase in major morbidity and 90-day mortality. In addition, more than one-third of these patients were prevented from receiving adjuvant chemotherapy secondary to postoperative morbidity. These findings are in line with a recent investigation on surgeons' barriers in performing simultaneous resection, with low support for cases involving major hepatectomy (20).

'LIVER FIRST' APPROACH

More recently, the 'liver first' (reverse strategy) has been proposed to treat SCRLM. Preoperative chemotherapy is administered, prior to hepatectomy,

followed by resection of the colorectal primary at a later date. Initially proposed in 2006, this approach produced impressive survival outcomes in 20 patients with advanced disease (21) and was particularly well suited for rectal cancers, with 7/8 patients with rectal tumours receiving a full course of pelvic radiotherapy shortly after hepatectomy, but prior to rectal surgery. The advantage of this strategy, as well as the combined strategy, is that the delay in addressing the systemic disease that drives overall survival is avoided. Whether this is with initial locoregional therapy of a primary rectal tumour or surgical resection, both can result in significant delays in initiation of systemic chemotherapy. Those opposed to the reverse approach argue that failure to treat the primary colorectal tumour will lead to complications such as bleeding, obstruction, or perforation. However, rates of primary tumour-related complications in asymptomatic patients treated with chemotherapy are quite low (16,22).

De Jong et al. (23) in a retrospective study assessing the feasibility of a 'liver first' approach showed that 76% of patients completed the strategy with concurrent extrahepatic disease, often the limiting factors preventing both stages of the cancer resection. The median overall survival rate was 33.1 months albeit with a higher recurrence rate (51.4%) after a median interval of 20.9 months. Understandably, the overall survival was much longer in patients completing both liver and bowel resection (45 months) (20). Two further systematic reviews on a 'liver first' strategy similarly showed a 74% feasibility rate (24,25). Interestingly, studies on survival differences between the 'primary first' versus 'liver first' approach have not shown differences in overall survival (26,27). Most of the earlier literature, however, did not consider the impact of *KRAS* mutation and the possible association of failure to complete the 'liver first' approach.

Brouquet et al. (28) compared three strategies for managing SCRLM, analysing 72 staged, 43 simultaneous, and 27 reverse approach cases (21). Patients who underwent the combined approach were less likely to receive six or more cycles of preoperative chemotherapy (P < 0.001). Those who underwent the 'liver first' approach were much more likely to receive preoperative bevacizumab (78%) compared with the staged and combined groups (31%; P < 0.001). Patients treated with the reverse approach were also more likely to have a rectal primary tumour and a higher number of CRLMs resected (median of 4). Among 41 patients intended for the 'liver first' strategy, 14 (34%) did not have resection of the primary tumour for reasons such as: 1) Progression of metastatic disease (64%); 2) complete response of a rectal primary tumour (14%) and in three patients, postoperative death after LR; 4) progression of primary tumour, and 5) loss of follow-up (one patient each). Two of the 41 patients (5%) had symptoms from their primary tumour requiring colostomy. The mortality and cumulative morbidity rates between each of the three strategies were comparable. Also, survival rates did not significantly differ. Multivariate analysis showed that greater tumour size over 3 cm and cumulative postoperative morbidity were independently associated with survival.

The published evidence suggests a 'liver first' approach is feasible in up to three quarters of patients with SCLM with reasonable survival rates, although the survival rates were comparable to a 'primary first' approach. The 'liver first' approach however is often warranted, especially for larger tumours in the liver at risk of progression and subsequent inoperability particularly when the primary tumour required neoadjuvant treatment. The survival benefit of the 'liver first' strategy is yet to be determined.

SYNCHRONOUS COLON RESECTION PLUS ABLATION

Thermal ablation of colorectal liver metastases with radiofrequency ablation (RFA) or microwave ablation (MWA) has the advantage of fewer complications and better post-procedural quality of life. Although RFA has higher rates of local liver and extrahepatic recurrence rates when compared to resection, tumours <3 cm may achieve comparable oncological outcomes to resection with a local recurrence rate of 3% at one year (29–31). Lei et al. (32) recently reported on 68 SCLM patients of which 45 underwent simultaneous ablation of CRLM and colonic resection. Patients with rectal tumours were higher in number in the ablation group compared to the resection group (64.44% vs. 39.13%). Significantly higher CRLM lesions (p = 0.042) were observed and located in multiple liver lobes (p = 0.41) in the ablation group. The survival outcomes were however comparable with a median OS of 35 months in the resection group and 39 months in the ablation group (p = 0.714) and a median DFS of 10 months and 13 months in the resection and ablation groups, respectively (p = 0.680). The transfusion requirements and postoperative length of stay were longer in the resection group.

Hof et al. (33) in a retrospective analysis of 47 patients undergoing synchronous colon resection and RFA of liver metastasis has demonstrated that patients considered for RFA as opposed to an LR were likely to have bilobar liver metastasis, at risk of insufficient future liver remnant function, or small metastases after response to neoadjuvant chemotherapy. The average number of ablated lesions per patient was 1.81, with an average CRLM size of 16.4 mm. A matched comparison of patients undergoing RFA ± LR treatment with no RFA and only LR showed comparable survival in the RFA group and the LR group with a 5-year overall survival of 49.2% and 56.3%, and median overall survival of 48.4 months (95% CI = 18.3–78.4) and 70.2 months (95% CI = 31.1–109.3), respectively (p = 0.782).

The size of the tumour (>3 cm), proximity to bile ducts and venous and arterial vasculature in the liver and mutant *RAS* mutation status are often considered poor prognostic factors affecting local tumour progression-free survival. For tumours in close proximity to bile ducts and vasculature irreversible electroporation (IRE) could be an option because the technology obviates the heat sink effect and does not damage biliary or vascular structures (34).

SUMMARY

In line with the current published data, we recommend that simultaneous resection be considered for patients with limited metastatic tumour burden in the liver and localized colorectal cancer, both in terms of number of lesions and required resections as well as the location of the liver metastases. Current evidence suggests avoiding resection of more than two adjacent segments (i.e. hemi-hepatectomy) for anatomical LR and preferably four or fewer metastases for non-anatomical LR (*Table 54.1*). The combination of ablation therapy (RFA and MWA) and hepatic resection has been proven a valid and safe modality without increased perioperative morbidity or mortality compared with resection alone. In order to avoid excessive complications preventing the possibility of adjuvant chemotherapy, simultaneous surgery should be restricted to patients with a good performance status and not in the setting of acute bowel obstruction. In addition, because of a potentially higher complication rate for patients undergoing rectal cancer surgery, simultaneous resection for these patients should be considered only in selected cases.

Table 54.1 Strategies for management of synchronous colorectal primary and liver metastasis

Simultaneous resection recommended
- Less than 5 liver metastases for non-anatomical liver resections
- Resections of no more than 2 adjacent liver segments for anatomical liver resections
- T1–T3 colorectal cancer
- Good performance status (ECOG 0–2)

Simultaneous resection not recommended
- More than 4 liver metastases or resection of more than 2 adjacent liver segments
- T4 colorectal cancer
- Pre-treatment of colon cancer with stent or acute bowel obstruction
- Presence of non-resectable lung metastases or extrahepatic disease
- ECOG ≥3
- Major liver resection with major colorectal resection (rectal cancers)

Reversed, 'liver first' approach recommended
- Large tumours in the liver at risk of progression and subsequent inoperability
- Smaller tumours in critical location (close to outflow or inflow) at risk of progression necessitating a major liver resection in the future

REFERENCES

1. Manfredi S, Lepage C, Hatem C, Coatmeur O, Faivre J, Bouvier A-M. Epidemiology and management of liver metastases from colorectal cancer. *Ann Surg* 2006;**244(2)**:254–9.

2. Abdalla EK, Adam R, Bilchik AJ, Jaeck D, Vauthey J-N, Mahvi D. Improving resectability of hepatic colorectal metastases: Expert consensus statement. *Ann Surg Oncol* 2006;**13(10)**:1271–80.

3. Choti MA, Sitzmann JV, Tiburi MF, Sumetchotimetha W, Rangsin R, Schulick RD, et al. Trends in long-term survival following liver resection for hepatic colorectal metastases. *Ann Surg* 2002;**235(6)**:759–66.

4. Reddy SK, Barbas AS, Clary BM. Synchronous colorectal liver metastases: Is it time to reconsider traditional paradigms of management? *Ann Surg Oncol* 2009;**16(9)**:2395–410.

5. Hillingsø JG, Wille-Jørgensen P. Staged or simultaneous resection of synchronous liver metastases from colorectal cancer — A systematic review. *Colorectal Dis* 2009;**11(1)**:3–10.

6. Chen J, Li Q, Wang C, Zhu H, Shi Y, Zhao G. Simultaneous vs. staged resection for synchronous colorectal liver metastases: A metanalysis. *Int J Colorectal Dis* 2011;**26(2)**:191–9.

7. Gavriilidis P, Sutcliffe RP, Hodson J, Marudanayagam R, Isaac J, Azoulay D, et al. Simultaneous versus delayed hepatectomy for synchronous colorectal liver metastases: A systematic review and metaanalysis. *HPB (Oxford)* 2018;**20(1)**:11–19.

8. Feng Q, Wei Y, Zhu D, Ye L, Lin Q, Li W, et al. Timing of hepatectomy for resectable synchronous colorectal liver metastases: For whom simultaneous resection is more suitable — A meta-analysis. *PLoS One* 2014;**9(8)**:e104348.

9. Veereman G, Robays J, Verleye L, Leroy R, Rolfo C, Van Cutsem E, et al. Pooled analysis of the surgical treatment for colorectal cancer liver metastases. *Crit Rev Oncol Hematol* 2015;**94(1)**:122–35.

10. Reddy SK, Pawlik TM, Zorzi D, Gleisner AL, Ribero D, Assumpcao L, et al. Simultaneous resections of colorectal cancer and synchronous liver metastases: A multi-institutional analysis. *Ann Surg Oncol* 2007;**14(12)**:3481–91.

11. Adam R, de Gramont A, Figueras J, Kokudo N, Kunstlinger F, Loyer E, et al. Managing synchronous liver metastases from colorectal cancer: A multidisciplinary international consensus. *Cancer Treat Rev* 2015;**41(9)**:729–41.

12. Martin RC 2nd, Augenstein V, Reuter NP, Scoggins CR, McMasters KM. Simultaneous versus staged resection for synchronous colorectal cancer liver metastases. *J Am Coll Surg* 2009;**208(5)**:842–50.

13. Muangkaew P, Cho JY, Han H-S, Yoon Y-S, Choi YR, Jang JY, et al. Outcomes of simultaneous major liver resection and colorectal surgery for colorectal liver metastases. *J Gastrointest Surg* 2016;**20(3)**:554–63.

14. Martin R, Paty P, Fong Y, Grace A, Cohen A, DeMatteo R, et al. Simultaneous liver and colorectal resections are safe for synchronous colorectal liver metastasis. *J Am Coll Surg* 2003;**197(2)**:233–41.

15. Boudjema K, Locher C, Sabbagh C, Ortega-Deballon P, Heyd B, Bachellier P, et al. Simultaneous versus delayed resection for initially resectable synchronous colorectal cancer liver metastases: A prospective, open-label, randomized controlled trial. *Ann Surg* 2021;**273(1)**:49–56.

16. Poultsides GA, Servais EL, Saltz LB, Patil S, Kemeny NE, Guillem JG, et al. Outcome of primary tumor in patients with synchronous stage IV colorectal cancer receiving combination chemotherapy without surgery as initial treatment. *J Clin Oncol* 2009;**27(20)**:3379–84.

17. Silberhumer GR, Paty PB, Temple LK, Araujo RLC, Denton B, Gonen M, et al. Simultaneous resection for rectal cancer with synchronous liver metastasis is a safe procedure. *Am J Surg* 2015;**209(6)**:935–42.

18. Yin Z, Liu C, Chen Y, Bai Y, Shang C, Yin R, et al. Timing of hepatectomy in resectable synchronous colorectal liver metastases (SCRLM): Simultaneous or delayed? *Hepatology* 2013;**57(6)**:2346–57.

19. Driedger MR, Yamashita TS, Starlinger P, Mathis KL, Smoot RL, Cleary SP, et al. Synchronous resection of colorectal cancer primary and liver metastases: An outcomes analysis. *HPB (Oxford)* 2021;**23(8)**:1277–84.

20. Griffiths C, Bogach J, Simunovic M, Parpia S, Ruo L, Hallet J, et al. Simultaneous resection of colorectal cancer with synchronous liver metastases; A practice survey. *HPB (Oxford)* 2020;**22(5)**:728–34.

21. Mentha G, Majno PE, Andres A, Rubbia-Brandt L, Morel P, Roth AD. Neoadjuvant chemotherapy and resection of advanced synchronous liver metastases before treatment of the colorectal primary. *Br J Surg* 2006;**93(7)**:872–8.

22. Benoist S, Pautrat K, Mitry E, Rougier P, Penna C, Nordlinger B. Treatment strategy for patients with colorectal cancer and synchronous irresectable liver metastases. *Br J Surg* 2005;**92(9)**:1155–60.

23. de Jong MC, van Dam RM, Maas M, Bemelmans MHA, Olde Damink SWM, Beets GL, et al. The liver-first approach for synchronous colorectal liver metastasis: A 5-year single-centre experience. *HPB (Oxford)* 2011;**13(10)**:745–52.

24. Jegatheeswaran S, Mason JM, Hancock HC, Siriwardena AK. The liver-first approach to the management of colorectal cancer with synchronous hepatic metastases: A systematic review. *JAMA Surg* 2013;**148(4)**:385–91.

25. Lam VW, Laurence JM, Pang T, Johnston E, Hollands MJ, Pleass HCC, et al. A systematic review of a liver-first approach in patients with colorectal cancer and synchronous colorectal liver metastases. *HPB (Oxford)* 2014;**16(2)**:101–8.

26. Welsh FK, Chandrakumaran K, John TG, Cresswell AB, Rees M. Propensity score-matched outcomes analysis of the liver-first approach for synchronous colorectal liver metastases. *Br J Surg* 2016;**103(5)**:600–6.

27. Okuno M, Hatano E, Kasai Y, Nishio T, Seo S, Taura K, et al. Feasibility of the liver-first approach for patients with initially unresectable and not optimally resectable synchronous colorectal liver metastases. *Surg Today* 2016;**46(6)**:721–8.

28. Brouquet A, Mortenson MM, Vauthey J-N, Rodriguez-Bigas MA, Overman MJ, Chang GJ, et al.

Surgical strategies for synchronous liver metastases in 156 consecutive patients: Classic, combined or reverse strategy? *J Am Coll Surg* 2010;**210**(**6**):934–41.

29. Loveman E, Jones J, Clegg AJ, Picot J, Colquitt JL, Mendes D, Breen DJ, et al. The clinical effectiveness and cost-effectiveness of ablative therapies in the management of liver metastases: Systematic review and economic evaluation. *Health Technol Assess* 2014;**18**(**7**):1–283.

30. Ko S, Jo H, Yun S, Park E, Kim S, Seo H-I. Comparative analysis of radiofrequency ablation and resection for resectable colorectal liver metastases. *World J Gastroenterol* 2014;**20**(**2**):525–31.

31. van Amerongen MJ, Jenniskens SFM, van den Boezem PB, Fütterer JJ, de Wilt JHW. Radiofrequency ablation compared to surgical resection for curative treatment of patients with colorectal liver metastases - A meta-analysis. *HPB (Oxford)* 2017;**19**(**9**):749–56.

32. Lei P, Ruan Y, Tan L, Wei H, Chen T. Laparoscopic colorectal resection combined with simultaneous thermal ablation or surgical resection of liver metastasis: A retrospective comparative study. *Int J Hyperthermia* 2020;**37**(**1**):137–43.

33. Hof J, Wertenbroek MWJLAE, Peeters PMJG, Widder J, Sieders E, de Jong KP. Outcomes after resection and/or radiofrequency ablation for recurrence after treatment of colorectal liver metastases. *Br J Surg* 2016;**103**(**8**):1055–62.

34. Distelmaier M, Barabasch A, Heil P, Kraemer NA, Isfort P, Keil Sebastian K, et al. Midterm safety and efficacy of irreversible electroporation of malignant liver tumors located close to major portal or hepatic veins. *Radiology* 2017;**285**(**3**):1023–31.

Chapter 55

Abscesses and Parasitic Infections of the Liver

Shams ul Bari

INTRODUCTION

The liver is a common site for a wide variety of parasitic infections. These include echinococcosis, amoebiasis, ascariasis and tuberculosis. These parasitic infections have been widely reported from tropical and subtropical countries and due to international travel, the number of cases reporting from developed countries is also increasing. In this chapter, the basic knowledge about the involvement of liver in some of the clinically-relevant parasitic infections will be discussed.

PYOGENIC LIVER ABSCESS

Pyogenic liver abscess is a suppurative infection of the liver parenchyma and accounts for 0.007–0.004% of all hospital admissions (1). Liver abscess is commonly seen in young, otherwise healthy patients secondary to an intra-abdominal infection. The infection spreads to the liver via the portal vein, hepatic artery, biliary tract or as a direct extension from sub-diaphragmatic abscess or empyema thoracis (1).

Previously, the most frequent cause of pyogenic liver abscess (PLA) was pyelephebitis, secondary to acute appendicitis (1). With current aggressive and successful approaches to the treatment of appendicitis, biliary tract disease has become the most frequent cause of pyogenic hepatic abscess which is usually seen in fifth and sixth decades (2). Bacteria such as *Escherichia coli*, Enterobacteria and anaerobes are the most common causative pathogens associated with PLA. During last two decades, *Klebsiella pneumoniae* has emerged as the predominant pathogen responsible for PLA in 50–88% cases. Biliary ascariasis has been found to be one of the common causes of liver abscess in areas with high infestation of *Ascaris lumbricoides* (2).

DIAGNOSIS OF LIVER ABSCESSES

Patients with a pyogenic liver abscess present with fever, abdominal pain, vomiting and tender hepatomegaly. The abscess may be single or multiple and may involve the right- or left-lobe, although the former is more common. The laboratory tests may show a leukocytosis, raised C-reactive protein and deranged liver function tests, but blood cultures are frequently unhelpful. Recently, antigen testing and the use of new potential markers such as pyruvate phosphate dikinase have been investigated for the diagnosis of liver abscesses.

Ultrasonography (US) and computed tomography (CT) are the main tools for the diagnosis of PLA but may not be able to differentiate between PLA and amoebic liver abscess (ALA). US has a sensitivity of 90%, and CT 97%, for the detection of liver abscesses. US is cost-effective compared with CT and has been found useful in patients managed by percutaneous drainage and for follow up of patients treated with antibiotics alone. On US, PLA appears as a hypoechoic lesion with irregular margins and non-uniform areas of increased echogenicity (*Figure 55.1*). On CT, PLA appears as a low-density lobulated lesion with poorly defined edges (*Figure 55.2*).

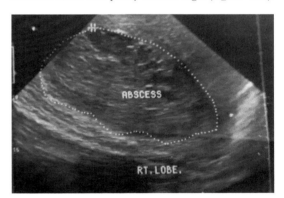

Figure 55.1 Labelled US image of a liver indicating the location of an abscess in the right lobe.

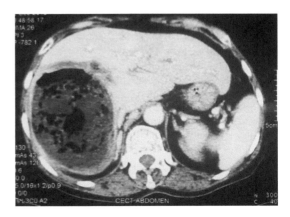

Figure 55.2 Axial CT scan showing a liver abscess in the right lobe.

DOI: 10.1201/9781003080060-55

Fine needle aspiration of an abscess cavity is the 'gold standard' for the diagnosis of PLA. The pus aspirated from PLA is usually purulent and foul smelling, due to infection with anaerobes (3,4).

Patients with pyogenic liver abscesses are managed with antibiotic therapy either alone, or in combination with percutaneous or surgical drainage. The selection of appropriate antibiotics depends on isolating the pathogen, results from laboratory culture and sensitivity assays and local epidemiology. A combination of ampicillin, gentamicin and metronidazole is recommended intravenously for 2 weeks, followed by a 4-week course of oral antibiotics (2). Most patients with a small abscess, either solitary or multiple, usually respond to antibiotic therapy. Patients with a solitary abscess over 6 cm in size, with US features suggesting impending perforation, and all patients with large multiple abscesses, need percutaneous or surgical drainage. Those with multiloculated abscess, ongoing sepsis despite antibiotics and percutaneous drainage, or those with thick pus, may only benefit from surgical drainage (3,4).

HYDATID DISEASE OF LIVER

Hydatid disease, or echinococcosis, is a parasitic infestation which is relatively common in sheep-rearing areas of the world. It is more prevalent in rural areas with poor sanitation facilities and poor living conditions. The definitive host of *Echinococcus granulosus* is the domestic dog and some other related carnivores including wolves and foxes. Humans are only accidental intermediate hosts. The infection is acquired by humans and other intermediate hosts such as grass-grazing animals after ingestion of vegetables, fruits, and drinking water contaminated with eggs excreted in the faeces of an infected carnivore or by handling pet dogs. An embryo with six hooks develops within the egg, which is known as the oncosphere or hexacanth embryo.

Once the oncosphere is released in the intermediate host it enters the portal circulation via the small intestine, and is carried to the liver where it develops into a larval stage - the hydatid cyst (5). Within this hydatid cyst, large numbers of viable protoscolices develop, which grow into adult worms in the intestines of definitive hosts within 5–7 weeks and the cycle is repeated (*Figure 55.3*). This type of cycle which includes a definitive and an intermediate host is the sexual cycle and the resulting disease is known as primary echinococcosis. New hydatid cysts can develop from any element of the larval stage of the parasite in the same intermediate host, as seen after the rupture of hydatid cysts into the peritoneal cavity. This is known as secondary echinococcosis (5).

Clinical features

Almost 75% of patients with hydatid cyst of the liver are asymptomatic and infection is detected accidentally (6). The cyst is generally over 5 cm in size when symptoms occur and the usual complaints are dull aching pain in the right upper quadrant, dyspepsia,

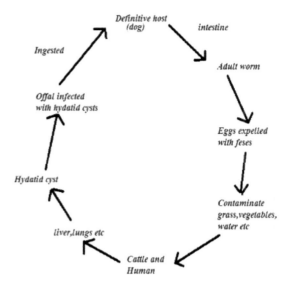

Figure 55.3 Diagrammatic representation of the life-cycle of *E. granulosus*.

and vomiting. Some patients may present due to a complication. Hepatomegaly is seen in 70% of patients and right upper quadrant tenderness is present in 20%. Occasionally, an infected child harbouring a large cyst may become cachectic, 'hydatid cachexia' (5).

Jaundice is an important clinical feature of patients with hydatid disease (7), and this may be due to: 1) Intra-ductal debris following the development of cysto-biliary communication; 2) a large hydatid cyst causing extrinsic compression of bile ducts; 3) sclerosing cholangitis seen in patients with previous history of hydatid liver surgery with use of scolicidal agents; 4) patients put on albendazole therapy, and 5) patients with alveolar disease caused by *Echinococcus multilocularis*.

Complications

More than 30% of patients with hepatic hydatid disease present with complications. Infection of the hydatid cyst, or rupture into the biliary tree, are the most common complications, but rupture into the peritoneal or pleural cavity, rupture into adjacent viscera including the gallbladder, intestines, pericardium, or vascular system and compression of the CBD or CHD and portal hypertension have all been reported.

Intrabiliary rupture

The incidence of biliary rupture ranges from 5–25% (8). This may be an internal rupture, where the laminar membrane gets separated from the pericyst, or external rupture in which the contents of cyst escape into the bile ducts, resulting in a cysto-biliary fistula and obstructive jaundice (9). The patients with external rupture present with biliary colic, cholangitis, and jaundice due to partial, intermittent, or complete ductal obstruction. Some patients may give a history of the passage of germinal membranes in the faeces (Hydatid enteria). In almost 90% of patients the rupture is silent or occult, probably due to bile refluxing into the cyst from an eroded duct and sterilizing the contents following which calcification may occur (9).

Intraperitoneal rupture of hydatid cyst liver

Intraperitoneal rupture of a hepatic hydatid cyst is a life-threatening complication, reported in 1–4% patients. It can present as diffuse peritonitis with shock, anaphylaxis, disseminated abdominal hydatidosis with silent distension (8), or rarely as dumb-bell hepato-peritoneal cyst formation due to herniation of a laminar membrane through a small tear in the pericyst (7).

Intrathoracic rupture

Rupture of a hepatic hydatid cyst into the thoracic cavity is an uncommon complication leading to pneumonitis, lung abscess and empyema. The hydatid cyst may sometimes erode into a bronchiole and lead to severe cough, dyspnoea, anaphylactic shock and expectoration of hydatid membranes and daughter cysts. Bile-tinged sputum is a pathognomonic sign of broncho biliary fistula (7) and these patients need an emergency thoracotomy to remove the parasite. The cyst in the liver can be managed through the diaphragm by simply enlarging the diaphragmatic defect.

Diagnosis of hydatid disease

The diagnosis of uncomplicated hydatid disease relies initially on a high index of clinical suspicion. A history of travel to an endemic area is very suggestive and an asymptomatic mass may be palpated in the right hypochondrium. An eosinophilia of more than 3% is seen in less than 50% patients, but transient elevations of gamma glutamyl transpeptidase or alkaline phosphatase and hyperamylasaemia are seen in patients with cysto-biliary rupture.

Serum immunoelectrophoresis is currently the most reliable immunodiagnostic test and has a sensitivity of 90%. The indirect haemagglutination (IHA) and complement fixation (CFT) tests have sensitivities of 85% and 70%, respectively. Enzyme-linked immunosorbent assay (ELISA) has a sensitivity of more than 90% with the advantage of low cost (5). A human basophil degranulation test has been introduced for rapid diagnosis. It has a sensitivity of almost 90% and becomes negative within a week after surgery. Excellent results have been obtained with Western blot analysis, particularly for *Echinococcus multilocularis* (5). These serological tests have little value during follow-up of patients as they remain positive for several years after surgery apart from the CFT which becomes negative 6 months after surgery or death of the parasite (7).

Standard radiographic examination may reveal calcification in the liver in approximately 50% of patients with a calcified or dead cyst, or elevation of right hemi diaphragm. Abdominal US has a sensitivity of 90% and is the investigation of choice as it defines the number, site,

dimensions and viability of cysts and their relationship to the biliary tree and liver vasculature, particularly the hepatic veins. The daughter cysts have a characteristic appearance within the main cyst cavity and look like radiating spokes of a wheel, the 'cartwheel sign'. US is an ideal modality for following the natural course of hydatid disease, screening of patients in endemic areas, monitoring the response in patients managed non-operatively and for postoperative follow-up. Practically all residual cavities disappear by 18 months, although in children they are replaced by fibrous tissue within 6 months (7).

CT has an almost 100% sensitivity in localizing and delineating the exact extent of a cyst. CT is the investigation of choice when the diagnosis is uncertain and when infection or rupture of the cyst is suspected. A detached laminar membrane from the pericyst is seen as a linear area of increased attenuation within the cyst, so called serpentine structures (*Figure 55.4*) and calcification of the cyst wall is well seen on CT. The daughter cysts have a typical appearance of radiating spokes in a rosette-like pattern (*Figure 55.5*) (10).

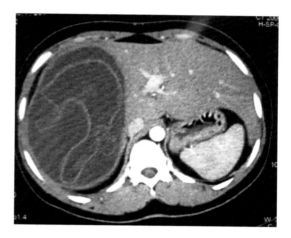

Figure 55.4 Axial CT image showing a detached laminated membrane.

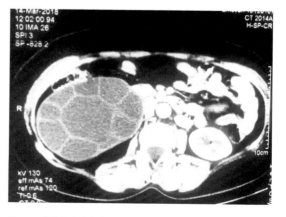

Figure 55.5 Axial CT image showing a multiloculated hydatid cyst in liver.

Endoscopic retrograde cholangiopancreatography (ERCP) and percutaneous transhepatic cholangiography (PTC) should be performed in all patients with obstructive jaundice and where rupture of hydatid cyst into the biliary tract is suspected. Although PTC is only diagnostic, ERCP is both diagnostic and therapeutic and should be performed preoperatively in all patients with evidence of hydatid material in the common bile duct (5,8). ERCP with endoscopic papillotomy is also done postoperatively in patients with: 1) A high output fistula (more than 1000 mL/24 hours); 2) biliary fistula persisting for more than 3 weeks; 3) postoperative evidence of hydatid membranes or daughter cysts in the CBD, and 4) postoperative jaundice.

Management of hydatid liver disease

The goals of treatment for hepatic hydatid cyst are complete elimination of the parasite, prevention of recurrence and minimizing morbidity and mortality. Therapeutic modalities available to treat hepatic hydatid cysts include both non-operative management and surgery. Non-operative methods include drug therapy and percutaneous aspiration under US guidance.

Operative management

Presently, surgery is the only viable treatment for hepatic hydatid disease. Indications for surgery include: 1) Cysts more than 4 cm in size; 2) infected and 3) ruptured cysts. If the patient has multiple cysts, only superficial and accessible cysts should be considered for surgery, and treatment of the remaining cysts can be delayed until they become superficial. Cysts smaller than 4 cm, cysts located deep within the liver substance, and calcified cysts are managed conservatively (7). Patients with centrally placed cysts should undergo US examination every 6 months and should be operated on only after the cysts reach the surface of the liver.

Radical operative procedures

These include pericystectomy procedures for peripherally placed cysts, pedunculated cysts and extrahepatic intra-abdominal cysts (11). It involves an *en bloc* excision of the intact cyst, including the pericyst, in the plane between the pericyst and liver parenchyma. Hepatic resection is indicated when the whole of one lobe is involved or if there are multiple cysts in one lobe, while wedge resection is indicated for peripherally located cysts. Since the integrity of the cyst is not breached in these procedures and chances of spillage is less, there is no need to aspirate cyst contents or use scolicidal agents. There is often considerable blood loss but the mortality rate is <5%. Biliary fistulae and recurrence rates of 10% and 2%, respectively, have been reported with radical procedures as compared to 25% and 16% in patients who undergo a conservative surgical procedure.

Conservative surgical method

Cystectomy is the most common conservative surgical method. It involves the evacuation of all the contents of the cyst including the germinal lining, daughter cysts, hydatid fluid and scoleces, leaving only the pericyst behind (*Figure 55.6*). This is followed by identification of any biliary communication, irrigation of the cavity with a scolicidal agent, and management of the residual cavity (11). Hypertonic saline 15%, chlorhexidine 10%, ethanol 80%, hydrogen peroxide 3%, povidone iodine 10%, silver nitrate 0.5% and cetrimide 0.5% have all been used as scolicidal agents. These scolicidal agents kill almost 80–90% of scoleces. Unfortunately, even the most effective scolicidal agents may not kill the protoscoleces, as they are unable to penetrate the wall of a daughter cyst, are not able to sterilize multilocular cysts, and can lead to inflammation and cholangitis if the cyst communicates with the biliary tract.

In patients with a biliary communication, the contents will be bile stained and in such cases injection of scolicidal agents should be avoided. In some cases, the contents are not bile stained, but after evacuation of the contents, a biliary communication becomes apparent due to a valvular mechanism which opens when the intra cystic pressure decreases after evacuation of the contents. Consequently, at the end of the procedure the cavity must be examined for any bile duct communication, which if found, has to be closed with a Vicryl suture.

There are several techniques for dealing with the residual cavity. These include: 1) Marsupialization for superficial infected cysts; 2) open drainage of the cyst cavity in case of small, superficial and large, shallow uninfected cysts; 3) saline tight closure of the cavity or capsulorraphy in patients with small, noncalcified non-infected cysts and univesicular cysts with no major biliary communication; 4) capitonnage (from the French for padding) for large cysts or calcified cysts; 5) external tube drainage of the cavity in infected cysts and cysts with biliary communication and omentopexy (11).

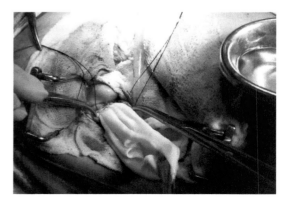

Figure 55.6 Laminated membrane being evacuated from a cyst during open surgery.

Management of bile duct communications

Intrabiliary communication should be suspected in patients with cysts more than 10 cm in size, cysts involving several segments of liver, degenerative cysts, patients with a history of biliary colic or cholangitis and where the US or ERCP demonstrates the presence of membranes and/or a cyst in the biliary tract. Several biochemical parameters may also predict a biliary communication. These include: 1) A raised serum bilirubin level >21 μmol/L; 2) alanine aminotransferase >28 IU/L; 3) ALP >165 IU/L and 4) LDH >194 IU/L. The presence of a biliary communication can also be demonstrated by: 1) Placing a white gauze in the cavity for a few minutes and checking for bile; 2) intraoperative cholangiography; 3) filling the cavity with saline and injecting air to look for air bubbles at the site of biliary leak and 4) by injection of methylene blue into the gallbladder or CBD (5).

In patients with small peripheral ducts, a simple Vicryl suture is appropriate. When a larger bile duct is involved, or hydatid debris is found in the CBD, the best approach is exploration with T-tube drainage and tension-free closure of the peripheral communication. If the CBD is markedly dilated, choledochoduodenostomy or Roux-en-Y hepaticojejunostomy is recommended (5). Where the papilla is obstructed by calcified debris an endoscopic or surgical spincteroplasty may be performed (8). In some patients where the cyst is close to the hilum and communicates with major ducts and where closure of communications would compromise biliary drainage, a Roux-en-Y hepaticojejunostomy will be required. A Roux-en-Y hepaticojejunostomy is also indicated in cases with major duct disruption within a cyst or where the confluence is damaged, and in these patients the jejunum is directly sutured to the duct opening within the cyst cavity.

Complications of hydatid surgery

Bile leakage, liver abscess, sub-phrenic abscess and wound infections are the early complications and recurrence is the late complication. Bile leakage is a relatively common but generally self-limiting problem due to an overlooked or inadequately managed cysto-biliary communication, obstruction of the distal bile duct by hydatid membranes or daughter cysts or iatrogenic injury to bile duct. Initial management should be conservative and the tube drain should be retained for 2–3 weeks as most bile leaks will resolve. If the biliary fistula continues, or is high output (>300 mL/day), the patient will need an endoscopic papillotomy which has a success rate of 90–100%. Some patients may need biliary decompression procedures such as T-tube drainage, trans-duodenal sphincterotomy, choledocho-duodenostomy or cysto-jejunostomy.

Recurrence usually occurs several years after the initial surgery and can be local, regional or distant. The recurrence is more frequent following conservative surgery, due to spillage of hydatid fluid and implantation of daughter cysts. Recurrence is substantially reduced by using pre- and postoperative albendazole (12).

Drug therapy in hydatid disease of liver

Mebendazole was the first drug to be used for hydatid disease at a dose of 40–60 mg/kg/day (12). Mebendazole causes death of germinal membrane cells and the cyst loses its ability to maintain homeostasis and integrity. Lately, albendazole was introduced with superior absorption and when albendazole is used preoperatively for 1 month, the majority of protoscoleces die but results improve with 3 months of continuous treatment. The usual dosage regimen suggested by Horton and endorsed by the WHO is three, 28-day courses of 10 mg/kg/day in divided doses separated by 2-week intervals (7,12).

Praziquantel in dose of 40–60 mg/kg/day is the most active and rapid scolicidal agent and is highly-effective against protoscoleces. It is the ideal agent for prophylaxis in the pre- and postoperative setting to prevent implantation of protoscoleces and recurrence, but is not as effective as albendazole in treating whole cysts as it is less active against the germinal layer (12). It has also been shown to be more effective in combination with albendazole than when used as a single agent.

Chemotherapy is effective in 30–40% of patients with *E. granulosus* infestation and is most effective in cysts less than 4 cm, cysts with thin walls, and in younger patients (12). Larger cysts with an intact laminated membrane and displaying endogenous vesiculization are more resistant and praziquentel is the only protoscolicidal effective agent against *Echinococcus multilocularis*.

Drug therapy as the primary treatment

1 Patients unfit for surgery
2 Recurrent disease
3 Disseminated or inoperable disease including patients with multiple peritoneal or liver cysts, multiorgan involvement, spinal, pelvic and long bone disease which may be unresectable or require mutilating surgery

Drug therapy as an adjuvant therapy

1 Postoperatively to prevent secondary echinococcosis after spillage during surgery
2 Preoperative therapy should be given for at least 1 month before surgery, as it decreases the viability of protoscoleces, reducing the chances of recurrence and anaphylaxis and cysts become flaccid making surgery easier
3 Drug therapy is also used as an adjuvant treatment for residual disease as in cases of spinal disease and as a concomitant therapy with percutaneous drainage

Percutaneous aspiration, injection, and re-aspiration (PAIR) technique

PAIR is a minimally-invasive procedure involving aspiration of cyst contents percutaneously under US guidance, followed by introduction of a protoscolicidal agent and finally re-aspiration (8). This reduces cyst size and volume and is indicated in patients with uncomplicated unilocular cysts, unfit or unwell patients, and patients with multiple previous surgical procedures. It is not recommended for patients with multilocular cysts, infected cysts, cysts with biliary communication, inaccessible cysts and cysts in technically difficult locations. Spillage, anaphylaxis and recurrence are the complications associated with the PAIR technique.

Laparoscopic hydatid liver surgery

The laparoscopic approach to hepatic hydatid cyst was introduced in 1993. Complete removal of the cyst, evacuation of contents, de-roofing and obliteration of the cyst cavity can be achieved (*Figure 55.7*). Laparoscopic surgery is minimally invasive, the hospital stay is shorter and wound-related complications are less frequent. It also allows for a detailed examination of the cyst cavity (7,12). The laparoscopic approach is not appropriate in complicated cysts or difficult locations and the risk of spillage and seeding is increased.

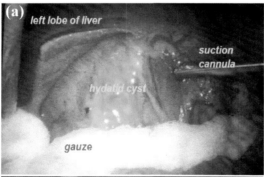
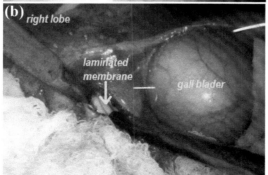

Figure 55.7 Labelled in-surgery image (a) and (b) showing a hydatid cyst in the left lobe of liver with a laparoscopic suction cannula inside the cavity.

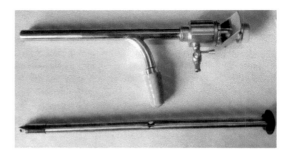

Figure 55.8 A Palanivelu hydatid system for use in laparoscopic surgery.

The components of the Palanivelu hydatid system (PHS) include a trocar, cannula and two reducers, of 3 and 5 mm (*Figure 55.8*). After the creation of the pneumoperitoneum the PHS trocar is introduced into the peritoneal cavity directly over the cyst. The trocar is removed and the cannula inserted into the cyst. With suction attached, the contents of the cyst, including fragments of the laminar membrane, daughter cysts and debris are evacuated (7).

TUBERCULAR LIVER ABSCESS

Tubercular liver abscess (TLA) is a rare clinical entity usually secondary to pulmonary or gastrointestinal tuberculosis (TB) (13). Primary involvement is rare due to the low tissue oxygen levels. Although tubercular liver abscess can occur in healthy individuals it is predominantly seen in unwell patients.

Three morphological types of hepatic tuberculosis are reported in the literature: 1) Liver involvement in systemic miliary TB; 2) primary hepatic miliary TB without involvement of other organs and 3) a primary nodular lesion or abscess. Haematogenous dissemination via the portal vein is the usual mode spread but lymphatic and biliary routes are also possible (14).

Hepatic TB is more common in males than females (2:1) and patients usually present with fever, abdominal pain, weight loss, jaundice and hepatomegaly (15) and a past history of TB and anti-tuberculous treatment (ATT) is not infrequent. Investigations are also generally non-specific, often with just a raised serum ALP. The Mantoux tuberculin skin test has a sensitivity of 65–94% in patients with active disease, which falls to 50% in critically ill patients with disseminated disease. X-ray findings are abnormal in 65–78%. US will demonstrate a round, heterogeneous, anechoic or hypo-echoic lesion with irregular margins and on CT a hypodense lesion with, or without, peripheral rim enhancement.

Although tubercular liver abscess has been diagnosed conventionally on the basis of histological samples obtained by laparotomy or US-guided biopsy, the definitive diagnosis is based on the demonstration of

M. tuberculosis bacilli in an aspirate or tissue biopsy or a positive result from culture or polymerase chain reaction (PCR) of abscess contents (14). The sensitivity for acid-fast staining and positive culture results varies from 0–45% and 10–60%, respectively (15). Recently the QuantiFERON TB gold test has been used with a sensitivity and a specificity of 75% and 81.3%, respectively (15). Granulomatous hepatitis and tubercular liver abscess are treated with standard anti-tubercular drug therapy.

AMOEBIASIS AND AMOEBIC LIVER ABSCESS

Amoebiasis is a parasitic infection caused by *Entamoeba histolytica*. It has a worldwide distribution and the incidence of infection is higher with poor living conditions and contaminated drinking water. Patients often give a history of travel to endemic areas. Liver abscess is the most common extra-intestinal manifestation of amoebiasis and the highest incidence at 21 per 100 000 per year is seen in Asian countries (5). Amoebic liver abscesses (ALA) predominantly affect men from 30–60 years of age and alcohol consumption, malnutrition and hypoalbuminemia are the main risk factors (3).

Patients with ALA often have a history of antecedent diarrhoea, a leukocytosis and deranged liver function tests. Serology can be useful in those with a history of travel to endemic areas, and currently indirect haemagglutination and gel diffusion precipitin (a rapid blood test that detects genus-specific, species-independent antibodies) are the most frequently used. US detects 90–95% of amoebic liver abscesses and CT has a sensitivity of 100% (2). CT is helpful in differentiating between pyogenic and amoebic liver abscess when sonography is inconclusive. Fine needle aspiration of ALAs is questionable and less useful as trophozoites are seen on microscopy in <25% of cases (4). Pus aspirated from an ALA is odourless, chocolate brown and thick, and referred to as 'anchovy paste' (3).

Metronidazole or tinidazole taken orally for a period of 10 days and 5 days, respectively, are the pharmacological agents of choice and should be followed by treatment with a luminal agent such as diloxanide furoate for a further 5–10 days to eradicate residual intestinal cysts. Most cases of ALA respond to medical treatment but non-responders should undergo drainage (1–3).

Therapeutic aspiration of amoebic liver abscesses should be considered when: 1) There is a high risk of rupture due to a cavity size greater than 5 cm; 2) location in the left lobe due to the high mortality following rupture into the pericardium; 3) failure of medical treatment and 4) when a pyogenic liver abscess cannot be excluded. Open surgical drainage should be avoided and only considered when the abscess is inaccessible, medical therapy fails or there is secondary infection (1–3).

SUMMARY

Due to its position in the gastrointestinal tract and its function, parasitic involvement of the liver is common and occurs in tropical and subtropical countries. International travel is responsible for the increasing number of cases reported from developed countries. The incidence of infections in non-endemic areas is also on the rise due to the extensive use of immunosuppressants in treating several chronic inflammatory disorders. For the diagnosis of parasitic liver involvement, a strong clinical suspicion is the key. Infections are generally asymptomatic and self-limited in well-nourished patients with normal immunity, but tend to be more aggressive and potentially fatal in immunocompromised individuals.

REFERENCES

1. Sifri CD, Madoff LC. Infections of the liver and biliary system (liver abscess, cholangitis, cholecystitis). In: Bennett JE, Dolin R, Blaser MJ (eds). *Principles and Practice of Infectious Diseases*, 8th edition, Elsevier Saunders, 2015, pp. 1270–9.
2. Bari S, Sheikh KA, Malik AA, Wani RA, Naqash SH. Percutaneous aspiration versus open drainage of liver abscess in children. *Pediatr Surg Int* 2007;**23(1)**:269–74.
3. Priyadarshi RN, Prakash V, Anand U, Kumar P, Jha AK, Kumar R. Ultrasound-guided percutaneous catheter drainage of various types of ruptured amoebic liver abscess: A report of 117 cases from a highly endemic zone of India. *Abdom Radiol (NY)* 2018;**44(3)**:877–85.
4. Blessmann J, Van LP, Nu PAT, Thi HD, Muller-Myhsok B, Buss H, et al. Epidemiology of amebiasis in a region of high incidence of amoebic liver abscess in Central Vietnam. *Am J Trop Med Hyg* 2002;**66(5)**:578–83.
5. Milicevic MN. Hydatid disease. In: Blumgart LH and Fong Y (eds). *Surgery of The Liver and Biliary Tract*, Vol. 2, WB Saunders, 2005, pp. 1167–97.
6. Barnes SA and Lillemoe KD. Liver abscess and hydatid cyst disease In: Apleton and Lange (eds). *Maingot's Abdominal Operations*, Vol. 2, 10th edition, Stamford, 1997, pp. 1513–44.
7. Malik AA and Bari SUL. Hydatid disease of liver clinical features and complications. In: Ajaz A Malik and Shams ul Bari (eds). *Human Abdominal Hydatidosis*, 1st edition. Springer Nature Singapore Ltd, 2019, pp. 15–22.
8. Zargar SA, Khuroo MS, Khan BA, Dar MY, Alai MS, Koul P. Intrabiliary rupture of hydatid cyst: Sonographic and cholangiographic appearances. *Gastrointest Radiol* 1992;**17(1)**:41–5.
9. al-Hashimi HM. Intrabiliary rupture of hydatid cyst the liver. *B J Surg* 1971;**58(3)**;228–32.
10. Pedrosa I, Saíz A, Arrazola J, Ferreirós J, Pedrosa CS. Hydatid disease: Radiologic and pathologic features and complications. *Radiographics* 2000;**20(3)**:795–817.
11. Malik AA, Bari S-UI, Amin R, Jan M. Surgical management of complicated hydatid cysts of the liver. *World J Gastrointest Surg* 2010;**2(3)**:78–84.
12. Bari S-UI, Hussain S, Malik AA, Rouf KA, Tufale AD, Zahoor AN. Role of albendazole in the man-

agement of hydatid cyst liver. *Saudi J Gastroenterol* 2011;**17(5)**:343–7.

13. Hersch C. Tuberculosis of the liver: A study of 200 cases. *S Afr Med J* 1964;**38**:857–63.

14. Rai R, Tripathi VD, Rangare V, Reddy DS, Patel P. Isolated tubercular liver abscess in an elderly diabetic successfully treated with systemic anti-tubercular drugs. *J Pak Med Assoc* 2012;**62(2)**: 170–2.

15. Kanagaraj A, Marthandam LR, Sriramakrishnan V, Rajesh A, Meenakumari P. Tuberculous liver abscess. *J Assoc Physicians India* 2008;**56**:647–8.

Chapter 56

Surgery for Portal Hypertension

Muhammad Umar Younis, Monis Jaleel Ahmed and Hemant Jitendra Vadeyar

INTRODUCTION

Portal hypertension is a common complication in patients with cirrhosis of the liver and can cause life-threatening gastrointestinal haemorrhage. In some countries, it is also seen in patients with other liver pathologies, including conditions such as non-cirrhotic portal fibrosis (NCPF) and extrahepatic portal vein obstruction (EHPVO). In the past, shunt surgery or devascularization was often required to treat uncontrollable haemorrhage in some of these patients. However, with advances in endoscopic, radiologic and medical management, the role of surgery has considerably reduced and is only applicable in rare situations. Nevertheless, with liver transplantation becoming established as the main treatment modality for cirrhosis of the liver, there is a newer role for the application of shunt surgery as a temporary or permanent component of liver transplantation. This chapter describes the evolution and principles of surgery for portal hypertension and also examines its role in the current era of liver transplantation.

SURGERY FOR PORTAL HYPERTENSION

Oesophageal varices develop in patients with portal hypertension and can cause life-threatening haemorrhage (1). Acute variceal bleeding is associated with a 20% mortality rate at 6 weeks (2). In most patients, portal hypertension is secondary to cirrhosis of the liver, but there are also a group of patients who develop portal hypertension in the absence of cirrhosis. These patients, such as those with EHPVO or NCPF, have normal liver function and therefore bleeding from oesophageal varices is the main factor responsible for the mortality in these patients. Overall, however, liver failure is the most common cause of mortality in patients with cirrhosis of liver and portal hypertension. Management of bleeding oesophageal varices has evolved over the past few decades to include pharmacologic, endoscopic, radiologic and surgical strategies. Liver transplantation has now become established as the treatment of choice for end-stage liver disease. While a detailed discussion of all the modalities is outside the scope of this chapter, the role of surgery in present day practice needs to be defined in relation to the available medical and endoscopic management techniques, transjugular intrahepatic portocaval shunts (TIPS) and liver transplantation.

SURGICAL OPTIONS FOR PORTAL HYPERTENSION

The first documented report of a successful portocaval shunt was described by the Russian surgeon Nikolai Vladimirovich Eck in September 1877 (3). Eck was a young surgeon working for Ivan Romanovich Tarkhanov in St. Petersburg. Eck successfully performed an end-to-side anastomosis of the portal vein to the vena cava in eight dogs by ligating the portal vein on the hepatic side of a portacaval anastomosis, in an attempt to disprove the notion that redirecting portal blood into systemic circulation was harmful. Although in this series only one dog survived, this did not deter Eck, and he persisted in this endeavour and was able to perform the same procedure in humans around 1890 (4). While the surgery itself was recognized as a means to control hematemesis and improve ascites, 'meat intoxication' later understood as hepatic encephalopathy, prevented it becoming an accepted clinical treatment. Ivan Petrovich Pavlov, famous for his conditioning dog experiments, extensively investigated this 'intoxication', documenting the negative nutritional and neurological implications (5). Vidal, Drummond, Morison and Talma, all well-known surgeons in their respective countries, contributed to the literature on portal hypertension in the early 1900s with case reports of shunts or devascularization techniques used to treat variceal haemorrhage or ascites. Although few patients survived these early treatments, the concepts of these great surgeons laid the groundwork for future developments.

Surgery in portal hypertension aims to achieve three objectives:

1 Reduction in the risk of haemorrhage from oesophageal and/or gastric varices
2 Reduction in sinusoidal pressure which in turn will aid in the reduction of ascites
3 Modulating portal inflow pressure during living donor liver transplantation to reduce the risk of small for size syndrome (SFSS)

The choice of surgical procedure, therefore, depends on the most important objective in a given patient since

DOI: 10.1201/9781003080060-56

the procedures differ in their ability to reliably achieve combinations of these objectives. There are two main types of surgical procedures:

1. Shunt procedures which aim to divert blood from the hyperdynamic portal circulation into the systemic circulation. These are further classified as:
   a. Non-selective shunts such as the portacaval shunt
   b. Partial or selective shunts such as the distal splenorenal shunt
2. Devascularization procedures which aim to reduce the risk of variceal haemorrhage by disconnecting the vascular channels around the lower oesophagus and stomach, usually accompanied by splenectomy. The commonest procedure is the Sugiura procedure (originally described by Sugiura and Futagawa as a two-stage procedure consisting of the initial thoracic component followed 3–4 weeks later by the abdominal operation). In current practice, this procedure is helpful for those rare patients who do not respond to medical therapy and are unsuitable for TIPS, shunt procedures or liver transplantation.

THE ROLE OF SHUNT PROCEDURES FOR PORTAL HYPERTENSION

Natural history of oesophageal varices

The natural history of varices suggests that a large majority of patients with varices do not experience any upper gastrointestinal (GI) haemorrhage (6). It is also known that the risk of bleeding is greatest in the first 1–2 years following identification of varices (7). Although the mortality rate in patients who bleed is almost 50% at 3-years, most patients die due to progressive liver failure, and variceal bleeding can be directly identified as the cause of patient mortality in about 20% of these patients (8,9). Re-bleeding rates after initial haemorrhage are also high at about 30% within the first 6 weeks.

The role of surgery as prophylaxis

There is currently no role for prophylactic shunt surgery for the prevention of variceal bleeding. This is because bleeding occurs in only a small percentage of patients with varices and because earlier trials comparing prophylactic shunt surgery with medical therapy demonstrated that although shunt surgery resulted in the successful prevention of variceal bleeding, it led to an increased mortality rate due to accelerated liver failure (10).

The role for surgery in the treatment of acute variceal bleeding

In most centres worldwide, endoscopic therapy is the first option for the treatment of bleeding oesophageal varices. Patients who do not respond to endoscopic therapy may then be referred for TIPS or for surgical treatment. Emergency surgical shunts are successful in controlling variceal haemorrhage in most instances, due to an immediate lowering of portal pressure, but they are associated with a high risk of mortality due to hepatic decompensation (11). In patients with a non-cirrhotic etiology such as NCPF or EHPVO, who bleed from oesophageal varices and fail to respond to endoscopic therapy, devascularization procedures may also have a role to play for control of haemorrhage (12). When shunt surgery is performed as an emergency treatment, a portacaval shunt is usually the quickest and most efficient option for rapid decompression and reduction of the portal pressure (13). However, if the patient is a potential candidate for future liver transplantation, a mesocaval shunt or a proximal lienorenal shunt can also successfully control variceal bleeding and help in the treatment of ascites. These procedures do not require dissection of the porta hepatis and hence do not complicate future liver transplantation.

The role of surgery for the prevention of recurrent haemorrhage after initial control

In view of the high risk of mortality and complications from emergency surgery for variceal bleeding and the ubiquitous availability of endoscopic therapy for these patients, the present role of shunt surgery is essentially restricted to preventing recurrent haemorrhage and as a bridge, pending a planned future liver transplant. Both TIPS and shunt surgery have been shown to be equally effective in preventing re-bleeding with similar encephalopathy and mortality rates, although TIPS is more cost effective (14).

The role of shunts in liver transplantation

Portosystemic shunts are being used in the setting of liver transplantation and have been shown to be beneficial in selected cases with both deceased donor (DDLT) and living donor liver transplantation (LDLT). In essence, two types of shunt procedures are performed in these settings. A temporary portocaval shunt (TPCS) is performed during a piggyback DDLT and has been shown to help in the dissection of the retro hepatic vena cava by reducing the portal venous pressure. It has been shown to improve the maintenance of haemodynamic stability, reduce blood transfusion requirements, preserve renal function and reduce the risk of primary non-function (PNF) (15). A hemi-portocaval shunt (HPCS) is performed during an LDLT and is a permanent shunt. This is done to regulate the pressure and flow in the portal system in some cases of LDLT and in cases where the relative graft weight is small compared with the patient's weight. This has been shown to help in preventing SFSS in these patients and results in an increase in 1-year graft and patient survival rates (15).

TYPES OF SHUNT PROCEDURES

Non-selective shunt procedures

In the present era, there is a limited role for non-selective shunts. They are sometimes performed as emergency procedures for variceal bleeding, as elective shunts for treatment of ascites, in patients with Budd–Chiari syndrome and as a bridge prior to liver transplantation.

The end-side portacaval shunt is the earliest shunt described and is the simplest and most effective of the shunt procedures. Studies have shown that the porta-caval shunt is efficient in controlling variceal haemor-rhage, but is associated with a high incidence of hepatic encephalopathy. Side-side portacaval shunt, mesocaval shunt or the proximal lieno-renal shunts are other types of non-selective shunts with the mesocaval and the proximal lienorenal shunts being the most popular pro-cedures. They are also particularly suitable as a bridge before eventual liver transplantation since they avoid dissection in the porta hepatis.

Selective shunt procedures

The 1980s saw a considerable body of work in which various surgical techniques for variceal decompression without accelerating liver failure were investigated. W Dean Warren who was the Joseph B. Whitehead Professor and Chairman of the Department of Surgery at Emory University, pioneered selective variceal decompression with the distal splenorenal shunt (16). The aim of this procedure is to maintain hepatopetal flow through the high pressure superior mesenteric venous system, while decompressing the splenoportal segment and thereby reducing variceal haemorrhage. Controlled trials have shown that there is a decrease in the rate of hepatic encephalopathy from selective versus non-selective shunts, but preservation of hepato-petal flow is still superior with sclerotherapy compared with a selective shunt. The selective shunts also confer no benefit in the treatment of ascites and indeed may worsen the production of ascitic fluid in some patients due to the disconnection of lymphatic channels during the dissection required and the persistence of the high sinusoidal pressure (17,18).

In 1967, Kiyoshi Inokuchi in Fukuoka, Japan went a step further, exploring innovative approaches to selective procedures and developed a left gastric venous caval shunt with splenectomy to provide postoperative portal perfusion and to avoid Eck's syndrome.

TECHNICAL ASPECTS OF COMMONLY PERFORMED SHUNT PROCEDURES

Portacaval shunt

This procedure involves an end-to-side or a side-to-side anastomosis between the portal vein (PV) and the inferior vena cava (IVC), with the side-to-side approach being the more commonly performed procedure. The traditional portacaval shunt is rarely performed in the present era, except in patients with ascites and uncon-trolled variceal haemorrhage who are not candidates for a future liver transplantation. This is technically a more straightforward operation compared with other shunts and can be constructed rapidly in a bleeding patient.

The steps of the operation are as follows:

1 A transverse upper abdominal incision is usually preferred
2 The common bile duct and a replaced right hepatic artery if present are held in a sling and retracted towards the left
3 The PV and the IVC are isolated and held in a sling
4 A side clamp is applied on both the PV and the IVC
5 An opening is made in both these vessels and a side-side anastomosis is created using a 6-0 Prolene running suture
6 The portal pressure is measured before and after construction of the shunt to demonstrate a signifi-cant reduction in the portal pressure at end of the surgery (*Figure 56.1*)

Mesocaval shunt

A mesocaval shunt is performed by anastomosis of the superior mesenteric vein (SMV) to the IVC using a conduit to bridge the gap between the two vessels. This procedure may be indicated in patients as a bridge to liver transplantation, or as definitive therapy when bleeding is not controlled by endoscopic methods, or by TIPS. A synthetic graft made from PTFE or Dacron, or a venous graft using the internal jugular vein, can be used as a conduit in this procedure. The long-term patency rates are likely to be better using a venous graft rather than a synthetic graft, but potential dilation and significantly increased flow rates are an issue.

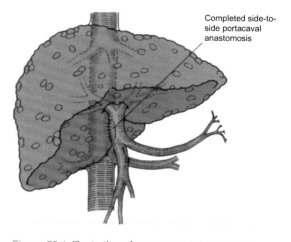

Completed side-to-side portacaval anastomosis

Figure 56.1 Illustration of a portacaval shunt procedure.

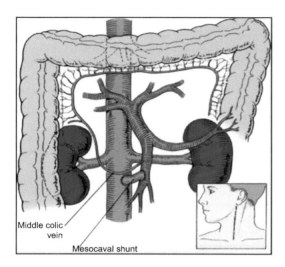

Figure 56.2 Labelled illustration of a mesocaval shunt procedure.

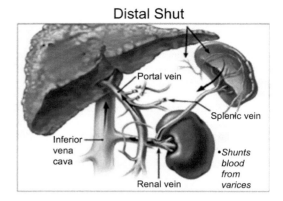

Figure 56.3 Labelled illustration of a distal splenorenal shunt procedure.

The steps of the operation are as follows:

1   A transverse upper abdominal incision is made
2   The SMV is identified by tracing the middle colic vein to its confluence with the SMV and a 2–3 cm segment of the SMV is isolated that is free of tributaries and is encircled
3   A segment of the IVC below the duodenum is isolated through the right colonic mesentery and encircled
4   An internal jugular vein (or 8 mm synthetic) graft is prepared and the proximal end is anastomosed end-side with the SMV using a 6-0 Prolene continuous suture
5   The distal end of the graft is anastomosed to the IVC in a similar manner using the shortest route and ensuring that the vein lies in a suitable position and is not twisted or under tension (*Figure 56.2*)
6   The flow is measured across the graft once it is constructed and should be approximately 1–2 L/min
7   The portal pressure is also measured and should be seen to reduce significantly after the flow across the anastomosis is established

Distal splenorenal shunt

A distal splenorenal shunt is a selective shunt and is performed by anastomosing the splenic vein to the left renal vein. In order to make the shunt a truly selective shunt, it is preferable to perform complete spleno-pancreatic disconnection and ligate the coronary (also known as the left gastric vein) vein.

The steps of the procedure are as follows:

1   A transverse upper abdominal incision is made
2   The lesser sac is entered through the gastrocolic omentum and the right gastroepiploic vein divided but the short gastric veins are left intact

3   The lower border of the pancreas is identified and is dissected to expose the splenic vein
4   The splenic vein is exposed along its length from the spleno-portal junction until the tail of the pancreas and all the tributaries of the splenic vein from the pancreas are ligated and divided to achieve spleno-pancreatic disconnection
5   The coronary vein is identified and divided close to its insertion into the splenic vein or the portal vein
6   A segment of the left renal vein is isolated and encircled
7   The splenic vein is divided close to its junction with the SMV
8   An end-side anastomosis is constructed between the splenic vein and the left renal vein using a continuous 6-0 Prolene suture (*Figure 56.3*)
9   Since this is a selective shunt and is primarily aimed at reducing variceal bleeding, the portal pressure gradient is unlikely to be reduced significantly by this procedure

SURGICAL DEVASCULARIZATION PROCEDURES

Surgical devascularization procedures were developed to treat bleeding oesophageal varices by disconnecting the varices from the high-pressure portal venous system, while preserving hepatopetal flow and thereby minimizing the risk of the hepatic encephalopathy seen after surgical shunts. The classical devascularization procedure is the Sugiura procedure, described by Sugiura and Futagawa in 1973 (19). The procedure consists of a transthoracic and an abdominal procedure performed through two separate incisions. The thoracic procedure involves extensive paraoesophageal devascularization up to the inferior pulmonary vein and oesophageal transection. The abdominal procedure includes splenectomy, devascularization of the abdominal esophagus and cardia, and a selective vagotomy and pyloroplasty (*Figure 56.4*). Although Sugiura showed excellent

or LDLT, respectively, and have been shown to be beneficial. A devascularization procedure should be considered in an emergency where a bleeding patient has failed all other modalities and is particularly useful in patients with non-cirrhotic causes of portal hypertension.

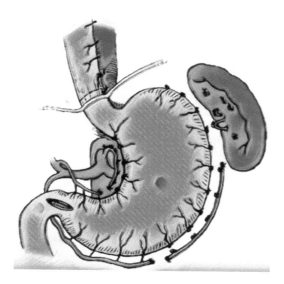

Figure 56.4 Labelled illustration of a Sugiura procedure, a splenectomy and devascularization.

results with his technique with minimal mortality, these results have not been replicated by others.

Hassab also described an effective procedure for gastric devascularization and splenectomy developed in Egypt in 1967 for his patients, the majority of who were infected with schistosomiasis. The spleen was removed, and the cardiac region of the stomach and abdominal section of the esophagus, including the supraphrenic veins, were devascularized. By ligating the left gastric and splenic arteries, portal blood flow was reduced, decompressing the portal system (20).

At the present time, this procedure should be considered for those rare patients whose bleeding is refractory to medical or endoscopic therapy and who are ineligible for a TIPS procedure or liver transplantation. It also has a role in patients with non-cirrhotic portal hypertension with conditions such as NCPF or EHPVO where bleeding from varices is the main risk factor for mortality.

SUMMARY

The treatment of bleeding varices and portal hypertension has changed dramatically over the past three decades. Most patients with bleeding varices can be successfully treated by endoscopic variceal ligation. In those patients who have intractable ascites or Budd–Chiari syndrome, TIPS has been shown to achieve excellent outcomes. The 'gold standard' for treatment of hepatic cirrhosis and portal hypertension is a liver transplant which should be considered in all patients. Surgical shunt procedures are reserved for patients where all other modalities of therapy have failed or as a bridge pending liver transplantation. A TPCS or a HPCS can be considered during a DDLT

REFERENCES

1. García-Pagán JC, Caca K, Bureau C, Laleman W, Appenrodt B, Luca A, et al. Early use of TIPS in patients with cirrhosis and variceal bleeding. *N Engl J Med* 2010;**362(25)**:2370–9.
2. Sarin SK, Kumar A, Angus PW, Baijal SS, Baik SK, Bayraktar Y, et al. Diagnosis and management of acute variceal bleeding: Asian Pacific Association for study of the liver recommendations. *Hepatology Int* 2011;**5(2)**:607–24.
3. Eck NV. On the question of ligature of the portal vein translated Child CG III. *Surg Gynecol Obstet* 1953;**96**: 375–6. Originally published, in Russian, in: *Voyenno-Med J* 1877;130:1–2.
4. Eck NV. On the question of ligature of the portal vein translated Child CG III. *Surg Gynecol Obstet* 1953;**96**:375–6.
5. Rocko JM, Swan KG. The Eck-Pavlov connection. *Am Surg* 1985;**51(11)**:641–4.
6. Henriksen JH, Juhl E, Matzen P, Ring-Larsen H, A Sgrensen TI, et al. Prophylaxis of first haemorrhage from oesophageal varices by sclerotherapy, propranolol or both in cirrhotic patients: A randomized multicenter trial. The PROVA study group. *Hepatology* 1991;**14(6)**:1016–24.
7. Siringo S, Bolondi L, Gaiani D, Sofia S, Zironi G, Rigamonti A, et al. Timing of the first variceal haemorrhage in cirrhotic patients: Prospective evaluation of doppler flowmetry, endoscopy and clinical parameters. *Hepatology* 1994;**20(1 Pt 1)**:66–73.
8. Sauerbruch T, Wotzka R, Köpcke W, Härlin M, Heldwein W, Bayerdörffer E, et al. Prophylactic sclerotherapy before the first episode of variceal haemorrhage in patients with cirrhosis. *N Engl J Med* 1988;**319(1)**:8–15.
9. Triger DR, Smart HL, Hosking SW, Johnson AG. Prophylactic sclerotherapy for oesophageal varices: Long-term results of a single-center trial. *Hepatology* 1991;**13(1)**:117–23.
10. Grace ND. Prevention of initial variceal haemorrhage. *Gastroenterol Clin North Am* 1992;**21(1)**:149–61.
11. D'amico G, Pagliaro L, Bosch J. The treatment of portal hypertension: A meta-analytic review. *Hepatology* 1995;**22(1)**:332–54.
12. Burroughs AK, Hamilton G, Phillips A, Mezzanotte G, McIntyre N, Hobbs KE. A comparison of sclerotherapy with staple transection of the esophagus for the emergency control of bleeding from esophageal varices. *N Engl J Med* 1989;**321(13)**:857–62.
13. Orloff MJ. Fifty-three years' experience with randomized clinical trials of emergency portacaval shunt for bleeding oesophageal varices in cirrhosis: 1958-2011. *JAMA Surg* 2014;**149(2)**:155–69.

14. Henderson JM, Boyer TD, Kutner MH, Galloway JR, Rikkers LF, Jeffers LJ, et al. Distal splenorenal shunt versus transjugular intrahepatic portal systematic shunt for variceal bleeding: A randomized trial. *Gastroenterology* 2006;**130**(**6**):1643–51.

15. Nacif LS, Zanini LY, Sartori VF, Kim V, Rocha-Santos V, Andraus W, et al. Intraoperative surgical portosystemic shunt in liver transplantation: Systematic review and meta-analysis. *Ann Transplant* 2018;**23**:721–32.

16. Warren WD, Zeppa R, Fomon JJ. Selective trans-splenic decompression of gastrooesophageal varices by distal splenorenal shunt. *Ann Surg* 1967;**166**(**3**):437–55.

17. Henderson JM, Kutner MH, Millikan Jr WJ, Galambos JT, Riepe SP, Brooks WS, et al. Endoscopic variceal sclerosis compared with distal spleno-renal shunt to prevent recurrent variceal bleeding in cirrhosis. A prospective, randomized trial. *Ann Intern Med* 1990;**112**(**4**):262–9.

18. Rikkers LF, Jin G, Burnett DA, Buchi KN, Cormier RA. Shunt surgery versus endoscopic sclerotherapy for variceal haemorrhage: Late results of a randomized trial. *Am J Surg* 1993;**165**(**1**):27–32.

19. Sugiura M, Futagawa S. A new technique for treating oesophageal varices. *J Thorac Cardiovasc Surg* 1973;**66**(**5**):677–85.

20. Hassab MA. Gastroesophageal decongestion and splenectomy in the treatment of oesophageal varices in bilharzial cirrhosis: Further studies with a report on 355 operations. *Surgery* 1967;**61**(**2**): 169–76.

Chapter 57

Sphincter of Oddi Dysfunction

Rajneesh Kumar Singh, Samir Mohindra and Radha Krishna Dhiman

INTRODUCTION

The sphincter of Oddi (SO) forms a high-pressure zone that regulates the flow of bile and pancreatic juice into the duodenum, regulates gallbladder emptying, and prevents reflux of duodenal contents (1). Non-adrenergic non-cholinergic nerve fibres are thought to mediate an inhibitory action on the SO (2). Nitric oxide donor drugs like amyl nitrite and nitroglycerin relax the sphincter (2,3). Cholecystokinin (CCK) which mediates the contraction of the gallbladder and relaxation of the SO is the most important peptide hormone (4,5).

SPHINCTER OF ODDI MANOMETRY

Despite all its shortcomings, manometry during endoscopic retrograde cholangio-pancreatography (ERCP) is still considered the 'gold standard' for the diagnosis of sphincter of Oddi dysfunction (SOD). Low compliance, water-perfused catheter systems and a pull-through technique have been used in the majority of studies. The primary manometry is for the biliary sphincter, but pancreatic manometry is advocated in specific clinical situations such as recurrent acute pancreatitis (6). There is consensus on using the basal pressure of 40 mmHg or more (for either biliary or pancreatic sphincters) as the criteria to diagnose SOD (6).

Aside from the general risks of ERCP and endoscopy, the main risk of ERCP for diagnosis of SOD is that of post-procedure pancreatitis (15–30%) (6–8).

CONVENTIONAL VIEWPOINT OF SPHINCTER OF ODDI DYSFUNCTION

Presentation

SOD refers to an altered function of the SO leading to an increased resistance to flow of bile/pancreatic juice, in the absence of any structural abnormality to explain the findings. Clinical manifestations include biliary or pancreatic type pain, dilatation of proximal ducts, altered enzyme values, delayed passage of contrast or radionuclide tracer or recurrent pancreatitis. To understand the modern view of SOD it is also important to first look at the older conventional definitions as summarized by the ROME-2 and -3 consensus meetings (9,10).

The diagnosis of SOD is usually suspected in one of the following clinical scenarios:

1. Recurrent biliary pain following cholecystectomy (post-cholecystectomy syndrome [PCS]), without any structural disease. In a systematic review, SOD accounted for 1.8–31% of patients, while it was much higher (25–47%) when reported from tertiary care centres (11)
2. Biliary pain in the presence of an intact gallbladder without stone disease
3. Idiopathic recurrent acute pancreatitis (RAP) has been associated with SOD in 15–72% of cases, based on manometry studies (10,12–16). Recently, however, doubts have been raised about the aetiological association of pancreatic SOD with RAP (17). An alternative view is that the manometry findings may be an epiphenomenon, possibly the 'consequence' of inflammation and fibrosis secondary to RAP

SOD also seems to be associated with other functional gastrointestinal (GI) disorders including irritable bowel syndrome (IBS), small intestinal dysmotility, pain perception disorders and psychosocial comorbidities (18–25). These associations are important because they may play a role in the outcome of treatment of SOD (26).

CLINICAL DEFINITIONS AS PER ROME 3 CONSENSUS GUIDELINES

The general diagnostic criteria for functional gallbladder disorders or SOD have been further characterized by the ROME-3 expert consensus (10). Biliary pain occurs in the epigastrium or right upper quadrant of the abdomen with the general characteristics (all are mandatory) and supportive characteristics (at least one is required) (*see Table 57.1*).

Diagnostic criteria for Biliary SOD (as per ROME-3 consensus guidelines) include: 1) Essential criteria include biliary pain as defined above and 2) a normal amylase/lipase. Altered LFTs temporally related to the pain on at least two occasions form a non-essential but supportive criterion (10).

Diagnostic criteria of Pancreatic SOD (as per ROME-3 consensus guidelines) include: 1) Essential criteria include pancreatic pain and 2) elevated amylase/lipase (10).

DOI: 10.1201/9781003080060-57

Table 57.1 Characteristics of biliary pain – as per ROME-3 consensus (10)

General characteristics (all are mandatory for the definition)

- Episodic pain and each episode lasting 30 minutes or longer (continuous pain is ruled out)
- Pain recurring at different intervals (not daily pain)
- Pain severity builds up to a steady level
- Moderate/severe enough to interfere with activities of daily living or need a visit to the hospital
- Not relieved by bowel movements
- Not relieved by antacids
- Not relieved by posture change
- Exclusion of any organic structural cause to explain the pain

Supportive characteristics (at least one is required for the definition)

- Pain awakens patient at night
- Radiation to back and/or right subscapular region
- Associated with nausea/vomiting

CLINICAL CLASSIFICATIONS
Milwaukee classification

Hogan and Geenen introduced the term 'sphincter of Oddi dysfunction' and proposed a clinical classification (Milwaukee classification) based on symptoms, imaging criteria and liver function tests (27).

Their SOD classification is as follows:

1 *Type 1*: Biliary type pain; abnormal LFT documented on at least two occasions; delayed drainage of ERCP contrast >45 min; dilated CBD >12 mm
2 *Type 2*: Patients have biliary type pain but have only one or two of the rest of the criteria; abnormal LFTs (two occasions); delayed drainage of ERCP contrast and/or dilated bile duct
3 *Type 3*: Patients with only biliary type pain and none of the other objective findings (27)

The Milwaukee classification was devised to stratify the need for manometry and further intervention. SOD type 1 was believed to be mainly due to SO stenosis, SOD type 2 was considered to be true muscular spasm and responsive to drugs such as CCK or amyl nitrite, and SOD type 3 was thought to be a 'functional' disorder and SO manometry was considered mandatory to confirm the diagnosis (27).

Later studies revealed only a moderate degree of concordance between the Milwaukee classification and the manometry findings. Abnormal manometry findings occur in the majority (65–95%) of biliary SOD type 1, 50–63% of biliary SOD type 2 and a smaller proportion (12–59%) of biliary SOD type 3 (13, 28).

INVESTIGATIONS

In the absence of another cause, a rise in the liver/pancreatic enzymes temporally related to an episode of biliary pain is suggestive of SOD. Ultrasound (US) examination of the abdomen is an important screening investigation to rule out other structural diseases such as gallstones (29). A hepatobiliary scintigraphy study (choledocho-scintigraphy) refers to Technetium-99m (Tc99m)-labelled iminodiacetic acid (HIDA) based scintigraphy, to study the delay in bile reaching the duodenum due to obstruction at the SO. There have been wide variations in techniques (30,31). Endoscopic ultrasound (EUS) is an important screening tool for structural causes of recurrent acute pancreatitis, before considering the diagnosis of pancreatic SOD. Magnetic resonance cholangiopancreatography (MRCP) is useful to rule out other structural diseases such as stones, tumours and chronic pancreatitis as the aetiology of the abdominal pain. Magnetic resonance imaging (MRI)/MRCP and EUS complement each other while considering various alternative or differential diagnosis of SOD and increase the diagnostic rate. Secretin-stimulated dynamic MRCP (ss-MRCP) is a test under evaluation. Dilatation of greater than 1 mm of the main pancreatic duct that persists for more than 7 min after a secretin injection at 1 IU/kg is considered to be suggestive of SOD (32). Functional MR cholangiography with biliary contrast media such as Gadoxetate is another promising test that merits further investigation (33,34).

EVALUATION OF PATIENTS WITH SUSPECTED SOD

An algorithm for the evaluation of post-cholecystectomy biliary pain (modified from the ROME-4 consensus) is shown in *Figure 57.1*. Initial screening, with a good history and examination should be done to consider, and if possible, exclude other differential diagnoses (10, 35–37). The initial work-up should include an US of the abdomen, upper GI endoscopy and blood investigations including liver function tests (LFTs) and pancreatic enzymes. Contrast-enhanced CT (CECT) scan, MRI/MRCP or EUS may be subsequently requested in specific instances and presently a HIDA scan is only routine in a small number of units. Other clinicians have followed the approach of a therapeutic trial of 'low-risk' treatments (such as proton-pump inhibitors (PPIs), calcium-channel blockers, spasmolytic dugs and even psychotropic drugs and antidepressants) prior to ERCP and manometry (38–41). Presently, however, these decisions are more influenced by the patient's presentation and clinician's experience, rather than evidence-based guidelines.

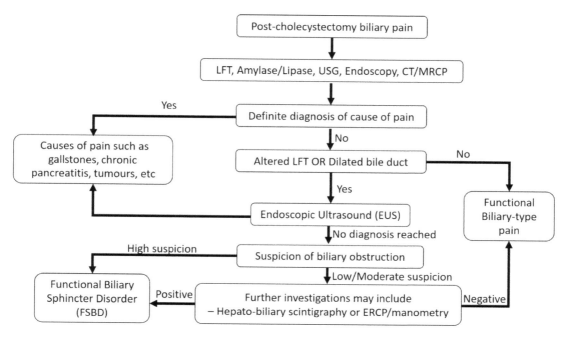

Figure 57.1 Decision-making algorithm for post-cholecystectomy biliary pain diagnosis. (Modified from ROME-4 consensus [37].)

There is a paucity of literature on the issue of biliary SOD in patients with an intact gallbladder (42–44). After excluding gallstones, gallbladder dyskinesia can be ruled out by cholescintigraphy (a gallbladder ejection fraction of less than 40% is diagnostic) and SOD may then be considered (9,45,46). Others have considered the diagnosis of SOD only in cases of non-response of symptoms following cholecystectomy (42).

The indications for sphincter of Oddi manometry remain controversial. Traditionally, it was not considered necessary for Milwaukee SOD type 1 patients but was advisable for SOD types 2 and 3 patients where there was a need to confirm the diagnosis prior to invasive interventions such as sphincterotomy (10). In view of the risks associated with ERCP manometry, other authors have proposed treatment protocols completely based on non-manometric investigations (41,43). At the present time, it is reasonable to say that manometry may be indicated in patients with disabling pain suspected to be of SOD origin, when other investigations have not revealed any organic pathology and conservative treatments have not had any effect on a patient's symptoms.

TREATMENT OF BILIARY SOD

Medical treatment

Even after several decades of research into the diagnosis and management of SOD, the role of medical treatment remains uncertain. One of the reasons to consider medical treatment of SOD is the relative 'low risk' of this approach compared with 'high risk' investigations and interventions such as ERCP with manometry and/ or sphincterotomy, especially in SOD types 2 and 3. Medical treatment includes anti-spasmodic drugs (nifedipine and nitrates) which reduce SO spasm and anti-depressants and neuro-modulatory agents to address the 'functional' and psychosocial dimensions of the pain (39, 47–50).

Botulinum toxin

Injection of botulinum toxin (BTX), an acetylcholine-release inhibitor, produces a transient response rate of about 64% (53–73%) that lasts for approximately 3–6 months and the majority of responders will have recurrent symptoms (51,52). Despite a number of limitations, studies have shown that a good clinical response to BTX injections correlates with outcomes following endoscopic sphincterotomy.

Endoscopic treatment

ERCP with sphincterotomy where the sphincter of Oddi is ablated (ES) is preferred as it is less invasive and has greater patient acceptance. Dual endoscopic sphincterotomy (DES) includes division of the septum between the pancreatic and bile ducts in the ampulla. Biliary SOD type 1 is considered to be SO stenosis and has consistently good outcomes after ES, with

77–100% of patients reporting relief after treatment (13,29,47,53–55). In biliary SOD type 2 the reported clinical response rates of ES vary widely (38–94%), with the best responses in those with high biliary pressures (26,28,47). In biliary SOD type 3, the response rates following ES are quite low (37%; range 8–62%) (26,47,53,56–58) and recent evidence suggests that there is no role for invasive interventions in SOD type 3.

Surgical treatment

Surgical transduodenal sphincteroplasty (TDS) and transampullary septectomy (TAS) were the standard of care for sphincter ablation until the advent of suitable endoscopic approaches (59–66). Currently, ES is favoured as the first choice of treatment because of better patient acceptance, its less invasive nature, the lower morbidity and a more rapid recovery (67,68). Surgical sphincteroplasty is usually reserved for re-stenosis following ES or when ES is not feasible due to altered anatomy as in Roux-en-Y gastric bypass or technical non-availability (47,69).

Treatment of pancreatic sod

Most of the literature pertaining to intervention for pancreatic SOD refers to RAP, that is congruous with pancreatic SOD type 2. Even though in the short-term, good results have been achieved after ES, these patients have a high rate of recurrent pain (up to 50%) and some have even been diagnosed with chronic pancreatitis during follow-up (70–74).

Predictors of response/ failure of endoscopic sphincterotomy

Apart from the classical parameters of increased basal SO pressures measured by manometry and the Milwaukee classification, other parameters that have been found to correlate with outcomes include: 1) Chronic narcotic use; 2) older age; 3) atypical pain; 4) gastroparesis; 5) pancreatic sphincter hypertension; 6) chronic pancreatitis and 7) other associated functional bowel disorders including IBS and psycho-social issues (27,68,75–78). Some factors correlating with symptom relapse after ES include: 1) Re-stenosis of SO; 2) incomplete sphincterotomy; 3) an initial placebo effect; 4) pain not due to SOD; 5) pancreatic SO hypertension and 6) chronic pancreatitis (66,75,78–81).

CONTEMPORARY VIEW OF SPHINCTER OF ODDI DYSFUNCTION

Background

The classical understanding of SOD where symptoms are due to SO obstruction has been challenged due to: 1) Lack of high concordance between manometric findings and symptoms; 2) poor reproducibility of SO manometry findings; 3) lack of relief in a significant proportion of patients despite having intervention based on typical manometry findings; 4) the benefit of sham treatments even with typical manometry findings; 5) recurrence of symptoms even after seemingly appropriate treatment and the association with other pain syndromes; 6) and functional GI disorders and psycho-social issues (22,28,79,82,83). The Evaluating Predictors and Interventions in Sphincter of Oddi Dysfunction (EPISOD) trial was a sham-controlled double-blind randomized controlled trial that studied ES versus sham treatment for patients with only post-cholecystectomy pain and biliary SOD type 3 (84). The outcome, including long-term follow up, demonstrated no benefit for ES or dual sphincterotomy (85). Several other studies from this dataset published subsequently, showed: 1) Poor reproducibility of the manometry findings; 2) questioned the completeness of the pancreatic sphincterotomy; 3) confirmed the high risk of post-ERCP pancreatitis in patients with suspected SOD; 4) documented the high psycho-social comorbidity in these patients and 5) quantified the therapeutic benefit of the placebo effect (25,86–90).

ROME-4 classification

The ROME-4 guidelines, published after the results of the EPISOD study, re-emphasized the difficulties in evaluation and treatment due to the fluctuating nature of symptoms in post-cholecystectomy patients and the placebo effects of the intervention treatments in suspected SOD (37). The Milwaukee classification was deemed outdated and that guidelines recommended should be abandoned. Type 1 SOD patients were classified as having an organic stenosis rather than functional SOD and the original type 3 SOD was no longer considered to be a distinct entity. The term 'suspected functional biliary sphincter disorder' (suspected FBSD) was introduced to include patients with prior type 2 SOD (with post-cholecystectomy pain and few objective findings). The new ROME-4 modified criteria for diagnosis of FBSD are shown in *Table 57.2*.

Table 57.2 ROME-4 modified criteria for diagnosis of FBSD

Diagnostic criteria

- Criteria for biliary pain as per ROME-3 consensus (with modifications as described above)
- Altered liver enzymes or dilated bile duct (not both)
- No structural abnormalities or bile duct stones to explain the symptoms

Supportive criteria

- Normal pancreatic enzymes (amylase/lipase)
- SO manometry abnormality
- Hepato-biliary scintigraphy study

Table 57.3 ROME-4 modified criteria for diagnosis of pancreatic SOD

Diagnostic criteria

- Documented recurrent acute pancreatitis (typical pancreatic pain with raised amylase/ lipase more than three times normal and/or imaging evidence of acute pancreatitis)
- Exclusion of other aetiologies of acute pancreatitis
- Negative EUS investigation
- Abnormal pancreatic sphincter manometry

Although the modified Milwaukee classification had proposed three groups of pancreatic SOD similar to biliary SOD, the ROME-4 consensus defined pancreatic SOD only in patients with documented RAP. The proposed ROME-4 criteria for pancreatic SOD are shown in *Table 57.3*.

Pain sensitization and psycho-social issues in SOD

Despite the lack of consensus, several studies have pointed out the association of SOD with other functional GI disorders, visceral hyperalgesia, somatization disorder and other psychosocial comorbidities (18,21,22,24,26,91,92). Other, more recent studies have provided data to the contrary. It is clear that more research is required to define and clarify these associations (25).

SUMMARY

Our understanding of SOD has changed significantly in the last decade and it is important to understand the Milwaukee classification, SO manometry and the ROME-3 and -4 consensus meeting guidelines. The Milwaukee classification objectively defined the clinical diagnosis and grouping of the different types of SOD. Over the following decades the advent of ERCP and SO manometry provided a 'gold standard' against which to weigh the clinical diagnosis, treatment and outcomes. There was very little high-quality published evidence at this point, and what was available was limited to a small number of expert centres, or of low-quality. There were only a few, small prospective controlled studies, prior to the EPISOD trial. A number of authors have highlighted problems with regard to the entity of SOD, including the reproducibility of manometry, the difficulties in predicting failure of treatment and issues with outcome assessment after ES. The ROME-4 consensus, together with high-quality data from the EPISOD trial, are the most recent efforts to define and clarify the entity of SOD. It is recommended that the previously defined types 1 and 3 SOD should no longer be considered as functional sphincter of Oddi disorders. The issue of pancreatic SOD in RAP needs further study to assess the association and develop a logical management strategy.

Though links between SOD, function GI disorders and psychosocial comorbidities have been pointed out by a number of authors, details remain poorly defined and contradictory results from recent studies have cast further doubt on the entity of SOD.

Patients labelled as SOD are likely to have a more complex aetiopathogenesis of their symptoms than was previously understood or accepted, and SOD may only be one component. More high-quality research and data are required to clarify our understanding of SOD.

REFERENCES

1. Geenen JE, Hogan WJ, Dodds WJ, Stewart ET, Arndorfer RC. Intraluminal pressure recording from the human sphincter of Oddi. *Gastroenterology* 1980;**78(2)**:317–24.
2. Ballal MA, Sanford PA. Physiology of the sphincter of Oddi-the present and the future? Part 1. *Saudi J Gastroenterol* 2000;**6(3)**:129–46.
3. Bar-Meir S, Halpern Z, Bardan E. Nitrate therapy in a patient with papillary dysfunction. *Am J Surg* 1983;**78(2)**:94–5.
4. Behar J. Physiology and pathophysiology of the biliary tract: The gallbladder and sphincter of Oddi—A review. *ISRN Physiol* 2013;**2013**:837630.
5. Ono K, Suzuki H, Hada R, Sasaki M, Endoh M. Gastrointestinal hormones and motility of The human sphincter of Oddi. *Nihon Heikatsukin Gakkai Zasshi* 1985;**21 Suppl**:69–75.
6. Pfau PR, Banerjee S, Barth BA, Desilets DJ, Kaul V, Kethu SR, et al. Sphincter of Oddi manometry. *Gastrointest Endosc* 2011;**74(6)**:1175–80.
7. Chen TS. Sphincter of Oddi Dysfunction. In: Lai KH. Mo LR, Wang HP (eds). *Biliopancreatic Endoscopy*. Springer, 2018, pp 213–24.
8. Toouli J. Sphincter of Oddi: Function, dysfunction, and its management. *J Gastroenterol Hepatol* 2009;**24 Suppl 3**:S57–62.
9. Corazziari E, Shaffer EA, Hogan WJ, Sherman S, Toouli J. Functional disorders of the biliary tract and pancreas. *Gut* 1999;**45 Suppl 2(Suppl 2)**:II48–II54.
10. Behar J, Corazziari E, Guelrud M, Hogan W, Sherman S, Toouli J. Functional gallbladder and sphincter of oddi disorders. *Gastroenterology* 2006;**130(5)**:1498–509.
11. Isherwood J, Oakland K, Khanna A. A systematic review of the aetiology and management of post cholecystectomy syndrome. *Surgeon* 2019;**17(1)**:33–42.
12. Geenen JE, Nash JA. The role of sphincter of Oddi manometry and biliary microscopy in evaluating idiopathic recurrent pancreatitis. *Endoscopy* 1998;**30(9)**:A237–41.
13. Sherman S, Troiano FP, Hawes RH, O'Connor KW, Lehman GA. Frequency of abnormal sphincter of Oddi manometry compared with the clinical suspicion of sphincter of Oddi dysfunction. *Am J Gastroenterol* 1991;**86(5)**:586–90.
14. Toouli J, Di Francesco V, Saccone G, Kollias J, Schloithe A, Shanks N. Division of the sphincter of

Oddi for treatment of dysfunction associated recurrent pancreatitis. *BJS* 1996;**83(9)**:1205–10.

15. Venu RP, Geenen JE, Hogan W, Stone J, Johnson GK, Soergel K. Idiopathic recurrent pancreatitis. An approach to diagnosis and treatment. *Dig Dis Sci* 1989;**34(1)**:56–60.

16. Cote GA, Imperiale TF, Schmidt SE, Fogel E, Lehman G, McHenry L, et al. Similar efficacies of biliary, with or without pancreatic, sphincterotomy in treatment of idiopathic recurrent acute pancreatitis. *Gastroenterology* 2012;**143(6)**:1502–9 e1.

17. Guda NM, Muddana V, Whitcomb DC, Levy P, Garg P, Cote G, et al. Recurrent acute pancreatitis: International State-of-the-Science Conference with recommendations. *Pancreas* 2018;**47(6)**:653–66.

18. Evans PR, Bak YT, Dowsett JF, Smith RC, Kellow JE. Small bowel dysmotility in patients with postcholecystectomy sphincter of Oddi dysfunction. *Dig Dis Sci* 1997;**42(7)**:1507–12.

19. Evans PR, Dowsett JF, Bak YT, Chan YK, Kellow JE. Abnormal sphincter of Oddi response to cholecystokinin in postcholecystectomy syndrome patients with irritable bowel syndrome. The irritable sphincter. *Dig Dis Sci* 1995;**40(5)**:1149–56.

20. Sanmiguel C, Soffer EE. Intestinal dysmotility and its relationship to sphincter of Oddi dysfunction. *Curr Hepatol Rep* 2004;**6(2)**:137–9.

21. Chun A, Desautels S, Slivka A, Mitrani C, Starz T, Di Lorenzo C, et al. Visceral algesia in irritable bowel syndrome, fibromyalgia, and sphincter of Oddi dysfunction, type III. *Dig Dis Sci* 1999;**44(3)**:631–6.

22. Desautels SG, Slivka A, Hutson WR, Chun A, Mitrani C, DiLorenzo C, et al. Postcholecystectomy pain syndrome: Pathophysiology of abdominal pain in sphincter of Oddi type III. *Gastroenterology* 1999;**116(4)**:900–5.

23. Kellow JE. Sphincter of Oddi dysfunction type III: Another manifestation of visceral hyperalgesia? *Gastroenterology* 1999;**116(4)**:996–1000.

24. Bennett E, Evans P, Dowsett J, Kellow J. Sphincter of Oddi dysfunction: Psychosocial distress correlates with manometric dyskinesia but not stenosis. *World J Gastroenterol* 2009;**15(48)**:6080–5.

25. Brawman-Mintzer O, Durkalski V, Wu Q, Romagnuolo J, Fogel E, Tarnasky P, et al. Psychosocial characteristics and pain burden of patients with suspected sphincter of Oddi dysfunction in the EPISOD multicenter trial. *Am J Gastroenterol* 2014;**109(3)**:436–42.

26. Linder, J. Incomplete response to endoscopic sphincterotomy in patients with sphincter of Oddi dysfunction: Evidence for a chronic pain disorder. *Am J Gastroenterol* 2003;**98(8)**:1738–43.

27. Hogan WJ, Geenen JE. Biliary dyskinesia. *Endoscopy* 1988;**20 Suppl 1**:179–83.

28. Geenen JE, Hogan WJ, Dodds WJ, Toouli J, Venu RP. The efficacy of endoscopic sphincterotomy after cholecystectomy in patients with sphincter-of-Oddi dysfunction. *NEJM* 1989;**320(2)**:82–7.

29. Hall TC, Dennison AR, Garcea G. The diagnosis and management of Sphincter of Oddi dysfunction: A systematic review. *Langenbecks Arch Surg* 2012; **397(6)**:889–98.

30. Corazziari E, Cicala M, Scopinaro F, Schillaci O, Habib IF, Pallotta N. Scintigraphic assessment of SO dysfunction. *Gut* 2003;**52(11)**:1655–6.

31. Craig AG, Peter D, Saccone GT, Ziesing P, Wycherley A, Toouli J. Scintigraphy versus manometry in patients with suspected biliary sphincter of Oddi dysfunction. *Gut* 2003;**52(3)**:352–7.

32. Pereira SP, Gillams A, Sgouros SN, Webster GJ, Hatfield AR. Prospective comparison of Secretin-stimulated magnetic resonance cholangiopancreatography with manometry in the diagnosis of sphincter of Oddi dysfunction types II and III. *Gut* 2007;**56(6)**:809–13.

33. Fidler JL, Knudsen JM, Collins DA, McGee KP, Lahr B, Thistle JL, et al. Prospective assessment of dynamic CT and MR cholangiography in functional biliary pain. *AJR Am J Roentgenol* 2013;**201(2)**:W271–82.

34. Corwin MT, Lamba R, McGahan JP. Functional MR cholangiography of the cystic duct and sphincter of Oddi using gadoxetate disodium: Is a 30-minute delay long enough? *J Magn Reson Imaging* 2013;**37(4)**:993–8.

35. Berger MY, Olde Hartman TC, Bohnen AM. Abdominal symptoms: Do they disappear after cholecystectomy? *Surg Endosc* 2003;**17(11)**:1723–8.

36. Black NA, Thompson E, Sanderson CF. Symptoms and health status before and six weeks after open cholecystectomy: A European cohort study. ECHSS Group. European Collaborative Health Services Study Group. *Gut* 1994;**35(9)**:1301–5.

37. Cotton PB, Elta GH, Carter CR, Pasricha PJ, Corazziari ES. Rome IV. Gallbladder and sphincter of Oddi Disorders. *Gastroenterology* 2016;**19**:S0016-5085(16)00224-9.

38. Cheon YK, Cho YD, Moon JH, Im HH, Jung Y, Lee JS, et al. Effects of vardenafil, a phosphodiesterase type-5 inhibitor, on sphincter of Oddi motility in patients with suspected biliary sphincter of Oddi dysfunction. *Gastrointest Endosc* 2009;**69(6)**:1111–6.

39. Vitton V, Ezzedine S, Gonzalez JM, Gasmi M, Grimaud JC, Barthet M. Medical treatment for sphincter of Oddi dysfunction: Can it replace endoscopic sphincterotomy? *World J Gastroenterol* 2012;**18(14)**:1610–5.

40. Khuroo MS, Zargar SA, Yattoo GN. Efficacy of nifedipine therapy in patients with sphincter of Oddi dysfunction: A prospective, double-blind, randomized, placebo-controlled, cross over trial. *Br J Clin Pharmacol* 1992;**33(5)**:477–85.

41. Kalaitzakis E, Ambrose T, Phillips-Hughes J, Collier J, Chapman RW. Management of patients with biliary sphincter of Oddi disorder without sphincter of Oddi manometry. *BMC Gastroenterology* 2010;**10**:124.

42. Choudhry U, Ruffolo T, Jamidar P, Hawes R, Lehman G. Sphincter of Oddi dysfunction in patients with intact gallbladder: Therapeutic response to endoscopic sphincterotomy. *Gastrointest Endosc* 1993;**39(4)**:492–5.

43. Heetun ZS, Zeb F, Cullen G, Courtney G, Aftab AR. Biliary sphincter of Oddi dysfunction: Response rates after ERCP and sphincterotomy in a 5-year ERCP series and proposal for new practical guidelines. *Eur J Gastroenterol Hepatol* 2011;**23(4)**:327–33.

44. Ruffolo TA, Sherman S, Lehman GA, Hawes RH. Gallbladder ejection fraction and its relationship to sphincter of Oddi dysfunction. *Dig Dis Sci* 1994;**39(2)**:289–92.

45. Delgado-Aros S, Cremonini F, Bredenoord AJ, Camilleri M. Systematic review and meta-analysis: Does gall-bladder ejection fraction on cholecystokinin cholescintigraphy predict outcome after cholecystectomy in suspected functional biliary pain? *Aliment Pharmacol Ther* 2003;**18(2)**:167–74.

46. DiBaise, J. Does gallbladder ejection fraction predict outcome after cholecystectomy for suspected chronic acalculous gallbladder dysfunction? A systematic review. *Am J Gastroenterol* 2003;**98(12)**:2605–11.

47. Sgouros SN, Pereira SP. Systematic review: Sphincter of Oddi dysfunction – non-invasive diagnostic methods and long-term outcome after endoscopic sphincterotomy. *Aliment Pharmacol Ther* 2006;**24(2)**:237–46.

48. Tzovaras G, Rowlands BJ. Diagnosis and treatment of sphincter of Oddi dysfunction. *BJS* 1998;**85(5)**:588–95.

49. Craig A, Toouli J. Sphincter of Oddi dysfunction: Is there a role for medical therapy? *Curr Gastroenterol Rep* 2002;**4(2)**:172–6.

50. Fazel A, Li SC, Burton FR. Octreotide relaxes the hypertensive sphincter of Oddi: Pathophysiological and therapeutic implications. *Am J Gastroenterol* 2002;**97(3)**:612–6.

51. Menon S, Kurien R, Mathew R. The role of intrasphincteric botulinum toxin injection in the management of functional biliary pain: A systematic review and meta-analysis. *Eur J Gastroenterol Hepatol* 2020;**32(8)**:984–9.

52. Wehrmann T, Schmitt TH, Arndt A, Lembcke B, Caspary WF, Seifert H. Endoscopic injection of botulinum toxin in patients with recurrent acute pancreatitis due to pancreatic sphincter of Oddi dysfunction. *Aliment Pharmacol Ther* 2000;**14(11)**:1469–77.

53. Rosenblatt ML, Catalano MF, Alcocer E, Geenen JE. Comparison of sphincter of Oddi manometry, fatty meal sonography, and hepatobiliary scintigraphy in the diagnosis of sphincter of Oddi dysfunction. *Gastrointest Endosc* 2001;**54(6)**:697–704.

54. Cicala M, Habib FI, Vavassori P, Pallotta N, Schillaci O, Costamagna G, et al. Outcome of endoscopic sphincterotomy in post cholecystectomy patients with sphincter of Oddi dysfunction as predicted by manometry and quantitative choledochoscintigraphy. *Gut* 2002;**50(5)**:665–8.

55. Thatcher BS, Sivak MV, Jr., Tedesco FJ, Vennes JA, Hutton SW, Achkar EA. Endoscopic sphincterotomy for suspected dysfunction of the sphincter of Oddi. *Gastrointest Endosc* 1987;**33(2)**:91–5.

56. Wehrmann T, Wiemer K, Lembcke B, Caspary WF, Jung M. Do patients with sphincter of Oddi dysfunction benefit from endoscopic sphincterotomy?

A 5-year prospective trial. *Eur J Gastroenterol Hepatol* 1996;**8(3)**:251–6.

57. Bozkurt T, Orth KH, Butsch B, Lux G. Long-term clinical outcome of post-cholecystectomy patients with biliary-type pain: results of manometry, non-invasive techniques and endoscopic sphincterotomy. *Eur J Gastroenterol Hepatol* 1996;**8(3)**:245–9.

58. Botoman VA, Kozarek RA, Novell LA, Patterson DJ, Ball TJ, Wechter DG, et al. Long-term outcome after endoscopic sphincterotomy in patients with biliary colic and suspected sphincter of Oddi dysfunction. *Gastrointest Endosc* 1994;**40(2 Pt 1)**:165–70.

59. Jones SA, Steedman RA, Keller TB, Smith LL. Transduodenal sphincteroplasty (not sphincterotomy) for biliary and pancreatic disease. Indications, contraindications, and results. *Am J Surg* 1969;**118(2)**:292–306.

60. Giannopoulos GA, Digalakis MK. Surgical pancreatic sphincteroplasty. Historic or history ? A review. *Acta chirurgica Belgica* 2010;**110(6)**:569–74.

61. Hästbacka J, Järvinen H, Kivilaakso E, Turunen MT. Results of sphincteroplasty in patients with spastic sphincter of Oddi. Predictive value of operative biliary manometry and provocation tests. *Scand J Gastroenterol* 1986;**21(5)**:516–20.

62. Miccini M, Amore Bonapasta S, Gregori M, Bononi M, Fornasari V, Tocchi A. Indications and results for transduodenal sphincteroplasty in the era of endoscopic sphincterotomy. *Am J Surg* 2010;**200(2)**:247–51.

63. Moody FG, Vecchio R, Calabuig R, Runkel N. Transduodenal sphincteroplasty with transampullary septectomy for stenosing papillitis. *Am J Surg* 1991;**161(2)**:213–8.

64. Morgan KA, Romagnuolo J, Adams DB. Transduodenal sphincteroplasty in the management of sphincter of Oddi dysfunction and pancreas divisum in the modern era. *J Am Col Surg* 2008;**206(5)**:908–14; discussion 14–7.

65. Stephens RV, Burdick GE. Microscopic transduodenal sphincteroplasty and transampullary septoplasty for papillary stenosis. *Am J Surg* 1986;**152(6)**:621–7.

66. Seifert E. Long-term follow-up after endoscopic sphincterotomy (EST). *Endoscopy* 1988;**20 Suppl 1**:232–5.

67. Small AJ, Kozarek RA. Sphincter of Oddi dysfunction. *Gastrointest Endosc Clin N Am* 2015;**25(4)**:749–63.

68. Leung WD, Sherman S. Endoscopic approach to the patient with motility disorders of the bile duct and sphincter of Oddi. *Gastrointest Endosc Clin N Am* 2013;**23(2)**:405–34.

69. Morgan KA, Glenn JB, Byrne TK, Adams DB. Sphincter of Oddi dysfunction after Roux-en-Y gastric bypass. *Surg Obes Relat Dis* 2009;**5(5)**:571–5.

70. Coyle WJ, Pineau BC, Tarnasky PR, Knapple WL, Aabakken L, Hoffman BJ, et al. Evaluation of unexplained acute and acute recurrent pancreatitis using endoscopic retrograde cholangiopancreatography, sphincter of Oddi manometry and endoscopic ultrasound. *Endoscopy* 2002;**34(8)**:617–23.

71. Jacob L, Geenen JE, Catalano MF, Geenen DJ. Prevention of pancreatitis in patients with idiopath-

ic recurrent pancreatitis: A prospective nonblinded randomized study using endoscopic stents. *Endoscopy* 2001;**33(7)**:559–62.

72. Kaw M, Brodmerkel GJ, Jr. ERCP, biliary crystal analysis, and sphincter of Oddi manometry in idiopathic recurrent pancreatitis. *Gastrointest Endosc* 2002;**55(2)**:157–62.

73. Okolo PI, 3rd, Pasricha PJ, Kalloo AN. What are the long-term results of endoscopic pancreatic sphincterotomy? *Gastrointest Endosc* 2000;**52(1)**:15–9.

74. Park SH, Watkins JL, Fogel EL, Sherman S, Lazzell L, Bucksot L, et al. Long-term outcome of endoscopic dual pancreatobiliary sphincterotomy in patients with manometry-documented sphincter of Oddi dysfunction and normal pancreatogram. *Gastrointest Endosc* 2003;**57(4)**:483–91.

75. Heinerman PM, Graf AH, Boeckl O. Does endoscopic sphincterotomy destroy the function of Oddi's sphincter? *Arch Surg* 1994;**129(8)**:876–80.

76. Koussayer T, Ducker TE, Clench MH, Mathias JR. Ampulla of Vater/duodenal wall spasm diagnosed by antroduodenal manometry. *Dig Dis Sci* 1995;**40(8)**:1710–9.

77. Freeman ML, Gill M, Overby C, Cen Y-Y. Predictors of outcomes after biliary and pancreatic sphincterotomy for sphincter of Oddi dysfunction. *J Clin Gastroenterol* 2007;**41(1)**:94–102.

78. Tarnasky PR, Hoffman B, Aabakken L, Knapple WL, Coyle W, Pineau B, et al. Sphincter of Oddi dysfunction is associated with chronic pancreatitis. *Am J Gastroenterol* 1997;**92(7)**:1125–9.

79. Varadarajulu S, Hawes R. Key issues in sphincter of Oddi dysfunction. *Gastrointest Endosc Clin N Am* 2003;**13(4)**:671–94.

80. Elton E, Howell DA, Parsons WG, Qaseem T, Hanson BL. Endoscopic pancreatic sphincterotomy: Indications, outcome, and a safe stentless technique. *Gastrointest Endosc* 1998;**47(3)**:240–9.

81. Elmi F, Silverman WB. Long-term biliary endoscopic sphincterotomy restenosis: Incidence, endoscopic management, and complications of retreatment. *Dig Dis Sci* 2010;**55(7)**:2102–7.

82. Toouli J, Roberts-Thomson IC, Kellow J, Dowsett J, Saccone GT, Evans P, et al. Manometry based randomised trial of endoscopic sphincterotomy for sphincter of Oddi dysfunction. *Gut* 2000;**46(1)**: 98–102.

83. Kovács Z, Kovács F, Pap Á, Czobor P. Sphincter of Oddi dysfunction: Does psychosocial distress play a role? *J Clin Psychol Med Settings* 2007;**14(2)**:138–44.

84. Cotton PB, Durkalski V, Romagnuolo J, Pauls Q, Fogel E, Tarnasky P, et al. Effect of endoscopic sphincterotomy for suspected sphincter of Oddi dysfunction on pain-related disability following cholecystectomy: The EPISOD randomized clinical trial. *JAMA* 2014;**311(20)**:2101–9.

85. Cotton PB, Pauls Q, Keith J, Thornhill A, Drossman D, Williams A, et al. The EPISOD study: Long-term outcomes. *Gastrointest Endosc* 2018;**87(1)**:205–10.

86. Sabour S. Sphincter of Oddi manometry: Methodological issues in reproducibility of measurements. *J Neurogastroenterol Motil* 2016;**22(3)**:541.

87. Suarez AL, Pauls Q, Durkalski-Mauldin V, Cotton PB. Sphincter of Oddi manometry: Reproducibility of measurements and effect of sphincterotomy in the EPISOD Study. *J Neurogastroenterol Motil* 2016;**22(3)**:477–82.

88. Romagnuolo J, Cotton PB, Durkalski V, Pauls Q, Brawman-Mintzer O, Drossman DA, et al. Can patient and pain characteristics predict manometric sphincter of Oddi dysfunction in patients with clinically suspected sphincter of Oddi dysfunction? *Gastrointest Endosc* 2014;**79(5)**:765–72.

89. Yaghoobi M, Pauls Q, Durkalski V, Romagnuolo J, Fogel EL, Tarnasky PR, et al. Incidence and predictors of post-ERCP pancreatitis in patients with suspected sphincter of Oddi dysfunction undergoing biliary or dual sphincterotomy: Results from the EPISOD prospective multicenter randomized sham-controlled study. *Endoscopy* 2015;**47(10)**:884–90.

90. Cotton PB. Why did the sham-treated EPISOD study subjects do so well? Important lessons for research and practice. *Gastrointest Endosc* 2019;**89(5)**:1054–5.

91. Wald A. Functional biliary-type pain: Update and controversies. *J Clin Gastroenterol* 2005;**39(5 Suppl 3)**:S217–22.

92. Abraham HD, Anderson C, Lee D. Somatization disorder in sphincter of Oddi dysfunction. *Psychosom Med* 1997;**59(5)**:553–7.

Bailey & Love's Essential Operations Bailey & Love's Essential Operations Bailey & Love's Essential Operations Bailey & Love's Essential Operations Bailey & Love's Essential Operations

SECTION 9 | BILIARY TRACT

Chapter
58

Common Bile Duct Stones

Rebecca Dalli and Jo E. Abela

INTRODUCTION

For a tube which is only 7 cm long and on average 4 mm wide, located in the right upper quadrant, the bile duct is affected by a remarkable range of pathologies and causes significant morbidity and occasional mortality. Stone disease of the bile duct (choledocholithiasis) is responsible for a very major disease burden which is prevalent across the world. Although subject to considerable variation in incidence, it places very high demands on most healthcare systems. In the United States alone, gallstone disease and its complications, cost a staggering 5 billion U.S. dollars annually (1).

ANATOMICAL CONSIDERATIONS

The extra-hepatic biliary tree usually consists of a fairly simple arrangement of fibro-muscular tubes and the saccular gallbladder. In cross section, the ducts are made of an outer fibro-areolar coat with sparse and mostly circular muscle fibres. The inner mucosal layer is a columnar epithelium with lobulated mucus glands. In the liver hilum, the short right- and slightly longer left-hepatic ducts join up at the confluence to form the common hepatic duct (CHD) which is soon joined by the cystic duct to form the common bile duct (CBD) (*Figure 58.1*).

In its supra-duodenal part in the free-edge of the lesser omentum, the CBD is the most lateral (rightward) structure to the right of the hepatic artery and overlying the portal vein. It then moves behind the second part of the duodenum where it overlies the inferior vena cava and enters a groove within the right side of the pancreatic head (the duct may embed completely in the pancreatic substance). The last part of its course is within the medial wall of the mid-section of the second part of the duodenum. Here it is joined by the main pancreatic duct forming the ampulla of Vater (*Figure 58.2*).

Ductal stones may be found throughout this course with impaction in the distal portion being a common occurrence. Variations of the extrahepatic biliary tree are very common (*Figure 58.3*).

Whilst a detailed description is beyond the scope of this chapter, it is useful to mention that abnormal cystic duct length and insertion may be observed in up to 25% of patients. The extrahepatic course and insertion

of the right posterior sectoral duct is particularly notorious, and the surgeon's appreciation of its variant is important during gallbladder surgery (2).

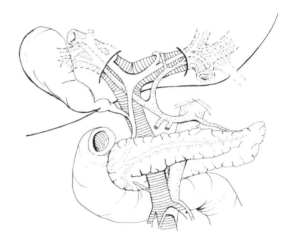

Figure 58.1 Illustration showing traditional biliary anatomy and the relationships of the common bile duct.

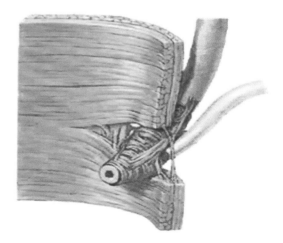

Figure 58.2 Ampulla of Vater showing the junction of CBD and pancreatic duct and the muscular sphincter.

DOI: 10.1201/9781003080060-58

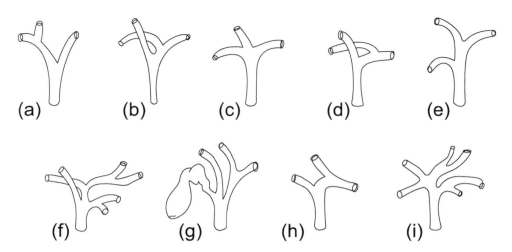

Figure 58.3 Illustrations of the common variations of bile duct anatomy at the hilum (1–9) with approximate frequency with which they occur: **(a)** (57%); **(b)** (16%); **(c)** (12%); **(d)** (5%); **(e)** (4%); **(f)** (2%); **(g)** (2%); **(h)** (1%); **(i)** (1%).

STONE AETIOLOGY

Gallstone formation is a multi-factorial process. The biochemical and biophysical factors are easy to understand and, in essence, follow this principle: stones form once a nidus is available and bile stasis is concomitant with super-concentration of solutes (most commonly cholesterol) in the relative absence of emulsifying bile salts. Thus, mucin may act as a suitable nidus and stasis may be observed in pregnancy or patients receiving total parenteral nutrition (TPN) for long periods. Super-concentration of bile is seen in obesity and dyslipidaemias, whereas lack of bile salts ensues from the impaired entero-hepatic circulation seen in Crohn's ileitis. Haemolytic syndromes result in high pigment concentrations in bile associated with the formation of pigment stones (*Figure 58.4*).

The effect of a strong genetic predisposition has been confirmed and gallstones are virtually unheard of in Africans of Masai extraction but are conversely seen in 70% of Pima Indians. First-degree relatives of gallstone patients have at least a three-fold higher risk (3).

The overwhelming majority of bile duct stones are secondary, originally developing in the gallbladder, from where they pass through a cystic duct which is usually,

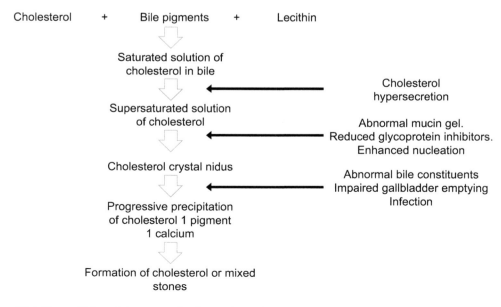

Figure 58.4 The multi-factorial process of gallstone formation.

but not invariably, wide. Some 15% of patients with symptomatic gallstones will have bile duct stones. The true incidence of bile duct stones in completely asymptomatic individuals may never be known although it is likely that most small duct stones will pass into the duodenum silently and harmlessly. Less than 2% of patients who have undergone cholecystectomy for symptomatic gallstones will have residual bile duct stones (4).

Primary bile duct stones are seen most commonly in South-East Asia, Africa and South America. They are relatively uncommon in the West but are seen in elderly patients with dilated or tortuous CBDs. They are thought to occur as a result of bacterial infection (*Escherichia coli*) and/or infection with parasites such as *Clonorchis sinensis* and *Lascaris lumbricoides*.

CLINICAL PRESENTATION

Gallstones tend to be commoner in the 4 F's, a useful *aide memoire*. Gallstone disease is more common in females, in their 40's and 50's, who have had pregnancies and are obese. Almost 20% of patients with bile duct stones are completely asymptomatic (5). Stones may be discovered incidentally in the course of investigations or another pathology when liver function tests (LFTs) are abnormal and radiological investigations reveal stones. Patients being investigated for right subcostal pain may, in addition to abnormal LFTs, be found to have a dilated biliary tree on ultrasound (US) examination which should alert the clinician to the possibility of bile duct stones. Following a cholecystectomy, residual duct stones may be discovered many months or even years after the surgery in approximately 1–2% of patients. It is not possible in a percentage of cases to differentiate between residual and primary duct stones.

CHOLANGITIS

Bile duct stones may present with right-sided subcostal pain, fever and jaundice. This symptom complex is commonly referred to as Charcot's triad and this is in keeping with ascending cholangitis. Whereas gallbladder pain tends to be severe and well-localized, bile duct pain is more usually mild and ill-defined. Nausea and vomiting are common associations. Cholangitis tends to give rise to a high fever, with a classical pattern of chills and rigours. Abdominal palpation may elicit Murphy's sign. The sign is named after John Benjamin Murphy (1857–1916), a Chicago surgeon who first described the hypersensitivity to deep palpation in the subcostal area when a patient with gallbladder disease takes a deep breath. Nausea and vomiting are common associations. Bile duct stones are an important cause of obstructive jaundice, most commonly due to one or more stones impacting in the distal CBD. This is not uncommonly

seen in the presence of an inflammatory or fibrotic stricture. In severe cases of cholangitis, the patient may rapidly become obtunded with the development of multi-organ dysfunction, hypotension, oliguria and respiratory distress.

ACUTE PANCREATITIS

The index admission may be acute pancreatitis with the classical presentation of epigastric and central abdominal pain with distention and radiation to the back. Nausea and vomiting are common but fever is not generally present at the initial presentation or at an early stage. Typically, a raised serum amylase or lipase of more than three times the upper limit of normal corroborates the diagnosis. Although less commonly used, serum lipase is felt to be superior because it is more specific and has a slower return to baseline.

MIRIZZI'S SYNDROME

Mirizzi's syndrome (described in detail in **Chapter 70**) usually presents with Charcot's triad and the diagnosis is radiological. Two main subsets were originally recognized. Mirizzi Type 1 occurs when a large stone in Hartmann's pouch is pressing on the CHD or CBD due to its size and there is an inevitable inflammatory reaction (*Figure 58.5*).

Mirizzi type 2 is diagnosed when a large stone which has impacted in Hartmann's pouch erodes and fistulates into the bile duct. Modifications have been made in recognition of the variable presentations and radiological findings and the most commonly used is the Csendes classification shown in *Table 58.1*.

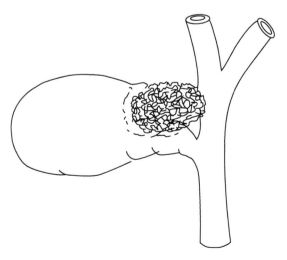

Figure 58.5 Illustration of Mirizzi syndrome type 1, note the large stone in Hartmann's pouch pressing on the CHD.

Table 58.1 Csendes classification of Mirizzi's syndrome

Type	Description
Type I	External compression on CBD
Type II	Cholecystocholedochal fistula affecting less than one third of the CBD
Type III	Cholecystocholedochal fistula affecting up to two thirds of the CBD
Type IV	Cholecystocholedochal fistula with complete destruction of CBD wall
Type V	Types I–IV with cholecystoenteric fistula

DIAGNOSIS

As previously mentioned, altered LFTs often alert clinicians to the possibility of bile duct stones. The pattern of derangement is not specific to stone disease but an obstructive picture, with elevations of the gamma glutamyl transferase (GGT) and alkaline phosphatase (ALP), are common. The list of alternative possible diagnoses however is long and includes: 1) Liver disease including steatosis and cirrhosis; 2) benign strictures from primary or secondary sclerosing cholangitis and IgG4-cholangiopathy and 3) malignant strictures resulting from cholangiocarcinoma, ampullary and pancreatic and duodenal lesions.

The basis for bile duct stone diagnosis has been radiology and will remain so for the foreseeable future. Both transabdominal ultrasonography (US) and computerized tomography (CT) are useful for the identification of dilated intra- and extrahepatic bile ducts. Whereas US excels in the diagnosis of gallbladder stones, bile duct stones (unless large or multiple) offer a serious challenge. CT scanning may be unreliable especially for the diagnosis of radiolucent stones but is the 'gold standard' for the diagnosis and assessment of patients with acute pancreatitis. CT-cholangiography can be used but has been replaced by magnetic resonance imaging (MRI) and, where available, magnetic resonance cholangiopancreatography (MRCP) is the current 'gold standard' non-invasive diagnostic test for ductal stones.

In the past, intra-operative cholangiography (IOC) was a routine step in the course of open cholecystectomy. In the minimally invasive era, most centres are tending to a selective use of IOC. This is possibly due to the perception that minimally invasive IOC requires complex laparoscopic skills and the overwhelming majority of surgical units have opted for a selective IOC strategy, given that MRCP is now much more freely available. Laparoscopy also allows the assessment of the bile duct by laparoscopic US in addition to direct visualization by choledochoscopy. Indeed, ultra-slim 3 mm endoscopes may be introduced into the CBD through the cystic duct (this may require pre-dilatation with a balloon catheter).

Peroral endoscopic techniques are very effective and reliable. In most surgical units worldwide, endoscopic retrograde cholangiopancreatography (ERCP) is the mainstay of therapy for bile duct stones. However, given the range and incidence of complications ERCP is no longer used diagnostically. Direct visualization of the bile ducts can be achieved during ERCP via through-the-scope solutions such as Spyglass™ (Boston Scientific, MS, US). In addition to ERCP, endoscopic ultrasonography (EUS) has become an established and safe diagnostic tool which is used in hepato-pancreatico-biliary (HPB) units for a wide range of pathologies. Although more invasive than conventional radiology techniques (US and MRCP) the risk is very low and it allows a very detailed assessment of the extrahepatic biliary tree and the pancreas. Therapeutic applications of EUS will be discussed later.

MANAGEMENT

Some 50 years ago, ERCP revolutionized the treatment of bile duct stones. Before the advent of this peroral minimally invasive stone removal technique, surgeons were reliant on open surgery in the form of bile-duct exploration, usually in the course of an open cholecystectomy and after confirmation by intraoperative cholangiography. More recently, improved laparoscopic optics and devices allow this open procedure to be performed laparoscopically.

Endoscopic retrograde cholangiopancreatography

ERCP is performed through a side-viewing endoscope which features a 'bridging' control to elevate and manipulate the position of accessories being used through the therapeutic channel. The safest technique involves passing a guidewire into the bile duct, via a cannula or sphincterotome inserted into the ampulla of Vater. Gentle injection of contrast material opacifies the biliary tree and bile duct stones will appear as filling defects. This process is not always straightforward due to a hooded configuration of the ampulla, an ampullary stenosis or a periampullary diverticulum and selective CBD cannulation may require an initial pre-cut using an endoscopic knife. Scarring of the duodenum and anatomical abnormalities, usually due to previous surgery, such as a distal gastrectomy or obesity surgery may also render ERCP difficult or occasionally impossible.

The sphincterotome is used to make a radial incision in the ampulla dividing the muscle fibres of the sphincter of Oddi. This facilitates the passage of a retrieval and/or crushing device (balloons, baskets and lithotripsy probes) into the biliary tree and stones up to 10 mm may be trawled into the duodenum using wires baskets or balloons. Larger stones may be broken up with hydraulic and/or laser lithotripsy techniques and the fragments subsequently removed. Plastic stents are left *in situ* when the operator elects to perform a staged approach with clearance over several sessions, typically 6 weeks apart. This approach is adopted when stones are very large or multiple, when the procedure is poorly tolerated and a different method of sedation or even a general anaesthetic is required. In elderly patients, it is considered safer.

The incidence of serious complications following stone extraction at ERCP when attempting to clear the duct is approximately 7% (6). Post-procedural cholangitis is treated with intravenous (IV) antibiotics but may require repeat ERCP and plastic stenting. Intra- and post-procedural haemorrhage may be managed with submucosal adrenaline injection, thermal therapy such as argon-plasma coagulation (APC) or the use of a heater-probe or haemostatic clips. Acute pancreatitis is usually self-limiting but may be severe. The risk of pancreatitis appears to be reduced by the administration of non-steroidal anti-inflammatory drugs (NSAIDs) immediately prior to the procedure. Visceral perforation in the absence of significant contamination is managed conservatively.

Open and laparoscopic bile-duct exploration

The open approach to a CBD exploration is usually through a right subcostal (Kocher's) incision or an upper midline incision. The laparoscopic approach is through the traditional 4-port placement and the steps for the two approaches are identical. After dissection of Calot's triangle, a trans-cystic cholangiogram is performed. If bile duct stones smaller than 5 mm (in size) are confirmed, trans-cystic clearance may be attempted using wire baskets. This can be done through a 3 mm choledochoscope, or through the cholangiogram cannula itself, under fluoroscopy. When the cystic duct anatomy is unfavourable (e.g. unyielding valve of Heister) or stones are larger than 5mm, formal bile duct exploration is performed. This is done via an oblique choledochotomy when the bile duct diameter is 8mm or more. For reasons mentioned in the next section, we do not recommend choledohotomy in smaller caliber ducts (these ducts qualify for rendezvous or post-operative ERCP). Choledochotomy allows easy passage for 5mm choledochoscopy, with direct visualization of the stones and enhanced engagement in baskets or balloons. Small stones and debris can be flushed into the duodenum especially when a sphincterotomy has been performed at a prior ERCP. IV administered sphincter relaxants such as hyoscine hydrocholoride and glucagon, may facilitate this process. Choledochotomy closure remains a matter of some controversy and there are a number of options. Primary closure alone, closure over a T-tube, closure over a trans-cystic drain, closure over an ERCP-type plastic stent or formation of choledocho-duodenostomy (although the latter may

be challenging to perform laparoscopically). In our laparoscopic practice, we prefer to achieve primary closure with a running 4/0 polydiaxonone suture over a 70 mm 7Fr straight plastic stent and we always drain the subhepatic space. The stent is removed at gastroscopy 6-weeks after the operation (7).

Other forms of treatment

Hybrid procedures employing laparoscopy and ERCP, the so called 'rendezvous' procedures, are also performed in some units. We reserve these for inadvertently discovered ductal stones in patients with small ducts of less than 5 mm where trans-cystic exploration has failed. In this situation, we prefer the hybrid approach because of the significant rate of stricture formation in very small ducts.

Extra-corporeal shock wave lithotripsy (ESWL) has been reported and is offered by some specialist centres and may be useful in the context of intra-hepatic ductal stones (8). Percutaneous trans-hepatic cholangiographic techniques are also available and we reserve this option for intra-hepatic stones where an endoscopic approach has been attempted but was unsuccessful (9). Novel EUS techniques allow the formation of endoscopic choledochoduodenostomy, by the deployment of covered self-expanding apposing stents. This allows large-caliber internal biliary drainage. This is a very recent development and there is a paucity of data regarding the specific indications and complication rates (10).

SUMMARY

Common bile duct stones present as a significant disease burden. They are associated with serious complications, including obstructive jaundice, ascending cholangitis and acute pancreatitis. Whereas abdominal US/CT examinations and blood tests are the initial line of investigation, MRCP and EUS are more accurate in confirming CBD stones. Various techniques and approaches are available for the treatment of CBD stones. Various techniques and approaches are available for the treatment of CBD stones including ERCP, open or minimally invasive bile duct exploration and hybrids thereof. Novel EUS techniques appear promising, but data on their medium- and long-term outcomes are still lacking.

REFERENCES

1. Stinton LM, Shaffer EA. Epidemiology of gallbladder disease: Cholelithiasis and cancer. *Gut Liver* 2012;**6(2)**:172–87.
2. Janssen BV, van Laarhoven S, Elshaer M, Cai H, Praseedom R, Wang T, Liauand SS, et al. Comprehensive classification of anatomical variants of the main biliary ducts, *BJS* 2021;**108(5)**:458–62.
3. Jones MW, Weir CB, Ghassemzadeh S. Gallstones (Cholelithiasis). Available from: www.ncbi.nlm.nih.

gov/books/NBK459370/. StatPearls Publishing, Treasure Island (Accessed 28 August 2024).

4. Williams E, Beckingham I, El Sayed G, et al. Updated guideline on the management of common bile duct stones, (CBDS). *Gut* 2017;**66**:765–82.

5. Rosseland AR, Glomsaker TB. Asymptomatic common bile duct stones. *Eur J Gastroenterol Hepatol* 2000;**11**:1171–3.

6. Szary NM, Al-Kawas FH. Complications of endoscopic retrograde cholangiopancreatography: How to avoid and manage them. *Gastroenterol Hepatol* 2013;**9(8)**:496–504.

7. Marks B, Al Samaraee A. Laparoscopic exploration of the common bile duct: A systematic review of the published evidence over the last 10 Years. *Am Surg* 2021;**87(3)**:404–18.

8. Muratori R, Azzaroli F, Buonfiglioli F, Alessandrelli F, Cecinato P, Mazzella G, et al. ESWL for difficult bile duct stones: A 15-year single centre experience. *World J Gastroenterol* 2010;**16(33)**:4159–63.

9. Güngören, FZ, Erol C, Seker M. et al. The efficacy of percutaneous treatment methods in bile duct stones. *Indian J Surg* 2023;**85**:863–67.

10. Jacques J, Privat J, Pinard F, Fumex F, Valats JC, Chaoui A, et al. Endoscopic ultrasound-guided choledochoduodenostomy with electrocautery-enhanced lumen-apposing stents: A retrospective analysis. *Endoscopy* 2019;**51(6)**:540–7.

Chapter
59

Biliary Strictures

Abhirup Banerjee and Sudeep R. Shah

INTRODUCTION

What is a biliary stricture?

A stricture is an abnormal narrowing in the biliary system that often results in clinically and physiologically relevant mechanical obstruction. Biliary strictures are usually diagnosed in patients whose liver function tests (LFTs) demonstrate a cholestatic pattern. These are usually triggered by the appearance of the features of obstructive jaundice (icterus, dark urine, pale stools) which leads to a range of investigations initially, usually blood tests and imaging. Occasionally, biliary strictures or dilatation may also be identified incidentally on imaging in patients without any, or only with minimal, derangement in their liver profiles who are being investigated or managed for other conditions.

Investigations: Blood tests and imaging

A rise in the conjugated (direct) component, and total levels, of serum bilirubin along with a concomitant rise in the levels of serum alkaline phosphatase (ALP) and gamma-glutamyl transferase (GGT) will suggest an obstructive cause.

An abrupt change in the calibre of the common bile duct (CBD) on imaging, as opposed to the smooth tapering towards the ampulla normally observed in the CBD, suggests a mid- or distal-biliary stricture. Stricturing disease can also be observed in the peri-hilar bile ducts frequently due to the development of a cholangiocarcinoma (Klatskin tumour) with, or without, involvement of the intra-hepatic biliary system.

A number of imaging modalities are at the disposal of the clinician to define the extent of disease and to look for an associated mass or other related pathology. These include ultrasonography (US), computed tomography (CT), magnetic resonance imaging (MRI), magnetic resonance cholangiopancreatography (MRCP), endoscopic retrograde cholangiopancreatography (ERCP), percutaneous transhepatic cholangiography (PTC), endoscopic ultrasound (EUS), cholangioscopy (Spyglass™ [Boston Scientific, MS, US]), and intraductal ultrasound (IDUS). Diagnostic accuracies vary but generally range between 60–80%. Tumour markers such as carcinoembryonic antigen (CEA) and carbohydrate antigen (CA) 19-9 can sometimes help and narrow down the diagnosis. CA 19-9 is a sialylated form of the Lewis blood group antigen which exists in serum as a mucin, a high molecular weight (>1 million Daltons) glycoprotein complex with a half-life of approximately 1 day. It is produced by ductal cells in the pancreas, biliary system, and epithelial cells in the stomach, colon, uterus, and salivary glands. It is however important to be aware of confounding variables as levels may be raised in a variety of benign conditions, especially in biliary obstruction from any cause, and it is negative in approximately 5–10% of the population (patients who lack the Lewis antigen A cannot synthesize CA 19-9) (1).

Options for tissue sampling

Tissue for diagnosis can be obtained by ERCP, PTC, EUS, and cholangioscopy in addition to being possible percutaneously under imaging guidance generally USG or CT. Fine needle biopsies (FNB) and Tru-cut biopsies (core needle biopsy) are preferred over cytology (fine needle aspiration cytology [FNAC] and biliary brushings) to help study the tissue architecture in more detail and perform genetic studies if indicated. For potentially malignant extrahepatic strictures, EUS-guided sampling is preferred to ERCP both for obtaining tissue and concomitantly imaging the abnormal area. If FNAC is performed, rapid on-site evaluation (ROSE) is recommended where available (FNB obviates the need for ROSE) (2). FNB also results in a higher yield of nucleic acids for genomic profiling. Tissue obtained can be subjected to histopathological examination using haematoxylin and eosin (H&E) staining, immunohistochemistry (IHC), and fluorescent in situ hybridization (FISH) to help arrive at a diagnosis.

Newer generation core needles with varying bevel geometries such as reverse bevel, Franseen, and fork-tip enable tissue sampling with higher diagnostic yields and are technically as easy to use as FNA needles (3,4). They also reduce the number of passes required to obtain a diagnosis. Histological yield is however variable and definitive results are often difficult to obtain. In patients with a history of repeated biliary interventions and particularly multiple stent exchanges, there is an inevitable reactive biliary atypia and making or refuting a diagnosis of malignancy can be extremely challenging for the pathologist.

For perihilar strictures, intraductal sampling should be favoured while EUS-FNAC/FNB or percutaneous sampling should be avoided. Lymph node sampling

DOI: 10.1201/9781003080060-59

Table 59.1 Aetiology of biliary strictures

Malignant, primary

- Pancreatic cancer
- Cholangiocarcinoma
- Gallbladder cancer
- Hepatocellular carcinoma
- Lymphoma
- Neuroendocrine tumour

Malignant, metastatic

- Colon cancer
- Breast cancer
- Gastric cancer
- Ovarian cancer
- Renal cell cancer
- Extrinsic compression from portal/hilar lymph nodes

Benign

- Stones: CBD, Mirizzi syndrome
- Chronic pancreatitis
- Primary sclerosing cholangitis
- Autoimmune (Immunoglobulin G [IgG] 4–mediated) pancreatitis
- IgG4-mediated cholangitis
- Eosinophilic cholangitis
- Xanthogranulomatous cholecystitis
- Sarcoidosis
- Recurrent pyogenic cholangitis
- Extrinsic compression by a pancreatic fluid collection
- Inflammatory pseudotumour
- TB, HIV (AIDS cholangiopathy), parasitic oriental cholangiohepatitis
- Radiation
- Trauma
- Vasculitis: SLE, ANCA-related

Benign (lower bile duct pathology)

- Papillary stenosis
- Sphincter of Oddi dysfunction (SOD)
- Duodenal diverticulum
- Chronic duodenal ulcer

Iatrogenic

- Cholecystectomy
- CBD exploration
- Hepaticojejunostomy
- Hepatectomy
- Gastrectomy
- Liver transplantation
- Local cancer treatment (chemoembolization, radiation therapy, microwave ablation, and radiofrequency ablation)

Vascular

- Portal hypertensive biliopathy
- Ischaemic biliary injury

Congenital

- Biliary atresia
- Agenesis
- Choledochal cyst

Abbreviations: ANCA: antineutrophilic cytoplasmic antibody; SLE: systemic lupus erythematosus.

may be performed by EUS-guided or percutaneous techniques.

Differentiating benign versus malignant disease

The aim of treatment in a patient with a biliary stricture, is to establish the diagnosis using all modalities available confirm or refute the presence of malignancy and re-establish uninterrupted flow of bile into the intestine.

Making the correct diagnosis is vital to ensure that malignancies are not missed while also preventing unnecessary interventions (including surgery) in benign aetiologies. Major surgery for a patient with a putative diagnosis of malignancy, especially if there is significant postoperative morbidity or mortality, is a frequent cause of medical litigation when benign disease is found on the definitive histopathology. However, in the presence of an indeterminate stricture, the underlying pathology is statistically more likely to be malignant than benign and sometimes it is impossible to exclude a tumour. In this situation a detailed, carefully documented consultation with appropriate counselling is essential.

Despite significant technical advances over the last two decades, establishing an unequivocal diagnosis for a biliary stricture in the absence of a mass-forming lesion frequently represents a significant challenge for the clinical team. Many of the common causes of biliary strictures are covered in Chapter 58 including malignancy, trauma, Mirizzi syndrome, bile duct stones, biliary parasitic disease and IPMN-B. In this chapter, we discuss some of the other causes of biliary strictures that must be kept in mind when evaluating these patients. We will also describe some general principles of management. Possible aetiologies of biliary strictures are listed in *Table 59.1*.

IATROGENIC BILIARY STRICTURES

The vast majority of iatrogenic bile duct strictures are the result of surgery on the gallbladder, principally following a laparoscopic cholecystectomy. This may be due to a partial narrowing of the bile duct due to an incorrectly placed clip at the time of cystic duct transection or secondary to diathermy-induced thermal injury or vascular complication leading to an ischaemic stricture (*Figure 59.1*). In the worst-case scenario, the common hepatic duct may be completely transected (*Figure 59.2*). The incidence of bile duct injury following laparoscopic cholecystectomy is reported to be 0.1–0.3%. The management of bile duct injuries detected intraoperatively or in the early postoperative period are discussed in **Chapter 62**. Bile duct strictures can also arise following liver transplantation and as a complication of other surgical procedures listed in *Table 59.1*, but a detailed discussion is beyond the scope of this chapter.

Obtaining a good quality cholangiogram, most commonly with an MRCP, and classifying the extent of injury (*Figure 59.3*) is essential for planning

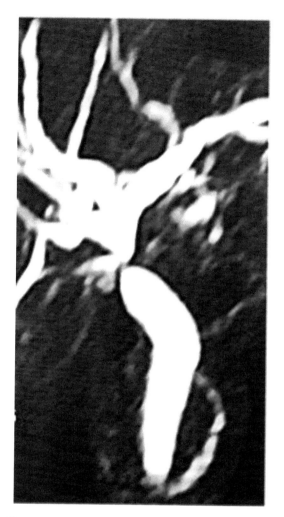

Figure 59.1 MRCP showing a tight ischaemic biliary stricture (arrow) following a laparoscopic cholecystectomy.

reconstructive surgery. Inadequate planning and suboptimal surgery risks subjecting the patient to months or sometimes years of repeated interventions prolonging their suffering.

PRIMARY SCLEROSING CHOLANGITIS

Definition and epidemiology

Primary sclerosing cholangitis (PSC) is a chronic cholestatic liver disease in which multifocal biliary strictures characterized by inflammation and concentric periductal fibrosis may involve the intra- and/or extra-hepatic biliary system. There is bilateral involvement in 70% of patients, intra-hepatic alone in 25%, and extra-hepatic alone in 5%. The alternating areas of normal but slightly dilated biliary segments may give rise to a 'beaded' appearance (*Figure 59.4*).

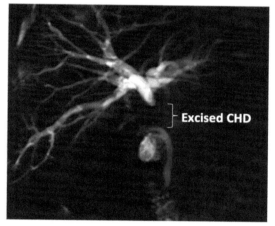

Figure 59.2 Accidental transection and excision of the common hepatic duct (CHD) noted on an MRCP following a laparoscopic cholecystectomy.

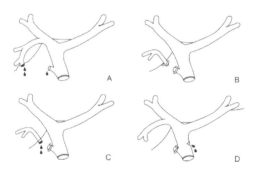

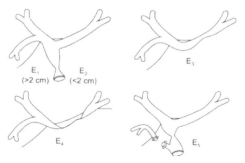

Figure 59.3 Strasberg modification of the Bismuth classification for bile duct injury. **(A)** Bile leak from cystic duct stump or minor biliary radicle in gallbladder fossa. **(B)** Occluded right posterior sectoral duct. **(C)** Bile leak from divided right posterior sectoral duct. **(D)** Bile leak from main bile duct without major tissue loss. **(E_1)** Transected main bile duct with a stricture more than 2 cm from the hilum. **(E_2)** Transected main bile duct with a stricture less than 2 cm from the hilum. **(E_3)** Stricture of the hilum with right and left ducts in communication. **(E_4)** Stricture at the hilum with separation of right and left ducts. **(E_5)** Stricture of the main bile duct and the right posterior sectoral duct. Adapted from (5).

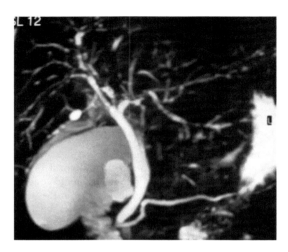

Figure 59.4 MRCP in a patient with PSC showing multiple intrahepatic biliary strictures and a 'beaded' appearance.

As the fibrosis progresses, the peripheral ducts become poorly visible, giving a 'pruned tree' appearance. The disease process may also involve the gallbladder and the cystic duct.

Men are predominantly affected (M : F = 2 : 1) with the peak incidence in the 3rd/4th decades. Approximately 60–90% of patients with PSC will also have concomitant inflammatory bowel disease (IBD), with ulcerative colitis (UC) being five times more common than Crohn's disease. The prevalence of PSC in UC is estimated to be approximately 4–5% and is more common in men with pancolitis as opposed to those with proctitis or left-sided colitis (5.5% vs 0.5%) (6). In the absence of IBD, there is a slight female preponderance. Secondary sclerosing cholangitis, as opposed to PSC, is characterized by a similar process but from an identifiable cause (e.g. choledocholithiasis).

Clinical presentation and investigations

Although half the patients with PSC are asymptomatic at diagnosis, fatigue and pruritis are commonly observed non-specific symptoms. Cholangitis may occur, while ongoing inflammation can eventually lead to cirrhosis and portal hypertension. At diagnosis, bilirubin levels are often normal while the transaminases may show a modest elevation. Liver profile predominantly demonstrates an elevated ALP and GGT. About one-tenth of patients may have elevated IgG4 levels and this may represent a distinct subset of patients that tend to manifest a more rapid progression of disease (7). However, unlike the typical patient with PSC, this subset does seem to respond to treatment with steroids and therefore all PSC patients should be tested at least once for elevated IgG4 levels.

An MRCP usually establishes the diagnosis of PSC in the appropriate clinical setting. It is generally not necessary to perform a liver biopsy unless there is suspected small-duct PSC or if overlap syndromes such as concomitant autoimmune hepatitis need to be excluded. The infrequent but typical 'onion-skin' pattern on histology comprises fibrous obliteration of small bile ducts with periductal concentric replacement by connective tissue (8).

Dominant strictures, defined at ERCP as a CBD stricture <1.5 mm or <1 mm in a duct within 2 cm of the biliary confluence, arise in up to 50% of patients during follow-up (9). Approximately 5% of patients with small-duct PSC disease will have a normal cholangiogram but nearly one quarter of them will develop large-duct PSC within 10 years.

The lifetime risk of developing a cholangiocarcinoma (CCA) in PSC is 10–20% with an annual incidence of 0.5–2%. Once a diagnosis of PSC has been made it is important to develop a surveillance plan including the risk stratification, staging, and management, (summarized in *Figure 59.5*). The main causes of mortality in PSC are cholangiocarcinoma (~30%), liver failure (~18%), complications of liver transplantation (~9%), and colorectal cancer (~8%).

Medical treatment

Although data from well-controlled trials are lacking, ursodeocycholic acid (UDCA) is the only medical treatment that may potentially be of some benefit, but it should not be routinely used for patients with a new diagnosis of PSC. High doses above 28 mg/kg/day have been demonstrated to result in harm rather than benefit (11).

Other drugs such as azathioprine, budesonide, methotrexate, MMF, prednisolone and vancomycin, have been tested but no obvious clinical benefit has been demonstrated. Symptomatic relief for PSC patients with pruritis should be prescribed in the form of skin emollients, antihistamines, or bile acid sequestrants such as cholestyramine. If these are ineffective, second-line options such as rifampin and naltrexone may be considered.

Endoscopy

Recent advances in endoscopy have focused on the treatment of dominant strictures as they are a common problem in patients with PSC and are potentially amenable to treatment at ERCP. Balloon dilatation is recommended for these strictures to relieve symptoms, but they must also be sampled with cytology, biopsies, and FISH to exclude CCA even though most of these strictures will prove to be benign. It must be kept in mind that half the malignancies in PSC are diagnosed within the first 4–6 months following the initial diagnosis. Bile duct stones are also routinely encountered in PSC and extraction reduces biliary outflow obstruction. Routine

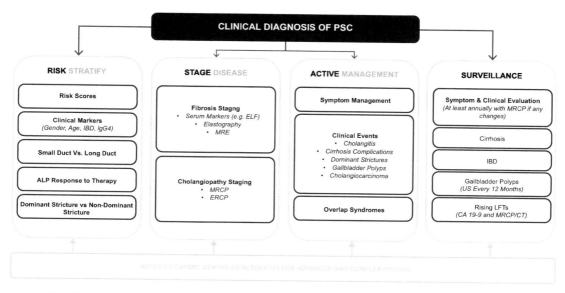

Figure 59.5 Algorithm for the management of suspected PSC. (Adapted from [10].)

stenting after dilatation of a dominant stricture is not considered to be necessary but short-term stents may be placed in those with severe stricturing disease.

Post-ERCP cholangitis is a significant and potentially life-threatening problem due to the difficulty in decompressing intra-hepatic areas of biliary obstruction. Even though there is a lack of prospective studies, a peri-procedural antibiotic course for 3–5 days is recommended.

The introduction of cholangioscopy has allowed for better and direct visualization and biopsies of dominant strictures with sensitivity and specificity of greater than 90%. This is particularly valuable in the setting of indeterminate strictures to ensure that a CCA is not missed, and it also helps to detect stones in the biliary system that were missed on cross-sectional imaging. Confocal laser microscopy and IDUS are other techniques that may offer an improved diagnostic yield.

Radiological and surgical options

Percutaneous transhepatic access and dilatation is an option in patients with intrahepatic strictures difficult to access at endoscopy or when there are very tight strictures that cannot be traversed at ERCP.

In the absence of effective medical treatment for PSC, the median time for progression from diagnosis until death or liver transplantation is approximately 10 years. Liver transplantation is the definitive treatment for patients with decompensated cirrhosis and in this setting, it is recommended over endoscopic or surgical drainage procedures. Even after liver transplantation, about 20% of patients will develop recurrent PSC within 5 years but the majority of this cohort do not experience significant morbidity or mortality (12).

IMMUNOGLOBULIN G4-RELATED SCLEROSING CHOLANGITIS

The manifestation of IgG4-related disease in the biliary tract may present in isolation or together with other complications of autoimmune disease (frequently associated with autoimmune pancreatitis). Immunoglobulin G4-related sclerosing cholangitis (IgG4-SC) is characterized by the presence of an obliterative phlebitis, storiform fibrosis, and IgG4+ plasma cells (greater than ten IgG4+ cells per high power field) on histology. A schematic classification of IgG4-SC by cholangiography is shown in *Figure 59.6*.

IgG4-SC responds to treatment with steroids within 8 weeks, is not associated with inflammatory bowel disease (IBD) and does not undergo malignant transformation. Apart from these, the other features that help differentiate IgG4-SC from PSC include continuous rather than multifocal bile duct strictures, a thick-walled GB and CBD, and concomitant involvement of other organs such as the pancreas or kidney.

GENERAL MANAGEMENT PRINCIPLES

Endoscopic options

An ERCP is often the first invasive procedure that a patient with a biliary stricture undergoes. This helps to obtain a good quality cholangiogram and potentially a histopathological diagnosis with the help of brushings, biopsies, or bile aspiration. The diagnostic yield of the above techniques varies widely, and a negative result should not stop further investigations and interventions, especially if the clinical suspicion of malignancy is high

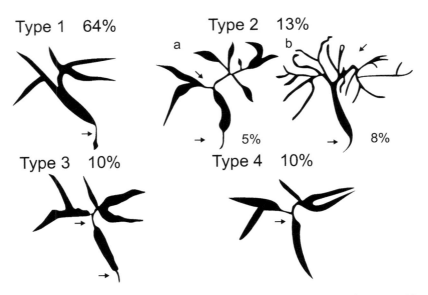

Figure 59.6 Types of biliary strictures in IgG4-SC. **Type 1**: Isolated stricture of the distal common bile duct. **Type 2**: Diffuse strictures of the intra- and extrahepatic bile ducts with (**Type 2a**) or without (**Type 2b**) pre-stenotic dilatation. **Type 3**: Hilar stricture and distal common bile duct stricture. **Type 4**: Isolated hilar stricture. Adapted from (13).

based on clinical presentation and radiological features. Strictures at, or above, the level of the common bile duct bifurcation are more difficult to navigate as compared to distal strictures and these patients often end up having percutaneous transhepatic cholangiography to sample and/or stent the stricture.

Apart from obtaining a diagnosis at ERCP, benign biliary strictures can be balloon dilated which may suffice as treatment although the procedure may need to be repeated if the stricture re-forms. Strictures due to chronic pancreatitis or post-cholecystectomy strictures can be treated by temporary insertion of multiple plastic biliary stents or by placement of a fully covered self-expandible metal stent (fcSEMS). The latter stents have a small but definite risk of migration, and this should be kept in mind while placing these. These too may need to be replaced at regular intervals depending on the benefit achieved with stenting. The treatment duration with stents ranges from 6–12 months before considering other options such as surgery.

In the absence of cholangitis, preoperative stenting may be avoided for distal malignant biliary strictures whereas hilar strictures almost always require preoperative drainage, usually via PTC. If extrahepatic strictures do need preoperative drainage, a 10 mm short fcSEMS is usually preferred. Longer stents can block off the cystic duct insertion into the CBD leading to acute cholecystitis.

Uncovered metal stents should only be placed after a diagnosis of malignancy is confirmed. In most centres, these would only be used if the intent of treatment is palliation. These generally become anchored to the bile ducts even in the absence of malignancy due to

tissue ingrowth into the mesh structure of the stent. The median patency of these stents is approximately 9 months. When these stents become permanently embedded, recurrent stent occlusion and chronic low-grade obstruction leading to secondary biliary cirrhosis or sclerosing cholangitis are important long-term considerations. Although removal can be performed, it is technically challenging, risky, and may not be possible. If these stents are inserted in patients with a benign pathology, they are very likely to require repeated ERCPs for recurrent stent blockage and cholangitis.

The experience with endoscopic ultrasound-guided biliary drainage (EUS-BD) is increasing and this provides an additional modality to obtaining biliary drainage into the stomach or duodenum from the gallbladder and the CHD/CBD in cases where conventional techniques have failed. Use of plastic stents, metals stents and lumen-apposing metal stents (LAMS) in isolation, or in combination, have shown promising results. These procedures should only be performed following a thorough multidisciplinary discussion and undertaken at a tertiary centre where there is an experienced operator and team familiar with the technique.

For unresectable malignant biliary strictures, photodynamic therapy (PDT) and radiofrequency ablation (RFA) are commercially available techniques that can be applied via PTBD or ERCP to improve survival (14). PDT involves the diffusion of a specific wavelength of light using a laser fibre resulting in activation of a photosensitizer (either porfimer sodium or a second-generation haematoporphyrin derivative) injected intravenously (IV) prior to the procedure. This generates reactive oxygen species that directly destroy the tumour cells.

Following PDT, the patient should avoid direct and indirect sunlight for 4–6 weeks to avoid severe cutaneous burns as a result of PDT-induced photosensitivity. RFA employs bipolar electrodes that delivers thermal energy resulting in coagulative necrosis in the stricture where there is contact with the RFA catheter.

Surgical treatment

Once a definitive diagnosis of a benign biliary stricture has been made, surgery is often the only option once all endoscopic options have been exhausted and the intended clinical benefit has not been achieved. A thorough knowledge of common and uncommon variations in biliary and vascular anatomy, (discussed in **Chapter 4**), is essential prior to embarking upon these operations. Multiple endoscopic and percutaneous interventions prior to an operative procedure can often make the surgical field extremely difficult to navigate and the preoperative delineation of biliary and vascular anatomy is crucial (*Figure 59.7*). For iatrogenic biliary strictures due to surgical misadventure, this is even more important due to the medico-legal implications. A Roux-en-Y hepaticojejunostomy is the most versatile reconstructive option and is employed by hepatobiliary surgeons across the world to surgically drain the biliary tree proximal to the strictured segment. Surgery for biliary strictures secondary to malignancy have been discussed in **Chapter 61**.

Despite the growing experience with minimally invasive surgery, most surgeons would adopt an open approach (either by using a reverse-L incision or by extending an existing subcostal incision from previous surgery) especially while approaching a biliary stricture at the hilum. Lowering the hilar plate is one of the most important steps in surgery for peri-hilar biliary strictures. This enables the surgeon to easily access the biliary bifurcation (*Figure 59.8A*) and if needed, a hepatotomy can also be performed to improve access (*Figure 59.8B*). The left hepatic duct has a longer extrahepatic course than the right hepatic duct and this is used to the surgeon's advantage during biliary reconstruction. The left hepatic duct can be opened along its length which facilitates creation of a wide anastomosis. Preoperatively placed biliary stents are often helpful in guiding the surgeon towards the bile duct in what is often a hostile surgical field.

A single layer duct-to-mucosa anastomosis is preferred between the bile duct and the Roux loop of jejunum that is usually brought up through a mesocolic window to the right of the middle colic vessels. A fine, delayed absorbable, monofilament suture such

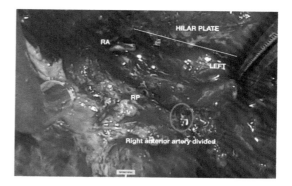

Figure 59.7 In-surgery labelled image showing a complex injury to the hilar bile ducts at a laparoscopic cholecystectomy noted at delayed exploration. Biliary stents can be seen protruding through the damaged right anterior (RA) and right posterior (RP) bile ducts. The right anterior hepatic artery (red circle) has been accidentally divided.

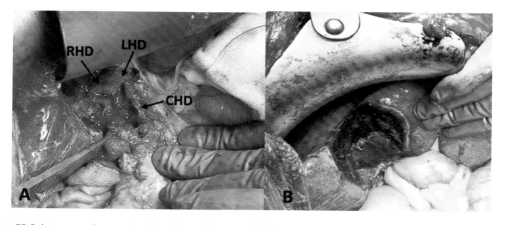

Figure 59.8 In-surgery image showing the confluence of the bile ducts has been opened showing the right and left hepatic ducts (RHD and LHD) after lowering the hilar plate. The upper end of the common hepatic duct (CHD) has also been laid open (A). Occasionally a hepatotomy may be required in patients with complex high biliary hilar strictures that are difficult to access even after lowering the hilar plate (B).

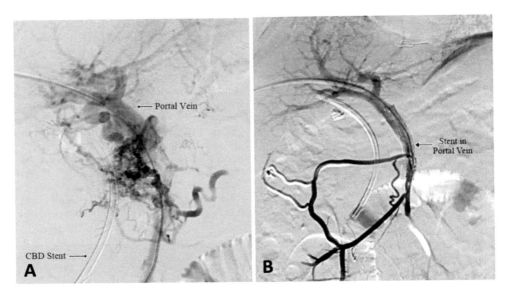

Figure 59.9 Portal biliopathy in a patient with chronic pancreatitis (A). Resolution of the portal cavernoma following placement of a stent in the portal vein enabling subsequent surgery (hepaticojejunostomy) (B) (15).

as 4-0 or 5-0 polydioxanone is preferred for biliary anastomoses depending on the location and thickness of the bile duct to be reconstructed. Depending on the clinical situation and location of the stricture, the bilio-enteric anastomosis can be performed in a side-to-side fashion. Alternatively, the lower end of the bile duct can be disconnected, and the stump secured with a running suture, following which an end-to-side bilio-enteric anastomosis can also be performed to the hepatic duct(s). Sometimes, multiple anastomoses (2–3) may be required if the stricturing process has led to disconnection of the bile ducts at the hilum.

For patients with portal biliopathy leading to a biliary stricture, an additional procedure may be required prior to embarking upon surgery to perform a biliary bypass. For example, in patients with extrahepatic portal venous obstruction (EHPVO) a surgical portal-systemic shunt may need to be performed prior to the biliary bypass (traditionally performed in two stages but can sometimes be undertaken as a one-stage procedure) (16). Alternatively in patients with extrinsic pathology, such as chronic pancreatitis, leading to occlusion of the portal venous system and formation of a portal cavernoma a portal vein stent can be placed percutaneously leading to resolution of the cavernoma making the surgery possible (*Figure 59.9*).

REFERENCES

1. Ballehaninna UK, Chamberlain RS. Serum CA 19-9 as a biomarker for pancreatic cancer: A comprehensive review. *Indian J Surg Oncol* 2011;**2(2)**: 88–100.

2. de Moura DTH, McCarty TR, Jirapinyo P, Ribeiro IB, Hathorn KE, Madruga-Neto AC, et al. Evaluation of endoscopic ultrasound fine-needle aspiration versus fine-needle biopsy and impact of rapid on-site evaluation for pancreatic masses. *Endosc Int Open* 2020;**8(6)**:E738–47.

3. Kandel P, Nassar A, Gomez V, Raimondo M, Woodward TA, Crook JE, et al. Comparison of endoscopic ultrasound-guided fine-needle biopsy versus fine-needle aspiration for genomic profilin and DNA yield in pancreatic cancer: A randomized crossover trial. *Endoscopy* 2021;**53(4)**:376–82.

4. Bang JY, Hebert-Magee S, Navaneethan U, Hasan MK, Hawes R, Varadarajulu S. EUS-guided fine needle biopsy of pancreatic masses can yield true histology. *Gut* 2018;**67(12)**:2081–4.

5. Strasberg SM, Hertl M, Soper NJ. An analysis of the problem of biliary injury during laparoscopic cholecystectomy. *J Am Coll Surg* 1995;**180(1)**:101–25.

6. Olsson R, Danielsson A, Järnerot G, Lindström E, Lööf L, Rolny P, et al. Prevalence of primary sclerosing cholangitis in patients with ulcerative colitis. *Gastroenterology* 1991;**100(5 Pt 1)**:1319–23.

7. Mendes FD, Jorgensen R, Keach J, Katzmann JA, Smyrk T, Donlinger J, et al. Elevated serum IgG4 concentration in patients with primary sclerosing cholangitis. *Am J Gastroenterol* 2006;**101(9)**:2070–5.

8. Lewis J. Pathological patterns of biliary disease. *ClinLiver Dis* 2017;**10(5)**:107–10.

9. Björnsson E, Lindqvist-Ottosson J, Asztely M, Olsson R. Dominant strictures in patients with primary sclerosing cholangitis. *Am J Gastroenterol* 2004;**99(3)**:502–8.

10. Chapman MH, Thorburn D, Hirschfield GM, Webster GGJ, Rushbrook SM, Alexander G, et al. British

Society of Gastroenterology and UK-PSC guidelines for the diagnosis and management of primary sclerosing cholangitis. *Gut* 2019;**68(8)**:1356–78.

11. Lindor KD, Kowdley KV, Luketic VAC, Harrison ME, McCashland T, Befeler AS, et al. High-dose ursodeoxycholic acid for the treatment of primary sclerosing cholangitis. *Hepatol Baltim Md* 2009;**50(3):**808–14.

12. Campsen J, Zimmerman MA, Trotter JF, Wachs M, Bak T, Steinberg T, et al. Clinically recurrent primary sclerosing cholangitis following liver transplantation: A time course. *Liver Transpl* 2008;**14(2)**: 181–5.

13. Kamisawa T, Nakazawa T, Tazuma S, Zen Y, Tanaka A, Ohara H, et al. Clinical practice guidelines for IgG4-related sclerosing cholangitis. *J Hepato-Biliary-Pancreat Sci* 2019;**26(1)**:9–42.

14. Wang AY, Yachimski PS. Endoscopic management of pancreatobiliary neoplasms. *Gastroenterology* 2018;**154(7)**:1947–63.

15. Banerjee A, Kulkarni AV, Shah SR. Percutaneous stenting of the portal vein prior to biliary bypass in a patient with chronic pancreatitis and portal biliopathy. *Indian J Gastroenterol* 2015;**34(3)**:261–3.

16. Dhiman RK, Saraswat VA, Valla DC, Chawla Y, Behera A, Varma V, et al. Portal cavernoma cholangiopathy: Consensus statement of a working party of the Indian national association for study of the liver. *J Clin Exp Hepatol* 2014;**4(1)**:2–14.

Chapter
60
Choledochal Cysts

Prateek Arora, Shreeyash Modak and G. V. Rao

INTRODUCTION

In 1723, the first description of a fusiform dilation of the common bile duct was published by Vater, but the first authenticated case of a choledochal cyst (CDC) was not reported until Douglas described the classical features in 1852. Pancreaticobiliary maljunction was recognized by Kozumi and Kodama during an autopsy in 1916 where congenital biliary dilation was found. These initial observations went largely unheeded and the importance overlooked until in 1969, Babbit described the concept of reflux causing pathological bile duct changes. He postulated that the pancreaticobiliary junction is located outside the duodenal wall, where the normal sphincter does not work. This permits reflux of pancreatic juice into the biliary tract with chronic damage to the bile duct wall. This is associated with the production of inflammatory substances including activated pancreatic enzymes, lysolecithin, secondary or unconjugated bile acids and a mutagen which chronically injures the epithelium, produces cholangitis and induces metaplasia and in some cases subsequent malignant changes.

Whilst 'bile duct cyst', 'biliary cyst' or a 'choledochal malformation' (1) are more appropriate terms, 'choledochal cyst' is enshrined in the medical literature as the common hepatic (CHD) and common bile duct (CBD) are the most common sites (2–4). There are no established size criteria for bile duct dilatation which is ubiquitously accepted as defining a CDC. Instead, the characteristic anatomical shape and presence of supportive factors form the basis of the diagnosis. Todani's classification is the most widely used and classifies CDCs with different aetiologies and management principles (*Figure 60.1*) (5). The presentation differs between age groups and resection is the rule, after discovery, in view of the malignant potential.

AETIOPATHOGENESIS

Pathological dilatation of the biliary tract in the majority of CDCs is widely accepted to be caused by the presence of an abnormal pancreaticobiliary junction (APBJ), where the common channel of both bile and pancreatic ducts extends outside the duodenal wall, thus escaping its sphincter mechanism (*Figure 60.2*) (6). Babbit hypothesized that the higher pancreatic ductal pressures lead to reflux of pancreatic enzymes into the biliary system causing

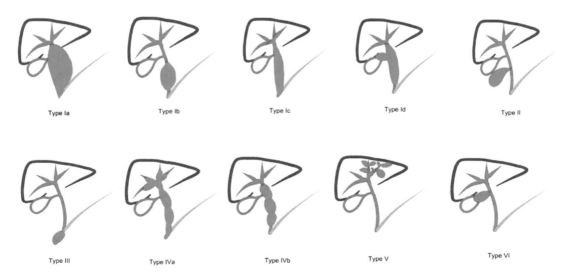

Figure 60.1 Todani's classification of choledochal cysts including **Types Id** and **VI**. Normal biliary system and pancreaticobiliary junction are depicted in green. The pancreatic duct is depicted in yellow and the affected biliary system by choledochal malformation and abnormal pancreaticobiliary junction is depicted in red.

DOI: 10.1201/9781003080060-60

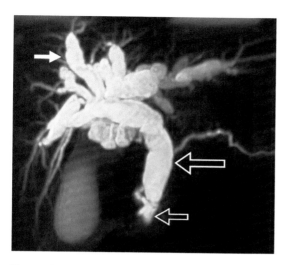

Figure 60.2 MRCP of a type IVa choledochal cyst. Solid arrow (white) marks the intrahepatic cystic biliary dilatations. Large arrow (outline) marks the extrahepatic biliary dilatations, and small arrow (outline) marks the long common channel between the distal common bile duct and pancreatic duct.

weakening of biliary ducts and resultant dilatation (7). This theory is supported by clinical findings including the presence of elevated amylase levels in choledochal cysts (8), higher CDC incidence in the Japanese population where APBJs are up to 1000 times more common and there is a female preponderance of both APBJ and CDC (9). APBJs are found in 1–3% of the population and are generally discovered when the size of the common channel exceeds 15 mm (10). Their identification and classification require anatomical characterization of the distal pancreaticobiliary ductal system, which is best done by endoscopic retrograde cholangiopancreatography (ERCP) but most commonly by magnetic resonance cholangiopancreatography (MRCP) (11) (*Figure 60.2*).

With, or without, biliary tract dilatation, APBJs are implicated in both benign and malignant pancreaticobiliary disorders ranging from gallbladder adenomyomatosis, pancreatitis, strictures in cholangiocarcinomas and carcinoma of the gallbladder (CAGB) (12). Not all CDCs can be explained by Babbit's hypothesis and a number of subtypes are not associated with APBJs. Raised intracholedochal pressure has been shown to correlate better than cyst amylase levels with the severity of dilatation in choledochal cysts (13). In neonatal CDCs, the fetal pancreas is yet to produce functional pancreatic enzymes (14). Alternate theories refer to functional, or mechanical, obstruction of the distal bile duct including oligoganglionosis and web formation respectively (14,15) and studies also suggest that choledochal cysts can be an 'acquired' defect in adults (16).

PRESENTATION

CDCs are most prevalent in the Far East especially Japan where the incidence of 1 per 1000 births, is considerably higher than in the West where it is to 1 : 10 000–150 000 with a female to male ratio of 3 : 1 (17). Incidental detection in prenatal scans is being reported but differentiation from biliary atresia is difficult. Re-evaluation shortly after birth is advised to confirm the diagnosis and elective surgery at 3–6 months of age is recommended. Neonates can present with jaundice, acholic stools and abdominal pain. Differentiation from biliary atresia can still be difficult even in neonates and exploration with intraoperative cholangiography is indicated (18).

More than 80% of CDCs present in the first decade of life with jaundice, right upper quadrant pain and an abdominal mass. At presentation, all three symptoms are present, however, is uncommon and two thirds of paediatric cases will have two of the three symptoms (3). As age increases, incidental detections and presentations with pancreaticobiliary complications such as pancreatitis, cholecystitis and cystolithiasis become increasingly common (19). Pancreatitis in CDCs is mild, recurrent and usually self-resolving, and the causation is multifactorial. The possibility of biliary tract malignancies also increases with age and can be a rare presenting feature in adults. Other rare presentations include neglected cases of biliary tract obstruction presenting with intrahepatic abscesses, biliary cirrhosis and portal hypertension in adults, and cyst rupture, haemorrhage from paracholedochal arteries or gastric outlet obstruction from a large choledochocoele in young children (3,19,20).

MALIGNANT CHANGE IN CHOLEDOCHAL CYSTS

APBJs lead to constant reflux of pancreatic enzymes which get activated by stagnated and deconjugated bile acids within the cyst, leading to a 'hyperplasia - carcinoma sequence' with activation of P53 and KRAS in both the dilated and non-dilated segments of the bile duct (*Figure 60.3*) (12).

APBJs are independently associated with higher rates of malignancy affecting the whole pancreaticobiliary system with cholangiocarcinomas being more common in cystic dilatations and gallbladder cancers (CAGB) being more common in non-dilated or minimal cylindrically dilated bile ducts (21). Thus, in an asymptomatic patient with APBJ and a non-dilated biliary system, the range of acceptable strategies includes regular follow-up, prophylactic cholecystectomy and prophylactic extrahepatic bile duct (EHBD) resection with a biliary diversion procedure (21). With time, the incidence of malignancy in CDCs rises from below 1% in the first decade to around 10% in adulthood reaching up to 40% in 6th–7th decades. Up to 70% are cholangiocarcinomas in EHBDs, the remainder being

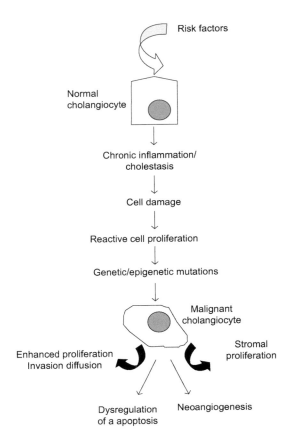

Figure 60.3 Pathway of malignant changs in choledochal cysts.

mostly CAGB (24%) and intrahepatic cholangiocarcinomas (2%) with rare liver or pancreatic malignancies presenting metachronously (22). Once malignant change has occurred in a CDC the overall survival is limited (23).

The possible development of malignancy, its increasing incidence with age, and poor prognosis once developed is a persuasive argument for considering excision of the affected EHBD with flow diversion surgery and explains why presently it is the standard surgical approach (24). Flow diversion alone with procedures like cystoduodenostomy were popular prior to the end of the 20th century. They are now unacceptable with the odds of developing a malignancy approximately four times higher than the risk associated with resectional procedures especially in Type 1 and 4 cysts (25). Where a bypass procedure has been performed, patients in all age groups require a further surgical procedure to resect the remaining cyst or cyst remnants. Resection of the EHBD dramatically decreases the incidence of malignancy, although it doesn't completely eliminate it as cancers can still develop in the intrahepatic biliary system and rarely the liver and pancreas (26).

CLASSIFICATION AND PRINCIPLES OF MANAGEMENT

Alonso-lej in1959 was the first person to classify CDCs and described three types based on the clinical presentation and anatomical distribution in 96 patients (27). After the discovery of intrahepatic cysts, Todani et al. added types IV and V and later revised the classification again by including APBJs (4,28). At present Todani's classification remains the most widely used (*Figure 60.1*). The six types differ in morphology, theories of causation and most importantly in the appropriate management strategies.

Types I and IV CDCs are the most common with an incidence of approximately 80% and 20% respectively (3). Type I CDCs are subdivided into Type Ia where there is cystic dilatation of the entire EHBD and the cystic duct arises from the cyst itself. Type Ib has an isolated focal segmental dilatation below the cystic duct insertion. Type Ic is a smooth fusiform dilatation of the extrahepatic biliary tree sometimes extending intrahepatically (4). Types Ia and Ic are associated with APBJ (28). Type Id is a recent addition where a cystic duct cyst with extrahepatic choledochal involvement presents a bicornuate cystic appearance (*Figure 60.4*) (29). Management for Type I CDC entails resection of the extrahepatic biliary system with flow diversion procedure as described.

Type II CDCs are very rare, constituting about 2% of cases (2). Type II refers to a cystic outpouching from the main bile duct most commonly above the cystic duct CBD junction (3). In view of the low risk of malignancy with this variant, they can be excised laparoscopically but in the presence of an APBJ, additional cholecystectomy or even EHBD resection is recommended. Type II cysts located in the pancreas can be drained into the

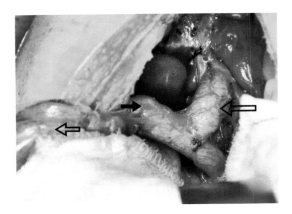

Figure 60.4 Intraoperative photograph showing Type Id choledochal malformation with typical bicornuate cystic malformation. The solid arrow indicates the dilated cystic duct, small arrow (outline) indicates the gallbladder and the large arrow (outline) indicates the dilated main bile duct.

duodenum (30) although differentiation from a dupli-cated gallbladder can be difficult and the final diagno-sis is frequently only confirmed following histological examination (31,32).

Type III CDCs or choledochocoeles are rare intra-mural distal bile duct cysts located in the duodenal wall with an incidence of 1–5% and they may be 'true' cysts or duodenal cysts (3). They are rarely associated with APBJ or malignancy, and present with biliary colic, cholangitis, or pancreatitis (33). An ERCP-guided endo-scopic biliary sphincterotomy (EBS) and cyst deroofing suffices and is associated with low morbidity. It is the preferred treatment although transduodenal cyst exci-sion and sphincteroplasty can be done if endoscopic treatment fails (2,3,33).

Multiple fusiform and cystic dilatations of both the intrahepatic and extrahepatic biliary systems are classified as Type IV which are more common than Type IVb which has multiple dilatations confined to the extrahepatic biliary system (4). Type IVa is sig-nificantly associated with APBJs and consequently has the highest risk of malignant transformation (28). More than 80% of Type IV CDCs are associated with membranous or septal stenosis in a major lobar bile duct and as a result are the most common Type to be associated with hepaticolithiasis (34). The majority of Type IV lesions are treated by excision of the EHBD with flow diversion and symptom relief is usually excel-lent with a marked improvement in the intrahepatic biliary dilatation (35). For significant and symptomatic intrahepatic disease, the management is the same as for Type V choledochal cysts.

Type V CDC or Caroli's disease, refers to multi-ple saccular dilatations affecting the intrahepatic ducts, which are discontinuous, and not associated with extrahepatic involvement [36]. Caroli's disease was first described in 1958 by the French gastroenterolo-gist Jacques Caroli. He noted that some patients had dilated bile ducts in their liver and that, in some cases, there was also hepatic fibrosis. These intrahepatic bili-ary dilatations surround the associated portal pedicles and appear as cysts surrounding a vascular structure, which can appear as a central 'dot sign' on computed tomography (CT), magnetic resonance (MR) and ultra-sound (US) scans (37). The level of congenital ductal plate malformation decides the presentation with larger intrahepatic bile duct involvement presenting as Caro-li's disease, and interlobular ductal plate malformation presenting as congenital hepatic fibrosis with or with-out renal involvement which is referred to as Caroli's syndrome (38). They are uncommon and are not asso-ciated with APBJ (28). They frequently cause biliary stasis, hepatolithiasis, liver atrophy and can undergo malignant degeneration forming cholangiocarcinomas, or to cirrhosis and portal hypertension which can be fatal without liver transplantation. Consequently, a localized segmental or lobar disease should be consid-ered for hepatic resection or a Roux-en-Y intrahepatic

cholangiojejunostomy if resection is not possible (39). Diffuse bilobar disease is a management dilemma and although liver transplantation is the logical treatment it is associated with a significant mortality and morbidity and only considered for symptomatic patients where conservative methods have failed and complications ensued (40).

Newer subtypes are being added to Todani's classi-fication with Type Id as described and Type VI refer-ring to cystic duct choledochal malformation alone (41). A symptomatic patient with doubtful dilatation of the main bile duct and an APBJ can be classified as having a 'forme fruste' choledochal cyst (42). The diagnosis, implications and treatment strategies are not clearly defined and patients usually undergo cholecystectomy and are placed on a surveillance program. If symptoms persist an EHBD resection with flow diversion surgery is the best option (43).

Of all the subtypes Type I and IV CDCs com-prises over 95% of all the cases and are most com-monly associated with APBJs and almost exclusively associated with development of malignancy (25). Type 1c and IVa CDCs behave in a similar fashion with a steadily increasing severity of dilatation and incidence of malignancy. This has led the authors to consider both Types I and IV as a part of same process and to consider them together as 'congenital choledochal cysts' with Types II, III and V being distinct and sepa-rate disease entities (44).

INVESTIGATION AND DIAGNOSIS

During the evaluation of a symptomatic patient a number of different scenarios may suggest a CDC: 1) When a dilated biliary system is encountered with no evidence of obstruction and relatively normal liver function tests; 2) when an abnormal biliary dilatation persists for a pronged period of time after relieving an obstructed biliary system; and 3) a characteristic pattern of biliary dilatation may also suggest the diag-nosis irrespective of biliary obstruction. The lack of strict size criteria for defining choledochal cysts can lead to diagnostic dilemma in borderline cases. A common bile duct diameter of up to 6 mm and further 2–3 mm dilatation post-cholecystectomy should be considered within normal limits in adults (45).

Imaging plays an important role in CDCs, includ-ing the investigation of an incidentally detected abnor-mal biliary tract dilation, diagnostic criteria, anatomical characterization, preoperative evaluation and postop-erative surveillance. All investigations that visualize the biliary system have some role in the management of choledochal cysts. These include: 1) US; 2) cross-sec-tional imaging with CT and MRCP; 3) functional imaging with hepatobiliary scintigraphy (HIDA scan-ning); and 4) MR and CT cholangiography. Invasive procedures include: 1) Percutaneous transhepatic chol-angiography (PTC); 2) intraoperative cholangiography

(IOC); 3) endoscopic ultrasound (EUS) and 4) endoscopic retrograde cholangiopancreatography (ERCP). Of all the available modalities, abdominal US, MRCP and CT are the most commonly used (46).

Abdominal US is non-invasive, inexpensive and repeatable and the investigation of choice for screening and follow-up after surgery for CDCs. Initial abdominal US will image the intrahepatic ducts, supraduodenal EHBDs, liver, gallbladder, associated pathologies and adjacent viscera (47). A suspicion of CDC on US is confirmed with a MRCP, which is presently the 'gold standard' for the diagnosis of biliary tract pathology due to the excellent delineation of the whole biliary tree and its non-invasive nature (*Figure 60.2*). MRCP provides a clear anatomical outline of the biliary tree and facilitates diagnoses and classification of any abnormalities which is invaluable during the work up for surgery (48). However, the definition of the most distal portion of the bile duct is variable and MRCP detects only 70% of APBJs. ERCP excels in APBJ delineation and is the most sensitive modality to detect a CDC but due to its invasive nature is only used for therapeutic purposes such as treatment of a choledochocoele, drainage to treat cholangitis, stone extraction, or biopsy where there is a suspected malignant mass (11). CT is sparingly used to assess other causes of biliary dilatation (48).

Blood tests are not useful for the diagnosis of CDCs apart from when mildly abnormal liver function tests (LFTs) are found with a dilated biliary tract. A leukocytosis with abnormal LFTs with, or without, raised amylase or lipase levels indicate the onset of cholangitis or pancreatitis respectively (19). Abnormally raised CA 19-9 levels in the absence of cholangitis may suggest malignant transformation but caution is required as CA 19-9 is also elevated by infection and jaundice (49).

SURGICAL MANAGEMENT

As the majority of the CDCs are Types I and IV, EHBD excision (including cholecystectomy) with Roux-en-Y hepaticojejunostomy is the most commonly performed surgical procedure. It is an elective procedure, and complications such as pancreatitis and cholangitis should be managed conservatively before definitive intervention (24). Preoperative delineation of the biliary anatomy is paramount to prevent pancreatic duct injury when mobilizing the lower end of CBD and at the hilum to prevent injury to ducts which join a significant way below the hilum.

The abdomen is entered via a right subcostal incision and is explored for rare but reported malignant deposits. The duodenum is Kocherized for better access to the pancreaticoduodenal complex, which helps in intrapancreatic CDC dissection and gives a safety margin in case of an intrapancreatic bleed. After thorough hepatoduodenal ligament exposure, the gallbladder is taken down, the cystic artery is ligated, traction is

applied to the CDC and circumferential bile duct dissection commenced. Rarely in patients with a history of recurrent attacks of cholangitis and dense pericholedochal adhesions, partial excision of the cyst with ablation of the mucosa or submucosal dissection on the medial and posterior aspect to prevent hepatic artery and portal venous injury respectively, known as Lilly's procedure is an acceptable alternative (50). Bipolar cautery should be used in circumferential dissection to take down small pericholedochal vessels and manage any neovascularization. Dissection proceeds distally into the pancreas terminating a few millimetres above the pancreatic duct or until the tapering of the cyst, whichever is more proximal. The bile duct is then transected distally and flushed with a soft-tip catheter to remove any debris. Superiorly it is important to dissect up to the hilum prior to transection and even to continue onto the left duct to provide for a wide anastomosis as these bile ducts are likely to be affected (even if not macroscopically obvious) and post-anastomotic stricture rates are high (51). To ensure the anastomosis is as technically straightforward as possible, a 'cuff' of duct can be left below the hilum, especially in laparoscopic procedures (52). Flushing intrahepatic ducts with a soft-tipped catheter to remove any debris and break soft membranes is important, particularly before commencing the anastomosis especially in Type IV lesions.

A Roux-en-Y hepaticojejunostomy is the standard method used for reconstruction due to the excellent results and the versatility of the technique (24). The anastomosis is mucosa-to-mucosa and commonly done with interrupted absorbable sutures (*Figures 60.5* and *60.6*).

Hepaticoduodenostomy (HD) is another acceptable and more physiological procedure performed in

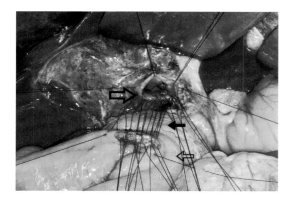

Figure 60.5 Intraoperative photograph showing an interrupted single layer end-to-side Roux en-Y hepaticojejunostomy with posterior layer pre-placed sutures *in situ*. The large arrow (outline) indicates the divided bile duct at hilum with right- and left- main duct septoplasty completed. The solid arrow (black) indicates the duodenum and the small arrow (outline) indicates the Roux loop. Sutures are 4-0 polydioxanone (PDS).

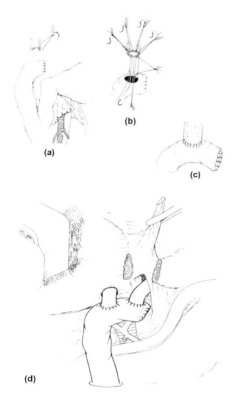

(a)

(b)

(c)

(d)

Figure 60.6 Illustrations of Roux-en-Y Choledochoje-junostomy Formation Post Choledochal Cyst Excision. This figure demonstrates the surgical steps involved in forming a Roux-en-Y choledochojejunostomy following the excision of a choledochal cyst, targeting the common hepatic duct and the area above the bile duct. First, a Roux limb of adequate length is created (a). Multiple fine interrupted sutures are then placed between the bile duct and the appropriately sized Roux limb enterotomy (b). The anastomosis is completed by securing these sutures (c). In cases where the excision of the choledochal cyst results in two separate bile duct openings, two separate anastomoses to the Roux limb can be performed (d).

infants where the duodenum is lax and easily mobil-ized to facilitate a tension-free anastomosis at the hilum while preserving the route for future endoscopic inter-ventions (53). However, studies have shown that HD is associated with higher rates of cholangitis, biliary gas-tritis and even a higher incidence of gastric cancer but no clear difference in morbidity related to surgery (54). Other methods such as jejunal interposition grafts and appendiceal conduits for reconstruction are described, but are not routinely, or widely, performed (55). Post-operative morbidity is reported to be 15–20% (56).

FOLLOW-UP

Postoperative histology generally reveals epithelial hyperplasia with round cell infiltration and fibrosis (57).

As EHBD resection does not completely eliminate the chances of malignancy and other benign complications especially in Type IV cysts and APBJs, a lifelong follow-up is advised. This is usually done with abdom-inal US, LFTs and CA 19-9 levels (19). A definite and ubiquitously accepted follow-up protocol does not exist.

SUMMARY

Choledochal cysts are abnormal pathological dilatations in the biliary ductal system. They are rare, but relatively more prevalent in females, and more common in Japan and Asia. They are usually diagnosed in children under 10 years of age, although up to 20% are diagnosed in adults. The majority are believed to be caused by reflux of pancreatic enzymes due to an abnormal pancreaticobiliary junction. CDCs usually present before adolescence with jaundice and palpation of an abdominal mass or pain, but many present in adulthood either symptomatically or as an incidental finding. CDCs are associated with the development of biliary calculi, protein plugs, strictures and complications such as cholangitis and pancreatitis are common. However, it is their tendency to undergo malignant transformation which mandates their resec-tion on discovery. The risk of malignant transforma-tion increases with age, and is more common in Types I and IV cysts. Imaging of the bile ducts reveals their characteristic anatomy which aids diagnosis and also helps with classification which is essential for surgical planning. Surgical excision of the affected extrahepatic biliary tract with flow diversion in an elective setting is usually required, which provides good symptom control and a significant reduction in the incidence of malignancy. Malignant change in bile duct epithelium can occur after cyst excision, sometimes after many years, and in areas of the biliary tree remote from the cyst including the gallbladder. All patients require lifelong follow-up.

REFERENCES

1. Makin E, Davenport M. Understanding choledochal malformation. *Arch Dis Child* 2012;**97(1)**:69–72.
2. Singham J, Yoshida EM, Scudamore CH. Choledo-chal cysts: Part 1 of 3: Classification and pathogene-sis. *Can J Surg* 2009;**52(5)**:434–40.
3. Soares KC, Arnaoutakis DJ, Kamel I, et al. Choled-ochal cysts: Presentation, clinical differentiation, and management. *J Am Coll Surg* 2014;**219(6)**:1167–80.
4. Todani T, Watanabe Y, Narusue M, et al. Congen-ital bile duct cysts: Classification, operative proce-dures, and review of thirty-seven cases including cancer arising from choledochal cyst. *Am J Surg* 1977;**134(2)**:263–9.
5. Todani T, Watanabe Y, Toki A, et al. Classification of congenital biliary cystic disease: Special reference to Type Ic and IVA cysts with primary ductal stric-ture. *J Hepatobiliary Pancreat Surg* 2003;**10(5)**:340–4.

6. Todani T, Arima E, Eto T, et al. Diagnostic criteria for pancreaticobiliary maljunction 2013. *J Hepatobiliary Pancreat Surg* 2014;**21(3)**:159–61.

7. Babbitt DP, Starshak RJ, Clemett AR. Choledochal-cyst: A concept of etiology. *Am J Roentgenol Radium Ther Nucl Med* 1973;**119(1)**:57–62.

8. Todani T, Urushihara N, Watanabe Y, et al. Pseudopancreatitis in choledochal cyst in children: Intraoperative study of amylase levels in the serum. *J Pediatr Surg* 1990;**25(3)**:303–6.

9. Ragot E, Mabrut JY, Ouaïssi M, et al; Working Group of the French Surgical Association. Pancreaticobiliary Maljunctions in European Patients with Bile Duct Cysts: Results of the Multicenter Study of the French Surgical Association (AFC). World J Surg 2017;**41(2)**:538–45.

10. Nagi B, Kochhar R, Bhasin D, et al. Endoscopic retrograde cholangiopancreatography in the evaluation of anomalous junction of the pancreaticobiliary duct and related disorders. *Abdom Imaging* 2003;**28(6)**:847–52.

11. Ono A, Arizono S, Isoda H, Togashi K. Imaging of pancreaticobiliary maljunction. *Radiographics* 2020;**40(2)**:378–92.

12. Funabiki T, Matsubara T, Miyakawa S, et al. Pancreaticobiliary maljunction and carcinogenesis to biliary and pancreatic malignancy. *Langenbecks Arch Surg* 2009;**394(1)**:159–69.

13. Turowski C, Knisely AS, Davenport M. Role of pressure and pancreatic reflux in the aetiology of choledochal malformation. *Br J Surg* 2011;**98(9)**:1319–26.

14. Schroeder D, Smith L, Prain HC. Antenatal diagnosis of choledochal cyst at 15 weeks' gestation: Etiologic implications and management. *J Pediatr Surg* 1989;**24(9)**:936–8.

15. Kusunoki M, Saitoh N, Yamamura T, et al. Choledochal cysts. Oligoganglionosis in the narrow portion of the choledochus. *Arch Surg* 1988;**123(8)**:984–6.

16. Han SJ, Hwang EH, Chung KS, et al. Acquired choledochal cyst from anomalous pancreatobiliary duct union. *J Pediatr Surg* 1997;**32(12)**:1735–8.

17. Hung MH, Lin LH, Chen DF, et al. Choledochal cysts in infants and children: Experiences over a 20-year period at a single institution. *Eur J Pediatr* 2011;**170(9)**:1179–85.

18. Mackenzie TC, Howell LJ, Flake AW, et al. The management of prenatally diagnosed choledochal cysts. *J Pediatr Surg* 2001;**36(8)**:1241–3.

19. Machado NO, Chopra PJ, Al-Zadjali A, et al. Choledochal cyst in adults: Etiopathogenesis, presentation, management, and outcome-case series and review. *Gastroenterol Res Pract* 2015;**2015**:602591.

20. Bhavsar MS, Vora HB, Giriyappa VH. Choledochal cysts: A review of literature. *Saudi J Gastroenterol* 2012;**18(4)**:230–6.

21. Tashiro S, Imaizumi T, Ohkawa H, et al; Committee for Registration of the Japanese Study Group on Pancreaticobiliary Maljunction. Pancreaticobiliary maljunction: Retrospective and nationwide survey in Japan. *J Hepatobiliary Pancreat Surg* 2003;**10(5)**:345–51.

22. Sastry AV, Abbadessa B, Wayne MG, et al. What is the incidence of biliary carcinoma in choledochal cysts, when do they develop, and how should it affect management? *World J Surg* 2015;**39(2)**:487–92.

23. Jan YY, Chen HM, Chen MF. Malignancy in choledochal cysts. *Hepatogastroenterology* 2000;**47(32)**:337–40.

24. Lipsett PA, Pitt HA. Surgical treatment of choledochal cysts. *J Hepatobiliary Pancreat Surg* 2003;**10(5)**:352–9.

25. Ten Hove A, de Meijer VE, Hulscher JBF, et al. Meta-analysis of risk of developing malignancy in congenital choledochal malformation. *Br J Surg* 2018;**105(5)**:482–90.

26. Tsuchida A, Kasuya K, Endo M, et al. High risk of bile duct carcinogenesis after primary resection of a congenital biliary dilatation. *Oncol Rep* 2003;**10(5)**:1183–7.

27. Alonso-Lej F, Rever WB JR, Pessagno DJ. Congenital choledochal cyst, with a report of 2, and an analysis of 94, cases. *Int Abstr Surg* 1959;**108(1)**:1–30.

28. Todani, T. Congenital choledochal dilatation: Classification, clinical features, and long-term results. *J Hep Bil Pancr Surg* 1994;**4**:276–82.

29. Michaelides M, Dimarelos V, Kostantinou D, et al. A new variant of Todani Type I choledochal cyst. Imaging evaluation. *Hippokratia* 2011;**15(2)**:174–7.

30. Khandelwal C, Anand U, Kumar B, et al. Diagnosis and management of choledochal cysts. *Indian J Surg* 2012;**74(1)**:29–34.

31. Chowdhury A, Tandup C, Aruni A, et al. Hepatic hilum-Type II choledochal cyst Masquerading as gallbladder duplication. *BMJ Case Rep* 2021;**14(2)**: e238971.

32. Bhojwani R, Jain N, Mishra S. Laparoscopic evaluation and resection of Type-II choledochal cyst arising from right hepatic duct mimicking gall bladder duplication. *J Minim Access Surg* 2018;**15(2)**:158–60.

33. Ziegler KM, Zyromski NJ. Choledochoceles: Are they choledochal cysts? *Adv Surg* 2011;**45**:211–24.

34. Lal R, Agarwal S, Shivhare R, et al. Type IV-A choledochal cysts: A challenge. *J Hepatobiliary Pancreat Surg* 2005;**12(2)**:129–34.

35. Kawarada Y, Das BC, Tabata M, et al. Surgical treatment of Type IV choledochal cysts. *J Hepatobiliary Pancreat Surg* 2009;**16(5)**:684–7.

36. Hamaoka M, Kozaka K, Matsui O, et al. Early detection of intrahepatic cholangiocarcinoma. *Jpn J Radiol* 2019;**37(10)**:669–84.

37. Levy AD, Rohrmann CA Jr, Murakata LA, et al. Caroli's disease: Radiologic spectrum with pathologic correlation. *AJR Am J Roentgenol* 2002;**179(4)**:1053–7.

38. Ananthakrishnan AN, Saeian K. Caroli's disease: Identification and treatment strategy. *Curr Gastroenterol Rep* 2007;**9(2)**:151–5.

39. Kassahun WT, Kahn T, Wittekind C, et al. Caroli's disease: Liver resection and liver transplantation. Experience in 33 patients. *Surgery* 2005;**138(5)**: 888–98.

40. Habib S, Shakil O, Couto OF, et al. Caroli's disease and orthotopic liver transplantation. *Liver Transpl* 2006;**12(3)**:416–21.

41. Conway WC, Telian SH, Wasif N, et al. Type VI biliary cyst: report of a case. *Surg Today* 2009;**39(1)**:77–9.

42. Lilly JR, Stellin GP, Karrer FM. Forme fruste choledochal cyst. *J Pediatr Surg* 1985;**20(4)**:449–51.

43. Shimotakahara A, Yamataka A, Kobayashi H, et al. Forme fruste choledochal cyst: Long-term follow-up with special reference to surgical technique. *J Pediatr Surg* 2003;**38(12)**:1833–6.

44. Visser BC, Suh I, Way LW, et al. Congenital choledochal cysts in adults. *Arch Surg* 2004;**139(8)**:855–60.

45. Park SM, Kim WS, Bae IH, et al. Common bile duct dilatation after cholecystectomy: A one-year prospective study. *J Korean Surg Soc* 2012;**83(2)**: 97–101.

46. Kim OH, Chung HJ, Choi BG. Imaging of the choledochal cyst. *Radiographics* 1995;**15(1)**:69–88.

47. She WH, Chung HY, Lan LC, et al. Management of choledochal cyst: 30 years of experience and results in a single center. *J Pediatr Surg* 2009;**44(12)**: 2307–11.

48. Lewis VA, Adam SZ, Nikolaidis P, et al. Imaging of choledochal cysts. *Abdom Imaging* 2015;**40(6)**: 1567–80.

49. La Pergola E, Zen Y, Davenport M. Congenital choledochal malformation: Search for a marker of epithelial instability. *J Pediatr Surg* 2016;**51(9)**:1445–9.

50. Lilly JR. The surgical treatment of choledochal cyst. *Surg Gynecol Obstet* 1979;**149(1)**:36–42.

51. Kim JH, Choi TY, Han JH, et al. Risk factors of postoperative anastomotic stricture after excision of choledochal cysts with hepaticojejunostomy. *J Gastrointest Surg* 2008;**12(5)**:822–8.

52. Senthilnathan P, Patel ND, Nair AS, et al. Laparoscopic management of choledochal cyst-technical modifications and outcome analysis. *World J Surg* 2015;**39(10)**:2550–6.

53. Patil V, Kanetkar V, Talpallikar MC. Hepaticoduodenostomy for biliary reconstruction after surgical resection of choledochal cyst: A 25-year experience. *Indian J Surg* 2015;**77(Suppl 2)**:240–4.

54. Narayanan SK, Chen Y, Narasimhan KL, et al. Hepaticoduodenostomy versus hepaticojejunostomy after resection of choledochal cyst: A systematic review and meta-analysis. *J Pediatr Surg* 2013;**48(11)**:2336–42.

55. Fu M, Wang Y, Zhang J. Evolution in the treatment of choledochus cyst. *J Pediatr Surg* 2000;**35(9)**: 1344–7.

56. Soares KC, Kim Y, Spolverato G, et al. Presentation and clinical outcomes of choledochal cysts in children and adults: A multi-institutional analysis. *JAMA Surg* 2015;**150(6)**:577–84.

57. Oguchi Y, Okada A, Nakamura T, et al. Histopathologic studies of congenital dilatation of the bile duct as related to an anomalous junction of the pancreaticobiliary ductal system: Clinical and experimental studies. *Surgery* 1988;**103(2)**:168–73.

Bailey & Love's Essential Operations Bailey & Love's Essential Operatic
SECTION 9 | BILIARY TRACT
Bailey & Love's Essential Operations Bailey & Love's Essential Operatic
Bailey & Love's Essential Operations Bailey & Love's Essential Operatic

Chapter 61

Biliary Malignancies

Emily Britton and Jia Hong-Dong

INTRODUCTION

Biliary malignancies encompass a spectrum of tumours, predominantly adenocarcinomas that arise from either the gallbladder mucosa or the epithelium of the bile duct. The cholangiocarcinomas (CCA) are classified as either intrahepatic cholangiocarcinoma or extrahepatic cholangiocarcinoma, and the group is further subdivided into perihilar cholangiocarcinoma previously known as Klatskin tumours and distal cholangiocarcinoma. Gerald Klatskin, (1910–1986) was the founder of the liver study unit at Yale School of Medicine, where he developed the technique of liver biopsy. Cholangiocarcinomas are comparatively rare compared with other malignancies, especially in high-income countries, but are increasing in incidence globally. The only potentially curative approach is complete surgical excision but unfortunately most patients present with either locally advanced or metastatic disease that precludes any surgical option. As a consequence, the prognosis is poor with survival at 5 years being less than 20% for gallbladder carcinoma and 25% for cholangiocarcinoma. Surgical approaches have become increasingly aggressive in an attempt to improve outcomes, but this is associated with a concomitant increase in morbidity and mortality for which justification in terms of clear survival benefit is lacking. Management can be both challenging and controversial. The best outcomes are achieved where the resources and experience of specialist multidisciplinary teams are utilized. This chapter summarizes the aetiology of biliary tract malignancies, preoperative and operative considerations, and extant controversies.

GALLBLADDER CARCINOMA

Epidemiology

Gallbladder carcinoma is the most common biliary malignancy, accounting for 60% of cases. In 2020, it accounted for 115 949 new diagnoses and 84 695 deaths (1). The incidence shows a marked geographical variation with rates up to 27 per 100 000 being observed in Latin America and Asia, whilst in resource rich areas where the population has a high proportion of individuals of European ancestry the incidence is less than 2 per 100 000 (2). *Figure 61.1* shows the incidence of both gallbladder carcinoma and CCA globally.

Historically the incidence has been reported as 3–6 times higher in women, which has been attributed to a higher predisposition to gallstones and hormonal influences in cholesterol cycling (2). However, is it much more common in those over 65 and age-standardized incidence rates from 2018 demonstrated a much lower difference with rates of 2.4 per 100 000 in women and 2.2 per 100 000 in men (3). Any condition, or exposure, that induces chronic inflammation and increased cell turnover increases the risk of carcinoma. The most recognized cause of biliary tract inflammation is gallstones, which are concurrent in up to 85% of cases, but less than 3% of those with gallstones will be diagnosed with gallbladder carcinoma (4). Notably, symptomatic, long standing, and large gallstones greater than 3 cm are associated with an increased incidence (3,5,6).

Other risk factors include (7,8):

- Gallbladder polyps
- Porcelain gallbladder
- Primary sclerosing cholangitis
- Chronic infections, notably with *Salmonella* or *Helicobacter* colonization
- Congenital abnormalities including choledochal or intrahepatic cysts, and an anomalous pancreaticobiliary duct junction
- Genetics (often *KRAS* and *p53* mutations) and family history
- Environmental mutagens in oil, chemical, textiles and mining industries
- Medications such as methyldopa, isoniazid, oral contraceptives and hormone replacement treatment
- Smoking, obesity, diabetes and poor diet

Polyps

Any protruding lesion of the gallbladder wall mucosa is generally reported as a gallbladder polyp. True adenomatous polyps may follow the established adenoma-carcinoma sequence of carcinogenesis, but cholesterol polyps or adenomyomatosis although remaining benign are indistinguishable on imaging. The risk of malignancy in adenomatous polyps increases with size (≥10 mm), growth rate and patient age. Current guidance is to offer laparoscopic cholecystectomy to appropriate patients when polyps ≥10 mm and surveillance if polyps are ≤5 mm (9). Management of polyps 6–9 mm is dependent on other risk factors, morphology and patient preference.

DOI: 10.1201/9781003080060-61

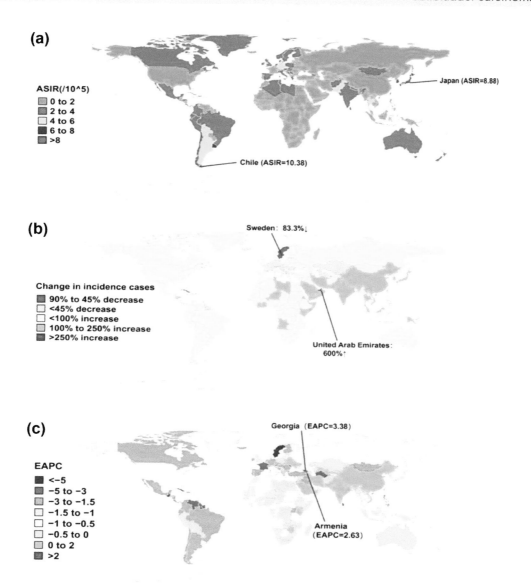

Figure 61.1 The global disease burden of gallbladder and biliary tract cancer (GBTC) is illustrated in 195 countries and territories, including the age-standardized incidence rate (ASIR) of GBTC in 2017 (a), the relative change in incident cases of GBTC between 1990 and 2017 (b) and the estimated annual percent change (EAPC) of ASIR for the GBTC from 1990 to 2017 (c). *Abbreviations:* ASIR: age-standardized incidence rate; EPAC: estimated annual percent change; GBTC: gallbladder and biliary tract cancer.

Porcelain gallbladder

Less than 1% of patients will have total or partial calcification of the gallbladder wall secondary to calcium deposition following chronic inflammation (10). Traditionally, it was believed to be associated with rates of malignancy of up to 33% but in the more recent literature it was reported to be <5%. There is some evidence that the risk of malignancy is higher in those with heterogenous or partial wall calcification (10). Appropriate symptomatic patients should be offered standard cholecystectomy and the management of asymptomatic patients is dependent on holistic assessment.

Pathology and staging

Adenocarcinomas arising from secretory cells lining the gallbladder lumen account for 90% of cases. Papillary adenocarcinomas from papillary cells involved in bile motility are much less frequent but have a better prognosis (3,4). Very rarely, pathological examination will demonstrate a squamous cell carcinoma, small-cell neuroendocrine carcinoma, lymphoma or sarcoma. Survival of the former two is exceptionally poor, but the latter are more favourable than adenocarcinoma (4).

Staging is determined using the American Joint Committee on Cancer (AJCC) tumour, node, metastasis (TNM) classification. The current 8th edition of which was published in 2018 and is shown in *Table 61.1*.

The gallbladder wall consists of mucosa, lamina propria, muscularis propria, subserosal connective tissue and on the inferior surface only, a serosal layer. On the superior hepatic surface, the subserosal connective tissue is continuous with the hepatic connective tissue, facilitating early vascular, neural and parenchymal infiltration (11). The current classification separates

Table 61.1 The AJCC (American Joint Committee on Cancer) gallbladder cancer staging system; This 8th edition was introduced in 2018

TNM system	
T: Primary tumour	
Tis	Carcinoma *in situ* – tumour only within the epithelium (the inner layer of the gallbladder)
T1	Tumour invades the lamina propria or muscularis
T1a	Limited to lamina propria
T1b	Invades muscularis
T2	Tumour invades the perimuscular fibrous tissue
T2a	Tumour invades the perimuscular fibrous tissue on the side of the peritoneum (the lining of the abdominal cavity)
T2b	Tumour invades the perimuscular fibrous tissue on the side of the liver, but has not invaded the liver
T3	Tumour invades the serosa (the outermost covering of the gallbladder) and/or directly invades the liver and/or one other adjacent structure (stomach, duodenum, colon, pancreas, omentum or extrahepatic bile ducts)
T4	Tumour invades the hepatic artery, main portal vein, or two or more extra-hepatic organs
N: Regional lymph node involvement	
N0	No regional lymph node metastasis
N1	Metastasis in 1–3 regional lymph nodes
N2	Metastasis in ≥4 regional lymph nodes
M: Distant metastasis	
M0	No distant metastasis
M1	Distant metastasis present
Stage groupings	
Stage 0	Tis, N0, M0
Stage I	T1, N0, M0
Stage II	
Stage IIa	T2a, N0, M0
Stage IIb	T2b, N0, M0
Stage III	
Stage IIIa	T3, N0, M0
Stage IIIb	T1-T3, N1, M0
Stage IV	
Stage IVa	T4, N0-N1, M0
Stage IVb	Any T, N2, M0 or any T, any N, M1

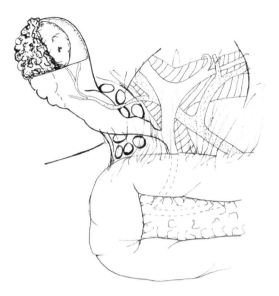

Figure 61.2 Illustration of a Type 2a tumour arising from, and invading, the peritoneal surface of the gallbladder.

T2a tumours where connective tissue invasion is on the peritoneal side (*Figure 61.2*) from T2b tumours where invasion is into the connective tissue on the hepatic side as the latter prognosis is expected to be worse.

PREOPERATIVE CONSIDERATIONS

There are no disease-specific symptoms caused by gallbladder carcinoma in its early stages. Approximately 50% of all cases and the vast majority of early-stage cases, are diagnosed on pathological inspection of a cholecystectomy specimen resected for cholelithiasis or cholecystitis (12). Of those that present clinically, 75% will have unresectable disease. The majority will report biliary type abdominal pain, nausea, vomiting or dyspepsia, some may be jaundiced with or without features of cholangitis, and a palpable mass may be present on clinical examination. A minority of patients will present with cachexia or ascites (4). Cross-sectional contrast enhanced imaging is essential for staging of patients with both new and post cholecystectomy diagnoses. Multiphasic computed tomography (CT) or magnetic resonance imaging (MRI) provide more accurate information on local disease vascular involvement than standard contrast enhanced abdominal CT. Fluorodeoxyglucose positron emission tomography (FDG-PET) can identify metastatic disease that precludes resection and changes management in around 20% of patients (13). It is important to complete staging imaging prior to any intervention necessary to relieve obstructive jaundice as the overlay of procedural inflammation hampers

interpretation. However, jaundice is normally a harbinger of advanced disease and very careful assessment, multidisciplinary team (MDT) discussion and diagnostic laparoscopy should be performed prior to any attempt at surgical resection.

Given the increased incidence with age, if the medical fitness of a patient for resection is questionable cardio-pulmonary exercise testing (CPEX) and the American College of Surgeons National Surgical Quality Improvement Program (NSQIP) risk calculator can be useful adjuncts for patient and MDT discussions (*see* **Chapters 6** and **19**).

It is not necessary to obtain a tissue diagnosis of malignancy for suspicious lesions on imaging that appear resectable and doing so risks seeding tumour cells to the peritoneum. However, tissue confirmation is required to deliver palliative chemotherapy and should be taken at surgery if the patient is inoperable. Contraindications to resection include peritoneal metastases, non-contiguous liver lesions, tumour involvement of the hepatic vasculature or biliary tree that would preclude a complete resection, and the presence of disease in distant lymph node groups.

OPERATIVE CONSIDERATIONS

Overall survival for patients that undergo incomplete surgical resection (R1/R2) is not significantly different to those with inoperable disease. Achieving an R0 resection is therefore critical although the appropriate extent of surgery that is necessary and justified to achieve this remains controversial. Typically, gallbladder carcinoma has been excised with a cholecystectomy, segment IVb and V resection and portal lymphadenectomy. At one end of the spectrum, some consider cholecystectomy alone sufficient for early-stage tumour, and at the other, surgeons support major multi-visceral resections in the quest for clear margins.

Staging laparoscopy

Staging laparoscopy in primary gallbladder carcinoma yields a diagnosis of disseminated disease in 20–30% of patients and is of clear benefit (14). Use in incidental gallbladder carcinoma is less established, but recent studies show yields in between 5–20% of patients (14,15). The prognostic value is highest in those with cholecystitis, positive resection margins, and a higher T stage. This can be performed pragmatically on the day of planned resection in low-risk patients.

Port site excision

It has been postulated that iatrogenic perforation of the gallbladder during dissection or extraction in incidental cases causes peritoneal seeding and high port site recurrence, so some surgeons have included port site excision at the time of completion surgery. There is no demonstrable survival benefit from this intervention (12).

Lymphadenectomy

Nodal involvement is an independent prognostic factor for survival and increases with T stage and over 60% of T2 tumours have positive nodes (15). Locoregional lymphadenectomy removing nodes in the porta hepatis and gastrohepatic ligament to allow a minimum examination of six lymph nodes is recommended. Suspicious nodes outside these areas should be sent intraoperatively for analysis by frozen section as a positive result would contraindicate proceeding to a formal resection.

Segmental liver resection

Resection of segments IVb and V remains routine practice in both primary tumours and as completion surgery in incidental tumours. T1a and T1b tumours are confined within the wall of the lamina propria and complete excision should be achieved by a standard cholecystectomy, however, current guidelines still recommend liver resection for T1b tumours. The largest and most recent multinational data comes from the Operative Management of Gallbladder Cancer (OMEGA) study which demonstrated no benefit of liver resection for T1 carcinomas (16) and performing completion surgery in these incidental tumours is therefore unnecessary. The same study demonstrated segmental liver resection improved recurrence-free survival (RFS) in all types of T2 carcinomas. There has been further debate over whether formal segmental resection is necessary in T2 cases or whether a 2–3 cm deep wedge excision is sufficient. A recent systematic review found that, although there was a RFS benefit in formal resection, it also carried a higher complication rate (17).

Extended and multi-visceral resections

Locally advanced disease is frequently inoperable, but in some cases of T3 and T4 tumours, excision of the biliary confluence and extended right hepatectomy can achieve complete resection and was previously believed to be justified. However, the OMEGA study demonstrated no RFS or overall survival (OS) benefit for these patients and the operations are associated with significant risks including liver insufficiency or failure (16,18).

Bile duct resection is performed in patients with a positive cystic duct margin either at previous cholecystectomy or on intraoperative frozen section, where there is direct invasion of the bile duct or fibrosis around the hepatoduodenal ligament compromises lymphadenectomy. Again, this increases the risk of complications without a clearly demonstrable survival benefit (16,18).

Hepatopancreatoduodenectomy (HPD) has been performed in patients with invasion of the hilum, distal bile duct or duodenum and extensive peripancreatic lymph node involvement. The decision to proceed was taken intraoperatively in almost 50% of cases in one study and the 3-year OS was reported to be 26%. However, mortality and morbidity are undoubtedly significantly higher, and the OMEGA study data did not demonstrate any survival benefit following these aggressive resections.

CHOLANGIOCARCINOMA

Cholangiocarcinomas (CCA) are a heterogenous group of cancers primarily classified by their anatomical location. Intrahepatic cholangiocarcinomas (iCCA) occur proximal to the second order bile ducts within the liver parenchyma, perihilar (pCCA) (previously Klatskin tumours), occur between second order ducts and the insertion of the cystic duct into the common bile duct, and distal cholangiocarcinomas (dCCA) arise within the common bile duct distal to the cystic duct insertion. Examining the incidence of the different varieties demonstrates that pCCA represent around 60% of cases, dCCA approximately 20–30%, and iCCA 10%.

Epidemiology

As with gallbladder carcinoma there is considerable geographical variation in incidence, with a similarly low incidence found in high-income Western countries, frequently less than 2 per 100 000 (15). The highest rates, often exceeding 100 per 100 000, occur in areas of Southeast Asia where liver flukes are endemic (19). An increasing incidence of iCCA in high-income countries has been reported recently, but it is unclear if this a true increase or a reflection of a greater availability and range of diagnostic modalities and more accurate reporting of intrahepatic lesions. An increase in chronic hepatic inflammation from a growing prevalence of obesity, alcohol or viral pathologies may however be responsible for a true increase in these primary liver tumours.

Parasites

The high rates of CCA in Southeast Asia are secondary to parasitic infection with members of the Opisthorchiidae family endemic to the region. *Opisthorchis viverrini* and *Clonorchis sinensis* are flatworm parasites carried in freshwater fish, which act as secondary hosts. When undercooked infected fish flesh is digested by humans, the larvae migrate through the ampulla of Vater into the common bile duct where they mature, reproduce, and can live without causing symptoms for many years. The endemic areas with the highest incidences are in Thailand, Taiwan, Korea, Eastern China and Russia (19).

Primary sclerosing cholangitis

In the West, the most common and best understood risk factor is primary sclerosing cholangitis (PSC). It is characterized by repeated inflammation and then stricture of both intra- and extrahepatic bile ducts causing a 'beaded' appearance that is pathognomonic (*Figure 61.3*).

In patients with PSC the risk of developing CCA is up to 600 times greater than the general population. The cumulative incidence for the development of an HPB malignancy, the majority of which are CCAs, is 20–25% for PSC patients (19). There is no unifying guidance for a surveillance protocol, due to issues with distinguishing between malignant and benign strictures on non-invasive imaging, and low sensitivity with relatively high risk in repeated endoscopic procedures. However, annual MRCP and CA 19-9 may be both pragmatic and life saving for patients (19).

Other risk factors include (19,20):

- Age >65 with peak incidence in 8th decade of life
- Male gender 1.5 times more commonly affected than women
- Hispanic or Asian heritage/ethnicity

Pathology

CCA can also be classified by its growth pattern into periductal infiltrating (*Figure 61.4*), mass-forming (*Figure 61.5*) and intraductal papillary lesions (19). The latter expand rather than constrict the duct, are more easily resectable and have a better prognosis regardless of anatomical location but are unfortunately also the rarest.

ICCA are predominantly mass forming with ~80% presenting as a single solid nodular lesion. They may be large with evidence of central necrosis or scarring as well as mucin production. As they advance, satellite lesions or multifocal intrahepatic lesions may be seen. Infiltrative lesions grow longitudinally along the walls of the bile ducts and portal tracts, causing stricturing

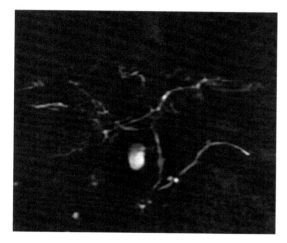

Figure 61.3 Typical MRCP image of primary sclerosing cholangitis with 'beaded' appearance of the intrahepatic ducts and diffuse widespread strictures. The intrahepatic ducts usually do not dilate due to the pathological process involving the whole of the biliary tract.

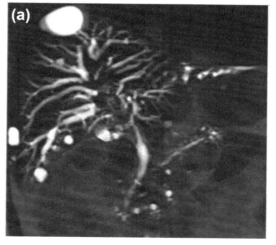

(a)

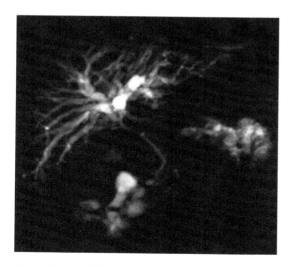

Figure 61.4 MRCP image showing a hilar cholangiocarcinoma (Klatskin tumour) demonstrating tight stricture and intrahepatic dilatation of intrahepatic ducts due to infiltrating tumour.

(b)

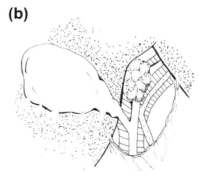

Figure 61.5 MRCP image (a) and illustration (b) of an apparent space-occupying lesion due to mass-forming variety of CCA.

and upstream biliary dilatation but no mass. The infiltrative variant accounts for ~75% of eCCA and focal segmental biliary dilatation should raise this suspicion. Six percent of iCCAs and 27% of eCCAs are slow growing polypoidal papillary lesions. Biliary intra-epithelial neoplasia is a precursor of infiltrative lesions and is graded 1–3 depending on cellular and nuclear atypia. Intraductal papillary neoplasms of the bile duct (IPNB) are precursors for papillary CCA (15). Of the CCAs 90–95% are adenocarcinomas that may be well, moderately, or poorly differentiated (19). The Bismuth-Corlette classification sub-divides pCCA based on their location and longitudinal extension and anticipates the necessary surgical resection and is summarized in *Table 61.2* and *Figure 61.6*.

Staging

Current staging is the AJCC TNM classification in its 8th edition (*Table 61.3*), with separate classification for iCCA, pCCA and dCCA. In iCCA, mass size and vascular involvement are key, in pCCA it is the relationships

Table 61.2 Bismuth-Corlette classification of perihilar cholangiocarcinoma (pCCA)

Type I	Distal to hepatic duct confluence
Type II	Extend to and involve the hepatic duct confluence
Type IIIa	Involve the hepatic duct confluence and proximal right hepatic duct
Type IIIb	Involve the hepatic duct confluence and proximal left hepatic duct
Type IV	Extend from the hepatic duct confluence bilaterally to the proximal hepatic ducts and segmental bile ducts
Type IV	Multicentric tumours
Type V	Junction of cystic duct and bile duct

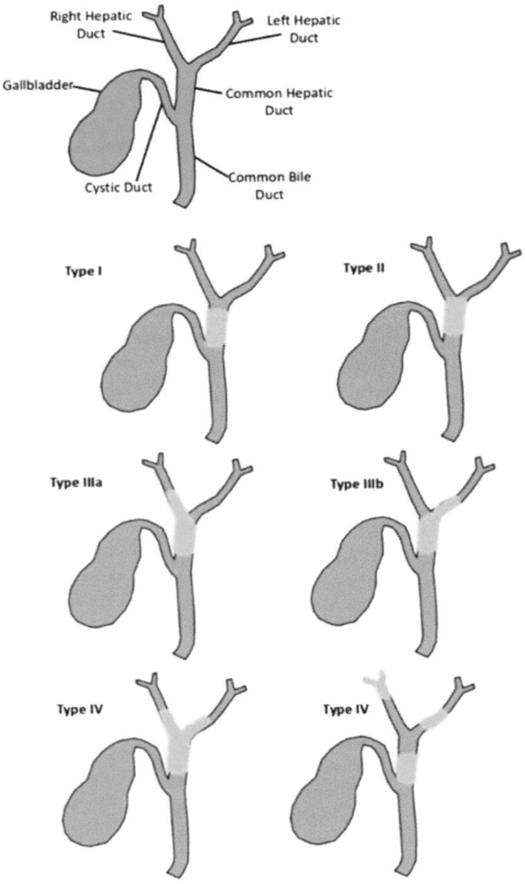

Table 61.3 Current staging of cholangiocarcinoma after the AJCC TNM classification 8th edition

T category (pT)	
Tis	Carcinoma *in situ* (intraductal tumour)
T1	Solitary, without vascular invasion
T1a	Solitary, **≤5 cm** without vascular invasion
T1b	Solitary, **>5 cm** without vascular invasion
T2	Solitary, with vascular invasion; or multiple, with or without vascular invasion
T2a	
T2b	
T3	Perforating the visceral peritoneum
T4	**Involving local extrahepatic structures by direct invasion**
N category (pN)	
N0	No regional lymph node metastasis
N1	Regional lymph node metastasis
AJCC stage groupings	
IA	**T1a N0 M0**
IB	**T1b N0 M0**
I	
II	T2 N0 M0
IIIA	T3 N0 M0
IIIB	**T4 N0 M0; any T, N1 M0**
III	
IV	Any T, any N, M1
IVA	
IVB	

Note: **Bold** text within the table indicates a change from the AJCC TNM classification 7th edition.

Figure 61.6 Illustrations of the Bismuth-Corlette classification of perihilar cholangiocarcinoma.

to inflow and outflow structures and in dCCA it is the depth of invasion of the bile duct wall (21).

PREOPERATIVE CONSIDERATIONS

Presentation

Whilst iCCAs are usually asymptomatic until they reach an advanced stage, they may produce abdominal discomfort, or pain, from stretching of the hepatic capsule, weight loss or fatigue. Patients are rarely jaundiced and up to a third of iCCAs are found incidentally on imaging (19). The presentation of eCCA is generally earlier due to outflow obstruction of the biliary tree. Worsening jaundice is present in 75–90% of patients, with, or without, concurrent cholangitis. dCCA mimic pancreatic and ampullary adenocarcinoma, although clinically the management is the same (19).

Tumour markers

Carbohydrate antigen 19-9 (CA 19-9) is the most frequently used biomarker in CCA for both diagnostic and prognostic purposes. CA 19-9 is a cell surface glycoprotein complex originally described in 1979 by Koprowski using a mouse monoclonal antibody in a colorectal cancer cell line. However, 5–10% of the population are Lewis antigen-negative (Lewis antigens are glycoproteins that are found on the surface of many cells and secreted in various body fluids) and do not produce any, or very low levels, of CA 19-9 from any cell (15). CA 19-9 is also raised in biliary obstruction and a multitude of other malignant and benign conditions (22). Carcinoembryonic antigen (CEA) is of well-established utility in colorectal adenocarcinomas and has shown higher accuracy in differentiating between PSC and CCA than CA 19-9 (23) and in differentiating between hepatocellular carcinoma and iCCA. Elevated levels of both CA 19-9 and CEA have been shown to be associated with significantly worse survival.

Imaging and investigations

Plain abdominal ultrasonography (US) is usually performed initially at presentation. It is insufficient for staging but may show a space-occupying lesion, biliary obstruction, or concurrent benign pathology such as gallstones and suggest which further investigations will be of most value.

Cross-sectional imaging using triple phase CT is the mainstay of staging as the superior vascular enhancement is critical for assessment of resectability. The arterial phase will normally show a degree of rim enhancement with gradual centripetal infilling on delayed images. The portal venous phase provides essential information on portal tract relationships or involvement. CT may also visualize segmental obstruction or lobar atrophy suggesting vascular involvement or long-standing biliary obstruction, or signs of fat infiltration or cirrhosis, and can also be used to calculate segment volumes. These are important considerations in determining the minimal acceptable volume of the predicted future liver remnant (FLR) if an extended resection is likely to be required.

MRI with hepatic-specific contrast and diffusion weighting provides accurate anatomical details of both ductal and vascular disease and variant anatomy. It can also identify, and in some cases, differentiate concurrent benign or malignant pathologies within the liver or gallbladder. The image reconstruction provided by MRCP can be useful for both diagnosis and surgical planning in eCCA, but is less useful in iCCA.

FDG-PET is better than CT or MRI in identifying distant metastases or lymph node involvement in eCCA but is of limited value in iCCA. Studies have shown that the management is changed as a result of findings following FDG-PET in 20–60% of cases (24). It has been investigated in an attempt to distinguish between malignant and benign pathology in PSC, but results have been disappointing and it cannot be relied upon as a screening tool.

Endoscopic retrograde cholangiopancreatography (ERCP) can be both diagnostic and therapeutic. It can provide important information about the precise location and length of stricture and also obtain a tissue diagnosis through brush cytology which has a high specificity (97%) (15), but low sensitivity (43%) or choledochoscopy and direct biopsy. Finally, in those requiring relief of obstructive jaundice, it also presents an opportunity for stenting. However, it is an invasive procedure and, in addition to the procedural risks of perforation and pancreatitis, it does by definition infect the biliary tree and lead to increased complications following surgery. The effectiveness and safety of preoperative biliary drainage in patients with cholangiocarcinoma remains controversial. Treatment must be decided on a case-to-case basis and will depend on the level of jaundice at presentation, the finding of the initial investigations, the level of symptoms and the planned surgical procedure. Symptoms can be very distressing and even in patients with inoperable disease stenting is justified. If a major resection is planned, it is essential to ensure that the proposed FLR is not only of sufficient volume but is functioning adequately which almost always requires preoperative drainage. Presently this is endoscopic in 75% of patients and radiological in 25%, but almost half of the endoscopic procedures experience complications. Drainage is often inadequate and needs to be repeated. It is also important to remember that following biliary drainage for CCA the 90-day mortality is approximately 35% and there is a risk of tumour seeding within the biliary tract.

Endoscopic ultrasound (EUS) is a more recent modality but can also provide very useful morphological assessment and sampling of regional lymph nodes with extra hepatic CCA, but it has a higher sensitivity for dCCA (91%) compared with pCCA (59%) (19). Its sensitivity is also higher for the detection of malignancy than ERCP, but EUS has the potential for tumour seeding outside the biliary tract due to the route of access when performing biopsies.

Portal venous embolization

An extended hepatectomy may be necessary in pCCA to achieve clearance. This can only be performed if the FLR is sufficient to avoid hepatic insufficiency or failure. A FLR of 25% of total preoperative volume is usually sufficient when the parenchyma is healthy, but if there is suspicion or evidence of background liver disease such as fibrosis, chronic cholestasis or cirrhosis the FLR must be >40% (15). Percutaneous embolization of selected intrahepatic portal tracts induces hypertrophy of the non-occluded segments within 4–6 weeks. The growth rate of diseased liver is lower than that of healthy liver, and if a large percentage increase is necessary in this context some specialist centres may perform an associating liver partition and portal vein ligation for staged hepatectomy (ALPPS) (25). The ALPPS procedure is performed in two stages usually 7–15 days apart. The initial stage involves ligation of the right portal vein and the splitting of the liver parenchyma at the site of the falciform ligament. The liver which is to be subsequently resected remains *in situ* receiving its blood supply from the right hepatic artery only. Biliary drainage via the right biliary duct and systemic outflow via the hepatic veins are preserved. The involved side of the liver is removed at the second stage of the procedure following ligation and transection of the residual structures in the right portal pedicle. The ALPSS procedure can induce growth of over 60% in a median time of 8 days and it may be used as a first-line approach or a salvage procedure when portal vein embolization (PVE) alone has not achieved sufficient growth. Unfortunately, while the ALPSS procedure produces significant and rapid hypertrophy of the proposed FLR, it is associated with significant morbidity and mortality. The original report of the ALPSS procedure in 2012 described division of the segment 4 portal pedicles and the middle hepatic vein during the parenchymal transection. This was performed to maximize FLR growth but can produce severe ischaemia and congestion of the right liver and abscess formation was not infrequent. Abscesses within the devascularized liver can result in severe sepsis, multi-organ failure, and mortality. To avoid these complications a number of modifications have been suggested including transections of only 80%, non-transection, laparoscopic hybrid procedures employing radio frequency ablation, preservation of the inflow to segment 4 and even ALPSS without portal vein ligation.

Jaundice and cholangitis

Cholangitis secondary to biliary obstruction is associated with an increased post operative mortality and

in these circumstances endoscopic or percutaneous drainage should be performed preoperatively. In the absence of cholangitis, the risk of complication or biliary infection from drainage procedures may outweigh its benefits, particularly if primary resection can be performed before bilirubin levels rise to unacceptable levels and liver function, particularly synthetic capacity, is compromised. If PVE is required to increase the FLR drainage of the proposed remnant it should always be performed (15).

OPERATIVE CONSIDERATIONS

Complete surgical excision is the only curative treatment. As with gallbladder carcinoma, survival following an incomplete resection is equivalent to unresectable disease. The surgery required to achieve this is personalized and determined by the anatomy of each tumour. Careful assessment both preoperatively and intraoperatively is required. The procedures required range from a non-anatomical liver resection to liver transplantation. Resections for CCA are associated with high rates of postoperative complications, morbidity and mortality and it is therefore also essential to ensure that patients are willing and fit enough to tolerate the surgery required (*see* **Chapters 6** and **19**). The best outcomes are achieved with the resources and experience of specialist multidisciplinary teams.

Typically, small iCCA that are peripherally located may be adequately cleared and an R0 margin achieved with a non-anatomical liver resection. Formal segmental or major liver resections are indicated when the mass is more centrally located, or when there are multiple lesions in the same lobe. In pCCA, Bismuth IIIb lesions typically require a left hepatectomy, while Bismuth I, II, and IIIa lesions usually require an extended right hepatectomy. Pancreaticoduodenectomy is the standard procedure for dCCA.

Staging laparoscopy

Staging laparoscopy with intraoperative US reduces the likelihood of an unnecessary laparotomy and is of particular benefit in high-risk patients with multicentric ICCA, and all CCA with a high CA 19-9 or a suspicion of vascular invasion or peritoneal disease (19).

Frozen section

The proximal and distal margins following bile duct resection should be sent for frozen section intraoperatively. This allows for extended resections to be undertaken if there is evidence of malignancy in those specimens confirming more extensive disease than predicted from preoperative and intraoperative imaging. Positive para-aortic lymph nodes make eCCA stage IV disease and preclude a curative resection. If there is clinical suspicion during exploration, an excision biopsy for frozen section should be performed prior to proceeding.

Lymph nodes

The extent of optimum lymphadenectomy is controversial and the subject of ongoing debate. Current AJCC recommendation is the retrieval of at least twelve lymph nodes for eCCA and six for iCCA. Routine practice is for a complete porta hepatis lymphadenectomy in all patients but the case for more extended lymph node dissection to include para-aortic lymph nodes in extra-hepatic CCA remains controversial and no survival benefit has been demonstrated to date. The Relay-HC trial aims to determine primarily if an extended lymphadenectomy improves overall survival compared with a standard lymphadenectomy and secondarily the impact on morbidity, mortality and disease-free survival (12).

Caudate lobe

The caudate lobe is pathologically involved in 40% of pCCA (12) and multiple studies have demonstrated that an *en bloc* excision for pCCA significantly increases the likelihood of achieving a curative resection and improves RFS and OS with no increase in morbidity. It should be the standard of care. The only situation when the value of caudate lobe excision should be questioned is when it is not obviously involved on preoperative and intraoperative imaging and the background liver is of poor quality and/or the proposed FLR volume is marginal.

Extended vascular resection

Portal venous resection and extended liver resections can improve resection rates and overall survival, but with an associated higher postoperative mortality (19). Arterial resections have so far demonstrated increased morbidity and mortality without conferring any demonstrable long-term survival benefit.

Hepatopancreaticoduodenectomy

Infiltrative CCA spreads longitudinally along periductal tissues and it can be difficult to achieve negative margins at both the distal and proximal ends of the bile duct. To address this issue, some units undertake HPD resections for eCCA but this approach is highly controversial. Studies have shown major complication rates of over 50% with only marginal increases in OS from 33.3% with hepatic resection alone to 36.8% following HPD. The trend towards more aggressive and extended surgical resections may have a place in highly selected fit patients with favourable tumour biology, but to-date there is no conclusive data from well-constructed trials. In view of the minimal benefits demonstrated from a small number of centres and the numbers required, identification of the indications and appropriate cohort for these major surgical procedures is likely to be extremely difficult.

Liver transplantation

Specialist centres in the USA have reported 5-year RFS of 65% within a protocol utilizing neoadjuvant chemoradiation followed by liver transplantation for patients with early stage but unresectable pCCA and all CCA in the context of PSC regardless of resectability (19). This is a better survival than that reported for resectable CCA at the same stages receiving standard surgical treatment.

NEOADJUVANT AND ADJUVANT TREATMENT

Upfront surgery is recommended for all suitably fit patients with resectable gallbladder carcinoma or cholangiocarcinoma on diagnosis. There is much interest in whether similar benefits to those seen for borderline resectable pancreatic adenocarcinoma might be achieved in the management of biliary tract malignancies. Presently there is limited and inconclusive data, but this is an area presently being investigated and likely to be the focus of a number of future trials.

A 6-month course of capecitabine is standard of care for all resected gallbladder carcinomas and cholangiocarcinomas based solely on data from the UK's multicentre capecitabine compared with observation in resected biliary tract cancer (BILCAP) randomized control trial. This showed an improved RFS and OS with capecitabine compared with surgery alone. Further studies assessing alternative regimes with or without radiotherapy are presently being conducted.

SUMMARY

Biliary malignancies comprise a heterogenous group of rare, but frequently fatal, tumours arising from either the gallbladder and intrahepatic or extrahepatic biliary tract. Their incidence is highest in lower-income regions of South Asia and South America and lowest in higher-income Western countries. The only curative treatment is complete surgical extirpation but unfortunately, as they are commonly asymptomatic in early stages, the majority of patients present with advanced and incurable disease. The prognosis is poor with less than a quarter of patients surviving 5 years from diagnosis. There are many areas of debate regarding the nature and extent of optimal surgical management for the minority of patients where potentially curative surgery is possible, and especially the place of extended resections with radical lymphadenectomy or vascular reconstructions.

REFERENCES

1. Sung H, Ferlay J, Siegel RL, Laversanne M, Soerjomataram I, Jemal A, et al. Global Cancer Statistics 2020: GLOBOCAN estimates of incidence and

mortality worldwide for 36 cancers in 185 countries. *CA Cancer J Clin* 2021;**71(3)**:209–49.

2. Schmidt MA, Marcano-Bonilla L, Roberts LR. Gallbladder cancer: Epidemiology and genetic risk associations. *Chin Clin Oncol* 2019;**8(4)**:31.

3. Rawla P, Sunkara T, Thandra KC, Barsouk A. Epidemiology of gallbladder cancer. *Clin Exp Hepatol* 2019;**5(2)**:93–102.

4. Halaseh SA, Halaseh S, Shakman R. A review of the etiology and epidemiology of gallbladder cancer: What you need to know. *Cureus* 2022;**14(8)**:e28260.

5. Alshahri TM, Abounozha S. Best evidence topic: Does the presence of a large gallstone carry a higher risk of gallbladder cancer? *Ann Med Surg (Lond)* 2021;**61**:93–6.

6. Sturm N, Schuhbaur JS, Huttner F, Perkhofer L, Ettrich TJ. Gallbladder cancer: Current multimodality treatment concepts and future directions. *Cancers (Basel)* 2022;**14(22)**:5580.

7. Pilgrim CH, Groeschl RT, Christians KK, Gamblin TC. Modern perspectives on factors predisposing to the development of gallbladder cancer. *HPB (Oxford)* 2013;**15(11)**:839–44.

8. Kellil T, Chaouch MA, Aloui E, Tormane MA, Taieb SK, Noomen F, et al. Incidence and preoperative predictor factors of gallbladder cancer before laparoscopic cholecystectomy: A systematic review. *J Gastrointest Cancer* 2021;**52(1)**:68–72.

9. Foley KG, Lahaye MJ, Thoeni RF, Soltes M, Dewhurst C, Barbu ST, et al. Management and follow-up of gallbladder polyps: Updated joint guidelines between the ESGAR, EAES, EFISDS and ESGE. *Eur Radiol* 2022;**32(5)**:3358–68.

10. Morimoto M, Matsuo T, Mori N. Management of porcelain gallbladder, its risk factors, and complications: A review. *Diagnostics (Basel)* 2021;**11(6)**:1073.

11. Sung YN, Song M, Lee JH, Song KB, Hwang DW, Ahn CS, et al. Validation of the 8th Edition of the American Joint Committee on Cancer Staging System for Gallbladder Cancer and Implications for the Follow-up of Patients without Node Dissection. *Cancer Res Treat* 2020;**52(2)**:455–68.

12. Washington K, Rocha F. Approach to resectable biliary cancers. *Curr Treat Options Oncol* 2021;**22(11)**:97.

13. Leung U, Pandit-Taskar N, Corvera CU, D'Angelica MI, Allen PJ, Kingham TP, et al. Impact of pre-operative positron emission tomography in gallbladder cancer. *HPB (Oxford)* 2014;**16(11)**:1023–30.

14. van Dooren M, de Savornin Lohman EAJ, Brekelmans E, Vissers PAJ, Erdmann JI, Braat AE, et al. The diagnostic value of staging laparoscopy in gallbladder cancer: A nationwide cohort study. *World J Surg Oncol* 2023;**21(1)**:6.

15. Valle JW, Kelley RK, Nervi B, Oh DY, Zhu AX. Biliary tract cancer. *Lancet* 2021;**397(10272)**:428–44.

16. Balakrishnan A, Barmpounakis P, Demiris N, Jah A, Spiers HVM, Talukder S, et al. Surgical outcomes of gallbladder cancer: The OMEGA retrospective, multicentre, international cohort study. *EClinicalMedicine* 2023;**59**:101951.

17. Chen Z, Yu J, Cao J, Lin C, Hu J, Zhang B, et al. Wedge resection versus segment IVb and V resection of the liver for T2 gallbladder cancer: A systematic review and meta-analysis. *Front Oncol* 2023;**13**:1186378.

18. Sun J, Xie TG, Ma ZY, Wu X, Li BL. Current status and progress in laparoscopic surgery for gallbladder carcinoma. *World J Gastroenterol* 2023;**29(16)**:2369–79.

19. Brindley PJ, Bachini M, Ilyas SI, Khan SA, Loukas A, Sirica AE, et al. Cholangiocarcinoma. *Nat Rev Dis Primers* 2021;**7(1)**:65.

20. Vithayathil M, Khan SA. Current epidemiology of cholangiocarcinoma in Western countries. *J Hepatol* 2022;**77(6)**:1690–8.

21. Liao X ZD. The 8th Edition American Joint Committee on Cancer Staging for Hepato-pancreato-biliary Cancer: A review and update. *Arch Pathol Lab Med* 2021;**145**:543–53.

22. Kim S, Park BK, Seo JH, Choi J, Choi JW, Lee CK, et al. Carbohydrate antigen 19-9 elevation without evidence of malignant or pancreatobiliary diseases. *Sci Rep* 2020;**10(1)**:8820.

23. Loosen SH, Roderburg C, Kauertz KL, Koch A, Vucur M, Schneider AT, et al. CEA but not CA19-9 is an independent prognostic factor in patients undergoing resection of cholangiocarcinoma. *Sci Rep* 2017;**7(1)**:16975.

24. Kiefer LS, Sekler J, Guckel B, Kraus MS, la Fougere C, Nikolaou K, et al. Impact of (18)F-FDG PET/CT on clinical management in patients with cholangiocellular carcinoma. *BJR Open* 2021;**3(1)**:20210008.

25. Charles J, Nezami N, Loya M, Shube S, Davis C, Hoots G, et al. Portal vein embolization: Rationale, techniques, and outcomes to maximize remnant liver hypertrophy with a focus on contemporary strategies. *Life (Basel)* 2023;**13(2)**:279.

Chapter

62

Iatrogenic Biliary Injuries

Keno Mentor, Wasfi Alrawashdeh and Steve White

INTRODUCTION

Bile duct injury (BDI) is one of the most serious and devastating complications of laparoscopic cholecystectomy. It has a profound impact on patients with increased morbidity, reduced survival and impaired quality of life in addition to its socio-economic impact. An interesting historical case, which demonstrates this clearly, involves prominent political figures during a crucial period in British history. Anthony Eden, the then foreign secretary, suffered with gallstone disease and intermittent obstructive jaundice. In selecting a surgeon to perform his cholecystectomy, he ignored the recommendation of advisors who suggested three of the most eminent surgeons of the time, in favour of Mr Basil Hume who had removed his appendix many years before. Hume was under intense pressure and was contacted directly by then prime minister Winston Churchill, who reminded him repeatedly of the importance of Mr Eden's position in government. Unsurprisingly, Hume suffered a nervous breakdown during the operation and transected the common bile duct. Hume was reported as commenting that Eden 'had two cystic ducts' – a clue as to the cause of the bile duct injury. Eden was then transported to Boston at great expense, where Dr Richard Cattell, a world-renowned biliary surgeon, successfully performed a hepaticojejunostomy. Eden initially recovered well from this procedure but had long-term problems with recurrent cholangitis due to anastomotic stricture. He abused multiple psychotropic drugs to control his symptoms, which significantly altered his mood and is widely regarded as one of the reasons for his aggressive response to the Suez Canal crisis of 1956, leading to the death of more than 3000 soldiers (1).

BDI is associated with 3.5–4.5% disease-specific mortality (2,3), and a four-fold increase in liver-associated mortality (4). In the long term, all-cause mortality is 8.8% higher in these patients compared to controls (5). Long-term complications such as cholangitis, biliary strictures and secondary biliary cirrhosis are common, and in some cases, patients may require liver transplantation to deal with the sequelae of BDI (6). Even the less complex cases of BDI requiring only endoscopic treatment are associated with significant short-term morbidity, long-term complications and costs (7,8). In addition to loss of productivity, patients suffering BDI have a significantly worse quality of life (QoL) which

persists beyond 5 years, even with successful treatment of the injury (3,9,10).

In addition, litigation resulting from BDI has a significant impact on surgeons and healthcare systems. According to one study from the UK, litigation following laparoscopic cholecystectomy resulted in 20.4 million GBP in payouts between 1995 and 2009 (11). In this study, BDI was the most frequent cause of litigation representing 43% of claims, and the most likely to succeed at an average cost of 102 827 GBP (168 337 USD). Similarly in the USA, 44% of litigations after laparoscopic cholecystectomy were related to BDI but attracting a much higher average payout of 1 068 545 USD (12).

In view of this wide-ranging impact of BDI, there is a large body of literature examining the different facets of BDI from mechanisms and risk factors to classification, management and assessment of the clinical and non-clinical outcomes. In this chapter, we will summarize and discuss the available data on these pertinent topics.

INCIDENCE

The incidence of BDI, following laparoscopic cholecystectomy, in large population-based studies ranges from 0.3–1.5% (13–16). This is in contrast to 0.2% after open cholecystectomy (17). One of the major factors contributing to this variation is the definition of BDI in each study. For example, a Swedish study reported a 1.5% incidence of BDI but included all postoperative bile leaks (16) whereas others with lower estimates used the need for reconstruction as a proxy for BDI (13). Nonetheless, data shows a significant increase in the incidence of BDI following the implementation of laparoscopic cholecystectomy in the early 1990s (18,19), although this reduced over subsequent years (20). In fact, more recent estimates from the last decade suggest that this is now equivalent to historical rates associated with open cholecystectomy according to a study based on National Surgical Quality Improvement Program (NSQIP) data (0.19%) (21). In addition to the incidence, data suggest that the pattern of BDI associated with laparoscopic cholecystectomy is also different to open procedures with a higher percentage of both transectional and hilar injuries in the laparoscopic era (22,23).

DOI: 10.1201/9781003080060-62

The incidence of associated arterial injuries varies widely (20–60%) depending on the method of investigation and accuracy of reporting. Over 90% of those involve the right hepatic artery (RHA) (2,24,25). They are more often associated with transectional and complex injuries of the biliary tree (26). Portal and other arterial injuries are rare. When isolated, some of those arterial injuries may not have any clinical consequences and remain undetected (27) presumably due to sufficient collateral circulation at the hilar plate (25).

MECHANISMS OF BILE DUCT INJURY

Early series of laparoscopic cholecystectomy reporting BDI revealed an association with the surgeon's overall experience (28,29), yet more recent data did not show such a clear relationship (30). Consequently, up to 30% of BDI are attributable to experienced surgeons (31) suggesting that learning curves are not the only factor contributing to BDI. Literature reporting the relationship between a surgeon's experience and BDI comes with a significant number of caveats as most of it belongs to the first decade of laparoscopic cholecystectomy and does not take into consideration the case mix complexity, which is a very important contributing factor. Hence, the question of whether BDI is avoidable or an inherent risk of cholecystectomy has been a matter of constant debate (32,33). Whilst an injury may result from partial or complete transection, clip application or thermal damage (34), it is increasingly appreciated that the factors contributing and leading to BDI encompass a complex mix of anatomical, disease related, technical and human factors. The recent decline in the incidence, along with improved understanding of the underlying mechanisms and initiatives addressing those factors (35,36), clearly demonstrate the ability to minimize the risk of BDI.

The anatomy of the biliary tree and its anomalies are covered elsewhere in this book. However, certain anomalies may increase the risk of biliary injury particularly an aberrant (low) insertion of the right posterior sectoral duct (37) which can make it vulnerable to injury during laparoscopic cholecystectomy. Acute cholecystitis is also a recognized risk factor for BDI in larger cohort studies (21,38), and in cases of severe inflammation, the common hepatic duct (CHD) can be drawn into and become adherent to Hartmann's pouch, causing the surgeon to mis-identify the main bile duct as the cystic duct (CD).

The role that the approach to identify and then secure the CD plays in bile duct injury is not clear. Whilst the most common method is metallic clips, others include ligature ties, locking clips, staplers and, in some series, energy devices alone. Although these have been compared in relation to bile leak, there is no data regarding the incidence of bile duct injury. Certain pitfalls should be considered, however, such as narrowing or injuring the common bile duct (CBD) when staplers are applied without an adequate distance from the CBD.

Nonetheless, misidentification remains the major factor in BDI. In an interesting analysis of 256 cases of BDI, Way et al. concluded that 97% of BDI stemmed from visual misperception related to unusual anatomical configuration and subconscious human assumptions. Only 3% resulted from technical errors, highlighting the complexity of events culminating in a BDI and therefore directing training on those critical stages of the procedure (39). Consequently, Strasburg introduced the concept of 'error traps' in laparoscopic cholecystectomy, defined as a 'method that works well in most circumstances but which is apt to fail under certain conditions' (40). In other words, these are meant to be 'safety nets' but can themselves increase the risk of biliary injury in certain circumstances. He described four of these 'error traps':

1 The 'infundibular view'
2 Fundus-down cholecystectomy in the face of severe inflammation
3 Failure to perceive the presence of an aberrant right hepatic duct (RHD) on cholangiography
4 Injury to the CBD in the case of a 'parallel union' cystic duct

Based on this cumulative work, several recommendations have been made to reduce the risk of BDI including among others: 1) The critical view of safety; 2) stop times; 3) subtotal cholecystectomy and 4) the debatable role of intraoperative cholangiography (35,36,41). These are discussed elsewhere.

CLASSIFICATION

Several classification systems have been proposed to describe the extent of biliary injury. These are useful when planning a management strategy and surgical repair, along with facilitating standardized nomenclature for research. The most popular system is that described by Strasburg, which also incorporated and expanded the previous Bismuth classification (42). Others include the Stewart-Way (26) and more recently Hannover classification (43). The Strasberg classification (*Figure 62.1*) does not provide details of any associated vascular injuries whilst the Stewart-Way (*Figure 62.2*) is a simplified classification that does include injury to the RHA in class III and IV, although it does not differentiate CHD injuries at or above the confluence of the left- and right-hepatic ducts. The Hannover classification provides a much more detailed description of both biliary and associated vascular injuries detailing 21 different patterns of injury, which perhaps limits its use. Importantly, none of these classifications differentiate between early- and late-presentation or include variables related to the physiology of the patient at the time of presentation, therefore missing several confounding factors that may contribute to decision making and overall prognosis.

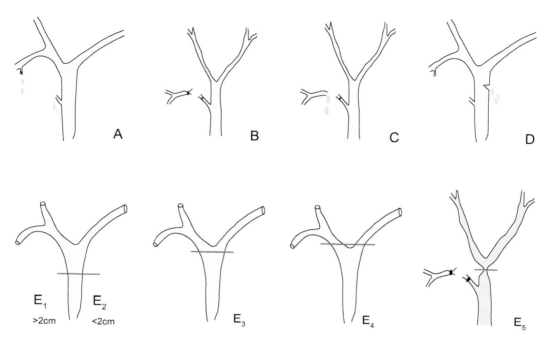

Figure 62.1 Bismuth-Strasberg classification of BDI. Bile leak from cystic duct or liver bed (A); occlusion of the right segmental duct (B); bile leak from divided right segmental duct (C); lateral injury to the CHD (D); main bile duct injury, >2 cm from the confluence (E_1); main bile duct injury, <2 cm from the confluence (E_2); hilar injury with intact confluence (E_3); confluence involved, right- and left-hepatic ducts are separated (E_4); injury of aberrant right sectoral duct with concomitant injury of main bile duct (E_5) (42).

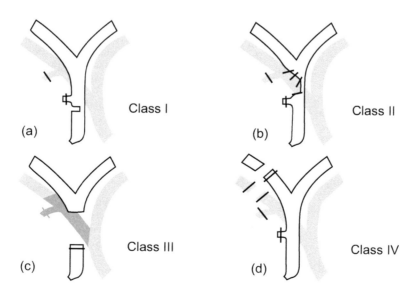

Figure 62.2 Stewart-Way classification of BDI injury. Class I: incision (incomplete transection) of the CBD (a). Class II: lateral damage to the CHD with resultant stricture and/or leak (b). Class III: complete transection of the main bile duct (c). Class IV: transection or leak of the RHD or posterolateral sectoral duct, often combined with injury to the RHA (d) (39).

PRESENTATION

The timing of presentation, or identification of BDI, has important implications for management as well as outcomes. A high index of suspicion must be maintained as early identification is associated with better outcomes (16).

There are four broad patterns of presentation:

1   *Immediate intraoperative identification.* Typically, only around 23–41% are identified intraoperatively although this may be higher for major injuries (16,44)

2   *Early postoperative presentation.* Patients in this group often present with varying symptoms including non-specific abdominal pain, bile leak, biliary peritonitis, sepsis and occasionally jaundice if there is an occluding injury (45). Any patient who becomes unwell or fails to thrive after laparoscopic cholecystectomy should raise the suspicion of BDI

3   *Delayed presentation.* Patients presenting several weeks after the injury more commonly manifest cholangitis, jaundice and abdominal pain (46)

4   *Late or very delayed presentation.* Some patients may have missed injuries that result in late strictures and walled-off collections, presenting months or years later with features of recurrent cholangitis, pain, sepsis or even biliary cirrhosis. Some of those may also be asymptomatic with simply mildly abnormal liver function tests (LFTs), incidental biliary dilatation or even atrophy of affected part of liver on imaging.

INVESTIGATIONS

The goals of investigation of a suspected BDI are to: 1) define the injury in relation to the biliary anatomy; 2) identify associated injuries such as vascular or bowel injury and other complications including collections and 3) determine the physiological status of the patient to guide the timing of operative repair allowing for optimization. Thorough investigation to precisely define the configuration of BDI in relation to the biliary anatomy before any attempted repair is crucial in both immediate and delayed presentations in order to select the appropriate operative strategy. This is especially important in more proximal injuries (Strasberg type E_2–E_4), where aberrant anatomy exists, and in cases with associated vascular injuries.

Immediate (intraoperative) presentation

For those cases where BDI is suspected at the time of surgery, an intraoperative cholangiogram (IOC) is usually the only investigation required if immediate repair by an experienced surgeon is to be undertaken (*Figure 62.3*).

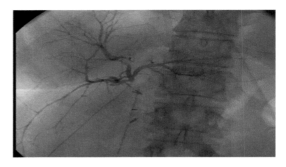

Figure 62.3 Intraoperative cholangiogram of complete bile duct transection.

Early postoperative or delayed presentation

If either the diagnosis or management of BDI is delayed, enough time may have lapsed for the development of biliary peritonitis and resultant deterioration in the physiological state of the patient. The scope of investigations may need to be more thorough, and plans made for temporising measures by percutaneous abdominal drainage or laparotomy with washout and later formal 'delayed' repair.

Laboratory investigations should include a standard resuscitation panel (arterial blood gas, renal function tests), markers of inflammation and sepsis (C-reactive protein, white cell count and blood culture) and LFTs. The latter can provide information as to the nature of the BDI with obstructive injuries causing significant increases in serum bilirubin and canalicular enzymes, while bile leak is usually associated with only a minimal increase in bilirubin, which is caused by peritoneal absorption. A disproportionate rise in transaminases may signify a co-existing vascular injury.

Although duplex ultrasound (US) can detect biliary dilatation and sub-hepatic collections suggestive of bile leak, contrast-enhanced computer tomography (CECT) four phase with optimally timed arterial and portal venous phases) is usually the first imaging modality undertaken as it is widely available and provides the clinician with more detailed information. In addition to identifying collections suggestive of bile leak and the level of injury in obstructive BDI, CECT can also exclude associated vascular injuries and, in patients with longer delays to presentation, hepatic atrophy or secondary biliary cirrhosis (47).

While CECT findings can suggest the level of BDI and potential bile leak, magnetic resonance cholangiopancreatography (MRCP) is the imaging modality of choice for non-invasive visualization of the biliary tree (*Figure 62.4*). With the addition of hepato-specific contrast agents (gadotexate disodium; Primovist® and Eovist®), which are excreted into the biliary tree, bile

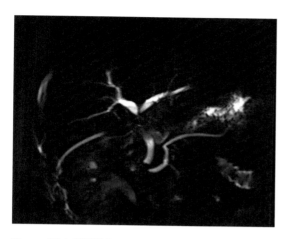

Figure 62.4 MRCP image of bile duct transection.

leaks can be more definitively diagnosed and the site of leak more precisely localized (48). This is important because accessory ducts can easily be missed at the time of hepaticojejunostomy, resulting in bile leak which can be difficult to manage. Magnetic resonance imaging (MRI) findings suggestive of bile leak include a collection with high-signal intensity on T2-weighted imaging and low T1-weighted signal intensity, which distinguishes bile from other sources of fluid (e.g. seroma, ascites). Extravasation of hepato-specific contrast during the delayed hepatobiliary excretion phase on T1-weighted imaging confirms the biliary source of the collection and can localize the site of injury (49). This modality may be less accurate in patients with an occlusive injury and obstructive jaundice, as excretion of hepato-specific contrast is impaired in the liver with cholestasis (50).

In patients where MRI is contraindicated, the presence of bile leak can be confirmed with hepatobiliary scintigraphy (hepatobiliary iminodiacetic acid [HIDA] scan) and biliary anatomy can be delineated with drip infusion cholangiography with CT (DIC-CT). However, DIC-CT use is associated with contrast-related adverse reactions in up to 2.2% of cases and is not popular, or widely used (51). In practice, where MRI is unavailable or contraindicated, a high bile content of abdominal drains is highly suggestive of a bile leak, while a dilated biliary tree on CECT signifies a BDI associated with obstruction. Endoscopic retrograde cholangiopancreatography (ERCP) and percutaneous transhepatic cholangiography (PTC) can be employed to localize the bile leak and delineate biliary anatomy if the transection is not complete.

ERCP and PTC have the advantage of potentially being able to add therapeutic procedures in addition to identifying and localizing bile leaks. In cases of a major BDI (Strasberg E), ERCP is more limited as

a diagnostic modality as it only enables visualization of the common bile duct distal to the injury. In these cases, PTC should be used to delineate proximal bile duct anatomy, which will be critical in planning surgical repair (52). PTC also has the advantage of being utilized to assess anastomotic patency and diagnose bile leak after surgical repair of the injury and can be useful to use as a postoperative stent across the hepaticojejunostomy if there are concerns about early integrity.

MANAGEMENT

The goal of management of BDI is to re-establish biliary-enteric communication while, in the long term, minimizing the risk of a stricture. This is best achieved with a tension-free repair in healthy, well-vascularized tissue in the absence of infection or inflammation in a patient with optimal systemic physiology (53). Preoperative preparation and the timing of repair should be directed to achieve these pre-requisite conditions before surgery is undertaken.

Timing of repair

In general, the timing of repair is less important than the availability of surgical expertise, and accurate delineation of biliary anatomy and the extent of the BDI (54). A recent multicentre study concluded that the timing of bile duct repair did not affect the rate of postoperative complications or overall outcome (55). However, the advantages of early hepato-pancreatico-biliary (HPB) specialist involvement have also been documented in multiple reports (56,57). Taken together, these findings suggest that the timing of surgery should be individualized and delayed if necessary to allow optimal preoperative investigation and physiological improvement at a specialist HPB centre.

Immediate (intraoperative) repair

When a BDI is recognized at the time of cholecystectomy and there is clear demonstration of biliary anatomy with IOC, immediate repair is preferable if HPB expertise exists. This can prevent further complications and spare the patient numerous investigations and other procedures. Any deviation from this ideal situation is best managed with a 'damage control' approach with control of major bleeding, placement of closed-system abdominal drains and exteriorization of transected bile ducts. This can be achieved by passing a small calibre tube into the proximal duct(s) and securing with a simple tie (*Figure 62.5*). In doing so, care should be taken not to cause further damage or devascularization of the remaining duct(s), as this would complicate subsequent repair. Prompt referral to an HPB specialist centre for further investigation and management should then be arranged.

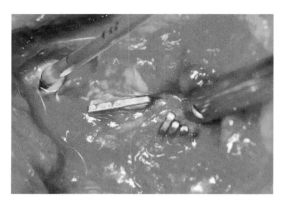

Figure 62.5 In-surgery image showing a feeding tube placed in a transected bile duct to divert bile (58).

Early postoperative or delayed repair

This is a heterogenous group of patients where the management strategy will depend on the extent of the injury, presence of complications (obstruction or bile leak) and the physiological status of the patient.

The patient's physiological state should be optimized with appropriate resuscitation and anti-microbial therapy guided by local microbiology protocols for empiric therapy. Uncontrolled biliary peritonitis can be managed with either emergency re-laparoscopy with washout and placement of drains if early in the postoperative period, or with image-guided percutaneous drainage. For minor self-limiting injuries, external drainage may be all that is required to allow spontaneous resolution of a bile leak. This conservative strategy requires serial abdominal examination and close monitoring of the patient's physiological state as delays in recognition and failure to act upon biliary peritonitis can be catastrophic.

BDI with obstructive jaundice usually occurs in the context of a proximal injury with complete occlusion of the bile duct with a clip. Where this is complicated by cholangitis, an external percutaneous transhepatic biliary drainage (PTBD) catheter should be placed to decompress the biliary tree and broad-spectrum antibiotics administered to control systemic sepsis. More than one drain may be needed if the occlusion is above the level of the biliary confluence. If the PTBD is positioned just proximal to the occluded duct, the surgeon also has a palpable landmark to locate the bile duct when repair is undertaken at a later stage.

PTBD can also be utilized in injuries with transected ducts with free bile leak by passing the catheter across the duct opening, facilitating simultaneous biliary diversion and drainage of the sub-hepatic space. Wider calibre abdominal drains may also be needed to achieve adequate control. As the peripheral biliary tree is often collapsed in this scenario, this strategy is more technically challenging. The liberal application

of PTBD for BDI is controversial. Advocates of this approach cite the numerous diagnostic and therapeutic functions possible from this single modality (58), while opponents argue that the risk of major bleeding and septic complications, which are as high as 2%, mandate a more selective approach (59).

Non-operative management of minor injuries

Minor injuries (Stewart-Way class 1, Strasberg A) can often be managed conservatively, facilitated by abdominal drainage. A period (2–3 weeks) of external drainage with a steadily decreasing bile leak volume indicates a spontaneously resolving biliary fistula often due to a leak from a duct of Luschka, which does not require further management.

Where drain volumes are persistently high, endoscopic or radiological techniques should be employed to reduce the flow across the bile duct defect, thereby facilitating spontaneous closure. ERCP is most often utilized in this clinical scenario by reducing the trans-papillary pressure gradient to facilitate preferential flow away from the bile duct injury. Endoscopic biliary sphincterotomy (EBS) and stent placement, in combination or alone is employed to achieve bile diversion. Extensive study has been conducted to examine the relative risks and benefits of various combinations of endoscopic therapy, including whether stenting and EBS should be done alone or in combination, the size and positioning of stents, and the duration of stent placement (60–62). The details of these investigations go beyond the scope of this text but in summary, there is currently no consensus on these technical considerations and the details of the endoscopic therapy employed will depend on local preference and expertise. Where ERCP is not possible because of previous surgery or technical difficulty, PTC should be employed to achieve bile diversion.

Surgical management with primary repair

Minor injuries which are recognized immediately at cholecystectomy may be amenable to simple primary repair. Segmental or accessory ducts less than 2–3 mm in diameter (Strasberg type A) can be ligated once the biliary anatomy has been definitively delineated with IOC. Small lacerations to the bile duct can be repaired with interrupted sutures taking care not to narrow the lumen in doing so. Repair over the well-known 'T-tube' assists in preventing narrowing both during the repair and in the postoperative period. Repair over a biliary stent can also be performed if the duct remains in continuity, which is then later removed endoscopically.

Primary repair of complete transections with end-to-end anastomosis (EEA) is controversial. The advantages of maintaining normal biliary anatomy and avoiding the complications of hepaticojejunostomy are offset by reports of high rates of long-term stricture

(56). However, these historical reports include EEA performed at non-specialist centres and under operative conditions which are unclear and unlikely to be ideal. Some authors argue that good long-term results can be achieved with EEA at specialist centres when loss of duct length and surrounding tissue damage is minimal (63,64). In practice, however, these conditions are rarely met, necessitating more extensive repairs with biliary-enteric reconstruction for most transection injuries.

Surgical management with biliary-enteric anastomosis

Major or proximal BDIs (Bismuth-Strasberg Types E_1–E_5) are best managed with a mucosa-to-mucosa hepaticojejunostomy with a tailored technical approach depending on the level of injury. Major injuries to the distal bile duct could be repaired with choledochoduodenostomy, but this technique is not often utilized because of increased risk of ascending cholangitis and bile leaks. These types of repairs often re-present at a later stage and require conversion to a hepaticojejunostomy. Furthermore, when anastomotic leak does occur from a choledochoduodenostomy, the resultant high volume duodenal fistula is more difficult to manage than a comparable leak from hepaticojejunostomy (65).

Proximal injuries, especially those close to, or involving, the biliary confluence (Bismuth-Strasberg Type E_2 & E_3), may require modification of the technique to achieve a tension-free hepaticojejunostomy that effectively drains both left- and right-biliary systems. A well-positioned PTBD catheter will aid the surgeon in locating the proximal duct. If this is not possible, lowering of the hilar plate inferior to segment 4B will expose the proximal biliary tree without compromising its blood supply (*Figure 62.6*). Extension of the choledochotomy into the more accessible left hepatic duct (Hepp-Couinaud approach) may be required to fashion an anastomosis of sufficient calibre.

Injuries which completely separate the left- and right-biliary systems require more complex reconstructions with separate anastomosis of each duct. If there is limited extrahepatic length of either or both ducts, a parenchymal dissection or excision of segment 4B is necessary to achieve sufficient length of the left and right hepatic ducts to facilitate a large enough choledochotomy for an effective side-to-side hepaticojejunostomy to each duct (*Figure 62.7*).

In the most severe form of injury where no ducts are available for anastomosis, a portoenterostomy with a loop of jejunum anastomosed to the exposed liver parenchyma should be performed as a rescue procedure. Alternatively, a hepatotomy can be performed to identify a viable duct and surrounding parenchyma resected to achieve an anastomosis. The long-term outcomes of portoenterostomy are very poor. For those that fail, two alternatives exist: 1) Either a major resection with biliary-enteric anastomosis to the liver remnant or 2) liver transplantation (66).

Vasculobiliary injuries

Because of extensive hepatic collateral arterial supply, the risk of hepatic ischaemia following RHA injury or ligation is low and is estimated to occur in 10% of cases (25). When it does occur, it usually manifests as hepatic abscesses or an incidental finding of atrophy of

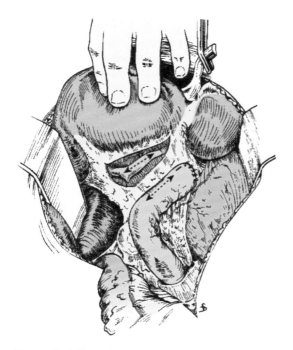

Figure 62.6 Illustration demonstrating a lowered hilar plate with exposed biliary confluence (arrow on green) and left hepatic duct (arrow on pink).

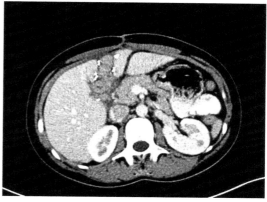

Figure 62.7 Postoperative axial CT scan showing segment 4b resection and hepaticojejunostomy. This case required two separate biliary-enteric anastomoses.

the right hemi-liver in the long-term (67). The benefit of RHA repair is unclear as the long-term risk of clinically relevant hepatic ischaemia is similar, whether or not repair is undertaken. In practice, repair is only advocated when the RHA injury is minor and can be repaired immediately. These conditions rarely exist, and the injured RHA is usually ligated to control acute haemorrhage.

In contrast, the effect of RHA injury on the long-term risk of biliary stricture formation following repair remains controversial. Multiple studies have reported conflicting results and a systematic review, which included the major series investigating this question, found no significant overall association of RHA injury with biliary stricture (68). These differences in reports probably reflect the confounding effect of other risk factors, including the level of the bile duct injury and the timing of repair. A sub-group analysis of those patients with RHA injury who have a delayed bile duct repair were found to have lower rates of biliary stricture (26,69,70). The underlying pathogenesis of this relationship is thought to be due to biliary ischaemia, which may not be apparent immediately after the injury, and subsequent anastomosis to biliary structures of questionable viability. For this reason, some authors advocate for delaying biliary repair for 3 months, and using adjuncts (PTBD, percutaneous drainage) to divert bile while awaiting repair. If early repair is undertaken, it should be at a higher level to ensure viability of the anastomosed tissue (69).

More severe vasculobiliary injuries (VBI) involving the portal vein and/or common hepatic artery are rare but have catastrophic consequences. Rapid hepatic ischaemia and infarction ensues, resulting in perioperative mortality rates as high as 35% despite attempts at vascular reconstruction. Right hepatectomy should be undertaken for acute infarction of the right hemi-liver but liver transplantation is frequently required in these cases (25,71).

Chronic biliary obstruction

Unrecognized prolonged biliary obstruction can cause progressive hepatic fibrosis culminating in secondary biliary cirrhosis (SBC). The incidence of SBC following BDI is 7–25% (72), but is probably overestimated because of referral bias inherent in reports from specialist centres. The average time interval for the development of SBC is 4 years but pathological changes are seen in the liver as early as 1 month after the original injury (73). Portal hypertension develops in as much as 20% of these cases and significantly increases mortality (26–36%) if bile duct repair is undertaken at this late stage (74). When liver failure develops, liver transplantation is required but is associated with mortality rates as high as 29% (6,75,76).

OUTCOMES

The success rates of BDI management have steadily increased as surgical, endoscopic and interventional radiological techniques have improved (77) but long-term sequelae can still have a profound effect on patient outcome.

Short-term outcomes following surgical repair of BDIs are associated with low perioperative mortality rates of 0–1.9% (45,77–79). When mortality does occur, it is most commonly as a result of pre-existing liver parenchymal disease, portal hypertension, significant comorbidity or profound sepsis. Morbidity occurs in 24% of patients and is associated with infective complications including surgical site sepsis, cholangitis and pneumonia (77). Where more severe complications such as anastomotic leak or intra-abdominal sepsis occur, they are usually amenable to minimally invasive procedures and re-operation is infrequently required (80).

Long-term outcome data of surgical repair of BDIs show similarly reassuring results with numerous authors reporting high success rates, with 85–95% of patients not requiring any further intervention (77). However, most of these reports have follow-up periods of <5 years, and there is evidence to suggest that biliary anastomotic stricture can develop beyond this period in up to 24% of patients (81). When stricture does occur, surgical reconstruction of the hepaticojejunostomy provides the most durable results but stricture can recur in up to 23% of cases (82,83). Percutaneous balloon dilatation of biliary anastomotic strictures provides a minimally invasive option, but up to three sessions are required to achieve acceptable patency rates comparable to that achieved with re-operation (84,85). These procedures are best reserved for patients who decline re-operation, have had multiple previous reconstructions or who are poor surgical candidates. Long-term stent or catheter placement (4–12 months) significantly improves patency rates (89% at 3-years) (77,84,85), but data beyond 5 years of follow-up is lacking. Novel biodegradable stents offer the potential for a single-procedure solution and have achieved 100% success rates but with a median follow-up of only 11 months (86).

The QoL measures of patients who undergo repair of BDI reported by different studies are conflicting, with a lack of consistency in design and inclusion of heterogenous patient groups (87). One study compared the physical, psychological and social QoL scores of patients who had a successful surgical BDI repair with patients who had uncomplicated laparoscopic cholecystectomy (LC) and with healthy controls. Of the three domains of QoL, only the psychological score was significantly different between groups (BDI repair 77% vs. LC 85%) while physical and social scores were similar. In contrast, data from a different study showed significant differences across all QoL domains in patients who experienced BDI compared to healthy controls, which was exacerbated by a longer duration of treatment (88).

The sequelae of BDI and the therapeutic modalities employed in its management have important implications for patient long-term QoL and significantly reduces overall survival compared to uncomplicated LC (HR 2.7) (14). In obtaining consent for cholecystectomy, the surgeon should take care to adequately inform the patient of the risks associated with this potentially serious outcome.

SUMMARY

BDI is a serious complication of cholecystectomy, which has profound implications for a patient's quality of life. The incidence of BDI initially increased with the adoption of LC but has steadily improved with better understanding of the underlying mechanisms leading to injury and the development of strategies to ameliorate risk factors.

Investigation of a BDI aims to accurately define the configuration and location of the BDI in relation to biliary and vascular anatomy, and is primarily based on CECT and MRI. ERCP and PTC are useful imaging adjuncts in situations where CT or MRI are contraindicated.

The management of BDI is best instituted at specialist hepatobiliary units and should be tailored to the level and extent of the injury. Minimally invasive modalities such as ERCP or PTC with the placement of biliary stents are effective for less severe injuries, but surgical repair with hepatojejunostomy is required in most cases to prevent long-term complications.

The short-term outcomes following BDI repair are good, but the rates of long-term biliary stricture are underestimated in non-specialist centres. Patient QoL measures following BDI are unclear but are likely worse for those patients who experience postoperative morbidity or who require repeat procedures (*Figure 62.8*).

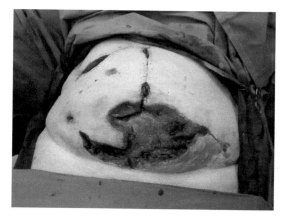

Figure 62.8 Potentially catastrophic outcome of BDI. This patient underwent multiple surgeries for a chronic bile leak and surgical site infection.

REFERENCES

1. Tebala GD, Nuzzo G. Iatrogenic biliary injury during cholecystectomy: Critical review of a historical case and its political consequences. *Dig Surg* 2021;**38(2)**:91–103.
2. Perera MT, Silva MA, Hegab B. Specialist early and immediate repair of post-laparoscopic cholecystectomy bile duct injuries is associated with an improved long-term outcome. *Ann Surg* 2011;**253(3)**:553–60.
3. Booij KAC, Reuver PR, Dieren S. Long-term impact of bile duct injury on morbidity, mortality, quality of life, and work related limitations. *Ann Surg* 2018;**268(1)**:143–50.
4. Tornqvist B, Zheng Z, Ye W. Long-term effects of iatrogenic bile duct injury during cholecystectomy. *Clin Gastroenterol Hepatol* 2009;**7(9)**:1013–8.
5. Halbert C, Altieri MS, Yang J. Long-term outcomes of patients with common bile duct injury following laparoscopic cholecystectomy. *Surg Endosc* 2016;**30(10)**:4294–9.
6. Tsaparas P, Machairas N, Ardiles V. Liver transplantation as last-resort treatment for patients with bile duct injuries following cholecystectomy: A multicenter analysis. *Ann Gastroenterol* 2021;**34(1)**:111–8.
7. Halle-Smith JM, Hodson J, Stevens LG. A comprehensive evaluation of the long-term clinical and economic impact of minor bile duct injury. *Surgery* 2020;**167(6)**:942–9.
8. Booij KA, Reuver PR, Yap K. Morbidity and mortality after minor bile duct injury following laparoscopic cholecystectomy. *Endoscopy* 2015;**47(1)**:40–6.
9. Boerma D, Rauws EA, Keulemans YC. Impaired quality of life 5 years after bile duct injury during laparoscopic cholecystectomy: A prospective analysis. *Ann Surg* 2001;**234(6)**:750–7.
10. de Reuver P, Sprangers M, Rauws E. Impact of bile duct injury after laparoscopic cholecystectomy on quality of life: A longitudinal study after multidisciplinary treatment. *Endoscopy* 2008;**40(8)**:637–43.
11. Alkhaffaf B, Decadt B. 15 years of litigation following laparoscopic cholecystectomy in England. *Ann Surg* 2010;**251(4)**:682–5.
12. Anandalwar SP, Choudhry AJ, Choudhry AJ. Litigation in laparoscopic cholecystectomies. *Am Surg* 2014;**80(6)**:E179–E181.
13. Waage A, Nilsson M. Iatrogenic bile duct injury: A population-based study of 152 776 cholecystectomies in the Swedish Inpatient Registry. *Arch Surg* 2006;**141(12)**:1207–13.
14. Flum DR, Cheadle A, Prela C. Bile duct injury during cholecystectomy and survival in medicare beneficiaries. *JAMA* 2003;**290(16)**:2168–73.
15. Sheffield KM, Riall TS, Han Y. Association between cholecystectomy with vs without intraoperative cholangiography and risk of common duct injury. *JAMA* 2013;**310(8)**:812–20.
16. Tornqvist B, Stromberg C, Persson G. Effect of intended intraoperative cholangiography and early detection of bile duct injury on survival after cholecystectomy: Population-based cohort study. *BMJ* 2012;**345**:e6457.

17. Roslyn JJ, Binns GS, Hughes EF. Open cholecystectomy. A contemporary analysis of 42,474 patients. *Ann Surg* 1993;**218**(2):129–37.

18. Adamsen S, Hansen OH, Funch-Jensen P. Bile duct injury during laparoscopic cholecystectomy: A prospective nationwide series. *J Am Coll Surg* 1997;**184**(6):571–8.

19. Rutledge R, Fakhry SM, Baker CC. The impact of laparoscopic cholecystectomy on the management and outcome of biliary tract disease in North Carolina: A statewide, population-based, time-series analysis. *J Am Coll Surg* 1996;**183**(1):31–45.

20. Pucher PH, Brunt LM, Davies N. Outcome trends and safety measures after 30 years of laparoscopic cholecystectomy: A systematic review and pooled data analysis. *Surg Endosc* 2018;**32**(5):2175–83.

21. Mangieri CW, Hendren BP, Strode MA. Bile duct injuries (BDI) in the advanced laparoscopic cholecystectomy era. *Surg Endosc* 2019;**33**(3):724-30

22. Misawa T, Saito R, Shiba H. Analysis of bile duct injuries (Stewart-Way classification) during laparoscopic cholecystectomy. *J Hepatobiliary Pancreat Surg* 2006;**13**(5):427–34.

23. Chaudhary A, Manisegran M, Chandra A. How do bile duct injuries sustained during laparoscopic cholecystectomy differ from those during open cholecystectomy? *J laparoendosc Adv Surg Tech A* 2001;**11**(4):187-91.

24. Pulitano C, Parks RW, Ireland H. Impact of concomitant arterial injury on the outcome of laparoscopic bile duct injury. *Am J Surg* 2011;**201**(2):238–44.

25. Strasberg SM, Helton WS. An analytical review of vasculobiliary injury in laparoscopic and open cholecystectomy. *HPB (Oxford)* 2011;**13**(1):1–14.

26. Stewart L, Robinson TN, Lee CM. Right hepatic artery injury associated with laparoscopic bile duct injury: Incidence, mechanism, and consequences. *J Gastrointest Surg* 2004;**8**(5):30–1.

27. Halasz NA. Cholecystectomy and hepatic artery injuries. *Arch Surg* 1991;**126**(2):137–8.

28. Hobbs MS, Mai Q, Knuiman MW. Surgeon experience and trends in intraoperative complications in laparoscopic cholecystectomy. *Br J Surg* 2006;**93**(7):844–53.

29. Deziel DJ, Millikan KW, Economou SG. Complications of laparoscopic cholecystectomy: A national survey of 4,292 hospitals and an analysis of 77,604 cases. *Am J Surg* 1993;**165**(1):9–14.

30. Abelson JS, Spiegel JD, Afaneh C, Mao J, Sedrakyan A, Yeo HL. Evaluating cumulative and annual surgeon volume in laparoscopic cholecystectomy. *Surgery* 2017;**161**(3):611–7.

31. Archer SB, Brown DW, Smith CD. Bile duct injury during laparoscopic cholecystectomy: Results of a national survey. *Ann Surg* 2001;**234**(4):58–9.

32. de Reuver P, Dijkgraaf M, Gevers S. Poor agreement among expert witnesses in bile duct injury malpractice litigation: an expert panel survey. *Ann Surg* 2008; **248**(5):815–20.

33. Gordon-Weeks A, Samarendra H, Bono J. Surgeons opinions of legal practice in bile duct injury following cholecystectomy. *HPB (Oxford)* 2017;**19** (8):721–6.

34. Davidoff AM, Pappas TN, Murray EA. Mechanisms of major biliary injury during laparoscopic cholecystectomy. *Ann Surg* 1992;**215**(3):196–202.

35. Brunt LM, Deziel DJ, Telem DA. Safe Cholecystectomy Multi-society Practice Guideline and State of the Art Consensus Conference on prevention of bile duct injury during cholecystectomy *Ann Surg* 2020;**272**(1):3–23.

36. Pucher PH, Brunt LM, Fanelli RD. SAGES expert Delphi consensus: Critical factors for safe surgical practice in laparoscopic cholecystectomy. *Surg Endosc* 2015;**29**(11):3074–85.

37. Babel N, Sakpal SV, Paragi P. Iatrogenic bile duct injury associated with anomalies of the right hepatic sectoral ducts: a misunderstood and underappreciated problem. *HPB Surg* 2009;**2009**: 153269.

38. Nuzzo G, Giuliante F, Giovannini I. Bile duct injury during laparoscopic cholecystectomy: results of an Italian national survey on 56 591 cholecystectomies. *Arch Surg* 2005;**140**(10):986–92.

39. Way LW, Stewart L, Gantert W. Causes and prevention of laparoscopic bile duct injuries: analysis of 252 cases from a human factors and cognitive psychology perspective. *Ann Surg* 2003;**237**(4):460–9.

40. Strasberg SM. Error traps and vasculo-biliary injury in laparoscopic and open cholecystectomy. *J Hepatobiliary Pancreat Surg* 2008;**15**(3):284–92.

41. Ausania F, Holmes LR, Ausania F, Iype S, Ricci P, White SA. Intraoperative cholangiography in the laparoscopic cholecystectomy era: Why are we still debating? *Surg Endosc* 2012;**26**(5):1193–200.

42. Strasberg SM, Hertl M, Soper NJ. An analysis of the problem of biliary injury during laparoscopic cholecystectomy. *J Am Coll Surg* 1995;**180**(1):101–25.

43. Bektas H, Schrem H, Winny M. Surgical treatment and outcome of iatrogenic bile duct lesions after cholecystectomy and the impact of different clinical classification systems. *Br J Surg* 2007;**94**(9):1119–27.

44. Stilling NM, Fristrup C, Wettergren A. Long-term outcome after early repair of iatrogenic bile duct injury. A national Danish multicentre study. *HPB (Oxford)* 2015;**17**(5):394–400.

45. de Reuver P, Grossmann I, Busch O. Referral pattern and timing of repair are risk factors for complications after reconstructive surgery for bile duct injury. *Ann Surg* 2007;**245**(5):763–70.

46. Ibrarullah M, Sankar S, Sreenivasan K. Management of bile duct injury at various stages of presentation: Experience from a tertiary care centre. *Indian J Surg* 2015;**77**(2):92–8.

47. Pesce A, Palmucci S, La Greca G, Puleo S. Iatrogenic bile duct injury: Impact and management challenges. *Clin Exp Gastroenterol* 2019;**12**:121–8.

48. Gupta RT, Brady CM, Lotz J, Boll DT, Merkle EM. Dynamic MR Imaging of the biliary system using hepatocyte-specific contrast agents. *Am J Roentgenol* 2010;**195**(2):405–13.

49. Mungai F, Berti V, Colagrande S. Bile leak after elective laparoscopic cholecystectomy: Role of MR imaging. *Radiology Case* 2013;**7**(1):25–32.

50. Thian YL, Riddell AM, Koh D-M. Liver-specific agents for contrast-enhanced MRI: role in

oncological imaging. *Cancer Imaging* 2013;**13(4)**: 567–79.

51. Hyodo T, Kumano S, Kushihata F, Okada M, Hirata M, Tsuda T, et al. CT and MR cholangiography: Advantages and pitfalls in perioperative evaluation of biliary tree. *Br J Radiol* 2012;**85(1015)**:887–96.

52. Rustagi T, Aslanian HR. Endoscopic management of biliary leaks after laparoscopic cholecystectomy. *J Clin Gastroenterol* 2014;**48(8)**:674–8.

53. Lillemoe, K. 2021 Repair of common bile duct injuries. Available from: https://medilib.ir/uptodate/show/3682, UptoDate online resource. (Accessed 29 August 2024).

54. Stewart L. Laparoscopic bile duct injuries: Timing of surgical repair does not influence success rate. A multivariate analysis of factors influencing surgical outcomes. *HPB (Oxford)* 2009;**11(6)**:516–22.

55. Rystedt JML, Kleeff J, Salvia R, Besselink MG, Prasad R, Lesurtel M, et al. Post cholecystectomy bile duct injury: Early, intermediate or late repair with hepaticojejunostomy – an E-AHPBA multi-center study. *HPB (Oxford)* 2019;**21(12)**:1641–7.

56. L S, Lw W. Bile duct injuries during laparoscopic cholecystectomy. Factors that influence the results of treatment. *Arch Surg* 1995;**130(10)**:1123–8.

57. Carroll BJ, Birth M, Phillips EH. Common bile duct injuries during laparoscopic cholecystectomy that result in litigation. *Surg Endosc* 1998;**12(4)**:310–4.

58. Jonas, E. 2020 Iatrogenic bile duct injury. Available from: https://eahpba.org/education-and-training/webinars/. Online training from E-AHPBA (Accessed 29 August 2024)

59. Thompson CM, Saad NE, Quazi RR, Darcy MD, Picus DD, Menias CO. Management of iatrogenic bile duct injuries: Role of the interventional radiologist. *RadioGraphics* 2013;**33(1)**:117–34.

60. Nawaz H, Papachristou GI. Endoscopic treatment for post-cholecystectomy bile leaks: update and recent advances. *Ann Gastroenterol* 2011;**24(3)**:161–3.

61. Kim KH, Kim TN. Endoscopic management of bile leakage after cholecystectomy: A single-center experience for 12 Years. *Clin Endosc* 2014;**47(3)**:248–53.

62. Brady PG, Taunk P. Endoscopic treatment of biliary leaks after laparoscopic cholecystectomy: Cut or plug? *Dig Dis Sci* 2018;**63(2)**:273–4.

63. Jablonska B, Lampe P, Olakowski M, Górka Z, Lekstan A, Gruszka T. Hepaticojejunostomy vs. end-to-end biliary reconstructions in the treatment of iatrogenic bile duct injuries. *J Gastrointest Surg* 2009;**13(6)**:1084–93.

64. de Reuver PR, Busch ORC, Rauws EA, Lameris JS, van Gulik ThM, Gouma DJ. Long-term results of a primary end-to-end anastomosis in peroperative detected bile duct injury. *J Gastrointest Surg* 2007;**11(3)**:296–302.

65. Karanikas M, Bozali F, Vamvakerou V, Markou M, Chasan ZTM, Efraimidou E, et al. Biliary tract injuries after lap cholecystectomy—types, surgical intervention and timing. *Ann Transl Med* 2016;4(9):163.

66. Mercado MA, Domínguez I. Classification and management of bile duct injuries. *World J Gastrointest Surg* 2011;**3(4)**:43–8.

67. Mathisen O, Søreide O, Bergan A. Laparoscopic cholecystectomy: Bile duct and vascular injuries: management and outcome. *Scand J Gastroenterol* 2002;**37(4)**:476–81.

68. Tzovaras G, Dervenis C. Vascular injuries in laparoscopic cholecystectomy: An underestimated problem. *Dig Surg* 2006;**23(5–6)**:370–4.

69. Alves A, Farges O, Nicolet J, Watrin T, Sauvanet A, Belghiti J. Incidence and consequence of an hepatic artery injury in patients with postcholecystectomy bile duct strictures. *Ann Surg* 2003;**238(1)**:93–6.

70. Winslow ER, Fialkowski EA, Linehan DC, Hawkins WG, Picus DD, Strasberg SM. 'Sideways': results of repair of biliary injuries using a policy of side-to-side hepaticojejunostomy. *Ann Surg* 2009;**249(3)**:426–34.

71. Strasberg SM, Gouma DJ. 'Extreme' vasculobiliary injuries: Association with fundus-down cholecystectomy in severely inflamed gallbladders. *HPB (Oxford)* 2012;**14(1)**:1–8.

72. Barbier L, Souche R, Slim K, Ah-Soune P. Long term consequences of bile duct injury after cholecystectomy. *J Visc Surg* 2014;**151(4)**:269–79.

73. Negi SS, Sakhuja P, Malhotra V, Chaudhary A. Factors predicting advanced hepatic fibrosis in patients with postcholecystectomy bile duct strictures. *Arch Surg* 2004;**139(3)**:299–303.

74. Chapman WC, Halevy A, Blumgart LH, Benjamin IS. Postcholecystectomy bile duct strictures: Management and outcome in 130 Patients. *Arch Surg* 1995;**130(6)**:597–604.

75. Ardiles V, McCormack L, Quiñonez E, Goldaracena N, Mattera J, Pekolj J, et al. Experience using liver transplantation for the treatment of severe bile duct injuries over 20 years in Argentina: Results from a National Survey. *HPB (Oxford)* 2011;**13(8)**:544–50.

76. de Santibañes E, Ardiles V, Gadano A, Palavecino M, Pekolj J, Ciardullo M. Liver transplantation: The last measure in the treatment of bile duct injuries. *World J Surg* 2008;**32(8)**:1714–21.

77. Pitt HA, Sherman S, Johnson MS, Hollenbeck AN, Lee J, Daum MR, et al. Improved outcomes of bile duct injuries in the 21st century. *Ann Surg* 2013;**258(3)**:490–9.

78. Lillemoe KD, Melton GB, Cameron JL, Pitt HA, Campbell KA, Talamini MA, et al. Postoperative bile duct strictures: Management and outcome in the 1990s. *Ann Surg* 2000;**232(3)**:430–41.

79. de Santibañes E, Palavecino M, Ardiles V, Pekolj J. Bile duct injuries: Management of late complications. *Surg Endosc* 2006;**20(11)**:1648–53.

80. Sicklick JK, Camp MS, Lillemoe KD, Melton GB, Yeo CJ, Campbell KA, et al. Surgical management of bile duct injuries sustained during laparoscopic cholecystectomy: perioperative results in 200 patients. *Ann Surg* 2005;**241(5)**:786–92.

81. Abdel Rafee A, El-Shobari M, Askar W, Sultan AM, El Nakeeb A. Long-term follow-up of 120 patients after hepaticojejunostomy for treatment of post-cholecystectomy bile duct injuries: A retrospective cohort study. *Int J Surg* 2015;**18**:205–10.

82. Pellegrini CA, Thomas MJ, Way LW. Recurrent biliary stricture: Patterns of recurrence and outcome of surgical therapy. *Am J Surg* 1984;**147(1)**:175–80.

83. Pitt HA, Miyamoto T, Parapatis SK, Tompkins RK, Longmire WP. Factors influencing outcome in patients with postoperative biliary strictures. *Am J Surg* 1982;**144(1)**:14–21.

84. Bang Y, Patil S, Singh J, Rabella P, Rao GV. Percutaneous biliary balloon dilatation and sequential upsizing of silastic transanastomotic stents for benign hepaticojejunostomy strictures: Long-term results. *HPB (Oxford)* 2018;**20**:S747.

85. Azeemuddin M, Turab N, Chaudhry MBH, Hamid S, Hasan M, Sayani R. Percutaneous Management of Biliary Enteric Anastomotic Strictures: An Institutional Review. *Cureus* 2018;**10(2)**: e2228.

86. Vaz OP, Al-Islam S, Khan ZA, Wilde N, Lowe B, Magilton A, et al. Bio-degradable stents: Primary experience in a tertiary hepatopancreaticobiliary center in the United Kingdom. *Cureus* 2021;**13(10)**:e19075.

87. Dominguez-Rosado I, Mercado MA, Kauffma C, Ramirez-del Val F, Elnecavé-Olaiz A, Zamora-Valdés D. Quality of life in bile duct injury: 1-, 5-, and 10-year outcomes after surgical repair. *J Gastrointest Surg* 2014;**18(12)**:2089–94.

88. Boerma D, Rauws EAJ, Keulemans YCA, Bergman JJGHM, Obertop H, Huibregtse K, et al. Impaired quality of life 5 Years after bile duct injury during laparoscopic cholecystectomy. *Ann Surg* 2001;**234(6)**:750–7.

Chapter
63
Management of Bile Leaks and Fistulae

Major Kenneth Lee and Charles M. Vollmer Jr.

INTRODUCTION

Iatrogenic injury to the biliary tree can complicate all aspects of hepato-pancreato-biliary (HPB) surgery and is a major source of postoperative morbidity. Due to the prevalence of gallstone disease, it is most commonly discussed as a complication of cholecystectomy. In these cases, it is almost always localized to the major bile duct, sectoral ducts, or subvesical ducts in close proximity to the cystic plate. It is the single most consequential complication as it typically requires invasive management that can result in prolonged hospitalization. Bile leak is also arguably the most significant issue following hepatectomy. It is less dramatic than liver failure but occurs more commonly and has more management considerations due to the inevitable complexity. Post-pancreatectomy bile leak is less well evaluated and nearly always reflects anastomotic failure at the hepaticojejunostomy. This chapter summarizes the aetiology and management of bile leak after hepatopancreatobiliary surgery excepting major bile duct injury following cholecystectomy which is covered in **Chapter 62**.

POST-CHOLECYSTECTOMY BILE LEAK

Aetiology

Cholecystectomy remains the most commonly performed general surgery procedure. Approximately 700 000 to 1 million cholecystectomies are performed annually in the United States. Bile leak occurs after 0.3–4% of cholecystectomies and remains the most significant source of morbidity (1–13). The majority of bile leaks following laparoscopic cholecystectomy are from two sources: 1) The cystic duct stump and small subvesical, non-essential ducts extending from the cystic plate to the gallbladder; 2) the ducts of Luschka named after the German anatomist Hubert von Luschka (1820–1875) who described the first case in 1863. Several classification systems have been developed to describe iatrogenic biliary injuries including the Bismuth, Strasberg/Washington University, Stewart and Way, McMahon, Neuhaus, and Hanover classifications (14–19). The Strasberg/Washington University classification is perhaps the most comprehensive and well known (15). It describes five anatomical patterns of bile leak and bile duct injury post-cholecystectomy

(Types A–E; *Figure 63.1*). Type A injuries are bile leaks from the cystic duct stump or ducts of Luschka. Types B and C are injuries to the right duct with occlusion (Type B) or a leak (Type C). Type D injuries involve a leak from the main bile duct involving less than 50% of its circumference. Type E injuries involve circumferential transection or stricture of the main bile duct occurring various distances from the biliary confluence, with Type E_5 being the most complex injuries and involving an injury to the common hepatic/bile duct as well as an injury to a separate right sectoral duct. Type A injuries are most common comprising approximately 85% percent of significant bile leaks. The majority are from the cystic duct stump while approximately 10–25% are from ducts of Luschka (8,15,20,21).

Many contemporary series reporting on bile leak after cholecystectomy have focused on the specific technique of subtotal cholecystectomy. Subtotal cholecystectomy involves removal of a portion of the gallbladder and has been increasingly utilized as a 'bail out' strategy in cholecystectomy (22) and it is particularly prone to bile leakage. Techniques for subtotal cholecystectomy have been broadly classified as 'fenestrating' or 'reconstituting' depending on whether the gallbladder remnant is left open or is closed (23). Fenestrating subtotal cholecystectomy is associated with the highest incidence of bile leakage (over 30%) due to the inability to secure the cystic duct orifice. Though the vast majority of these leaks are minor rather than major bile duct injuries, there may be an increase in the incidence of bile leaks as these procedures become more commonplace.

Endoscopic management

Approximately 85% of bile leaks are relatively minor with preservation of biliary-enteric continuity. These can present as small collections in the gallbladder fossa postoperatively or as bilious effluent from a surgical or percutaneous drain. In these cases, conservative management can result in self-resolution without any invasive intervention. However, management with endoscopic retrograde cholangiopancreatography (ERCP) has become first-line therapy for minor bile leaks with high rates of success (5,24). The principle underlying endoscopic therapy is elimination of the transpapillary pressure gradient maintained by the sphincter of Oddi. This promotes preferential

DOI: 10.1201/9781003080060-63

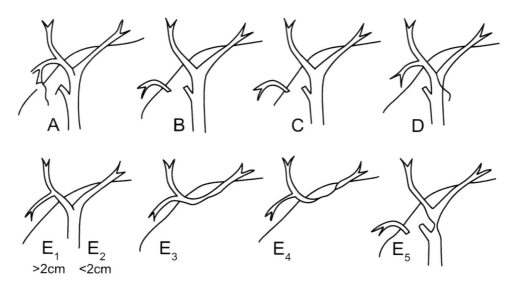

Figure 63.1 Strasberg/Washington University classification of bile duct injuries. Type **(A)** injuries originate from the cystic duct or from small bile ducts in proximity to the cystic plate. Types **(B)** and **(C)** injuries involve division of a typically aberrant right hepatic duct with or without occlusion. Type **(D)** injuries are lateral injuries to the extrahepatic bile duct without complete transection. Types **(E$_1$-E$_5$)** injuries involve circumferential injury to the major bile duct at varying levels.

drainage of bile into the duodenum and away from the site of bile leakage to facilitate resolution. This can be achieved with either sphincterotomy or transpapillary stent placement (1,25–28). Endoscopic management also provides an opportunity to eliminate any obstructive issue such as retained stones. Success rates of endoscopic therapy for minor bile leaks exceed 90% with no reported failures in some series (1,4,25).

Several controversies exist in endoscopic management of bile leaks. The initial consideration in these instances is whether invasive intervention is mandated. Deciding on the timing at which to consider endoscopic therapy can be difficult and large series suggest that the success rate and adverse event rate with endoscopic therapy are similar whether these procedures are performed 'emergently,' 'urgently,' or 'expectantly' (29–31). In these studies, the expectant group refers to patients treated any more than 3 days after recognition of a bile leak. This is a relatively early time point in the course of some patients especially after complex cholecystectomies. There are few studies examining the outcome of prolonged observation due to the availability and efficacy of endoscopic therapy. It has been suggested that bile leaks totalling <200 mL/day which downtrend quickly will likely resolve without intervention, but that is not an algorithm which is often followed (3).

Once endoscopic therapy is chosen, the method of biliary decompression is the next consideration. Sphincterotomy alone and transpapillary stenting are the options. Early studies suggested that endoscopic sphincterotomy may have higher healing rates than biliary stenting (9,32,33). However, endoscopic

sphincterotomy as a sole modality can require lengthy sphincterotomies associated with increased rates of complications including bleeding, pancreatitis, perforation, and cholangitis (25). For these reasons, many prefer transpapillary stenting. Stents are generally left in place for 4–6 weeks at which point a repeat ERCP can be performed to evaluate the bile leak or the stent can be removed with standard oesophagogastroduodenoscopy.

A third uncertainty regards the management of refractory leaks that fail initial endoscopic therapy. Transpapillary stenting will often successfully rescue patients treated with sphincterotomy alone (34), but the management of patients that fail stent placement is less clear. Placement of multiple plastic stents or fully covered metal stents are both options (24,35). Fully covered metal stents are associated with stent migration and stent occlusion (36,37) but have very high efficacy rates and do appear to be more effective at resolving refractory leaks than plastic stents (35,38) (*Figure 63.2*). Fully covered metal stents have shown efficacy rates between 90% and 100% in the management of refractory leaks (36,37,39–42).

The role of interventional radiology

The role for interventional radiology in resolution of post-cholecystectomy bile leaks is relatively minimal. Though percutaneous drainage is frequently needed to prevent sepsis, therapeutic measures used to resolve the leak are uncommon. Small case series have reported successful coil embolization of cystic duct stumps through established percutaneous tracts several

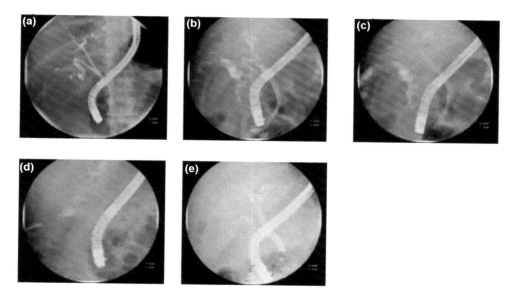

Figure 63.2 Endoscopic resolution of bile leak. This figure demonstrates a bile leak after a subtotal cholecystec-tomy (a) that was initially treated with up to three endoscopic plastic stents (b, c). These failed to resolve the leak which was then treated with a covered metal stent (d). This ultimately resolved the leak (e).

weeks after drain placement (43, 44). This technique has generally been limited to unique and refractory circumstances.

Percutaneous strategies are more commonly required in cases of aberrant anatomy such as Roux-en-Y gastric bypass patients where endoscopic therapy is technically challenging. In this setting, percutaneous access to the intrahepatic ducts allows for placement of internal-external catheters that promote flow across the site of leakage. Endoscopic therapy is preferred over percutaneous routes for a number of reasons including the need for an external catheter in the latter approach. The morbidity of percutaneous drainage has also historically been greater with major complications including: 1) Bleeding (haemobilia, haemoperitoneum, subcapsular liver haematoma); 2) sepsis; 3) cholangitis; 4) bile leak, and 5) pleural complications (45). The average rates of major complications in percutaneous biliary drainage have declined and are now relatively low (46).

Surgical management

Because of the efficacy of endoscopic therapy, surgery is rarely required to resolve bile leaks that do not involve major bile duct transection which are covered elsewhere (**Chapter 62**). However, bile leaks are often unrecognized, and patients can present with diffuse collections and bile peritonitis and surgery can be required in these cases. The primary goal of these procedures is to irrigate bile and control the leak with wide drainage. Depending on the timing and site, the porta hepatis can be explored and minor leaks may be able to be

secured surgically. Historical series reported early in the laparoscopic cholecystectomy experience have detailed surgical correction of cystic duct leaks primarily through open operative approaches (11,47,48). The morbidity of an open exploration for this purpose is now somewhat difficult to justify.

POST-HEPATECTOMY BILE LEAK

Aetiology

Though bile leaks due to cholecystectomy are far more prevalent, those that occur after liver resection are typically associated with greater morbidity (49). Initial reports on post-hepatectomy bile leak suffered from inconsistencies in definition and terminology. Post-hepatectomy bile leak has now been formally defined by the International Study Group for Liver Surgery (ISGLS) (50) (*Table 63.1*). It is defined as discharge of fluid with an elevated bilirubin level in the abdomen or in an abdominal drain on or after postoperative day 3. A grading system of severity was used to stratify clinical relevance of the leak. Grade A leaks require little change in patient management, Grade B leaks are prolonged or require a change in management but without re-laparotomy, and Grade C leaks require re-laparotomy. Multiple factors probably contribute to the development of post-hepatectomy bile leaks. Unrecognized transected ducts from the surgical procedure are frequent culprits. Biliary stones or strictures can increase intraductal pressure and facilitate leaks, and there is also the suggestion that elevated sphincter of Oddi tone after hepatectomy can contribute (51,52).

Table 63.1 ISGLS definition and severity grading for bile leakage (50)

Definition of bile leakage	Bile leakage is defined as fluid with an increased bilirubin concentration (>3 times serum concentration measured at the same time) in an abdominal drain or intra-abdominal fluid on, or after, postoperative day 3 or the need for radiologic/surgical intervention (i.e. interventional drainage) because of biliary collections
Severity grading	**Details**
Grade A	Bile leakage requiring no, or little, change in patients' clinical management
Grade B	Bile leakage requiring a change in the patient's clinical management but manageable without re-laparotomy or Grade A bile leakage lasting for >1 week
Grade C	Bile leakage requiring re-laparotomy

Leaks can arise from various sites including the cut edge of the liver, the cystic duct stump, or sectoral/major bile ducts.

The incidence of bile leakage after hepatic resection is 3.6–12% (53–61). An American College of Surgeons (ACS) National Surgical Quality Improvement Program (NSQIP) study included 6859 patients and reported a bile leak incidence of 7.7% using ISGLS criteria (53). Grade A leaks were most common (52.5%), followed by Grade B leaks (38.5%) with Grade C leaks being the least frequent (9.1%). Studies have identified various risk factors that may be associated with increased rates of bile leakage. These include: 1) The extent of resection; 2) operative approach; 3) post-resection cholangiograms, and 4) vessel sealing strategies (55,62,63). In the aforementioned ACS-NSQIP study the following were all significantly associated with postoperative bile leak: 1) Major hepatectomy; 2) malignant indication; 3) neoadjuvant therapy; 4) longer operative time; 5) concomitant biliary-enteric reconstruction; 6) preoperative biliary stenting and 7) the presence of a surgical drain Other reports have suggested increased bile leak rates with particular procedures including left hepatectomy (64) or central hepatectomies which create broad transection planes with large raw surfaces and approach the hepatic hilum (54,65,66). Various risk mitigation strategies have been employed to prevent post-hepatectomy bile leaks including nasobiliary drainage, sealants, and completion cholangiograms (54,59,67) although no single strategy has become universal.

Endoscopic management

The threshold for invasive management of post-procedural bile leaks is much higher in hepatectomy than cholecystectomy and conservative management is far more common (54,56,66,68,69). Approximately 75% of bile leaks after hepatectomy will resolve without an invasive intervention (54,56,66,69,70). Several factors can predict the likelihood of a prolonged bile leak. Most consistently referenced is the site of the leak, with those from central/hilar structures or from peripheral but excluded ducts less likely to resolve spontaneously (54,64,66).

Endoscopic therapy remains the standard approach in patients with persistent bile leakage after hepatic resection without biliary-enteric reconstruction. The success rate of endoscopic management in liver resection appears to be inferior to that seen in cholecystectomy. Larger series suggest that resolution of bile leaks occur approximately 75% of the time (65,71,72) though rates as high as 95–100% have been reported (51,73). Multiple procedures are often required (72) and in virtually all series, endoscopic stent placement was preferred over sphincterotomy alone (51,71–74).

The site of bile leakage affects both the endoscopic strategy and outcome. Peripheral leaks are difficult to access and are typically treated with transpapillary stenting. By contrast, attempts are made to reach more central leaks and to cover the leak site with endoprostheses (72,73). There is a suggestion that therapeutic success rates may be higher in cases where bridging stents are successfully deployed (71). It seems clear that the site of a leak influences the likelihood of endoscopic success, but the specifics have been somewhat inconsistently described. Some series suggest that smaller, peripheral bile leaks are more likely to resolve (51,65,72) while in one large series, these peripheral leaks responded far less often (71).

The role of interventional radiology and surgery

Post-hepatectomy bile leakage frequently requires percutaneous drainage to prevent sepsis, but percutaneous techniques are rarely employed as active measures in resolving leaks. As noted earlier, aberrant anatomy in which ERCP is not feasible can mandate percutaneous biliary drainage. Mosconi et al. reported a 79% resolution of bile leaks with percutaneous transhepatic management, although multiple percutaneous treatments were required in 54% of patients (75). Success rates were relatively poor in liver transplant patients and more complex percutaneous strategies are limited to case reports and small series. There are several reports of ethanol ablation for the treatment of peripheral bile leaks (65,76–81). Ethanol ablation involves injection of absolute ethanol through surgical drains or percutaneous catheters. These procedures are to be considered carefully and require ERCP or fistulography, as communication of the leak with the biliary tree can result in irreversible damage to the bile ducts. Percutaneous transhepatic portal vein embolization has also been described in case reports but is not widely used (82).

Surgery is rarely the treatment of choice for post-hepatectomy bile leaks. It is typically employed in situations where endoscopic therapy is not feasible, or has failed, and often in patients whose clinical scenario is complicated by abdominal sepsis. Procedures typically involve wide drainage for control of intra-abdominal sepsis as well as suture closure of the bile leak site when feasible. Relatively high rates of mortality have historically been noted in patients that undergo surgery after failed endoscopic therapy (71,72).

POST-PANCREATECTOMY BILE LEAK

Excluding anomalous events, bile leaks in pancreatic resection result from anastomotic leakage at the hepaticojejunostomy site after pancreatoduodenectomy. Though terminology has been problematic, the previously presented ISGLS criteria provide standard definitions that can promote consistency (50). The reported incidence of bile leak following pancreatoduodenectomy is 2–8% (83–92). Technical factors are likely to be the dominant issue and bile duct ischaemia may contribute. Potential risk factors include: 1) Older age; 2) obesity; 3) prior ERCP; 4) preoperative chemotherapy; 5) longer operative time; 6) pancreatic fistula; 7) small calibre bile duct; 8) malnutrition, and 9) sepsis (84,85,88–90,93). There are accumulating studies evaluating the effects of a minimally invasive approach to bile leaks and other complications, but there is little high-quality evidence due to a lack of randomized controlled trials (94–96). A particularly notable risk factor is pancreatic fistula, as the combination of bile leak and pancreatic leak is associated with significant risk of mortality that approaches 35% (85,86,89,97).

Prior to 2012, there was a single study from Japan characterizing hepaticojejunostomy leaks (91). Several studies have since been published, but there are differing conclusions regarding the management of this issue. In contrast to cholecystectomy and hepatectomy, endoscopic approaches in this setting are unusual given the concern for worsened anastomotic disruption. There are essentially three management options:

1 Asymptomatic, lower-volume leaks controlled with surgical drains are typically managed conservatively and generally resolve (85–88)
2 Higher output leaks that are difficult to control can be treated with either percutaneous biliary drainage or re-exploration
3 Percutaneous biliary drainage tubes can often be placed across the anastomosis to control the leak and facilitate anastomotic healing (*Figure 63.3*) (89,92)

The principal goal in re-exploration is to control the leak and resolve biliary sepsis with wide drainage. Various revisional strategies have been reported including revision of the hepaticojejunostomy and placement of 'T tubes' (84,86). Whether to proceed with percutaneous transhepatic drainage or re-exploration depends upon many factors including timing, patient stability, extent of disruption, and whether there is a concomitant pancreatic fistula.

SUMMARY

Iatrogenic injury to the biliary tree can complicate all aspects of hepatopancreatobiliary surgery and is a major source of postoperative morbidity. It promotes sepsis, prolongs hospitalization, increases cost, and typically results in invasive procedures that carry risk. Bile leaks occurring after cholecystectomy typically originate from the cystic duct stump or from subvesical ducts of Luschka and qualify as minor. Those that occur after hepatectomy can occur from multiple sites

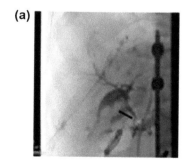
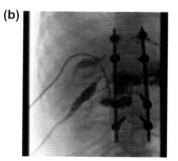

Figure 63.3 Percutaneous biliary drainage for treatment of a hepaticojejunostomy leak. This patient developed high output bilious drainage from a percutaneous drain 2 weeks after a pancreatoduodenectomy. A percutaneous cholangiogram demonstrated a leak (black line) from the hepaticojejunostomy (a). This was treated with a percutaneous transhepatic catheter placed across the anastomosis, as seen in (b).

in the biliary tree. Endoscopic therapy is the primary treatment modality for post-cholecystectomy and post-hepatectomy bile leaks. It is highly effective after cholecystectomy, and repeated endoscopic attempts are generally made even in cases of initial failure. While less reliable after hepatectomy, endoscopic management remains the principal strategy and is typically successful. Following cholecystectomy or hepatectomy, interventional radiology is often necessary to prevent sepsis due to bile leaks but has a more limited therapeutic role otherwise. There is a role for percutaneous transhepatic drains in post-pancreatectomy bile leaks. These drains can decompress the biliary tree and promote healing of an anastomotic disruption. Surgical management was previously a mainstay in the management of post-procedural bile leaks but is now largely restricted to situations with uncontrolled sepsis. Attempts can be made at securing the site of leakage but are often unsatisfactory.

REFERENCES

1. Kaffes AJ, Hourigan L, De Luca N, Byth K, Williams SJ, Bourke MJ. Impact of endoscopic intervention in 100 patients with suspected postcholecystectomy bile leak. *Gastrointest Endosc* 2005;**61(2)**:269–75.
2. Agarwal N, Sharma BC, Garg S, Kumar R, Sarin SK. Endoscopic management of postoperative bile leaks. *Hepatobiliary Pancreat Dis Int* 2006;**5(2)**:273–7.
3. Ahmad F, Saunders RN, Lloyd GM, Lloyd DM, Robertson GS. An algorithm for the management of bile leak following laparoscopic cholecystectomy. *Ann R Coll Surg Engl* 2007;**89(1)**:51–6.
4. Sandha GS, Bourke MJ, Haber GB, Kortan PP. Endoscopic therapy for bile leak based on a new classification: Results in 207 patients. *Gastrointest Endosc* 2004;**60(4)**:567–74.
5. Kim KH, Kim TN. Endoscopic management of bile leakage after cholecystectomy: A single-center experience for 12 years. *Clin Endosc* 2014;**47(3)**:248–53.
6. Binmoeller KF, Katon RM, Shneidman R. Endoscopic management of postoperative biliary leaks: Review of 77 cases and report of two cases with biloma formation. *Am J Gastroenterol* 1991;**86(2)**:227–31.
7. Bjorkman DJ, Carr-Locke DL, Lichtenstein DR, Ferrari AP, Slivka A, Van Dam J, et al. Postsurgical bile leaks: Endoscopic obliteration of the transpapillary pressure gradient is enough. *Am J Gastroenterol* 1995;**90(12)**:2128–33.
8. Barkun AN, Rezieg M, Mehta SN, Pavone E, Landry S, Barkun JS, et al. Postcholecystectomy biliary leaks in the laparoscopic era: Risk factors, presentation, and management. McGill Gallstone Treatment Group. *Gastrointest Endosc* 1997;**45(3)**:277–82.
9. Davids PH, Rauws EA, Tytgat GN, Huibregtse K. Postoperative bile leakage: Endoscopic management. *Gut* 1992;**33(8)**:1118–22.
10. Misra M, Schif J, Rendon G, Rothschild J, Schwaitzberg S. Laparoscopic cholecystectomy after the

11. Wills VL, Jorgensen JO, Hunt DR. Role of relaparoscopy in the management of minor bile leakage after laparoscopic cholecystectomy. *Br J Surg* 2000;**87(2)**:176–80.
12. Braghetto I, Bastias J, Csendes A, Debandi A. Intraperitoneal bile collections after laparoscopic cholecystectomy: Causes, clinical presentation, diagnosis, and treatment. *Surg Endosc* 2000;**14(11)**:1037–41.
13. Lien HH, Huang CS, Shi MY, Chen DF, Wang NY, Tai FC, et al. Management of bile leakage after laparoscopic cholecystectomy based on etiological classification. *Surg Today* 2004;**34(4)**:326–30.
14. Bismuth H, Majno PE. Biliary strictures: Classification based on the principles of surgical treatment. *World J Surg* 2001;**25(10)**:1241–4.
15. Strasberg SM, Hertl M, Soper NJ. An analysis of the problem of biliary injury during laparoscopic cholecystectomy. *J Am Coll Surg* 1995;**180(1)**: 101–25.
16. Stewart L, Way LW. Bile duct injuries during laparoscopic cholecystectomy. Factors that influence the results of treatment. *Arch Surg* 1995;**130(10)**: 1123–8.
17. McMahon AJ, Fullarton G, Baxter JN, O'Dwyer PJ. Bile duct injury and bile leakage in laparoscopic cholecystectomy. *Br J Surg* 1995;**82(3)**:307–13.
18. Schmidt SC, Settmacher U, Langrehr JM, Neuhaus P. Management and outcome of patients with combined bile duct and hepatic arterial injuries after laparoscopic cholecystectomy. *Surgery* 2004;**135(6)**: 613–8.
19. Bektas H, Schrem H, Winny M, Klempnauer J. Surgical treatment and outcome of iatrogenic bile duct lesions after cholecystectomy and the impact of different clinical classification systems. *Br J Surg* 2007;**94(9)**:1119–27.
20. Schnelldorfer T, Sarr MG, Adams DB. What is the duct of Luschka? A systematic review. *J Gastrointest Surg* 2012;**16(3)**:656–62.
21. Ryan ME, Geenen JE, Lehman GA, Aliperti G, Freeman ML, Silverman WB, et al. Endoscopic intervention for biliary leaks after laparoscopic cholecystectomy: A multicenter review. *Gastrointest Endosc* 1998;**47(3)**:261–6.
22. Sabour AF, Matsushima K, Love BE, Alicuben ET, Schellenberg MA, Inaba K, et al. Nationwide trends in the use of subtotal cholecystectomy for acute cholecystitis. *Surgery* 2020;**167(3)**:569–74.
23. Strasberg SM, Pucci MJ, Brunt LM, Deziel DJ. Subtotal cholecystectomy-'Fenestrating' vs 'Reconstituting' subtypes and the prevention of bile duct injury: Definition of the optimal procedure in difficult operative conditions. *J Am Coll Surg* 2016;**222(1)**:89–96.
24. Ahmad DS, Faulx A. Management of postcholecystectomy biliary complications: A narrative review. *Am J Gastroenterol* 2020;**115(8)**:1191–8.
25. Rainio M, Lindstrom O, Udd M, Haapamaki C, Nordin A, Kylanpaa L. Endoscopic therapy biliary injury after cholecystectomy. *Dig Dis Sci* 2018;**63(2)**:474–80.
26. Mavrogiannis C, Liatsos C, Papanikolaou IS, Karagiannis S, Galanis P, Romanos A. Biliary stenting alone versus biliary stenting plus sphincterotomy for

the treatment of post-laparoscopic cholecystectomy biliary leaks: A prospective randomized study. *Eur J Gastroenterol Hepatol* 2006;**18(4)**:405–9.

27. Tewani SK, Turner BG, Chuttani R, Pleskow DK, Sawhney MS. Location of bile leak predicts the success of ERCP performed for postoperative bile leaks. *Gastrointest Endosc* 2013;**77(4)**:601–8.

28. Llach J, Bordas JM, Elizalde JI, Enrico C, Gines A, Pellise M, et al. Sphincterotomy in the treatment of biliary leakage. *Hepatogastroenterology* 2002;**49(48)**:1496–8.

29. Abbas A, Sethi S, Brady P, Taunk P. Endoscopic management of postcholecystectomy biliary leak: When and how? A nationwide study. *Gastrointest Endosc* 2019;**90(2)**:233–41 e1.

30. Coelho-Prabhu N, Baron TH. Assessment of need for repeat ERCP during biliary stent removal after clinical resolution of postcholecystectomy bile leak. *Am J Gastroenterol* 2010;**105(1)**:100–5.

31. Adler DG, Papachristou GI, Taylor LJ, McVay T, Birch M, Francis G, et al. Clinical outcomes in patients with bile leaks treated via ERCP with regard to the timing of ERCP: A large multicenter study. *Gastrointest Endosc* 2017;**85(4)**:766–72.

32. Del Olmo L, Merono E, Moreira VF, Garcia T, Garcia-Plaza A. Successful treatment of postoperative external biliary fistulas by endoscopic sphincterotomy. *Gastrointest Endosc* 1988;**34(4)**:307–9.

33. Libby ED, Branch MS, Cotton PB. Cystic duct leak after laparoscopic cholecystectomy despite preoperative sphincterotomy. *Gastrointest Endosc* 1995;**41(5)**:511–4.

34. Brady PG, Taunk P. Endoscopic treatment of biliary leaks after laparoscopic cholecystectomy: Cut or plug? *Dig Dis Sci* 2018;**63(2)**:273–4.

35. Canena J, Horta D, Coimbra J, Meireles L, Russo P, Marques I, et al. Outcomes of endoscopic management of primary and refractory postcholecystectomy biliary leaks in a multicentre review of 178 patients. *BMC Gastroenterol* 2015;**15**:105.

36. Lalezari D, Singh I, Reicher S, Eysselein VE. Evaluation of fully covered self-expanding metal stents in benign biliary strictures and bile leaks. *World J Gastrointest Endosc* 2013;**5(7)**:332–9.

37. Wang AY, Ellen K, Berg CL, Schmitt TM, Kahaleh M. Fully covered self-expandable metallic stents in the management of complex biliary leaks: Preliminary data: A case series. *Endoscopy* 2009;**41(9)**:781–6.

38. Canena J, Liberato M, Meireles L, Marques I, Romao C, Coutinho AP, et al. A non-randomized study in consecutive patients with postcholecystectomy refractory biliary leaks who were managed endoscopically with the use of multiple plastic stents or fully covered self-expandable metal stents (with videos). *Gastrointest Endosc* 2015;**82(1)**:70–8.

39. Baron TH. Covered self-expandable metal stents for benign biliary tract diseases. *Curr Opin Gastroenterol* 2011;**27(3)**:262–7.

40. Canena J, Liberato M, Horta D, Romao C, Coutinho A. Short-term stenting using fully covered self-expandable metal stents for treatment of refractory

biliary leaks, postsphincterotomy bleeding, and perforations. *Surg Endosc* 2013;**27(1)**:313–24.

41. Akbar A, Irani S, Baron TH, Topazian M, Petersen BT, Gostout CJ, et al. Use of covered self-expandable metal stents for endoscopic management of benign biliary disease not related to stricture (with video). *Gastrointest Endosc* 2012;**76(1)**:196–201.

42. Pausawasadi N, Soontornmanokul T, Rerknimitr R. Role of fully covered self-expandable metal stent for treatment of benign biliary strictures and bile leaks. *Korean J Radiol* 2012;**13(Suppl 1)**:S67–73.

43. Nezami N, Jarmakani H, Arici M, Latich I, Mojibian H, Ayyagari RR, et al. Selective trans-catheter coil embolization of cystic duct stump in post-cholecystectomy bile leak. *Dig Dis Sci* 2019;**64(11)**:3314–20.

44. Rai V, Beckley A, Fabre A, Bellows CF. Successful treatment of persistent postcholecystectomy bile leak using percutaneous cystic duct coiling. *Case Rep Surg* 2015;**2015**:273198.

45. Zhu Y, Hickey R. The role of the interventional radiologist in bile leak diagnosis and management. *Semin Intervent Radiol* 2021;**38(3)**:309–20.

46. Saad WE, Wallace MJ, Wojak JC, Kundu S, Cardella JF. Quality improvement guidelines for percutaneous transhepatic cholangiography, biliary drainage, and percutaneous cholecystostomy. *J Vasc Interv Radiol* 2010;**21(6)**:789–95.

47. Woods MS, Shellito JL, Santoscoy GS, Hagan RC, Kilgore WR, Traverso LW, et al. Cystic duct leaks in laparoscopic cholecystectomy. *Am J Surg* 1994;**168(6)**:560–3; discussion 3–5.

48. Wise Unger S, Glick GL, Landeros M. Cystic duct leak after laparoscopic cholecystectomy. A multi-institutional study. *Surg Endosc* 1996;**10(12)**:1189–93.

49. Guillaud A, Pery C, Campillo B, Lourdais A, Sulpice L, Boudjema K. Incidence and predictive factors of clinically relevant bile leakage in the modern era of liver resections. *HPB (Oxford)* 2013;**15(3)**:224–9.

50. Koch M, Garden OJ, Padbury R, Rahbari NN, Adam R, Capussotti L, et al. Bile leakage after hepatobiliary and pancreatic surgery: A definition and grading of severity by the International Study Group of Liver Surgery. *Surgery* 2011;**149(5)**:680–8.

51. Yun SU, Cheon YK, Shim CS, Lee TY, Yu HM, Chung HA, et al. The outcome of endoscopic management of bile leakage after hepatobiliary surgery. *Korean J Intern Med* 2017;**32(1)**:79–84.

52. Ijichi M, Takayama T, Toyoda H, Sano K, Kubota K, Makuuchi M. Randomized trial of the usefulness of a bile leakage test during hepatic resection. *Arch Surg* 2000;**135(12)**:1395–400.

53. Martin AN, Narayanan S, Turrentine FE, Bauer TW, Adams RB, Stukenborg GJ, et al. Clinical factors and postoperative impact of bile leak after liver resection. *J Gastrointest Surg* 2018;**22(4)**:661–7.

54. Yamashita Y, Hamatsu T, Rikimaru T, Tanaka S, Shirabe K, Shimada M, et al. Bile leakage after hepatic resection. *Ann Surg* 2001;**233(1)**:45–50.

55. Lam CM, Lo CM, Liu CL, Fan ST. Biliary complications during liver resection. *World J Surg* 2001;**25(10)**:1273–6.

56. Capussotti L, Ferrero A, Vigano L, Sgotto E, Muratore A, Polastri R. Bile leakage and liver resection: Where is the risk? *Arch Surg* 2006;**141(7)**:690–4.

57. Ishii H, Ochiai T, Murayama Y, Komatsu S, Shiozaki A, Kuriu Y, et al. Risk factors and management of postoperative bile leakage after hepatectomy without bilioenteric anastomosis. *Dig Surg* 2011;**28(3)**:198–204.

58. Yoshioka R, Saiura A, Koga R, Seki M, Kishi Y, Yamamoto J. Predictive factors for bile leakage after hepatectomy: Analysis of 505 consecutive patients. *World J Surg* 2011;**35(8)**:1898–903.

59. Zimmitti G, Vauthey JN, Shindoh J, Tzeng CW, Roses RE, Ribero D, et al. Systematic use of an intraoperative air leak test at the time of major liver resection reduces the rate of postoperative biliary complications. *J Am Coll Surg* 2013;**217(6)**:1028–37.

60. Brauer DG, Nywening TM, Jaques DP, Doyle MB, Chapman WC, Fields RC, et al. Operative site drainage after hepatectomy: A propensity score matched analysis using the American College of Surgeons NSQIP Targeted Hepatectomy Database. *J Am Coll Surg* 2016;**223(6)**:774–83 e2.

61. Erdogan D, Busch OR, van Delden OM, Rauws EA, Gouma DJ, van Gulik TM. Incidence and management of bile leakage after partial liver resection. *Dig Surg* 2008;**25(1)**:60–6.

62. Alexiou VG, Tsitsias T, Mavros MN, Robertson GS, Pawlik TM. Technology-assisted versus clamp-crush liver resection: A systematic review and meta-analysis. *Surg Innov* 2013;**20(4)**:414–28.

63. Kaibori M, Ishizaki M, Matsui K, Kwon AH. Intraoperative indocyanine green-fluorescent imaging for prevention of bile leakage after hepatic resection. *Surgery* 2011;**150(1)**:91–8.

64. Lo CM, Fan ST, Liu CL, Lai EC, Wong J. Biliary complications after hepatic resection: Risk factors, management, and outcome. *Arch Surg* 1998; **133(2)**:156–61.

65. Sakamoto K, Tamesa T, Yukio T, Tokuhisa Y, Maeda Y, Oka M. Risk factors and managements of bile leakage after hepatectomy. *World J Surg* 2016;**40(1)**:182–9.

66. Nagano Y, Togo S, Tanaka K, Masui H, Endo I, Sekido H, et al. Risk factors and management of bile leakage after hepatic resection. *World J Surg* 2003;**27(6)**:695–8.

67. Kubo S, Sakai K, Kinoshita H, Hirohashi K. Intraoperative cholangiography using a balloon catheter in liver surgery. **World J Surg** 1986;**10(5)**:844–50.

68. Vigano L, Ferrero A, Sgotto E, Tesoriere RL, Calgaro M, Capussotti L. Bile leak after hepatectomy: Predictive factors of spontaneous healing. *Am J Surg* 2008;**196(2)**:195–200.

69. Tanaka S, Hirohashi K, Tanaka H, Shuto T, Lee SH, Kubo S, et al. Incidence and management of bile leakage after hepatic resection for malignant hepatic tumors. *J Am Coll Surg* 2002;**195(4)**:484–9.

70. Imamura H, Seyama Y, Kokudo N, Maema A, Sugawara Y, Sano K, et al. One thousand fifty-six hepatectomies without mortality in 8 years. *Arch Surg* 2003;**138(11)**:1198–206.

71. Schaible A, Schemmer P, Hackert T, Rupp C, Schulze Schleithoff AE, Gotthardt DN, et al. Location of a biliary leak after liver resection determines success of endoscopic treatment. *Surg Endosc* 2017;**31(4)**:1814–20.

72. Dechene A, Jochum C, Fingas C, Paul A, Heider D, Syn WK, et al. Endoscopic management is the treatment of choice for bile leaks after liver resection. *Gastrointest Endosc* 2014;**80(4)**:626–33 e1.

73. Bhattacharjya S, Puleston J, Davidson BR, Dooley JS. Outcome of early endoscopic biliary drainage in the management of bile leaks after hepatic resection. *Gastrointest Endosc* 2003;**57(4)**:526–30.

74. Lau JY, Leung KL, Chung SC, Lau WY. Endoscopic management of major bile leaks complicating hepatic resections for hepatocellular carcinoma. *Gastrointest Endosc* 1999;**50(1)**:99–101.

75. Mosconi C, Calandri M, Mirarchi M, Vara G, Breatta AD, Cappelli A, et al. Percutaneous management of postoperative bile leak after hepato-pancreato-biliary surgery: A multi-center experience. *HPB (Oxford)* 2021;**23(10)**:1518–24.

76. Kyokane T, Nagino M, Sano T, Nimura Y. Ethanol ablation for segmental bile duct leakage after hepatobiliary resection. *Surgery* 2002;**131(1)**:111–3.

77. Matsumoto T, Iwaki K, Hagino Y, Kawano K, Kitano S, Tomonari K, et al. Ethanol injection therapy of an isolated bile duct associated with a biliary-cutaneous fistula. *J Gastroenterol Hepatol* 2002;**17(7)**:807–10.

78. Shimizu T, Yoshida H, Mamada Y, Taniai N, Matsumoto S, Mizuguchi Y, et al. Postoperative bile leakage managed successfully by intrahepatic biliary ablation with ethanol. *World J Gastroenterol* 2006;**12(21)**:3450–2.

79. Kataoka M, Ooeda Y, Yoshioka S, Wakatsuki K, Tonooka T, Kawamoto J, et al. Percutaneous transhepatic ethanol ablation for postoperative bile leakage after a hepatectomy. *Hepatogastroenterology* 2011;**58(107–108)**:988–91.

80. Sakaguchi T, Shibasaki Y, Morita Y, Oishi K, Suzuki A, Fukumoto K, et al. Postoperative bile leakage managed by interventional intrabiliary ethanol ablation. *Hepatogastroenterology* 2011;**58(105)**:157–60.

81. Ito A, Ebata T, Yokoyama Y, Igami T, Mizuno T, Yamaguchi J, et al. Ethanol ablation for refractory bile leakage after complex hepatectomy. *Br J Surg* 2018;**105(8)**:1036–43.

82. Kubo N, Shirabe K. Treatment strategy for isolated bile leakage after hepatectomy: Literature review. *Ann Gastroenterol Surg* 2020;**4(1)**:47–55.

83. El Nakeeb A, El Sorogy M, Hamed H, Said R, Elrefai M, Ezzat H, et al. Biliary leakage following pancreaticoduodenectomy: Prevalence, risk factors and management. *Hepatobiliary Pancreat Dis Int* 2019;**18(1)**: 67–72.

84. Duconseil P, Turrini O, Ewald J, Berdah SV, Moutardier V, Delpero JR. Biliary complications after pancreaticoduodenectomy: Skinny bile ducts are surgeons' enemies. *World J Surg* 2014;**38(11)**:2946–51.

85. Andrianello S, Marchegiani G, Malleo G, Pollini T, Bonamini D, Salvia R, et al. Biliary fistula after

pancreaticoduodenectomy: Data from 1618 consecutive pancreaticoduodenectomies. *HPB (Oxford)* 2017;**19**(**3**):264–9.

86. Malgras B, Duron S, Gaujoux S, Dokmak S, Aussilhou B, Rebours V, et al. Early biliary complications following pancreaticoduodenectomy: Prevalence and risk factors. *HPB (Oxford)* 2016;**18**(**4**):367–74.

87. House MG, Cameron JL, Schulick RD, Campbell KA, Sauter PK, Coleman J, et al. Incidence and outcome of biliary strictures after pancreaticoduodenectomy. *Ann Surg* 2006;**243**(**5**):571–6.

88. de Castro SM, Kuhlmann KF, Busch OR, van Delden OM, Lameris JS, van Gulik TM, et al. Incidence and management of biliary leakage after hepaticojejunostomy. *J Gastrointest Surg* 2005;**9**(**8**):1163–71.

89. Jester AL, Chung CW, Becerra DC, Molly Kilbane E, House MG, Zyromski NJ, et al. The impact of hepaticojejunostomy leaks after pancreatoduodenectomy: A devastating source of morbidity and mortality. *J Gastrointest Surg* 2017;**21**(**6**):1017–24.

90. Antolovic D, Koch M, Galindo L, Wolff S, Music E, Kienle P, et al. Hepaticojejunostomy—analysis of risk factors for postoperative bile leaks and surgical complications. *J Gastrointest Surg* 2007;**11**(**5**): 555–61.

91. Suzuki Y, Fujino Y, Tanioka Y, Ajiki T, Hiraoka K, Takada M, et al. Factors influencing hepaticojejunostomy leak following pancreaticoduodenal resection; importance of anastomotic leak test. *Hepatogastroenterology* 2003;**50**(**49**):254–7.

92. Burkhart RA, Relles D, Pineda DM, Gabale S, Sauter PK, Rosato EL, et al. Defining treatment and outcomes of hepaticojejunostomy failure following pancreaticoduodenectomy. *J Gastrointest Surg* 2013;**17**(**3**):451–60.

93. Kadaba RS, Bowers KA, Khorsandi S, Hutchins RR, Abraham AT, Sarker SJ, et al. Complications of biliary-enteric anastomoses. *Ann R Coll Surg Engl* 2017;**99**(**3**):210–5.

94. Shi Y, Jin J, Qiu W, Weng Y, Wang J, Zhao S, et al. Short-term outcomes after robot-assisted vs open pancreaticoduodenectomy after the learning curve. *JAMA Surg* 2020;**155**(**5**):389–94.

95. Doula C, Kostakis ID, Damaskos C, Machairas N, Vardakostas DV, Feretis T, et al. Comparison between minimally invasive and open pancreaticoduodenectomy: A systematic review. *Surg Laparosc Endosc Percutan Tech* 2016;**26**(**1**):6–16.

96. Nickel F, Haney CM, Kowalewski KF, Probst P, Limen EF, Kalkum E, et al. Laparoscopic versus open pancreaticoduodenectomy: A systematic review and meta-analysis of randomized controlled trials. *Ann Surg* 2020;**271**(**1**):54–66.

97. Herzog T, Belyaev O, Hessam S, Uhl W, Chromik AM. Management of isolated bile leaks after pancreatic resections. *J Invest Surg* 2014;**27**(**5**):273–81.

Bailey & Love's Essential Operations Bailey & Love's Essential Operatic
Bailey & Love's Essential Operations Bailey & Love's Essential Operatic
SECTION 9 | BILIARY TRACT
Bailey & Love's Essential Operations Bailey & Love's Essential Operatic

Chapter 64

Intraductal Papillary Neoplasm of the Bile Duct and Biliary Cysts

Noel Cassar

INTRADUCTAL PAPILLARY NEOPLASM OF THE BILE DUCT

Introduction

Removing a pre-malignant lesion before malignant transformation and the development of invasive cancer, is a major goal of preventive surgery. This is especially pertinent if the cancer is an aggressive one like cholangiocarcinoma, which is associated with a poor overall 5-year survival rate of 5–15% (1).

Intraductal papillary neoplasm of the bile duct (IPN-B) is a precursor of CCA (2), and it can be seen as the histopathological equivalent of intraductal papillary mucinous neoplasm of the pancreas (IPMN) (3). Previously, IPN-B were known by other terminologies including biliary papillomatosis (4), biliary papillary adenoma (5), and non-invasive papillary carcinoma of the biliary tract (5). Up to a third of these neoplasms produce significant amounts of mucin, and they are then referred to as intraductal papillary mucinous neoplasm of the bile duct (IPMN-B) (6).

Histopathophysiology of IPN-B

IPN-Bs can occur anywhere within the biliary tract when there is papillary proliferation of atypical biliary epithelial cells with central fibrovascular cores (7). IPN-Bs are found predominantly within the extrahepatic ducts in Western populations, but occur more frequently at the hilum, or within the intrahepatic ducts in Asia, where there is a higher incidence of hepatolithiasis (8) and the flatworm *Clonorchis sinensis* (9). In a systematic review and meta-analysis of studies incorporating IPN-B, Gordon-Weeks et al. found that in four studies of 253 patients with IPN-B, hepatolithiasis and *C. sinensis* were each found in 27% of patients (10) and IPN-B is multifocal in up to 41% of patients (10–12).

IPN-B usually spreads longitudinally along the biliary epithelium, penetrating the duct wall as the stage progresses, providing a potential window for surgical resection before malignant transformation with the development of CCA (13). IPN-B is believed to follow the adenoma to carcinoma sequence, as following resection,

invasive carcinoma has been found in 40–94% of resected tumours (14). Several studies have also demonstrated the accumulation of genetic mutations in invasive malignancy, further corroborating this theory (15).

Histologically, IPN-Bs are classified based on the degree of dysplasia: 1) Low-grade dysplasia; 2) high-grade dysplasia and 3) high-grade dysplasia with an invasive component (16) and on the epithelial subtype which include: 4) pancreaticobiliary; 5) intestinal; 6) gastric and 7) oncocytic (17,18) (*see Table 64.1*). This is similar to IPMN of the pancreas. However, IPN-Bs are more frequently associated with invasive malignancy than pancreatic IPMNs (44.4% vs. 6.8%) (19). Pancreaticobiliary and intestinal subtypes are the most common (5,10,20,21) and the former is the subtype most frequently associated with invasive malignancy and expression of the mucin core protein MUC-1 (5). It is more common is Western countries, while the intestinal subtype is more common in Asian countries and expresses the mucin core protein MUC-2 (5,10).

The morphological appearance of IPN-B is also varied. Radiologically it can appear as a focal polypoidal lesion, a frond-like neoplasm (with or without mural nodules), a flat plaque-like lesion or an infiltrative mass (9). Absence of a mass in the presence of upstream bile duct dilatation is also possible (9).

Regarding tumour location, up to half of the IPN-Bs are found in the intrahepatic portion of the biliary tract, with the rest distributed evenly between hilar and distal segments of the bile duct, although there remains some controversy in the literature regarding the anatomical site (10,22) and interestingly within the liver, 75% occur on the left (10). The fact that hepatolithiasis are found mainly in the left side of the liver (8) suggests a causative association between hepatolithiasis and IPN-B. It is thought that hepatolithiasis causes cholangitis, followed by periductal inflammation and reparative hyperplasia which may lead to IPN-B, dysplasia and ultimately CCA (23).

Clinical features of IPN-B and treatment

The clinical presentation of IPN-B varies, and patients can be completely asymptomatic, with the lesions

DOI: 10.1201/9781003080060-64

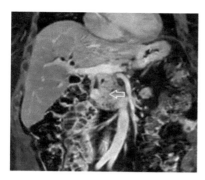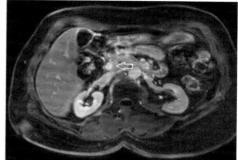

Figure 64.1 Coronal and axial cross-sectional imaging showing a hyper-enhancing lesion in the distal bile duct (white open arrow).

discovered incidentally on imaging. In one such patient treated by the author; a 67-year-old female underwent imaging after routine bloods tests which revealed an obstructive pattern to the liver function tests. Computed tomography (CT) and magnetic resonance imaging (MRI) showed a filing defect in her lower common bile duct associated with an enhancing polypoidal lesion. There was no indication of invasion beyond the wall (*Figure 64.1*) and the lesion was thought to represent an IPN-B of the distal extrahepatic bile duct. The patient underwent a Whipple's pancreaticoduodenectomy and histopathology confirming the IPN-B with no invasive or malignant component. The patient remains well 2-year postoperatively and this type of a presentation has been described in up to 12% of patients (10). Symptomatic patients will present with abdominal pain and jaundice in 42% and 33% of patients respectively, with jaundice thought to occur from obstruction, or intermittent obstruction, caused by a variable degree of mucin production (10). Tumour markers have not been shown to be helpful in the diagnosis of IPN-B (19).

Whether symptomatic or not, surgery to remove the lesion should be undertaken if feasible to reduce the chance of invasive transformation or to eradicate the lesion at an early stage if malignant change has already occurred. The extent of resection will depend on the location. For intrahepatic lesions, a hepatectomy is the appropriate treatment and for lesions of the distal bile duct a Whipple's pancreaticoduodenectomy should be performed. Hilar lesions will need a radical resection of the biliary tree and an extended liver resection, if required, to achieve tumour clearance with a reconstruction employing a Roux-en-Y hepaticojejunostomy. Invasive CCA in the setting of IPN-B carries a median survival of 52.3 months compared with 28 months for conventional CCA (13), supporting radical surgical resection (*Table 64.1*).

BILIARY CYSTS

Introduction

Biliary cysts refer to dilatations of bile ducts anywhere along the biliary tract (24). Biliary cyst is the preferred

Table 64.1 Summary of the presentation, management and treatment of IPN-B

Definition	Papillary proliferation of atypical biliary epithelial cells with central fibrovascular cores anywhere along the biliary tree
Location	• Intrahepatic • Extrahepatic (hilar and distal bile duct)
Presenting features	• Jaundice • Abdominal pain • Asymptomatic
Classification	**Grade of Dysplasia** • Low-grade • High-grade • High-grade with invasive component **Epithelial Subtypes** • Pancreatobiliary • Intestinal • Gastric • Oncocytic
Treatment	Radical resection

term as opposed to choledochal cyst, as the latter implies that dilatation is limited to the common bile duct. Presentation is usually in childhood, but up to 20% will be diagnosed as an adult (25). Biliary cysts, although very rare with an incidence of 1 in 100 000 live births in the Western world (25) represents an important spectrum of disease due to their association with malignancy. This entity is more common in Asian populations with frequency of up to 1 in 13 000 live births (25).

Aetiology

The most commonly accepted theory regarding the aetiology of biliary cysts is that an anomalous pancreaticobiliary union, or bilio-pancreatic maljunction causes reflux of pancreatic fluid into the bile duct causing weakening of the wall, chronic inflammation and cystic

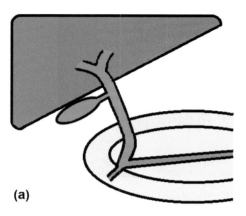
(a)

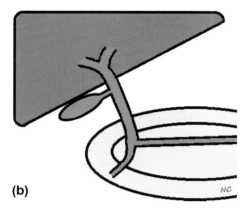
(b)

Figure 64.2 Illustrative anatomy of the bilio-pancreatic junction. Normal (a), note that the junction occurs in the wall of the duodenum, at the ampulla of Vater. Abnormal (b), note that the junction occurs outside the duodenum, and the common channel is longer than usual.

changes (26). Identifying this maljunction is crucial to the diagnosis of a biliary cyst. It results in a longer common channel than usual, with the junction of the bile and pancreatic ducts occurring proximal to and outside the duodenal wall (*Figure 64.2*) and a common channel longer than 15 mm is considered abnormal (27). The Japanese Study Group on Pancreaticobiliary Maljunction (JSPBM) has further classified this malunion into stenotic, non-stenotic, dilated and complex types (28).

Other theories which have been proposed regarding causation include abnormal autonomic innervation of the extrahepatic biliary tree and abnormal canalization of the bile duct during embryogenesis causing distal obstruction. The latter causes increased pressure in the bile duct followed by a weakening of its walls (29).

Presentation and risk of malignancy

Malignancy is rare in children and in a review of 78 studies totalling 5780 patients from 1996–2010, Sastry et al. (30) found that only 0.4% of patients with choledochal cysts developed a malignancy before the age of 18. Conversely, the incidence of malignancy in adults was 11.4%, with median age, at diagnosis, of 42 years (30). The incidence of malignancy increased with each decade, with 10.6% of patients between 31–40 years having malignancy as compared to 38.2% patients over the age of 60 (30). Types 1 and 4 choledochal cysts are the most common type and are the ones most frequently associated with malignancy. Of malignancies associated with biliary cysts, 70.4% were found to be CCAs, 23.5% were gallbladder carcinoma, with other miscellaneous malignancies making up the remaining 6.1% (30).

Biliary cysts can present with abdominal pain, jaundice, right upper quadrant mass, pancreatitis or cholangitis, but with the ever-increasing use of cross-sectional imaging, up to 36% of patients with

biliary cysts are detected incidentally and are asymptomatic (31). The investigation of choice is magnetic resonance cholangiopancreatography (MRCP) as it will delineate the biliary tree and show any cystic dilatations. Endoscopic retrograde cholangiopancreatography (ERCP) has traditionally been the 'gold standard', but is invasive and associated with potentially serious complications (31).

Classification

Todani et al (32) modified the original Alonso-Lej classification (33) to include the intrahepatic dilatations (Caroli's disease) producing the most frequently used classification system (*Table 64.2*).

Type 1 choledochal cyst

This is the most common type of biliary cyst, being found in up to 70% of patients who have choledochal cysts (29). It is associated with a 7.6% incidence of malignancy. Todani et al. mention three types of Type 1 choledochal cysts (29,32):

1 *Type 1A cyst* is a saccular dilatation of the extrahepatic biliary tree with the gallbladder arising out of it with dilatation of both the common hepatic and the bile ducts
2 *Type 1B cyst* is a focal dilatation of the common bile duct
3 *Type 1C* is a fusiform dilatation (as opposed to saccular) of the extrahepatic biliary tree

The treatment of a Type 1 choledochal cyst is excision of the extrahepatic biliary and reconstruction with a Roux-en-Y hepaticojejunostomy, which can be done minimally invasively. Duan et al. (34) published a series of 31 adult patients with choledochal cysts treated laparoscopically with good outcomes compared with open surgery and no perioperative mortality (*Figure 64.3*).

Table 64.2 Overview of biliary cysts as classified by Todani et al. (32)

Type	Description	Frequency	Malignancy risk	Treatment
1	Dilatation of the extrahepatic biliary tree	70%	High	Excision of bile duct and hepaticojejunostomy
2	Diverticulum of the common bile duct	2%	Low	Excision of the diverticulum
3	Choledochocoele	1%	Low	ERCP
4A	Extrahepatic biliary tree dilatation with involvement of the intrahepatic ducts	24%	High	As per Type 1 +/– hepatic resection (see text)
4B	Segmental dilatation of the extrahepatic biliary tree			As per Type 1
5	Cystic dilatation of the intrahepatic biliary tree – Caroli's disease	3%	Low	Hepatic resection or liver transplantation

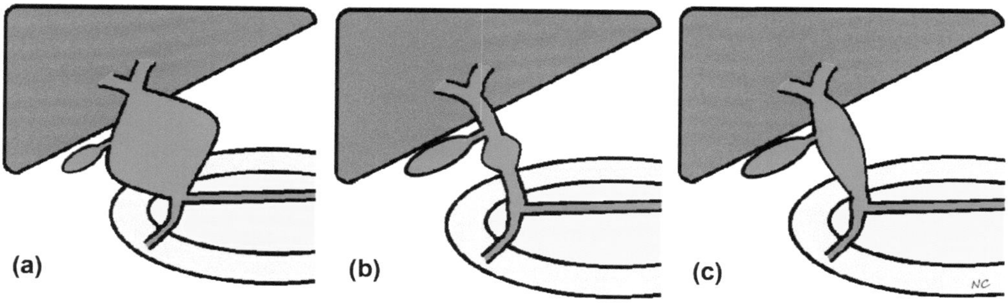

(a)   **(b)**   **(c)**

Figure 64.3 Illustrations of Type 1 choledochal cysts, Type 1A **(a)** Saccular dilatation of the extrahepatic biliary tree, note that the gallbladder arises from it. Type 1B **(b)** Localized dilatation of the bile duct and Type 1C **(c)** Fusiform dilatation of the extrahepatic tree.

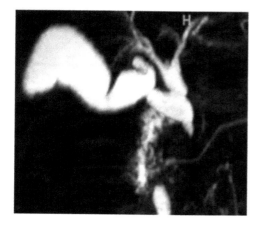

Figure 64.4 MRCP of a 42-year-old man who presented with signs and symptoms of cholangitis and was diagnosed with a Type 1B choledochal cyst.

Drainage operations on the cyst without excision should not be considered standard of care, as the chance of malignancy remains, and the procedure renders subsequent surgery more difficult (35).

Figure 64.4 shows the MRCP of a 42-year-old man who presented with signs and symptoms of cholangitis and was diagnosed with a Type 1B choledochal cyst. This was treated by the author with excision of the extrahepatic biliary tree and hepaticojejunostomy. He is doing well three years after the operation.

Type 2 choledochal cyst

This is an isolated true diverticulum of the common bile duct (29,32) and occurs in 2% of patients with choledochal cysts. Treatment involves cholecystectomy and excision of the diverticulum. The rate of malignant transformation is low at 4% (30) (*Figure 64.5*).

Type 3 choledochal cyst

This can also be termed a choledochocoele and refers to a dilatation of the intraduodenal portion of the common bile duct (29,32). This type of cystic dilatation is the least common variety and only a very small number cases of malignant transformation have ever been reported, and radical excision is not recommended (36). Suggested treatment is deroofing of the cyst at ERCP (36,37) (*Figure 64.6*).

Type 4 choledochal cyst

This is the second most common type of biliary cyst, occurring in up 24% of patients with choledochal cysts,

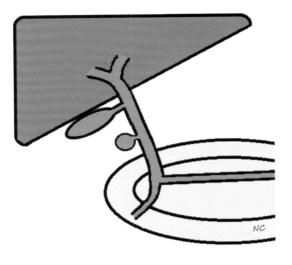

Figure 64.5 Illustration of Type 2 choledochal cyst, consisting of a diverticulum of the common bile duct.

Figure 64.6 Illustration of Type 3 choledochal cyst, consisting of a choledochocoele.

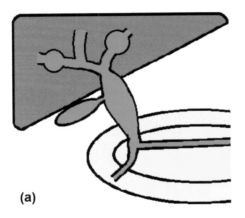

(a)

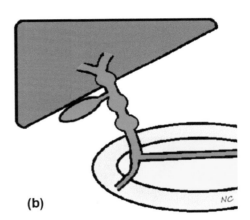

(b)

Figure 64.7 Illustrations of Type 4 choledochal cysts. Type 4A (a) Extrahepatic biliary tree dilatation together with dilated intrahepatic biliary tree. Type 4B (b) segmental dilatation of the extrahepatic biliary tree.

and similarly to Type 1 cysts have an increased risk of malignant transformation (30) with 9% of resected specimens found to harbour malignancy (30).

Type 4A cysts are those having cystic dilatations of the extrahepatic ducts with involvement of the intrahepatic ducts, whilst Type 4B cysts are those having segmental dilatations of only the extrahepatic ducts (29,32). The extrahepatic component should be treated as per Type 1 cysts, with excision of the duct and hepaticojejunostomy (24). A transduodenal sphincteroplasty might be required if there is an associated choledochocoele (24). The treatment of the intrahepatic component of a Type 4A cyst will depend on the context and must be on a case-to-case basis especially if there is hepatolithiasis, strictures, cholangitis, abscess formation or any

suspicion of malignancy. In the latter instance a hepatic resection may be necessary (*Figure 64.7*).

Type 5 choledochal cyst: Caroli's disease

Caroli's disease is the presence of multiple intrahepatic cystic dilatations and treatment depends on whether the disease is limited to one lobe, is bilobar and/or multifocal (29,32). Patients with Caroli's disease often present with recurrent episodes of cholangitis, stone formation or features of malignancy if a CCA has developed. The picture may be further complicated by the presence of congenital hepatic fibrosis or secondary biliary cirrhosis.

Type 5 biliary cysts are found in 3% of patients with a choledochal cyst and malignant transformation occurs in 2.5% of patients (30). In the case of complicated

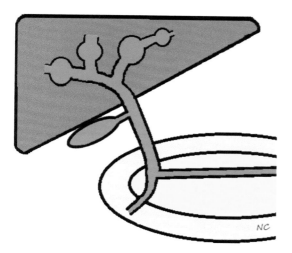

Figure 64.8 Illustration of Type 5 choledochal cyst: Caroli's disease.

Caroli disease limited to a segment or lobe of the liver, a limited hepatic resection is curative (24), however, if the disease is bilobar a more extensive liver resection or even liver transplantation may be required (24) (*Figure 64.8*).

Follow-up

Even after successful resection of a choledochal cyst the lifelong risk of biliary malignancy remains and has been documented at 0.7% which is higher than that of the general population (35,38). Malignancies have been detected between 1–19 years after surgery occurring at the site of anastomoses in 35% of patients (38). These patients consequently need long-term clinical and radiologically follow-up after excision with regular review and cross-sectional imaging.

SUMMARY

IPN-B is a premalignant lesion and CCA development is not uncommon. It can occur anywhere along the biliary tract and histologically it is seen as papillary proliferation of atypical biliary epithelial cells with central fibrovascular cores. In Asian countries, there is a causal association with hepatolithiasis and *Clonorchis sinensis*. Epithelial subtypes include intestinal, gastric, oncocytic and pancreaticobiliary, with the latter most commonly associated with the development of malignancy. Precursor lesions tend to grow longitudinally along the bile duct before becoming invasive, providing a potential window for radical curative removal of the neoplasm. Patients may present with jaundice or abdominal pain, although less commonly they may be asymptomatic.

Biliary cysts refer to dilatations of the biliary tree and although they usually occur in childhood, up to 20% present in later life. Patients present with abdominal pain, jaundice, cholangitis or, like IPN-B, may be

asymptomatic. There are five types of biliary cysts, depending on their location and configuration. There is a risk of malignancy mainly associated with the more common Types I and IV cysts and the chance of malignancy increases with age. Surgical drainage of the cysts is not acceptable, and where appropriate in patients who are fit, radical resection of the cysts greatly reduces the risk of malignancy.

REFERENCES

1. Vignone A, Biancaniello F, Casadio M, et al. Emerging therapies for advanced cholangiocarcinoma: An updated literature review. *J Clin Med* 2021;**10(21)**:4901.
2. Mondal D, Silva MA, Soonawalla Z, et al. Intraductal papillary neoplasm of the bile duct (IPN-B): Also a disease of western Caucasian patients. A literature review and case series. *Clin Radiol* 2016;**71(1)**:e79–87.
3. Zen Y, Fujii T, Itatsu K, et al. Biliary papillary tumors share pathological features with intraductal papillary mucinous neoplasm of the pancreas. *Hepatology* 2006;**44(5)**:1333–43.
4. Naknuma Y, M. Sasaki M, A. Ishikawa A, Chen TC, Huang SF. Biliary papillary neoplasm of the liver. *Histol Histopathol* 2002;**17**:851–61
5. Chatterjee A, Vendrami CL, Nikolaidis P, et al. Uncommon intraluminal tumors of the gallbladder and biliary tract: Spectrum of imaging appearances. *RadioGraphics* 2019;**39(2)**:388–412.
6. Nakanuma Y. A novel approach to biliary tract pathology based on similiarities to pancreatic counterparts: is the biliary tract an incomplete pancreas? *Pathol Int* 2010;**60**:419–29.
7. Wan XS, Xu YY, Qian JY, et al. Intraductal papillary neoplasm of the bile duct. *World J Gastroenterol* 2013;**19(46)**:8595–604.
8. Tyson GL, El-Serag HB. Risk factors for cholangiocarcinoma. *Hepatology* 2011;**54(1)**:173–84.
9. Chang JI, Lee K, Kim D, et al. Clinical characteristics of *Clonorchis sinensis*-associated Cholangiocarcinoma: A large-scale, single-center study. *Front Med (Lausanne)* 2021;**8**:675207.
10. Gordon-Weeks AN, Jones K, Harriss E, et al. Systematic review and meta-analysis of current experience in treating IPNB: Clinical and pathological correlates. *Ann Surg* 2016;**263(4)**:656–63.
11. Kang MJ, Jang J-Y, Lee KB, et al. Impact of macroscopic morphology, multifocality, and mucin secretion on survival outcome of intraductal papillary neoplasm of the bile duct. *J Gastrointest* 2013;**17**:931–8.
12. Ueda M, Miura Y, Kunihiro O, et al. MUC1 overexpression is the most reliable marker of invasive carcinoma in intraductal papillary-mucinous tumor (IPMT). *Hepatogastroenterology* 2005;**52(62)**:398–403.
13. Saxena A, Chua TC, Chu FC, et al. Improved outcomes after aggressive surgical resection of hilar cholangiocarcinoma: A critical analysis of recurrence and survival. *Am J Surg* 2011;**202(3)**:310–14.
14. Lee SS, Kim MH, Lee SK, et al. Clinicopathologic review of 58 patients with biliary papillomatosis. *Cancer* 2004;**100(4)**:783–93.

15. Nakanishi Y, Zen Y, Kondo S, et al. Expression of cell cycle-related molecules in biliary premalignant lesions: Biliary intraepithelial neoplasia and biliary intraductal papillary neoplasm. *Hum Pathol* 2008;**39(8)**:1153–61.

16. Aslam A, Wasnik AP, Shi J, et al. Intraductal papillary neoplasm of the bile duct (IPNB): CT and MRI appearance with radiology-pathology correlation. *Clin Imaging* 2020;**66**:10–17.

17. Park HJ, Kim SY, Kim HJ, et al. Intraductal papillary neoplasm of the bile duct: Clinical, imaging, and pathologic features. *Am J Roentgenol* 2018;**211(1)**:67–75.

18. Ainechi S, Lee H. Updates on precancerous lesions of the biliary tract: Biliary precancerous lesion. *Arch Path Lab* 2016;**140(11)**:1285–89.

19. Minagawa N, Sato N, Mori Y, et al. A comparison between intraductal papillary neoplasms of the biliary tract (BT-IPMNs) and intraductal papillary mucinous neoplasms of the pancreas (P-IPMNs) reveals distinct clinical manifestations and outcomes. *Eur J Surg Oncol* 2013;**39(6)**:554–8.

20. Barton JG, Barrett DA, Maricevich MA, et al. Intraductal papillary mucinous neoplasm of the biliary tract: a real disease? *HPB (Oxford)* 2009;**11(8)**:684–91.

21. Choi SC, Lee JK, Jung JH, et al. The clinicopathological features of biliary intraductal papillary neoplasms according to the location of tumors. *J Gastroenterol Hepatol* 2010;**25(4)**:725–30.

22. Nakagawa T, Arisaka Y, Ajiki T, et al. Intraductal tubulopapillary neoplasm of the bile duct: A case report and review of the published work. *Hepatol Res* 2016;**46(7)**:713–8.

23. Kim HJ, Kim JS, Joo MK, et al. Hepatolithiasis and intrahepatic cholangiocarcinoma: A review. *World J Gastroenterol* 2015;**28**;21(48):13418–31.

24. Croome KP, Nagorney DM. Bile Duct Cysts in Adults. In: Jarnagin WR (Ed). Blumgart's *Surgery of the Liver, Biliary Tract and Pancreas*, 6th edn. London: Elsevier, 2016, Chapter 46, pp 752–64.

25. Soares KC, Arnaoutakis DJ, Kamel I, et al. Choledochal cysts: Presentation, clinical differentiation, and management. *J Am Coll Surg* 2014;**219(6)**:1167– 80.

26. Miyano T, Suruga K, Suda K. "The choledocho-pancreatic long common channel disorders" in relation to the etiology of congenital biliary dilatation and other biliary tract disease. *Ann Acad Med Singap* 1981;**10(4)**:419–26.

27. Liu QY, Nguyen V. Endoscopic approach to the patient with congenital anomalies of the biliary tract. *Gastrointest Endosc Clin N Am* 2013;**23(2)**: 505–18.

28. Urushihara N. Classification of Pancreaticobiliary Maljunction and Congenital Biliary Dilatation. In: Kamisawa, T., Ando, H. (eds) *Pancreaticobiliary Maljunction and Congenital Biliary Dilatation*. New York: Springer, 2018.

29. Yamashita H, Otani T, Shioiri T, et al. Smallest Todani's type II choledochal cyst. *Dig Liver Dis* 2003;**35(7)**:498–502.

30. Sastry AV, Abbadessa B, Wayne MG, et al. What is the incidence of biliary carcinoma in choledochal cysts, when do they develop, and how should it affect management? *World J Surg* 2015;**39(2)**: 487–92.

31. Dhupar R, Gulack B, Geller DA, et al. The changing presentation of choledochal cyst disease: An incidental diagnosis. *HPB Surg* 2009;**2009**:103739.

32. Todani T, Watanabe Y, Narusue M, et al. Congenital bile duct cysts: Classification, operative procedures, and review of thirty-seven cases including cancer arising from choledochal cyst. *Am J Surg* 1977;**134(2)**:263–9.

33. Alonso-Lej F, Rever WB, Jr, Pessagno DJ. Congenital choledochal cyst, with a report of 2, and an analysis of 94, cases. *Int Abstr Surg* 1959;**108**:1–30.

34. Duan X, Mao X, Jiang B, et al. Totally laparoscopic cyst excision and Roux-en-Y hepaticojejunostomy for choledochal cyst in adults: A single-institute experience of 5 years. *Surg Laparosc Endosc Percutan Tech* 2015;**25(2)**:e65–8.

35. He XD, Wang L, Liu W, et al. The risk of carcinogenesis in congenital choledochal cyst patients: An analysis of 214 cases. *Ann Hepatol* 2014;**13(6)**: 819–26.

36. Lopez RR, Pinson CW, Campbell JR, et al. Variation in management based on type of choledochal cyst. *Am J Surg* 1991;**161(5)**:612–5.

37. Khandelwal C, Anand U, Kumar B, et al. Diagnosis and management of choledochal cysts. *Indian J Surg* 2012;**74(5)**:401–6.

38. Watanabe Y, Toki A, Todani T. Bile duct cancer developed after cyst excision for choledochal cyst. *J Hepatobiliary Pancreat Surg* 1999;**6(3)**:207–12.

Chapter 65

Biliary Parasitic Disease

Vikram Kate and Raja R. Kalayarasan

INTRODUCTION

Parasitic infestations, although a global issue, have a disproportionate impact on healthcare systems in developing countries (1). Parasites commonly infest the intestines and biliary tract involvement occurs when it acts as the natural habitat for the parasite, or when parasites enter due to ectopic migration. As biliary tract infestation by parasites is an important cause of a range of hepatobiliary complications, including cholangiocarcinoma, it is crucial to be aware of its diverse clinical manifestations and treatment options (2). This chapter focuses on primary biliary parasites and biliary complications from the common infestations such as ascariasis, and hydatid cyst.

FASCIOLIASIS

Fascioliasis or distomatosis is a parasitic infestation caused by the digenetic trematodes *Fasciola hepatica* or *Fasciola gigantica*. *F. hepatica* infection is more widely distributed around the world than *F. gigantica*, which is only commonly reported from the tropical regions of Africa, the Middle East and Asia (3). As contaminated water and poor public health are important predisposing factors for the infestation, fascioliasis is endemic in developing countries. The World Health Organization (WHO) has included human fascioliasis in the priorities among 'neglected tropical diseases' and it is now considered an important human parasitic disease instead of a secondary zoonotic disease (4).

Pathogenesis

Humans become infected by consuming contaminated raw freshwater plants like watercress, lettuce, and dandelion leaves (*Figure 65.1*). In the bile ducts, the parasites mature and become adult flukes which produce eggs that are excreted in the faeces. Occasionally the larvae migrate to locations other than the liver resulting in ectopic fascioliasis. Common ectopic sites in the abdomen are the pancreas, spleen, appendix and abdominal wall.

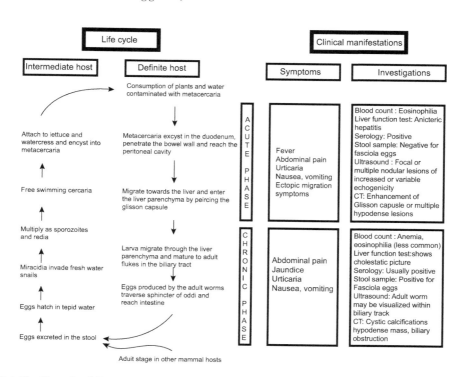

Figure 65.1 The lifecycle of *Fasciola* species: Clinical manifestations and diagnostic modalities.

DOI: 10.1201/9781003080060-65

In humans, the prepatent period, defined as the time from the ingestion of metacercariae to the first appearance of the first eggs in the faeces, lasts for 3–4 months (5). The clinical manifestations are primarily due to the migration and destruction of host tissue. *F. gigantica* is more pathogenic than *F. hepatica* due to its larger size and biomass (6) but the clinical manifestations of these two species are broadly similar.

Clinical features

Symptoms in the acute or hepatic phase include fever, upper abdominal pain, loss of appetite, nausea and vomiting and acute-phase symptoms often mimic cholecystitis (7). Pancreatic duct obstruction and pancreatitis is a common manifestation of pancreatic fascioliasis. Fever, jaundice and abdominal pain in the chronic or biliary phase are due to biliary inflammation, hyperplasia, fibrotic bile duct thickening and biliary obstruction induced by adult flukes in the biliary tract (8).

Diagnosis

While clinicians in endemic areas may suspect liver fluke infection based on clinical presentation, confirmation of the diagnosis requires direct parasitological, indirect immunological or imaging techniques. Hypereosinophilia is present in almost all patients with acute infection except those in the early phase of the disease, but is a less common finding in chronic infection (9). Raised aspartate and alanine aminotransferase levels with a normal bilirubin is a common finding during acute infection. In chronic infection, bilirubin, alkaline phosphatase and gamma-glutamyl transferase levels are elevated due to cholestasis.

SeroFluke (a new highly stable, sensitive and specific lateral flow immunological assay for the serodiagnosis of human fasciolosis) is the serological assay with the maximum sensitivity and specificity. It uses a recombinant cathepsin L1 from *F. hepatica*, along with protein A and mAb MM3 as detector reagents in the test and control lines (10).

Coprological tests refer to the analysis of stool samples for detection of *Fasciola* eggs, and analysis of stool samples on 3 consecutive days is recommended to improve the sensitivity. Quantitative coprological techniques like the Kato-Katz method are useful in epidemiological studies and for monitoring treatment response (11). A 400 eggs per gram (EPG) threshold is commonly used to diagnose a high infection burden.

Ultrasound (US) of the abdomen is a commonly used investigation but its sensitivity is poor in respect of the diagnosis of fascioliasis. Findings in the acute hepatic phase include focal or multiple areas of increased or variable echogenicity. When affected areas are cystic, they may mimic hydatid disease, abscesses or malignancy. Contrast-enhanced computed tomography (CECT) performed shortly after infection may show contrast enhancement of the Glisson capsule

because of inflammation caused by penetration of the juvenile larva. Multiple, small, clustered, ill or well-defined necrotic hypodense areas that, unlike pyogenic abscess, do not merge to form a large abscess cavity is a common finding in the acute phase (12). Biliary dilation with irregularly thickened ductal walls can be observed in the biliary phase and magnetic resonance cholangiopancreatography (MRCP) will demonstrate the biliary dilatation with hypointense tubular or crescent-like filling defects representing adult flukes in the bile ducts or gallbladder (13).

Treatment

Triclabendazole (a member of the benzimidazole family of antihelmintics) given at a dose of 10 mg/kg is the drug of choice for the treatment of both acute- and chronic-phase infections (14). A single dose achieves a cure rate close to 90%, and administering a second dose will improve this to almost 100% without significant adverse effects. Unfortunately, the widespread use of triclabendazole in animals has resulted in the emergence of resistant fluke strains.

Endoscopic or surgical intervention is primarily required in patients with chronic infection presenting with biliary obstruction. While administration of anti-parasite drugs can kill the parasites, they remain in the biliary tract for a few days till they are cleared, causing persistent biliary obstruction and symptoms. Occasionally, especially in nonendemic areas, a complex cystic mass in the liver might be mistaken for malignancy potentially resulting in an unnecessary liver resection.

CLONORCHIASIS AND OPISTHORCHIASIS

Clonorchiasis is an infection caused by *Clonorchis sinensis*, whereas *Opisthorchis viverrini* and *Opisthorchis felineus* cause opisthorchiasis (15). Of the three parasites, *C. sinensis* is the most frequent and is endemic in East Asia, including most parts of Eastern China, Russia and the Far East including Korea, Taiwan and Northern Vietnam (15,16). *O. viverrini* is the next most common parasite and is endemic in Northern Thailand, Laos, Southern Vietnam and Cambodia. In some European countries including Romania, Russia, Ukraine, Moldova and Kazakhstan, *O. felineus* infection is endemic (16). These parasites are endemic where dietary habits and environmental conditions favour their breeding and transmission. As both *C. sinensis* and *O. viverrini* are implicated in the development of cholangiocarcinoma, they are classified as group one carcinogens by the WHO (17). Despite minor differences in epidemiology and pathogenicity, both clonorchiasis and opisthorchiasis have similar clinical manifestations and will be discussed together.

Pathogenesis

The lifecycle of *C. sinensis* and both the species of *Opisthorchis* are remarkably similar. The snail, mainly *Bithynia* species (a genus of small freshwater snails with an operculum), is the first intermediate host, infected by eggs released from the mammalian hosts (*Figure 65.2*). During the acute phase of the infection, symptoms are due to inflammatory reactions incited by the parasite in the biliary tract. Intrahepatic biliary obstruction is the dominant manifestation in the chronic phase and occurs due to inflammation-induced ductal fibrosis, the formation of intrahepatic pigment stones due to bile stasis and the adult flukes and eggs acting as a nidus for the formation of stones (18). Ductal and periductal fibrosis with bile cholestasis can result in biliary cirrhosis. The chemical, mechanical, and immunological irritation by the adult worms results in inflammation, epithelial hyperplasia, goblet cell metaplasia, adenomatous hyperplasia, dysplasia and the development of cholangiocarcinoma (19,20).

Clinical presentation

Most patients are asymptomatic during the acute phase of infection although some may develop: 1) Fever; 2) upper abdominal pain; 3) a rash; 4) nausea; 5) flatulence and 6) malaise. In the chronic phase, patients present with hepatobiliary complications such as: 1) cholecystitis; 2) recurrent pyogenic cholangitis; 3) liver abscess; 4) obstructive jaundice; 5) cirrhosis, and 6) portal hypertension. Pancreatic stones and pancreatitis occur in patients with adult flukes in the main pancreatic duct. Intrahepatic cholangiocarcinoma is the most feared complication as flukes often reside in the second-order bile ducts.

Diagnosis

The 'gold standard' investigation for diagnosis is the detection of eggs in stool or bile aspirates using the Kato-Katz technique (a diagnostic technique for the detection of helminth eggs in stools using a light microscope) or a similar examination technique (21). The sensitivity of faecal examination can be improved by using immunological tests to detect parasite eggshell antigens or molecular methods such as conventional or real-time polymerase chain reaction (PCR) to detect parasite DNA (22). Currently, the use of an enzyme-linked immunosorbent assay (ELISA) to detect antibodies against crude somatic extracts or excretory-secretory proteins of the parasite is the most widely used serological test, and antigen-based tests are helpful to determine treatment efficacy.

Imaging studies are useful to evaluate hepatobiliary manifestations. US demonstrates thickened and echogenic intrahepatic duct with minimal intrahepatic dilatation (23). and the gallbladder may contain worms seen as echogenic floating objects or debris in

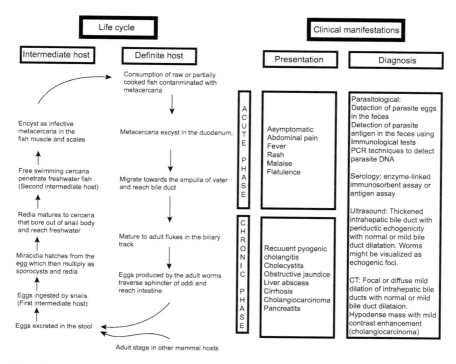

Figure 65.2 The lifecycle of *Clonorchis* and *Opisthorchis* species: Clinical manifestations and diagnostic modalities.

the dependant portion. The common bile duct is usually of normal size or mildly dilated, and in patients with a low burden of infection CT will show dilated small peripheral ducts. In patients with a heavy worm burden, however, there will be diffuse dilatation of the intrahepatic ducts out to the periphery of the liver. The characteristic pattern of mild intrahepatic dilatation helps to differentiate clonorchiasis and opisthorchiasis from stone disease or tumours (12,13). Patients with intrahepatic cholangiocarcinoma have a hypodense mass with delayed contrast enhancement and marked intrahepatic biliary dilatation.

Treatment

Praziquantel is the drug of choice for both clonorchiasis and opisthorchiasis (24). The recommended dose for *C. sinensis* and *O. felineus* is 25 mg/kg given three times orally in 1 day with a 5-hour intervals between the doses (total dose, 75 mg/kg). For *O. viverrine,* a total dose of 75 mg/kg is given in unequal divided doses (50 mg/kg followed by 25 mg/kg) orally with a 4-hour interval between the doses. Biliary complications are treated using endoscopic, percutaneous or surgical procedures as appropriate but should always be combined with pharmacotherapy as intervention alone may not remove all the adult worms. For patients with cholangiocarcinoma, liver resection is the only potentially curative option.

ASCARIASIS

Ascariasis caused by the nematode *Ascaris lumbricoides* is one of the most common parasites infesting the gastrointestinal (GI) tract (25). Although *A. lumbricoides* infection is globally distributed, improvements in sanitation have reduced its prevalence in developed nations. Nevertheless, it remains a common problem in developing countries especially among children. Adult worms typically reside in the small intestine, especially the jejunum. In patients with a heavy infestation, adult worms migrate cranially to the duodenum and enter the biliary tract through the papilla of Vater resulting in biliary ascariasis. In endemic regions, ascariasis accounts for up to 10–30% of biliary tract disease which is a major cause of acariasis-related hospital admissions.

Pathogenesis

Humans acquire infection by ingesting food or drinks contaminated with Ascaris eggs which have been excreted in faeces. Gastric juice dissolves the eggs in the stomach, releasing rhabdoid larva, which migrate to the intestine (26). The larvae penetrate the intestinal mucosa and reach the liver via the portal vein. The larvae may go to the right heart, lungs and ascend the respiratory tract to reach the pharynx from where they are again swallowed and in the small bowel mature into adult worms (26). The time taken from ingestion

to maturation is approximately 4 months. Biliary manifestations are seen in patients with a heavy worm burden where the adult worms migrate to the biliary tract and initiate acute symptoms. These symptoms usually resolve when the worm migrates back to the intestine although in some patients, the worm ascends to the intrahepatic bile duct resulting in cholecystitis and cholangitis. Often, the worms trapped in the bile duct perish and act as a nidus for the formation of sludge and stones. Intrahepatic stones and inflammation-induced biliary stricture frequently result in recurrent pyogenic cholangitis.

Clinical presentation

Migration of worms to the duodenum manifests as pain in the right hypochondrium associated with nausea and vomiting, and often the vomit contains live adult worms confirming proximal migration. Fever, jaundice and abdominal pain suggestive of cholangitis indicates the entry of worms into the bile duct (27). Acalculous cholecystitis in biliary ascariasis is usually due to obstruction of the cystic duct and rarely due to entry of worms into the gallbladder. Liver abscess as a presenting feature is observed in a few patients with intrahepatic stones and recurrent pyogenic cholangitis resulting in biliary cirrhosis and end-stage liver disease have been reported from endemic countries (27).

Diagnosis

As worms intermittently move in and out of the biliary tract, the diagnosis of biliary ascariasis requires a high index of clinical suspicion. In patients with a heavy intestinal infestation, the adult worms can be seen as a 'bull's-eye' within the intestinal lumen (*Figure 65.3a*). The characteristic finding on abdominal US are echogenic tubular structures on a long axis with a relatively hypoechoic centre representing the worm's alimentary canal (28). On the transverse section, worms in the bile duct appear as a 'bull's-eye' echo (29). The absence of posterior acoustic shadowing and slow writhing movement differentiates echogenic worms from stones. US is also helpful to monitor the movement of worms out of the biliary tract. MRCP is more valuable than CT to demonstrate worms which will be seen as linear, hyperintense tubular structures with a central hypointense area.

Treatment

Management depends upon the clinical presentation. In patients presenting with cholecystitis and cholangitis, the first line of treatment is antibiotics, antipyretics, oral anthelmintics and adequate hydration (30). While multiple oral anthelmintics are available, albendazole is the preferred agent and oral anthelmintics aim to treat intestinal ascariasis and prevent reinfection of the biliary tract. They are usually ineffective against worms already present in the biliary tract due to the poor

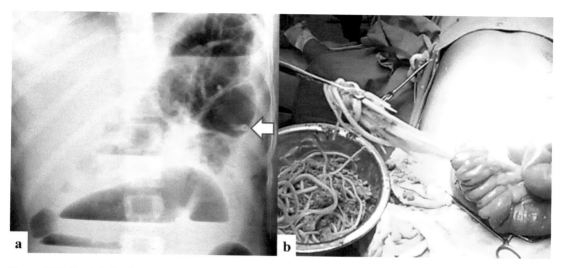

Figure 65.3 Erect abdominal radiograph showing multiple air-fluid levels due to Ascaris-induced intestinal obstruction with adult worms seen as 'bull's-eye' within the intestinal lumen (arrow) (a). An impacted worm bolus being removed after making an enterotomy (b).

enterohepatic circulation of the drug and the success of conservative treatment depends on the spontaneous exit of worms from the biliary tract. Endoscopic retrograde cholangiography (ERC) and worm extraction is preferred for patients with persistent symptoms and US showing worms in the biliary tract. Surgery is indicated if endoscopic extraction fails, and the preferred surgical treatment is choledochotomy and extraction of worms with or without a T-tube. In patients with a heavy intestinal infestation causing bowel obstruction, enterotomy and removal of worms is recommended (*Figure 65.3b*).

HYDATID CYST WITH CYSTOBILIARY COMMUNICATION

Hydatid cysts are caused by the larval stage of the adult parasite tapeworm *Echinococcus granulosus*. The liver is the primary site of involvement and biliary communication is the most common complication. The true incidence of cystobiliary communication is not known with any certainty, principally due to the lack of consensus regarding the definition. The majority of patients will have a minor biliary communication with reported incidences ranging from 5–40%, with major cystobiliary communication occurring in 5–10% of cases (31). Risk factors for cystobiliary communication are: 1) Multiple cysts; 2) multilocular cysts; 3) degenerated cysts; 4) cysts close to the hilum and 5) large cysts more than 10 cm in size. Patients with minor biliary communication are usually asymptomatic and manifest clinically due to a bile leak in the postoperative period. Major biliary communication, defined as a fistula size >5 mm, results in the passage of the cyst contents into the bile duct causing obstructive jaundice

or cholangitis (32). In asymptomatic patients, a raised alkaline phosphatase is a most reliable preoperative predictor of biliary communication. Symptomatic patients will have raised bilirubin and aminotransferase levels and in patients with a major cystobiliary fistula, US scanning and an abdominal CT may demonstrate the communication. Air within a cyst after ERC and stenting of the bile duct is also highly suggestive of a cystobiliary communication (*Figure 65.4a*).

Surgery is the mainstay of treatment in symptomatic patients as percutaneous interventions are contraindicated in the presence of suspected or confirmed cystobiliary communication (33). In patients who present with cholangitis, ERC with stenting is indicated to evacuate the cyst contents and treat cholangitis. Conservative surgical options like cystectomy and partial pericystectomy are commonly performed but after evacuation of the cyst contents, the cavity should be inspected for evidence of a biliary communication. Sometimes the ERC-placed stent can be seen within the cyst cavity demonstrating the site of the communication (*Figure 65.4b*) and leaving a dry gauze pack in the residual cyst cavity for few minutes may reveal a bile leak. Alternatively, intraoperative cholangiography or injection of methylene blue through the cystic duct can be used to reveal small calibre or overlooked biliary communications or leaks. As methylene blue stains the cyst wall in patients with a biliary communication, the authors prefer to use 1% propofol, a lyophilic intravenous anaesthetic prepared as an emulsion in long chain triglyceride, which has a 'milk-like' consistency and is safe and very easy to see. Intraoperatively detected small biliary communications should be suture closed using delayed absorbable sutures like polydioxanone

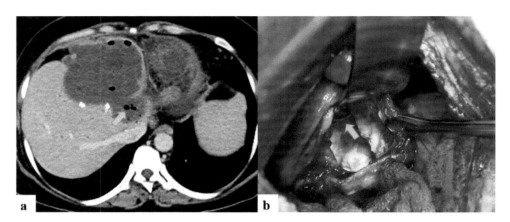

Figure 65.4 Hydatid cyst with cystobiliary communication. Axial CT abdominal scan showing air within cyst following ERC and stenting of the bile duct (a). Intraoperative picture of stent visualized within the cyst cavity (b).

to prevent the development of a postoperative biliary fistula. A Roux-en-Y hepaticojejunostomy is preferred for the treatment of major cystobiliary communication involving a sectoral or hepatic duct (34). Radical treatment options like cystopericystectomy or anatomic liver resection have a lower incidence of postoperative bile leaks but are associated with more perioperative morbidity and hence are reserved for patients with peripherally located cysts or a major cystobiliary communication (35).

SUMMARY

Parasitic infestations of the biliary tract are an important cause of biliary complications, especially in tropical countries. Fascioliasis presents with biliary symptoms in the chronic phase of infection. While triclabendazole is an effective drug to treat acute and chronic phases of fascioliasis, endoscopic or surgical intervention is required in patients presenting with biliary obstruction. Clonorchiasis caused by *C. sinensis* and closely related *Opisthorchis* species (*O. viverrini* and *O. felineus*) is an important cause of intrahepatic stones and intrahepatic cholangiocarcinoma. Infection with *A. lumbricoides* can present with biliary obstruction due to ectopic migration of the worm. Endoscopic or surgical intervention may be required in patients with persistent biliary symptoms. Cystobiliary communication is the most common complication of a hydatid cyst and surgery is the mainstay of treatment when the communication is major.

REFERENCES

1. Torgerson PR, Devleesschauwer B, Praet N, et al. World Health Organization rstimates of the Global and Regional Disease Burden of 11 Foodborne Parasitic Diseases, 2010: A Data Synthesis. *PLoS Med* 2015;**12(12)**:1001920.

2. Lübbert C, Schneitler S. Parasitic and infectious diseases of the biliary tract in migrants and international travelers. *Expert Rev Gastroenterol Hepatol* 2016;**10(11)**:1211–25.

3. Webb CM, Cabada MM. Recent developments in the epidemiology, diagnosis, and treatment of *Fasciola* infection. *Curr Opin Infect Dis* 2018;**31(5)**:409–14.

4. Savioli L, Daumerie D. 2013. Sustaining the drive to overcome the global impact of neglected tropical diseases: Second WHO report on neglected diseases. Available from: https://www.who.int/publications/i/item/9789241564540. WHO. (Accessed 28 August 2024).

5. Valero MA, De Renzi M, Panova M, et al. Crowding effect on adult growth, pre-patent period and egg shedding of *Fasciola hepatica*. *Parasitology* 2006;**133(Pt 4)**:453–63.

6. Valero MA, Bargues MD, Khoubbane M, et al. Higher physiopathogenicity by *Fasciola gigantica* than by the genetically close *F. hepatica*: Experimental long-term follow-up of biochemical markers. *Trans R Soc Trop Med Hyg* 2016;**110(1)**:55–66.

7. Harrington D, Lamberton PHL, McGregor A. Human liver flukes. *Lancet Gastroenterol Hepatol* 2017;**2(9)**:680–9.

8. Marcos LA, Terashima A, Yi P, et al. Mechanisms of liver fibrosis associated with experimental *Fasciola hepatica* infection: Roles of Fas2 proteinase and hepatic stellate cell activation. *J Parasitol* 2011;**97(1)**:82–7.

9. Kaya M, Bestas R, Cetin S. Clinical presentation and management of *Fasciola hepatica* infection: Single-center experience. *World J Gastroenterol* 2011;**17(44)**:4899–904.

10. Martínez-Sernández V, Muiño L, Perteguer MJ, et al. Development and evaluation of a new lateral flow immunoassay for serodiagnosis of human fasciolosis. *PLoS Negl Trop Dis* 2011;**5(11)**:e1376.

11. Zárate-Rendón DA, Vlaminck J, Levecke B, et al. Comparison of Kato-Katz thick smear, mini-FLO TAC, and Flukefinde for the detection and quantification of *Fasciola hepatica* eggs in artificially spiked human stool. *Am J Trop Med Hyg* 2019;**101(1)**:59–61.

12. Lim JH, Kim SY, Park CM. Parasitic diseases of the biliary tract. *AJR Am J Roentgenol* 2007;**188(6)**:1596–603.

13. Kabaalioglu A, Cubuk M, Senol U, et al. Fascioliasis: US, CT, and MRI findings with new observations. *Abdom Imaging* 2000;**25(4)**:400–4.

14. Keiser J, Utzinger J. Food-borne trematodiasis: Current chemotherapy and advances with artemisinins and synthetic trioxolanes. *Trends Parasitol* 2007;**23(11)**:555–62.

15. Petney TN, Andrews RH, Saijuntha W, et al. The zoonotic, fish-borne liver flukes *Clonorchis sinensis*, *Opisthorchis felineus* and *Opisthorchis viverrini*. *Int J Parasitol* 2013;**43(12–13)**:1031–46.

16. Fedorova OS, Kovshirina YV, Kovshirina AE, et al. *Opisthorchis felineus* infection and cholangiocarcinoma in the Russian Federation: A review of medical statistics. *Parasitol Int* 2017;**66(4)**:365–71.

17. Hong ST, Fang Y. *Clonorchis sinensis* and clonorchiasis, an update. *Parasitol Int* 2012;**61(1)**:17–24.

18. Attwood HD, Chou ST. The longevity of *Clonorchis sinensis*. *Pathology* 1978;**10(2)**:153–6.

19. Gouveia MJ, Pakharukova MY, Laha T, et al. Infection with *Opisthorchis felineus* induces intraepithelial neoplasia of the biliary tract in a rodent model. *Carcinogenesis* 2017;**38(9)**:929–37.

20. Prueksapanich P, Piyachaturawat P, Aumpansub P, et al. Liver fluke-associated biliary tract cancer. *Gut Liver* 2018;**12(3)**:236–45.

21. Qian MB, Yap P, Yang YC, et al. Accuracy of the Kato-Katz method and formalin-ether concentration technique for the diagnosis of *Clonorchis sinensis*, and implication for assessing drug efficacy. *Parasit Vectors* 2013;**6(1)**:314.

22. Cai XQ, Yu HQ, Bai JS, et al. development of a TaqMan based real-time PCR assay for detection of *Clonorchis sinensis* DNA in human stool samples and fishes. *Parasitol Int* 2012;**61(1)**:183–6.

23. Lim JH, Mairiang E, Ahn GH. Biliary parasitic diseases including clonorchiasis, opisthorchiasis and fascioliasis. *Abdom Imaging* 2008;**33(2)**:157–65.

24. Sayasone S, Meister I, Andrews JR, et al. Efficacy and safety of praziquantel against light infections of *Opisthorchis viverrini*: A randomized parallel single-blind dose-ranging Trial. *Clin Infect Dis* 2017;**64(4)**:451–8.

25. Khuroo MS. Ascariasis. *Gastroenterol Clin North Am* 1996;**25(3)**:553–77.

26. Crompton DW. Ascaris and ascariasis. *Adv Parasitol* 2001;**48**:285–375.

27. Khuroo MS, Zargar SA. Biliary ascariasis. A common cause of biliary and pancreatic disease in an endemic area. *Gastroenterology* 1985;**88(2)**:418–23.

28. Al Absi M, Qais AM, Al Katta M, et al. Biliary ascariasis: The value of ultrasound in the diagnosis and management. *Ann Saudi Med* 2007;**27(3)**:161–5.

29. Wu S. Sonographic findings of ascaris lumbricoides in the gastrointestinal and biliary tracts. *Ultrasound Q* 2009;**25(4)**:207–9.

30. Khuroo MS, Rather AA, Khuroo NS, et al. Hepatobiliary and pancreatic ascariasis. *World J Gastroenterol* 2016;**22(33)**:7507–17.

31. Ramia JM, Figueras J, De la Plaza R, et al. Cysto-biliary communication in liver hydatidosis. *Langenbecks Arch Surg* 2012;**397(6)**:881–7.

32. Toumi O, Ammar H, Gupta R, et al. Management of liver hydatid cyst with cystobiliary communication and acute cholangitis: A 27-year experience. *Eur J Trauma Emerg Surg* 2019;**45(6)**:1115–19.

33. Gupta N, Javed A, Puri S, et al. Hepatic hydatid: PAIR, drain or resect? *J Gastrointest Surg* 2011;**15(10)**:1829–36.

34. Bayrak M, Altintas Y. Current approaches in the surgical treatment of liver hydatid disease: Single center experience. *BMC Surg* 2019;**19(1)**:95.

35. Deo KB, Kumar R, Tiwari G, et al. Surgical management of hepatic hydatid cysts – conservative versus radical surgery. *HPB (Oxford)* 2020;**22(10)**:1457–62.

Bailey & Love's Essential Operations Bailey & Love's Essential Operatio
Bailey & Love's Essential Operations Bailey & Love's Essential Operatio
Bailey & Love's Essential Operations Bailey & Love's Essential Operatio

SECTION 9 | BILIARY TRACT

Chapter 66

Biliary Pseudotumours

Georgi Atanasov and Markus Trochsler

INTRODUCTION

Pseudotumours can be the consequence of iatrogenic or traumatic injuries, although they are more commonly associated with infectious and inflammatory processes and autoimmune disorders. Biliary inflammatory pseudotumours (BIP) are benign lesions located within the biliary tree (intra hepatic or extra hepatic) and are most often at the porta hepatis or the distal common bile duct (CBD) (1,2). Inflammatory pseudotumours have been described in almost every organ or location in the human body, however, the mesentery, omentum and lungs are the most common sites (3). The definitive diagnosis of BIP is classically by histopathology. Little is known about the morphology of the immunological cellular infiltrates associated with the mass-forming desmoplastic nature of the lesions, and the aetiology of the underlying molecular pathways that significantly contribute to facilitating the inflammation reaction (4). Emerging data from the literature, however, does identify the clinical significance of IgG4-associated autoimmune diseases, contributing significantly to the mass-forming effect in the affected organ or at the anatomical site (5). In addition, the iatrogenically induced (post-surgery or post-interventional procedure) abnormalities of the liver and biliary tree represent a diagnostic challenge. The available published data confirms that pseudotumours have the capacity to mimic the morphological features of both benign and malignant lesions, especially on diagnostic clinical imaging. In some cases, the clinical symptoms generated by these pseudotumours resemble the biological behaviour of malignant lesions posing additional challenges for clinicians.

The clinical significance of BIP and their ability to masquerade as malignant lesions means the affected patients are frequently investigated and considered for major surgical interventions with the inevitable treatment-related morbidity and mortality associated with a major hepatobiliary procedure Although medical professionals should always consider the possibility of BIP in patients with mass-forming ill-defined lesions, in whom a malignant process cannot be excluded, formal curative surgical options must be considered and weighed against an individual patient's risk of complications.

INCIDENCE

Inflammatory pseudotumours involving the biliary tree are rare and the published data consists of single case reports and limited retrospective single centre case series (5). Due to the paucity of published data, the actual incidence of BIP is unknown and reports regarding the prevalence of post-interventional or post-surgical iatrogenic BIP is virtually non-existent. The only published data is in the form of case reports detailing radiological findings after hepatic injury (6–9).

Knoeffel et al. studied 33 consecutive patients who underwent curative surgical tumour resection for presumed malignancies involving the hepatic hilum and reported an incidence of 18% for BIP (10) while 27 of the 33 surgical specimens demonstrated malignant lesions. Six of the 33 (18.2%) showed only fibrosing cholangitis mimicking a mass-forming lesion, also known as 'Klatskin-mimicking' lesions. In another retrospective analysis, Corvera et al. studied the outcome of 275 patients with proximal biliary strictures and presumed malignancy, who received formal curative intent surgery (11). Despite the preoperative suspicion of a malignant process, 22 out of 275 (8%) patients had a final histological diagnosis of a benign stricture within a mass-forming lesion diagnosed as BIP. All 22 cases had undergone major abdominal surgery including resection and reconstruction of the extrahepatic biliary tree. In addition, 10 of the cases received *en bloc* partial hepatectomy, which was necessary to facilitate a curative oncological approach for the presumed malignant lesion. After confirmation of benign tissue, the authors re-examined the specimens and found that granulomatous disease, nonspecific fibrosis and inflammation, lymphoplasmacytic sclerosing pancreatitis and cholangitis, and primary sclerosing cholangitis were responsible for the tumour-mimicking and mass-forming character of the BIP lesions.

AETIOLOGY

In the majority of patients, with the exception of iatrogenic injury, the aetiology of BIP remains unclear. The most common non-iatrogenic, pathogenetic mechanisms are related to chronic bacterial, viral and parasitic infections, predominantly on the background of an established but clinically unremarkable low-grade

DOI: 10.1201/9781003080060-66

immunosuppression (12–14). In addition, autoimmune diseases have increasingly been reported as causative pathologies producing BIP and are now increasingly recognized (15).

Epstein–Barr virus is often confirmed histologically in pseudotumour specimens and current scientific evidence strongly supports its causal involvement in the pathogenesis of this chronic process (16–19). Common pathogenetic hypotheses also report the importance of recurrent episodes of acute cholangitis, secondary to bacterial translocation and portal venous infections, and obliterative phlebitis (20,21). Recurrent episodes of pyogenic cholangitis, causally involved in the occurrence of significant strictures in the biliary tree, are also associated with the presence of inflammatory pseudo-tumours (22–24). Latent subclinical infections with tuberculosis are coupled with pseudotumour formation (25–28) and Agarwal et al. noted the significance of pulmonary parenchymal pseudotumoural tuberculosis in patients in whom clinical and radiological resolution followed anti-tuberculosis therapy alone (27). Sfeir et al. showed that *Mycobacterium avium* complex, followed by *Mycobacterium tuberculosis* complex were the most frequent pathogens isolated in the specimens of patients with a mycobacterial spindle cell pseudotumour (14). Mass-forming infection affecting the lymph nodes is the hallmark of tuberculosis and while parenchymal masses are rare, clinicians should remember that tuberculosis can initiate mass-forming infections in most areas of the body, including the biliary tract.

IgG4-ASSOCIATED AUTOIMMUNE DISEASES MIMICKING MASS FORMING LESIONS

In recent years, the clinical importance of IgG4-associated autoimmune diseases has been recognized. Autoimmune pancreatitis with a prevalence of approximately 2.2 per 100 000 people constitute the best example of these immunological disorders (28). IgG4-associated autoimmune diseases can affect every organ system, and the extra hepatic and intra hepatic biliary tree represents one of the most frequently affected anatomical sites (29,30). These disorders can result in pronounced inflammatory reactions which cause swelling and the formation of a pseudotumorous mass at the affected site. The histological appearance of this inflammatory reaction is heterogeneous though the presence of lymphocytes and IgG4-positive plasma cells is characteristic. Autoimmune molecular pathways mediate the typical occurrence of the so called 'storiform fibrosis' (the name 'storiform' originates from the Latin word '*storea*' (woven) meaning whorled, like a 'straw mat') and obliterative with vessel-occluding phlebitis (31). In this setting, the elevated plasma levels of IgG4 antibodies are not pathogenic. However, Th1 and Th2 lymphocytes play a crucial role in orchestrating the autoimmune process (31,32). Guidelines for the

state-of-the-art treatment of IgG4-related pathologies are built upon retrospective studies or limited number of prospective, one-armed clinical trials. IgG4-positive syndromes respond well to glucocorticosteroids treatment with Stone et al. reporting clinical remission rates as high as 98% (33). Most clinical experience in treating IgG4-associated autoimmune diseases has been accumulated in the setting of autoimmune pancreatitis (32,33). Of note, clinical remission can occur in affected patients in up to 74 % of the cases, even without treatment (34).

HISTOPATHOLOGICAL CHARACTERISTICS

Heterogeneous immunological cellular infiltrates invade the solid mass of pseudotumours, causing a profound desmoplastic reaction (3, 11). Coffin et al. identified plasma cells, eosinophils and lymphocytes (11) in a retrospective analysis of 84 patients with inflammatory pseudotumours originating from the abdomen, retroperitoneum, or pelvis in 61 patients, the head and neck, including upper respiratory tract in 12 patients, the trunk in eight patients and the extremities in three cases. Due to the pronounced inflammatory nature of the lesions, a causal involvement of various subtypes of infiltrating monocytes and macrophages in different polarization modes (M1 or M2 polarization states) seems plausible although there remains a paucity of clear scientific data.

IATROGENIC PSEUDOTUMOURS

Focal lesions may be identified on surveillance imaging following surgical procedures on the liver, biliary tree and pancreas. Residual fluid collection or even haematoma within the postoperative bed can exhibit a heterogeneous appearance on imaging. Typical characteristics distinguishing these lesions from solid tumours are that surgical tissue or three-dimensional organ architectural defects usually extend to the margin of the affected organ, and no enhancement is observed on computed tomography (CT) after intravenous (IV) contrast medium. The use of packing material or specific surgical packing techniques may also hinder the interpretation of radiological imaging. Packing using the greater omentum to fill defects, a common approach in liver and pancreatic surgery, typically resembles focal homogenous fat attenuation on CT (35). The application of various agents for surgical haemostasis including the use of haemostatic compounds, such as Surgicel™ (J&J Med Tech, New Jersey, USA) may mimic the macroscopic appearance of a focal gas-containing area on imaging (36) (*Figure 66.1*) and these findings might be mistaken for biliary or postoperative abscess. Adequate communication with the surgeon, the presence of surgical metallic clips at the resection surface, and the history from the patient are helpful in obtaining the correct diagnosis.

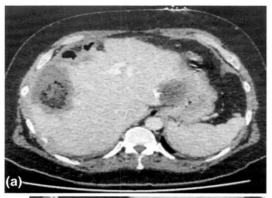

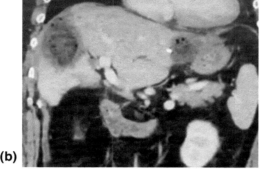

Figure 66.1 Postoperative CT imaging findings; axial (a) and coronal (b) following liver resection. Images show a collection at the surgical site, which might mimic postoperative abscess formation. In this case, surgical haemostasis using Surgicel™ (J&J Med Tech, New Jersey, USA) was performed. On imaging, this corresponds directly to the area of presumed abscess formation. Arrows show focal gas-containing area and pseudotumour formation.

Injury from the use of a surgical retractor may occur in patients who require prolonged mechanical liver retraction. This can be seen in patients undergoing laparoscopic or open abdominal surgery. Different surgical systems are used worldwide and the most common are the laparoscopic Nathanson liver retractor (Mediflex Surgical Products, NY, USA), Omni-Tract® (Integra LifeSciences, NJ, USA) and the Rochard retractor system (Surtex Instruments, Surrey, UK). Mild parenchymal injuries to the liver and bile ducts occur frequently, but generally resolve spontaneously without specific management and elevated liver enzymes normalize within a few days. Retractor injuries do not typically produce a mass effect or loss of vascular signal on imaging although they can imitate and be mistaken for an ill-defined neoplastic process. Yassa et al. reported the occurrence of hypoattenuating areas in the liver on non-contrast CT following retractor injuries and the same lesions were shown to have heterogeneous enhancement on contrast-enhanced CT (CECT) (37).

Percutaneous intervention involving the bile ducts and liver, including ultrasound (US) or CT-guided biopsies or percutaneous transhepatic cholangiography (PTC), especially with drain insertion into the biliary tree, may lead to focal post-interventional abnormalities (38). Even after standard laparoscopic procedures such as laparoscopic cholecystectomy with clipping of the cystic duct, migration of the surgical clips into the bile ducts has been demonstrated in a small number of patients (39) (*Figure 66.2*). The most common post procedural complication is acute bleeding and haematoma formation and because the haematoma is within adjacent and viable tissues and organs, most frequently the liver, contrast enhancement may sometimes be detected on clinical imaging. In this setting, follow-up imaging with documentation of the decrease in size of the lesion may help to distinguish a haematoma from other solid lesions or tumours.

Transarterial chemoembolization (TACE) of the liver is an established approach to deliver localized chemotherapy to intrahepatic malignancies, combined with selective embolization of the tumour vasculature (40). The most common indications are palliative treatment for unresectable liver cancer, or as 'bridging therapy' for hepatocellular carcinoma patients on a transplant waiting list. Some of the post-interventional findings, which may occur as a complication following the procedure, pose diagnostic challenges due to pseudotumour formation and post-procedural CT imaging often reveals unusual findings. Necrosis following embolization of the tumour vessels with gas appearance is recognized (41) and this process can mimic biliary or hepatic abscesses or tumours. The absence of marked fluid collections at the lesion site and the history of previous intervention should suggest the correct diagnosis and allow appropriate management (42).

The occurrence of pancreatic head pseudotumours is well documented following endoscopic retrograde cholangiopancreatography (ERCP), especially when a papillotomy has been performed (43). Papillotomy involves division of the muscle fibres of the ampulla of Vater with electrocautery in order to improve bile drainage and allow the passage or retrieval of stones from the CBD. It is performed using a diathermy wire through a duodenoscope during ERCP and De Vries et al. studied the outcome of patients undergoing ERCP and interventional papillotomy (43) with pre- and post-procedure CT. Pseudotumours were detected in 17% of papillotomy patients compared with patients who had not undergone a papillotomy where no pseudotumours were detected.

While the intraperitoneal location of the liver and biliary tree means that trauma-induced inflammatory pseudotumours after foreign body ingestion are uncommon, there are case reports that detail penetration through the wall of the GI tract (44–46). Most often these pseudotumours occur in the left liver lobe, however cases of a toothpick in the right liver lobe or a migrated

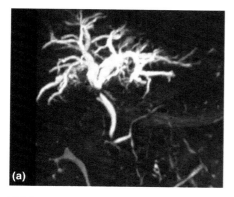

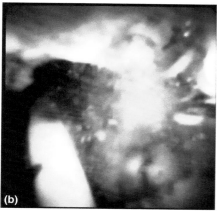

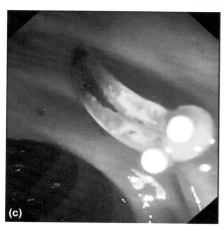

Figure 66.2 Pseudotumour formation caused by a migrated surgical clipping material into the biliary tree leading to obstruction of the bile duct and mimicking hilar cholangiocarcinoma. MRCP showing a lesion (structure), directly after the confluence of the left- and right-hepatic duct, highly suspicious for a Klatskin tumour (a) (39). ERCP and cholangioscopy revealing a Hem-a-lok® (Teleflex, NC, USA) surgical clip used at the time of laparoscopic cholecystectomy, that has migrated into the main bile duct (b) (39). Using ERCP, the clip has been mobilized into the duodenum prior to removal (c) (39).

fishbone with a concomitant plasma alpha-fetoprotein (AFP) increase have been documented (45–49).

CLINICAL SYMPTOMS AND DIAGNOSIS

There are myriad presenting complaints of patients who have developed pseudotumours and these will depend on the specific underlying cause and anatomical situation. The most common complaints are upper abdominal distension and right-sided or right upper quadrant abdominal pain. Fever is common in patients with abscess manifestation, or cholangitic and septic complications. In patients with deranged liver enzymes and elevated plasma bilirubin, clinical jaundice may occur. Appropriate imaging with a CECT and/or magnetic resonance imaging (MRI), are the established diagnostic modalities to further define the morphology of the lesion and the underlying cause. In some patients with chronically prolonged inflammation, elevated levels of tumour biomarkers such as AFP, cancer antigen 19-9 (CA 19-9) and carcinoembryonic antigen (CEA) can be detected (50–52). Correct and thorough patient examination and eliciting a history of previous interventions or surgical procedures involving the hepatobiliary tract are of key importance.

CLINICAL MANAGEMENT AND PRACTICAL CONSIDERATIONS

A meticulous work-up is required for most cases where pseudotumour formation is considered and a malignant process has to be excluded. *Table 66.1* illustrates some practical considerations regarding the timing and use of different imaging modalities and *Figure 66.3* is a decision-making algorithm outlining the suggested diagnostic pathway.

A thorough and exact medical history is of key importance and should always include detailed questioning about previous surgical procedures with an emphasis on abdominal operations. In this setting, old medical notes detailing any procedures are crucial as they will contain details concerning the use of foreign material, surgical clips, haemostatic agents and theatre checklists. Prior to considering surgical exploration, adequate imaging is essential to gain as much information as possible about the lesion under investigation. US is useful to determine the extent of any vasculature, echo or shadowing effects, and the density of tissues or presumed foreign bodies. An X-ray provides an easily accessible and good overview and might help in uncovering packing material or foreign bodies especially if metallic. A CT of the abdomen with IV contrast, especially a triple phase CT with additional arterial and portal venous phases, is the modality of choice to detect contrast extravasation, infiltration of adjacent tissues and organs, arterial enhancement with neoplastic lesions, such as hepatocellular and

Table 66.1 Practical considerations for the use of different management modalities in the work-up process for Pseudotumours

Management tools	Indications/Practical considerations
Past medical history	• Previous abdominal operations • Use of foreign material • Surgical clips • Haemostatic material • Theatre nurse count sheets
US	• Extent of vasculature • Echo or shadowing effects • Densities of tissues • Foreign body
X-ray	• Good overview • Approximate location • Signs of contained or free perforation/free gas • Packing material • Foreign body
CT (contrast-enhanced [CECT], oral contrast)	• Infiltration of adjacent tissues and organs • Features concerning for malignancy • Contrast extravasation • Signs of contained or free perforation/free gas • Rim enhancement with contrast/abscess • Arterial enhancement • Hypodense or isodense lesions • Pneumobilia
MRI/MRCP	• Bile duct anatomy • Infiltration of adjacent tissues and organs • Features concerning for malignancy • Helpful for depicting small processes • Limitations: Presence of metallic implants and foreign bodies
PET-CT	• Assessment of metabolic activity of the lesion • Features concerning for malignancy • Limitations: Chronic inflammatory processes might also exhibit increased metabolic activity
EUS	• Detailed morphology, anatomy and disease extent • Vasculature • Tissue biopsies • Limitations: Invasive procedure and associated risks
Surgery (laparoscopic / open)	• Tissue biopsy or resection • Potential cure in case of malignancy • Symptomatic relief • Limitations: Invasive procedure and associated risks

cholangiocarcinoma, hypodense or isodense lesions and pneumobilia.

Further options for abdominal imaging include MRI, MRCP (magnetic resonance cholangio pancreatography) and positron emission CT (PET-CT). MRCP is the 'gold standard' for delineating biliary anatomy, MRI can be helpful to further examine involved tissues and low volume and small processes and lesions involving the biliary tree, liver and pancreas. MRI is limited in some instances due to the presence of metallic implants and foreign bodies which should be considered where this is likely from a previous surgical procedure. The use of fluorodeoxyglucose (FDG) positron emission tomography (PET) (FDG-PET) provides a reliable tool to assess the metabolic activity of the lesion. In case of malignant transformation, the FDG uptake and activity in the vicinity of the lesion are likely to be increased when compared with the normal adjacent parenchyma but inflammatory processes also frequently show increased avidity. Endoscopic ultrasound (EUS) is a minimally invasive procedure and is very valuable in providing detailed imaging of the morphology, anatomy and disease extent of the involved upper GI tract. In addition, there is the option to obtain representative tissue samples for histological examination. As the *ultima ratio*, a laparoscopic or open surgical exploration with tissue biopsy or resection is warranted

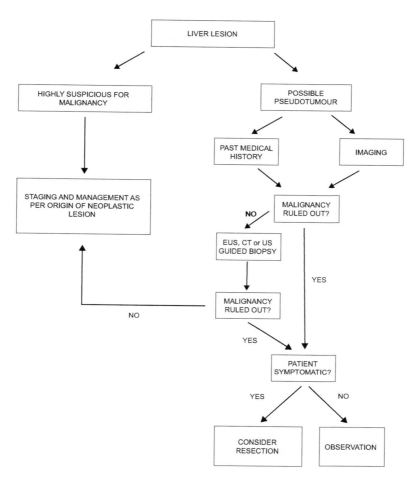

Figure 66.3 Decision-making algorithm outlining a diagnostic pathway for pseudotumour identification and treatment.

in cases where a malignancy cannot be ruled out or in symptomatic patients.

SUMMARY

In the clinical setting, BIPs represent a major problem for clinicians due to their potential to mimic malignant processes, especially if located at the liver hilum, distal CBD or the region of the pancreatic head. This diagnostic dilemma not infrequently results in major, unnecessary abdominal surgery with its significant associated morbidity and mortality. The possibility of pseudotumour formation in the setting of iatrogenic injury or trauma should always be considered and it is essential to consider the probability of BIP in any patient with a tumorous mass or poorly defined processes affecting the liver, biliary tree or pancreas. Patients should be investigated and considered for surgical management. If, after a thorough history, optimal work-up and clinical imaging, malignancy cannot be excluded, a

laparoscopy or formal exploration is justified. In patients with pseudotumours, in whom underlying infection, septic or autoimmune complications are confirmed as a primary source for the pseudotumour occurrence, and a malignant process is ruled out, a disease specific and individually tailored therapeutic approach should be considered the treatment of choice.

REFERENCES

1. Nonomura A, Minato H, Shimizu K, et al. Hepatic hilar inflammatory pseudotumor mimicking cholangiocarcinoma with cholangitis and phlebitis: A variant of primary sclerosing cholangitis? *Pathol Res Pract* 1997;**193**(**7**):519–25.
2. Amankonah TD, Strom CB, Vierl ing JM, et al. Inflammatory pseudotumor of the liver as the first manifestation of Crohn's disease. *Am J Gastroenterol* 2001;**96**(**8**):2520–22.
3. Coffin CM, Humphrey PA, Dehner, LP. Extrapulmonary inflammatory myofibroblastic tumor: A

clinical and pathological survey. *Semin Diagn Pathol* 1998;**15(2)**:85–101.

4. Tang N, Jiao Y, Wang Y, She C, Wang J, Wei Z, Liu B. Inflammatory demyelinating pseudotumor with liver dysfunction: IgG4 related disease with primary biliary cholangitis. *Am J Med Sci* 2020;**360(4)**:410–13.

5. Sasahira N, Kawabe T, Nakamura A, et al. Inflammatory pseudotumor of the liver and peripheral eosinophilia in autoimmune pancreatitis. *World J Gastroenterol* 2005;**11(6)**:922–5.

6. Katabathina VS, Dasyam AK, Dasyam N, Hosseinzadeh K. Adult bile duct strictures: Role of MR imaging and MR cholangiopancreatography in characterization. *Radiographics* 2014;**34(3)**:565–86.

7. Thanage R, Jain S, Sonthalia N, Udgirkar S, Chandnani S, Contractor Q , Rathi P. An enigmatic liver mass in a child. *Euroasian J Hepatogastroenterol* 2019;**9(2)**:104–7.

8. Blachar A, Federle MP, Sosna J. Liver lesions with hepatic capsular retraction. *Semin Ultrasound CT MR* 2009;**30(5)**:426–35.

9. Sok D, Boerma EJ, Tan PB. A remarkable subhepatic tumour. *Neth J Surg* 1989;**41(5)**:114–6.

10. Knoefel WT, Prenzel KL, Peiper M, et al. Klatskin tumors and Klatskin mimicking lesions of the biliary tree. *Eur J Surg Oncol* 2003;**29(8)**:658–61.

11. Corvera CU, Blumgart LH, Darvishian H, et al. Clinical and pathologic features of proximal biliary strictures masquerading as hilar cholangiocarcinoma. *J Am Coll Surg* 2005;**201(6)**:862–9.

12. Bai S, Maykel JA, Yang MX. Inflammatory pseudotumor associated with HSV infection of rectal vascular endothelium in a patient with HIV: A case report and literature review. *BMC Infect Dis* 2020;**20(1)**:234.

13. Chesdachai S, Udompap P, Li F, Lake JR, Kc M. Pulmonary mycobacterium spindle cell pseudotumor in patient with liver transplant. *Am J Med Sci* 2020;**359(1)**:42–50.

14. Sfeir MM, Schuetz A, Van Besien K, Borczuk AC, Soave R, Jenkins SG, Walsh TJ, Small CB. Mycobacterial spindle cell pseudotumour: Epidemiology and clinical outcomes. *J Clin Pathol* 2018;**71(7)**:626–30.

15. Lee HE, Zhang L. Immunoglobulin G4-related hepatobiliary disease. *Semin Diagn Pathol* 2019;**36(6)**: 423–33.

16. Van Baeten C, Van Dorpe J. Splenic Epstein-Barr virus-associated inflammatory pseudotumor. *Arch Pathol Lab Med* 2017;**141(5)**:722–7.

17. Kazemimood R, Saei Hamedani F, Sharif A, Gaitonde S, Wiley E, Giulianotti PC, Groth JV. A rare case of Epstein-Barr virus negative inflammatory pseudotumor-like follicular dendritic cell sarcoma presenting as a solitary colonic mass in a 53-Year-Old Woman: Case report and review of literature. *Appl Immunohistochem Mol Morphol* 2017;**25(5)**: e30–e33.

18. You Y, Shao H, Bui K, Bui M, Klapman J, Cui Q, Coppola D. Epstein-Barr virus positive inflammatory pseudotumor of the liver: Report of a challenging case and review of the literature. *Ann Clin Lab Sci* 2014;**44(4)**:489–98.

19. Deyrup AT. Epstein-Barr virus-associated epithelial and mesenchymal neoplasms. *Hum Pathol* 2008;**39(4)**:473–83.

20. Yoon KH, Ha HK, Lee JS, et al. Inflammatory pseudotumor of the liver in patients with recurrent pyogenic cholangitis: CT: Histopathologic correlation. *Radiology* 1999;**211(2)**:373–9.

21. Someren A. Inflammatory pseudotumor of liver with occlusive phlebitis: Report of a case in a child and review of the literature. *Am J Clin Pathol* 1978;**69(2)**: 176–81.

22. Zen Y. The pathology of IgG4-related disease in the bile duct and pancreas. *Semin Liver Dis* 2016; **36(3)**:242–56.

23. Bae SK, Abiru S, Kamohara Y, Hashimoto S, Otani M, Saeki A, Nagaoka S, Yamasaki K, Komori A, Ito M, Fujioka H, Yatsuhashi H. Hepatic inflammatory pseudotumor associated with xanthogranulomatous cholangitis mimicking cholangiocarcinoma. *Intern Med* 2015;**54(7)**:771–5.

24. Mittal PK, Moreno CC, Kalb B, Mittal A, Camacho JC, Maddu K, Kitajima HD, Quigley BC, Kokabi N, Small WC. Primary biliary tract malignancies: MRI spectrum and mimics with histopathological correlation. *Abdom Imaging* 2015;**40(6)**:1520–57.

25. Kanhere HA, Trochsler MI, Pierides J, Maddern GJ. Atypical mycobacterial infection mimicking metastatic cholangiocarcinoma. *J Surg Case Rep* 2013;**2013(6)**:rjt038.

26. Pickhardt PJ, Bhalla S. Unusual non neoplastic peritoneal and subperitoneal conditions: CT findings. *Radiographics* 2005;**25(3)**:719–30.

27. Agarwal R, Srinivas R, Aggarwal AN. Parenchymal pseudotumoral tuberculosis: Case series and systematic review of literature. *Respir Med* 2008;**102(3)**:382–9.

28. Kanno A, Ikeda E, Ando K, Nagai H, Miwata T, Kawasaki Y, Tada Y, Yokoyama K, Numao N, Ushio J, Tamada K, Lefor AK, Yamamoto H. The diagnosis of autoimmune pancreatitis using endoscopic ultrasonography. *Diagnostics (Basel)* 2020;**10(12)**:1005.

29. Rebours V, Lévy P. Pancreatic and biliary tract involvement in IgG4-related disease. *Presse Med* 2020;**49(1)**:104015.

30. Lee SL, DuBois JJ. Hepatic inflammatory pseudotumor: Case report, review of the literature, and a proposal for morphologic classification. *Pediatr Surg Int* 2001;**17(7)**:555–9.

31. Demir AM, Aydin F, Acar B, Kurt T, Poyraz A, Kiremitci S, Gülleroglu B, Azili MN, Bayrakci US. IgG4-related disease and ANCA positive vasculitis in childhood: A case-based review. *Clin Rheumatol* 2021;**40(9)**:3817–25.

32. Wu Z, MacPhee IA, Oliveira DB. Reactive oxygen species in the initiation of IL-4 driven autoimmunity as a potential therapeutic target. *Curr Pharm Des* 2004;**10(8)**:899–913.

33. Stone JH, Zen Y, Deshpande V: IgG4-related disease. *N Engl J Med* 2012;**366**:539–51.

34. Hart PA, Topazian MD, Witzig TE, et al. Treatment of relapsing autoimmune pancreatitis with immunomodulators and rituximab: The Mayo Clinic experience. *Gut* 2013;**62**:1607–15.

35. Kamisawa T, Shimosegawa T, Okazaki K, et al. Standard steroid treatment for autoimmune pancreatitis. *Gut* 2009;**58**:1504–7.

36. Fultz PJ, Hampton WR, Skucas J, Sickel JZ. Differential diagnosis of fat-containing lesions with abdominal and pelvic CT. *Radiographics* 1993;**13(6)**:1265–80.

37. Arnold AC, Sodickson A. Postoperative Surgicel mimicking abscesses following cholecystectomy and liver biopsy. *Emerg Radiol* 2008;**15(3)**:183–5.

38. Yassa NA, Peters JH. CT of focal hepatic injury due to surgical retractor. *AJR Am J Roentgenol* 1996;**166(3)**:599–602.

39. Truniger Samuel, Peter Ueli. Schmerzloser Ikterus bei extrahepatischer Cholestase. *Swiss Med Forum* 2021;**21(0708)**:135–7.

40. Filippone A, Iezzi R, Di Fabio F, Cianci R, Grassedonio E, Storto ML. Multidetector-row computed tomography of focal liver lesions treated by radiofrequency ablation: Spectrum of finding at long-term follow-up. *J Comput Assist Tomogr* 2007;**31(1)**:42–52.

41. Atanasov G, Dino K, Schierle K, Dietel C, Aust G, Pratschke J, Seehofer D, Schmelzle M, Hau HM. Recipient hepatic tumor-associated immunologic infiltrates predict outcomes after liver transplantation for hepatocellular carcinoma. *Ann Transplant* 2020;**25**:e919414.

42. Scholz A, Langer M, Langer R, Felix R, Neuhaus P. Intra-arterial chemoembolization of non-resectable hepatocellular carcinoma [in German]. *Rofo* 1991;**154(3)**:258–61.

43. Sakamoto N, Monzawa S, Nagano H, Nishizaki H, Arai Y, Sugimura K. Acute tumor lysis syndrome caused by transcatheter oily chemoembolization in a patient with a large hepatocellular carcinoma. *Cardiovasc Intervent Radiol* 2007;**30(3)**:508–11.

44. de Vries JH, Duijm LE, Dekker W, Guit GL, Ferwerda J, Scholten ET. CT before and after ERCP: Detection of pancreatic pseudotumor, asymptomatic retroperitoneal perforation, and duodenal diverticulum. *Gastrointest Endosc* 1997;**45(3)**:231–5.

45. Nishimoto, Yuko Suita, Sachiyo Taguchi, Tomoaki Noguchi, Shin-IchiIeiri, Satoshi. Hepatic foreign body – a sewing needle – in a child. *Asian J Surg* 2003;**26(4)**:231–3.

46. Aftab Z, Ali SM, Koliyadan S, Al-Kindi N. Foreign body in the liver: Case report and review of literature. *Qatar Med J* 2015;**2015(1)**:5.

47. Singhal V. Chintamani, P. Lubhana, R. Durkhere, S. Bhandari. Liver abscess secondary to a broken needle migration: A case report. *BMC Surg* 2003;**3**:8.

48. Patnana M, Sevrukov AB, Elsayes KM, et al. Inflammatory pseudotumor: The great mimicker. *AJR Am J Roentgenol* 2012;**198(3)**:W217–27.

49. Endo S, Watanabe Y, Abe Y, Shinkawa T, Tamiya S, Nishihara K, Nakano T. Hepatic inflammatory pseudotumor associated with primary biliary cholangitis and elevated alpha-fetoprotein lectin 3 fraction mimicking hepatocellular carcinoma. *Surg Case Rep* 2018;**4(1)**:114.

50. Perera MT, Wijesuriya SR, Kumarage SK, Ariyaratne MH, Deen KI. Inflammatory pseudotumour of the liver caused by a migrated fish bone. *Ceylon Med J* 2007;**52(4)**:141–2.

51. Misao T, Satoh K, Nakano H, Yamamoto Y. Pulmonary inflammatory pseudotumor with rapid growth and serum carcinoembryonic antigen elevation. *Jpn J Thorac Cardiovasc Surg* 2003;**51(3)**:104–6.

52. Shirai Y, Shiba H, Fujiwara Y, Eto K, Misawa T, Yanaga K. Hepatic inflammatory pseudotumor with elevated serum CA19-9 level mimicking liver metastasis rom rectal cancer: Report of a case. *Int Surg* 2013;**98(4)**:324–9.

Chapter
67

Gallstone Disease

Helen Pham and Arthur Richardson

INTRODUCTION

Cholelithiasis (gallstones) are common and occur in 5–25% of the adult population. Symptomatic gallstone disease is one of the most common gastrointestinal (GI) complaints accounting for more than 225 000 admissions per year (1). The prevalence of cholelithiasis has geographical variability and is seen to be higher in Western countries with a prevalence rate estimated to be 15–20%. Worldwide, it is higher in Caucasian, Native American and Hispanic populations, and lowest in African and Asian populations at 5%. In higher-income countries, there has been an increase in prevalence rates possibly due to high carbohydrate, high fat diets and increasingly sedentary behaviour (2). This chapter focuses on risk factors for developing gallstones, common presentations and diagnosis of gallstone disease.

CLASSIFICATION

Gallstones are classified depending on their predominant composition. Cholesterol stones represent the majority of gallstones and account for up to 80% of stones although the majority have mixed compositions and also contain bilirubinate salts and calcium palmitate. Cholesterol stones form due to an imbalance of cholesterol solubility in bile, supersaturation of bile and gallbladder hypomotility. The presence of cholesterol and supersaturated bile is lithogenic and is modified by endogenous factors such as low bile salts, gallbladder hypomotility, changes in biliary-intestinal microbiome, abnormal lipid transport and increased cholesterol levels. Macroscopically, cholesterol stones are yellow in colour and variable in size and shape.

Pigment stones occur due to abnormal bilirubin metabolism and can be further classified as brown pigment stones (15–20%) or black stones (<5%). Brown stones are composed of bilirubin and calcium, commonly resulting from infection and biliary stasis. They can form in any part of the biliary tract and occur due to excess bacterial β-glucuronidase resulting in hydrolysis of bilirubin glucuronide into free bilirubin and glucuronic acid, which binds to calcium to form stones in the presence of mucin gel traps. Brown pigment stones are frequent in Asia and are associated with conditions such as primary sclerosing cholangitis, strictures, or infections such as recurrent pyogenic cholangitis. Black pigment stones are composed of calcium bilirubinate and mucin glycoproteins and are associated with haemolysis in conditions such as haemolytic anaemias, chronic liver disease and ileal resection or bypass.

RISK FACTORS

Several factors are associated with an increased risk of developing gallstones, summarized in *Table 67.1*.

Table 67.1 Risk factors for developing gallstones

Risk factor	Details
Age and female sex	• Increasing age is associated with gallstone formation • More common in women compared to men in all age groups
Genetics	• Genetic factors affect the development of gallstones • More common in first degree female relatives compared to matched controls (3) • In a Swedish study, genetic factors accounted for a 25% risk of developing symptomatic gallstone disease (4)
Diabetes mellitus	• Mechanism is unclear, but hepatic insulin resistance appears to play a role in the predisposition to gallstones • Elevated low-density lipoprotein cholesterol associated with an increased risk of gallstones
Pregnancy	• Pregnancy associated with an increased risk of cholesterol gallstones due to increased oestrogen that results in biliary stasis and sludge formation • 20% of patients, gallstones persist after delivery

(Continued)

DOI: 10.1201/9781003080060-67

Table 67.1 (*Continued*) Risk factors for developing gallstones

Risk factor	Details
Obesity and physical inactivity	• Obesity is a risk factor for the development of cholesterol gallstones • Younger women have a reported threefold increase in incidence • Physical inactivity is a risk factor for obesity, large prospective studies have demonstrated that higher physical activity levels had a reduced risk of gallstone formation with a RR of 0.75 (5)
Rapid weight loss	• Patients who experience rapid weight loss, most commonly due to obesity surgery, have higher rates of gallstones • Thought to be due to changes in bile composition during periods of weight loss and an increase in the concentration of calcium which promotes cholesterol nucleation
Medications	• Fibrates • Somatostatin analogues • Oestrogen therapy • Ceftriaxone • Thiazide diuretics
Total parenteral nutrition (TPN)	• Lack of enteral stimulation leads to biliary stasis and the formation of microlithiasis • In critically ill patients, biliary sludge is present on US in up to 50% of patients after prolonged TPN and in many cases resolves after TPN is stopped
Ileal Crohn's disease	Associated with the formation of pigment stones due to: • Altered enterohepatic bilirubin circulation
Cirrhosis	Associated with risk of pigment stones due to: • Abnormal bile salt metabolism • High oestrogen levels • Impaired gallbladder contraction
Spinal cord injury	Patients with spinal cord injury are at high risk of gallstone formation due to: • Reduced gallbladder motility • Decreased enterohepatic circulation • Abnormal biliary lipid secretion (6)

NATURAL HISTORY

The majority of patients with gallstones are asymptomatic and the diagnosis is often made incidentally. The majority remain asymptomatic for the remainder of their lives and only 10–15% of patients go on to present with biliary colic in the following 10–15 years. Those who initially present with symptoms have a 2–3% per year risk of developing complicated gallstone disease such as cholecystitis, pancreatitis or choledocholithiasis. For those patients who develop complicated gallstone disease, there is a 30% risk of recurrence within 12 months.

PRESENTATION

Biliary colic

Patients with gallbladder stones can present with biliary colic which manifests as characteristic episodic attacks of epigastric or right upper abdominal quadrant (RUQ) pain lasting for 20–30 minutes with radiation to the back. This is typically precipitated by a fatty meal, often associated with nausea or vomiting and improves with administration of analgesics. These symptoms are due to contraction of the gallbladder in response to neural or hormonal stimulation. This can cause gallbladder outlet obstruction due to a stone lodging in the neck of the gallbladder and when the stone dislodges symptoms resolve. Patients with biliary colic often have a normal full blood count (FBC), liver function tests (LFTs) and lipase. Symptomatic patients should undergo imaging to confirm the presence of gallstones or sludge.

In asymptomatic gallstone patients, the majority can be managed expectantly and if symptoms subsequently develop, patients can then be referred for a cholecystectomy. It has been demonstrated that prophylactic cholecystectomy, in patients with asymptomatic gallstones, is not beneficial as the risk of developing life-threatening sequelae is low. This approach nevertheless has to take into account the age and fitness of the patient. In younger, very fit patients, the risks and benefits should be discussed. In cases where patients are at risk of developing symptoms, such as those following bariatric surgery or patients at risk of developing gallbladder malignancy, cholecystectomy may be considered. In general, fit patients with symptomatic gallbladder disease should be treated surgically and elective laparoscopic cholecystectomy is the treatment of choice.

Cholecystitis

Acute cholecystitis is the most common complication of gallstone disease, characterized by inflammation of the gallbladder and may occur due to persistent outlet obstruction resulting in an increased intraluminal pressure. This is associated with: 1) RUQ pain lasting for more than 6 hours; 2) fever and 3) nausea or vomiting. Acute cholecystitis is often associated with a positive Murphy's sign, pyrexia is common and an enlarged palpable gallbladder is present in one-third of patients. The diagnosis of acute cholecystitis relies on clinical examination and diagnostic imaging which are outlined in the 2018 Tokyo guidelines (7) (*Table 67.2*).

Table 67.2 Diagnostic criteria for acute cholecystitis (Tokyo guidelines) (7)

A: Local signs of inflammation

- Murphy's sign
- RUQ pain/tenderness

B: Systemic signs of inflammation

- Fever
- Elevated CRP
- Leucocytosis

C: Imaging findings

- Findings characteristic of cholecystitis

Diagnosis

Suspected diagnosis = A + B

Definite diagnosis = A + B + C

Abbreviations: CRP: C-reactive protein; RUQ: right upper abdominal quadrant.

Other complications

Severe complications occur in 10–30% of patients with cholecystitis, including empyema of the gallbladder, mucocele and gallbladder perforation. Gallstones are the most common cause of acute pancreatitis due to intermittent obstruction of the pancreatic duct. When an impacted gallstone compresses the bile duct, this can lead to obstructive jaundice due to Mirizzi's syndrome. A fistulous tract may develop between the gallbladder and bowel. This may occur in up to 1% of patients and passage of large stones through the fistula can manifest as gallstone ileus.

DIAGNOSIS

Laboratory tests

Patients with gallstone disease should have a FBC, electrolytes, and LFTs with particular attention being paid to the bilirubin and alkaline phosphatase levels to look for the obstructive sequelae of gallstone disease. Other inflammatory markers such as C-reactive protein and coagulation studies can be performed when indicated. In addition, serum amylase and lipase should be performed to exclude pancreatitis.

Transabdominal ultrasound

Transabdominal US (TAUS) is indicated in all patients with suspected gallstone disease and is considered the investigation of choice. It is non-invasive, readily available, and inexpensive. On US, gallstones appear as echogenic foci (*Figure 67.1a*) with posterior acoustic shadowing (*Figure 67.1b*). US has been reported to have a sensitivity of 84% and specificity of 99% for the detection of gallstones (8) and can identify stones as small as 1.5–2 mm in diameter (9). The limitations

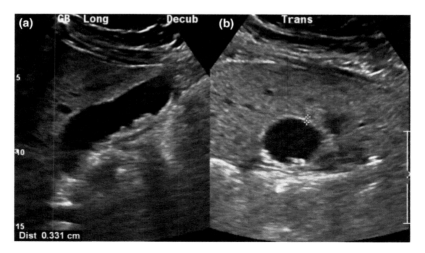

Figure 67.1 Transabdominal US of gallbladder demonstrating dependent stones (a) and associated acoustic shadowing (b).

of TAUS include obesity, operator experience and previous surgery. In cholecystitis, the typical findings include gallbladder wall thickening of greater than 3 mm, pericholecystic fluid and a positive Murphy's sign when the gallbladder is compressed by the transducer. TAUS has a sensitivity of 94% and specificity of 78% for the diagnosis of acute cholecystitis.

Computed tomography

Computed tomography (CT) has a role in complicated cholecystitis such as empyema of the gallbladder, emphysematous cholecystitis or gallbladder perforation. It is not recommended in the routine diagnosis of gallstone disease as it is less sensitive than US for the detection of gallstones ranging from 55–80% (10). Additionally, less than 10% of gallstones are radio-opaque so gallstones may be missed completely on CT scanning (*Figure 67.2*).

Endoscopic ultrasound

Using endoscopy, an US transducer, which is located at the tip of the endoscope, is placed at the gastric antrum which allows visualization of the gallbladder. Use of endoscopic US (EUS) is indicated in patients with an unconfirmed diagnosis but suspected gallstone disease. EUS has been shown to be more sensitive in the detection of small stones and microlithiasis with a sensitivity and specificity of 96% and 86%, respectively (11). EUS may be useful in obese patients and those with abnormal anatomy but requires specialized training and equipment which may not be widely available.

Magnetic resonance cholangiopancreatography

Magnetic resonance cholangiopancreatography (MRCP) is useful for the visualization of the biliary tree and pancreatic ducts but is not recommended for the routine detection of gallstones. As well as bile duct dilation, MRCP can detect bile duct stones with a sensitivity of 85%. Its limitations include overall cost, patient claustrophobia and contraindication in patients with pacemakers (*Figure 67.3*).

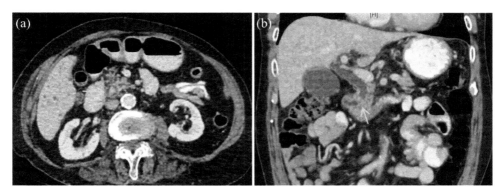

Figure 67.2 CT image of abdomen with portal-venous phase of choledocholithiasis and common bile dilation (yellow arrow). Axial (a) and coronal (b) CT images.

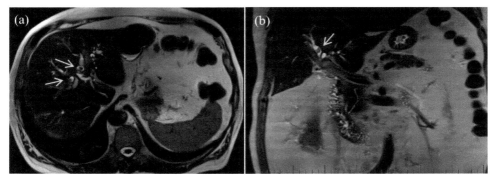

Figure 67.3 MRCP demonstrating bilateral hepatolithiasis on T2 HASTE multi-breath-hold (yellow arrows); axial (a) and coronal (b) views.

CHOLEDOCHOLITHIASIS

Choledocholithiasis can occur due to migration of stones from the gallbladder (secondary stones) or less commonly, stones that formed within the bile duct (primary stones). Up to 20% of patients with gallstone disease present with choledocholithiasis and elderly patients are at increased risk. Symptomatic choledocholithiasis may be due to acute blockage of the bile duct which is characterized by epigastric or right upper quadrant pain and may be associated with obstructive jaundice. In 10% of cases, common bile duct stones are found incidentally. Patients who present with choledocholithiasis may have abnormal liver function tests with increased bilirubin, and increased serum transaminases due to hepatocyte stress and necrosis in the first 24 hours. This is followed by a gradual rise in cholestatic enzymes, typically exhibiting a slower rise in levels than liver transaminases. TAUS may be performed to detect the presence of bile duct stones but is more likely to detect biliary tree dilation which may be an indirect indicator of choledocholithiasis. Its sensitivity in detecting bile duct stones is low, ranging from 38–82%. EUS and MRCP are the more accurate imaging modalities for detecting bile duct stones with both having a sensitivity of 93–95% and specificity of 96–97% (12). Endoscopic retrograde cholangiography (ERCP) is indicated if there is detection of choledocholithiasis on imaging, preoperative jaundice, or presentation with cholangitis. ERCP is the treatment of choice for choledocholithiasis as it permits sphincterotomy and stone extraction but has associated complications such as bleeding, perforation and pancreatitis. In most cases, cholecystectomy is routinely performed in these patients to prevent further migration of stones into the bile duct.

HEPATOLITHIASIS

Intrahepatic bile duct stones, or hepatolithiasis usually occur as a consequence of bile duct strictures which can be the result of bile duct injury, or sclerosing cholangitis as well as in cholestatic conditions such as Caroli's disease. In Asian countries, hepatolithiasis is associated with recurrent pyogenic cholangitis and parasitic infections. Frequently it is found incidentally in asymptomatic patients but can present with acute cholangitis. Less commonly, patients develop long-term complications such as liver atrophy, biliary cirrhosis, intrahepatic abscesses or the development of cholangiocarcinoma. TAUS and MRCP (*Figure 67.3*) are commonly used to identify hepatolithiasis and biliary duct dilation. Areas of biliary dilation, pneumobilia, segmental liver atrophy and decreased flow may identify the location of the stones. MRCP permits identification of biliary strictures and the potential concurrent diagnosis of cholangiocarcinoma must be considered in these cases.

Treatment of hepatolithiasis is determined based on individual factors and the location of the stones. Non-invasive management options include radiological or endoscopic treatment. Peroral or percutaneous transhepatic lithotripsy where stone fragmentation occurs under visualization can be considered in some cases but long-term efficacy is limited due to stone recurrence. The success rates of complete stone removal range from 64–85% dependent on the approach (13). Hepatectomy is considered in patients with unilateral stone disease particularly when hepatic atrophy or biliary strictures are present. The advantage of surgical treatment allows for removal of hepatic stones as well as pathological ducts which reduces the risk of recurrence and the formation of cholangiocarcinoma.

SUMMARY

Gallstones are a common GI condition and occur in 5–20% of the world's population. The classification of gallstones is based on stone type, and their formation is associated with a variety of modifiable and non-modifiable risk factors. Gallstone disease can present in a variety of ways including biliary colic, cholecystitis and its complications including, gallstone pancreatitis, choledocholithiasis and hepatolithiasis.

REFERENCES

1. Peery AF, et al. Burden of gastrointestinal disease in the United States: 2012 Update. *Gastroenterology* 2012;**143(5)**:1179–1187.e3.
2. Tsai TC, Joynt KE, Orav, EJ., Gawande AA, Jha AK. Variation in surgical-readmission rates and quality of hospital care. *N Engl J Med* 2013;**369(12)**:1134–42.
3. Sarin SK, Negi VS, Dwan R, SasanS, Saraya A. High familial prevalence of gallstones in the first-degree relatives of gallstone patients. *Hepatology* 1995;**22(1)**:138–41.
4. Katsika D, Grjibovski A, Einarsson C, Lammert F, Lichtenstin P, Marschall HU. Genetic and Environmental Influences on Symptomatic Gallstone Disease: A Swedish Study of 43,141 Twin Pairs. *Hepatology* 2005;**41(5)**:1138–43.
5. Aune D, Leitzmann M, Vatten LJ. Physical activity and the risk of gallbladder disease: A systematic review and meta-analysis of cohort studies. *JPAH* 2016;**13(7)**:788–95.
6. Rotter KP, Larraín CG. Gallstones in spinal cord injury (SCI): A late medical complication? *Spinal Cord* 2003;**41(2)**:105–8.
7. Yokoe M, Hata J, Takada T, Strasberg SM, Asbun HJ, Wakabayashi G, et al. Tokyo Guidelines 2018: Diagnostic criteria and severity grading of acute cholecystitis (with videos). *J Hepatobiliary Pancreat Sci* 2018;**25(1)**:41–54.
8. Shea JA, Berlin JA, Escarce JJ, Clarke JR, Kinosian BP, Cabana MD, et al. Revised estimates of diagnostic test sensitivity and specificity in suspected biliary tract disease. *Arch Intern Med* 1994;**154(22)**:2573–81.
9. Garra BS, et al. Visibility of gallstone fragments at US and fluoroscopy: Implications for monitoring gallstone lithotripsy. *Radiology* 1990;**174(2)**:343–7.

10. Benarroch-Gampel J, Boyd CA, Sheffield KM, Townsend CM, Riall TS. Overuse of CT in patients with complicated gallstone disease. *J Am Coll Surg* 2011;**213**(**4**):524–30.

11. Dahan P, Andant C, Lévy P, Amouyal P, Amouyal G, Dumont M, et al. Prospective evaluation of endoscopic ultrasonography and microscopic examination of duodenal bile in the diagnosis of cholecystolithiasis in 45 patients with normal conventional ultrasonography. *Gut* 1996;**38**(**2**):277–81.

12. Giljaca V, Gurusamy KS, Takwoingi Y, Higgie D, Poropat G, Davor Š, et al. Endoscopic ultrasound versus magnetic resonance cholangiopancreatography for common bile duct stones. *Cochrane Database Syst Rev* 2015; **2015**(**2**):CD01154913.

13. Huang M-H, Chen C-H, Yan J-C, Yang CC, Yeh Y-H, Chou D-A, et al. Long-term outcome of percutaneous transhepatic cholangioscopic lithotomy for hepatolithiasis. *Am J Gastroenterol* 2003;**98**(**12**): 2655–62.

Bailey & Love's Essential Operations Bailey & Love's Essential Operation
Bailey & Love's Essential Operations Bailey & Love's Essential Operation
Bailey & Love's Essential Operations Bailey & Love's Essential Operation

SECTION 10 | GALLBLADDER

Chapter

68

Cholecystitis

Jack A. Helliwell and Mark A. Taylor

INTRODUCTION

Acute cholecystitis (ACC) is characterized by acute inflammation of the gallbladder and in 90–95% of cases it is caused by obstruction of the cystic duct by gallstones. Gallstones are common globally with an annual incidence of 0.6% of individuals in the Western world (*see* **Chapter 67**). The prevalence of cholelithiasis (gallstones) is variable throughout the world and in certain ethnic groups the incidence is significantly increased. The prevalence is 10–15% in adult Caucasians in developed countries (1–3) but in some groups, including Pima Indians, the prevalence can be as high as 60–70%. In the USA and Europe 80% of the gallstones are composed primarily of cholesterol and a number of risk factors have been identified. The prevalence of gallstones is 2–3 times higher in women than men which is largely a result of the significantly increased incidence during the reproductive years. The frequency of cholecystitis is highest in people aged 50–69 years old (4).

Complications related to gallstones are experienced by around 20% of patients, with an annual incidence of 1–4%. The management of gallstone disease represents a substantial workload for acute surgical services and a major burden on all healthcare systems around the world. Cholecystitis accounts for 3–10% of cases of abdominal pain worldwide (4) and in 2012 caused an estimated 651 829 emergency department visits and 389 180 hospital admissions in the USA with a mortality rate of 7 in 10 000 people (5). In 5–10% of cases, ACC occurs without the presence of gallstones, described as acalculous cholecystitis. The underlying cause of this is not well understood and is thought to involve multiple factors. Some of the factors associated with acalculous cholecystitis include: 1) Critical illness; 2) diabetes; 3) HIV infection and 4) total parenteral nutrition (TPN). Typically, patients are older and may have complications related to atherosclerosis. Although it has traditionally been predominantly linked to critical illness, up to 88% of patients will be admitted from home.

RISK FACTORS

Cholelithiasis, the presence of gallstones in the gallbladder, is the most common cause of acute cholecystitis. Several factors contribute to the development of gallstones and, subsequently, the onset of acute cholecystitis, summarized in *Table 68.1*.

Table 68.1 Factors that contribute to the development of gallstones and, subsequently, the onset of acute cholecystitis

Factor	Details

Genetic susceptibility	• Genetic factors play a crucial role in gallstone formation
	• Familial studies revealed that relatives of gallstone patients have an almost five times higher risk of developing gallstones
	• Several genes have been associated with gallstones disease including those encoding:
	  o Apolipoproteins E (APOE) and B (APOB)
	  o Cholesterol ester transporting protein (CETP)
	  o Cholecystokinin receptor A (CCKAR) (6)

Increasing age	• The risk of gallstone formation rises with increasing age, particularly after the age of 40 years
Gender	• Women are more susceptible than men to the development of gallstones • Increased risk in women is attributed to higher levels of oestrogen, which reduces gallbladder motility, facilitating bile stasis and the formation of stones and sludge • Effect is particularly notable during pregnancy, where endogenous oestrogen levels are raised, and approximately 5–30% of women may develop biliary sludge with the risk related to the number of pregnancies • Hormone replacement therapy in postmenopausal women and oral contraceptives have also been shown to increase the risk for the formation of gallstones
Obesity	• Obesity represents a significant risk factor for gallstone formation • Excess body weight can lead to alterations in bile composition and metabolism, promoting the formation of gallstones (3)

(Continued)

DOI: 10.1201/9781003080060-68

Table 68.1 (*Continued*) Factors that contribute to the development of gallstones and, subsequently, the onset of acute cholecystitis

Factor	Details
Extreme weight loss	● Such as following bariatric surgery
Medications	● Several medications have been associated with an increased risk of gallstone formation

Somatostatin analogues	● Somatostatin (SST) is a cyclic polypeptide derived from an SST precursor protein
	● STT inhibits the secretion of:
	  o Growth hormone
	  o Prolactin
	  o Thyrotropin
	  o Cholecystokinin
	  o Gastric inhibitory peptide
	  o Gastrin
	  o Motilin
	  o Neurotensin
	  o Secretin
	  o Glucagon
	  o Insulin
	  o Pancreatic polypeptides
	● Drugs such as octreotide and lanreotide can impair gallbladder and small bowel motility, influencing gallstone formation

Ceftriaxone	● An antibiotic in the cephalosporin group (cephalosporins are a class of bactericidal β-lactam antibiotics originally derived from the fungus *Acremonium*, previously known as *Cephalosporium*) ● Associated with the development of biliary sludge due to its excretion in bile and subsequent precipitation as a calcium ceftriaxone salt

Glucagon-like peptide-1 receptor agonists	● GLP-1 receptor agonists (GLP-1-RA), incretin mimetics, or GLP-1 analogues, are agonists of the GLP-1 receptor and may be associated with an increased risk of gallbladder disease due to:
	  o Reduced gallbladder motility
	  o Delayed gallbladder emptying following suppression of cholecystokinin secretion

PATHOGENESIS

ACC is primarily caused by obstruction of the gallbladder outlet due to gallstones, resulting in a sequence of events leading to inflammation. Initial episodes with short-term obstruction of the cystic duct causes biliary colic. This can be relieved as the stone spontaneously dislodges which is common. However, if the stone becomes impacted at the neck of the gallbladder, it increases the intralumenal pressure, which when coupled with cholesterol supersaturated bile, triggers an acute inflammatory response. In approximately 20% of cases, this inflammation can lead to secondary bacterial infection with enteric organisms (1). The pathogenesis of acute calculous cholecystitis can be categorized into three distinct phases. During phase one, there is an initial increase in blood flow to the gallbladder wall, with oedema, acute inflammation and bacterial translocation. Phase two is characterized by an increased pressure in the gallbladder wall, resulting in reduced blood flow, venous congestion, ischaemia, and patchy mucosal necrosis. This may subsequently lead to gallbladder perforation at a site of ischaemic

gangrene, leading to biliary peritonitis. During phase three, active evidence of repairing inflammation, proliferative fibrosis, and intra-mural abscesses can be observed. Repeated episodes of ACC may lead to the development of chronic cholecystitis, where fibrosis leads to a shrunken gallbladder and chronic inflammation becomes prominent. In some cases, this chronic condition can lead to the development of a fistula between the gallbladder and adjacent organs including the common bile duct, duodenum, abdominal wall or colon. Acalculous cholecystitis, on the other hand, is believed to result from bile stasis and disturbed gallbladder circulation. Bile stasis, caused by fasting or ileus, leads to inspissation of bile, which becomes directly toxic to the gallbladder epithelium. Disturbed gallbladder circulation can occur in critically ill patients due to a low-flow state and vasospasm induced by vasopressors. The combination of bile stasis and ischaemia caused by this reduced gallbladder circulation can subsequently lead to secondary bacterial infection. In up to 50% of patients, acalculous cholecystitis can progress to more severe complications, such as gangrene, gallbladder empyema and perforation.

DIAGNOSIS

Clinical presentation

The most frequent presentation of ACC is characterized by pain in the right upper quadrant, associated with nausea or vomiting. Upon clinical examination, tenderness in the right upper quadrant is typically observed. An important diagnostic sign is Murphy's sign (named after John Benjamin Murphy 1857–1916 who described eliciting his sign as a 'deep grip' palpation under the right costal margin with the patient upright in a seated position on deep inspiration), where firm palpation of the right upper quadrant causes the patient to involuntarily cease inspiration. Patients may also exhibit systemic signs of inflammation, such as fever, anorexia and back or shoulder pain.

For patients suspected of having acute cholecystitis, the initial work-up should include a comprehensive assessment. Blood tests can help in the initial evaluation of suspected cases and should include a full blood count (FBC) and C-reactive protein (CRP) to assess for the presence of an inflammatory response, urea and electrolytes (U&Es), liver function tests (LFTs), and amylase/lipase to exclude pancreatitis. Additionally, a chest radiograph is important to exclude right lower lobe consolidation or visceral perforation. An electrocardiograph (ECG) helps to eliminate cardiac causes. Patients with ACC typically display a significant leucocytosis and a raised alkaline phosphatase (ALP) indicating ductal occlusion. In severe cases, a raised bilirubin may be present due to an inflamed gallbladder compressing the bile duct.

The diagnosis of acute cholecystitis, according to the 2018 Tokyo guidelines (TG-18) (7), relies on a combination of clinical findings and imaging (*Table 68.2*). The sensitivity and specificity of the TG-18 criteria for ACC are 83–85%, and 37–50%, respectively.

Investigation

Ultrasonography

A transabdominal ultrasound (TAUS) is the preferred initial imaging modality for most cases of suspected ACC due to its cost-effectiveness, widespread availability, and lack of the use of ionizing radiation. It is also one of the most accurate imaging modalities with a sensitivity of 81% and a specificity of 80% for acute cholecystitis. Sonograms obtained through ultrasound (US) can visualize the presence of gallstones or sludge as well as gallbladder wall thickness and distension. They also provide valuable information about associated findings such as impacted stones or bile duct dilatation suggestive of possible concurrent choledocholithiasis (*Figure 68.1*).

Hepatic iminodiacetic acid scan

If the results of TAUS are inconclusive, further imaging options are available. The hepatic iminodiacetic acid (HIDA) scan is a diagnostic nuclear medicine test that involves injection of a radiotracer. The radiotracer is excreted with the bile, and the scan can help visualize gallbladder filling in the presence of a patent cystic duct, ruling out acute cholecystitis. The HIDA scan boasts a high sensitivity of 96% and specificity of 90% for diagnosing ACC but its use is limited due to the availability and practicality of nuclear medicine imaging. As an alternative, more commonly used imaging techniques

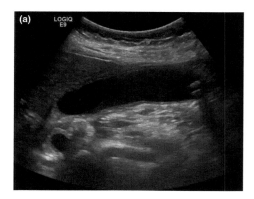

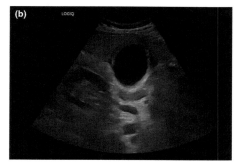

Table 68.2 Diagnostic criteria for ACC (Tokyo guidelines) (7)

A: Local signs of inflammation

- Murphy's sign
- RUQ mass, pain, or tenderness

B: Systemic signs of inflammation

- Fever
- Elevated CRP
- Elevated WBC count

C: Imaging findings

- Imaging findings characteristic of ACC

Diagnosis

Suspected diagnosis = A + B

Definite diagnosis = A + B + C

Abbreviations: CRP: C-reactive protein; RUQ: right upper abdominal quadrant; WBC: white blood count.

Figure 68.1 US scans demonstrating cholecystitis with mild mural oedema and obstructing stone (a) and thickened gallbladder and pericholecystic fluid (b).

are computed tomography (CT) or magnetic resonance cholangiopancreatography (MRCP).

Computed tomography

CT scans can provide valuable findings indicative of acute cholecystitis, such as gallbladder distension, wall thickening, subserosal oedema, mucosal enhancement, or pericholecystic fat stranding (*Figure 68.2*). In a 2012

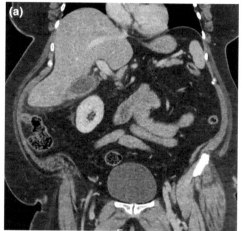

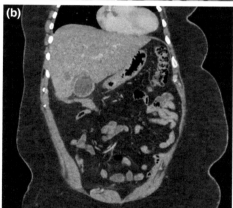

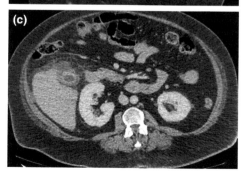

Figure 68.2 Coronal CT scans demonstrating severe cholecystitis (a) and severe cholecystitis with adjacent liver abscess (b). Axial CT scan demonstrating severe cholecystitis with fluid tracking around the liver (c).

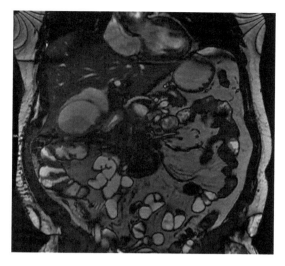

Figure 68.3 Coronal MRI scan showing inflamed and very thickened gallbladder with a large collection and contiguous involvement of the liver.

meta-analysis of 5859 patients, CT demonstrated a sensitivity of 94% and a specificity of 59% for diagnosing ACC (8). It is important to note that the detection of gallstones on CT imaging depends on their composition. Around 20% of gallstones possess a similar attenuation to bile, rendering them undetectable on CT scans.

Magnetic resonance cholangiopancreatography

MRCP provides detailed images of the biliary tree and pancreatic ducts. It may provide imaging findings suggestive of acute cholecystitis, such as gallstones lodged in the neck of the gallbladder and gallbladder wall thickening (*Figure 68.3*). MRCP is primarily used to exclude concurrent choledocholithiasis in cases where there is abnormal LFTs results or evidence of dilated bile ducts on US.

Differential diagnoses

When a patient presents with right upper quadrant pain, there are several other conditions which must be considered within the list of differential diagnoses, summarized in *Table 68.3*.

MANAGEMENT

The standard approach to treating ACC involves early laparoscopic cholecystectomy (ELC). However, in practice, a significant number of patients will initially receive conservative management, followed by a delayed, interval cholecystectomy. There are a number of reasons for this approach, including limited immediate surgeon availability, competing caseload for theatre time, and the relatively high success rate of non-operative management in resolving the acute symptoms.

Table 68.3 Conditions to consider when making a differential diagnosis

Biliary colic	• Manifests as right upper quadrant pain, typically triggered by eating • Unlike acute cholecystitis, it does not initially involve an inflammatory response, and therefore there is no fever and inflammatory markers are normal • US findings usually reveal the presence of gallstones with no evidence of gallbladder wall thickening or pericholecystic fluid
Acute cholangitis	• Presents with right upper quadrant pain • Fever and jaundice occurs when gallstones obstruct the common bile duct, leading to a superadded infection • US typically shows gallstones along with dilated intrahepatic and extrahepatic biliary ducts, indicating common bile duct obstruction
Acute pancreatitis	• Characterized by epigastric pain or right upper quadrant pain that may radiate to the back • Blood tests usually reveal elevated levels of amylase or lipase, indicating pancreatic inflammation

Non-operative management

Non-operative management consists of intravenous (IV) antibiotics, fluids, analgesics and anti-emetics. While ACC is primarily an inflammatory process, approximately 20% of cases may also involve secondary bacterial infection. Hence, antibiotics covering Gram-negative and anaerobic organisms are administered. Around 90% of patients show improvement within a few days of non-operative management but patients undergoing this approach experience prolonged hospital stays and remain at risk of recurrent episodes of cholecystitis while waiting for cholecystectomy.

Operative management

For most cases of acute cholecystitis, ELC is the preferred treatment approach. The definition of 'early' varies among surgeons and is debated in the literature, but the generally accepted definition is within 72 hours from admission. While operating after 72 hours is possible, it is generally not recommended. A review from 2020 of over 100 000 cholecystectomies revealed that patients who underwent cholecystectomy within 72 hours of admission had a lower conversion rate to open procedure (9). A 2013 open-label randomized controlled trial compared patients undergoing surgery within 24-hours of admission to those initially treated with antibiotics before undergoing cholecystectomy between 7–45 days after admission (10). Early cholecystectomy was associated with significantly lower postoperative complications, shorter hospital stays, and reduced total hospital costs.

Gallbladder drainage

Gallbladder drainage with a percutaneous cholecystostomy tube (PCT) represents an option to temporize the acute presentation in some instances. This is typically reserved for high-risk patients who have not responded to conservative treatment and are deemed unsuitable for immediate surgery. The PCT is inserted using US or CT guidance and the catheter tip is placed into the gallbladder. This facilitates decompression of the gallbladder, collection of samples for culture and drainage of infected bile, stabilizing the patient and providing time to optimize conditions for potential cholecystectomy. Quite often such an intervention may be all that is required and given the risk factors in this group of individuals a cholecystectomy is frequently not performed. A number of trials have compared cholecystostomy with emergency cholecystectomy for cholecystitis and have demonstrated the superiority of drainage in respect of morbidity and mortality. In 2013, Anderson et al. (11) examined their data from 1998–2010 and concluded that patients treated by cholecystostomy had a reduced risk of complications but an increased risk of death, longer lengths of stay, and higher total charges. In the same year, Simorov et al. published a paper entitled 'Emergent cholecystostomy is superior to open cholecystectomy in extremely ill patients with acalculous cholecystitis: A large multicentre outcome study' (11). Relevant studies are shown in *Table 68.4* (10–14). The issue remains controversial but in cases where surgery is not possible, due to comorbidities, or the condition of the patient due to their acute illness, cholecystostomy often represents an important option.

In 2012, the CHOCOLATE trial (15), a randomized controlled multicentre study comparing laparoscopic cholecystectomy with percutaneous drainage to determine the best treatment for acute calculous cholecystitis in high-risk patients concluded that laparoscopic cholecystectomy, compared with percutaneous catheter drainage, reduced the rate of major complications in high-risk patients with acute cholecystitis. Primary and secondary endpoints from the trial are summarized in *Table 68.5.*

Table 68.4 Trials comparing percutaneous cholecystostomy with emergency cholecystectomy

Study group	Time frame	Summary/Title
Anderson et al. 2013 (10)	1998–2010	A nationwide examination of outcomes of percutaneous cholecystostomy compared with cholecystectomy for ACC
Simorov et al. 2013 (11)	2007–2011	Emergent cholecystostomy is superior to open cholecystectomy in extremely ill patients with acalculous cholecystitis: A large multicentre outcome study
McGillcuddy et al. 2012 (12)	2000–2009	Non-operative management of ACC in the elderly
Melloul et al. 2011 (13)	2001–2007	Percutaneous drainage versus emergency cholecystectomy for the treatment of ACC in critically ill patients. Does it matter?
Abi-Haidar et al. 2012 (14)	2001–2010	Revisiting percutaneous cholecystostomy for ACC based on a 10-year experience

Table 68.5 Primary and secondary endpoints for participants allocated to laparoscopic cholecystectomy or percutaneous catheter drainage: Values are numbers (percentages) unless stated otherwise (15)

Outcomes	Cholecystectomy group (n = 66)	Drainage group (n = 68)	Risk ratio (95% CI)	P value
Primary endpoints				
Death	2 (3)	6 (9)	0.34 (0.07–1.64)	0.27
Major complications	8 (12)	44 (65)	0.19 (0.10–0.37)	<0.001
Secondary endpoints				
Death	2 (3)	6 (9)	0.34 (0.07–1.64)	0.27
Directly or indirectly related to cholecystitis	0	3 (4)		
Unrelated to cholecystitis	2 (3)	2 (3)		
Unknown cause	0	1 (20)		
Infectious and cardiopulmonary complications	5 (8)	3 (4)	0.97 (0.89–1.05)	0.49
Intra-abdominal abscess	4 (6)	2 (3)		
Pneumonia	2 (3)	1 (2)		
Myocardial infarction	0	0		
Pulmonary embolus	0	0		
Need for reintervention	8 (12)	45 (66)	0.18 (0.09–0.36)	<0.001
Surgical intervention	3 (5)	32 (47)	0.10 (0.03–0.30)	<0.001
Emergency cholecystectomy	NA	11 (16)		
Clinical deterioration	NA	2 (3)		
Recurrent cholecystitis	NA	9 (13)		
Elective cholecystectomy	2 (2)	20 (29)		
Recurrent gallstone related disease	NA	15 (22)		
Dysfunctional drain	NA	1 (2)		

FURTHER CONSIDERATIONS

Acute cholecystitis in older patients

Even in the context of older patients, the favoured strategy for addressing ACC is ELC when feasible. A study carried out in England examined a cohort of 47 500 patients aged 80 years or older, drawn from a national hospital database. While the study revealed a higher 30-day mortality rate among those who underwent early cholecystectomy compared to those who underwent delayed cholecystectomy (11.9% vs. 9.9%), there was a more substantial increase in mortality at 1 year for patients who received delayed cholecystectomy (20.8% vs. 27.1%; P<0.001) (16). Nevertheless, certain elderly patients with ACC might not be considered suitable candidates for surgery due to their concurrent medical conditions. A thorough risk evaluation is essential and should encompass elements such as mortality rates associated with both conservative and surgical treatment approaches, the probability of gallstone-related complications, life-expectancy, and an assessment of frailty through the use of frailty scores. For cases where surgery is not appropriate, and medical interventions are ineffective, the option of percutaneous cholecystostomy should be considered (11–16).

Acute cholecystitis during pregnancy

The incidence of ACC in pregnancy varies, with reports indicating a range from one case per 16 000 pregnancies to one case per 10 000 pregnancies. It stands as the second most common reason for non-obstetrical abdominal surgery after appendicitis. When considering the most suitable approach to managing ACC during pregnancy, several factors must be considered including: 1) The risk of complications from cholecystitis; 2) limitations in medication options based on trimester; 3) the risk of recurrence; 4) the possibility of associated complications during pregnancy and 5) the proximity to delivery or fetal maturity. Generally, laparoscopic cholecystectomy is recommended as first-line management at any trimester during pregnancy, in line with guidelines from the World Journal of Emergency General Surgery (WJEGS) and American College of Obstetrics and Gynaecologists (ACOG). Current data indicates a relatively low-risk of obstetric complications among patients undergoing non-obstetric surgical interventions. The alternative is non-operative management with IV antibiotics. However, this carries the risk of potential fetal drug toxicity and is associated with higher incidence of spontaneous abortion, threatened abortion, and premature birth when compared with those who undergo cholecystectomy. Despite the aforementioned recommendations and findings, present data indicates that roughly 60% of pregnant women with ACC receive non-operative management (17).

Acute cholecystitis in patients with cirrhosis

In patients with cirrhosis, surgical interventions carry additional risk, primarily due to the increased incidence of bleeding and other serious complications. There is a paucity of clinical data to provide definitive guidance for managing ACC in patients with liver cirrhosis. The current body of evidence suggests that cholecystectomy is safer than non-operative management for patients with a Child-Pugh score A or B, as well as those possessing a model for end-stage liver disease (**MELD**) score below 15. Nevertheless, clinicians must factor in additional clinical variables when assessing the best course of action in these patients, including age, other medical comorbidities, and the presence of ascites. In cases of advanced cirrhosis and severe portal hypertension, the risk associated with surgery is significant. Technical challenges may arise, such as difficulty safely dissecting Calot's triangle and the gallbladder hilum, the presence of neovascularization or a portal cavernoma, and difficulties in controlling bleeding originating from the liver bed. An analysis of data from the American College of Surgeons (ACS) National Surgical Quality Improvement Programme (NSQIP) revealed that among patients with a MELD score $\geq$15, the mortality rate was 3.2%. In the same analysis, the presence of ascites and a MELD score >20 was associated with an even more pronounced risk of postoperative complications of 66.7%, along with a mortality risk of 33.3%. When surgical risk becomes excessively high, consideration may be given to alternatives such as internal drainage via endoscopic retrograde cholangiopancreatography (ERCP) or endoscopic US (EUS)-guided transduodenal drainage, depending on the experience of the available clinicians (18–21).

SUMMARY

ACC is one of the most common, surgically treatable, diseases worldwide. It is usually mild, often self-limiting or settles rapidly with conservative management with antibiotics and fluid. It can however be life-threatening especially when it occurs in elderly patients or those with significant comorbidities. In addition, although generally mild, the global incidence represents a significant resource issue and ACC is a burden on all healthcare systems. A number of guidelines are available from 2018 Tokyo (TG-18) (7), American Association for the Surgery of Trauma (AAST) (22), ACS-NSQIP (23), the CHOCOLATE study and the World Society of Emergency Surgery (WSES) (20). These aid the diagnosis and management of ACC but must be interpreted in the context of available staff and resources in the patient's healthcare system. *Figure 68.4* outlines a proposed management pathway. ELC is the preferred option in fit patients within 72 hours of the onset of symptoms. This will reduce hospital length of stay, minimize disruption to the patient and manage workload most efficiently with reduced costs. In very fit patients with mild symptoms whose investigations suggest limited inflammation, cholecystectomy can be performed within 7 days.

The management of high-risk patients, either due to comorbidities or their illness, requires clinical judgement and the implementation of guidelines. Local protocols should be in place to ensure that care is standardized and appropriate with sufficient resource

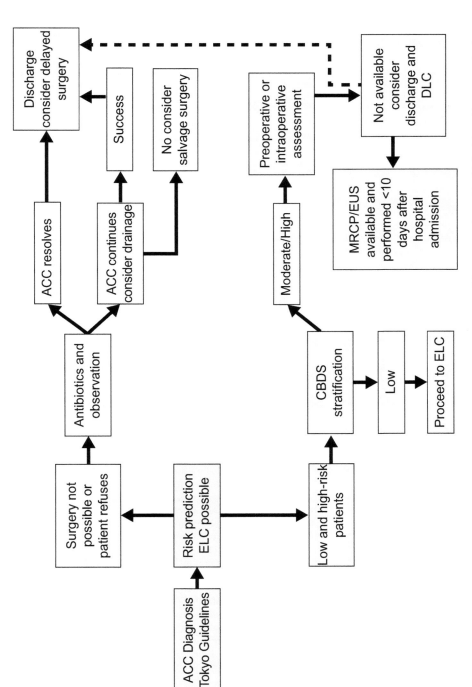

Figure 68.4 Suggested management pathway for acute cholecystitis. *Abbreviations:* ACC: acute cholecystitis; DLC: delayed laparoscopic cholecystectomy; CBDS: common bile duct stones.

to facilitate necessary investigations. Although surgery is the definitive treatment, depending on the patient's condition at presentation, antibiotics and minimally invasive drainage are often an attractive and potentially lifesaving option.

REFERENCES

1. Shaffer EA. Gallstone disease: Epidemiology of gallbladder stone disease. *Best Pract Res Clin Gastroenterol* 2006;**20(6)**:981–96.
2. Stinton LM, Myers RP, Shaffer EA. Epidemiology of gallstones. *Gastroenterol Clin North Am* 2010;**39(2)**:157–69, vii.
3. Kimura Y, Takada T, Kawarada Y, Nimura Y, Hirata K, Sekimoto M, et al. Definitions, pathophysiology, and epidemiology of acute cholangitis and cholecystitis: Tokyo Guidelines. *J Hepatobiliary Pancreat Surg* 2007;**14(1)**:15–26.
4. Peery AF, Crockett SD, Barritt AS, Dellon ES, Eluri S, Gangarosa LM, et al. Burden of gastrointestinal, liver, and pancreatic diseases in the United States. *Gastroenterology* 2015;**149(7)**:1731–41.e3.
5. Lim J, Wirth J, Wu K, Giovannucci E, Kraft P, Turman C, et al. Obesity, adiposity, and risk of symptomatic gallstone disease according to genetic susceptibility. *Clin Gastroenterol Hepatol* 2022;**20(5)**:e1083–e1120.
6. Yokoe M, Hata J, Takada T. Tokyo Guidelines 2018: Diagnostic criteria and severity grading of acute cholecystitis (with videos). *J HepatoBiliary Pancreat Sci* 2018;**25(1)**:41–54.
7. Kiewiet JJ, Leeuwenburgh MM, Bipat S, Bossuyt PM, Stoker J, Boermeester MA. A systematic review and meta-analysis of diagnostic performance of imaging in acute cholecystitis. *Radiology* 2012;**264(3)**:708–20.
8. Kirkendoll SD, Kelly E, Kramer K, Alouidor R, Winston E, Putnam T, et al. Optimal timing of cholecystectomy for acute cholecystitis: A retrospective cohort study. *Cureus* 2022;**14(8)**:e28548.
9. Gutt CN, Encke J, Köninger J, Harnoss J-C, Weigand K, Kipfmüller K, et al. Acute cholecystitis: Early versus delayed cholecystectomy, a multicenter randomized trial (ACDC Study, NCT00447304). *Ann Surg* 2013;**258(3)**:385–93.
10. Anderson JE, Chang DC, Talamini MA. A nationwide examination of outcomes of percutaneous cholecystostomy compared with cholecystectomy for acute cholecystitis, 1998–2010. *Surg Endosc* 2013;**27(9)**:3406–11.
11. Simorov A, Ranade A, Parcells J, Shaligram A, Shostrom V, et al. Emergent cholecystostomy is superior to open cholecystectomy in extremely ill patients with acalculous cholecystitis: A large multicenter outcome study. *Am J Surg* 2013:**206(6)**:935–41.
12. McGillicuddy EA, Schuster KM, Barre K, Suarez L, Hall MR, Kaml GJ, et al. Non-operative management of acute cholecystitis in the elderly. *B J Surg* 2012;**99(9)**:1254–61.
13. Melloul E, Denys A, Demartines N, Calmes J-M, Schäfer M, et al. Percutaneous drainage versus emergency cholecystectomy for the treatment of acute cholecystitis in critically ill patients: Does it matter? *World J Surg* 2011;**35**:826–33.
14. Abi-Haidar Y, Sanchez V, Williams SA, Itani KM. Revisiting percutaneous cholecystostomy for acute cholecystitis based on a 10-year experience. *Arch Surg* 2012;**147(5)**:416–22.
15. Loozen CS, van Santvoort HC, van Duijvendijk P, Besselink MG, Gouma DJ, Nieuwenhuijzen GA, et al. Laparoscopic cholecystectomy versus percutaneous catheter drainage for acute cholecystitis in high-risk patients (CHOCOLATE): Multicentre randomised clinical trial. *BMJ* 2018;**363**:k3965.
16. Wiggins T, Markar SR, Mackenzie H, Jamel S, Askari A, Faiz O, et al. Evolution in the management of acute cholecystitis in the elderly: Population-based cohort study. *Surg Endosc* 2018;**32(10)**:4078–86.
17. Rios-Diaz AJ, Oliver EA, Bevilacqua LA, Metcalfe D, Yeo CJ, Berghella V, et al. Is it safe to manage acute cholecystitis nonoperatively during pregnancy? A nationwide analysis of morbidity according to management strategy. *Ann Surg* 2020;**272(3)**:449–56.
18. Pinheiro RS, Waisberg DR, Lai Q, Andraus W, Nacif LS, Rocha-Santos V, et al. Laparoscopic cholecystectomy and cirrhosis: Patient selection and technical considerations. *Ann Laparoscopic Endo Surgery* 2017;**2(3)**: doi: 10.21037/ales.2017.01.08.
19. Hanna K, Zangbar B, Kirsch J, Bronstein M, Okumura K, Gogna S, et al. Non-operative management of cirrhotic patients with acute calculous cholecystitis: How effective is it? *Am J Surg* 2023;**226(5)**:668–74.
20. James TW, Krafft M, Croglio M, Nasr J, Baron T. EUS-guided gallbladder drainage in patients with cirrhosis: Results of a multicenter retrospective study. *Endosc Int Open* 2019;**7(9)**:E1099–E1104.
21. Schuster KM, O'Connor R, Cripps M, Kuhlenschmidt K, Taveras L, Kaafarani HM, et al. Revision of the AAST grading scale for acute cholecystitis with comparison to physiologic measures of severity. *J Trauma Acute Care Surg* 2022;**92(4)**:664–74.
22. Massoumi RL, Trevino CM, Webb TP. Postoperative complications of laparoscopic cholecystectomy for acute cholecystitis: A comparison to the ACS-NSQIP Risk Calculator and the Tokyo Guidelines. *World J Surg* 2017;**41**:935–39.
23. Pisano M, Allievi N, Gurusamy K, Borzellino G, Cimbanassi S, Boerna D, et al. 2020 World Society of Emergency Surgery updated guidelines for the diagnosis and treatment of acute calculus cholecystitis. *World J Emerg Surg* 2020;**15(1)**:61.

Chapter 69

Gallbladder Cancer

Kurt Carabott and Hou-Bao Liu

INTRODUCTION

Gallbladder cancer (GBC) is a rare but highly lethal malignancy. It is the 6th most common gastrointestinal (GI) malignancy but the most common biliary malignancy with over 115 000 new cases diagnosed worldwide in 2020. The highest incidence rates of GBC are observed in South Central Asia, North Africa and South America but the global incidence has decreased over the past three decades (1). The established risk factors for GBC are:

- Gallstones
- Gallbladder polyps >10 mm
- Porcelain gallbladder
- Primary sclerosing cholangitis
- Chronic *Salmonella* or *Helicobacter* infections
- Congenital biliary anomalies
- Obesity
- Carcinogen exposure (e.g. cigarettes, aflatoxin)
- Family history

PATHOLOGY AND STAGING OF GALLBLADDER CANCER

GBCs are staged according to the American Joint Committee on Cancer (AJCC) 8th edition staging system (*Table 69.1*) (2). TNM stage is the main determinant of the prognosis in GBC, with higher stage disease exhibiting worse prognosis. The T classification is shown in *Figure 69.1*.

Ninety per cent of all GBCs are adenocarcinomas. Other rarer malignant gallbladder tumours include squamous/adenosquamous, neuroendocrine, sarcoma/adenosarcoma and melanoma. GBCs are aggressive cancers, with direct and lymphatic spread accounting for early hepatic invasion and hepatic metastases. GBCs may also spread directly to the extrahepatic biliary tree, giving a clinical picture resembling extrahepatic cholangiocarcinoma, or may invade the GI tract, causing bowel obstruction. Lymphatic spread may occur with T1b tumours or above, once invasion of the muscular layer of the gallbladder has taken place. The regional lymph node groups commonly affected by GBC are the cystic duct, common bile duct, retroportal, proper and common hepatic artery nodes (*Figure 69.2*). Malignant extra-regional lymph nodes are considered metastatic.

MODE OF DISCOVERY

GBC may be discovered:

1 *Preoperatively*: Symptomatic patients may have GBC suspected or confirmed during clinical work-up or GBC may be discovered during the investigation of another pathology
2 *Intraoperatively*: The surgeon may encounter GBC during laparoscopic cholecystectomy for presumed benign disease
3 *Postoperatively (primary)*: GBC may be diagnosed on histology following laparoscopic cholecystectomy for presumed benign disease

Intraoperatively and postoperatively discovered GBC are collectively termed 'incidental' GBC.

Table 69.1 AJCC 8th edition staging system for gallbladder cancer

T Category	
Tx	Primary tumour cannot be assessed
Tis	Carcinoma in situ
T1	
T1a	Tumour invades the lamina propria
T1b	Tumour invades the muscular layer
T2	
T2a	Tumour invades the perimuscular connective tissue on the peritoneal side, without involvement of the serosa (visceral peritoneum)
T2b	Tumour invades the perimuscular connective tissue on the hepatic side, with no extension into the liver

(Continued)

DOI: 10.1201/9781003080060-69

Table 69.1 (*Continued*) AJCC 8th edition staging system for gallbladder cancer

T Category	
T3	Tumour perforates the serosa (visceral peritoneum) and/or directly invades the liver and/or one other adjacent organ or structure, such as the stomach, duodenum, colon, pancreas, omentum, or extrahepatic bile ducts
T4	Tumour invades the main portal vein or hepatic artery or invades two or more extrahepatic organs or structures
N Category	
Nx	Regional lymph nodes cannot be assessed
N0	No regional lymph node metastases
N1	Metastases to 1–3 regional lymph nodes
N2	Metastases to ≥4 regional lymph nodes
M Category	
M0	No distant metastases
M1	Distant metastases
Stage	
0	Tis, N0, M0
I	T1, N0, M0
IIA	T2a, N0, M0
IIB	T2b, N0, M0
IIIA	T3, N0, M0
IIIB	T1–3, N1, M0
IVA	T4, N0–1, M0
IVB	Any T, Any N, M1

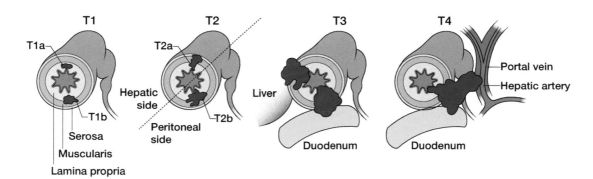

Figure 69.1 T stage classification of gallbladder cancer based on the AJCC 8th edition. Four drawings of the gallbladder transected in a vertical plane with each showing different T stages of gallbladder cancer (T1–T4) with tumour invasion into different layers of the gallbladder and/or liver, duodenum and portal vein/hepatic artery.

MANAGEMENT APPROACH

Preoperative diagnosis

For symptomatic patients, early-stage disease may cause abdominal pain and discomfort, which are frequently attributed to biliary colic or cholecystitis. Patients with more advanced disease may present with jaundice, weight loss and an abdominal mass. These symptoms are associated with lower resectability rates and poorer survival. Jaundice caused by GBC is a particularly ominous sign, but the presence of jaundice does not necessarily preclude surgery. Patients presenting with jaundice may be effectively treated by endoscopic or radiological biliary stenting while full

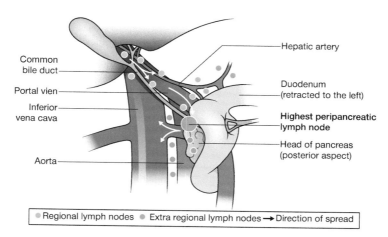

Figure 69.2 Illustration showing regional and extra-regional nodes in gallbladder cancer. A Kocher manoeuvre of the duodenum is shown, and the highest peripancreatic lymph node is highlighted. The direction of lymph node spread is demonstrated by arrows.

staging and assessment of resectability is completed. Ultrasound (US) is usually the initial modality used to investigate symptoms of suspected biliary origin. US has a low sensitivity for diagnosing GBC but may demonstrate high-risk features for malignancy such as large polyps greater than 10 mm in size, sessile polyps or focal gallbladder thickening above 4 mm, irregular inner or outer surfaces or hilar biliary obstruction. Contrast-enhanced US may improve both the sensitivity and specificity for GBC. Preoperative biopsy and tissue diagnosis of potentially resectable GBC is generally unnecessary.

Intraoperative diagnosis

The surgeon may suspect GBC if a gallbladder mass or focal gallbladder thickening is encountered at laparoscopic cholecystectomy. Other intraoperative risk factors for GBC are: 1) Gallbladder perforation; 2) conversion to open procedure; 3) cholecystitis without gallstones and 4) the presence of gallbladder polyps. When GBC is suspected intraoperatively, the diagnosis should be confirmed by frozen section at the time of surgery and if malignancy is confirmed, surgery should generally be aborted at this stage. The reasons against proceeding to a more extensive resection at index surgery include: 1) The patient's condition and inability to withstand major resection; 2) lack of consent; 3) limitation of technical skill and organizational set-up; 4) lack of information about tumour stage and 5) risk of biliary or vascular injuries in the presence of inflammation. Furthermore, extended resections are ideally performed in experienced hepatobiliary centres, where morbidity and mortality rates are lower.

Postoperative diagnosis

Postoperative diagnosis of GBC accounts for up to 60% of cases of GBC, with cancer being discovered on histology of the gallbladder following cholecystectomy for presumed benign disease. GBC is detected incidentally in 0.2–1.6% of laparoscopic cholecystectomies (3). Under these circumstances, it is imperative to scrutinize the index surgical note and intraoperative events (*Table 69.2*). Intraoperative bile spillage leads

Table 69.2 Clinical and prognostic operative variables to consider in incidental gallbladder assessment

Indication	• Biliary colic • Cholecystitis • Gallbladder polyps
Approach	• Laparoscopic • Open • Laparoscopic converted to open
Intraoperative difficulty	• Partial/subtotal cholecystectomy • Fibrotic gallbladder • Perforation/bile spillage
Gallbladder extraction	• Port site used • ? Use of extraction bag
Other findings	• Liver or peritoneal nodules
Specimen pathology	• Cystic node status (if taken) • Cystic duct margin involvement • T-stage • Tumour on hepatic or peritoneal side

almost inevitably to tumour recurrence and poor outcomes after repeat resection. The surgical approach during index cholecystectomy has no effect on patient outcome. Careful consideration of these factors can assist in planning the delivery of systemic therapy within the patient management pathway.

STAGING

Complete tumour staging should be performed for both incidental and non-incidental GBC. High-quality computed tomography (CT) of the chest, abdomen and pelvis represents the cornerstone of locoregional and distant staging of GBC and can accurately determine resectability. The accuracy of CT in assessing the T and N stages is more variable. Contrast-enhanced magnetic resonance imaging (ceMRI) is complimentary to CT and improves T-stage assessment, together achieving almost 100% accuracy. Fluorodeoxyglucose positron emission tomography (FDG-PET) has a limited role as a diagnostic test but may be a useful tool for GBC staging and will alter patient management in up to 25% of cases. FDG-PET accurately identifies lymph node and distant metastases, particularly in higher T-stage disease. In incidental GBC, postoperative FDG-PET detects residual disease in approximately half of cases, with half of these being disseminated disease. Nevertheless, the exact role of FDG-PET in GBC is controversial, mainly owing to the inability to discriminate between inflammation and malignancy. Staging laparoscopy (SL) for primary GBC is recommended and may alter management in approximately 20% of cases. For incidental GBCs, SL has a lower yield for detection of metastatic disease and using SL selectively for cases of margin-positive tumours and T3 tumours and above improves detection rates.

TIMING OF RE-RESECTION

The ideal timing of re-resection after incidentally discovered GBC remains controversial but appears to be 4–8 weeks following the index cholecystectomy. Earlier re-operation gives inadequate time for postoperative inflammation to settle and makes the repeat surgery more hazardous, while re-operation after 8 weeks may lead to disease progression. It should be emphasized that tumour biology plays a more important role in outcomes than timing. It may therefore be appropriate to delay re-resection beyond 8 weeks in patients with high-risk of disease recurrence and limit repeat surgery to patients whose disease does not progress within this timeframe.

SURGICAL APPROACH BY T STAGE

The involvement of surgical margins by tumour is one of the most important factors affecting survival after surgery. Thus, GBC is considered resectable when complete excision with negative margins (R0) can be achieved. Unfortunately, only about 25% of patients have resectable disease at the time of diagnosis. The absolute contraindications for surgery are:

- Liver or peritoneal metastases
- Distant metastases
- Malignant ascites
- Extra-regional malignant lymph nodes
- Portal vein or hepatic artery encasement
- 'Frozen' hepatoduodenal ligament
- Patients unfit for a major liver resection

Relative contradications to surgery are less clear but include the presence of jaundice and immunocompromized or immunosuppressed patients.

T1 disease

Early T1a GBC that has not yet invaded the muscular layer has an excellent prognosis. Lymph node positivity rate is 1.8% and 5-year survival following simple cholecystectomy approaches 100% (4). Simple cholecystectomy with negative margins therefore represents definitive treatment for T1a disease and no further extended resection is indicated. Conversely, T1b GBC is associated with lymph node positivity rates of up to 20% and consequently, a higher rate of disease recurrence following simple cholecystectomy alone. The current standard of care is extended cholecystectomy with partial, or complete, segment IVb/V resection and hepatoduodenal lymphadenectomy. Nevertheless, there is some controversy regarding the necessity of extended cholecystectomy for T1b tumours with some studies showing no differences in recurrence and overall survival (OS) rates between simple and extended cholecystectomy. This controversy is reflected in international guidelines, with Western guidelines recommending hepatic resection and lymphadenectomy (5,6), and Eastern guidelines recommending simple cholecystectomy (7). The optimal strategy for T1b GBC thus remains to be elucidated by further studies.

T2 disease

Lymph node positivity rates are higher in T2 disease than in T1 disease, with approximately half of T2 patients having lymph node metastases. Patients with T2 disease undergoing simple cholecystectomy have a 5-year OS of approximately 40%. Extended cholecystectomy with partial, or complete, segment IV/V resection and hepatoduodenal lymphadenectomy improves survival outcomes and is therefore considered appropriate for T2 tumours. Hepatic side (T2b) tumours have higher rates of vascular, perineural and lymph node involvement and lower OS than do peritoneal side (T2a) tumours. Nevertheless, it remains unclear whether altering the surgical strategy to simple cholecystectomy for T2a tumours and extended cholecystectomy for T2b tumours improves survival outcomes. In the absence of further data, extended resection should be undertaken for all T2 GBCs.

T3 and T4 disease

Achieving negative margins in T3 tumours often requires extensive hepatic resection up to, and including, a right hepatectomy or trisectionectomy, bile duct excision and/or extra-biliary organ resection. These patients have high rates of positive margins, residual tumour, lymph node positivity and a poor overall prognosis following a radical resection. Upfront major liver resections are associated with high morbidity and mortality with poor survival outcomes. An appropriate strategy for this subset of patients may be administering neoadjuvant therapy in the context of a clinical trial and performing the least extensive liver resection to achieve an R0 resection. Portal vein, hepatic artery and multiorgan involvement associated with T4 disease precludes curative surgery in any form.

TECHNICAL ASPECTS OF SURGERY

Technique of extended cholecystectomy (segment IVb/V resection)

The aims of a segment IVb/V resection are to remove a rim of liver tissue surrounding the gallbladder bed, taking the gallbladder *en bloc* for preoperatively diagnosed GBC and to perform a complete lymphadenectomy. An adequate 'extended cholecystectomy' liver resection may be achieved by non-anatomical resection of segments IVb/V taking a rim of 2–3 cm around the gallbladder bed or an anatomical resection of IVB/V (*Figure 69.3*). Neither of these two approaches has been shown to be superior and achieving an R0 resection is the most important factor.

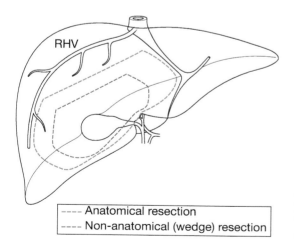

RHV

---- Anatomical resection
---- Non-anatomical (wedge) resection

Figure 69.3 Liver with surface margins of an anatomical segment IVb/V resection and a non-anatomical (wedge) segment IV/V resection outlined. The red dotted line shows the margins of an anatomical segment IVb/V resection. The green dotted line shows the margins of a non-anatomical (wedge) segment IV/V resection. *Abbreviation:* RHV: right hepatic vein.

Incision and exploration

Adequate access can be obtained by various incisions including right subcostal, upper midline, Chevron and reverse L incisions. Upon abdominal entry, it is imperative to carefully assess for peritoneal as well as liver metastases. Intraoperative ultrasound (IOUS) should be used to detect intrahepatic lesions too small to have been detected on preoperative imaging and any evidence of disseminated disease precludes curative surgery. Liver mobilization is not necessary but partial division of the falciform ligaments and right triangular ligaments may facilitate liver resection. At this stage, if a cholecystectomy was previously performed, the cystic duct stump may be excised and sent for frozen section analysis.

Lymphadenectomy

Lymphadenectomy is performed for all T1b tumours and above. Malignant extra-regional nodes need to be excluded as this constitutes metastatic disease. The procedure is started by performing an extensive Kocher manoeuvre which exposes the highest peripancreatic lymph node (HPLN) at the junction of the common bile duct and superior aspect of the pancreas, which is the border between regional and extra-regional nodes (*see Figure 69.2*). The HPLN is sent for frozen section analysis. At this point, retropancreatic and aortocaval nodes are also sampled and sent for frozen section analysis and the procedure is abandoned if any of these lymph nodes demonstrate evidence of malignant involvement. Regional lymphadenectomy is commenced by sharply incising the peritoneum overlying the hepatoduodenal ligament just above the duodenum. The right gastric vessels are divided. The anterior aspect of the common bile duct and common hepatic duct are cleared of lymphatic tissue from the superior border of the pancreas up to the inferior surface of the liver. Lymphadenectomy is then continued circumferentially around the bile duct and portal vein, aided by medial retraction of the bile duct. The lymphadenectomy next proceeds to the left side of the hepatoduodenal ligament and the hepatic artery and its branches are circumferentially cleared of all lymphatic tissue from the right side of the coeliac axis up to the inferior border of the liver. Lymphadenectomy normally proceeds in a caudo-cranial direction and the result is skeletonization of the common bile duct, hepatic duct, portal vein and full length of hepatic artery and branches (*Figure 69.4*). The 8th edition of the *AJCC Cancer Staging Manual* recommends a minimum lymph node yield of six nodes for accurate disease staging (2).

Liver resection

If a cholecystectomy was not previously performed, the hepatocystic triangle is dissected at this point, the cystic duct is divided, and the edge sent for frozen section analysis. Attention is needed to avoid spillage of bile.

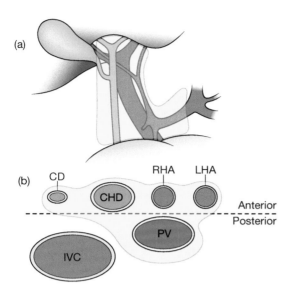

(a)

(b)

Figure 69.4 Illustration showing extent of lymph-adenectomy recommended in gallbladder cancer resection (highlighted in yellow). Hepatoduodenal ligament: coronal plane (a); Hepatoduodenal ligament: axial plane (b). *Abbreviations:* CD: cystic duct; CHD: common hepatic duct; IVC: inferior vena cava; LHA: left hepatic artery; PV: portal vein; RHA: right hepatic artery.

The steps involved in anatomical resection of segments IVb and V are shown in *Figure 69.5*. The hepatic transection margins are marked with electrocautery using anatomical landmarks and IOUS guidance. The hilum of the liver is lowered to avoid damage to the hilar structures and the liver resection is carried along four separate transection margins:

1 *Left margin*: Starts just to the right of the falciform ligament. As the liver is divided from inferior to superior, portal inflow branches to segment IVb will be encountered, and these are ligated and divided. Segment IVa branches should be recognized and preserved *(Figure 69.5a)*

2 *Right margin*: Follows a path parallel to the right scissura, just to the left of the course of the right hepatic vein. It is imperative to ensure preservation of the right hepatic vein during right margin transection, dividing only the venous branches to segment V *(Figure 69.5b)*

3 *Superior margin*: Undertaken at the level of the portal bifurcation, which separates segment IVa from IVb and segment VIII from segment V. At this margin, 1–3 terminal branches of the middle hepatic vein will be encountered, and these must be secured and divided. Further transection will lead to the segment V inflow portal pedicle, which may be test clamped and divided. The segment V inflow should be accurately identified to avoid injury to the right anterior or segment VIII portal pedicles *(Figure 69.5c)*

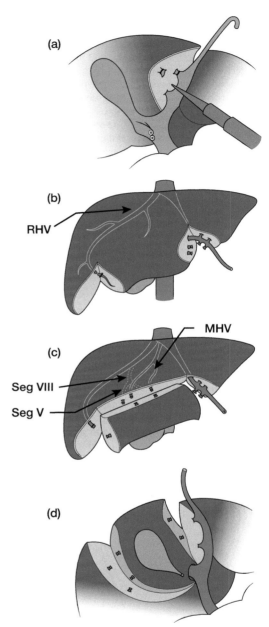

Figure 69.5 Illustrations demonstrating the technique of anatomical resection of segment IVb/V. Left margin on the right of the falciform ligament with division of segment IVb inflow (a). Right margin parallel to the right hepatic vein (RHV) with division of branches to segment V (b). Superior margin on a plane level to the portal bifurcation with division of branches of middle hepatic vein (MHV) and inflow to segment V, preserving inflow to segment VIII (c). Inferior margin (d). The previous margins are progressed and joined at a level just above the hepatic hilum.

4   *Inferior margin*: The superior, left and right transection margins are carried down and joined to the inferior margin just above the hilar plate *(Figure 69.5d)*

For a non-anatomical segment IVb/V resection, the transection margins are marked closer to the gallbladder bed, taking approximately a 2–3 cm margin from the gallbladder bed in every direction. The surgical principles are the same as anatomical IVb/V resection, but more terminal portal pedicle and hepatic vein branches are encountered during hepatic dissection. The instrument used for liver transection, use of Pringle manoeuvre and use of postoperative drains are at the discretion of the surgeon.

Extrahepatic biliary tree resection

Routine extrahepatic biliary tree (EHBT) resection has not been shown to improve outcomes of GBC surgery. Studies have demonstrated that non-selective EHBT resection resulted in similar lymph node yields and is associated with higher morbidity related to the bilio-enteric anastomosis and a worse overall survival. A selective approach to EHBT resection solely for achieving R0 resection is therefore appropriate. EHBT resection is indicated when the cystic duct margin is positive for malignancy on histological analysis or when there is gross tumour invasion into the EHBT. In this setting, following a Kocher manoeuvre of the duodenum, the EHBT can be divided distally above the duodenum, dissected cranially up to the biliary confluence and divided at this level. Reconstruction is performed using a Roux-en-Y hepaticojejunostomy.

Port site resection

Routine port site excision following laparoscopic cholecystectomy for incidental GBC has not been shown to improve survival outcomes. Port site excision should not therefore be routinely performed.

Minimally invasive resection

The current standard approach to re-operation for GBC is the open approach. Widespread adoption of the minimally invasive approach has been inhibited by fears of increased rates of port-site recurrence and oncological inadequacy. The presently available data do not support these assumptions, with minimally invasive resections showing similar survival outcomes to the open approach. Better short-term outcomes include a reduced hospital stay and earlier recovery. Minimally invasive extended cholecystectomy is therefore feasible in expert hepato-pancreatico-biliary (HPB) centres but is not presently the standard approach owing to the paucity of high-quality data.

NEOADJUVANT AND ADJUVANT THERAPY

There is presently no Level I evidence to support use of neoadjuvant therapy (NAT) for GBC and data is extrapolated from studies assessing the use of systemic therapy in the adjuvant or advanced (palliative) setting. Nevertheless, selective NAT for high-risk patients may be appropriate in the following settings: 1) Patients with high T stage; 2) positive lymph nodes; 3) residual disease after cholecystectomy, 4) preoperative jaundice and 5) bile spillage. Adjuvant chemotherapy is recommended for resected GBC of any stage. Current guidelines recommend adjuvant capecitabine, based on the results of the Capecitabine compared with Observation in Resected Biliary Tract Cancer (BILCAP) trial, which showed improved survival outcomes on per-protocol analysis in the adjuvant capecitabine groups (8). Multiple chemotherapy regimens are used in clinical practice and the results of the multinational ACTICCA-1 trial investigating adjuvant gemcitabine plus cisplatin versus capecitabine are awaited (9). The trial is investigating adjuvant chemoradiotherapy using capecitabine plus gemcitabine and radiotherapy for GBC. It is well-tolerated, and may decrease local tumour recurrence rates particularly in patients with an R1 resection and improve survival as demonstrated in one phase II trial (10). Despite limited evidence, adjuvant chemoradiotherapy may be considered for patients with R1 resections. It should be noted that all these trials combine GBCs with other biliary tract cancers, and GBC represents only up to one third of all patients recruited. Further studies are needed and any decisions regarding treatment sequencing are ideally taken in the context of the multidisciplinary team.

UNRESECTABLE OR METASTATIC GALL BLADDER CANCER

Patients who cannot undergo curative resection require biopsy to confirm the diagnosis and molecular testing. Combination gemcitabine, cisplatin and durvalumab improves survival and is currently the preferred first-line regimen based on the results of the ABC-02 (11) and TOPAZ-1 trials (12). FOLFOX is considered the preferred second-line regimen (13). Patients developing obstructive jaundice or duodenal obstruction may be effectively palliated by endoscopic/radiological biliary stenting and duodenal stenting respectively.

FOLLOW-UP

Following R0/R1 GBC resection, current NCCN guidelines (5) recommend 3–6-monthly cross-sectional imaging for the first 2 years then 6–12-monthly for 5 years or as clinically indicated, following the protocol from the BILCAP trial (8). CEA and CA 19-9 follow-up, as clinically indicated, is also recommended.

SUMMARY

Gallbladder cancer is an uncommon malignancy that exhibits early local invasion and lymphatic spread.

Early GBC is usually diagnosed incidentally after laparoscopic cholecystectomy for presumed benign disease but may sometimes be identified pre- or intra operatively. Surgical resectability is defined as the ability to achieve a negative-margin (R0) resection. Very early T1a disease has an excellent prognosis, and the definitive treatment is laparoscopic cholecystectomy. Higher T stages are associated with a greater degree of direct invasion and lymph node metastases and may necessitate extended cholecystectomy via anatomical or non-anatomical resection of liver segments IVb and V or major liver resection plus hepatoduodenal lymphadenectomy with extrahepatic biliary tree resection in selected cases. More extensive resections such as right hepatectomy or right tri-sectionectomy are sometimes necessary to achieve an R0 resection.

REFERENCES

1. Globocan 2020. Gallbladder Available from: https://gco.iarc.fr/today/data/factsheets/cancers/12-Gallbladder-fact-sheet.pdf. International Agency for Research of Cancer, World Health Organization. (Accessed 28 August 2024).
2. Zhu AX, Pawlik TM, Kooby DA, Schefter TE, Vauthey JN. Gallbladder. In: Amin MB (ed). *AJCC Cancer Staging Manual*, 8th edition, American College of Surgeons, 2018. pp. 303–9.
3. Kellil T, Chaouch MA, Aloui E, Tormane MA, Taieb SK, Noomen F, et al. Incidence and preoperative predictor factors of gallbladder cancer before laparoscopic cholecystectomy: A systematic review. *J Gastrointest Cancer* 2021;**52(1)**:68–72.
4. Lee SE, Jan J-Y, Lim C-S, Kang NJ, Kim S-W. Systematic review on the surgical treatment for T1 gallbladder cancer. *World J Gastroenterol* 2011;**17(2)**:174.
5. Benson AB, D'Angelica MI, Abrams T, Abbott DE, Ahmed A, Anaya DA, et al. NCCN Guideline s® Insights: Biliary Tract Cancers, Version 2.2023. *J Natl Compr Canc Netw* 2023;**21(7)**:694–704.
6. Vogel A, Bridgewater J, Edeline J, Kelley RK, Klümpen HJ, Malka D, et al. Biliary tract cancer: ESMO Clinical Practice Guideline for diagnosis, treatment and follow-up. *Ann Oncol* 2023;**34(2)**:127–40.
7. Nagino M, Hirano S, Yoshitomi H, Aoki T, Uesaka K, Unno M, et al. Clinical practice guidelines for the management of biliary tract cancers 2019: The 3rd English edition. *J Hepatobiliary Pancreat Sci* 2021;**28(1)**:26–54.
8. Primrose JN, Fox RP, Palmer DH, Malik HZ, Prasad R, Mirza D, et al. Capecitabine compared with observation in resected biliary tract cancer (BILCAP): A randomised, controlled, multicentre, phase 3 study. *Lancet Oncol* 2019;**20(5)**:663–73.
9. Stein A, Arnold D, Bridgewater J, Goldstein D, Jensen LH, Klümpen HJ, et al. Adjuvant chemotherapy with gemcitabine and cisplatin compared to observation after curative intent resection of cholangiocarcinoma and muscle invasive gallbladder carcinoma (ACTICCA-1 trial): A randomized, multidisciplinary, multinational phase III trial. *BMC Cancer* 2015;**15(1)**:564.
10. Ben-Josef E, Guthrie KA, El-Khoueiry AB, Corless CL, Zalupski MM, Lowy AM, et al. SWOG S0809: A Phase II Intergroup Trial of Adjuvant Capecitabine and Gemcitabine Followed by Radiotherapy and Concurrent Capecitabine in Extrahepatic Cholangiocarcinoma and Gallbladder Carcinoma. *J Clin Oncol* 2015;**33(24)**:2617–22.
11. Valle J, Wasan H, Palmer DH, Cunningham D, Anthoney A, Maraveyas A, et al. Cisplatin plus gemcitabine versus gemcitabine for biliary tract cancer. *N Engl J Med* 2010;**362(14)**:1273–81.
12. Oh DY, Ruth He A, Qin S, Chen LT, Okusaka T, Vogel A, et al. Durvalumab plus gemcitabine and cisplatin in advanced biliary tract cancer. *NEJM Evid* 2022;**1(8)**:DOI:10.1056/EVIDoa2200015.
13. Lamarca A, Palmer DH, Wasan HS, Ross PJ, Ma YT, Arora A, et al. Second-line FOLFOX chemotherapy versus active symptom control for advanced biliary tract cancer (ABC-06): A phase 3, open-label, randomised, controlled trial. *Lancet Oncol* 2021;**22(5)**:690–701.

Chapter 70

Mirizzi Syndrome

Adam Peckham-Cooper and Giles Toogood

INTRODUCTION

Named after the Argentinean surgeon Pablo Luis Mirizzi, who first described it in 1948, Mirizzi syndrome describes a partial obstruction of the common bile duct secondary to an impacted gallstone. This chapter outlines the diagnosis of the condition and the range of conservative, non-surgical and surgical options to manage patients presenting with this complex problem. The most widely accepted classification system is one proposed by Csendes in 1989 (1) (*Table 70.1*) and describes five Mirizzi types.

Table 70.1 Csendes classification system of Mirizzi syndrome (1)

Type I	External compression of the common bile duct (CBD) as a result of an impacted gallstone in the cystic duct or neck of the gallbladder
Type II	Erosion of a gallstone into the CBD causing a cholecystocholedochal fistula (fistula less than $1/3$ of the circumference of the CBD)
Type III	Erosion of a gallstone into the CBD causing a cholecystocholedochal fistula (fistula $1/3$–$2/3$ of the circumference of the CBD)
Type IV	Erosion of a gallstone into the CBD causing a cholecystocholedochal fistula involving the whole circumference of the CBD
Type V	Any type plus a cholecystoenteric fistula either causing or not causing a gallstone ileus

A diagrammatic summary is shown in *Figure 70.1*. Diagnosis and management options are dependent on the type and degree of fistulation, but conservative, endoscopic and laparoscopic or open surgical techniques can be considered.

PATHOPHYSIOLOGY OF MIRIZZI SYNDROME

Mirizzi syndrome is typically the result of long-standing gallstones and remains a rare but serious sequalae of calculous disease. Reported incidence and prevalence varies in the literature but ranges from 0.06–5.7%

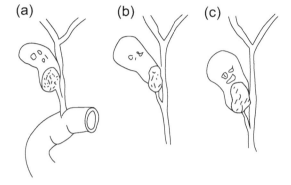

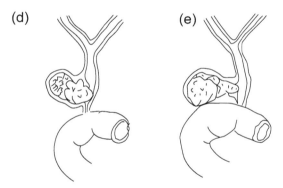

Figure 70.1 Csendes classification of Mirizzi syndrome: Type I (a), Type II (b), Type III (c), Type IV (d), Type V (e).

of patients undergoing cholecystectomy and 1.07% of those patients undergoing endoscopic retrograde cholangiopancreatography (ERCP) (2). The pathophysiology of Mirizzi syndrome results from a gallstone or gallstones becoming lodged within the cystic duct or gallbladder neck, resulting in external compression and a subsequent inflammatory response, pressure ulcer and/or necrosis of the biliary tree leading to erosion into surrounding structures. Beltran et al. (3) reported various anatomical variations which may precipitate and predispose patient to developing Mirizzi syndrome. These are summarized in *Table 70.2*.

Prevalence data for Mirizzi syndrome remains limited with high-quality epidemiological studies absent. However, studies suggest that the syndrome is more commonly seen in females presenting with a mean age

DOI: 10.1201/9781003080060-70

Table 70.2 Variant anatomy pre-disposing to Mirizzi syndrome (3)

1	Atrophic gallbladder with either thick or thin wall, with impacted gallstones at the infundibulum or at Hartmann's pouch
2	Obliterated cystic duct
3	Long cystic duct running parallel to the CBD with a low insertion point
4	A normal anatomically variant short cystic duct

of 50–70 years and is more common in certain geographical regions, such as South America and Asia when compared to North America and Europe (4). Morbidity and mortality remain high despite modern imaging and interventional/surgical treatment modalities with estimates quoting 5–31% (5).

The clinical presentation of Mirizzi syndrome can be deceptive, often mimicking other gallbladder-related conditions such as acute cholecystitis or choledocholithiasis. Patients may present with right upper quadrant abdominal pain (50–100%), recurrent episodes of jaundice (60–100%) and fever and recurrent cholangitis in patients with known or suspected gallstone disease. A leucocytosis and obstructive pattern of liver function tests (high bilirubin and high alkaline phosphatase) are typical (4,6). Given the complex nature of the disease and high-risk interventions required, both preoperative diagnosis and proper surgical, and interventional, planning are essential to optimize the management of this disease. Challenges, however, remain with only 8–62.5% of patients having a preoperative diagnosis (7).

Gallbladder cancer and Mirizzi syndrome

Mirizzi syndrome is associated with a significant increased incidence of gallbladder cancer when compared with uncomplicated cholelithiasis. Gallbladder carcinoma has been associated with all stages of Mirizzi syndrome, however, the majority seem to be found in those diagnosed with Type II pathology. A range of 6–24% of those patients diagnosed preoperatively with Mirizzi syndrome are associated with gallbladder cancer and as such a high level of clinical suspicion is required. Known risk factors for gallbladder cancer include long-standing gallstone disease and stasis, and as such, it is perhaps not surprising that Mirizzi syndrome has such a significant crossover in terms of presentation, underlying pathology and aetiology (3).

DIAGNOSIS

Advanced imaging techniques, including ultrasonography, magnetic resonance cholangiopancreatography

(MRCP), computed tomography (CT) and ERCP all play a pivotal role in delineating the underlying diagnosis and expected anatomy in Mirizzi syndrome. However, even with modern imaging techniques, the preoperative diagnosis remains challenging and the diagnosis of Mirizzi syndrome is often made intraoperatively. Safe and effective preoperative planning is essential and as such imaging remains central to the diagnostic and management pathway. There is good evidence that a bimodal approach using at least two imaging modalities increases sensitivity and specificity in these cases but there remains no clear consensus on which modalities or combinations are superior (8,9).

Ultrasound

Focussed abdominal ultrasound (US) remains the best modality for the diagnosis of gallstones and is associated with a 90.9–100% specificity. US can detect stones as small as 2 mm and is inexpensive, non-invasive and accessible globally in a wide range of different healthcare settings. Radiological findings raising the suspicion of Mirizzi syndrome include a contracted gallbladder, impacted cystic duct stones, common hepatic duct and intrahepatic duct dilatation above the site of obstruction and a normal or reduced size CBD size distal to the point of obstruction. Joseph et al. (10) suggested that the 'tri-duct sign' represented by the presence of cystic duct, common hepatic duct and portal vein dilatation is helpful in the ultrasonographic diagnosis of Mirizzi syndrome, but this is rare and US reporting is extremely operator dependent.

Sensitivity is reported to range from 8.3–57% with diagnostic challenges including body habitus, inflammation and obstructed views secondary to overlying bowel gas. (11). However, US remains the most appropriate investigation for patients with suspected gallstones and is helpful in guiding subsequent management.

Computed tomography

CT is reported to be as accurate as US for the diagnosis of Mirizzi syndrome with studies demonstrating a sensitivity of 42–50%. The value of CT is however limited by the difficultly in identifying stones. CT is a useful adjunct helping to differentiate between Mirizzi syndrome, cholangiocarcinoma and other malignant processes which are known to mimic it diagnostically and clinically. Care in interpretation is required though to identify non-specific signs, or the over-reporting of periductal inflammation as gallbladder cancer, and multidisciplinary input is recommended (11)

Magnetic resonance cholangiopancreatography

Magnetic resonance cholangiopancreatography (MRCP) remains the 'gold standard' non-invasive, repeatable and multi-layer cross-sectional imaging modality with a reported sensitivity of 63–89% and specificity of 93.5% (12). The pathognomonic features of Mirizzi syndrome include extrinsic narrowing of the common hepatic duct, a gallstone in the cystic duct or dilated common hepatic and intrahepatic ducts, all of which are routinely visible on MRCP. It can fully display the number, distribution and size of stones, any distortion of the configuration of the bile duct and the associated level of obstruction. MRCP is also good at recognizing anatomical variants that might predispose patients to Mirizzi syndrome (*see Table 70.2*). A limitation to the use of MRCP, however is the lower availability and associated costs particularly in low- and middle-income countries. Perhaps more significantly it is unable to reliably view the degree of fistulation, making preoperative Csendes classification difficult (13,14).

Endoscopic retrograde cholangiopancreatography

Whilst invasive, ERCP forms both a diagnostic and interventional option for the management of Mirizzi syndrome. It provides a robust method of assessing the biliary ductal anatomy providing a cholangiogram that illustrates the relationship between the CBD, cystic duct and gallbladder. Furthermore, ERCP can differentiate between benign and malignant lesions and obtain tissue samples where required. Therapeutic ERCP is useful, potentially retrieving bile duct stones post-sphincterotomy where feasible, and/or placing stents to relieve obstruction and allow biliary drainage. *Figure 70.2* shows an example of a typical cholangiogram seen in a patient presenting with Mirizzi syndrome.

A study by Wu et al. in 2020 (15) analysed the predictive value of ERCP for the delineation of cholecystocholedochal fistulae. The authors suggest that gallbladder opacification and pus in the CBD are both predictive factors for the presence of a fistula, but

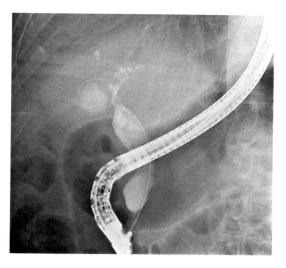

Figure 70.2 ERCP cholangiogram showing a large gallstone causing extrinsic bile duct obstruction.

interestingly, evidence of a long CBD stricture (>2 cm) was a negative indicator.

Other modalities

Percutaneous transhepatic cholangiography offers an alternative approach for both diagnostic and intervention to relieve obstructive symptoms preoperatively, particularly in those patients where endoscopic treatment has failed or may not be possible. Endoscopic ultrasound (EUS) can be used either independently or as an adjunct to ERCP to evaluate the bile duct and delineate an underlying cause of biliary strictures, however despite its increasing prevalence and availability, only one single patient case report is available describing its utility (16). *Figures 70.3* and *70.4*

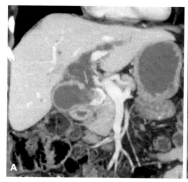
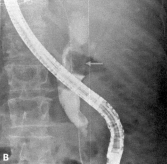
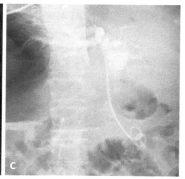

Figure 70.3 Intraoperative images illustrating **Case 1**. Coronal portal venous phase CT demonstrating a large gallstone eroding through the gallbladder neck into the proximal CBD. Discontinuity in the wall of the gallbladder and bile duct at the site of erosion (arrow). The upstream biliary tree is dilated **(A)**. ERCP demonstrating a large filling defect in the proximal CBD secondary to the large, eroded stone **(B)**. ERCP with two pigtail stents *in situ* to aid biliary drainage whilst awaiting more definitive treatment **(C)**.

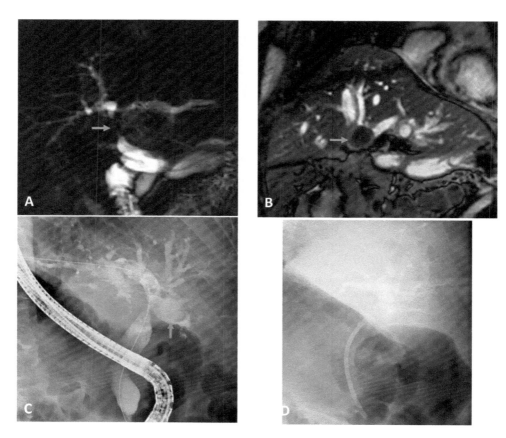

Figure 70.4 Intraoperative images illustrating **Case 2**. Coronal T2-weighted MIP image **(A)** and coronal true fast imaging with steady-state free precession (TRUFISP) MRI image **(B)** demonstrating a hilar stricture secondary to a large stone in the gallbladder neck with upstream intrahepatic duct dilatation. ERCP images **(C)** and **(D)** showing the large, calcified stone (blue arrow) and secondary hilar stricture (orange arrow) with contrast extending superiorly above the stricture into the intrahepatic ducts. A plastic biliary stent was inserted to relieve the obstruction whilst awaiting more definitive management.

illustrate two complex Mirizzi syndrome cases (Cases 1 and 2) and the benefits of mixed modality imaging in delineating anatomy and pathology. Note that in both cases, temporary therapeutic intervention with ERCP and stent placement was performed whilst patients awaited more definitive management.

MANAGEMENT

Non-surgical

The primary management for Mirizzi syndrome remains surgical intervention. However, non-surgical treatment options are available, and can be useful especially for those patients who are not surgical candidates or as an adjunct preoperatively as an aid to future, safe operative treatment in patients waiting for surgery (see *Table 70.3*).

Surgical

The surgical management, much like the diagnosis of Mirizzi syndrome, can be challenging with the anatomy and pathology of the affected area often distorted, complex and fibrous in nature. Case difficulty is confounded by low incidence rates resulting in surgeons having difficulty accumulating personal experience, with patients often referred to specialist centres.

The primary goal of any surgical intervention for Mirizzi syndrome is to relieve the biliary obstruction, remove the impacted stone, and repair or remove any associated biliary tract defects. Preoperative surgical planning and decision making is crucial and should involve a surgeon, gastrointestinal (GI) radiologist and, where applicable, an advanced endoscopist. Morbidity and mortality remain high as a direct result of the complex pathology with some studies quoting up to a 17%

Table 70.3 Non-surgical management options for Mirizzi syndrome

Pain management	Patients with Mirizzi syndrome often experience severe abdominal pain directly relating to the inflammatory process and compression of the biliary tree. Pain management is an important aspect of non-surgical management and should be based on the traditional analgesic ladder. Non-steroidal analgesics may also prove beneficial as a result of their direct anti-inflammatory activity
Antibiotics	Antibiotics are typically prescribed as prophylaxis or for the treatment of cholangitis resulting directly from bile duct obstruction. Antibiotic use should be judicial and regimen choice based on local hospital policy and guidance
ERCP	ERCP is a minimally invasive procedure that can be used to relieve biliary obstruction in Mirizzi syndrome. During the procedure, a flexible endoscope is inserted into the duodenum, and a catheter is used to inject contrast dye into the biliary tree. This allows visualization of the impacted stone and the placement of a stent to relieve the obstruction
Percutaneous transhepatic cholangiography (PTC)	PTC is another minimally invasive procedure that can be used to relieve biliary obstruction. Under US control a radiologically guided needle is inserted through the skin and into the liver giving access to the biliary tree. Contrast is then injected into the biliary tree allowing visualization of the impacted stone and subsequent placement of a stent or drain will relieve the obstruction
Nutritional support	Patients with Mirizzi syndrome may experience nausea, vomiting, decreased appetite and non-specific symptoms associated with a low-grade chronic cholangitis leading to nutritional deficiency. Nutritional support with dietary supplements, or supported feeding, may improve the patient's nutritional status, optimize preoperative prehabilitation and reduce poor outcomes and complications

incidence of iatrogenic surgical CBD injury (3). The surgical approach itself will depend on the severity of the condition and the extent of the disease as outlined by the Csendes classification (7). The surgical options are outlined.

Cholecystectomy

The standard treatment for uncomplicated gallstone disease is cholecystectomy and in some cases of Mirizzi syndrome, cholecystectomy alone may be sufficient to relieve the biliary obstruction. Mirizzi syndrome Type I is, anecdotally, often over reported on preoperative radiology. As such there is frequently a plane of dissection remaining between the medial gallbladder wall and lateral margin of common hepatic duct. With careful and cautious dissection, and in the absence of fistulation, a laparoscopic cholecystectomy can be completed without involvement or repair of the bile duct being required. In more severe cases, cholecystectomy may not be possible due to inflammation and fibrosis of the surrounding tissue and a more major surgical intervention and reconstruction will be necessary.

Subtotal cholecystectomy and fistula patch repair with remnant gallbladder plus or minus the insertion of T-tube

A subtotal cholecystectomy is performed using a 'fundus first' approach. The central portion of the infundibulum is left intact. The fistulous opening in the bile duct is then repaired using the remnant gallbladder

'flap' as a patch, taking care not to narrow the bile duct. A T-tube can be placed either above or below the 'flap' to facilitate drainage (17,18). This technique is often possible when dealing with Mirizzi syndrome Types II and III.

Hepaticoduodenostomy

Following removal of the gallbladder any fistulation to the bile duct is identified and assessed. Further debridement in a linear orientation may be required. Following full Kocherization of the duodenum to allow the upper aspect of the duodenum to lie tension-free against the dilated CBD, a longitudinal incision can be made in the duodenum abutting the CBD. A side-to-side anastomosis is performed transversely producing a diamond-shaped anastomosis with a good-sized orifice of at least 2 cm (19,20). Although well described, particularly across the Asian subcontinent, this would not be the authors' recommendation particularly when repairing a Type III and IV Mirizzi syndrome. It is our belief that a full Roux-en-Y hepaticojejunostomy offers a better long-term drainage solution with no possibility of 'sump' syndrome and as such results in improved patient outcomes. This remains experiential with limited case numbers in the literature preventing robust comparison trials and data.

Roux-en-Y hepaticojejunostomy

A Roux-en-Y hepaticojejunostomy allows a new biliary drainage route to be constructed by anastomosing the common hepatic duct to a loop of jejunum when vascularity or viability of the hepatic duct, or the quality of the tissues available for duct repair, is questionable. After careful dissection and division of the extrahepatic duct and removal of the fistula, a Roux-en-Y jejunal limb is prepared by transecting the jejunum at 20–30 cm distal to the ligament of Treitz. The Roux limb is delivered to the right upper quadrant in a retro colic fashion and ensuring a tension-free jejunal limb with sufficient length is vital. A small orifice (5 mm) on the anti-mesenteric side of the Roux limb is created ensuring the diameter of the jejunal orifice is smaller than the width of the hepatic duct. A single-layer, end-to-side hepaticojejunostomy anastomosis can then be formed using interrupted sutures with needles passing through the bile duct from out-to-in, and then through the jejunum from in-to-out. The biliary limb can then be anastomosed to a distal jejunal loop with a side-side small bowel anastomosis (21). Debate around the advantages and disadvantages of the options for biliary reconstruction continues with advocates for both Roux-en-Y hepaticojejunostomy or hepaticoduodenostomy. Hepaticoduodenostomy is considered a more physiological procedure, is simpler to perform and has a lower complication rate when compared with a Roux-en-Y (anastomotic leak, small bowel obstruction). It is however associated with a higher risk of bile reflux and cholangitis and concern remains about the associated increased risk of cholangiocarcinoma. Of note, the evidence base supporting the debate relies on data relating to reconstructive techniques following choledochal cyst surgery and only single centre experience is reported in relation to Mirizzi syndrome pathology and outcomes (19).

Minimally invasive versus open approach

Open surgical approaches remain the mainstay of Mirizzi syndrome surgical management and a laparoscopic approach remains controversial. Minimally invasive techniques are generally only feasible and appropriate in the early stages of Mirizzi syndrome (Csendes Grade 1) and are contraindicated if there is any preoperative evidence suggesting a cholecystocholedochal fistulae (22). Preoperative diagnosis and accurate staging was reported to be the most important predicative factor related to success (23) conversion, complications, and reoperation rates remain as high as 41%, 20%, and 6%, respectively in most published case series (24). The most recent systematic review assessing the evidence for laparoscopic surgery in Mirizzi syndrome by Gulla et al. (2022) summarized 221 minimally invasive cases (25). Sixty-percent of Type 1 ($n = 105$) and 80% of Type II ($n = 40$) Mirizzi cases were completed successfully laparoscopically. However, a mean conversion rate

of 26% was reported with an 18% complication rate. The authors concluded that minimally invasive techniques are safe and feasible and associated with a reduced length of stay, shorter operating times and less blood loss. Patient selection remains critical and as such these data remain skewed in favour of an amenable patient cohort. No randomized trial data exist comparing the different approaches at this time.

However, advances in robotic technologies and surgical techniques may overcome some of the limitations of conventional laparoscopic surgery allowing improved views, fine dissection and advanced suturing. Evidence is largely anecdotal from very small single centre case reports and case series, however, early data suggest a lower rate of conversion and complications associated with robotic-assisted surgery when compared with traditional laparoscopic strategies (26).

FUTURE DEVELOPMENT AND TRENDS

A number of publications and reports outline new and novel strategies for both the diagnosis and management of Mirizzi syndrome with a focus on improving outcomes. Indeed, several different classification systems which support different management approaches based on alternative scoring outcomes have been suggested (27,28). Some authors suggest research should be undertaken to achieve the 'unification of classification and diagnostic algorithms' which it is felt would be beneficial and improve outcomes (29). The Csendes classification, however, remains at this stage the 'gold standard'. An example of a diagnostic decision-making algorithm using this classification is shown in *Figure 70.5*.

Newer diagnostic methods such as intraductal US have also shown promise but are not widely available, are expensive and rely on considerable operator expertise. Moreover, the additional time spent undertaking intraductal US is considered to outweigh the potential benefits. Nevertheless, a 97% sensitivity and 100% specificity for the diagnosis of Mirizzi syndrome is reported, which is significantly better than any alternative single diagnostic modality presently available (30). Therapeutically, laser-assisted bile duct exploration by the laparoendoscopy (LABEL) technique with access through the trans-infundibular route has reported positive outcomes in selected cases. Fragmentation of large or impacted stones allows complete CBD exploration and stone clearance, and avoids the need for choledochotomy and/or fistulotomy (31,32). Similarly, new endoscopic techniques and instrumentation, such as the Spyglass™ system (Boston Scientific, MS, US) allow laser lithotripsy and fragment retrieval via ERCP and case studies describe the use of this technique to obviate the need for surgical intervention (32).

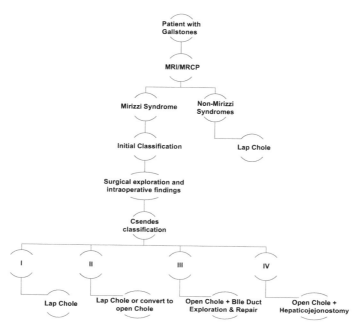

Figure 70.5 Decision-making algorithm to aid treatment of gallstones. (Adapted from Gomez et al. [6].)

REFERENCES

1. Csendes A, Diaz JC, Burdiles P, Maluenda F, Nava O. Mirizzi syndrome and cholecystobiliary fistula: A unifying classification. *B J Surg* 1989;**76(11)**:1139–43.
2. Antoniou SA, Antoniou GA, Makridis C. Laparoscopic treatment of Mirizzi syndrome: A systematic review. *Surg Endosc* 2010;**24(1)**:33–9.
3. Beltrán MA. Mirizzi syndrome: History, current knowledge and proposal of a simplified classification. *World J Gastroenterol* 2012;**18(34)**:4639–50.
4. Shirah BH, Shirah HA, Albeladi KB. Mirizzi syndrome: Necessity for safe approach in dealing with diagnostic and treatment challenges. *Ann Hepatobiliary Pancreat Surg* 2017;**21(3)**:122.
5. Pak S, Valencia D, Sheehy B, Agbim U, Askaroglu Y, Dee C, et al. Ticking bomb: Asymptomatic Mirizzi syndrome. *Cureus* 2017;**9(11)**:e1854.
6. Gomez D, Rahman SH, Toogood GJ, Prasad KR, Lodge JPA, Guillou PJ, et al. Mirizzi's syndrome – results from a large Western experience. *HPB (Oxford)* 2006;**8(6)**:474–9.
7. Lai W, Yang J, Xu N, Chen JH, Yang C, Yao HH. Surgical strategies for Mirizzi syndrome: A ten-year single center experience. *World J Gastrointest Surg* 2022;**14(2)**:107–19.
8. Yun EJ, Choi CS, Yoon DY, Seo YL, Chang SK, Kim JS, et al. Combination of magnetic resonance cholangiopancreatography and computed tomography for preoperative diagnosis of the Mirizzi syndrome. *J Comput Assist Tomogr* 2009;**33(4)**:636–40.
9. Chen H, Siwo EA, Khu M, Tian Y. Current trends in the management of Mirizzi Syndrome: A review of literature. *Medicine (Baltimore)* 2018; *97(4)*:e9691.
10. Joseph S, Carvajal S, Odwin C. Sonographic diagnosis of Mirizzi's syndrome. *J Clin Ultrasound* 1985; **13(3)**:199–201.
11. Valderrama-Treviño AI, Granados-Romero JJ, Espejel-Deloiza M, Chernitzky-Camaño J, Mera BB, Estrada-Mata AG, et al. Updates in Mirizzi syndrome. *Hepatobiliary Surg Nutr* 2017;**6(3)**:170.
12. Testini M, Massimiliano G, Luca D, Alessandro P, Gurrado A. Management of Mirizzi syndrome in emergency. *J Laparoendosc Adv Surg Tech A* 2016;**27(1)**:28–32.
13. Kwon AH, Inui H. Preoperative diagnosis and efficacy of laparoscopic procedures in the treatment of Mirizzi syndrome. *J Am Coll Surg* 2007;**204(3)**:409–15.
14. Piccinni G, Sciusco A, De Luca GM, Gurrado A, Pasculli A, Testini M. Minimally invasive treatment of Mirizzi's syndrome: Is there a safe way? Report of a case series. *Ann Hepatol* 2014;**13(5)**:558–64.
15. Wu CH, Liu NJ, Yeh CN, Wang SY, Jan YY. Predicting cholecystocholedochal fistulas in patients with Mirizzi syndrome undergoing endoscopic retrograde cholangiopancreatography. *World J Gastroenterol* 2020;**26(40)**:6241–9.
16. Rayapudi K, Gholami P, Olyaee M. Mirizzi syndrome with endoscopic ultrasound image. *Case Rep Gastroenterol* 2013;**7(2)**:202–7.
17. Minta P. Plastic repair of a defect in the wall of the common bile duct with the wall of the gallbladder (Polish). *Wiadomosci Lekarskie* 1974;**27(8)**:737–9.
18. Chourdakis CN, Androulakakis PA, Lekakos NL. Repair of cholecystocholedochal fistulas using gallbladder patching. *Arch Surg* 1976;**111(2)**:197–9.

19. Carvalho GL, De Abreu Fernandes G, Lima DL, Belarmino De Góes GH. Type IV Mirizzi Syndrome treated with hepaticoduodenostomy and minilaparoscopy. *CRSLS* 2016;e2016.00057.

20. Weledji EP, Mbengawoh NZ, Zouna F. Impacted common bile duct stone managed by hepaticoduodenostomy. *Case Rep Gastroenterol* 2022;**16**:675–9.

21. Moris D, Papalampros A, Vailas M, Petrou A, Kontos M, Felekouras E. The hepaticojejunostomy technique with intra-anastomotic stent in biliary diseases and its evolution throughout the years: A technical analysis. *Gastroenterol Res Pract* 2016;**2016**:3692096.

22. Erben Y, Benavente-Chenhalls LA, Donohue JM, Que FG, Kendrick ML, Reid-Lombardo KM, Farnell MB, Nagorney DM. Diagnosis and treatment of Mirizzi syndrome: 23-year Mayo Clinic experience. *J Am Coll Surg* 2011;**213**(1):114–9.

23. Antoniou SA, Antoniou GA, Makridis C. Laparoscopic treatment of Mirizzi syndrome: A systematic review. *Surg Endosc* 2010;**24**(1):33–9.

24. Payá-Llorente C, Vázquez-Tarragón A, Alberola-Soler A, Martínez-Pérez A, Martínez-López E, Santarrufina-Martínez S, et al. Mirizzi syndrome: A new insight provided by a novel classification. *Ann Hepatobiliary Pancreat Surg* 2017;**21**(2):67.

25. Gulla A, Jasaite M, Bilotaite L, Strupas K. Mirizzi syndrome: Is there a place for minimally invasive surgery? *Visc Med* 2022;**38**(6):369–75.

26. D'Hondt M, Wicherts DA. Robotic biliary surgery for benign and malignant bile duct obstruction: A case series. *J Robot Surg* 2023;**17**(1):55–62.

27. Payá-Llorente C, Vázquez-Tarragón A, Albero la-Soler A, Martínez-Pérez A, Martínez-López E, Santarrufina-Martínez S, et al. Mirizzi syndrome: A new insight provided by a novel classification. *Ann Hepatobiliary Pancreat Surg* 2017;**21**(2):67.

28. Klekowski J, Piekarska A, Góral M, Kozula M, Chabowski M. The current approach to the diagnosis and classification of Mirizzi syndrome. *Diagnostics (Basel)* 2021;**11**(9):1660.

29. Wehrmann T, Riphaus A, Martchencko K, Kokabpick S, Pauka H, Stergiou N, et al. Intraductal ultrasonography in the diagnosis of Mirizzi syndrome. *Endoscopy* 2006;**38**(7):717–22.

30. Quang PV, Lai VT, Cuong DC, Duc NM. Laparoscopic treatment of Mirizzi syndrome with subtotal cholecystectomy and electrohydraulic lithotripsy: A case report. *Radiol Case Rep* 2023;**18**(8):2667–72.

31. Senra F, Navaratne L, Acosta A, Martínez-Isla A. Laparoscopic management of type II Mirizzi syndrome. *Surg Endosc* 2020;**34**(5):2303.

32. Hua L, Bull N, Fox A. Totally endoscopic management of type III Mirizzi syndrome using spyglass cholangioscopy. *ANZ J Surg* 2023;**93**(7–8):2014–16.

Chapter 71

Laparoscopic Cholecystectomy

David J. Brough and Nicholas O'Rourke

INTRODUCTION

Laparoscopic cholecystectomy was first performed in the 1980s, beginning a paradigm shift in abdominal surgery. It led to the global uptake of the minimal access techniques that we use today. In Australia, more than 55 000 laparoscopic cholecystectomies are performed annually. With widespread adoption, there remains the risk of bile duct injury, the 'bête noire' of biliary surgery. This chapter outlines the principles and techniques of safe laparoscopic cholecystectomy.

Erich Muhe of Boblingen, Germany performed the first laparoscopic cholecystectomy in September 1985 after being inspired by the development of laparoscopic surgery by the German gynaecologist Kurt Semm (1,2). Coincidentally, this occurred just over 100 years after Carl Langenbuch in Berlin performed the first open cholecystectomy in July 1882 (3). Despite Muhe's enthusiasm for this new technique, his presentation of 94 laparoscopic cholecystectomies at the Congress of the German Surgical Society (GSS) conference in April 1986 was poorly received, possibly because of his awkward approach, needing to look directly through the laparoscope.

With the introduction of video laparoscopy and two-handed surgery in the mid-1980s, French pioneers Philippe Mouret, Francois Dubois and Jacques Perrisat further developed and promoted this new procedure in Europe, as did Eddie Reddick and Doug Olsen in the United States (4–6). While surgeons advocated for the role of the laparoscopic technique in cholecystectomy

early in its development there was significant resistance for several years. In 1990, Hans Troidl from Germany published a series of 100 laparoscopic cholecystectomies at the German Society of Surgery which resulted in him being removed from the programme (7).

After this initial scepticism subsided and surgeons reflected on the potential advantages, there was a ubiquitous worldwide uptake of the laparoscopic approach to cholecystectomy. It has been variously described as an 'explosion' or a 'revolution' or even the cause of a 'renaissance' in general surgery, but it is now unanimously accepted as the most appropriate approach to the performance of a wide range of procedures. Surgeons who became early adopters of the laparoscopic technique were impressed by the dramatic reduction in postoperative pain, the shorter hospital stays, and the often much earlier return to normal activity (8–12). Interestingly, this 'revolution' was not accompanied by robust evidence and early randomized control trials actually failed to demonstrate superior outcomes (13–18). Despite this, laparoscopic cholecystectomy continued its worldwide uptake and has become the 'gold standard' for management of symptomatic gallstone disease. The authors note with interest, that the 21st edition of *Bailey and Love's Short Practice of Surgery* back in 1991 carried only a four-line reference to laparoscopic cholecystectomy (19).

Unfortunately, accompanying this initial surge of gallbladders removed laparoscopically, was a worrying rise in the incidence of significant bile duct injuries. Often surgeons felt compelled to perform laparoscopic cholecystectomies with minimal laparoscopic experience, often with little, or no, training and a poor understanding of the instrumentation with the two-dimensional image (20). During the 1990s, this led to significant new complications related to vascular and bowel trauma from laparoscopic access, as well as an increased bile duct injury rate (21–29). The learning curve for laparoscopic cholecystectomy was starkly outlined by the Southern Surgeons Club with 90% of bile duct injuries occurring within the first 30 operations performed by individual surgeons. While the rates of bile duct injury have since decreased, they still occur too frequently, often with devastating consequences for patients (30–33).

There are however significant advantages to the laparoscopic approach and the techniques and

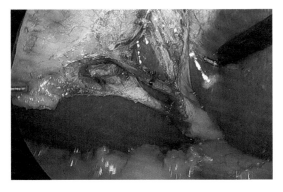

Figure 71.1 Intraoperative image showing the critical view of safety at laparoscopic cholecystectomy (anterior).

DOI: 10.1201/9781003080060-71

equipment provided surgeons with the tools and inspiration to develop approaches for other intra-abdominal procedures including appendicectomy, hernia repair, colectomy and ultimately complex liver and pancreatic surgery (34–38). At the Royal Brisbane Hospital we have a long history of minimally invasive hepatopancreaticobiliary surgery including laparoscopic cholecystectomy for acute cholecystitis and the laparoscopic management of bile duct stones (39,40).

INDICATIONS AND CONTRAINDICATIONS FOR LAPAROSCOPIC CHOLECYSTECTOMY

Indications for a laparoscopic approach are similar to those for an open cholecystectomy (*Table 71.1*). The decision to proceed laparoscopically, rather than open, nevertheless still depends on the surgeon's skill set and experience. Rarely, anaesthetic concerns preclude the use of laparoscopy in frail patients or those where a raised intra-abdominal pressure has to be avoided. General anaesthetic is preferred as operating under regional anaesthesia such as an epidural can be challenging due to diaphragmatic pain following the pneumoperitoneum (41,42). Gallbladder cancer has previously been considered a contraindication to laparoscopic surgery (43) however, improvements in instrumentation and techniques allow experienced surgeons to offer combined liver resection, nodal dissection and even bile duct excision for appropriate cancers. For early gallbladder carcinoma (T1 and T2), the laparoscopic approach offers non-inferior oncological outcomes, a shorter hospital stay and similar overall survival rates compared with the open approach (44–47).

PREOPERATIVE EVALUATION

Patients being worked up for elective or emergency laparoscopic cholecystectomy should all have liver function tests (LFT's) performed in addition to an abdominal ultrasound (US). These investigations provide critical information, guiding patient selection and indicate when further investigations should be performed. With gallstones, an elevation of LFT's can suggest biliary obstruction. US is essential for confirming cholelithiasis but can also measure gallbladder wall thickness, detect pericholecystic fluid, assess the diameter of the common hepatic duct and occasionally identify choledocholithiasis. US can also examine the liver morphology which may be important in patients with undiagnosed chronic liver disease.

In centres where magnetic resonance imaging (MRI) is available, if there is a suggestion of ductal stones a preoperative magnetic resonance cholangiopancreatogram (MRCP) to define the biliary anatomy and assess the bile duct stone load should be organized (*Figure 71.2*). This information guides our decision-making regarding the need for preoperative endoscopic retrograde cholangiopancreatography (ERCP) or laparoscopic common bile duct (CBD) exploration (48–51). Our preference is to plan a transcystic exploration at laparoscopic cholecystectomy, if a low stone load and suitable anatomy, particularly cystic duct diameter is identified on MRCP (*Figures 71.3*, *71.4* and *71.5*). While comprehensive laparoscopic management of common duct stones falls outside the scope of this chapter, the authors note the benefit of managing both the gallbladder and common duct stones at the same operation. Additionally, with the rise of bariatric surgery and Roux-en-Y gastric bypass, endoscopic access to the ampulla may be impossible and often the only option for duct stones may be laparoscopic CBD exploration.

Table 71.1 Summary of indications for laparoscopic cholecystectomy

Symptomatic cholelithiasis	• Biliary pain (colic) • Cholecystitis (acute and chronic)
Complications of cholelithiasis	• Choledocholithiasis • Gallstone pancreatitis • Mirrizi syndrome • Choledochoduodenal fistula
Other indications	• Acalculous cholecystitis • Gallbladder polyps • Early gallbladder carcinomas • Primary infective cholecystitis (Enterobacteriaceae including *Salmonella*) • Gallbladder torsion • Prophylactic in some circumstances for patients with asymptomatic cholelithiasis

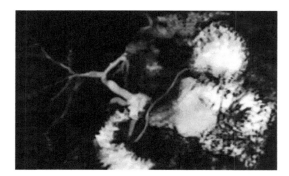

Figure 71.2 A normal MRCP post cholecystectomy demonstrating still fluid without the need for intravenous contrast. There is a clear depiction of the biliary tree, cystic duct CBD junction and pancreatic duct.

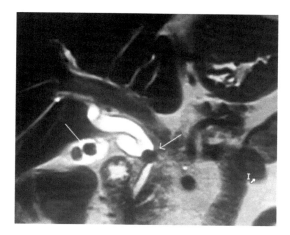

Figure 71.3 Abnormal MRCP showing a large CBD stone at the CBD cystic duct junction (middle arrow).

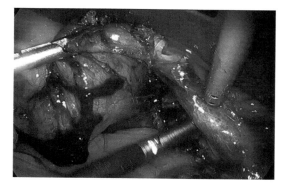

Figure 71.4 Intraoperative image of cystic ductotomy using the laparoscopic instruments to 'milk out' the stone.

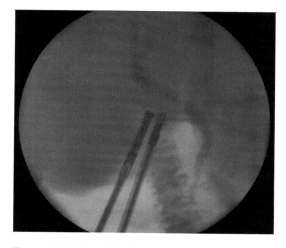

Figure 71.5 Completion intraoperative cholangiogram demonstrating a clear CBD with no filling defects.

Case study 1

A 50-year-old man presented with pain and jaundice. The MRCP demonstrated a gallstone impacted at the cystic duct CBD junction. This was successfully managed laparoscopically with a cystic ductotomy and 'milking' the stone from the CBD. (*Figures 71.3*, *71.4* and *71.5*).

TIMING OF LAPAROSCOPIC CHOLECYSTECTOMY

The traditional teaching was to delay cholecystectomy after patients presented with acute cholecystitis or pancreatitis but there is now good evidence to support early cholecystectomy (52–55). In acute cholecystitis, surgery is easier in the first few days, and generally most difficult between days 7–10. With gallstone pancreatitis, patients with mild-to-moderate, pancreatitis should have their cholecystectomy during the index admission. Performing delayed cholecystectomy puts the patient at risk of a second episode of biliary pancreatitis, often worse than their first and does not reduce the risk of intraoperative or postoperative complications (56,57).

Laparoscopic cholecystectomy can safely be performed throughout each trimester of pregnancy (58). The indication should be reserved for complications of gallstones such as acute cholecystitis, gallstone pancreatitis or choledocholithiasis. Selective intra-operative cholangiogram can be done without known adverse harm to the mother or foetus. The authors have experience of successful laparoscopic cholecystectomies in pregnant patients up to 33-weeks of gestation.

PREDICTING THE DIFFICULT GALLBLADDER

Most laparoscopic cholecystectomies are uncomplicated, however as with all surgical procedures some can be technically extremely challenging (*Table 71.2*). There have been multiple guidelines published by distinguished groups from different countries on laparoscopic cholecystectomy (59,60). *Table 71.3*

Table 71.2 Patient and disease factors predicting a difficult laparoscopic cholecystectomy

Patient factors	• Elderly
	• Male
	• Cirrhosis
	• Diabetes
	• Previous open upper abdominal surgery
	• Obesity
Disease factors	• Acute cholecystitis
	• Present or past cholangitis
	• Shrunken or intrahepatic gallbladder

Table 71.3 Guidelines and scoring systems for laparoscopic cholecystectomy and their clinical applicability (both pre-operative and inta-operative) (59,60,62–67)

Guideline	Scoring system	Clinical application
The SAGES safe cholecystectomy program	Six surgical principles that surgeons can employ to adopt a universal culture of safety for cholecystectomy to minimize the risk of bile duct injury	These principles should be adhered to in all cholecystectomies
Tokyo Guidelines 2018 (TG-18) diagnostic criteria and severity grading of acute cholecystitis	Severity of grading of acute cholecystitis: Grade I (mild), Grade II (moderate) and Grade III (severe)	TG-18 is the third revision of the Tokyo Guidelines (previous 2013 and 2007). These criteria were unchanged from the TG-13 after voting at the A-PHPBA Conference at Yokohama in 2017. TG-18 provides surgeons with a rapid diagnosis and grading of acute cholecystitis. Grade III are associated with higher rates of conversion to open, bile duct injuries, longer operative times, hospital stays and overall mortality
Other scoring systems	Parkland grading scale for cholecystitis, Nassar, American Association for Surgery of Trauma (AAST), North Shore grading system	Simple grading systems that relate to intraoperative gallbladder appearance. Higher grades reflect more difficult operations

highlights some of these key guidelines and indicates their clinical applicability. One of the most recent publications is the excellent SAGES safe cholecystectomy guidelines after a task force was established in 2014 to emphasize safe surgical principles in laparoscopic cholecystectomy and readers are encouraged to explore these guidelines (60). Scoring systems exist and can be based on preoperative features or intraoperative appearance at the initial laparoscopy (61–67). Surgeons should not be embarrassed by referring difficult cases to specialist centres, even after inserting a laparoscope. It is essential that hepato-pancreatico-biliary (HPB) surgeons remain supportive and not critical of colleagues referring patients with potentially high risk pathology.

CIRRHOSIS

The word cirrhosis comes from the Greek word *kirrhós* meaning 'tawny' due to the appearance in chronic liver disease. While cirrhosis is a histological diagnosis, blood tests and imaging (US, computed tomography [CT] and MR) can often be suggestive. When planned, the benefit of laparoscopic over open cholecystectomy in cirrhosis has been well established through randomized controlled trials and multiple meta-analyses (68–70). Surgeons should, however, approach these cases with care and have a low-threshold for using advanced bipolar energy devices such as the LigaSure™ (Medtronic, Minnesota, USA) in these cases.

The unexpected intraoperative finding of cirrhosis is not uncommon. In Child-Pugh Grade A cirrhosis (*see* **Chapter 43**) without portal hypertension, the risks are minimal, and surgeons can usually proceed as planned.

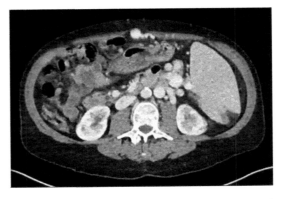

Figure 71.6 Axial CT demonstrating significant portal hypertension with large varices including caput medusae.

With more severe cirrhosis or portal hypertension, specialist HPB referral is indicated, as bleeding or postoperative liver failure can occur. Preoperative cross-sectional imaging is critical in all patients with portal hypertension to assess for umbilical vein recanalization and caput medusae which would indicate that umbilical access should be avoided (*Figure 71.6*).

EQUIPMENT

There is considerable variability in laparoscopic equipment, based on surgeon preferences and financial constraints. Our standard equipment includes a 10 mm Hasson port (umbilical access), three 5 mm standard ports, toothed graspers, hook diathermy, suction irrigation and Hem-a-lok® (Teleflex, USA) or LIGACLIP™ (J&J Med Tech, NJ, USA). For cholangiography, a 4Fr end-hole ureteric catheter is used inside an Olsen-Reddick® cholangiogram clamp (Karl Storz SE & Co, Tuttlingen, Germany). When cannulating smaller cystic ducts, an epidural catheter can be used.

Our preference is to use iodixanol contrast diluted to 50% with 0.9% sodium chloride. If the patient has a documented severe iodine contrast allergy, we will use gadolinium contrast which is non-iodine based. Contrast injected into the biliary tree rarely causes severe reactions unlike agents which have to be given intravenously. A Nathanson basket (Cook Medical, USA) or Choledochoscope (Olympus, USA) should be available for transcystic CBD explorations.

PRINCIPLES

During a laparoscopic cholecystectomy, the aim is to remove the entire gallbladder without perforating the wall while preserving the biliary tree and avoiding injury to other organs and vascular structures. This is usually straightforward but both acute and chronic inflammation and their sequalae can render the operation hazardous and sometimes the removal of the stones alone with or without partial or subtotal cholecystectomy is prudent.

Most guidelines recommend perioperative antibiotics for all biliary surgery despite meta-analyses having failed to demonstrate any benefit in reducing surgical site infection in uncomplicated cases (71,72). For acute cholecystitis, antibiotics should be used, noting that approximately 40–70% have positive bile cultures (73). Extended antibiotic use should be used in patients with an empyema, when gallstones have been spilled or following a bile duct exploration.

SURGICAL TECHNIQUE

Set-up

While surgical techniques for laparoscopic cholecystectomy vary, what follows describes our preference. The patient is supine, both arms abducted at 90° with the surgeon on the patient's right and the assistant on the left. The monitor is positioned above the patient's head. The initial access is via the umbilicus using an open Hasson trocar technique, although an optical access trocar in the left upper abdomen may be used, if periumbilical adhesions are suspected. Ideally, this should be placed through the rectus muscle where the layers are more defined, and the risk of intra-abdominal injury is reduced.

Port placement is shown in *Figure 71.7*. A pneumoperitoneum with carbon dioxide insufflation is achieved with a setting of 12–15 mmHg. Three accessory 5 mm ports are placed, one in the epigastrium, one in the right iliac fossa in the mid clavicular line and one in the right upper quadrant in the mid axillary line. A total 5 mm port approach can also be used (74).

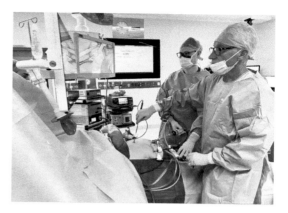

Figure 71.7 The author's operative set-up for laparoscopic cholecystectomy.

Dissection of the hepatocystic triangle

The fundus is grasped by the assistant and retracted antero-cephalically to expose the porta hepatis and hepatocystic triangle of Calot. In the original description by Calot in 1891, the triangle was described as bounded medially by the hepatic duct, laterally by the cystic duct and superiorly by the cystic artery.

The surgeon grasps Hartmann's pouch with their left hand with a bullnose grasper (or toothed grasper in acute cholecystitis) and dissects with their right-hand opening the peritoneum below Hartmann's pouch. Hartmann's pouch was originally described in 1884 and named after Henri Albert Hartmann, who believed it was a rare diverticulum where the wall of the gallbladder neck joins the cystic duct. Whether this is a constant anatomical feature or a product of pathological change to the gallbladder is controversial but there is a clear association with the presence of stones.

Our preferred method of dissection is with a monopolar hook diathermy, dissecting the postero-lateral aspect first, as this allows elevation of the lower gallbladder. The surgeon looks for the cystic duct and cystic artery and ideally identifies and defines both as coming up from the porta hepatis onto the gallbladder surface. The spaces between the cystic duct, cystic artery and gallbladder bed are defined, achieving the critical view of safety (*Figure 71.1*).

Rouvière's sulcus (or Gans incisura) was initially described in 1924 by Henri Rouviere, a French anatomist. It is a 2–5 cm fissure on the liver between the right lobe and caudate process and an important landmark in laparoscopic cholecystectomy. This anatomical cleft in the right lobe of the liver overlies the posterior sectoral duct and is present in 70% of the population. Dissection should be kept anterior to this landmark to avoid bile duct injury (75).

In cases where the gallbladder is tense due to acute cholecystitis or a mucocele, using the lateral port, one can cannulate the distended gallbladder with a trocar and aspirate the liquid contents using a sucker (*Figure 71.8*). Inflammatory changes may warrant the use of a suction irrigation device, so called hydro-dissection, which is often helpful in acute cholecystitis.

Critical view of safety

In 1995, Steven Strasberg from the Washington University School of Medicine described the 'critical view of safety' in an attempt to codify the anatomy that is dissected and reduce the incidence of bile duct injury (76). The criteria for the critical view of safety can be seen in *Table 71.4*. A key to obtaining the critical view is the axiom that 'one can never do too much posterior dissection'. Unlike at open surgery, where assessing the posterior attachments of the gallbladder is difficult, the laparoscopic approach, especially with a 30° scope, affords an excellent view of the posterior peritoneal attachments. When these are divided, it allows better separation of the gallbladder from its bed and makes anterior dissection simpler although sometimes

despite these manoeuvres, the critical view is hard to define. Dense adhesions of cystic duct to common hepatic duct can lead to the classic mistake of CBD transection with inadvertent dissection on the medial aspect of the common duct, where the planes are easier to dissect and the common duct is mistaken for the cystic duct (77). If the anatomy remains unclear, rather than risk bile duct injury, a decision should be made to call for assistance. Other options include cholangiography, further blunt hydro-dissection, opening the gallbladder or converting to an open procedure. It is important to remember that removal of the gallbladder is not mandatory and although the stones need to be removed, the gallbladder can be subsequently left open or closed with a suture. Suturing in this situation however can be difficult and potentially dangerous if the anatomy remains uncertain. A drain must be left, and persistent bile drainage may warrant subsequent ERCP. Steven Strasberg has also codified these 'bailout options' with the concepts of fenestration or reconstitution of the gallbladder remnant (*Figures 71.9* and *71.10*) (78). Please see the author's flow diagram of safe intraoperative decision-making (*Figure 71.11*).

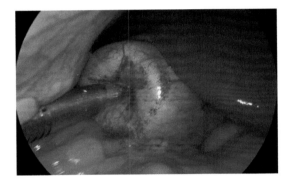

Figure 71.8 Intraoperative image showing decompression of a tense and distended gallbladder in acute cholecystitis when the fundus cannot be easily grasped.

Table 71.4 Criteria required to achieve the 'critical view of safety'

Clearance of hepatocystic triangle	Hepatocystic triangle is cleared of tissue, so visibility of cystic structures and plate is unimpeded, and the surgeon is certain no other structures are in the hepatocystic triangle
Two structures connected to gallbladder	Only two structures (cystic artery and cystic duct) should be clearly seen entering the gallbladder
Cystic plate	Approximately one-third of the cystic plate is visibly clear

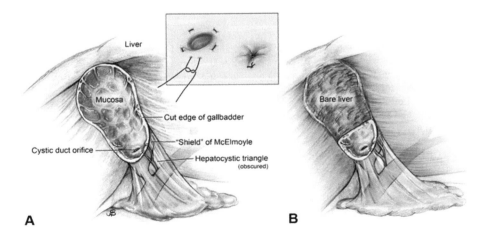

Figure 71.9 Labelled illustrations showing a subtotal fenestrating cholecystectomy (A) cut-away view with insert indicating suture position and (B) Final view of fenestrating cholecystectomy prior to suture insertion.

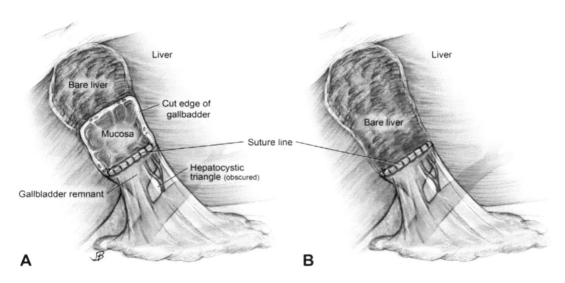

Figure 71.10 Labelled illustrations showing a subtotal reconstituting cholecystectomy (A) cut-away view and (B) Final view of reconstituting cholecystectomy after suture closure of remnant.

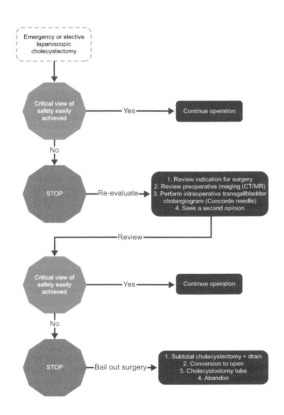

Figure 71.11 Flow diagram demonstrating safe intra-operative decision-making for laparoscopic cholecystectomy.

The surgeon must always remember that a bile duct injury reduces a patient's life expectancy by at least 10 years (and possibly more for the surgeon!) and if concerns remain about the ability to perform the cholecystectomy a drain should be inserted, the procedure abandoned, and the patient referred to a specialist centre.

Intraoperative cholangiography

The Argentinian Pablo Luis Mirizzi performed the first intraoperative cholangiogram on the 6 June, 1931 which he described a year later with the heading '*La Lipiodo Radiografis de las Vias Biliares*' translated as 'The lipiodol x-rays of the biliary conduits' (79). Since the original description, cholangiography has had its proponents and detractors but we are enthusiasts for routine cholangiography and like the reassurance of a biliary roadmap, and the prognostic help of a clear biliary tree (*Figures 71.12* and *71.13*). It adds expense, time and radiation but does enhance the skill set useful in trans-cystic exploration. Detractors point out the possibility of inadvertent choledochotomy, with inadequate dissection, but this is better than clipping and division of the bile duct. Previous studies have demonstrated a reduced inci-dence of bile duct injury when cholangiography is used during laparoscopic cholecystectomy but recent system-atic reviews have not replicated this (80–84). When an intraoperative cholangiogram (IOC) is performed and interpreted correctly, surgeons can avoid severe bile duct injuries with complete bile duct excision.

Another rarely mentioned benefit of operative cholan-giography is the definition of the cystic remnant. This can be substantial in size and dilate over time giving more symp-toms with the occasional need for redo-cholecystectomy.

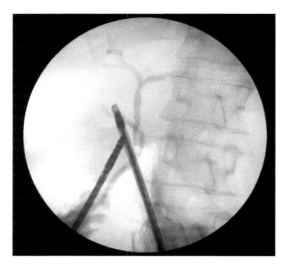

Figure 71.12 Normal intraoperative cholangiogram (IOC) demonstrating a long, spiral cystic duct, entire filling of the biliary tree, normal diameter CBD, free flow of contrast into the second part of the duodenum and no filling defects.

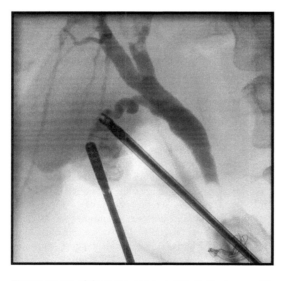

Figure 71.13 IOC demonstrating bile duct stones with a dilated biliary tree. Note the meniscus around the large stone in the distal CBD and more stones visible in the left hepatic duct. The patient was referred for postoperative ERCP.

Our practice is to 'milk' the cystic duct up to the cystic ductotomy as this allows any small stones to be removed (*Figure 71.14*).

If bile duct stones are seen on operative cholangiography, there are several options available to the surgeon and decisions can be made on the basis of the cholangiogram appearance (85).

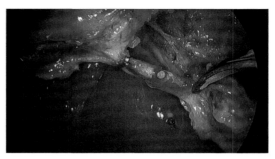

Figure 71.14 Intraoperative view of a cystic duct stone after the bile duct had been swept with forceps.

Indocyanine green fluorescent cholangiography

There is growing enthusiasm for the use of indocyanine green (ICG) fluorescent cholangiography at laparoscopic cholecystectomy (86–89). The authors note it can be helpful in the elective non-inflamed setting but can be difficult to interpret in acute cholecystitis or where tissues are inflamed. It certainly is not as accurate as standard operative cholangiography and further evidence is required to support its routine use.

Detaching the gallbladder from the liver

The gallbladder is taken off the gallbladder fossa with hook diathermy using both the hook and the heel while the assistant helps by providing countertraction. This plane is usually clear but dense adhesions can lead to gallbladder perforation or entering the liver where the middle hepatic vein can be superficial, running just beneath the gallbladder bed.

Once detached, the assistant can then use the gallbladder as a visceral retractor (if not perforated) to retract the colon and duodenum, allowing the surgeon to wash and visualize the gallbladder bed and porta hepatis.

The gallbladder fossa is then thoroughly inspected to ensure that there are no bile leaks, and that haemostasis is complete. For haemostasis we often turn the diathermy up to 80–120 on the coagulation setting to cauterize the liver bed while using the suction irrigation to obtain a clear view of the operative field.

Prevention of bile leaks

Approximately 50% of bile leaks following laparoscopic cholecystectomy are from inadequately controlled cystic duct stumps. Clips must be secure and cover the entire stump downstream from any defects. Larger cystic ducts can be controlled with large Hem-a-lok® non-absorbable polymer clips, endo-loops or suture ligation. Copious saline lavage after cholecystectomy combined with 'underwater laparoscopy' is useful to

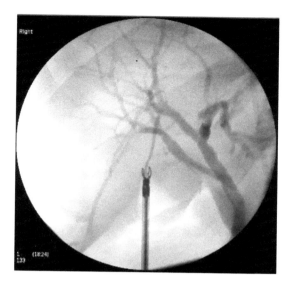

Figure 71.15 IOC view through an accessory duct (duct of Luschka).

check for bile leaks that can occur from the cystic duct or accessory ductules in the gallbladder bed (*Figure 71.15*). When these ducts are sizable, a cholangiogram can be performed through them to confirm their size and anatomy and they may be occluded with clips or sutures.

Closure following laparoscopic cholecystectomy

The gallbladder is removed via the umbilical port site in a retrieval bag. The incision may need to be extended to remove large stones or thick-walled gallbladders. The fascia at the umbilicus is typically closed with an absorbable suture such as an 0-0 polyglycolide-trimethylene carbonate suture (Maxon®, Medtronic Inc, Ireland) and the port-sites with an absorbable suture such as a 3-0 poliglecaprone suture (Monocryl®, J&J Med Tech, NJ, USA). Dose-adjusted local anaesthetic is injected at the port-sites.

Non-standard techniques

Multiple surgical approaches have been described for laparoscopic cholecystectomy including other minimally invasive surgery techniques such as natural orifice surgery (NOTES), single-incision laparoscopic (SILS) cholecystectomy and needlescopic cholecystectomy. Centres offering the transvaginal cholecystectomy technique found decreased postoperative pain but did not demonstrate any significant advantage over standard laparoscopic cholecystectomy (90). SILS was briefly popular in the early 2000's, boasting a small and single incision using a multiport set-up. In cholecystectomy, this technique offers slightly improved cosmesis, but

increased incisional hernia rates and challenging ergonomics. It has also failed to show superiority over the conventional four-port laparoscopic cholecystectomy (91–93). The use of 2–3 mm accessory ports ('needlescopic cholecystectomy') has been possible for some time but has not had widespread uptake due to lack of rigidity of the instruments and the minimal potential benefit.

Subtotal/partial cholecystectomy

While there are multiple techniques which can be used to perform a subtotal or partial cholecystectomy, we prefer to open the gallbladder, remove the stones and resect the body and fundus. The authors do not advocate trying to close the cystic duct orifice as blind suturing under these circumstances can cause an inadvertent vascular or biliary injury. We routinely leave a 19Fr Blake's drain in the gallbladder fossa accepting that there will be a bile leak.

In the event of a subtotal or partial cholecystectomy, patients may present at a later date with gallstone disease related to a remnant gallbladder (*Figure 71.16*). Importantly, surgeons should not criticize the original procedure but praise the surgeon for doing the safest operation for that patient under those circumstances. Redo cholecystectomy should be performed by HPB surgeons, and an intraoperative cholangiogram is recommended.

Case study 2

A 66-year-old female presented with recurrent biliary pain 10 years after a laparoscopic cholecystectomy and ERCP. The MRCP demonstrated a remnant cystic duct measuring over 20 mm. Recurrent biliary pain resolved after laparoscopic removal of the cystic duct stump remnant seen at MRCP.

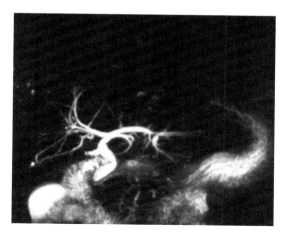

Figure 71.16 MRCP showing a remnant cystic duct measuring 23 mm, there were no stones.

SPECIFIC PROBLEMS

Bleeding

Uncontrollable brisk bleeding is the only indication for rapid conversion. Major bleeding during laparoscopic cholecystectomy can be from a trocar-related vascular injury, the hepatic artery or portal vein or the middle hepatic vein in the gallbladder bed. Most bleeding can be controlled with pressure, help from a suction irrigation and better retraction (*Figure 71.17*). Clips should not be placed blindly in the porta, and arteries should be clearly identified prior to clipping or closure with an energy device such as Ligasure™ (94). Diathermy on high (80–120 coagulation) can be useful for gallbladder bed oozing, but a bleeding middle hepatic vein, with visible endothelium may require suture. Haemostatic agents can help, with temporary pressure from a gauze square or even the gallbladder.

Gallbladder perforation with bile/ stone spillage

Gallbladder perforation with spillage of contents is not uncommon during laparoscopic cholecystectomy. Copious saline lavage and retrieval of all visible stones should be attempted. To achieve complete clearance of spilled stones a 10 mL sucker can be used or a small gauze square introduced as a mat on which to place stones. Particular attention should be paid to spilt stones adjacent to the diaphragm as delayed subphrenic abscess formation, due to spilled stones, is not uncommon and can be very difficult to treat definitively (*Figure 71.18*). We have also seen spilt stones causing an inflammatory biliary stricture and they are the most common cause of biliary pseudotumours (*see* **Chapter 66**) (95).

Biliary injuries

For biliary injury classification, management and options please *see* **Chapter 62**. IOC can help identify bile duct injury intraoperatively as seen in *Figure 71.19* (not our case).

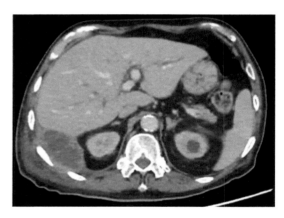

Figure 71.18 Axial CT demonstrating a sub-hepatic collection relating to the delayed presentation of a gallstone abscess more than 12 months after an emergency laparoscopic cholecystectomy with perforation and gallstone spillage.

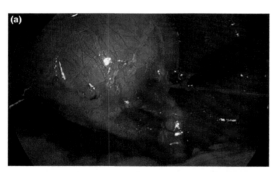

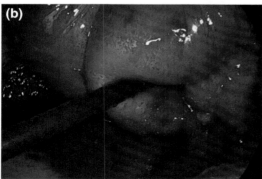

Figure 71.17 Intraoperative view of a cystic artery bleed with pressure applied using the gallbladder (a) then successfully clipped (b).

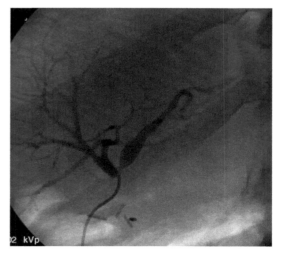

Figure 71.19 IOC demonstrating a major bile duct injury (Strasberg E4) after the CBD was clipped and cut following misidentification as the 'cystic duct'.

Table 71.5 Complications of laparoscopic cholecystectomy

Intraoperative	Early	Late

• Pneumoperitoneum-related
  ○ CO_2 embolism
  ○ Vasovagal reflex
  ○ Cardiac arrhythmias
  ○ Hypercapnic acidosis
• Trocar-related
  ○ Abdominal wall bleeding
  ○ Haematoma
  ○ Visceral injury
  ○ Vascular injury
• Haemorrhage
• Bile duct injury
• Visceral injury
	• Haemorrhage
	• Bile duct injury/bile leak
	• Retained bile duct stones
	• Intra-abdominal infection
	• Wound infection
	• Visceral injury
	• Pancreatitis
		• Port-site hernia
		• Biliary stricture
		• Dropped gallstone and abscess formation.
		• Post-cholecystectomy syndrome

Complications following laparoscopic cholecystectomy

Most laparoscopic cholecystectomies are uncompli-cated and therefore associated morbidity is minimal. A summary of surgical complications related to laparoscopic cholecystectomy is shown in *Table 71.5*. Importantly, patients undergoing a laparoscopic chole-cystectomy who do not follow the typical postoperative course should alert surgeons to the possibility of a complication and the need to identify the cause, exclude biliary peritonitis or perform a re-look laparoscopy if there is any doubt about the underlying cause.

POSTOPERATIVE CARE AND SYMPTOMS POST-CHOLECYSTECTOMY

Most patients are suitable for discharge 6 hours after their day-case laparoscopic cholecystectomy, but a small number may need overnight admission for 24 hours (96–98). Narcotic analgesia should be avoided, and non-steroid anti-inflammatory analgesia is preferred. All specimens should be routinely sent for histopathology.

Diarrhoea, post-cholecystectomy is reported and seems more common when functioning gallbladders are removed. Bowel frequency will usually resolve with time however, some patients suffer ongoing symptoms often induced by fatty foods and cholestyramine can be useful in these patients (99).

Patients returning to the surgeon after laparoscopic cholecystectomy with new or persistent symptoms remain a challenge. The nature of these symptoms is the key to establishing a diagnosis and surgeons need to be aware of, and exclude, conditions such as common duct stones, biliary strictures, occult hepato-pancreati-co-biliary malignancies, gallbladder remnant problems and chronic abscesses.

In 2013, Lamberts and colleagues reported that up to 40% of patients have pain, up to 5-years after cholecystectomy, yet around 90% of patients described their operation as successful (100). The term 'post-cholecystectomy syndrome' is used variably in the liter-ature to describe myriad symptoms including persistent upper abdominal pain similar to the pain experienced prior to cholecystectomy, nausea, dyspepsia, flatulence, bloating and an alteration in bowel habit. In addition to the variability of description there is considerable cross-over with functional gastrointestinal disorders (FGID) such as irritable bowel syndrome, functional abdominal bloating, functional dyspepsia and visceral hypersensi-tivity syndrome which makes identifying and reporting the true incidence difficult.

SUMMARY

Laparoscopic cholecystectomy remains the 'gold standard' for the management of gallbladder disease. It is a safe, low-risk and effective operation and in most patients the procedure is uneventful. The risk of bile duct injury remains a concern, and it is the responsi-bility of every surgeon to recognize situations where the bile duct could be at risk. When cholecystectomy is difficult and the anatomy cannot be fully appreciated, it must be remembered that 'bailing is not failing'. There needs to be a culture where surgeons feel comfortable to refer patients for a specialist opinion prior to causing bile duct injury. This decision can be preoperative or intraoperative without embarrassment.

REFERENCES

1. Mühe E. The first laparoscopic cholecystectomy. *Langenbecks Archiv für Chirurgie* 1986;**369**:804.
2. Reynolds W Jr. The first laparoscopic cholecystec-tomy. *JSLS* 2001;**5**:89–94.
3. Hardy KJ. Carl Langenbuch and the Lazarus Hos-pital: Events and circumstances surrounding the first cholecystectomy. *Aust N Z J Surg* 1993;**63**:56–64.
4. Reddick EJ, Olsen DO. Laparoscopic laser chole-cystectomy. A comparison with mini-lap cholecys-tectomy. *Surg Endosc* 1989;**3**:131–3.

5. Dubois F, Icard P, Berthelot G, et al. Coelioscopic cholecystectomy. Preliminary report of 36 cases. *Ann Surg* 1990;**211**:60–2.

6. Perissat J, Collet D, Belliard R. Gallstones: Laparoscopic treatment cholecystectomy, cholecystostomy, and lithotripsy. Our own technique. *Surg Endosc* 1990;**4**:1–5.

7. Alkatout I, Mechler U, Mettler L, et al. The development of laparoscopy: A historical overview. *Front Surg* 2021;**8**:799442.

8. Cuschieri A, Dubois F, Mouiel J, et al. The European experience with laparoscopic cholecystectomy. *Am J Surg* 1991;**161**:385–7.

9. Meyers WC. A prospective analysis of 1518 laparoscopic cholecystectomies: The southern surgeons club. *N Engl J Med* 1991;**324**:1073–78.

10. Peters JH, Ellison EC, Innes JT, et al. Safety and efficacy of laparoscopic cholecystectomy. A prospective analysis of 100 initial patients. *Ann Surg* 1991;**213**:3–12.

11. Grace PA, Quereshi A, Coleman J, et al. Reduced postoperative hospitalization after laparoscopic cholecystectomy. *Br J Surg* 1991;**78**:160–2.

12. Strasberg SM, Clavien PA. Overview of therapeutic modalities for the treatment of gallstone diseases. *Am J Surg* 1993;**165**:420–6.

13. Barkun JS, Barkun AN, Sampalis JS, et al. Randomised controlled trial of laparoscopic versus minicholecystectomy. The McGill Gallstone Treatment Group. *Lancet* 1992;**340**:1116–9.

14. McMahon AJ, Russell IT, Baxter JN, et al. Laparoscopic versus minilaparotomy cholecystectomy: A randomised trial. *Lancet* 1994;**343**:135–138.

15. Berggren U, Gordh T, Grama D, et al. Laparoscopic versus open cholecystectomy: hospitalization, sick leave, analgesia and trauma responses. *Br J Surg* 1994;**81**:1362–5.

16. McGinn FP, Miles AJ, Uglow M, et al. Randomized trial of laparoscopic cholecystectomy and mini-cholecystectomy. *Br J Surg* 1995;**82**:1374–7.

17. Majeed AW, Troy G, Nicholl JP, et al. Randomised, prospective, single-blind comparison of laparoscopic versus small-incision cholecystectomy. *Lancet* 1996;**347**:989–4.

18. Ros A, Gustafsson L, Krook H, et al. Laparoscopic cholecystectomy versus mini-laparotomy cholecystectomy: A prospective, randomized, single-blind study. *Ann Surg* 2001;**234**:741–9.

19. Bailey H, Love RJM, Mann CV, Russell RCG. *Bailey & Love's Short Practice of Surgery*, 18th edn. London: Chapman and Hall Medical; 1991.

20. Davidoff AM, Pappas TN, Murray EA, et al. Mechanisms of major biliary injury during laparoscopic cholecystectomy. *Ann Surg* 1992;**215**:196–202.

21. Deziel DJ, Millikan KW, Economou SG, et al. Complications of laparoscopic cholecystectomy: A national survey of 4,292 hospitals and an analysis of 77,604 cases. *Am J Surg* 1993;**165**:9–14.

22. McMahon AJ, Fullarton G, Baxter JN, et al. Bile duct injury and bile leakage in laparoscopic cholecystectomy. *Br J Surg* 1995;**82**:307–13.

23. Richardson MC, Bell G, Fullarton GM. Incidence and nature of bile duct injuries following laparoscopic cholecystectomy: An audit of 5913 cases. West of Scotland Laparoscopic Cholecystectomy Audit Group. *Br J Surg* 1996;**83**:1356–60.

24. Shea JA, Healey MJ, Berlin JA, et al. Mortality and complications associated with laparoscopic cholecystectomy. A meta-analysis. *Ann Surg* 1996;**224**:609–20.

25. MacFadyen BV Jr, Vecchio R, Ricardo AE, et al. Bile duct injury after laparoscopic cholecystectomy. The United States experience. *Surg Endosc* 1998;**12**:315–21.

26. Champault G, Cazacu F, Taffinder N. Serious trocar accidents in laparoscopic surgery: A French survey of 103,852 operations. *Surg Laparosc Endosc* 1996;**6**:367–70.

27. Hashizume M, Sugimachi K. Needle and trocar injury during laparoscopic surgery in Japan. *Surg Endosc* 1997;**11**:1198–201.

28. Bonjer HJ, Hazebroek EJ, Kazemier G, et al. Open versus closed establishment of pneumoperitoneum in laparoscopic surgery. *Br J Surg* 1997;**84**:599–602.

29. Schäfer M, Lauper M, Krähenbühl L. Trocar and Veress needle injuries during laparoscopy. *Surg Endosc* 2001;**15**:275–280.

30. Rothman JP, Burcharth J, Pommergaard H-C, et al. The quality of cholecystectomy in Denmark has improved over 6-year period. *Langenbecks Arch Surg* 2015;**400**:735–40.

31. Rystedt J, Lindell G, Montgomery A. Bile duct injuries associated with 55,134 cholecystectomies: Treatment and outcome from a national perspective. *World J Surg* 2016;**40**:73–80.

32. Stilling NM, Fristrup C, Wettergren A, et al. Long term outcome after early repair of iatrogenic bile duct injury. A national Danish multicentre study. *HPB (Oxford)* 2015;**17**:394–400.

33. Sturesson C, Hemmingsson O, Månsson C, et al. Quality-of-life after bile duct injury repaired by hepaticojejunostomy: A national cohort study. *Scand J Gastroenterol* 2020;**55**:1087–92.

34. Stoker DL, Spiegelhalter DJ, Singh R, et al. Laparoscopic versus open inguinal hernia repair: randomised prospective trial. *Lancet* 1994;**343**:1243–45.

35. Lumley JW, Fielding GA, Rhodes M, et al. Laparoscopic-assisted colorectal surgery. Lessons learned from 240 consecutive patients. *Dis Colon Rectum* 1996;**39**:155–9.

36. O'Rourke N, Fielding G. Laparoscopic right hepatectomy: Surgical technique. *J Gastrointest Surg* 2004;**8**:213–6.

37. Gagner M, Pomp A. Laparoscopic pylorus-preserving pancreatoduodenectomy. *Surg Endosc* 1994;**8**:408–10.

38. Taylor C, O'Rourke N, Nathanson L, et al. Laparoscopic distal pancreatectomy: The Brisbane experience of forty-six cases. *HPB (Oxford)* 2008;**10**:38–42.

39. O'Rourke NA, Fielding GA. Laparoscopic cholecystectomy for acute cholecystitis. *ANZ J Surg* 1992; **62**:944–6.

40. O'Rourke NA, Askew AR, Cowen AE, et al. The role of ERCP and endoscopic sphincterotomy in

SECTION 10 | GALLBLADDER

References   **579**

the era of laparoscopic cholecystectomy. *Aust N Z J Surg* 1993;**63**:3–7.

41. Pursnani KG, Bazza Y, Calleja M, et al. Laparoscopic cholecystectomy under epidural anesthesia in patients with chronic respiratory disease. *Surg Endosc* 1998;**12**:1082–84.

42. Yu G, Wen Q, Qiu L, et al. Laparoscopic cholecystectomy under spinal anaesthesia vs. general anaesthesia: A meta-analysis of randomized controlled trials. *BMC Anesthesiol* 2015;**15**:176.

43. Miyazaki M, Yoshitomi H, Miyakawa S, et al. Clinical practice guidelines for the management of biliary tract cancers 2015: The 2nd English edition. *J Hepatobiliary Pancreat Sci* 2015;**22**:249–73.

44. Agarwal AK, Javed A, Kalayarasan R, et al. Minimally invasive versus the conventional open surgical approach of a radical cholecystectomy for gallbladder cancer: A retrospective comparative study. *HPB (Oxford)* 2015;**17**:536–41.

45. Jang JY, Han H-S, Yoon Y-S, et al. Retrospective comparison of outcomes of laparoscopic and open surgery for T2 gallbladder cancer: Thirteen-year experience. *Surg Oncol* 2019;**29**:142–7.

46. Ahmed SH, Usmani SUR, Mushtaq R, et al. Role of laparoscopic surgery in the management of gallbladder cancer: Systematic review & meta-analysis. *Am J Surg* 2023;**225(6)**:975–87

47. Ong CT, Leung K, Nussbaum DP, et al. Open versus laparoscopic portal lymphadenectomy in gallbladder cancer: Is there a difference in lymph node yield? *HPB* 2018;**20**:505–13.

48. Rhodes M, Nathanson L, O'Rourke N, et al. Laparoscopic exploration of the common bile duct: Lessons learned from 129 consecutive cases. *Br J Surg* 1995;**82**:666–8.

49. Martin IJ, Bailey IS, Rhodes M, et al. Towards T-tube free laparoscopic bile duct exploration: A methodologic evolution during 300 consecutive procedures. *Ann Surg* 1998;**228**:29–34.

50. Cuschieri A, Lezoche E, Morino M, et al. E.A.E.S. multicenter prospective randomized trial comparing two-stage vs single-stage management of patients with gallstone disease and ductal calculi. *Surg Endosc* 1999;**13**:952–7.

51. Nathanson LK, O'Rourke NA, Martin IJ, et al. Postoperative ERCP versus laparoscopic choledochotomy for clearance of selected bile duct calculi: A randomized trial. *Ann Surg* 2005;**242**:188–92.

52. Gurusamy K, Samraj K, Gluud C, et al. Meta-analysis of randomized controlled trials on the safety and effectiveness of early versus delayed laparoscopic cholecystectomy for acute holecystitis. *Br J Surg* 2010;**97**:141–50.

53. Gutt CN, Encke J, Köninger J, et al. Acute cholecystitis: Early versus delayed cholecystectomy, a multicenter randomized trial (ACDC study, NCT00447304). *Ann Surg* 2013;**258**:385–93.

54. Wu X-D, Tian X, Liu M-M, et al. Meta-analysis comparing early versus delayed laparoscopic cholecystectomy for acute cholecystitis. *Br J Surg* 2015;**102**:1302–13.

55. Roulin D, Saadi A, Di Mare L, et al. Early versus delayed cholecystectomy for acute cholecystitis, are the 72 hours Still the Rule? A randomized trial. *Ann Surg* 2016;**264**:717–22.

56. Jee SL, Jarmin R, Lim KF, et al. Outcomes of early versus delayed cholecystectomy in patients with mild to moderate acute biliary pancreatitis: A randomized prospective study. *Asian J Surg* 2018;**41**:47–54.

57. Moody N, Adiamah A, Yanni F, et al. Meta-analysis of randomized clinical trials of early versus delayed cholecystectomy for mild gallstone pancreatitis. *Br J Surg* 2019;**106**:1442–51.

58. Kenington JC, Pellino G, Iqbal MR, Ahmed N, Halahakoon VC, Zaborowski AM, et al. Guidelines on general surgical emergencies in pregnancy *Br J Surg* 2024;**111(3)**:znae051.

59. Wakabayashi G, Iwashita Y, Hibi T, et al. Tokyo Guidelines 2018: Surgical management of acute cholecystitis: Safe steps in laparoscopic cholecystectomy for acute cholecystitis (with videos). *J Hepatobiliary Pancreat Sci* 2018;**25**:73–86.

60. Strategies for minimizing bile duct injuries: Adopting a universal culture of safety in Cholecystectomy. 2014. Available from: https://www.sages.org/safe-cholecystectomy-program/ The SAGES Safe Cholecystectomy Program (Accessed 28 August 2024).

61. Bourgouin S, Mancini J, Monchal T, et al. How to predict difficult laparoscopic cholecystectomy? Proposal for a simple preoperative scoring system. *Am J Surg* 2016;**212**:873–81.

62. Madni TD, Leshikar DE, Minshall CT, et al. The Parkland grading scale for cholecystitis. *Am J Surg* 2018;**215**:625–30.

63. Wennmacker SZ, Bhimani N, van Dijk AH, et al. Predicting operative difficulty of laparoscopic cholecystectomy in patients with acute biliary presentations. *ANZ J Surg* 2019;**89**:1451–6.

64. Tranter-Entwistle I, Eglinton T, Hugh TJ, et al. Use of prospective video analysis to understand the impact of technical difficulty on operative process during laparoscopic cholecystectomy. *HPB (Oxford)* 2022;**24**:2096–103.

65. Hernandez M, Murphy B, Aho JM, et al. Validation of the AAST EGS acute cholecystitis grade and comparison with the Tokyo guidelines. *Surgery* 2018;**163**:739–46.

66. Griffiths EA, Hodson J, Vohra RS, et al. Utilisation of an operative difficulty grading scale for laparoscopic cholecystectomy. *Surg Endosc* 2019;**33**:110–21.

67. Schuster KM, O'Connor R, Cripps M, et al. Revision of the AAST grading scale for acute cholecystitis with comparison to physiologic measures of severity. *J Trauma Acute Care Surg* 2022;**92**:664–74.

68. Ji W, Li L-T, Wang Z-M, et al. A randomized controlled trial of laparoscopic versus open cholecystectomy in patients with cirrhotic portal hypertension. *World J Gastroenterol* 2005;**11**:2513–17.

69. Laurence JM, Tran PD, Richardson AJ, et al. Laparoscopic or open cholecystectomy in cirrhosis:

A systematic review of outcomes and meta-analysis of randomized trials. *HPB (Oxford)* 2012;**14**: 153–61.

70. de Goede B, Klitsie PJ, Hagen SM, et al. Meta-analysis of laparoscopic versus open cholecystectomy for patients with liver cirrhosis and symptomatic cholecystolithiasis. *Br J Surg* 2013;**100**:209–16.

71. Pasquali S, Boal M, Griffiths EA, et al. Meta-analysis of perioperative antibiotics in patients undergoing laparoscopic cholecystectomy. *Br J Surg* 2016;**103**:27–34.

72. Gomez-Ospina JC, Zapata-Copete JA, Bejarano M, et al. Antibiotic prophylaxis in elective laparoscopic cholecystectomy: A systematic review and network meta-analysis. *J Gastrointest Surg* 2018;**22**: 1193–203.

73. Asai K, Watanabe M, Kusachi S, et al. Bacteriological analysis of bile in acute cholecystitis according to the Tokyo guidelines. *J Hepatobiliary Pancreat Sci* 2012;**19**:476–86.

74. Bender K, Lewin J, O'Rourke H, et al. Total 5-mm port approach: A feasible technique for both elective and emergency laparoscopic cholecystectomy. *ANZ J Surg* 2018;**88**:E751–E755.

75. Hugh TB, Kelly MD, Mekisic A. Rouvière's sulcus: A useful landmark in laparoscopic cholecystectomy. *Br J Surg* 1997;**84**:1253–4.

76. Strasberg SM, Hertl M, Soper NJ. An analysis of the problem of biliary injury during laparoscopic cholecystectomy. *J Am Coll Surg* 1995;**180**: 101–25.

77. Way LW, Stewart L, Gantert W, et al. Causes and prevention of laparoscopic bile duct injuries: Analysis of 252 cases from a human factors and cognitive psychology perspective. *Ann Surg* 2003;**237**:460–9.

78. Strasberg SM, Pucci MJ, Brunt LM, et al. Subtotal cholecystectomy: 'Fenestrating' vs 'Reconstituting' subtypes and the prevention of bile duct injury: Definition of the optimal procedure in difficult operative conditions. *J Am Coll Surg* 2016;**222**: 89–96.

79. Mirizzi PI. La colangiografia durante las operaciones de las vias biliares. *Bol Soc Chir BAires* 1932;**16**:1133.

80. Fletcher DR, Hobbs MS, Tan P, et al. Complications of cholecystectomy: Risks of the laparoscopic approach and protective effects of operative cholangiography: A population-based study. *Ann Surg* 1999;**229**:449–57.

81. Flum DR, Flowers C, Veenstra DL. A cost-effectiveness analysis of intraoperative cholangiography in the prevention of bile duct injury during laparoscopic cholecystectomy. *J Am Coll Surg* 2003;**196**: 385–93.

82. Buddingh KT, Weersma RK, Savenije RAJ, et al. Lower rate of major bile duct injury and increased intraoperative management of common bile duct stones after implementation of routine intraoperative cholangiography. *J Am Coll Surg* 2011;**213**:267–74.

83. Ford JA, Soop M, Du J, et al. Systematic review of intraoperative cholangiography in cholecystectomy. *Br J Surg* 2012;**99**:160–7.

84. Kovács N, Németh D, Földi M, et al. Selective intraoperative cholangiography should be considered over routine intraoperative cholangiography during cholecystectomy: A systematic review and meta-analysis. *Surg Endosc* 2022;**36**:7126–39.

85. Puhalla H, Flint N, O'Rourke N. Surgery for common bile duct stones: A lost surgical skill; still worthwhile in the minimally invasive century? *Langenbecks Arch Surg* 2015;**400**:119–27.

86. Ishizawa T, Bandai Y, Ijichi M, et al. Fluorescent cholangiography illuminating the biliary tree during laparoscopic cholecystectomy. *Br J Surg* 2010;**97**:1369–77.

87. Vlek SL, van Dam DA, Rubinstein SM, et al. Biliary tract visualization using near-infrared imaging with indocyanine green during laparoscopic cholecystectomy: Results of a systematic review. *Surg Endosc* 2017;**31**:2731–42.

88. Wang X, Teh CSC, Ishizawa T, et al. Consensus Guidelines for the Use of Fluorescence Imaging in Hepatobiliary Surgery. *Ann Surg* 2021;**274**:97–106.

89. van den Bos J, Schols RM, Boni L, et al. Near-infrared fluorescence cholangiography assisted laparoscopic cholecystectomy (FALCON): An international multicentre randomized controlled trial. *Surg Endosc* 2023;**37(6)**:4574–84.

90. Bulian DR, Knuth J, Cerasani N, et al. Transvaginal/transumbilical hybrid—NOTES—versus 3-trocar needlescopic cholecystectomy: Short-term results of a randomized clinical trial. *Ann Surg* 2015;**261**:451–8.

91. Markar SR, Karthikesalingam A, Thrumurthy S, et al. Single-incision laparoscopic surgery (SILS) vs. conventional multiport cholecystectomy: Systematic review and meta-analysis. *Surg Endosc* 2012;**26**: 1205–13.

92. Tranchart H, Ketoff S, Lainas P, et al. Single incision laparoscopic cholecystectomy: For what benefit? *HPB (Oxford)* 2013;**15**:433–8.

93. Hoyuela C, Juvany M, Guillaumes S, et al. Long term incisional hernia rate after single-incision laparoscopic cholecystectomy is significantly higher than that after standard three-port laparoscopy: A cohort study. *Hernia* 2019;**23**:1205–13.

94. Riccardi M, Dughayli M, Baidoun F. Open cholecystectomy for the new learner: Obstacles and challenges. *JSLS* 2021;**25(2)**:e2021.00026.

95. Stevens S, Rivas H, Cacchione RN, et al. Jaundice due to extrabiliary gallstones. *JSLS* 2003;**7**:277–9.

96. Lau H, Brooks DC. Contemporary outcomes of ambulatory laparoscopic cholecystectomy in a major teaching hospital. *World J Surg* 2002;**26**:1117–21.

97. Briggs CD, Irving GB, Mann CD, et al. Introduction of a day-case laparoscopic cholecystectomy service in the UK: A critical analysis of factors influencing same-day discharge and contact with primary care providers. *Ann R Coll Surg Engl* 2009;**91**:583–90.

98. Solodkyy A, Hakeem AR, Oswald N, et al. 'True Day Case' laparoscopic cholecystectomy in a

high-volume specialist unit and review of factors contributing to unexpected overnight stay. *Minim Invasive Surg* 2018;**2018**: 1260358.

99. O'Rourke NA, van Rensburg AJ. Post Cholecystectomy Symptoms. In: Cox MR, Eslick GD, Padbury R (eds) *The Management of Gallstone Disease: A Practical and Evidence-Based Approach.* New York: Springer International Publishing, 2018, pp. 205–19.

100. Lamberts MP, Den Oudsten BL, Keus F, et al. Patient-reported outcomes of symptomatic cholelithiasis patients following cholecystectomy after at least 5 years of follow-up: A long-term prospective cohort study. *Surg Endosc* 2014;**28**:3443–50.

Bailey & Love's Essential Operations Bailey & Love's Essential Operatio
Bailey & Love's Essential Operations Bailey & Love's Essential Operatio
Bailey & Love's Essential Operations Bailey & Love's Essential Operatio

SECTION 10 | GALLBLADDER

Chapter 72

Open Cholecystectomy

Paul M. Cromwell and Kevin C. Conlon

INTRODUCTION

Cholecystectomy is one of the commonest procedures performed by general surgeons and the history of the procedure dates back almost 150 years. The first successful cholecystectomy was performed in Berlin in 1882 by Carl Langenbuch. His patient was a 43-year-old man who had suffered from biliary colic for 16 years. Although he was discharged after 6 weeks, pain-free and gaining weight, cholecystectomy was often more perilous, with mortality rates as high as 20% in the early years of the 20th century. However, surgical methods such as placing the patient in the Trendelenburg position, common bile duct (CBD) exploration, perioperative investigations and perioperative antibiotics have significantly improved outcomes. The concept of 'laparoscopy' was first coined by Hans Christian Jacobaeus in 1910, but it was not until 1987 that a French surgeon Philip Mouret in Lyon performed the first laparoscopic cholecystectomy. The minimally invasive technique was subsequently introduced into the United States in 1988 and rapidly became accepted worldwide. It was rapidly adopted by surgeons through the mid-1990s (1) and as the vast majority of patients are candidates for a minimally invasive approach, the original open procedure has been largely supplanted. Nonetheless, there remain clear indications for an open approach, and surgeons need to be familiar with the technique and its pitfalls.

MODERN ERA

The indications for cholecystectomy are dealt with in **Chapter 71**. In brief, a cholecystectomy is performed in the setting of proven disease of the gallbladder, such as: 1) Symptomatic cholelithiasis; 2) gallstone pancreatitis; 3) biliary dyskinesia (detected on HIDA scan); 4) acalculous cholecystitis; 5) high-risk gallbladder polyps. The laparoscopic technique has been demonstrated to result in shorter hospital stays, lower wound infection rates and a lower incidence of pneumonia when compared with the open approach, and meta-analyses have demonstrated no difference in bile leakage rates, intraoperative blood loss or operative times compared to open cholecystectomy (2,3). Currently, 96% of cholecystectomies performed in the UK and Ireland for benign disease are completed laparoscopically (4).

INDICATIONS FOR OPEN CHOLECYSTECTOMY

At present, less than 5% of cholecystectomies performed for benign gallbladder disease in the UK are open procedures (4), while in the United States, this is somewhat higher ranging from 8.1–9.5% (5,6). Indications for a planned open cholecystectomy include: 1) Extensive upper abdominal surgery with adhesions; 2) gallbladder cancer; 3) cirrhosis; 4) right upper quadrant stoma or 5) as part of a larger procedure such as pancreaticoduodenectomy. This approach may also be necessary for the critically ill patient with acute cholecystitis as the impact of decreased cardiac return and high ventilation pressures can preclude the use of a pneumoperitoneum. Patient selection is important if severe cholecystitis is suspected, given the increased risk of significant vascular or biliary injury and a percutaneous cholecystostomy can be an effective treatment of acute cholecystitis and should be considered (7–9).

CONVERSION TO OPEN SURGERY

In current surgical practice, perhaps the most common reason for performing an open cholecystectomy is converting from a laparoscopic approach to an open incision due to technical issues or complications (10). Conversion should not itself be seen as a complication but as a responsible decision to avoid adverse outcomes such as bile duct injury. Preoperative risk factors for conversion to the open approach include: 1) Male sex; 2) increasing age; 3) leucocytosis; 4) duration of symptoms and 5) obesity (10). There have been no randomized trials on the merits of converting to an open cholecystectomy in the difficult laparoscopic gallbladder, however, common indications are extensive inflammation, adhesions, anatomical variances, bile duct injury, retained bile duct stones, concern for malignancy or uncontrolled bleeding. When faced with these hostile conditions, the laparoscopic surgeon should be confident in their ability to perform an open approach. Unfortunately, as the number of open procedures has decreased, it has become more difficult for senior surgical residents to gain expertise with open cholecystectomy during their training and as a result, new consultant surgeons are at risk of becoming less proficient in the technique (11). When confronted with the difficult laparoscopic gallbladder, guidelines now

DOI: 10.1201/9781003080060-72

recommend performing the most appropriate 'bail-out' procedure according to the surgeon's judgment, as outlined (12).

SUBTOTAL CHOLECYSTECTOMY

An alternative to performing a full cholecystectomy when faced with scenarios of a 'hostile environment' where the anatomy cannot be identified with certainty, is to perform a subtotal cholecystectomy. Recent data suggests that the use of this approach has increased in the United States, with cases increasing from 0.1–0.52% and 0.12–0.28% of all laparoscopic and open chole-cystectomies, respectively (13). The technique involves making an incision into the gallbladder, aspirating the contents, removing as much of the gallbladder wall as possible and securing the cystic duct orifice with a purse-string suture, ligature or stapling device. It can be performed through either a laparoscopic or open approach. There is no precise nomenclature in the literature, and the terms partial cholecystectomy and subtotal cholecystectomy are currently used interchangeably. Some studies refer to removing any portion of a gallbladder as a subtotal cholecystectomy. In contrast, others suggest that only if the gallbladder is excised down to Hartmann's pouch and secured should it be called a subtotal cholecystectomy (14,15). Common indications for subtotal cholecystectomy include severe or gangrenous cholecystitis and scarred intrahepatic gallbladders. In an attempt to complete a cholecystec-tomy safely without an accidental bile duct injury, this technique is usually performed as a 'bail-out' procedure. The reported rate of bile duct injury in subtotal chole-cystectomy is 0.08%, however, the reported rate of bile leak (18%) and retained stones (3%) are higher when compared to total cholecystectomy (0.3% and 0.3%, respectively) (15). The open subtotal cholecystectomy technique, including the concept of fenestration versus reconstituting methods, is described (14).

OPEN CHOLECYSTECTOMY OPERATIVE TECHNIQUE

The procedure is performed under general anaesthesia with the use of a suitable muscle relaxant.

Positioning

The patient is positioned supine on the operating table and can have both arms by the sides or extended to right angles to the body, depending on the surgeon's preference. An orogastric tube is inserted after intu-bation to deflate the stomach. An operating table that allows a C-arm to be centred under the patient is necessary should an intraoperative cholangiogram (IOC) be required. To improve exposure the patient can be tilted head-up. The operating surgeon stands on the right of the patient with the first assistant directly opposite.

Incision

The skin should be prepped and appropriate thrombo-embolic prophylaxis and intravenous antibiotics should be administered before incision. We prefer a right subcostal 'Kocher' incision, which should be made at 1–2 finger breaths below the right costal margin. In a patient with a palpable liver edge, this incision can be made at two finger breaths below the liver's edge. We would only select an upper midline incision when the patient has other abdominal pathology that needs to be addressed during the procedure. The incision, which should be adequate for exposure, is continued down through the anterior rectus sheath. The rectus muscle can be divided using electrocautery, and the incision continued into the peritoneal cavity.

RETRACTION

Upon entering the peritoneal cavity, the abdomen is explored to exclude any other intra-abdominal pathol-ogy. The liver is palpated and air allowed to enter the sub-phrenic space. The falciform ligament is divided and the round ligament ligated. A table-mounted, self-retaining retractor such as a Thompson® (Thomp-son Surgical Instruments, MI, USA) or Bookwalter® (Surgical Holdings, UK) combined with an Alexis® (Applied Medical, CA, USA) type wound protecting retractor can be used to aid exposure.

Adhesions from the gallbladder to adjacent surfaces such as the colon or duodenum may be present and should be divided with a combination of sharp scissors or electrocautery. Once divided, moist 30 x 30 cm gauze swabs can retract the colon, stomach and duodenum inferiorly and medially. The optimal exposure should result in the gallbladder in the centre of the wound and the bowel safely retracted from the operating field. The gauze swabs may have to be held in place with an assis-tant's left hand (*Figure 72.1*).

A Kelly clamp should be placed on the fundus of the gallbladder and in a tense, acutely inflamed gall-bladder, the contents may need to be aspirated with a needle and syringe before application of the Kelly clamp. A second Kelly clamp should then be applied to the gallbladder above Hartmann's pouch and used to retract this portion of the gallbladder towards the right lower quadrant.

The two main operative methods are a retrograde approach commencing the dissection at the triangle of Calot working towards the fundus of the gallbladder and an antegrade approach commencing at the fundus and working 'down' towards the triangle of Calot.

Retrograde approach

The surgeon should palpate the foramen of Winslow with their finger and thumb for evidence of calculi in the common duct or thickening of the head of the pancreas. A small moist swab placed behind the

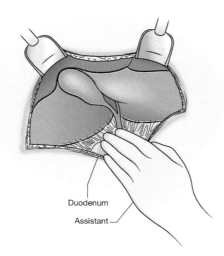

Duodenum

Assistant

Figure 72.1 Illustration of an initial optimal exposure.

gallbladder can prevent the inadvertent spillage of bile or calculi. Grasping the under surface of the gallbladder with a Kelly clamp provides, as noted previously, anterior and lateral traction. This clamp should be placed well up onto the under surface away from the neck, especially when the gallbladder is distended, to avoid incorporating the common bile duct into the clamp. The peritoneum is divided on the inferior surface of the gallbladder about 3 mm from the liver edge, and dissection is continued down to the hepatoduodenal ligament using diathermy or sharp scissors. The neck of the gallbladder can now be freed up with electrocautery or blunt gauze dissection to identify the region of the cystic duct. A Kelly clamp can now be placed on the infundibulum or neck of the gallbladder to provide traction, and the peritoneum is opened up on the superior surface of the gallbladder. The cystic node and fatty tissue can be displaced using blunt dissection to define the cystic duct clearly. It is important that the so called 'critical view' is obtained. Care should be taken while using electrocautery close to the hepatoduodenal ligament to avoid inadvertent damage to the common hepatic or common bile ducts.

A right-angle clamp can be passed behind the cystic duct to carefully isolate the duct from the surrounding tissues and common bile duct. Care is used to avoid excessive traction as this might 'tent up' the common duct and lead to inadvertent injury. This is a particular risk in either the very thin patient or those with a short cystic duct. A ligature can be passed around the cystic duct and the cystic artery is then isolated close to the gallbladder using the right-angle clamp or Kittner dissector. Careful dissection prevents injury or ligation of the right hepatic artery. The cystic duct should now be thoroughly palpated to ensure no calculi will remain

in the cystic duct stump or pass into the common bile duct. The gallbladder can now be dissected off the liver for approximately 2–3 cm to completely expose the 'critical view'. This is achieved by clearing the hepatocystic triangle of fat and fibrous tissue to dissect the lower part of the gallbladder off the cystic plate. There should be a clear view of only two structures entering the gallbladder, the cystic duct and the cystic artery. There are a number of variations in the anatomy of the cystic duct (*Figure 72.2*), right hepatic duct (*Figure 72.3*) and right segmental sector ducts (*Figure 72.4*). Once the anatomy has been confirmed, the surgeon can now divide the cystic duct and artery. Our preference is to deal with the cystic duct first. It can be divided between two curved clamps making sure to leave a cuff of tissue away from its confluence with the common hepatic duct. IOC can be performed routinely or selectively through the cystic duct stump. When complete, the cystic duct stump can be ligated with a transfixing suture and reinforced with a metal haemoclip. The cystic artery should be divided between two clamps and ligated away from the common hepatic duct. Reinforcing metal clips can also be used on the cystic artery. Care should be taken to ensure that the right hepatic artery has not been mistaken for the cystic artery as anatomical anomalies can occur in the region (*Figure 72.5*). If the cystic artery stump ligature slips, take care if applying a haemostatic clamp to control the haemorrhage as the common hepatic duct can inadvertently be clamped due to an obscured field. This can result in duct injury or the formation of a stricture.

Now that the cystic duct and cystic artery have been safely secured, the gallbladder can be dissected from the cystic plate. The clamp on the infundibulum of the gallbladder can be retracted anterior and superior with the surgeon's left hand, and the areolar tissue between the gallbladder and the liver can be dissected using electrocautery. In the non-inflamed gallbladder, dissection in this plane will avoid injury to the liver, the branches of the right hepatic artery or small intrahepatic ductules. When the gallbladder has been excised, if choledocholithiasis has been seen on IOC or confirmed on prior imaging, the surgeon can proceed to the common bile duct exploration. If bile or calculi have been spilt into the abdomen, care should be taken to remove visible calculi to avoid abscess formation. The abdomen should be irrigated with warm saline prior to closure.

Antegrade approach (fundus down)

In contrast to the retrograde approach, the antegrade technique begins at the fundus of the gallbladder and is continued in a top-down fashion towards the porta hepatis. A Kelly clamp is placed on the fundus of the gallbladder and used by the surgeon or assistant to provide anterior and medial traction. The peritoneum surrounding the gallbladder is incised about 3 mm from the liver inferiorly and superiorly using electrocautery. The areolar tissue connecting the gallbladder to the

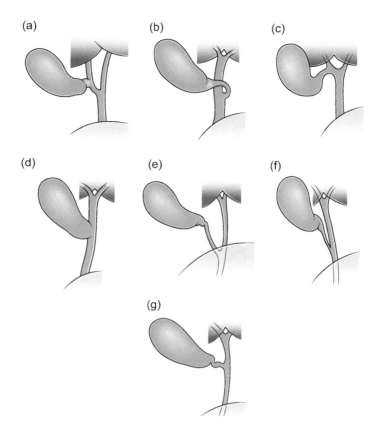

Figure 72.2 Hepatic and cystic duct union abnormalities (a); Low right hepatic duct (b); Anterior spiral (c); High right hepatic duct (d); Absent cystic duct (e&f); Low union (g); Normal.

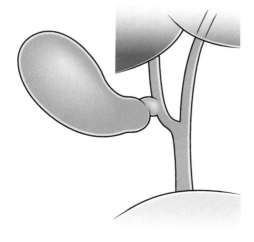

Figure 72.3 Labelled illustration of a right hepatic duct anomaly.

liver can then be divided with electrocautery, again care should be exercised as one approaches the neck of the gallbladder to avoid injury to the extra hepatic biliary system. Extreme care must be taken in the acutely inflamed gallbladder as dissection inferiorly along a thickened and contracted cystic plate can result in an inadvertent bile duct or vascular injury due to its relationship to the right portal pedicle. Once the gallbladder is fully dissected from the liver, gentle inferior and lateral traction can help expose the triangle of Calot with isolation of the cystic duct and cystic artery performed in a similar fashion as the retrograde approach (*Figure 72.6*).

Subtotal cholecystectomy technique

This method is usually reserved for cases of severe inflammation and is considered a 'bail-out' procedure. The indications for this method are discussed. Dissection begins in an antegrade (fundus down) approach as inflammation around the porta hepatis is severe, anatomy is unclear and dissection deemed too high-risk for bile duct or other major injury. Dissection should be

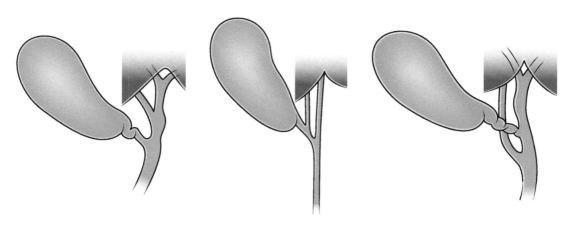

Figure 72.4 Accessory hepatic Duct variations (a) joining common hepatic duct, (b) joining cystic duct, (c) joining common hepatic duct.

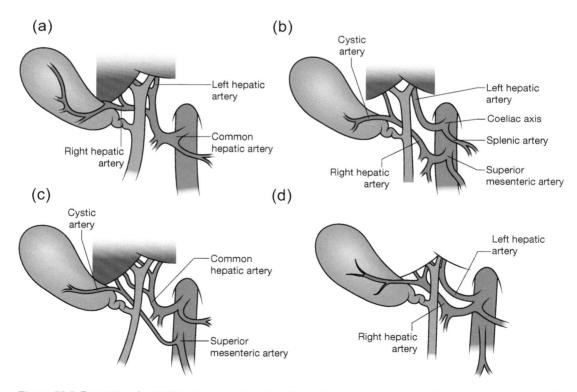

Figure 72.5 Examples of variations in the cystic artery, illustrating the potential risk of injury to the right hepatic artery: (a), (b), (c) and (d).

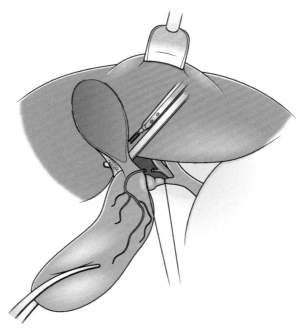

Figure 72.6 Illustration showing an antegrade technique.

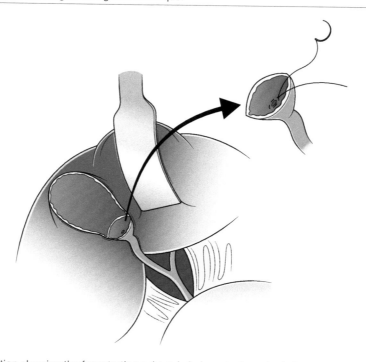

Figure 72.7 Illustration showing the fenestrating subtotal cholecystectomy technique.

continued inferiorly to attempt to remove as much of
the gallbladder as possible. Moist packs are used and
placed around the gallbladder to protect the peritoneal
cavity from contamination. The gallbladder is then
opened, aspirated and calculi, if present, are removed.

At this point, the surgeon can choose to fenestrate
or reconstitute the gallbladder remnant (14). To
fenestrate the gallbladder remnant (*Figure 72.7*), the
gallbladder's free-edge is left open and a purse-string
suture is secured around the gallbladder neck, care

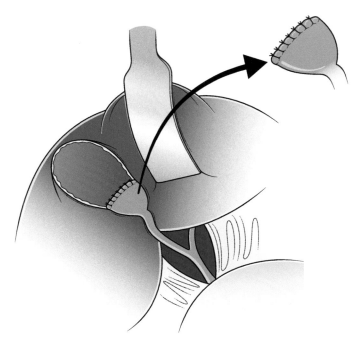

Figure 72.8 Illustration showing the reconstituting subtotal cholecystectomy technique.

being taken not to involve the cystic duct or bile duct. The remaining gallbladder mucosa is then ablated with either electrocautery or argon beam. If necessary, the anterior wall of the gallbladder can be excised while leaving the posterior wall behind. This can reduce the risk of vascular or biliary injury during posterior dissection. In addition, the cystic duct orifice can be occluded, as detailed. To reconstitute the gallbladder remnant, a running monofilament suture is used to close the upper edge of the gallbladder wall (*Figure 72.8*). A sub-hepatic closed suction drain should be placed due to the high risk of bile leak.

The fenestrating technique is, in theory, less likely to reform into a functioning gallbladder lumen which reduces the risk of a second procedure, although evidence regarding this is contradictory in systematic reviews (15,16). Proponents of the reconstituting approach would suggest this method should reduce the risk of bile leak, although no significant difference in bile leak has been demonstrated (15,16). There is some evidence that a fenestrating laparoscopic subtotal cholecystectomy can result in a higher rate of open conversion, retained stones, subhepatic collection, surgical site infection (SSI) and postoperative ERCP (16). There is currently insufficient data to determine which technique is superior when performing the open approach.

Closure

For the right subcostal incision, the anterior and posterior fascia are closed in two layers using a running

long-lasting absorbable monofilament suture such as 0 Polydioxanone (PDS) suture. The skin is then sutured closed with a running monofilament suture in a subcuticular fashion such as 4/0 Monocryl® (J&J Med Tech, NJ, USA).

POSTOPERATIVE CARE

The orogastric tube can be removed at the end of the procedure. Antibiotics are usually only required if the patient has an ongoing infection. The patient can start with sips of water early and progress their oral intake as tolerated. The expected length of stay is 2–3 days. In a routine open cholecystectomy, neither a nasogastric tube nor an intra-abdominal drain is required. However, in a complicated cholecystectomy, a surgically placed drain left in the sub-hepatic bed may be indicated to detect early postoperative bleeding or bile leak. The drain should be left in for several days as bile leaks may not become clinically apparent on the first postoperative day.

REFERENCES

1. Yannos S, Athanasios P, Christoforides C, Evangelos F. History of biliary surgery. *World J Surg* 2013;**37**(5):1006–12.
2. Keus F, De Jong JAF, Gooszen HG, Van Laarhoven CJHM. Laparoscopic versus open cholecystectomy for patients with symptomatic cholecystolithiasis. *Cochrane Database Syst Rev* 2006;(**4**):CD006231.

3. Coccolini F, Catena F, Pisano M, Gheza F, Fagiuoli S, Di Saverio S, et al. Open versus laparoscopic cholecystectomy in acute cholecystitis. Systematic review and meta-analysis. *Int J Surg* 2015;**18**: 196–204.

4. Vohra RS, Pasquali S, Kirkham AJ, Marriott P, Johnstone M, Spreadborough P, et al. Population-based cohort study of outcomes following cholecystectomy for benign gallbladder diseases. *Br J Surg* 2016;**103(12)**:1704–15.

5. Randall JA, Chen S, Brody F. Cholecystectomy outcomes in the Veterans Affairs Surgical Quality Improvement Program (2006–2017). *J Laparoendosc Adv Surg Tech* 2021;**31(3)**:251–60.

6. Csikesz N, Ricciardi R, Tseng JF, Shah SA. Current status of surgical management of acute cholecystitis in the United States. *World J Surg* 2008;**32(10)**: 2230–6.

7. Strasberg SM, Gouma DJ. 'Extreme' vasculobiliary injuries: Association with fundus-down cholecystectomy in severely inflamed gallbladders. *HPB (Oxford)* 2012;**14(1)**:1–8.

8. Horn T, Christensen SD, Kirkegård J, Larsen LP, Knudsen AR, Mortensen F V. Percutaneous cholecystostomy is an effective treatment option for acute calculous cholecystitis: A 10-year experience. *HPB (Oxford)* 2015;**17(4)**:326–31.

9. Simorov A, Ranade A, Parcells J, Shaligram A, Shostrom V, Boilesen E, et al. Emergent cholecystostomy is superior to open cholecystectomy in extremely ill patients with acalculous cholecystitis: A large multicenter outcome study. *Am J Surg* 2013;**206(6)**: 935–41.

10. Panni RZ, Strasberg SM. Preoperative predictors of conversion as indicators of local inflammation in acute cholecystitis: strategies for future studies to develop quantitative predictors. *J Hepatobiliary Pancreat Sci* 2018;**25(1)**:101–8.

11. St. John A, Caturegli I, Kubicki NS, Kavic SM. The rise of minimally invasive surgery: 16 Year analysis of the progressive replacement of open surgery with laparoscopy. *JSLS J Soc Laparosc Robot Surg* 2020;**24(4)**:e2020.00076.

12. Wakabayashi G, Iwashita Y, Hibi T, Takada T, Strasberg SM, Asbun HJ, et al. Tokyo Guidelines 2018: Surgical management of acute cholecystitis: Safe steps in laparoscopic cholecystectomy for acute cholecystitis. *J Hepatobiliary Pancreat Sci* 2018;**25(1)**:73–86.

13. Sabour AF, Matsushima K, Love BE, Alicuben ET, Schellenberg MA, Inaba K, et al. Nationwide trends in the use of subtotal cholecystectomy for acute cholecystitis. In: *Surgery*. Maryland Heights, MO: Mosby Inc, 2020. pp. 569–74.

14. Strasberg SM, Pucci MJ, Brunt LM, Deziel DJ. Subtotal cholecystectomy 'Fenestrating' vs 'Reconstituting' subtypes and the prevention of bile duct injury: Definition of the optimal procedure in difficult operative conditions. *J Am Coll Surg* 2016;**222(1)**:89–96.

15. Elshaer M, Gravante G, Thomas K, Sorge R, Al-Hamali S, Ebdewi H. Subtotal cholecystectomy for 'Difficult gallbladders': Systematic review and meta-analysis. *JAMA Surg* 2015;**150(2)**:159–68.

16. Koo JGA, Chan YH, Shelat VG. Laparoscopic subtotal cholecystectomy: Comparison of reconstituting and fenestrating techniques. *Surg Endosc* 2021;**35(3)**: 1014–24.

Chapter

73

Duodenal Tumours

Brendan P. Lovasik and David A. Kooby

INTRODUCTION

Duodenal tumours are encountered relatively infrequently and may be benign or malignant in behaviour. Appropriate surgical therapy for duodenal tumours can range from endoscopic piecemeal removal to radical surgical resection. The surgical approach is typically governed by tumour type, tumour size, and tumour location within the duodenum. This chapter reviews the relevant anatomy of the duodenum, its most common tumour types, and surgical strategies employed to treat these tumours.

ANATOMY

The duodenum represents the first part of the small bowel and is typically divided into four segments. The superior portion (D1) lies intraperitoneally between the pylorus and the neck of the gallbladder, anterior to the portal triad. The descending portion (D2) extends from the end of D1 to the 4th lumbar vertebral body (L4). The pancreatic and biliary ducts (pancreatobiliary tract) terminate at the ampulla of Vater on the posteromedial aspect of D2. The inferior portion (D3) extends from the right side of L4 to the left side of the aorta, crossed anteriorly by the superior mesenteric vessels and root of the small intestine mesentery. The second and third portions are bordered by the head of the pancreas anteriorly and by the right renal hilum posteriorly. The ascending portion (D4) extends superolaterally from the aorta and becomes intraperitoneal as it reaches the ligament of Treitz at the duodenojejunal junction. The unique location and relationship of the duodenum pose challenges when approaches to tumours are required (*Figure 73.1*). Lesions in D1 are most readily accessible, but reconstruction should address pyloric drainage and gastric emptying, and lesions in D2 should be assessed for proximity to the ampulla of Vater. The aperture and confluence of the common bile and main pancreatic ducts can occur in three ways. In 60% of patients the pancreatic duct and common bile duct merge to form a 3–5 mm common pancreatobiliary main duct. The pancreatic duct and common bile ducts can remain separate but form a 'double-barrelled' opening of the pancreatic and biliary ducts at the papilla which occurs in almost 40% of patients. Finally, in 1–2% of patients there may be entirely separate duodenal openings for the pancreatic and biliary ducts. Preoperative biliary drainage should be considered in patients with high-grade biliary obstruction (>150 mg/L of bilirubin), where there is a need for neoadjuvant therapy or when there are debilitating symptoms such as pruritis, cholangitis, and malabsorption (1). Tumours in both D3 and D4 can be locally invasive into the mesenteric root, rendering them unresectable. The arterial supply of D1 is provided by the supraduodenal artery (from the common hepatic artery) and superior pancreatoduodenal artery (from the gastroduodenal artery) (*Figure 73.1a*). The remaining three parts of the duodenum are supplied by anterior and posterior arcades from the

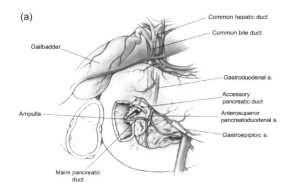

(a)

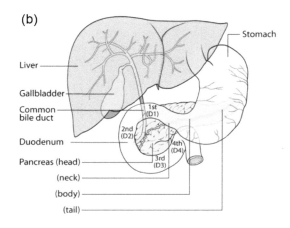

(b)

Figure 73.1 Labelled illustrations showing key anatomical relationships of the duodenum in the retroperitoneum. Main arterial and venous blood supply (a) and relative position to the stomach, liver, gallbladder and pancreas (b).

DOI: 10.1201/9781003080060-73

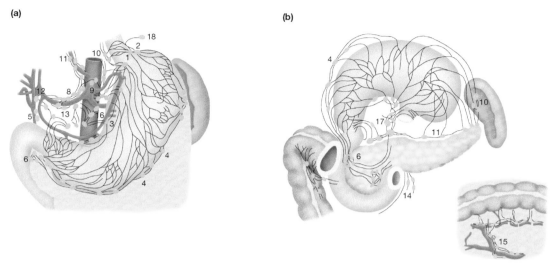

Figure 73.2 Lymphatic drainage of the stomach and duodenum and nodal stations by the Japanese classification (a) the anterior view of the stomach and duodenum (b) the posterior view.

right gastroepiploic and superior pancreatoduodenal arteries (from the gastroduodenal artery). The venous drainage of the duodenum largely follows the arterial supply (*Figure 73.1a*). Lymphatics originate as lacteals within the mucosa and form collecting lymphatic trunks to enter the anterior and posterior pancreatoduodenal lymph nodes, followed by secondary drainage to the coeliac and superior mesenteric nodes (*Figure 73.2a,b*).

BENIGN TUMOURS OF THE DUODENUM

Duodenal adenoma

Duodenal adenomas represent the overwhelming majority of duodenal tumours. Between 66–80% of patients diagnosed as having duodenal adenomas are asymptomatic at the time of diagnosis and they are detected due to the increasing use of screening and staging endoscopy. Most adenomas are flat or sessile solitary lesions with pearly villous surfaces, with a mean age at diagnosis in the seventh decade and an equal incidence among men and women. Approximately 40% of duodenal adenomas are sporadic, and the remaining 60% are associated with genetic polyposis syndromes such as familial adenomatous polyposis (FAP) or Peutz–Jeghers syndrome.

No definitive guidelines have been established, or consensus developed, regarding surveillance protocols or the lesion size of ampullary adenomas which mandates surgical removal. The emerging evidence for the prediction of advanced histology relies upon a variety of factors including the presence of high-grade dysplasia, the size of the adenoma, the extent of involved duodenal circumference, and the relation to the ampulla of Vater. Among patients with a preoperative diagnosis of a duodenal adenoma, final pathological analysis of the resected specimen resulted in upstaging to adenocarcinoma in around one-third of cases (2).

Other benign duodenal tumours

Other subtypes of benign duodenal tumours are less common. Surveillance is typically unnecessary for most benign lesions and resection is reserved for those causing symptomatic obstruction or haemorrhage. Duodenal lipomas and leiomyomas are usually incidentally discovered on endoscopy and biopsy is recommended to rule out sarcoma. Hamartomas are associated with Peutz–Jeghers syndrome and present as intermittent abdominal pain or intussusception. These lesions have been described as having a lobular or nodular appearance, whitish colour and whitish spots on the surface. Endoscopic removal is indicated as there is a small risk of malignant transformation (3). Duodenal haemangiomas are associated with Turner's and Osler–Weber–Rendu syndromes, and patients may present with anaemia secondary to bleeding from these lesions. Endoscopic ablation is often successful as definitive management. Symptomatic Brunner's gland tumours are extremely rare with a prevalence of less than 1 in 10 000 in an autopsy series. Brunner's gland tumours represent hyperplastic or adenomatous transformation of the physiologic mucosal-based glands. They usually follow a benign course but dysplasia and malignancy have occasionally been reported.

MALIGNANT TUMOURS OF THE DUODENUM

Adenocarcinoma

Adenocarcinoma is the most common malignant tumour of the duodenum. Although uncommon, adenocarcinoma of the duodenum accounts for 45–65% of all small bowel cancers. Adenocarcinomas are believed to progress through stepwise accumulation of genetic mutations, including APC, KRAS, and *p53*. Median disease-free survival is 53 months, with 1-, 3- and 5-year overall survival rates of 84%, 67% and 51%, respectively (4). When clinically indicated, operative resection affords the best chance for meaningful survival, and either pancreaticoduodenectomy or segmental resection can be considered. Pancreatoduodenectomy has been associated with a greater number of lymph nodes excised but not improved survival, and the data suggests that segmental resection is an appropriate strategy as long as negative margins can be obtained (5). Lymph node positivity is one of the most important prognostic indicators and a wide lymphadenectomy should be routinely performed. Factors associated with worse outcomes in adenocarcinoma include: 1) Advanced patient age; 2) the presence of distant metastasis; 3) the presence of lymph node metastasis; 4) increasing lymph node ratio; 5) a higher number of lymph nodes harvested; 6) high tumour grade; 7) increasing tumour (T) stage; 8) positive margin status; 9) the presence of lymphovascular or perineural invasion and 10) increasing overall cancer stage. Although data are limited in respect of guiding adjuvant therapy options, oxaliplatin-based chemotherapy is typically offered to high-risk patients, including those with positive lymph nodes. In some series, adjuvant radiation is associated with improved local control but no survival benefit (6).

Gastrointestinal stromal tumours

Gastrointestinal (GI) stromal tumours (GISTs) are malignant mesenchymal tumours originating from the interstitial cells of Cajal, which reside in muscular layers of the alimentary tract and function as the intestinal pacemaker cells. These tumours usually stain positively for CD117 (c-kit) and demonstrate spindle cell histology (7). Appropriate surgical therapy for GISTs is resection with grossly negative margins. Aggressive wide resection margins and lymph node dissection are not necessary in most settings, as submucosal spread and local lymph node involvement are rare for this tumour type (8). Local recurrence is influenced by the presence of positive resection margins but not by the type of surgical resection (limited resection or pancreaticoduodenectomy), as the two procedures have similar disease-free survival rates (9). Imatinib can be used as adjuvant therapy for either local or metastatic GIST, usually at a dose of 400 mg/day.

Neoadjuvant imatinib has been used in an attempt to reduce tumour burden, promote organ-preserving operations, and increase R0 resection rates (10–12). While there are no specific guidelines regarding the use of neoadjuvant imatinib for duodenal GISTs, the authors advocate the use of neoadjuvant imatinib for large tumours, tumours involving segments D2–D4 requiring complex resections, or locally advanced/resectable metastatic disease. During neoadjuvant therapy, patients are staged with cross-sectional imaging every 2–3 months and the timing of surgery is the point of peak response before secondary resistance is acquired, typically around 3–12 months (11).

Duodenal neuroendocrine tumours

Duodenal neuroendocrine tumours (D-NETs) arise from the peripheral endocrine system and enterochromaffin cells within the small bowel and typically present as hemispherical elevated submucosal tumours. D-NETs represent only 1–3% of all duodenal tumours and approximately 5–8% of all GI-NETs. While 90% of D-NETs are non-functional, up to 10% of them are functional with secretion of GI-active hormones. Functional D-NETs are divided into five functional subtypes based on the hormonal secretion, with the majority being duodenal gastrinomas (55–60% of all functional D-NETs), non-functional serotonin-containing tumours (20–25%), and somatostatin-producing tumours (15%). D-NETs are graded according to the World Health Organization (WHO) classification into low, intermediate, and high grades based on the proliferative rate of the tumour (mitotic count and Ki-67 immunohistochemistry index). Most patients with non-metastatic D-NETs greater than 1 cm in size or functional NETs of any size should be considered for resection. Small nonfunctional D-NETs less than 1 cm or multifocal lesions can be closely observed. Given their lack of prognostic value, the type of resection and extent of lymph node retrieval should be tailored to the patient's clinical picture and safety profile (13).

Lymphoma

Duodenal lymphoma is an uncommon malignant tumour of the duodenum. These tumours result from malignant transformation of lymphoid aggregates in the lamina propria, particularly in patients with inflammatory bowel disease, systemic lupus erythematosus, acquired immunodeficiency syndrome (AIDS), and other autoimmune and inflammatory disorders (14). Patients may present with nonspecific symptoms including fever, abdominal pain, diarrhoea and weight loss. Cross-sectional imaging of the abdomen may demonstrate bowel wall thickening, obstruction or mucosal ulceration. GI lymphomas are very responsive to chemotherapy and do not generally require surgical resection which is reserved for the management of complications such as perforation and haemorrhage (14).

GENETIC SYNDROMES

Familial adenomatous polyposis

Duodenal adenomas occur in up to 90% of patients with FAP, most commonly at the ampulla, peri-ampullary region or distal duodenum. The lifetime risk of duodenal cancer in patients with FAP is estimated to be 3–5% (15). Severity of duodenal adenomatosis is graded using the Spigelman classification, a 5-grade scale (stage 0–IV) based on adenoma number (1–4, 5–20, or >20), size (<5 mm, 5–10 mm, or >10 mm), histological type (tubular, tubulovillous, or villous) and severity of dysplasia (mild, moderate or severe). In addition to the typical indications for resection of spontaneous duodenal adenomas, resection is recommended for Spigelman stage IV adenomas.

Hereditary nonpolyposis colorectal cancer (Lynch syndrome)

Hereditary nonpolyposis colorectal cancer (HNPCC) carries an increased risk of small bowel adenocarcinoma related to the loss of mismatch repair genes, with a lifetime risk of small bowel adenocarcinoma of approximately 4.2% (16) with the duodenum being the most frequently involved site (50–80% of cases) (17). The relatively low prevalence of duodenal pathology does not support routine duodenal surveillance of HNPCC patients (16).

Peutz-Jeghers syndrome

Duodenal polyps are associated with Peutz–Jeghers syndrome, a rare autosomal dominant syndrome which is characterized by GI hamartomatous polyps and mucocutaneous pigmentation. Polyps are commonly discovered in adolescence and early adulthood due to polyp-related complications like abdominal pain, bowel obstruction, intussusception and overt, or occult, GI bleeding (18). Malignant degeneration of these polyps is caused by loss of the *STK11* tumour suppressor gene and leads to relatively high-rates of small bowel adenocarcinoma with a lifetime risk of 13% (19). Screening for GI cancers include yearly complete blood counts, faecal occult blood testing, and GI tumour markers, as well as abdominal US examination every 6 months and upper GI endoscopy every 3 years.

Multiple endocrine neoplasia type 1

Duodenal gastrinomas are associated with multiple endocrine neoplasia type-1 (MEN1) and may be associated with Zollinger-Ellison syndrome (ZES), a gastrin-secreting D-NET phenotype. Recommended duodenal neoplasia screening of MEN1 patients consists of annual cross-sectional imaging; magnetic resonance imaging (MRI), computed tomography (CT) or endoscopic ultrasound (EUS) (20).

SURGICAL APPROACHES

The surgical management of duodenal tumours varies based on: 1) classification of malignancy; 2) tumour size; 3) location within the duodenum; 4) involvement of neighbouring structures; and 5) the presence of lymph node involvement. Four major surgical procedures exist for the removal of duodenal tumours: 1) Transduodenal excision; 2) local full-thickness 'wedge' resection; 3) pancreas-sparing segmental duodenectomy, and 4) pancreaticoduodenectomy (*Figure 73.3*). Most open surgical approaches to the duodenum begin with the retroperitoneal exposure through a midline, right subcostal or bilateral subcostal incision. Minimally invasive surgery (MIS) duodenal procedures, including laparoscopic and robotic approaches, are suitable options but can be challenging due to limited exposure of the retroperitoneum and technical shortcomings of laparoscopic surgery for reconstructing the duodenum. While data is limited on MIS duodenal operations, reports and case series demonstrate that laparoscopic and robotic approaches are both feasible and safe in

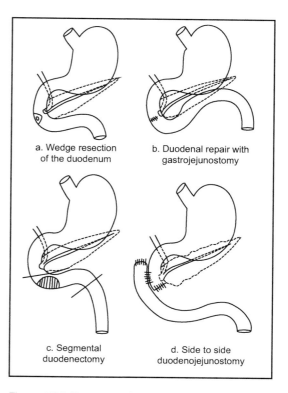

a. Wedge resection of the duodenum

b. Duodenal repair with gastrojejunostomy

c. Segmental duodenectomy

d. Side to side duodenojejunostomy

Figure 73.3 Four operative approaches to duodenal tumours. Wedge resection of the duodenum (a). Duodenal repair with gastrojejunostomy (b). Segmental duodenectomy (c). Side-to-side duodenojejunostomy (d).

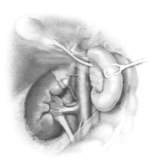

Figure 73.4 Duodenal mobilization from the retroperi-toneum (Kocher manoeuver).

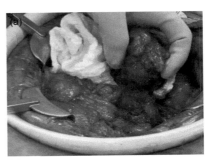

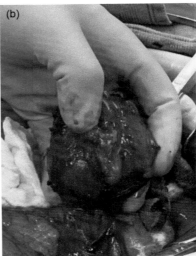

the hands of experienced MIS surgeons (21,22). All procedures performed on the first or second portion of the duodenum require elevation of the duodenum from the retroperitoneum, the eponymous Kocher manoeuvre, with the distal landmark close to the ligament of Treitz, the proximal landmark at the foramen of Winslow, and extended medially to the superior mesenteric artery take-off on the anterior aorta (*Figure 73.4*). Exposure of the third or fourth portions of the duodenum can be obtained from an incision through the transverse mesocolon or gastro-colic omentum into the lesser sac or from mobilization of the right colon via right medial-visceral rotation.

Transduodenal excision

Transduodenal excision is most commonly performed for benign and appropriate low-grade malignant tumours located in the antimesenteric wall of the duodenum. Once adequately mobilized (*Figure 73.5a*), suture fixation and needle tip electrocautery are used to open the duode-num and circumferentially enter the submucosal plane. The surgical margins may be evaluated by frozen section as needed, though the macroscopic boundaries of most adenomas are typically visible and sufficient (*Figure 73.5b*). The mucosal defect is closed with absorbable suture, and the duodenotomy is repaired transversely in two layers taking care to imbricate the ends of the suture line to minimize the potential for a leak (*Figure 73.5c*).

Segmental duodenal 'wedge' resection

Segmental duodenal resection is used for tumours involving the wall of the duodenum not amenable to transduodenal excision (medial or those involving the mesentery). Prior to division of the duodenum, cannulating the common bile duct with a 5Fr Fogarty catheter through the cystic duct stump after

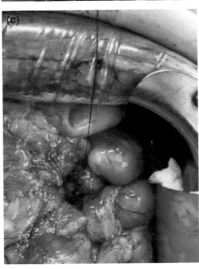

Figure 73.5 Intraoperative images showing the steps in a transduodenal excision of a large GIST tumour in the D2 segment. First grasping the tumour and elevation of the antimesenteric duodenum following mobilization from the retroperitoneum (a). Local excision of the tumour; exposed mucosa seen in the lower half of the image (b). Two-layer closure of the duodenum following resection (c).

cholecystectomy assists with establishing the location of the ampulla relative to medial lesions. A linear cutting stapler can be used to divide the duodenum, with bipolar electrocautery used to divide the duodenal mesentery and small perforating branches emanating from the head of the pancreas. Suture ligation should be used liberally, as any degree of postoperative pancreatitis may cause sealed arterioles to bleed. Continuity is restored with a two-layer duodenojejunostomy.

Ampullectomy

Two surgical procedures are commonly used for the treatment of ampullary tumours, ampullectomy and pancreaticoduodenectomy. Ampullectomy, a local resection of the ampulla of Vater, is a suitable strategy for the management of early periampullary tumours due to its lower complication profile and reduced perioperative morbidity compared with pancreatoduodenectomy. However, ampullectomy has been associated with higher rates of local recurrence than pancreatectomy due to the less radical resection, and does not accomplish regional lymphadenectomy (23,24). Ampullectomy may be favored for low- and high-grade dysplasia, ampullary adenomas without high-risk features, malignant disease with low depth-of-invasion (pTis or pT1), small ampullary lesions less than 1–2 cm in size, no clinical or radiographical evidence of lymph node metastasis, and in patients with high operative risk for a radical resection (25). Following an extensive Kocher manoeuvre, a duodenotomy is performed over the lesion, and silk stay sutures are placed circumferentially in the duodenal wall to expose the ampulla. The authors prefer to place 5-French paediatric feeding tubes, which are flexible and atraumatic, in the biliary and pancreatic ducts to confirm their positions. The mucosa is incised 5–10 mm away from visible adenomatous change with needle tip cautery to expose the submucosal plane, and it is carried circumferentially around the lesion (*Figure 73.6*). The duodenal mucosa is re-approximated to the common bile duct and pancreatic duct mucosa using absorbable monofilament interrupted sutures beginning at 12 o'clock and continuing in a clockwise fashion. The duodenotomy is then closed transversely with sutures or a surgical stapler, or it can be converted to a Billroth II gastrojejunostomy. While less morbid than pancreaticoduodenectomy, ampullectomy is still associated with significant postoperative complications. In the largest series comparing open ampullectomy versus pancreaticoduodenectomy, patients who underwent ampullectomy demonstrated lower rates of perioperative morbidity (33 vs. 52%) and lower rates of common complications such as delayed gastric emptying (0 vs.16%) and pancreatic leak (0% vs. 20.7%) (26).

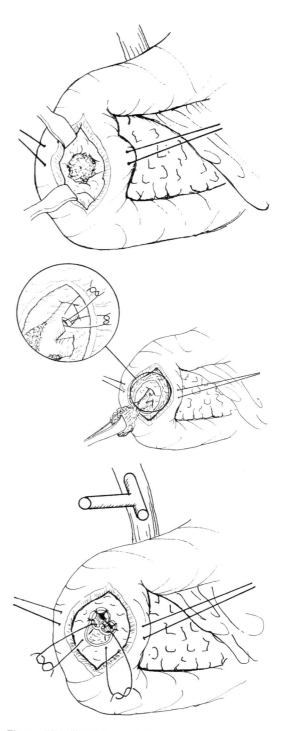

Figure 73.6 Illustrations of the ampullectomy procedure, demonstrating duodenotomy with stay-suture retraction (a) and resection of the ampulla (b). Reconstruction of the biliary and pancreatic ducts with interrupted monofilament sutures (c).

Pancreatoduodenectomy

Pancreaticoduodenectomy may be the appropriate surgical approach for patients with duodenal tumours that have extensive or multifocal involvement of the duodenum and neighbouring structures, or for patients with tumours with malignant potential requiring radical resection and lymphadenectomy. The available data indicate that local resection is associated with lower morbidity than pancreaticoduodenectomy, but at the expense of higher recurrence rates and inferior survival, at least in the setting of invasive disease (23,24). A more radical surgical approach is preferred for invasive tumours, including well-differentiated T1 lesions, as long as the patient is a reasonable candidate for a pancreaticoduodenectomy. However, the decision to perform pancreatoduodenectomy should take into consideration the risks of perioperative morbidity ranging from 30–60% and overall mortality ranging from 2–15% (27). There is limited available literature regarding standard versus pylorus-preserving pancreatoduodenectomy in the context of primary duodenal pathology.

ENDOSCOPIC APPROACHES

Endoscopic mucosal resection and endoscopic submucosal dissection

Endoscopic mucosal resection (EMR) is indicated for adenomas less than 20 mm in size and less than 33% of the duodenal circumference. When compared to those undergoing surgery, patients undergoing EMR had fewer haemorrhagic complications, shorter procedure times, and reduced hospital stays. Nevertheless, long-term surveillance is needed after EMR due to a high recurrence rate (28). A submucosal injection of lifting solution is performed, raising the lesion on a cushion of submucosal fluid which separates the mucosal and muscle layers, followed by snare resection of the mucosa. Lesions up to 20 mm in diameter may to be resected in a single piece, with piecemeal resection required for larger lesions (29). Endoscopic submucosal dissection (ESD) can achieve *en-bloc* resection of tumours larger than 1 cm in diameter, but is associated with a higher rate of complications including bleeding and perforation. ESD involves a submucosal injection to lift the lesion in a similar fashion to EMR, followed by a mucosal incision using an electrosurgical knife and the submucosal plane dissection to remove the lesion *en bloc*.

SUMMARY

Duodenal tumours represent a broad spectrum of uncommon benign and malignant neoplasms. The tumour biology, location of the tumour in the duodenum, and type of surgical resection are important considerations for surgeons, especially given the proximity to the ampulla of Vater and the mesenteric root.

A thoughtful approach to the diagnosis and treatment of duodenal tumours is needed to ensure that patients with these complex pathologies are treated optimally.

REFERENCES

1. Fang Y, Gurusamy KS, Wang Q, et al. Pre-operative biliary drainage for obstructive jaundice. *Cochrane Database Syst Rev* 2012;**(9)**:CD005444.
2. Eng NL, Mustin DE, Lovasik BP, et al. Relationship between cancer diagnosis and complications following pancreatoduodenectomy for duodenal adenoma. *Ann Surg Oncol* 2021;**28(2)**:1097–105.
3. Abbass R, Rigaux J, Al-Kawas FH. Nonampullary duodenal polyps: Characteristics and endoscopic management. *Gastrointest Endosc* 2010;**71(4)**:754–9.
4. Solaini L, Jamieson NB, Metcalfe M, et al. Outcome after surgical resection for duodenal adenocarcinoma in the UK. *Br J Surg* 2015;**102(6)**:676–81.
5. Cloyd JM, Norton JA, Visser BC, Poultsides GA. Does the extent of resection impact survival for duodenal adenocarcinoma? Analysis of 1,611 cases. *Ann Surg Oncol* 2015;**22(2)**:573–80.
6. Cloyd JM, George E, Visser BC. Duodenal adenocarcinoma: Advances in diagnosis and surgical management. *World J Gastrointest Surg* 2016;**8(3)**:212–21.
7. Miettinen M, Kopczynski J, Makhlouf HR, et al. Gastrointestinal stromal tumors, intramural leiomyomas, and leiomyosarcomas in the duodenum: A clinicopathologic, immunohistochemical, and molecular genetic study of 167 cases. *Am J Surg Pathol* 2003;**27(5)**:625–641.
8. Lau S, Tam KF, Kam CK, et al. Imaging of gastrointestinal stromal tumour (GIST). *Clin Radiol* 2004;**59(6)**:487–98.
9. Goh BK, Chow PK, Kesavan S, Yap WM, Wong WK. Outcome after surgical treatment of suspected gastrointestinal stromal tumors involving the duodenum: Is limited resection appropriate? *J Surg Oncol* 2008;**97(5)**:388–91.
10. Iwatsuki M, Harada K, Iwagami S, et al. Neoadjuvant and adjuvant therapy for gastrointestinal stromal tumors. *Ann Gastroenterol Surg* 2019;**3(1)**:43–49.
11. Rutkowski P, Gronchi A, Hohenberger P, et al. Neoadjuvant imatinib in locally advanced gastrointestinal stromal tumors (GIST): The EORTC STBSG experience. *Ann Surg Oncol* 2013;**20(9)**:2937–43.
12. Tielen R, Verhoef C, van Coevorden F, et al. Surgical treatment of locally advanced, non-metastatic, gastrointestinal stromal tumours after treatment with imatinib. *Eur J Surg Oncol* 2013;**39(2)**:150–5.
13. Gamboa AC, Liu Y, Lee RM, et al. Duodenal neuroendocrine tumors: Somewhere between the pancreas and small bowel? *J Surg Oncol* 2019;**120(8)**:1293–301.
14. Matysiak-Budnik T, Fabiani B, Hennequin C, et al. Gastrointestinal lymphomas: French Intergroup clinical practice recommendations for diagnosis, treatment and follow-up (SNFGE, FFCD, GERCOR, UNICANCER, SFCD, SFED, SFRO, SFH). *Dig Liver Dis* 2018;**50(2)**:124–31.

15. Bulow S, Bjork J, Christensen IJ, et al. Duodenal adenomatosis in familial adenomatous polyposis. *Gut* 2004;**53(3)**:381–6.

16. ten Kate GL, Kleibeuker JH, Nagengast FM, et al. Is surveillance of the small bowel indicated for Lynch syndrome families? *Gut* 2007;**56(9)**:1198–201.

17. Hammoudi N, Dhooge M, Coriat R, et al. Duodenal tumor risk in Lynch syndrome. *Dig Liver Dis* 2019;**51(2)**:299–303.

18. Kopacova M, Tacheci I, Rejchrt S, Bures J. Peutz-Jeghers syndrome: Diagnostic and therapeutic approach. *World J Gastroenterol* 2009;**15(43)**:5397–408.

19. Giardiello FM, Brensinger JD, Tersmette AC, et al. Very high risk of cancer in familial Peutz-Jeghers syndrome. *Gastroenterology* 2000;**119(6)**:1447–53.

20. Thakker RV, Newey PJ, Walls GV, et al. Clinical practice guidelines for multiple endocrine neoplasia type 1 (MEN1). *J Clin Endocrinol Metab* 2012;**97(9)**: 2990–3011.

21. Downs-Canner S, Van der Vliet WJ, Thoolen SJ, et al. Robotic surgery for benign duodenal tumors. *J Gastrointest Surg* 2015;**19(2)**:306–12.

22. Linn YL, Wang Z, Goh BKP. Robotic transduodenal ampullectomy: Case report and review of the literature. *Ann Hepatobiliary Pancreat Surg* 2021;**25(1)**: 150–4.

23. Grobmyer SR, Stasik CN, Draganov P, et al. Contemporary results with ampullectomy for 29 'benign' neoplasms of the ampulla. *J Am Coll Surg* 2008;**206(3)**:466–71.

24. Roggin KK, Yeh JJ, Ferrone CR, et al. Limitations of ampullectomy in the treatment of non familial ampullary neoplasms. *Ann Surg Oncol* 2005;**12(12)**: 971–80.

25. Yoon YS, Kim SW, Park SJ, et al. Clinicopathologic analysis of early ampullary cancers with a focus on the feasibility of ampullectomy. *Ann Surg* 2005;**242(1)**: 92–100.

26. Winter JM, Cameron JL, Olino K, et al. Clinico-pathologic analysis of ampullary neoplasms in 450 patients: Implications for surgical strategy and long-term prognosis. *J Gastrointest Surg* 2010;**14(2)**:379–87.

27. Ho CK, Kleeff J, Friess H, Buchler MW. Complications of pancreatic surgery. *HPB (Oxford)* 2005;**7(2)**:99–108.

28. Bartel MJ, Puri R, Brahmbhatt B, et al. Endoscopic and surgical management of nonampullary duodenal neoplasms. *Surg Endosc* 2018;**32(6)**:2859–69.

29. Basford PJ, Bhandari P. Endoscopic management of nonampullary duodenal polyps. *Therap Adv Gastroenterol* 2012;**5(2)**:127–38.

Chapter
74

Splenectomy

Fiona Hand and Sarah Thomasset

INTRODUCTION

Globally, the incidence of splenectomy is approximately 6.4–7.1 per 100 000 people per year, with trauma and haematological disorders being the most common indications (1). There is evidence, however, that the incidence of splenectomy for most indications has fallen over recent decades (2). The two main functions of the spleen are: 1) Production of antibodies and 2) filtration of the blood whereby defective components are removed. The white pulp of the spleen accounts for approximately 25% of splenic tissue and consists entirely of lymphoid tissue containing B- and T-cell lymphocytes. The surrounding red pulp is mainly composed of venous sinuses which ultimately drain into the splenic vein where the blood is cleared of old or defective or effete red blood cells and microorganisms.

ELECTIVE SPLENECTOMY

The most common conditions for which an elective splenectomy may be undertaken are shown in *Table 74.1*. Broadly speaking, haematological indications can be either for autoimmune or genetic disorders that cause abnormalities of erythrocyte structure. In terms of autoimmune disorders, surgery is most frequently performed for immune thrombocytopenic purpura (ITP). This is characterized by antibody induced platelet destruction and treatments include glucocorticoids, intravenous immunoglobulin and platelet transfusions, with rituximab and thrombopoetin-receptor agonists also demonstrating a beneficial response. However, for those with medically refractory ITP, elective splenectomy is the cornerstone of treatment (3). Similarly, elective splenectomy is indicated in certain cases of autoimmune induced thrombotic thrombocytopenic purpura (TTP). TTP is defined by thrombotic microangiopathy secondary to alterations in Von Willebrand factor homeostasis and characterized by fever, thrombocytopenia, microangiopathic haemolytic anaemia, renal dysfunction and neurological symptoms. While treatment with plasma infusion is sufficient for treatment of hereditary TTP, daily plasma exchange may be needed for cases of acquired TTP. Treatment with immunomodulators such as corticosteroids, rituximab, vincristine, cyclosporine and cyclophosphamide may all be needed to eliminate autoantibodies and produce a sustained response but in 20% of patients an elective splenectomy will be required (4).

Autoimmune haemolytic anaemia can be primary or secondary to another underlying illness and occurs when antibodies target erythrocytes resulting in haemolysis. Standard treatment consists of corticosteroids, rituximab and azathioprine with splenectomy indicated when medical treatment fails (5). A small number of patients with rheumatoid arthritis (1–3%) exhibit a triad of splenomegaly, neutropenia and rheumatoid arthritis, known as Felty's syndrome. Decreased granulogenesis and increased granulocyte destruction results in neutropenia which in turn contributes to increased opportunistic infections. Elective splenectomy results in resolution of the neutropenia in 80% of patients (6).

With regard to disorders of erythrocyte structure, sickle cell anaemia is a genetically inherited disorder which results in reduced elasticity and deformation of erythrocytes resulting in the typical 'sickle' shape. Characterized by anaemia, painful vaso-occlusive episodes and splenic sequestration, sickle cell anaemia can ultimately lead to hypersplenism and splenic infarction. Medical treatments include blood transfusion and hydroxycarbamide, however in cases refractory to medical treatment an elective splenectomy is needed (7).

Table 74.1 Conditions in which elective splenectomy may be indicated

Haematological disorders

- Immune thrombocytopenic purpura (ITP)
- Thrombotic thrombocytopenic purpura (TTP)
- Autoimmune haemolytic anaemia
- Sickle cell anaemia
- Thalassaemia
- Hereditary spherocytosis

Haematological malignancies

- Chronic lymphocytic leukaemia
- Chronic myeloid leukaemia
- Hairy cell leukaemia
- Non-Hodgkin's lymphoma

Non-haematological malignancy

- Distal pancreatic cancers
- Primary splenic angiosarcoma
- Oligometastatic disease

Benign splenic disease

- Hydatid disease
- Bacterial abscess

DOI: 10.1201/9781003080060-74

Thalassaemias are disorders characterized by an abnormal number or absence of haemoglobin subunits resulting in anaemia. Treatment is with blood transfusion and iron chelation therapy with splenectomy reserved for patients with transfusion dependant hypersplenism (8). Hereditary spherocytosis (HS), a genetically inherited abnormality in the cytoskeleton of erythrocytes, leads to splenomegaly, jaundice, anaemia and pigmented gallstones. Elective splenectomy in the setting of HS is curative and a simultaneous cholecystectomy should also be considered.

Elective splenectomy is also indicated in a number of malignant conditions. Haematological malignancies such as chronic lymphocytic leukaemia, chronic myeloid leukaemia, hairy cell leukaemia and non-Hodgkin's lymphoma may all present with splenomegaly and pancytopenia which resolves with elective splenectomy (9–11). In addition, when undertaking a distal pancreatectomy for pancreatic tail malignancies an *en-bloc* splenectomy is also often undertaken for oncological completeness (12). Primary splenic angiosarcoma is a rare malignancy with a poor prognosis (13). It is associated with splenic rupture and haemoperitoneum and a splenectomy provides the only chance of cure (14). In contrast to this, splenic metastases most commonly arising from breast, colorectal, lung, ovarian or melanoma primaries are commonly asymptomatic and in cases of oligometastatic disease, a splenectomy may be indicated (15–17). Hydatid disease caused by *Echinococcus granulosus* affecting the spleen, is the most common infectious indication for elective splenectomy. Treatment is with albendazole and resection of the parasitic cysts. Resection must be undertaken without cyst rupture so as to avoid dissemination and potential anaphylaxis (18). A splenectomy may also occasionally be considered for bacterial abscesses of the spleen, in cases where antimicrobial therapy and targeted drainage have been unsuccessful.

EMERGENCY SPLENECTOMY

The most common indication for an emergency splenectomy is abdominal trauma, usually resulting from an injury sustained following blunt trauma, and less often penetrating injuries. Other less common causes of splenic rupture requiring an emergency splenectomy include: 1) Iatrogenic injury; 2) infections such as malaria, infectious mononucleosis and cytomegalovirus; and 3) haematological disorders, including acute myeloid leukaemia and lymphoma.

Splenic trauma is often graded according to the system described by the American Association for the Surgery of Trauma (AAST) (*Table 74.2*) (19). Historically, splenectomy was frequently performed in the trauma setting, however, over the last few decades increasing evidence supports non-operative management (NOM) for certain groups (20). NOM consists of close monitoring, sometimes in combination with splenic artery

embolization, the main advantages being preservation of splenic function and prevention of overwhelming post splenectomy sepsis (OPSI). Splenic artery embolization can, however, give rise to complications, including splenic infarction, abscess formation, bleeding and coil migration and failure of NOM occurs in 4–15% of cases (20). Delayed splenic rupture (DSR), ongoing bleeding and pseudoaneurysms can occur. The incidence of DSR is approximately 1–2% and usually occurs 4–8 days after the trauma.

The absolute indication for an emergency splenectomy following trauma is when a splenic injury causes haemodynamic instability which does not respond to resuscitation with intravenous fluids and blood transfusion. It may also be required when NOM fails, indicated by the development of haemodynamic instability, a fall in haemoglobin levels or the need for repeated blood transfusions. A number of patients, presenting following abdominal trauma, will have concomitant injuries which are in themselves an indication for laparotomy. In this situation the spleen should be assessed intraoperatively and a decision made as to whether splenectomy is required. Splenic conservation methods, for example suture repair, mesh repair and topical haemostatic agents, have been described (21). Such techniques may have a role in Grade 1 or 2 injuries when the primary indication for a laparotomy has been another injury, but in the case of a haemodynamically compromised patient, or when NOM has failed, we recommend a splenectomy is performed. The overall

Table 74.2 American Association for the Surgery of Trauma (AAST) splenic grading system (2018 revision) (19)

Grade	CT findings
1	• Subcapsular <10% surface area • Parenchymal laceration <1 cm • Capsular tear
2	• Subcapsular 10–50% surface area • Intraparenchymal <5 cm • Parenchymal laceration 1–3 cm
3	• Subcapsular >50% surface area • Ruptured subcapsular or intraparenchymal haematoma ≥5 cm • Parenchymal laceration >3 cm
4	• Any injury in the presence of a splenic vascular injury or active bleeding confined within the splenic capsule • Parenchymal laceration involving segmental or hilar vessels producing >25% devascularization
5	• Any injury in the presence of a splenic vascular injury with active bleeding extending beyond the spleen into the peritoneum • Shattered spleen

hospital mortality of splenectomy in trauma is approximately 2%, with the incidence of postoperative bleeding ranging from 1.6–3%, but this is associated with a mortality rate of around 20% (22). Occasionally an emergency splenectomy may be considered in a patient with left-sided portal hypertension caused by splenic vein stenosis or occlusion, often in the context of prior pancreatitis. Patients may present with evidence of upper gastrointestinal (GI) bleeding from a ruptured gastric varix and potential treatment options include: 1) Endoscopic sclerotherapy; 2) splenic artery embolization and 3) occasionally splenectomy.

OPEN SPLENECTOMY

With the patient supine and the arms extended, an open splenectomy may be performed via an upper midline or left subcostal incision depending on surgeon preference. Packs are placed behind the spleen in order to elevate it and bring it towards the midline. In order to expose the gastrocolic ligament the colon must be retracted inferiorly and the stomach cranially. The gastrocolic ligament is divided along its avascular plane to enter the lesser sac and to identify the splenic artery as it courses along the superior border of the pancreas. In cases of splenomegaly, it may be prudent to ligate the splenic artery, followed by the vein, at this juncture prior to further mobilization. Ligation of the splenic artery and vein is usually performed using ties and transfixion sutures. The spleen is systematically freed from its surrounding ligamentous attachments. The gastrosplenic ligament containing the short gastric arteries and the lienocolic ligament are both divided to free the spleen medially. This allows elevation of the spleen and exposure of the splenorenal ligament. In cases where the spleen is normal in size, the splenic artery and vein may be ligated and divided at this point. Once the spleen has been removed, the abdomen must be inspected for accessory spleens (present in up to 15% of cases) (23). Care must also be taken during a splenectomy to avoid damaging the pancreatic tail which can give rise to a pancreatic fistula. In a trauma setting, a midline laparotomy is undertaken and the abdomen is initially packed. If a splenic injury is suspected, the last packs to be removed are those from the left upper quadrant. Clot is manually evacuated and often the various peritoneal attachments observed in an elective splenectomy have already torn. A hand is inserted over the spleen to retract it towards the midline. Ideally, each major splenic vessel is individually identified and ligated separately. However, if the spleen is shattered or the patient is in extremis, a clamp or stapler can be placed across the entire splenic hilum and the spleen rapidly removed to gain control. The principles of damage control surgery should be considered, with ongoing resuscitation, rapid control of haemorrhage and correction of any coagulopathy.

MINIMALLY INVASIVE SPLENECTOMY

Minimally invasive splenectomy using either a laparoscopic or robotic approach has become the standard technique in the elective setting. Regardless of the platform used, comparative perioperative outcomes can be achieved, although there is reportedly less blood loss and a lower rate of conversion to open with robotic splenectomy (24,25). The patient is placed in the right lateral decubitus position with the hip flexed and the left arm draped across the upper thorax, suspended on an arm board. The surgeon and assistant stand to face the patient on the patients' right side with monitors placed to face the surgeon. Once a pneumoperitoneum has been established, four trocars are placed under the left costal margin in a curvilinear line. The camera is usually inserted into the anterior axillary line port with the other four utilized as working ports. The splenic flexure is mobilized inferomedially with the surgeon's energy device of choice which allows the gastrosplenic ligament to be identified. Division of this ligament along with the short gastric vessels follows and facilitates medialization of the stomach and exposure of the splenic hilum and lienorenal ligament containing the splenic artery and vein. The spleen is then mobilized medially, freeing peritoneal attachments until the posterior peritoneum is opened allowing access to the splenic artery and vein from behind. The vessels are divided, often using an endoscopic vascular stapler taking care to protect the tail of the pancreas. The specimen is placed in an endobag and retrieved. Once removed, a final laparoscopy is performed to ensure haemostasis and check for accessory spleens.

PARTIAL SPLENECTOMY

Owing to the increased incidence of infection following splenectomy, partial splenectomy has gained popularity particularly for benign tumours such as hamartomas, haemangiomas and haematological conditions (26,27). However, for centrally located tumours, a partial splenectomy may not be possible due to the terminal blood supply of the spleen. Partial splenectomy is most commonly performed, employing a minimally invasive platform and the patient positioning and operating room set-up are the same as for a total splenectomy. In performing a partial splenectomy however, hilar dissection is of importance with particular attention paid to the splenic artery and vein which need to be preserved. The vessels supplying the region of the spleen to be removed are dissected out carefully and a clamp placed to confirm the blood supply and create an area of demarcation. Once confirmed, the artery and vein are then ligated in continuity and the line of demarcation is used as a guide for the parenchymal transection using a cautery device (28). Once the specimen is removed in an endobag, the cut surface is carefully inspected for bleeding. Haemostatic agents may be used on the resection margin to minimize ooze if needed (29).

SPLENIC PRESERVATION DURING PANCREATIC SURGERY

Increasing awareness of the haematopoietic and immunological functions of the spleen has meant that where possible, splenic preservation during a distal pancreatectomy is advised. As minimally invasive approaches are now the 'gold standard' for distal pancreatectomy,

in patients without confirmed malignancy, the spleen should be left *in situ* to avoid postoperative complications, particularly OPSI (30). During distal pancreatectomy, the spleen may be preserved using either the Kimura technique (*Figure 74.1a*) where both the splenic artery and vein are preserved (31) or the Warshaw technique (*Figure 74.1b*) in which the splenic artery and vein are divided with perfusion to the spleen maintained via the left gastroepiploic artery and short gastric vessels (32). In performing the Kimura procedure, the splenic artery and vein must be meticulously dissected from

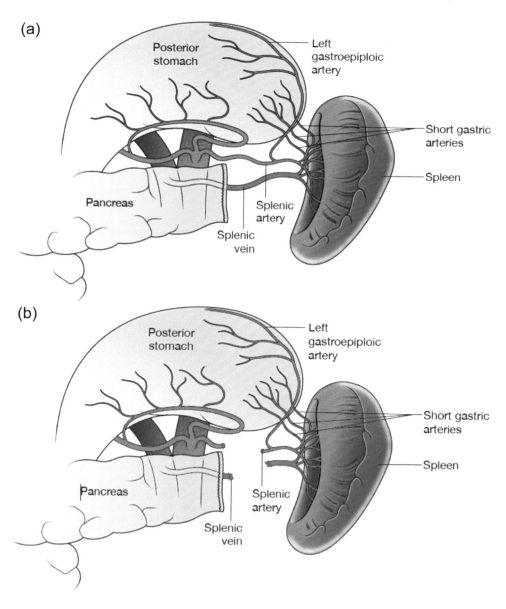

Figure 74.1 Labelled illustrations demonstrating splenic preservation during distal pancreatectomy using the Kimura technique (a) and Warshaw technique (b).

the pancreas. This is best performed by dividing the pancreatic parenchyma proximally and anterior to the vessels in the first instance. Dissection then proceeds laterally from right-to-left so as to visualize the short perforating arterial and venous branches dividing them as they arise. However, in patients with chronic pancreatitis or obesity, this dissection plane can prove difficult, with inadvertent damage to the splenic vein being the most common reason to abandon splenic preservation.

Performing the Warshaw procedure, the spleen is first visualized to assess for colour and size as in cases of splenomegaly, the spleen is unlikely to survive on the reduced blood supply left following the use of this technique (33). The lesser sac is entered taking care to preserve the left gastroepiploic vessels which will supply the spleen postoperatively, along with the short gastric vessels (34). Dissection is undertaken at the inferior border of the pancreas, in the region of the planned medial transection line, to reveal the splenic vein. The pancreatic body is further separated from the retroperitoneum towards the upper border of the pancreas until the splenic artery is visible and a tunnel created behind the pancreas. The splenic vessels and pancreas are then divided at this point. The distal pancreas can then be gently lifted and loose tissue in the retroperitoneal space divided up to the splenic hilum. At this point, the distal ends of the splenic artery and vein can be divided and the specimen extracted (35). The Kimura technique is more frequently utilized by surgeons despite a number of systematic reviews failing to demonstrate the superiority of either approach (36,37). While the Warshaw procedure is associated with less blood loss and a shorter operative time, the Kimura procedure is associated with a lower incidence of gastric varices and splenic infarction (38–40). More recently, a pan European study demonstrated equivalent major complication, splenic ischaemia and secondary splenectomy rates for both techniques although a longer operative time with less blood loss was noted with the Kimura procedure (41).

POST-SPLENECTOMY CONSIDERATIONS

Asplenic patients are particularly susceptible to infection with the encapsulated bacteria *Neisseria meningitidis*, *Streptococcus pneumonia* and *Haemophilus influenza* B, which can result in OPSI (42). OPSI is a potentially fatal event following splenectomy, affecting 0.9% of adults and 5% of children within the first 2-years postoperatively (43,44). For this reason, patients undergoing elective splenectomy should be vaccinated against these pathogens at least 2-weeks preoperatively, although optimal timing is 4–6 weeks prior to surgery. In the emergency setting, postoperative vaccines are most effective at least 14 days after surgery. Antibiotic prophylaxis should be offered to all patients in the first 3 years after splenectomy, and

lifelong prophylaxis should be offered to patients considered at high risk of pneumococcal infection. Patient education is very important, to ensure compliance with vaccinations, prophylactic antibiotics and rapid medical assessment when infection is suspected (21).

SUMMARY

Splenectomy remains an important surgical procedure for a number of elective and emergency indications which have been discussed above. Open splenectomy remains the approach of choice in the emergency setting, but electively minimally invasive techniques, laparoscopic splenectomy and more recently robotic splenectomy, are now more frequently performed. Partial splenectomy may be considered, particularly for benign tumours and some haematological conditions. Often the spleen can be preserved during distal pancreatic surgery. Post-splenectomy, there is a risk of developing overwhelming post-splenectomy sepsis and vaccinations against encapsulated bacteria, antibiotic prophylaxis and education are essential and will reduce this risk.

REFERENCES

1. Morgenstern L. A history of splenectomy. In: Hiatt JR, Phillips EH, Morgenstern L, (eds). *Surgical Diseases of the Spleen*. New York: Springer, 1997, pp 3–14.
2. Rose AT, Newman MI, Debelak J, et al. The incidence of splenectomy is decreasing: Lessons learned from the trauma experience. *Am Surg* 2000;**66(5)**:481–6.
3. Chaturvedi S, Arnold DM, McCrae KR. Splenectomy for immune thrombocytopenia: Down but not out. *Blood* 2018;**131(11)**:1172–82.
4. Saha M, McDaniel JK, Zheng XL. Thrombotic thrombocytopenic purpura: Pathogenesis, diagnosis and potential novel therapeutics. *J Thromb Haemost* 2017;**15(10)**:1889–1900.
5. Zanella A, Barcellini W. Treatment of autoimmune hemolytic anemias. *Haematologica* 2014;**99(10)**:1547–54.
6. Bullock J, Rizvi SAA, Saleh AM, et al. Rheumatoid arthritis: A brief overview of the treatment. *Med Princ Pract* 2018;**27(6)**:501–7.
7. Owusu-Ofori S, Remmington T. Splenectomy versus conservative management for acute sequestration crises in people with sickle cell disease. *Cochrane Database Syst Rev* 2017;**11**:CD003425.
8. Mathew ME, Sharma A, Aravindakshan R. Splenectomy for people with thalassaemia major or intermedia. *Cochrane Database Syst Rev* 2016;(**6**):CD010517.
9. Petroianu A. Subtotal splenectomy for the treatment of chronic lymphocytic leukemia. *Blood Cancer J* 2015;**5**:e289.
10. Chihara D, Kreitman RJ. Treatment of hairy cell leukemia. *Expert Rev Hematol* 2020;**13(10)**:1107–17.

11. Yoong Y, Kurtin PJ, Allmer C, et al. Efficacy of splenectomy for patients with mantle cell non-Hodgkin's
lymphoma. *Leuk Lymphoma* 2001;**42(6)**:1235–41.

12. Lillemoe KD, Kaushal S, Cameron JL, Sohn TA,
Pitt HA, Yeo CJ. Distal pancreatectomy: Indications and outcomes in 235 patients. *Ann Surg*
1999;**229(5)**:693–8.

13. Batouli A, Fairbrother SW, Silverman JF, et al. Primary splenic angiosarcoma: Clinical and imaging
manifestations of this rare aggressive neoplasm. *Curr
Probl Diagn Radiol* 2016;**45(4)**:284–7.

14. Özcan B, Çevener M, Kargi AO, et al. Primary
splenic angiosarcoma diagnosed after splenectomy for
spontaneous rupture. *Turk J Surg* 2018;**34(1)**:68–70.

15. Efared B, Mazti A, Atsame-Ebang G, et al.
An unusual site of metastasis: Splenic metas-
tastasis from a colon cancer. *J Surg Case Rep*
2016;**2016(11)**:rjw175.

16. El Fadli M, Kerrou K, Alaoui Mhamdi H, et al.
Breast cancer metastasis to the spleen: A case report
and literature review. *Oxf Med Case Reports* 2017;
2017(12):omx069.

17. Durmus Y, Isçi Bostanci E, Duru Çöteli AS, Kay-
ikçioglu F, Boran N. Metastasis patterns of the
spleen and association with survival outcomes in
advanced ovarian-tubal-peritoneal epithelial cancer.
Arch Gynecol Obstet 2019;**300(5)**:1367–75.

18. Mejri A, Arfaoui K, Ayadi MF, Aloui B, Yaakoubi
J. Primitive isolated hydatid cyst of the spleen: total
splenectomy versus spleen saving surgical modalities.
BMC Surg 2021;**21(1)**:46.

19. American Association for the Surgery of Trauma.
Injury scoring scale, 2023 Available from: www.aast.
org/resources-detail/injury-scoring-scale. (Accessed
28 August 2024).

20. Coccolini F, Montori G, Catena F, et al. Splenic
trauma: WSES Classification and Guidelines for
Adult and Pediatric Patients. *WJES* 2017;**12**:40.

21. Jones C. Surgery of the spleen. *Surgery (Oxford)*.
2022;**40(4)**:274–6.

22. Qu Y, Ren S, Li C, et al. Management of postoperative complications following splenectomy. *Int Surg*
2013;**98**:55–60.

23. Vikse J, Sanna B, Henry BM, et al. The prevalence and morphometry of an accessory spleen:
A meta-analysis and systematic review of 22,487
patients. *Int J Surg* 2017;**45**:18–28.

24. Bhattacharya P, Phelan L, Fisher S, Hajibandeh S,
Hajibandeh S. Robotic vs. laparoscopic splenectomy
in management of non-traumatic splenic pathologies: A systematic review and meta-analysis. *Am Surg*
2022;**88(1)**:38–47.

25. Peng F, Lai L, Luo M, et al. Comparison of early
postoperative results between robot-assisted and laparoscopic splenectomy for non-traumatic splenic diseases rather than portal hypertensive hypersplenism:
A meta-analysis. *Asian J Surg* 2020;**43(1)**:36–43.

26. Wang L, Xu J, Li F, et al. Partial splenectomy is superior to total splenectomy for selected
patients with hemangiomas or cysts. *World J Surg*
2017;**41(5)**:1281–86.

27. Wang X, Wang M, Zhang H, Peng B. Laparoscopic partial splenectomy is safe and effective in
patients with focal benign splenic lesion. *Surg Endosc*
2014;**28(12)**:3273–8.

28. Di Mauro D, Fasano A, Gelsomino M, Manzelli
A. Laparoscopic partial splenectomy using the harmonic scalpel for parenchymal transection: Two
case reports and review of the literature. *Acta Biomed*
2021;**92**:e2021137.

29. Costamagna D, Rizzi S, Zampogna A, Alonzo
A. Open partial splenectomy for trauma using
GIA-Stapler and FloSeal matrix haemostatic agent.
BMJ Case Rep 2010;**2010**:bcr0120102601.

30. Asbun HJ, Moekotte AL, Vissers FL, et al. The
Miami International Evidence-Based Guidelines on
Minimally Invasive Pancreas Resection. *Ann Surg*
2020;**271(1)**:1–14.

31. Kimura W, Fuse A, Hirai I, et al. Spleen-preserving distal pancreatectomy with preservation of the
splenic artery and vein for intraductal papillary-mucinous tumor (Ipmt): Three interesting cases. *Hepatogastroenterology* 2003;**50(54)**:2242–45.

32. Warshaw AL. Conservation of the spleen with distal
pancreatectomy. *Arch Surg* 1988;**123(5)**:550–3.

33. Warshaw AL. Distal pancreatectomy with preservation of the spleen. *J Hepatobiliary Pancreat Sci*
2010;**17(6)**:808–12.

34. Romero-Torres R. The true splenic blood supply
and its surgical applications. *Hepatogastroenterology*
1998;**45(21)**:885–8.

35. Wang L, Cheng Y, Xu J et al. Warshaw technique
in laparoscopic spleen-preserving distal pancre
atectomy: Surgical strategy and late outcomes of
splenic preservation. *Biomed Res Intl* 2019;**2019**:
4074369.

36. Elabbasy F, Gadde R, Hanna MM, Sleeman D,
Livingstone A, Yakoub D. Minimally invasive
spleen-preserving distal pancreatectomy: Does
splenic vessel preservation have better postoperative
outcomes? A systematic review and meta-analysis.
Hepatobiliary Pancreat Dis Int 2015;**14(4)**:346–53.

37. Song J, He Z, Ma S, Ma C, Yu T, Li J. Clinical
comparison of spleen-preserving distal pancreatectomy with or without splenic vessel preservation: A
systematic review and meta-analysis. *J Laparoendosc
Adv Surg Tech A* 2019;**29(3)**:323–32.

38. Paiella S, De Pastena M, Korrel M, et al. Long term
outcome after minimally invasive and open Warshaw
and Kimura techniques for spleen-preserving distal
pancreatectomy: International multicenter retrospective study. *Eur J Surg Oncol* 2019;**45(9)**: 1668–73.

39. Yongfei H, Javed AA, Burkhart R, et al. Geographical variation and trends in outcomes of laparoscopic spleen-preserving distal pancreatectomy with or
without splenic vessel preservation: A meta-analysis.
Int J Surg 2017;**45**:47–55.

40. Yu X, Li H, Jin C, et al. Splenic vessel preservation
versus Warshaw's technique during spleen-preserving distal pancreatectomy: A meta-analysis and systematic review. *Langenbecks Arch Surg* 2015;**400(2)**:
183–91.

41. Korrel M, Lof S, Sarireh BA, et al. Short-term outcomes after spleen-preserving minimally invasive distal pancreatectomy with or without preservation of splenic vessels: A pan-European retrospective study in high-volume centers. *Ann Surg* 2023;**277(1)**:e119-e125.

42. Tahir F, Ahmed J, Malik F. Post-splenectomy sepsis: A review of the literature. *Cureus* 2020;**12(2)**:e6898.

43. Casciani F, Trudeau MT, Vollmer CM. Perioperative immunization for splenectomy and the surgeon's responsibility: A review. *JAMA Surg* 2020;**155(11)**: 1068–77.

44. Theilacker C, Ludewig K, Serr A, et al. Overwhelming postsplenectomy infection: A prospective multicenter cohort study. *Clin Infect Dis* 2016;62(7): 871–8.

Chapter 75

Control of Splenic Bleeding

Ishtiyaq Bukhari, Seok Ling Ong and Andrew Tsang

INTRODUCTION

The spleen is present in all vertebrate animals apart from lampreys and hagfish and has the ubiquitous function of removing effete blood components and producing white cells and antibodies (1). Smooth muscle is absent in the capsule and trabeculae of the spleen in birds, reptiles and fish but is highly developed in mammals such as horses, pigs and dogs. The special location and morphology of the spleen make it one of the most frequently injured abdominal organs. Splenic bleeding can occur following blunt or penetrating trauma, spontaneously due to infectious diseases (malaria and mononucleosis) or involvement with lymphoma and following iatrogenic injury during surgical, endoscopic or interventional radiological procedures (2). The fragile nature and abundant blood supply mean that bleeding is frequently life threatening. Prompt recognition and treatment is essential to reduce morbidity and mortality. For hundreds of years surgery was the treatment of choice, but this changed with the recognition of the spleen's important immunological function which ushered in the era of research aimed at developing techniques for splenic preservation.

HISTORICAL APPROACHES TO SPLENIC BLEEDING

Over the centuries a myriad of functions has been attributed to the spleen. The central text of Rabbinic Judaism, the Talmud, refers to the spleen as the source of humour. The Greek word melaina kholé (μέλαινα χολή) which translates into English as 'black bile' is the root of the word 'melancholy'. Black bile emanating from the spleen was believed to cause depression. *Galen (130–210 AD)* was the first scientist and philosopher to assign specific parts of the soul to locations in the body and he also introduced the concept of the spleen as a filter. The human spleen is surrounded by a capsule composed of dense fibrous tissue, elastic fibres, and smooth muscle but their rudimentary nature, compared with some other mammals, is responsible for its fragile nature. It is understandable therefore that historically most surgical texts recommended splenectomy following trauma irrespective of the nature or severity (3). This approach was a retrograde step as many writings as early as the 16th century describe 'splenotomy' (incision of the spleen), 'splenorrhaphy' (suture), 'splenopexy' (fixation and partial removal). Today the approach is again aimed at splenic preservation wherever possible (4).

ANATOMY OF THE SPLEEN

The spleen is bean shaped, approximately 12 cm in length and located in the left upper quadrant (LUQ) (*Figure 75.1a*). Its axis lies parallel to the 10th rib and the smooth convex superior surface is applied to the concave surface of the diaphragm. Its capsule allows for considerable expansion, and apart from the hilum,

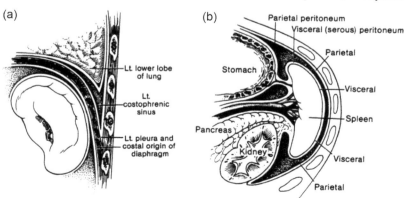

(a)   (b)

Figure 75.1 Important anatomical relationships of the spleen, coronal section showing relation of spleen to left lung, pleura and diaphragm (a) and peritoneal coverings and visceral peritoneal folds forming ligaments of attachment with other organs (b).

DOI: 10.1201/9781003080060-75

it is completely invested in visceral peritoneum (*Figure 75.1b*).

Its relationships are important as they indicate which other organs might be involved following significant blunt or penetrating trauma (5). Its medial aspect is shaped by the splenic flexure of the colon, the stomach and the left kidney. Surrounding ligaments attach the spleen to the greater curve of the stomach (the gastrosplenic ligament containing the short gastric and gastroepiploic vessels), the left kidney (the splenorenal ligament containing the splenic artery and vein) and the splenic flexure of the colon (the phrenocolic ligament also known as the sustentaculum lienis or Hensing's ligament after Friedrich Wilhelm Hensing (1719–1745), the German professor of medicine in Giessen.

IMMUNE FUNCTION

The spleen performs innate and adaptive functions (antibody and cell-mediated immune responses) of the immune system facilitated by its organized morphology (6). Its physical structure is designed to allow the filtering and removal of effete blood components, cellular debris and microorganisms. It is the most important organ for the antibacterial and antifungal immune response, and it facilitates low probability interactions between antigen presenting cells (APCs) and direct, cell-cell interaction between the antigen-specific receptor of the reactive T cell and the target cell. APCs unique to the spleen regulate the T- and B-cell responses to these antigenic targets in the blood.

INCIDENCE OF SPLENIC BLEEDING

The true incidence of splenic bleeding from all causes is almost impossible to quantify and the reporting of iatrogenic splenic injuries is so variable that comparisons are difficult. The principal mechanism producing traumatic rupture continues to be road traffic accidents, followed by direct blows to the abdomen during contact sports, cycling, skiing and horse riding. Traumatic bleeding appears to be most common in males (twice the incidence of females) from 18–34 years of age. A number of conditions are responsible for non-traumatic rupture including: 1) Neoplastic (30%); 2) infectious (30%); 3) inflammatory conditions (15%); 4) medication and medical treatment (10%); 5) mechanical (7%) and 6) idiopathic (7%).

Splenectomies, which make up 20% of treatment, are performed as a result of:

- Iatrogenic injury following colonoscopy
- Upper gastrointestinal (GI) procedures (particularly those involving mobilization of the stomach)
- Colonic surgery (especially transverse and left colon resections)
- ERCP
- Left nephrectomy and/or adrenalectomy
- Percutaneous nephrolithotomy

- Vascular operations involving the abdominal aorta
- Gynaecological operations
- Left lung biopsy
- Chest-drain insertion
- Spinal surgery (rare)
- Cardiopulmonary resuscitation (rare)

Re-do procedures and anatomical proximity significantly increase the risk of injury. The risk factors for an iatrogenic splenic injury can be categorized as patient-related factors and surgeon/procedure-related factors. Patient-related factors include splenomegaly, adhesions around the spleen from previous surgical procedures and an inflammatory process in the LUQ. Surgeon-related factors include undue traction, direct injury, inadequate exposure, inexperience and access to the LUQ (7,8).

CLINICAL PRESENTATION

The clinical manifestations of splenic bleeding are typically the consequence of peritoneal irritation or hypovolaemic shock if the blood loss is very rapid (9). In patients where the blood loss is minimal or prolonged, symptoms may be mild with just LUQ pain or tenderness. Delayed haemorrhage can also result from a subcapsular haematoma which ruptures often leading to massive blood loss. A ruptured spleen usually involves the superior pole or diaphragmatic surface and there are frequently corresponding rib fractures. The most dramatic splenic ruptures are those involving the hilum, especially when the splenic pedicle is torn. When splenic injuries are associated with damage to other intra-abdominal organs, symptoms will be mixed and generally more complicated to assess and investigate (10). Iatrogenic splenic injuries that occur and are recognized intraoperatively are often obvious, but they may manifest at a later stage with varying severity ranging from localized symptoms such as LUQ pain or Kehr's sign, originally described by the German surgeon Hans Kehr, 1862–1916 (it is a traditional example of referred pain with irritation of the diaphragm due to blood in the peritoneal cavity causing supraclavicular pain) to systemic signs of shock and haemorrhage.

DIAGNOSIS

In a patient with a suspected splenic injury, or rupture, the choice of imaging modality will depend on the haemodynamic condition of the patient. Where the patient is haemodynamically stable and/or responds to volume resuscitation, cross-sectional imaging with computed tomography (CT) of the abdomen and pelvis with IV contrast in arterial and delayed portovenous phases (CECT) is the 'gold standard' investigation. If the presentation is following trauma, a CECT must include the splenic parenchyma and consider the possibility of an associated vascular injury and the involvement of other hollow, and solid, intra-abdominal organs.

Iatrogenic splenic injuries are generally recognized intraoperatively from physical signs such as a capsular tear or laceration with haemorrhage. Missed injuries and injuries sustained during percutaneous and endoscopic procedures when suspected will need further investigation to confirm the diagnosis and to grade the severity of the injury (9,10)

CLASSIFICATION OF SPLENIC INJURIES

The American Association for the Surgery of Trauma (AAST) organ injury severity score (OIS) remains the most commonly used classification for splenic trauma. It was originally devised to facilitate comparisons between different series of patients. Its ease of use saw its widespread adoption and it is now used routinely to classify splenic injuries and guide management algorithms. It is based on the morphology of the splenic injury and was updated in 2018 (*Table 75.1*) but it is important to note that the AAST grading system was devised for the assessment of splenic injuries following trauma (9,10). Examples of CT scans showing splenic injuries, Grade I to Grade V are shown in *Figure 75.2*.

The World Society of Emergency Surgery (WSES) have also developed a classification system which describes three categories: 1) Minor (WSES class I); 2) Moderate (WSES classes II and III); 3) Severe (WSES class IV) and has the advantage of being applicable to paediatric patients (*Table 75.2*).

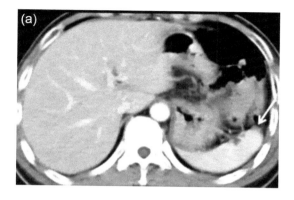

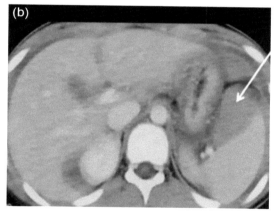

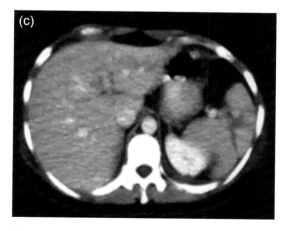

Table 75.1 AAST grading of splenic injuries: For multiple injuries the grade is advanced by one category up to Grade 3

Grade	CT diagnostic criteria
I	• Subcapsular haematoma <10% surface area • Depth of parenchymal laceration <1 cm • Capsular tear
II	• Subcapsular haematoma = 10–50% surface area • Intraparenchymal haematoma <5 cm • Depth of parenchymal laceration = 1–3 cm not involving trabecular vessel
III	• Subcapsular haematoma >50% surface area, or expanding • Ruptured subcapsular or intraparenchymal haematoma ≥5 cm • Depth of parenchymal laceration >3 cm or including trabecular vessel
IV	• With a splenic vascular injury or active bleeding confined within the splenic capsule • Major devascularization • Parenchymal laceration involving segmental or hilar vessels producing >25% devascularization
V	• With a splenic vascular injury with active bleeding extending beyond the spleen into the peritoneum or hilar injury that completely devascularizes the spleen • Completely shattered spleen

Figure 75.2 Axial CT scans showing examples of AAST grading of splenic injuries. Grade 1 (a). Grade II (b). Grade III (c).

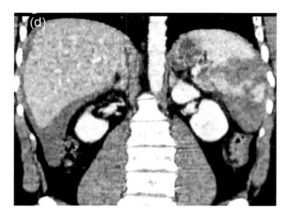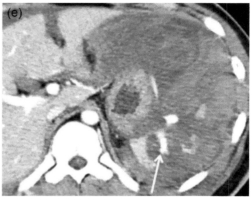

Figure 75.2 (*Continued*) Grade IV (d). Grade V (e).

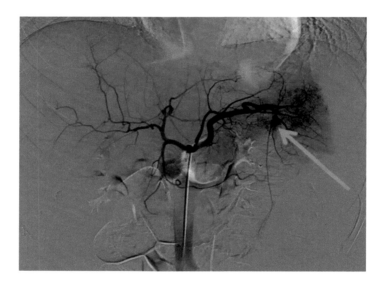

Figure 75.3 Splenic angiogram indicating the site of bleeding (red arrow).

Table 75.2 WSES grading of splenic injuries

	WSES grade	Mechanism of injury	AAST	Haemodynamic status	CT scan	First-line treatment adults	First-line treatment paediatric
Minor	WSES 1	Blunt/ penetrating	1–2	Stable	Yes + local exploration in SW	NOM + serial evaluation Consider angiography +/– embolization	NOM + serial evaluation Consider angiography +/– embolization
Moderate	WSES 2	Blunt/ penetrating	3	Stable		Angiography and embolization	
	WSES 3	Blunt/ penetrating	4–5	Stable			
Severe	WSES 4	Blunt/ penetrating	1–5	Unstable	No	OM	OM

MANAGEMENT

Factors that influence the management of iatrogenic splenic injury include; 1) Severity/grade of injury; 2) the timing of injury recognition; 3) availability of interventional radiology support; and 4) haemodynamic stability.

Haemodynamic instability in adults is defined by: 1) An admission systolic blood pressure <90 mmHg with evidence of skin vasoconstriction; 2) an altered level of consciousness and/or shortness of breath; 3) systolic blood pressure >90 mmHg but requiring bolus infusions/transfusions and/or 4) vasopressor drugs and/or 5) an admission base excess ≥5 mmol/L and/or 6) shock index >1 and/or 7) transfusion requirement of at least 4–6 units of packed red blood cells within the first 24 hours.

Splenic injuries are mainly parenchymal tears usually between segments perpendicular to the splenic axis and hilar vascular involvement is rare. As the majority of injuries do not directly involve an intersegmental blood vessel, bleeding will frequently stop spontaneously forming the basis for non-operative management (NOM). Splenic conservation should be favoured unless haemodynamic stability cannot be achieved without splenectomy. Patients who are haemodynamically stable after initial resuscitation, who are not peritonitic and do not have associated injuries requiring surgical intervention are managed with splenic conservation. In high-volume centres with supportive facilities NOM of splenic injuries is successful in almost 90% of the cases. The advantages of NOM over emergency splenectomy are lower hospital costs, avoidance of non-therapeutic laparotomies, lower rates of intra-abdominal complications and of blood transfusion, lower mortality with the maintenance of the immunological function, and the prevention of overwhelming post-splenectomy infection (OPSI) (11,12). Splenectomy is detailed in **Chapter 74** and will not be discussed in detail here.

NON-OPERATIVE MANAGEMENT (NOM)

Most splenic injuries of minor severity are managed conservatively with adequate resuscitation, correction of any coagulation defects and close monitoring (13–15). Haemodynamic instability, despite initial resuscitation, is an indication for a more radical approach in the form of splenectomy. In all patients it is important to follow trauma guidance (Advanced Trauma Life Support [ATLS], WSES) for the initial management. Initial A–E assessment, fluid resuscitation, blood transfusion if indicated and activation of massive transfusion protocols in some patients. After confirmation of the diagnosis and grading of the splenic laceration, the patient should be admitted to a high dependency unit for close monitoring, (with advice to limit mobilization in the initial phase), have a urinary catheter inserted and strict fluid balance maintained. If an iatrogenic injury

is recognized intraoperatively, the surgeon should liaise with the anaesthetist and ensure haemodynamic stability before deciding whether a conservative approach is possible. Reasons for the failure of NOM include age, the grade of injury, concomitant organ injury and vascular abnormalities. NOM is not always successful and if abdominal pain and peritoneal irritation worsen, transfusion requirements exceed 4 U in 24 hours, there is evidence of a continued fall in haematocrit which does not respond quickly to blood transfusion or signs develop suggesting damage to other abdominal organs, the patient should be considered for radiological or surgical management or transfer to a specialist HPB unit. Failure of NOM is usually manifest within 96 hours but may be delayed and occur from 6–20 days due to continued low-grade bleeding, secondary haemorrhage or infection.

MANAGEMENT FOLLOWING FAILURE OF NOM BY ANGIOEMBOLIZATION

Sclafani first described splenic artery embolization (SAE) to treat traumatic splenic bleeding in 1981 (16). Angioembolization has the advantage of identifying the source of bleeding (*Figure 75.3*) which can help clinicians decide on an appropriate management plan while also being potentially therapeutic. Since Sclafani's original report, SAE has been increasingly used to treat splenic bleeding and there is now a substantial body of research supporting its safety and effectiveness. Recent studies have demonstrated that SAE is effective in up to 97% of cases (17,18). Compared with a spleen-preserving operative approach, angioembolization is minimally invasive with the advantages of improved recovery, can be performed under local anaesthetic and hospital stays and costs are reduced. Traumatic or iatrogenic splenic injuries not detected during surgery, and where active bleeding is suspected, are often amenable to radiological intervention. If a CT scan shows an active arterial blush demonstrating active haemorrhage, then angioembolization is the mainstay of treatment (19). A standard angiographic technique is typically used with access obtained via a femoral approach with a micropuncture kit, after which the coeliac artery is selected with a curved or reversed curve catheter (Cobra™ [Cook Medical, IN, USA] or Simmons 1 or 2, respectively). Prior to selecting the splenic artery, a coeliac arteriogram should be performed with particular attention to the splenic artery but also the left gastric artery as it is often an important collateral feeder to the spleen. The main splenic artery is then catheterized, and a splenic arteriogram performed. If a distal embolization procedure is to be performed, a microcatheter and wire combination, for example a Renegade™ STS catheter and Fathom™ 0.016 inch wire (Boston Scientific, MS, USA) are placed as distally, and near to, the injured vessel as possible. Typically, a microcatheter with a standard, rather than high-flow lumen is used, due to the fact that a deployable coil may be used during the embolization procedure. High-flow lumen microcatheters may allow partial coiling within the lumen, causing blockage of the microcatheter. Their size may also allow premature deployment inside the catheter if coils with mechanical detachment mechanisms are used (Interlock™, Boston Scientific, MS, USA). As the spleen is generally considered to have an end-organ vascular supply, it is important to place the microcatheter as distally as possible before embolization to preserve as much native supply to the spleen. Once the microcatheter is properly positioned, embolization can be performed with a variety of agents: Gelfoam® (Pfizer, NY, USA), particles, or coils can be used in isolation or together (20). Complications following SAE, are uncommon but can be difficult to recognize and manage in the context of a significant splenic injury. The most common complication is postembolization syndrome (PES) which is associated with abdominal pain and an intermittent fever. PES usually results from ischaemic and/or necrotic splenic tissue, oedema, capsular pain, release of inflammatory mediators (prostaglandin E2 and interleukin) and endogenous pyrogens and diaphragmatic irritation. Symptoms depend on the volume of spleen embolized, and it is recommended that, where possible, this is limited to <70%. Abdominal pain can be treated conservatively, and antibiotics should be given to prevent any necrotic tissue becoming infected.

ALTERNATIVE NON-OPERATIVE APPROACHES

In addition to angioembolization there are a number of other approaches including abdominal drainage and autologous blood transfusion which can also be performed under local anaesthetic. Patients with an isolated splenic injury are suitable and blood is collected in a cell-salvage device, treated and reinfused. This technique is not appropriate if bleeding continues for more than 6 hours, or the collected blood is severely haemolyzed or infected. Other non-vascular interventions include ultrasound (US) and CT-guided procedures. US-guided microwave and radiofrequency ablation have been investigated to achieve haemostasis in patients with splenic bleeding and US combined with microbubble cavitation technology is a promising new non-invasive option.

FOLLOW-UP AND REPEAT IMAGING FOLLOWING NOM AND SPLEEN PRESERVING SURGERY

Follow-up imaging with CECT scan 48–72 hours following admission for splenic injuries WSES Class II/AAST Grade III or higher treated with NOM is recommended to ensure the early recognition of vascular complications. Following spleen preserving

surgical procedures the patient should be monitored clinically and biochemically and should have follow-up scans (US/CT) to detect any collections or vascular complications with particular care taken to exclude splenic artery pseudoaneurysm formation.

SURGICAL TREATMENT

Surgical operation is a very effective treatment for splenic bleeding. Basic principles apply and success relies on: 1) The rapid diagnosis of the source of bleeding; 2) identification of the appropriate surgical approach and 3) performance by experienced surgeons to reduce the operative time and consequent blood loss. Complete splenectomy is an established procedure, and often the simplest approach, but is associated with significant postoperative complications and immunocompromise. Laparoscopy is valuable in borderline cases and can occasionally facilitate therapeutic manoeuvres. Simple measures like pressure with a gauze, followed by topical haemostatic agents, are the first line of treatment. The range of topical haemostatic agents that are available is shown in *Table 75.3*. The most common agent used in the authors' centre is Floseal® (Baxter, USA), Surgicel® (J&J Med Tech, NJ, USA) and Veriset™ (Medtronic, MI, USA) are rarely used for splenic injury and are only effective in very superficial, and small, capsular tears.

Floseal® haemostatic matrix is a high-viscosity cross-linked gelatin-thrombin haemostatic matrix. It contains the gelatin matrix in the form of cross-linked bovine gelatin granules and human thrombin and acts during both the early and late phases of the coagulation cascade. Floseal® should be applied at the deepest part of the laceration and come in contact with the whole bleeding surface. Following application of Floseal®, a damp gauze is applied over the agent for

Table 75.3 Topical agents available to aid splenic haemostasis

Biologically active agents	Dry matrix agents
• Topical thrombin agents (Evithrom® [J&J Med Tech, NJ, USA]) • Bovine albumin-glutaraldehyde tissue adhesives (Bio-Glue® [Artivion, Inc. GA, USA]) • Fibrin sealants/glues (Crosseal™ [J&J Med Tech, NJ, USA]) • Gelatin/Thrombin sealants (Floseal®)	• Absorbable gelatin matrix (Gelfoam®) • Microporous polysaccharide spores derived from potato starch (Arista™ [BD, NJ, USA]) • Microfibrillar collagen (Avitene™ [BD, NJ, USA]) • Oxidized regenerated methylcellulose (Surgicel®)

approximately 2 minutes to hold it in place. The gelatin granules expand by 10–20% within 10 minutes which helps reduce blood flow and creates a tamponade effect. The unique spherical gelatin granules allow high concentrations of thrombin to surround the particles and react with the patient's endogenous fibrinogen to form a mechanically stable clot. Once haemostasis is achieved, excess product should be removed by gentle irrigation. Biologically active agents enhance coagulation at the bleeding site and dry matrix agents are passive substrates which promote haemostasis.

If the laceration is of higher grade and topical haemostatic agents fail to control the haemorrhage, the patient may require a splenectomy. Other spleen preserving treatment modalities are often of limited value in clinical practice due to lack of equipment or unfamiliarity of surgeons with the technical aspects. These operative approaches should only be used if the surgeon is fully conversant with the techniques and experienced in their use. Patient safety should not be compromised albeit with the laudable intention of preserving immune function and appropriate help should be sought if available.

Argon beam coagulation

If available, and if the surgical team is familiar with the equipment, it can be very effective in controlling bleeding from a broader superficial surface. Argon plasma coagulation is a monopolar electrosurgical technique which uses argon discharges at atmospheric pressure to coagulate tissue (*see* **Chapter 10** for a detailed description).

Pledgeted mattress sutures

This technique can be used to repair and salvage an injured spleen. The spleen is mobilized into the midline (*Figure 75.4*) and assessed as to whether repair is suitable and possible. The adult splenic capsule does not hold sutures well and a number of techniques attempt to overcome this using reinforcing tissue or material (20). A monofilament suture, preferably on a straight needle supported by a bolster (strips of Teflon™, omentum or posterior rectus sheath) on both sides of the laceration can be used (*Figure 75.5*).

Absorbable mesh wrap

Polyglycolic mesh wrap is another technique reported to be useful in splenic salvage. The injured spleen is passed through an enlarged hole in the mesh fashioned for this purpose. The mesh is then wrapped around the spleen and sutured to itself to provide tamponade. More recent reports also suggested incorporating methylcellulose into the mesh to help 'bulk it up'. In this technique, multiple layers of methylcellulose are placed directly onto the injured surfaces, after which the mesh is secured around the spleen, enhancing the tamponade effect (*Figure 75.6*). Previous concerns of possible mesh infection, especially in the setting of

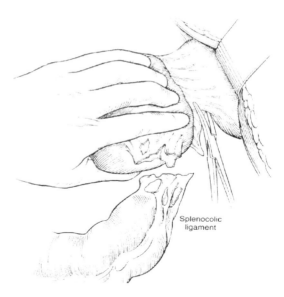

Figure 75.4 Labelled illustration of a mobilization of the spleen into the midline by division of the splenocolic ligament and splenorenal (lienorenal) ligaments.

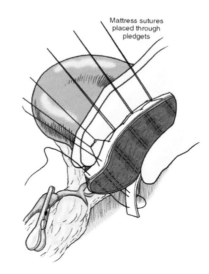

Figure 75.5 Labelled illustration of the method of using pledgeted mattress sutures to control splenic bleeding.

hollow viscus injury, have proved to be unfounded based on large series of patients (21). The need to place an LUQ or pelvic abdominal drain should be guided by the operative findings and should be left to the discretion of the operating surgeon at the time of intervention. Postoperatively patients should be closely monitored for any signs of haemodynamic deterioration. If these measures fail or the patient becomes haemodynamically unstable at any point, splenectomy is indicated, and the procedure is described in detail in **Chapter 74**.

Novel approaches

A number of additional approaches have been attempted with the aim of combining the advantage of minimally invasive approaches with spleen preserving surgery. These include laparoscopic devascularization of inferior pole of the spleen (22) and/or the creation of a pneumoperitoneum to aid haemostasis. Presently there are insufficient data to support the use of these procedures.

SUMMARY

The National Audit Office estimates that 20 000 cases of major trauma (MT) occur in England each year resulting in 5 400 deaths (23). Although this is predominantly in patients under 40 years of age, the MT population identified in the UK is becoming more elderly, and the predominant mechanism that precipitates MT is a fall from <2 m. Splenic bleeding is one of the most frequent causes of mortality due to its blood supply, morphology and vulnerable location. Early and rapid assessment of haemodynamic status is crucial to facilitate rapid appropriate management. The suspicion of splenic injury in a stable patient requires an urgent CECT which is the 'gold standard' for non-invasive diagnostic imaging of blunt abdominal trauma.

The subsequent management should always aim to preserve the spleen where possible and safe. A number of NOM techniques are available ranging from conservative treatment, through angioembolization, to spleen-preserving surgical procedures. With today's equipment and expertise, splenic preservation is possible in most patients and splenectomy is reserved for haemodynamically unstable patients where other methods have failed and/or there are associated injuries to other abdominal organs. A suggested management algorithm is shown in *Figure 75.7*.

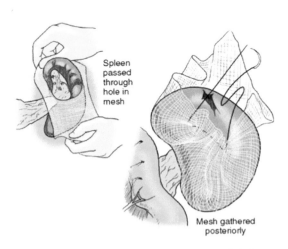

Spleen passed through hole in mesh

Mesh gathered posteriorly

Figure 75.6 Basic medical keys – managing injuries to the spleen.

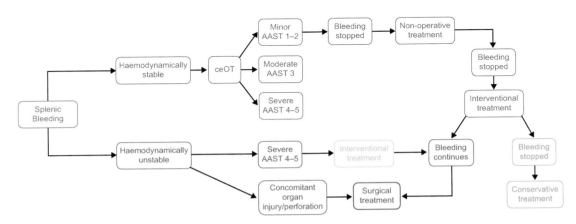

Figure 75.7 Suggested management decision-making pathway for the treatment of splenic bleeding following AAST grading.

REFERENCES

1. Brendolan A, Rosado MM, Carsetti R, Selleri L, Dear TN. Development and function of the mammalian spleen. *Bioessays* 2007;**29(2)**:166–77.

2. Khan RN, Jindal V. Systematic review of atraumatic splenic rupture *Br J Surg* 2009;**96**:1114–21.

3. Roy P, Mukherjee R, Parik M. Splenic trauma in the twenty-first century: Changing trends in management. *Ann R Coll Surg Engl* 2018;**100(8)**:1–7.

4. David A, McClusky III, BA, Skandalakis LJ, Colborn GL, Skandalakis JE. Tribute to a triad: History of splenic anatomy, physiology, and surgery: Part 2. *World J Surg* 1999;**23**:514–26.

5. Vishy Mahadevan. Anatomy of the pancreas and spleen. *Surgery (Oxford)* 2019;**37**:297–301.

6. Lewis SM, Williams A, Eisenbarth SC. Structure and function of the immune system in the spleen. *Sci Immunol* 2019;**4(33)**:eaau6085.

7. Akoury T, Whetstone DR. 2023. Splenic Rupture. Available from: https://www.ncbi.nlm.nih.gov/books/NBK525951/ StatPearls Publishing (Accessed 28 August 2024).

8. Wiik Larsen J, Søreide K, Søreide JA, Tjosevik K, Kvaløy JT, Thorsen K. Epidemiology of abdominal trauma: An age- and sex-adjusted incidence analysis with mortality patterns. *Injury* 2022;**53(10)**:3130–38.

9. Coccolini F, Fugazzola P, Morganti L, Ceresoli M, Magnone S, Montori G, et al. The World Society of Emergency Surgery (WSES) Spleen Trauma Classification: A useful tool in the management of splenic trauma. *World J Emerg Surg* 2019;**14**:30.

10. Podda M, De Simone B, Ceresoli M, Virdis F, Favi F, Wiik Larsen J, et al. Follow-up strategies for patients with splenic trauma managed non-operatively: The 2022 World Society of Emergency Surgery consensus document. *World J Emerg Surg* 2022;**17(1)**:52.

11. Gupta AK, Vazquez OA. Overwhelming post-splenectomy infection syndrome: Variability in timing with similar presentation. *Cureus* 2020;**12(8)**:e9914.

12. Grace M. Lee; Preventing infections in children and adults with asplenia. *Hematology Am Soc Hematol Educ Program* 2020;**2020(1)**:328–35.

13. Beuran M, Gheju I, Venter MD, Marian RC, Smarandache R. Non-operative management of splenic trauma. *J Med Life* 2012;**5(1)**:47–58.

14. Pachter HL, Guth AA, Hofstetter SR, Spencer FC. Changing patterns in the management of splenic trauma: The impact of nonoperative management. *Ann Surg* 1998;**227(5)**:708–17.

15. Spijkerman R, Teuben MPJ, Hoosain F, Taylor LP, Hardcastle TC, Blokhuis TJ, et al. Non-operative management for penetrating splenic trauma: How far can we go to save splenic function? *World J Emerg Surg* 2017;**12**:33.

16. Sclafani SJ. The role of angiographic hemostasis in salvage of the injured spleen. *Radiology* 1981;**141**:645–50.

17. Lin BC, Wu CH, Wong YC, et al. Splenic artery embolization changes the management of blunt splenic injury: An observational analysis of 680 patients graded by the revised 2018 AAST-OIS. *Surg Endosc* 2023;**37**:371–81.

18. van der Vlies CH, Hoekstra J, Ponsen KJ, Reekers JA, van Delden OM, Goslings JC. Impact of splenic artery embolization on the success rate of nonoperative management for blunt splenic injury. *Cardiovasc Intervent Radiol* 2012;**35(1)**:76–81.

19. Elabbasy F, Gadde R, Hanna MM, Sleeman D, Livingstone A, Yakoub D. Minimally invasive spleen-preserving distal pancreatectomy: Does splenic vessel preservation have better postoperative outcomes? A systematic review and meta-analysis. *Hepatobiliary Pancreat Dis Int* 2015;**14(4)**:346–53.

20. Yilmaz TH, Ndofor BC, Smith MD, Degiannis E. A heuristic approach and heretic view on the technical issues and pitfalls in the management of penetrating abdominal injuries. *Scand J Trauma Resusc Emerg Med* 2010;**18**:40.

21. Lange DA, Zaret P, Merlotti GJ, Robin AP, Sheaf C, Barrett JA. The use of absorbable mesh in splenic trauma. *J Trauma* 1988;**28(3)**:269–75.

22. Basso N, Silecchia G, Raparelli L, Pizzuto G, and Picconi T. Laparoscopic splenectomy for ruptured spleen: Lessons learned from a case. *J Laparoendosc Adv Surg Tech* A 2003;**2**:109–112.

23. Jesani H, Jesani L, Rangaraj A, and Rasheed A splenic trauma, the way forward in reducing splenectomy: Our 15-year experience. *Ann R Coll Surg Engl* 2020;**102(4)**:263–70.

Chapter 76   Splenic Tumours

Debanshu Bhaduri

INTRODUCTION

Historically the spleen has been an enigmatic organ and its nature and functions defied understanding for centuries. Despite being an integral part of the reticuloendothelial system, the spleen shows an innate resistance to becoming involved in neoplastic processes. Primary and secondary tumour involvement of the spleen is reported only occasionally despite the constant progress and ever-increasing sophistication of imaging technologies. Although the cornerstone of treatment for symptomatic splenic tumours remains surgery, the occurrence of overwhelming post-splenectomy infection (OPSI), albeit infrequent, remains an area of concern and partial splenectomy in selected cases should be considered.

In this chapter, the various space-occupying lesions affecting the spleen together with their aetiopathology are discussed and an outline of the methods of classification, evaluation and management are outlined.

HISTORICAL BACKGROUND

Several factors conspired to ensure that the spleen remained mysterious through hundreds of years of medical evolution. Ensconced in its own space in the left upper quadrant of the abdomen in close proximity to the stomach, colon, pancreas and left kidney and adrenal, the spleen has no connection or direct involvement with any of its immediate neighbours. Once considered a gland, it puzzled clinicians that 'no secretions emanated from it' (1). Its distinctive purple colour convinced ancient anatomists that it was the 'centre of rage', thus originating the phrase 'venting one's spleen' for an angry outburst. Considered to harbour 'black bile' (one of Galen's four humours), and apparently without any route for its exit, an excess of this black bile was supposed to lead to unpredictable moods and behaviour (1).

The spleen was initially thought to be the source of blood (rather than the bone marrow), because of the abundance of haematological formed elements found within it (1). Prior to the advent of advanced imaging, splenic tumours were usually discovered as an incidental finding at post-mortem. Rarely, a neoplasm of the spleen would become large enough to cause mechanical, or space occupying symptoms and thus reveal itself.

EPIDEMIOLOGY

There have been very few reports of splenic tumours of primary or secondary origin and the majority of the available data is from incidentally discovered lesions found post-mortem. Primary lymphomatous involvement of the spleen accounts for less than 1% of all lymphomas (2). Metastases to the spleen were identified by Berge in 312 out of 7165 post-mortems (4.35%), the largest reported series to-date and half of the patients had metastases in at least five other viscera (3). This is in-line with the prevalence reported in early studies which ranges between 2.3–7.1% (4). An incidence of metastases for solid tumours of 0.6% at post-mortem and 1.1% at splenectomy has been reported in a large clinicopathological study. Only 8% of these patients had reported symptoms, demonstrating not only the low frequency of splenic metastases but also that clinical presentation is very uncommon (5). A study from Germany demonstrated that males were more often affected, and the median age was 62-years (range 26–88 years). Only 3 of 29 364 such patients had primary splenic tumours (6). Of the very rare malignant lesions, involvement of the spleen as part of a systemic haematological malignancy is most frequent. Less frequent are the metastatic non-haematological tumours, chiefly from the breast, colon, lung, ovary and stomach (3). Melanomas are also known to metastasize to the spleen (7) and the lowest reported incidence is for primary, malignant non-lymphoid tumours.

AETIOPATHOLOGY

The reasons for an organ like the spleen, which is highly vascularized, being so rarely involved with secondary tumours remains a subject of debate and a number hypotheses have been posited. Anatomically, the lack of afferent lymphatics and the acute angulation of the splenic artery at its origin from the coeliac trunk trifurcation could mechanically interfere with tumour emboli. Dynamically, the rhythmic contraction of the spleen could produce an unfavourable milieu for tumour cells to adhere and implant and immunologically, the concentration of lymphoid tissue *per se* may have high anti-tumour activity (8).

Splenic masses have been broadly classified into solid and cystic. Cystic masses can be further divided into 'true' cysts and false or 'pseudocysts'. Solid masses

DOI: 10.1201/9781003080060-76

Table 76.1 Classification of splenic masses (10)

Solid masses	Cystic masses
Lymphoid	**Primary or 'true'**
● Hodgkin	● Parasitic
● Non-Hodgkin	● Nonparasitic
Non-lymphoid	● Congenital
● Benign	● Neoplastic
● Malignant (primary	**False or 'pseudocysts'**
or metastatic)	● Post-traumatic
	● Other

can be either lymphoid or non-lymphoid in nature. (*Table 76.1*) (9).

CYSTS OF THE SPLEEN

Cysts of the spleen commonly present in the second or the third decade of life and 30–45% are asymptomatic abdominal masses. Cysts are defined as 'true' or 'primary' and 'false' or 'secondary' or 'pseudocysts'.

PRIMARY OR TRUE CYSTS

These cysts are defined by the presence of an epithelial lining. A majority of these cysts are parasitic and in two thirds of these parasitic cysts, the offending organism is *Echinococcus*, usually *E. granulosus* (hydatid cysts).

Of the spleen, 10% of all cysts and 25% of non-parasitic primary cysts are congenital with the majority being discovered in children or young adults (9). The suggested aetiology is invagination or inclusion of the mesothelium lined splenic capsule during embryogenesis, which subsequently proliferates and undergoes metaplasia (10). A second possible cause is suggested by the finding that the squamous epithelium is keratinised, suggesting that these cysts may actually be neoplastic not metaplastic (11).

Neoplastic cysts can be epidermoid, dermoid or endodermoid although the latter are not true cysts. Epidermoid and dermoid cysts are very rare, and contain elements derived from all three layers, epithelium, mesothelium and endothelium.

SECONDARY CYSTS OR PSEUDOCYSTS

Seventy-five per cent of non-parasitic cysts of the spleen are pseudocysts, which by definition have no true epithelial lining. The majority of these pseudocysts follow trauma and frequently the event is subtle enough to pass unnoticed (12). These cysts occur mainly in the young and early middle age and there is a female preponderance which remains unexplained, although hormones and pregnancy induced changes are suspected (9). Although poorly understood, it is

hypothesized that following a traumatic event which leads to intra-splenic haemorrhage (with, or without, capsular laceration) the resulting haematoma becomes encapsulated and following resorption of the contained blood there is persistence of the false cyst wall. Eventually, this false cyst wall gets thickened, fibrosed and heavily calcified (13,14).

CLINICAL PRESENTATION OF SPLENIC CYSTS

Splenic cysts are rare entities and the majority are asymptomatic, especially if they are <5 cm in diameter. They are usually discovered during autopsies or while evaluating the abdomen for other pathologies. There may, or may not, be a history of trauma or exposure to animal hosts such as *Echinococcus*. Other symptoms such as left upper quadrant fullness, a dull aching pain, and symptoms related to visceral compression are mechanical and relate to organomegaly. Compressive symptoms usually only appear once the spleen weighs in excess of 3–4 kg (14). These could be intestinal and gastric obstruction, or poorly controlled hypertension due to compression of the left renal artery. Referred pain to the left shoulder tip and vague urinary complaints are due to left renal or ureteropelvic compression. Respiratory complaints include dyspnoea, left pleuritic chest pain or left lobar pneumonia are reported and splenomegaly can also result in hypersplenism with its attendant myeloid or erythroid related complications. A rare, but potentially lethal, complication is splenic rupture, a disastrous event heralded by the sudden onset of acute abdominal pain and exsanguinating haemorrhage which is unfortunately inevitable in most major splenic ruptures. There is also the risk of anaphylactic shock if the cyst was due to hydatid disease.

SOLID TUMOURS OF THE SPLEEN

Most solid tumours of the spleen produce the same symptoms as cystic lesions and the range is so diverse that no single symptom or clinically useful symptom complex can be identified as (14). Solid tumours of the spleen are either lymphoid or nonlymphoid.

LYMPHOID TUMOURS

The spleen is rarely the primary site of a lymphoid neoplasm but involvement as part of disseminated disease is much more frequent. Both non-Hodgkin's lymphoma (NHL) and Hodgkin's disease can involve the spleen which principally affects the white pulp. The involvement of the spleen may be diffuse, as in the nodular variant of lymphoma, or localized, manifesting as large, irregular tumours (9) such as seen in diffuse large B-cell lymphoma (DLBCL). DLBCL is also the most common lymphoma of primary splenic origin (*Figure 76.1*). The diagnosis of a primary splenic lymphoma relies on imaging characteristics, and is defined by organ-confined disease with, or without, hilar lymph nodes with no recurrence following splenectomy (15). Staging laparotomy, which included multi-site abdominal nodal and visceral biopsies together with splenectomy, was the standard oncological approach before the early 1990s. This was inevitably associated with a certain amount of morbidity and with more sophisticated radiological and nuclear medicine modalities including the advent of the fluorodeoxyglucose positron emission tomography (FDG-PET) scan, staging laparotomy is no longer required. Apart from the lymphomas, the other lymphoid tumours involving the spleen are exceedingly rare but include Castleman's tumour (a nonclonal lymphoproliferative disorder) (16), plasmacytoma, reactive lymphoid hyperplasia (17) and inflammatory pseudotumours (19). In addition to space-occupying features, nonspecific symptoms can occur with lymphoid lesions including fever, night sweats, weight loss and generalized pruritus.

NON-LYMPHOID TUMOURS OF THE SPLEEN

These may be primary, or metastatic, with the latter being far more common.

Metastatic tumours

Metastases may involve the spleen primarily from breast, lung, colon, ovary, melanoma and stomach (4) (*Figures 76.2* and *76.3*). It is very unusual for the spleen to be the first site of metastases, but it is most frequently described from an endometrial primary (19–22). Symptoms, if present are related to the size of the spleen, with compression or distortion of related structures

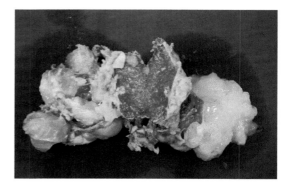

Figure 76.2 Postoperative image of a pseudomyxoma peritonei metastasis to spleen specimen (*Photo courtesy of Dr Taher Chharchhodwala*).

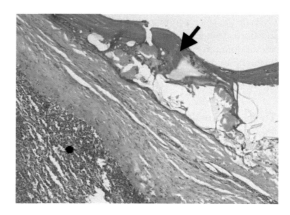

Figure 76.3 Tissue sample image taken from a pseudomyxoma peritonei due to low grade appendiceal mucinous neoplasm involving spleen. Note cystic area in the spleen containing predominantly acellular mucin (thick arrow). Left lower area (circle) shows unremarkable spleen (H&E stain; 40x magnification) (*Photo courtesy of Dr Taher Chharchhodwala*). *Abbreviation*: H&E: haematoxylin and eosin.

and hypersplenism with the attendant haematological abnormalities. In most cases, however, the splenic symptoms are overshadowed by the symptoms caused by the burden of the primary malignancy at its site of origin or the metastatic involvement of other sites.

Primary non-lymphoid tumours

Non-lymphoid tumours can be benign, or malignant, and are very unusual. The majority being vascular in origin.

BENIGN TUMOURS OF VASCULAR ORIGIN

Haemangiomas

Most haemangiomas are found incidentally during post-mortem or in spleens removed for other reasons

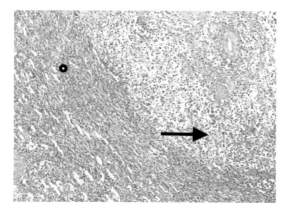

Figure 76.1 Tissue sample image from a splenic large β-cell non-Hodgkin lymphoma. Note the large paler neoplastic cells (thick arrow) present in splenic parenchyma. Normal appearing splenic parenchyma is seen adjacent (circle) (H&E stain; 100x magnification) (*Photo courtesy of Dr Taher Chharchhodwala*). *Abbreviation*: H&E: haematoxylin and eosin.

(9). Macroscopically, they can be single or multiple and may rarely become sufficiently large to occupy the entire organ. Microscopically the majority are cavernous haemangiomas although the capillary variant is also recognized (14).

Lymphangiomas

Lymphangiomas may be single (23) or multiple (24), can be associated with lymphangiomas in other sites and rarely occur as a component of cystic hygromas of the upper body (25). Lymphangiomas are less common than haemangiomas and are thought to be congenital malformations of the lymphatic system. The malformations may be filled with proteinaceous material leading to a massive increase in the size and weight of the spleen with most symptoms being related to this (4).

Littoral cell angiomas

Littoral cell angiomas are very rare benign vascular tumours arising from the red pulp of the spleen. Patients usually manifest with splenomegaly (4).

BENIGN TUMOURS OF NON-VASCULAR ORIGIN

Benign tumours of non-vascular origin are exceedingly uncommon and include hamartomas, lipomas, angiolipomas and myolipomas.

Hamartomas

A splenic hamartoma is a very rare, benign malformation, composed of an aberrant agglomerate of cells and tissues probably due to a developmental error. It occurs equally in males and females and was first described by Rokitansky as a 'splenoma'. They can occur at any age, but are most often discovered in the elderly with the majority being discovered incidentally at post-mortem (26). Splenic hamartomas are dark tumour-like growths which are usually exophytic and occasionally a large hamartoma will be detected on abdominal examination and confirmed on computed tomography (CT) or a magnetic resonance image (MRI). Symptoms, if present, are a result of compression, hypersplenism or rupture (14).

MALIGNANT PRIMARY NON-LYMPHOID TUMOURS

Malignant vascular tumours

Primary malignant vascular tumours of the spleen, although the commonest non-lymphoid primary malignancies of the spleen, are exceedingly rare.

Haemangiosarcoma

Haemangiosarcomas are the most common of the primary cancers of the spleen and this extremely aggressive malignancy was previously known as angiosarcoma (27), but was reclassified to differentiate it from lymphangiosarcomas. Angiosarcomas came to prominence in the late 20th century due to their possible occurrence as an occupational hazard associated with monomeric vinyl chloride, arsenic or thorium dioxide (14). This devastating malignancy metastasizes at a very early stage to the liver, lymph nodes, bone marrow and lungs. Clinical presentation is generally due to rapid onset splenomegaly and profound cancer cachexia (4). They may occasionally present in extremis following spontaneous rupture with no previous symptoms (5,28) or occasionally with malignant ascites or pleural effusions (4,14). There can also be angiopathic haemolytic anaemia (29) a process of red blood cell destruction within the microvasculature accompanied by thrombocytopenia due to platelet activation and consumption which has a very grave prognosis (30). Macroscopically haemangiosarcoma manifests as a highly variegated spleen with areas of necrosis, haemorrhage and spongy tumour nodules in the red pulp. Microscopically, the diagnosis can be confirmed by the demonstration of vascular channels with malignant appearing, budding endothelial cells and solid spindle cell sheets (14).

Other non-lymphoid primary splenic tumours include malignant fibrous histiocytosis (MFH), Kaposi's sarcoma, hemangioendothelial sarcoma and malignant hemangiopericytoma. However, the incidence of these cancers is so low that reports are generally considered to be anecdotal (14).

EVALUATION OF SPLENIC TUMOURS

The clinical presence of splenomegaly and haematological evaluation showing surrogate evidence of hypersplenism in the form of anaemia, leucopaenia and thrombocytopaenia may suggest a splenic tumour but confirmation invariably requires imaging. Ultrasound (US) will demonstrate a space-occupying lesion, either in isolation, or accompanied by lesions in other viscera, and will confirm whether the lesion is cystic or solid. If cystic, US examination will also reveal whether the lesion is unilocular or multilocular with clear or turbid contents. Gaseous bowel loops, especially the transverse colon or the splenic flexure, may obscure or prevent clear US images and the 'gold standard' is a contrast enhanced CT (CECT) scan of the abdomen (31). Haemangiomas will show early peripheral enhancement followed by centripetal filling during the delayed phases and MRI may also be diagnostic. Recently, 3D CT cinematic rendering has been evaluated for better delineation of splenic parenchymal lesions (32–35). Because of the chances of haemorrhage, percutaneous image-guided biopsies of splenic tumours are rarely performed, although a small number of units do still undertake them in the context of a defined protocol (36.37). In case of metastases involving the spleen, it is usually safer to obtain tissue diagnosis from other less vascular viscera or from the parietes. There have been a few reports of elevation of serum tumour

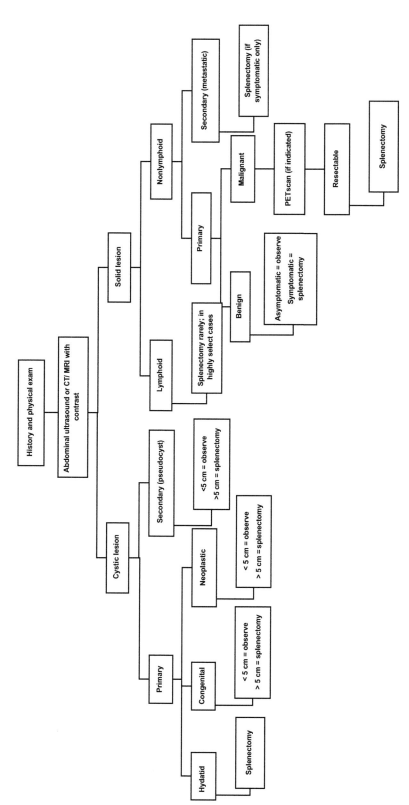

Figure 76.5 Modified decision-making algorithm for the work-up, diagnosis and management of solid and cystic lesions. (Adapted from [9].) *Abbreviations:* CT: computed tomography; MRI: magnetic resonance imaging; PET: positron emission tomography.

markers including carcinoembryonic antigen (CEA) and carbohydrate antigen (CA) 19-9 in certain primary cysts of the spleen. Some inner cyst wall linings show an anti-CA 19-9 immunoreactivity (38,39). A final diagnosis is usually obtained during post-mortem or following splenectomy, performed either for the tumour or with the tumour found incidentally during histopathological evaluation of a spleen removed for other reasons. Immunohistochemistry is used to further subclassify tumours in some cases (*Figure 76.4*).

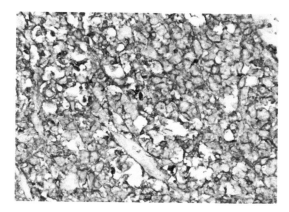

Figure 76.4 Tissue sample image from a diffuse, large β-cell lymphoma. Note the large lymphoid cells are CD20 diffuse membranous positive. (IHC; CD20; 100x magnification) (*Photo courtesy of Dr Taher Chharchhodwala*). *Abbreviations*: IHC: immunohistochemistry; CD20: cluster of differentiation 20.

MANAGEMENT OF SPLENIC TUMOURS

Figure 76.5 shows a decision-making algorithm for the management of splenic tumours.

Splenic cysts

As a general rule, benign cysts of the spleen <5 cm are observed. Cysts ≥5 cm or cysts with symptoms need to be excised, usually by performing a splenectomy. In highly selected cases, partial splenectomy can be considered. Both open, and laparoscopic, methods are possible. The results are equivalent and the approach should reflect institutional expertise and operator experience. It is prudent to vaccinate against the encapsulated organisms pneumococcus, meningococcus and influenza at least 2 weeks prior to total splenectomy and preferably 4 weeks prior, to decrease the chances of OPSI (40).

Solid tumours of the spleen

The role of splenectomy in lymphoid neoplasms has significantly decreased but occasionally there is still a role when there are intractable symptoms caused by massive splenomegaly in marginal zone lymphomas (41), although with the advent of FDG-PET for the staging of lymphomas even this indication is controversial (42,43). In non-lymphoid benign neoplasms, only tumours >5 cm or those with significant symptoms should be considered for splenectomy. Centrally located lesions are not suitable for partial resections. In non-lymphoid malignant primary tumour splenectomy with or without hilar dissection, should only be offered to those patients where the disease is restricted to the spleen and partial splenectomy is not appropriate. In patients with metastatic tumours, splenectomy is rare and reserved for rupture requiring emergency management or hypersplenism caused by splenic deposits. In cases of primary peritoneal or ovarian cancer, however, splenectomy may be a necessary part of the overall surgical planning to achieve adequate cytoreduction.

SUMMARY

The spleen is very rarely involved in secondary or primary neoplastic processes for reasons which are not yet clearly understood. Benign and malignant primary tumours can occur but are unusual, and metastases to the spleen are most often from lymphoid cancers. Metastases from solid tumours may involve the spleen, but this is usually concomitant with the involvement of multiple additional sites. CECT scanning is an excellent modality for the assessment of splenic tumours although a final, definitive diagnosis in the case of a primary tumour may only be possible on histopathology. Asymptomatic, small, benign tumours may be observed while symptomatic larger tumours may need to be removed depending on the clinical indications.

REFERENCES

1. Wilkins BS. Historical review. The spleen. *Br J Haematol* 2002;**117(2)**:265–74.
2. Spier CM. Malignant lymphoma with primary presentation in the spleen. A study of 20 patients. *Arch Pathol Lab Med* 1985;**109**:1076–80.
3. Berge T. Splenic metastases. Frequencies and patterns. *Acta Pathol Microbiol Scand A* 1974;**82**: 499–506.
4. Silver DS, Pointer DT Jr, Slakey DP. Solid tumors of the spleen: Evaluation and management. *Am Coll Surg* 2017;**224(6)**:1104–11.
5. Lam KY, Tang V. Metastatic tumors to the spleen: A 25-year clinicopathologic study. *Arch Pathol Lab Med* 2000;**124**:526–30.
6. Sauer J, Sobolewski K, Dommisch K. Splenic metastases – not a frequent problem, but an underestimate location of metastases: Epidemiology and course. *J Cancer Res Clin Oncol* 2009;**135**:667–71.
7. Marymount JH Jr, Gross S. Patterns of metastatic carcinoma in the spleen. *Am J Clin Pathol* 1963; **40**:58–66.

8. Compérat E, Bardier-Dupas A, Camparo P, et al. Splenic metastases: Clinicopathologic presentation, differential diagnosis, and pathogenesis. *Arch Pathol Lab Med* 2007;**131**:965–9.

9. Pointer DT, Slakey DP. Cysts and Tumors of the Spleen. In: Yeo GJ, Gross SD, and Kimmel S (eds). *Shackelford's Surgery of the Alimentary Tract* Vol 2. 8th edition, London: Elsevier, 2019, Chapter 142, pp. 1655–57.

10. Ough YD, Nash HR, Wood DA. Mesothelial cysts of the spleen with squamous metaplasia. *Am J Clin Pathol* 1981;**76(5)**:666–9.

11. Tsakraklides V, Hadley TW. Epidermoid cysts of the spleen. *Arch Pathol* 1973;**96(4)**:251–4.

12. Boesby S. Spontaneous rupture of benign non-parasitic cyst of the spleen. *Ugeskr Laeger* 1977;**134(49)**: 2596–7.

13. Dawes LG, Malangoni MA. Cystic masses of the spleen. *Am Surg* 1986;**52**:333.

14. Morgenstern L, Rosenberg J, Geller, SA. Tumors of the spleen. *World J Surg* 1985;**9**:468–76.

15. Dasgupta T, Coombes B, Brasfield RD. Primary malignant neoplasms of the spleen. *Surg Gynecol Obstet* 1965;**120**:947–60.

16. Gaba AR, Stein RS, Sweet DL, Variakojis, D. Multicentric giant lymph node hyperplasia. *Am J Clin Pathol* 1978;**69**:86–90.

17. Burke JS, Osborne BM Localized reactive lymphoid hyperplasia of the spleen simulating malignant lymphoma: A report of seven cases. *Am J Surg Pathol* 1983;**7(4)**:373–80.

18. Cotelingam JD, Jaffe ES. Inflammatory pseudotumor of the spleen. *Am J Surg Pathol* 1984;**8**:375–80.

19. Jorgensen LN, Chirintz H. Solitary metastatic endometrial carcinoma of the spleen. *Acta Obstet Gynecol Scand* 1988;**67(1)**:91–92.

20. Giuliani A, Caporale A, Di Bari M, et al. Isolated splenic metastasis from endometrial carcinoma. *J Exp Clin Cancer Res* 1999;**18**:93–96.

21. Gilks CB, Acker BD, Clement PB. Recurrent endometrial carcinoma: Presentation as a splenic mass mimicking malignant lymphoma. *Gynecol Oncol* 1989;**33**:209–11.

22. Hadjileonitis C, Amplianitis I, Valsamides C, et al. Solitary splenic metastasis of endometrial carcinoma ten years after hysterectomy. Case report and review of the literature. *Eur J Gynaecol Oncol* 2004;**25**:233–5.

23. Pearl GS, Nassar VH. Cystic lymphangioma of the spleen. *South Med J* 1979;**72(6)**:667–9.

24. Chan KW, Saw D. Distinctive, multiple lymphangiomas of spleen. *J Pathol* 1980;**131**:75–81.

25. Avigad S, Jaffe R, Frand M, Izhak Y, Rotem Y. Lymphangiomatosis with splenic involvement. *JAMA* 1976;**236**:2315–7.

26. Rokitansky K. Uber splenome. *Lehrbuch der Patho Anat* 1861.

27. Aranha GV, Gold J, Grage TB. Hemangiosarcoma of the spleen: Report of a case and review of previously reported cases. *J Surg Oncol* 1976;**8(6)**:481–7.

28. Alpert LI, Benisch B. Hemangioendothelioma of the liver associated with microangiopathic hemolytic anemia. *Am J Med* 1970;**48(5)**:624–8.

29. Autry JR, Weitzner S. Hemangiosarcoma of spleen with spontaneous rupture. *Cancer* 1975;**35(2)**:534–9.

30. Chen KTK, Bolles JC, Gilbert EF. Angiosarcoma of the spleen: A report of two cases and review of the literature. *Arch Pathol Lab Med* 1979;**103(3)**:122–4.

31. Robertson F, Leander P, Ekberg O. Radiology of the spleen. *Eur Radiol* 2001;**11(1)**:80–95.

32. Rowe SP, Chu LC, Fishman EK. 3D CT cinematic rendering of the spleen: Potential role in problem solving. *Diagn Interv Imaging* 2019;**100(9)**:477–83.

33. Dappa E, Higashigaito K, Fornaro J, et al. Cinematic rendering: An alternative to volume rendering for 3D computed tomography imaging. *Insights Imaging* 2016;**7**:849-856.

34. Eid M, DeCecco CN, Nance JW Jr. et al. Cinematic rendering CT: A novel, lifelike 3D visualization technique. *AJR Am J Roentgenol* 2017; **209**:370–9.

35. Johnson PT, Schneider R, Lugo-Fagundo C, et al. MDCT angiography with 3D rendering: A novel cinematic rendering algorithm for enhanced anatomic detail. *AJR Am J Roentgenol* 2017;**209**:309–12.

36. Olson MC, Atwell TD, Harmsen WS, et al. Safety and accuracy of percutaneous image-guided core biopsy of the spleen. *Am J Roentgenol* 2016;**206**: 655–9.

37. Gomez-Rubio M, Lopez-Cano A, Rendon P, et al. Safety and diagnostic accuracy of percutaneous ultrasound-guided biopsy of the spleen: A multicenter study. *J Clin Ultrasound* 2009;**37**:445–50.

38. Madia C, Lumachi F, Veroux M, et al. Giant splenic epithelial cyst with elevated tumor markers CEA and CA 19-9: An incidental association? *Anticancer Res* 2003;**23**:773–6.

39. Trompetas V, Panagopoulos E, Priovolou-Papaevangelou M, Ramantanis G. Giant benign true cyst of the spleen with high serum levels of CA 19-9. *Eur J Gastroenterol Hepatol* 2002;**14**:85–8.

40. Brigden ML, Patullo AL. Prevention and management of overwhelming postsplenectomy infection: An update. *Crit Care Med* 1999;**27(4)**:836–42.

41. Thieblemont C, Felman P, Callet-Bauchu E, et al. Splenic marginal-zone lymphoma: A distinct clinical and pathological entity. *Lancet Oncol* 2003;**4**:95–103.

42. Kalpadakis C, Pangalis GA, Vassilakopoulos TP, et al. Treatment of splenic marginal zone lymphoma: Should splenectomy be abandoned? *Leuk Lymphoma* 2014;**55(7)**:1463-70.

43. Martin P, Rutherford S, Leonard JP: Splenic lymphomas: Is there still a role for splenectomy? *Oncology (Williston Park)* 2012;**26(2)**:204–6.

Chapter 77

Liver Transplantation

Raaj Praseedom

INTRODUCTION

The liver is an essential organ and its failure or removal is rapidly fatal. It is responsible for a myriad of functions including: 1) The removal of toxic products which have resulted from normal metabolism (for example bilirubin and ammonia); 2) the breakdown and clearance of drugs; 3) the synthesis of a wide range of molecules including proteins, enzymes and clotting products and 4) antigen recognition and the subsequent immune response (1). Liver transplantation is the replacement of a diseased liver with a healthy organ from another person (allograft). Liver transplantation is a treatment option for end-stage liver disease and acute liver failure, although availability of donor organs remains a significant issue (2). Presently, the most common surgical procedure is orthotopic transplantation, where the patient's own liver is removed and replaced with an organ from a suitable donor with the reconstruction replicating the patient's original anatomy. Liver transplantation is a complex and lengthy procedure performed by large teams in specialist units. This chapter will explain the current indications for liver transplantation and highlight the different stages of the procedure together with the operative details required for a successful transplant.

INDICATIONS

The conditions considered for liver transplantation in adults fall into the broad categories summarized in *Table 77.1*.

The selection for liver transplantation in patients with these conditions (*Table 77.1*) is primarily based on the risk of death without a transplant (3). Selection criteria vary from country to country and different scoring systems are used, such as the UK model for end-stage liver disease (UKELD) and transplant benefit score (TBS) in the UK, and model for end-stage liver disease (MELD) in the USA (4). These scoring systems consider clinical factors such as: 1) The presence of diuretic resistant ascites; 2) hepatic encephalopathy; 3) laboratory parameters including bilirubin, creatinine, international normalized ratio (INR), sodium values and 4) symptoms such as intractable itching affecting quality of life.

Table 77.1 Summary of conditions considered for liver transplantation

Condition	Causes
Acute liver failure	• Paracetamol overdose • Prescription medications • Hepatitis • Autoimmune disease • Veno-occlusive disease
Chronic liver disease	• Cirrhosis secondary to any cause • Biliary atresia
Liver tumours	• Hepatocellular carcinoma • Hepatoblastoma
Variant syndromes	• Hepatopulmonary syndrome • Polycystic liver • Metabolic diseases

CADAVERIC DONOR HEPATECTOMY

Before commencing the operation, the donor details including the blood group, virology, certification of brain stem death and consent for organ donation should be checked. The donor is opened with an incision from the supra-sternal notch to the symphysis, and the chest and abdomen explored for any malignancy. The falciform ligament is divided cranially to the supra-hepatic inferior vena cava (IVC) and the left and right lobes are fully mobilized by dividing the corresponding triangular ligaments. The gallbladder is either removed or flushed clear of bile and the bile duct is divided. The hepatic artery is then identified. Approximately 30% of patients will be found to have anomalous hepatic arterial anatomy. The gastroduodenal artery is ligated and divided. The hepatic artery is then dissected towards the coeliac axis at least up to the origin of the splenic artery. The portal vein is then dissected to just behind the neck of the pancreas. The crus of the diaphragm is divided to facilitate slinging of the supra-coeliac aorta ready for cross-clamping. A 5 cm segment of infra-renal aorta and a 5 cm segment of infra-renal IVC are isolated. The inferior mesenteric vein (IMV) is also isolated for portal perfusion and the donor is then fully heparinized with 50 000 units. Appropriately sized perfusion cannulae are placed into the isolated aorta and the IMV connected to ice-cold organ perfusion fluid. Another

DOI: 10.1201/9781003080060-77

clamped cannula is placed in the isolated IVC to drain the blood and perfusion fluid. The supra-coeliac aorta is now cross-clamped followed by commencing the perfusion through the aorta and IMV. The clamp on the IVC is removed to allow drainage out to an external container. The abdomen is then filled with cold saline and crushed ice to cool the peritoneal cavity and organs. Once the perfusate fluid in the IVC drain clears, the perfusion is stopped and the liver is removed by dividing the supra-hepatic cava, the infra-hepatic IVC above the renal veins and the coeliac axis, which is harvested with a cuff of aorta. Additional vessels such as iliac arteries and veins are removed depending on the need for reconstruction in the recipient. It is important for individual teams (liver, kidney, pancreas, intestinal and cardiac) to be respectful of the donor, to each other and work collaboratively for the benefit of the various recipients. The liver is then flushed through the portal vein, hepatic artery, and the bile duct on the back table prior to packing it in the organ transport box (5).

LIVE DONOR HEPATECTOMY

An adult live donor right hepatectomy may be carried out by an open, laparoscopic or robotic technique (6,7). In the open technique, access to the abdomen is through a right subcostal, 'reverse L' incision. The falciform ligament is divided up to the supra-hepatic IVC and the gallbladder is removed fundus first. The right hepatic artery is dissected ready for transection and the right portal vein is encircled and prepared for transection. The right lobe is now fully mobilized by dividing the right triangular ligament and dissecting the retro-hepatic IVC by dividing the small caudate veins, while larger accessory veins should be isolated for re-anastomosing in the recipient. The right hepatic vein is slung and the hepatic parenchyma is transected (ensuring that the central venous pressure (CVP) is low during this phase) along the principal plain on the middle hepatic vein (MHV) aiming to leave the MHV in the donor in the majority of cases. Large segment 5, segment 8 and inferior hepatic veins should be isolated for reconstruction in the recipient.

At the end of the parenchymal transection, the right hepatic duct is divided in most instances as a single right duct. The right hepatic artery, portal vein and the right hepatic vein are clamped, and divided in that order, to remove the graft which is perfused on the back table. The right hepatic vein, right hepatic artery, right portal vein and right hepatic duct stumps are suture ligated in the donor. A completion cholangiogram may be obtained if there are any concerns, particularly when there is variant anatomy. The cut surface of the liver is treated appropriately and the abdomen closed with a subphrenic drain. The donor graft segments 5 and 8 (and any accessory veins) can now be reconstructed

using vein grafts on the bench. Liver donor hepatectomy is associated with a 1 in 200 perioperative mortality and the usual morbidity associated with a standard right hepatectomy.

BENCH PREPARATION OF THE GRAFT

In the recipient centre, the liver is unpacked but kept in ice cold perfusate and prepared for implantation. Any excess diaphragm, adrenal gland and other fibrofatty tissue is excised. The IVC is cleaned of excess surrounding tissue, checked for leaks and any suture holes closed. The hepatic artery and portal are similarly prepared. The liver is then packed back in cold perfusion solution and kept in the ice box until implantation.

RECIPIENT OPERATION

Preoperative checks

It is important to make sure that the donor organs are matched to the recipient in terms of blood group compatibility. Donor virology should be checked, and the recipient radiology reviewed prior to sending for the recipient in theatre. In most centres these procedures are part of the standard WHO checklist and team briefing procedures (8).

Surgical equipment

Liver transplant trays should have a full vascular set including microvascular instruments. Liver transplant theatres should have access to perfusion fluids such as University of Wisconsin solution (UW solution) and sterile crushed ice. The liver transplant procedure is best carried out using surgical loupes and headlights.

Anaesthesia and monitoring

Liver transplantation is carried out under general anaesthesia without additional regional anaesthesia (spinal or epidural) to avoid the risk of bleeding around the spinal cord consequent upon the inevitable coagulopathy.

Recipients require peripheral and central venous access (for filling and monitoring), a temperature probe and an arterial line (9). In patients expected to require a veno-venous bypass, additional lines need to be inserted into the jugular veins. Recipients with renal dysfunction and those where massive blood loss is anticipated would benefit from dialysis access and intraoperative filtration. Other specialized monitoring equipment include a dynamic trans-oesophageal echocardiography (TOE) probe and a Swan-Ganz catheter. Liver transplant theatres should be equipped with a cell saver, rapid transfuser with warmer, and facilities for thromboelastography (TEG).

Incision

The incision for a liver transplant is variable, but 'reverse L' and 'Mercedes-Benz' incisions are the most frequently performed. Once the abdomen is opened, a fixed traction subcostal retractor may be used to gain optimal exposure.

Explant hepatectomy

The hepatic hilum is initially dissected and the left- and right-hepatic arteries are identified and divided. The common bile duct is divided between ligatures, and the portal vein is then cleaned-off its surrounding fibrofatty neural and lymphatic tissue. Meticulous dissection is required to obtain a usable recipient hepatic artery and bile duct (*Figure 77.1*) for later anastomosis to the donor liver artery and duct. The next part of the recipient hepatectomy involves mobilization of the liver from its attachments. Initially, this is best achieved by fully dividing the falciform ligament cranially up to the supra-hepatic IVC to visualize the junction of the hepatic veins with the IVC. The left lobe is mobilized by dividing the left triangular ligament followed by division of the lesser omentum to expose the caudate lobe and the left side of the retro-hepatic IVC. The lesser omentum sometimes contains an accessory, or replaced, left hepatic artery from the left gastric artery, which may be divided. The right lobe is mobilized by incising the right triangular ligament starting from the right side of

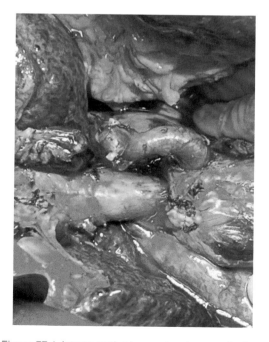

Figure 77.1 Intraoperative image showing a meticulous dissection to expose the portal vein and hepatic artery.

the right hepatic vein. Dissection is continued over the Gerota's fascia fully exposing the bare area of the liver up to the right edge of the IVC, avoiding the adrenal gland. At this stage the recipient liver may be removed in one of two different ways. The classical technique is by removing the retro-hepatic IVC along with the diseased liver. The alternative technique, known as 'piggyback' is by dissecting the liver off the IVC thereby preserving the native IVC. A liver transplant surgeon may prefer one or the other of these two techniques but should be competent in both.

In the classical technique, the infra-hepatic IVC is encircled followed by retrocaval dissection up to the pericardial diaphragm. The classical technique of removing the recipient IVC is only possible if the patient can tolerate cross-clamping of the IVC. In patients who are unable to tolerate an IVC cross-clamp, a veno-venous bypass between the femoral vein, and the internal jugular vein, may be required to prevent intractable haemodynamic instability. The alternative 'piggyback' technique preserves the recipient inferior vena cava by dissecting the liver off the retro-hepatic IVC. In this technique, the dissection is kept anterior to the vena cava and all the small caudate and inferior hepatic veins are ligated and divided. This technique is mandatory in living-donor liver transplants, and cadaveric liver transplants where a split liver graft is offered without a donor IVC. At the end of a caval preserving recipient hepatectomy, the right hepatic vein and the confluence of the middle- and left-hepatic veins are clamped and divided. Depending on the type of donor graft, any of these hepatic vein stumps or the side of the recipient IVC may be used for venous outflow from the donor graft (10). The diseased native liver is now removed by clamping and dividing the portal vein, followed by transection of the infra- and supra-hepatic IVC between appropriate vascular clamps in that order. If carrying out an IVC-preserving hepatectomy, then the diseased native liver is removed by clamping and dividing the portal vein, followed by clamping and dividing the hepatic veins.

Veno-venous bypass

The indications for veno-venous bypass include donor haemodynamic instability upon cross-clamping during a classical liver transplant, prophylactically in patients with renal dysfunction and in those circumstances where there is major haemorrhage due to severe portal hypertension (11). A right- or left-groin incision is performed centred on the saphenofemoral junction and the long saphenous vein at its junction with the femoral vein is isolated. If additional portal bypass is required, then a segment of portal vein should also be isolated. Alternatively, portal bypass may be achieved through the IMV. Appropriately sized cannulae are placed in the femoral vein through the saphenofemoral junction and the portal vein, which are then connected to a Y connector and the flow is sent to the neck veins through an external perfusion pump. The groin cannula may also be placed percutaneously under ultrasound (US) guidance avoiding the surgical incision. The most feared complication of a veno-venous bypass is life threatening air embolism but it is also associated with major bleeding from inadvertently pulled out cannulae and connectors. Percutaneous insertion of cannulae both in the groin and neck are associated with complications such as bleeding, inadvertent arterial injury and pneumothorax. Following removal of the recipient liver, the donor organ is now anastomosed in the following order: 1) The top-end of the donor IVC is anastomosed end-to-end, to the divided supra-hepatic cava in the recipient. 2) The bottom-end of the donor cava is anastomosed end-to-end, to the cut infra-hepatic recipient cava (*Figure 77.2*). Prior to finishing this anastomosis, the liver is flushed with a bag of colloid solution through the portal vein and drained through the nearly complete infra-hepatic caval anastomosis, to wash out the potassium-rich preservation fluid and avoid cardiac arrest at reperfusion. 3) The donor and recipient portal veins are then trimmed to length and an end-to-end anastomosis performed. 4) Reperfusion is undertaken by removing the supra-hepatic, infra-hepatic and portal vein clamps in that order. 5) Haemostasis is quickly achieved, and an end-to-end hepatic artery anastomosis is carried out as soon as possible to limit the secondary warm ischaemic time. 6) Arterial reperfusion is achieved by removing the hepatic artery clamp-off (*Figure 77.3*) (7). An end-to-end, bile duct to bile duct anastomosis is now performed. In certain situations, such as with recipient primary sclerosing cholangitis (PSC), when a re-transplant is being performed, or when there is a major size discrepancy between the donor and recipient ducts, a 70 cm Roux-en-Y hepaticojejunostomy may be carried

out instead. 8) Following haemostasis, the abdomen is closed after inserting subphrenic and subhepatic drains.

SURGICAL COMPLICATIONS

Intraoperative complications

These include major haemorrhage and coagulopathy particularly in those with severe portal hypertension

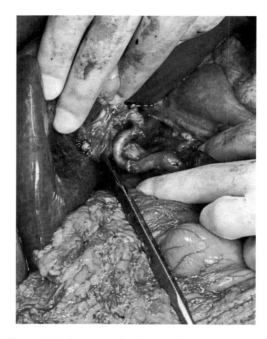

Figure 77.3 Intraoperative image showing an arterial reperfusion following clamp removal.

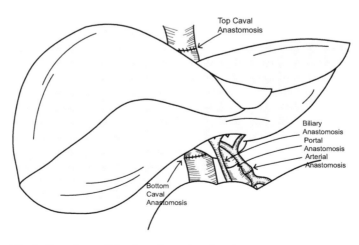

Figure 77.2 Labelled illustration of a graft implantation using the classical method, after removal of the recipient IVC.

and previous upper abdominal surgery including re-do liver transplants (12).

Immediate postoperative surgical complications

Reactionary and secondary haemorrhage may require exploratory laparotomy or interventional radiology for control. Bile leaks from the biliary anastomosis, missed ducts and the cut surface in split, or live, donor grafts may lead to sepsis and hepatic artery thrombosis or bleeding. Hepatic artery thrombosis is life threatening and is best managed in the early postoperative period by re-transplantation if possible. Hepatic artery narrowing may be dealt with by percutaneous angioplasty. Hepatic venous outflow obstruction usually manifests with increased ascitic losses which may be very significant (potentially several litres over 24 hours), elevated prothrombin time (PT), pedal oedema and renal dysfunction. This is usually related to a technical issue and seen with both classical and IVC preserving 'piggyback' liver transplants. Occasionally it may be possible to angioplasty the obstruction and deploy a stent, but long-term results are poor and these patients generally require a further transplant.

Late postoperative surgical complications

Late surgical complications include biliary strictures, both anastomotic and non-anastomotic. Significant anastomotic strictures may be treated either by endoscopic retrograde cholangiopancreatography (ERCP)-dilatation with, or without, stenting or more commonly by re-operation and a formal biliary bypass with a 70 cm Roux-en-Y hepaticojejunostomy. Late hepatic arterial stenosis may be treated with angioplasty but late hepatic artery thrombosis is often associated with intra-hepatic biliary stricturing, which leads to cholangitis and liver abscesses and often requires re-transplantation.

LIVER SPLITTING

The liver may be split into a right lobe for an adult (segments 1 and 4–8) and a left lateral segment for a child (segments 2 and 3) or alternatively may be split into right (segments 5–8) and left lobes (segments 1–4). Preservation of caudate lobe function is important in recipients with a borderline graft-recipient weight ratio to achieve better results. A split liver should not be confused with a 'cut down' liver where the donor graft is cut down to size and the excised segments are discarded and not transplanted. The liver may be split on the back table or in the donor prior to cross-clamping which is known as an *in-situ* split (13).

The most common split is a right lobe, left lateral segment split and is carried out on the back table at the recipient centre. Once full bench preparation has been carried out, the hepatic arteries are dissected to the hilum, clearly demonstrating the right- and left-hepatic arterial origins and the portal vein is similarly dissected. The parenchymal transection is performed 1 cm to the right of the falciform ligament using a finger fracture technique with a haemostat. All small vessels and biliary radicles are carefully ligated on both sides. The main IVC is kept with the right lobe graft and the left hepatic vein is transected from its confluence with the MHV. The resulting defect in the MHV is suture closed without narrowing the MHV. Towards the end of parenchymal transection, the left hepatic duct is transected and the stump of the left hepatic duct on the right side is closed with a suture. Depending on the requirements of the individual recipients, the left hepatic artery and left portal vein are transected from the main hepatic artery and main portal vein.

LIVER TRANSPLANT OUTCOMES

In the UK, 1-year patient survival for first elective deceased donor liver transplantation from all indications is 94%. Long-term 5- and 10-year survival depends on the indications for transplantation, but on average are 80% and 60% respectively (14,15).

REFERENCES

1. Squires JE, McKiernan P, Squires RH. Acute liver failure: An update. *Clin Liver Dis* 2018;**22(4)**:773–805.
2. Bodzin AS, Baker TB. Liver transplantation today: Where we are now and where we are going? *Liver Transpl* 2018;**24(10)**:1470–5.
3. Mahmud N. Selection for liver transplantation: Indications and evaluation. *Curr Hepatol Rep* 2020;**19**: 203–12.
4. Klein KB, Stafinski TD, Menon D. Predicting survival after liver transplantation based on pre-transplant MELD score: A systematic review of the literature. *PloS One* 2013;**8(12)**:e80661.
5. Marques HP, Barros I, Li J, Murad SD, di Benedetto F. Current update in domino liver transplantation. *Int Surg J* 2020;**82**:163–8.
6. Broering D, Sturdevant ML, Zidan A. Robotic donor hepatectomy: A major breakthrough in living donor liver transplantation. *AJT* 2022;**22(1)**:14–23.
7. Berardi G, Tomassini F, Troisi RI. Comparison between minimally invasive and open living donor hepatectomy: A systematic review and meta-analysis. *Liver Transpl* 2015;**21(6)**:738–52.
8. Zarrinpar A, Busuttil RW. Liver transplantation: Past, present and future. *Nat Rev Gastroenterol Hepatol* 2013;**10(7)**:434–40.
9. Brezeanu LN, Brezeanu RC, Diculescu M, Droc G. Anaesthesia for liver transplantation: An update. *J Crit Care Med* 2020;**6(2)**:91–100.
10. Markin NW, Ringenberg KJ, Kassel CA, Walcutt CR, Chacon MM. 2018 Clinical update in liver transplantation. *JCVA* 2019;**33(12)**:3239–48.

11. Lapisatepun W, Lapisatepun W, Agopian V, Xia VW. Venovenous bypass during liver transplantation: A new look at an old technique. *Transplant Proc* 2020;**52(3)**:905–9.

12. Craig EV, Heller MT. Complications of liver transplant. *Abdom Radiol* 2021;**46**:43–67.

13. Gavriilidis P, Roberts KJ, Azoulay D. Right lobe split liver graft versus whole liver transplantation: A systematic review by updated traditional and cumulative meta-analysis. *Dig Liver Dis* 2018;**50(12)**:1274–82.

14. Fodor M, Zoller H, Oberhuber R, Sucher R, Seehofer D, Cillo U, Line PD, Tilg H, Schneeberger S. The need to update endpoints and outcome analysis in the rapidly changing field of liver transplantation. *Transplantation* 2022;**106(5)**:938–49.

15. Yong JN, Lim WH, Ng CH, Tan DJ, Xiao J, Tay PW, Lin SY, Syn N, Chew N, Nah B, Dan YY. Outcomes of nonalcoholic steatohepatitis after liver transplantation: An updated meta-analysis and systematic review. *CGH* 2023;**21(1)**:45–54.

Chapter
78

Pancreatic Transplantation

M. Zeeshan Akhtar, Michael Silva and Peter J. Friend

INTRODUCTION

The first pancreas transplant was performed in 1966 by Lillehei and Kelly at the University of Minnesota (1). Today, over 50 000 pancreas transplants have been performed globally and transplant is considered the treatment of choice for patients with type 1 diabetes mellitus (T1DM) with hypoglycaemic unawareness. Improvements in patient management has resulted in the expanding indications for both simultaneous pancreas kidney and isolated pancreas transplantation. However, the pancreas remains one of the most challenging organs to successfully transplant and a constant assessment of risks of surgery and immunosuppression needs to be made and weighed against the clinical benefit associated with the long-term tight glycaemic control offered by pancreas transplantation. With an estimated 15% of healthcare costs in the West being diabetes-related and the healthcare costs of a typical patient with T1DM being over $52 000 by the age of 40, pancreas transplantation remains both of significant clinical and economic importance (2).

THE CLINICAL NEED AND INDICATIONS FOR PANCREAS TRANSPLANTATION

In addition to the economic argument for pancreas transplantation, the goal of diabetes management is to prevent the sequela of downstream disease, namely retinopathy, neuropathy, nephropathy and associated cardiovascular disease. Tight glycaemic control has been consistently shown to be essential in disease prevention as highlighted by the landmark diabetes control and complications (DCCT) trial (3). In addition, it is critical for any artificial, or augmented insulin secreting therapy to be able to prevent over treatment, the issue encountered by some with T1DM who go on to experience the life-threatening complication of hypoglycaemic unawareness. Both insulin pumps and pancreas transplantation have the ability to provide so called 'closed-loop systems' allowing for the tight autoregulation of glycaemic control, with pancreas transplant offering the most physiological and biological response system.

Pancreas transplantation achieves, on average, insulin independence in 82% of cases. Of the pancreas transplants performed, 90% are as simultaneous kidney pancreas transplants (SPK) whereas 4% are pancreas after kidney (PAK) and 6% are as pancreas alone transplants (PTA) (4). Unlike heart, liver and lung transplantation, pancreas transplantation is not a 'life-saving' procedure, and therefore clinical judgement needs to be exercised as to how to maximize patient and graft outcomes. Most pancreas transplant programmes necessitate that to be considered for pancreas transplantation, potential recipients have a minimum of three factors:

1 T1DM
2 T1DM is associated with secondary complications
3 Patients are able to pass evaluation for fitness for surgery

A careful assessment of the balance of risk and benefit needs to be sought when considering pancreas transplantation. In a young patient with no complications and tightly controlled diabetes, the risk may be too great to transplant. That said, in patients between 50–60 years of age with advanced complications of T1DM, it is unlikely that a transplant will be able to prevent the downstream complications of diabetes from manifesting. It is the identification of a 'sweet spot' which is required where the downstream complications can be prevented, whilst offsetting at least some of the associated risks.

When considering patients for SPK, PAK or PTA, the patients creatine clearance (CrCl) must be considered (*Table 78.1*).

SPK transplants are typically considered for recipients between the ages of 20–40 who are dialysis dependent. Pre-emptive transplantation can be considered in selected cases where patients are predicted to be dialysis dependent in the next 12–18 months who have complications such as macroglobulinaemia and proteinuria and supported by associated histological changes on biopsy. It is important to remember that after 20 years living with T1DM, 30–40% of patients will have

Table 78.1 Renal creatinine clearance and the recommended pancreas transplant type

CrCl (mL/min)	Recommended transplant type
<40 mL/min	SPK
>40 mL/min	PAK
>70 mL/min	PTA

DOI: 10.1201/9781003080060-78

end-stage renal failure. In the context of a living-donor kidney option being available for a potential SPK recipient, most centres would advocate an initial living-donor kidney with a deceased-donor pancreas transplant at a later stage. This strategy has better outcomes after the living-kidney donation including the improved ability of the recipient to autoregulate fluid balance. This makes pancreas transplantation surgery and subsequent perioperative management less complicated and safer.

PTA is typically reserved for patients who have unstable diabetes, most likely those with T1DM who have hypoglycaemic unawareness. Living-related pancreas transplantation have been performed previously, but the risks to the donor are too high for most centres to consider performing this routinely.

PATIENT AND DONOR SELECTION

There are a range of factors to consider in patient selection and significant associated work-up *(see Table 78.2)*. In addition to their insulin-treated diabetes a potential recipient needs to have the physiological reserve to undertake the extensive surgery and long-term immunosuppression. An extensive work-up consisting of interviews and consultations regarding potential cardiovascular, respiratory, endocrine, immunological problems, and when required genitourinary medicine are required. A careful history and work-up should also be considered for patients at risk of graft thrombosis, one of the most feared complications of pancreas transplantation.

Recipients are considered unsuitable candidates for transplantation where there is insufficient cardiovascular reserve, usually revealed during stress testing, echocardiography and in selective cases angiography. Active untreated sepsis, active hepatitis B, ongoing substance abuse and significant, or irreversible, hepatic or pulmonary dysfunction would also be considered by most centres to be contraindications for pancreas transplantation. HIV is no longer considered an absolute contraindication (5).

Most centres only consider pancreas allografts from after brain-death (DBD) donors although some centres have transplanted pancreases from donation after cardiac-death (DCD) donors. DCD donors considered for pancreas transplantation are typically younger (6). Pancreases should not be used from donors with established diabetes or evidence of fatty infiltration, calcification

Table 78.2 Evaluation of the recipient of a pancreas transplant

Factors to consider	Details
History and examination	• Performed by a nephrologist, endocrinologist and transplant surgeon • Clearance of visual status including acuity • Quality-of-life questionnaire and transplant coordinator/social worker clearance • Assessment of vaccination status, including COVID • Additional consultations from specialists including gynaecology, podiatry, psychology, neurology and gastroenterology may be required
Cardiovascular, respiratory and peripheral vascular work-up	• Electrocardiogram, chest X-ray and exercise testing (either via treadmill or dobutamine-induced) are considered standard • Additional specific testing may be required in the form of a 24-hour tape, aortography and pulmonary function testing
Metabolic and endocrine	• Fasting blood glucose • Glycohaemoglobin • Fasting lipid panel • C-peptide levels • Oral or intravenous glucose challenges
Genitourinary and renal evaluations	• Electrolytes and serum blood urea nitrogen and creatinine levels • Urinalysis with cultures and estimated or calculated protein/creatinine excretion • Voiding cystourethrogram when indicated • Kidney biopsy and calcineurin inhibitor challenge test • Hormonal profiles as indicated • Evaluation for erectile dysfunction
Serology and immunology	• ABO blood type and human leukocyte antigens (HLA) tissue type • Cytotoxic antibodies • Viral titres
Other laboratory tests	• Full blood count with differential • Abdominal ultrasound • Mammography in females over 35 • Colonoscopy/occult blood testing as per national protocol • For patients with gastric symptom issues consider a gastric emptying scan or nerve conduction studies

Table 78.3 Relative, and absolute, donor contraindications for whole pancreas transplantation

Relative contra indications	Absolute contraindications
• History of massive transfusion • Prior splenectomy • Mild-to-moderate obesity: <150% IBW; BMI >27.5 • Aberrant hepatic arterial anatomy • Positive VDR or RPR • Prolonged length of hospital-stay • Donor age >45 years • Cardiovascular or CVA as the cause of brain-death • Mild-to-moderate fatty infiltration of the pancreas, pancreatic oedema, or atherosclerosis • Donor instability • Mild pancreatic trauma	• History of T1DM, T2DM or gestational diabetes • Previous pancreatic surgery or moderate-to-severe pancreatic trauma • Severe obesity: >150% IBW; BMI >30 • Pancreatitis (active acute or chronic) • Significant intra-abdominal contamination • Major (active) infection • Chronic alcohol abuse • Recent history of IV drug abuse or high-risk sexual behaviour • Prolonged hypotension or hypoxaemia with evidence of significant end-organ (kidney, liver) damage • Severe atherosclerosis, fatty infiltration, or pancreatic oedema • Inexperienced organ retrieval team

Abbreviations: BMI: body mass index; CVA: cerebrovascular accident; IBW: ideal body weight; IV: intravenous; RPR: rapid plasma regain; T1DM: Type 1 diabetes mellitus; T2DM: Type 2 diabetes mellitus; VDR: venereal disease research laboratory.

Warm phase	**Exposure and mobilization of colon** 1. Standard abdominal exposure with thoracoabdominal incision. 2. Mobilization of the right colon exposing the left renal vein, anterior duodenal dissection is performed to mobilize the colonic mesentery off the anterior aspect of the pancreas.	**Hilar dissection** 1. Hilar dissection is performed to identify the bile duct (which is transected in the warm or cold phase), identify the GDA and trace the common hepatic artery to the splenic.	**Exposing the pancreas** 1. Dissection of the greater curvature is performed taking the short gastrics. The splenic flexure of the colin is taken down. The colonic mesentery is mobilized to expose the pancreas 2. The inferior and superior pancreatic dissection is performed. 3. The transection point on the gastric portion is identified and the distal duodenum is mobilized.
Cold phase	**Separating the liver from the pancreas** 1. After cross clamp and cold perfusion, the liver is safely removed from the abdominal cavity first. Care must be taken to leave an adequate stump of the GDA for liver side. In addition, the splenic should be carefully transected. The splenic vein should be divided the level of the coronary vein to allow for adequate length for both the liver and the pancreas.	**Completing mobilization and removal** 1. The gastric and duodenal sections are transected with a stapling device. 2. The spleen is mobilized and used as a handle to mobilize the pancreas from the retroperitoneum. 3. The colonic and small bowel mesentery are divided leaving a good length to ensure the inferior pancreaticoduodenal is left intact. 4. Care is taken to ensure a good length of the SMA with an aortic patch is removed to complete the explantation of the pancreas.	**Obtaining the Y graft** 1. Careful dissection of the internal and external iliac artery is performed to facilitate formation of the 'Y' graft on the backtable. In addition, the iliac vein is removed to facilitate portal vein extension.

Figure 78.1 Summary of the steps required in the completion of pancreas procurement in a brain-dead organ donor. The exact steps will vary according to surgical preference and practice. Warm phase refers to the portion of the donor operation prior to application of the cross-clamp and cold flush.

or fibrosis determined either through pre-procurement imaging or at the time of organ procurement itself. Globally, most centres are reluctant to accept grafts from donors who are older than 50–55 years of age. *Table 78.3* summarizes the relative, and absolute, donor contraindications to transplantation.

PANCREAS PROCUREMENT AND 'BACK BENCHING'

Hyperglycaemia is often observed in the donor and it has been shown that administering an insulin sliding-scale to establish euglycaemia can improve postoperative outcomes following pancreas transplantation (7). In addition, maintaining haemodynamic stability, cardiac function, oxygenation and electrolytes are critical, while ensuring pancreatic oedema is minimized by avoiding aggressive fluid resuscitation. Hyperamylasemia is often observed in the donor and is not a reason for discarding a potential pancreas allograft.

Multiple techniques have been described for pancreas procurement and *Figure 78.1* outlines the basic steps of the pancreas procurement process. Multiple anatomical anomalies may be encountered during the procurement process which may mean pancreas transplant is not possible. The most common anatomical variation preventing pancreas transplantation is a replaced, or accessory, right hepatic artery, particularly if its path runs through the pancreatic head with a proximal inferior pancreaticoduodenal (IPDA) branch.

Where a true conflict exists preventing the safe transplant of both organs the liver takes priority, although in our experience this situation rarely occurs. Another consideration during procurement is to perform *in situ* perfusion of the portal vein directly rather than through the inferior mesenteric vein (IMV) to prevent pancreatic oedema. Where this cannot be performed, portal vein flush should be performed on an explant of the liver as is frequently done during DCD donation. Some surgeons prefer to explant the pancreas and liver *en bloc* and separate them on the 'back table' or 'bench'. Where the liver is not being procured, the hepatic artery and portal vein can be tied high in the hilum of the liver, providing additional length and a common cuff of aorta containing both the inferior mesenteric artery (SMA) and the coeliac axis. The 'gold standard' preservation solution for pancreas allografts is University of Wisconsin solution.

Figure 78.2 summarizes the process for 'back benching' of the pancreas. The key aspect is to inspect the pancreas carefully to confirm the organ is suitable for transplant, paying attention to the degree of steatosis, nodularity and fibrosis. It is also important to ensure there is sufficient length of the donor portal vein, splenic artery and SMA to allow for reconstruction. The donor iliac artery and vein should be sent with the pancreas to facilitate the reconstruction. The back bench dissection of a pancreas requires meticulous attention to detail. It has been our practice to leave the gastricduodenal artery (GDA) open until the reconstruction is complete to check for back perfusion through the GDA when flushing the Y graft to ensure the IPDA is open. Where the IPDA is occluded, perfusion to the pancreatic head and duodenal segment cannot be guaranteed and serious consideration should be given to discarding the organ.

OPERATIVE AND PREOPERATIVE MANAGEMENT OF PATIENTS

Today the most common surgical technique for transplantation of the pancreas is to perform whole organ transplantation with the donor duodenum as

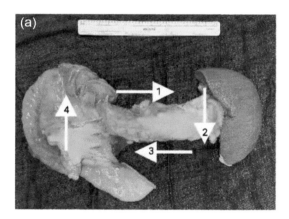

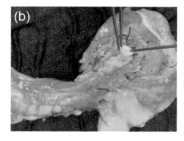 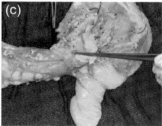 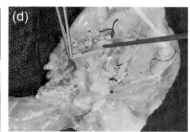

Figure 78.2 Demonstration of the surgical procedures required during the 'back bench' preparation of the pancreas, ahead of transplantation. Labelled image (a) shows steps 1–4 which involve the anterior pancreas: 1) Dissect the superior pancreatic border dissecting loose areolar tissue; 2) remove the spleen from the pancreas; 3) work along the inferior aspect of the pancreas dissecting loose areolar tissue and tying vessels including the inferior mesenteric vein which will be encountered. Trim the jejunal end back and restaple the end; 4) evaluate the small and large bowel mesentery. Oversew the mesentery length left so to ensure the inferior pancreatico-duodenal artery is not compromised (a). Steps 5–8 involve the posterior pancreas: 5) Dissect out the SMA creating good length for reconstruction (b); 6) dissect out the splenic artery preparing for reconstruction (c); 6) Step 7 dissect out the portal vein tying off adjacent neuro-lymphatic tissue (d). Final step: 8) The door iliac vessels are prepared and used to construct a 'Y' graft with the splenic artery and SMA of the pancreas allograft.

highlighted in *Figure 78.3*. The site most commonly used for transplantation is the pelvis with the Y graft being anastomosed to the common, or external, iliac artery and the portal vein being anastomosed to the common iliac vein. Historically, the operation has moved away from segmental transplantation of the pancreas which carried a much higher complication rate. A number of groups have explored the role of portal venous drainage which is commonly practiced in some centres where the superior mesenteric vein (SMV) or sizeable tributary is used. Systemic insulin levels are poorer in the portal venous group with no advantage being demonstrated over systemic drainage in preventing secondary complications.

There has been widespread debate in the literature regarding enteric or bladder drainage of the pancreas allograft. The advantage of bladder drainage is that it offers a readily accessible route to biopsy the donor duodenal segment, if rejection is suspected. However, there are a number of complications associated with bladder drainage, most notably the long-term effects on management of bicarbonate homeostasis, with excessive bicarbonate loss occurring in the urine. It is estimated that 40% of bladder-drained pancreases are eventually converted to being enterically drained for this reason (8). In addition, enteric drainage which is the practice in our centre for SPK transplantation appears to be more physiological and internationally more centres are moving away from bladder drainage (9). Nevertheless, in the event of a PTA transplant the argument for bladder drainage becomes more compelling, with potential conversion to enteric drainage, in the event of significant bicarbonate loss.

Many centres perform a two layered side-to-side bowel anastomosis for the enteric drainage of the

allograft, typically performed 40–60 cm from the duodenojejunal flexure. Some centres choose to perform a Roux loop, aiming to exclude the segment leading to the pancreatic graft (10). We routinely perform a side-to-side anastomosis but if a leak occurs, or the anastomosis is felt to be high risk for any reason, conversion to a Roux loop can be performed prophylactically, or as a salvage procedure. It has been our standard practice to consider performing a feeding jejunostomy in selective cases for patients with known, and profoundly delayed, gastric emptying to facilitate early nutrition.

Anaesthetic considerations during pancreas transplantation should focus on a number of established goals including the avoidance of excessive glucose administration, tight glycaemic control and minimizing crystalloid use. Fluid administration differs for kidney and pancreas transplantation and excessive fluids should not be administered to avoid pancreatic oedema. Aggressive fluid administration intraoperatively is usually required during isolated kidney transplantation. Many centres, including our own, administer intraoperative heparin prior to clamping of any vessels. A thromboelastogram (TEG) will help assess the coagulation state of the recipient and determine whether any further heparin is required during the procedure and in the postoperative period (11).

Postoperatively patients should be managed in either a high-dependency or intensive care unit and careful monitoring of electrolytes, glycaemic status, thrombosis and bleeding risk is required. Thrombosis of the allograft is encountered in 5–10% of cases, usually indicated by a sudden rise in glucose levels. It is our practice to administer antiplatelet agents alongside heparin but this must be guided by repeated TEGs. If thrombosis is suspected, an urgent ultrasound is performed and surgical re-exploration may be necessary. In the early postoperative period, bleeding can manifest with hypotension, tachycardia and decreased urine output. Not all patients with bleeding require exploration, as administration of blood and correction of any coagulopathy may be sufficient. Ongoing or unstable bleeding will necessitate exploration and a careful balance exists when managing bleeding and thrombosis risks in pancreas transplantation. Infection is also a common complication of pancreas transplantation, occurring in 10–15% of cases.

Other major risks in the postoperative period include leaks from the intestinal anastomosis which is usually a consequence of ischaemia of the duodenal segment. Mechanical obstruction also occurs and in any patient with excessively delayed return of bowel function or high nasogastric (NG) output, this complication should always be considered. For those who route the enteric anastomosis through the colonic mesentery, the small bowel can herniate through the mesenteric defect which may present with bowel obstruction. Graft pancreatitis is encountered in approximately 35% of cases and is most accurately assessed by computed

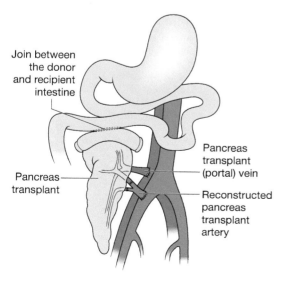

Join between the donor and recipient intestine

Pancreas transplant

Pancreas transplant (portal) vein

Reconstructed pancreas transplant artery

Figure 78.3 Labelled illustration of a transplanted pancreas demonstrating enteric drainage.

tomography (CT) scanning. Re-exploration and wash-out may be required for sizeable peri-pancreatic collections which become infected.

Longer-term vascular complications include pseudoaneurysm formation, which typically occurs in the Y graft and can result in catastrophic haemorrhage. Patients in which an enlarging pseudoaneurysm is identified should be placed on surveillance with imaging. In the case of allografts which are no longer functioning, a covered stent can be placed in the iliac artery to exclude the pseudoaneurysm (12).

Rejection can be challenging to diagnose, and where there is bladder drainage, cystoscopy and biopsy can be performed. Alternatively, if another organ from the same donor has been transplanted, as for SPK transplant, a biopsy of the kidney may reveal rejection which would be sufficient evidence to initiate treatment. Some centres empirically treat patients with suspected rejection, considering the risk of pancreatic biopsy to be too high. However, many high-volume centres perform core- and fine-needle allograft biopsies with low complication rates.

SUMMARY

The pancreas is one of the most complex abdominal organs to transplant. All stages of the process, from recipient selection through to donor selection, management, organ procurement, preservation and transplantation, present unique challenges. Pancreas transplantation is successful in the majority of cases, but has an inevitable associated risk and unlike organs such as the heart and liver, the pancreas is not a 'life-saving' organ transplant. Nevertheless, appropriately selected patients who can withstand the stress of surgery, can undergo a life-changing transplant, providing them with an insulin-free life, and when combined with a kidney transplant, cessation of dialysis.

REFERENCES

1. Kelly WD, Lillehei RC, Merkel FK, Idezuki Y, Goetz FC. Allotransplantation of the pancreas and duodenum along with the kidney in diabetic nephropathy. *Surgery* 1967;**61**(**6**):827–37.
2. American Diabetes Association. Economic costs of diabetes in the US in 2017. *Diabetes Care* 2018;**41**(**5**):917–28.
3. Keen H. The Diabetes Control and Complications Trial (DCCT). *Health Trends* 1994;**26**(**2**):41–3. PMID: 10137725.
4. Gruessner AC, Sutherland DE. Pancreas transplant outcomes for United States (US) cases as reported to the United Network for Organ Sharing (UNOS) and the International Pancreas Transplant Registry (IPTR). *Clin Transpl* 2008:45–56.
5. Akhtar MZ, Patel N, Devaney A, Sinha S, Shankar S, Vaidya A, Friend PJ. Simultaneous pancreas kidney transplantation in the HIV-positive patient. *Transplant Proc* 2011;**43**(**10**):3903–4. doi: 10.1016/j.transproceed.2011.08.093.
6. Siskind E, Akerman M, Maloney C, Huntoon K, Alex A, Siskind T, et al. Pancreas transplantation from donors after cardiac death: An update of the UNOS database. *Pancreas* 2014;**43**(**4**):544–7.
7. Shapey IM, Summers A, Yiannoullou P, Bannard-Smith J, Augustine T, Rutter MK, et al. Insulin therapy in organ donation and transplantation. *Diabetes Obes Metab* 2019;**21**(**7**):1521–28.
8. Adler JT, Zaborek N, Redfield RR 3rd, Kaufman DB, Odorico JS, Sollinger HW. Enteric conversion after bladder-drained pancreas transplantation is not associated with worse allograft survival. *Am J Transplant* 2019;**19**(**9**):2543–2549. doi: 10.1111/ajt.15341. PMID: 30838785.
9. van de Linde P, van der Boog PJ, Baranski AG, de Fijter JW, Ringers J, Schaapherder AF. Pancreas transplantation: Advantages of both enteric and bladder drainage combined in a two-step approach. *Clin Transplant* 2006;**20**(**2**):253–7. doi: 10.1111/j.1399-0012.2005.00477.x. PMID: 16640535.
10. Losanoff JE, Harland RC, Thistlethwaite JR, Garfinkel MR, Williams JW, Milner J, Millis JM. Omega jejunoduodenal anastomosis for pancreas transplant. *J Am Coll Surg* 2006;**202**(**6**):1021–4. doi: 10.1016/j.jamcollsurg.2006.02.025. PMID: 16735221.
11. Burke GW 3rd, Ciancio G, Figueiro J, Buigas R, Olson L, Roth D, Kupin W, Miller J. Hypercoagulable state associated with kidney-pancreas transplantation. Thromboelastogram-directed anti-coagulation and implications for future therapy. *Clin Transplant* 2004;**18**(**4**):423–8. doi: 10.1111/j.1399-0012.2004.00183.x. PMID: 15233820.
12. Akhtar MZ, Jones A, Sideso E, Sinha S, Vaidya A, Darby C. Management of a ruptured mycotic pseudo-aneurysm following pancreas-kidney transplantation. *Ann Transplant* 2011;**16**(**4**):122–5. doi: 10.12659/aot.882229. PMID: 22210432.

ailey & Love's Essential Operations Bailey & Love's Essential Operations
ailey & Love's Essential Operations Bailey & Love's Essential Operations
ailey & Love's Essential Operations Bailey & Love's Essential Operations

Index

- Note: Page numbers in *italics* refer to figures and tables.
- See also cross-references in *italics* either refer to entries within the *same* main entry, or are general cross-references (e.g. *see also specific...*).
- *vs* denotes differential diagnosis, or comparisons.

*For Product Safety Concerns and Information please contact
our EU representative GPSR@taylorandfrancis.com Taylor & Francis
Verlag GmbH, Kaufingerstraße 24, 80331 München, Germany*

T - #0255 - 160425 - C700 - 254/178/33 - PB - 9780367468798 - Gloss Lamination